Williams Hematology
The Red Cell and Its Diseases

For St.
who shares your
career long interest
in les globules rouges.

October 2021

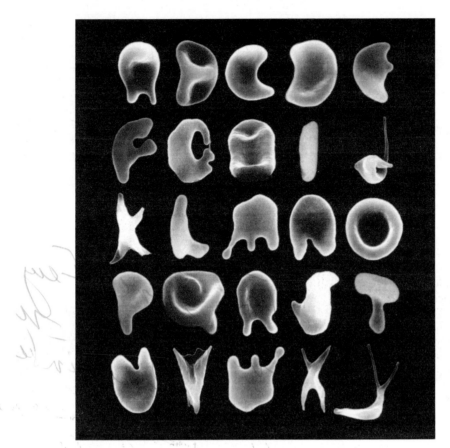

Plate 1. The alphabet made of poikilocytes from a single patient with sickle cell anemia and B-thalassemia trait. Note the electron dense areas in the cells that are in the patient who is homozygous for hemoglobin S, as a reflection of the para-crystallization of that hemoglobin in a low oxygen environment (venous blood). The patient with B-thalassemia trait from whom many of these cells were imaged was a physician whose family arrived to the United States originally from the United Kingdom with no apparent recent Mediterranean heritage. As a result of Rome's invasion of Britain on several occasions between 55 B.C.E. and 43 A.D., troops from current Italy, Spain, Egypt, and Syria garrisoned their married local Britons. *(Reproduced with permission from Lichtman MA, Shafer MS, Felgar RE, et al: Lichtman's Atlas of Hematology 2016. New York, NY: McGraw Hill; 2017.)*

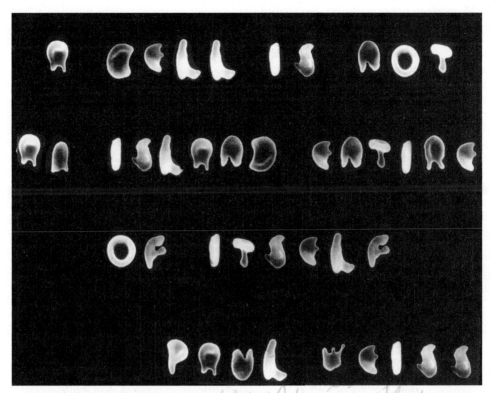

Plate 2. Paul Alfred Weiss (1898-1989) was an American cell and neurobiologist who had emigrated from Austria and specialized in morphogenesis, cell development, and differentiation. He encouraged cross-disciplinary interactions among scientist and was elected to the National Academy of Sciences. He was one of the earliest scientists to propose that the cell microenvironment (né stroma) had important influences on the parenchymal cells it held in its grasp as highlighted in this aphorism he coined, here spelled out with misshapen red cells. *(Reproduced with permission from Lichtman MA, Shafer MS, Felgar RE, et al: Lichtman's Atlas of Hematology 2016. New York, NY: McGraw Hill; 2017.)*

COVER IMAGE DESCRIPTION

The nine abnormal red cells depicted on the cover show the amazing plasticity of the red cell. Consider the membrane reorganization required to maintain these deviations from a biconcave disk.

In veins, the shear rate is low, and normal red cells remain close to a biconcave disk shape. They, also, may overlap tightly at very low flow rates into stacks (rouleaux). When subjected to increased shear rates in the arterial circulation, rouleaux would be dispersed and the red cells deform. At high flow velocities the red cell tends to elongate parallel to the direction of flow. The cytoplasm moves in what has been considered eddy flow. This eddy flow results from the shear flow of the blood being transmitted to the cytoplasm through a motion of the membrane around the elongated red cell, called *tank-tread motion* or *tank-treading*. In a blood capillary with diameters smaller than their own diameter, red cells are folded.

The markedly deformed red cells shown on the cover image were each found in the blood of a patient with a red cell disease (eg, hemoglobin SS, beta-thalassemia, or another red cell disorder). After enucleation, red cells leave the marrow through very narrow, temporary, apertures in the marrow sinus wall that separates hematopoietic cords from the marrow sinus network requiring marked deformation upon egress. Red cells navigate the confinements of capillary dimensions, squeeze through the inter-endothelial cell spaces of the splenic sinus walls, and navigate other physical constraints. Abnormal red cells may be shunted around those constricted dimensions.

The shapes of seven of the nine images approximate an animal form, if one's imagination is permitted to operate. In the upper-left corner is a slightly deformed (thickened edge) discocyte and in its biconcavity rests a triangular-shaped extremely small microcytic, but the latter, strikingly, retains its biconcavity. The other images are that of a simulated dinosaur (aka *Erythrosurus Rochesteriensis*), an octopus (although with more than eight limbs), a severely deformed red cell with a retained concavity and a large hole perforating its cytoplasm, a flying goose, a snail, dancing penguins, a shark, and a duckling, each with their own irregularities requiring extraordinary membrane adaptations. Several have para-crystallization of hemoglobin SS as a deforming force (eg, shark shape).

The distortions that can be maintained by abnormal red cells are extraordinary to consider and certain patterns, discerned on a careful examination of the blood film can be, and frequently are, important diagnostic clues to the nature of the underlying disease. In the absence of a crystallizing hemoglobin or a mutant gene that results in a membrane protein misconfiguration, it is possible that acquired alterations in the spectrin-based membrane protein network is altered so as to maintain abnormal bends and distortions of the red cell surface.

These images and those in Plates 1 and 2 were captured by Patricia A. Santillo, Senior Technologist, Electron Microscopy Laboratory, Hematology Unit at the University of Rochester Medical Center and have been used with permission from *Lichtman's Atlas of Hematology*. *www.accessmedicine.com*

Williams Hematology
The Red Cell and Its Diseases

Josef T. Prchal, MD
Professor of Hematology and Malignant
Hematology
Adjunct in Genetics and Pathology
University of Utah & Huntsman Cancer Institute
Salt Lake City, Utah
1. interní klinika VFN a Ústav patologické fyziologie
1. LF School of Medicine
Universita Karlova, Prague, Czech Republic

Marshall A. Lichtman, MD, MACP
Professor Emeritus of Medicine and of Biochemistry
and Biophysics
Dean Emeritus, School of Medicine and Dentistry
James P. Wilmot Cancer Institute
University of Rochester Medical Center
Rochester, New York

New York   Chicago   San Francisco   Athens   London   Madrid   Mexico City
Milan   New Delhi   Singapore   Sydney   Toronto

1 2 3 4 5 6 7 8 9   LWI   26 25 24 23 22 21

ISBN 978-1-264-26907-5
MHID 1-264-26907-2

> ### Notice
>
> Medicine is an ever-changing science. As new research and clinical experience broaden our knowledge, changes in treatment and drug therapy are required. The authors and the publisher of this work have checked with sources believed to be reliable in their efforts to provide information that is complete and generally in accord with the standards accepted at the time of publication. However, in view of the possibility of human error or changes in medical sciences, neither the authors nor the publisher nor any other party who has been involved in the preparation or publication of this work warrants that the information contained herein is in every respect accurate or complete, and they disclaim all responsibility for any errors or omissions or for the results obtained from use of the information contained in this work. Readers are encouraged to confirm the information contained herein with other sources. For example and in particular, readers are advised to check the product information sheet included in the package of each drug they plan to administer to be certain that the information contained in this work is accurate and that changes have not been made in the recommended dose or in the contraindications for administration. This recommendation is of particular importance in connection with new or infrequently used drugs.

This book was set in Minion Pro by KnowledgeWorks Global Ltd.
The editors were Jason Malley and Harriet Lebowitz.
The production supervisor was Richard Ruzycka.
The cover designer was W2 Design.
Project management was provided by Warishree Pant, KnowledgeWorks Global Ltd.
Production services were provided by KnowledgeWorks Global Ltd.

This book is printed on acid-free paper.

Library of Congress Cataloging-in-Publication Data

Names: Prchal, Josef T., editor. | Lichtman, Marshall A., editor.
Title: Williams hematology. The red cell and its diseases / [edited by]
   Josef T. Prchal, Marshall A. Lichtman.
Other titles: Red cell and its diseases
Description: New York : McGraw Hill, [2022] | Includes bibliographical
   references and index. | Summary: "An up to date consideration of the
   structure, function, and disorders of the red cell, to provide
   clinicians with new foundations for the development of therapies for red
   cell diseases"—Provided by publisher.
Identifiers: LCCN 2021013270 | ISBN 9781264269075 (paperback : alk. paper)
   | ISBN 1264269072 (paperback : alk. paper) | ISBN 9781264269082 (ebook)
Subjects: MESH: Erythrocytes—pathology | Hematologic Diseases |
   Erythrocytes—physiology
Classification: LCC RB145 | NLM WH 150 | DDC 616.1/5—dc23
LC record available at https://lccn.loc.gov/2021013270

McGraw Hill books are available at special quantity discounts to use as premiums and sales promotions, or for use in corporate training programs. To contact a representative please visit the Contact Us pages at www.mhprofessional.com.

CONTENTS

CONTRIBUTORS

Karl E. Anderson, MD
Professor of Medicine
Division of Gastroenterology
The University of Texas Medical Branch at Galveston
Galveston, Texas

Kelty R. Baker, MD, FACP [52]
President
Kelty R. Baker, M.D. P.A.
Houston, Texas

Marije Bartels, MD, PhD
Pediatric Hematologist
Van Creveldkliniek
University Medical Center Utrecht
Utrecht University
Utrecht, The Netherlands

Jaime Caro, MD
Professor of Medicine, Emeritus
Division of Hematology
Cardeza Foundation for Hematological Research
Sidney Kimmel Medical College
Philadelphia, Pennsylvania

Theresa L. Coetzer, PhD
Department of Molecular Medicine and Haematology
School of Pathology
Faculty of Health Sciences
University of the Witwatersrand
Johannesburg, South Africa

Claudia S. Cohn, MD
Associate Professor
Laboratory Medicine and Pathology
University of Minnesota
Minneapolis, Minnesota

Ross M. Fasano, MD
Center for Transfusion and Cellular Therapies
Department of Pathology and Laboratory Medicine
Emory University School of Medicine
Atlanta, Georgia

Tomas Ganz, PhD, MD
Departments of Medicine and Pathology
David Geffen School of Medicine
University of California, Los Angeles
Los Angeles, California

Victor R. Gordeuk, MD
Professor of Medicine
University of Illinois
Chicago, Illinois

Ralph Green, MD, PhD, FRCPath
Professor of Pathology and Medicine
Department of Pathology and Laboratory Medicine
University of California, Davis
Sacramento, California

Xylina T. Gregg, MD
Utah Cancer Specialists
Salt Lake City, Utah

Michael R. Grever, MD
Professor Emeritus
Division of Hematology
Department of Internal Medicine
The Ohio State University
Columbus, Ohio

Amel Hamdi, PhD
Department of Physiology
Lady Davis Institute
McGill University
Montreal, Quebec, Canada

Xiangrong He, MD
Clinical Fellow
Laboratory Medicine and Pathology
Mayo Clinic
Rochester, Minnesota

Jeanne E. Hendrickson, MD
Professor
Departments of Laboratory Medicine and Pediatrics
Yale University School of Medicine
New Haven, Connecticut

Paul C. Herrmann, MD, PhD
Professor and Chair
Department of Pathology and Human Anatomy
Loma Linda University School of Medicine
Loma Linda, California

Achille Iolascon, MD, PhD
Professor of Medical Genetics
Department of Molecular Medicine and Medical Biotechnology
University of Naples Federico II
Naples, Italy

Rami Khoriaty, MD
Assistant Professor, Department of Internal Medicine
Assistant Professor, Department of Cell and Developmental Biology
Section Head, Classical Hematology
Core Member, Rogel Cancer Center
University of Michigan
Ann Arbor, Michigan

Abdullah Kutlar, MD
Professor of Medicine
Augusta University
Augusta, Georgia

Marshall A. Lichtman, MD, MACP
Professor Emeritus of Medicine and of Biochemistry and Biophysics
Dean Emeritus, School of Medicine and Dentistry
James P. Wilmot Cancer Institute
University of Rochester Medical Center
Rochester, New York

Christine Lomas-Francis, MSc, FIBMS
Immunohematology and Genomics
New York Blood Center
Long Island City, New York

Gerard Lozanski, MD
Professor of Pathology Clinical
Department of Pathology
The Ohio State University
Columbus, Ohio

Naomi L.C. Luban, MD
Professor of Pediatrics and Pathology
School of Medicine and Health Sciences
George Washington University;
Medical Director, Office of Human Subjects Protection
Senior Hematologist
Children's National Hospital
Washington, DC

Jeffrey McCullough, MD
Global Blood Advisor
Edina, Minnesota;
Emeritus Professor
Laboratory Medicine and Pathology
University of Minnesota
Minneapolis, Minnesota

Ananya Datta Mitra, MD
Section of Hematopathology
Department of Pathology and Laboratory Medicine
University of California, Davis Health, School of Medicine
Sacramento, California

Joel Moake, MD
Professor of Medicine Emeritus
Baylor College of Medicine
Senior Research Scientist
Department of Bioengineering
Rice University
Houston, Texas

Mohandas Narla, DSc
Laboratory of Red Cell Physiology
New York Blood Center
New York, New York

Diana Morlote, MD
Assistant Professor
Hematopathology and Molecular Genetics Pathology
Division of Genomics and Bioinformatics
Department of Pathology
The University of Alabama at Birmingham
Birmingham, Alabama

Srikanth Nagalla, MBBS, MS
Chief of Benign Hematology
Miami Cancer Institute
Miami, Florida

Charles H. Packman, MD
Professor of Medicine
Department of Hematologic Oncology and Blood Disorders
Levine Cancer Institute
University of North Carolina School of Medicine
Charlotte, North Carolina

Charles J. Parker, MD
Professor of Medicine
Department of Medicine
Division of Hematology and Hematologic Malignancies
University of Utah School of Medicine
Salt Lake City, Utah

John D. Phillips, PhD
Division of Hematology
Department of Medicine
University of Utah School of Medicine
Salt Lake City, Utah

Josef T. Prchal, MD
Professor of Hematology and Malignant Hematology
Adjunct in Genetics and Pathology
University of Utah & Huntsman Cancer Institute
Salt Lake City, Utah
1. interní klinika VFN a Ústav patologické fyziologie, 1. LF School of Medicine
Universita Karlova, Prague, Czech Republic

Vishnu V.B. Reddy, MD
Section Head, UAB Hospital Hematology Bone Marrow Lab
Director, Hematopathology Fellowship Program
Division of Laboratory Medicine
Professor, Department of Pathology
The University of Alabama at Birmingham
Birmingham, Alabama

Roberta Russo, PhD
Assistant Professor of Medical Genetics
Department of Molecular Medicine and Medical Biotechnology
CEINGE
Biotecnologie Avanzate
University of Naples Federico II
Naples, Italy

George B. Segel, MD
Emeritus Professor of Pediatric
Professor of Medicine
James P. Wilmot Cancer Institute
University of Rochester Medical Center
Rochester, New York

Vivien A. Sheehan, MD, PhD
Assistant Professor of Pediatrics
Baylor College of Medicine
Houston, Texas

Sujit Sheth, MD
Department of Pediatrics
Weill Cornell Medicine
New York, New York

Swee Lay Thein, MD
National Heart, Lung, and Blood Institute
The National Institutes of Health
Bethesda, Maryland

Perumal Thiagarajan, MD
Professor of Medicine and Pathology
Baylor College of Medicine
Director of Transfusion Medicine and Hematology Laboratory
Michael E. DeBakey VA Medical Center
Houston, Texas

Eduard J. van Beers, MD, PhD
Hematologist
Van Creveldkliniek
University Medical Center Utrecht
Utrecht University
Utrecht, The Netherlands

Richard van Wijk, PhD
Associate Professor
Central Diagnostic Laboratory
University Medical Center Utrecht
Utrecht University
Utrecht, The Netherlands

Neal S. Young, MD
Chief, Hematology Branch
National Heart, Lung, and Blood Institute
Mark Hatfield Clinical Research Center
National Institutes of Health
Bethesda, Maryland

PREFACE

The discovery of the ruddy globules (red cells) is attributed to Jan Swammerdam (1637-1680) in Amsterdam; but, it was Antonj van Leeuwenhoek (1632-1723) of Delft, who as a result of his ability to grind lenses with greater magnifying power (x 275), made a more detailed description of red cells, delineating their gross structure.

The biochemistry, physiology, and biophysics of the red cell have been studied intensively over three centuries and, although considered a "simple" structure, since it is anucleate and after one day in the circulation has no cytoplasmic organelles, its mysteries have been slow to be unraveled. The process of enucleation of the erythroblast in the hematopoietic space and the movement of the anucleate cell from the hematopoietic space to the marrow sinus and from there to the systemic circulation, accomplished by a cell without an intrinsic apparatus to support amoeboid motility, and the determinants of its average life span of approximately 120 days are still being elucidated. Its structural and biophysical properties, biochemical pathways, and the relationship among those features have been of continued interest to scientists. Its absence of interfering granules, containing proteolytic enzymes, organelles, and other complexities have allowed the isolation of highly purified red cell membranes and the early exploration of the biochemical and biophysical features of cell membranes, applicable to other cells, including the characteristics of membrane transport of various molecules. The nature of the structure and function of hemoglobin and the exploration of the glycolytic pathway, the hexose monophosphate shunt, and the Luebering-Rapoport pathway were other rewards reaped from the study of red cells.

Much is known, but as our mentor, friend, and colleague, Ernest Beutler, cautioned Ph.D. graduates at a Scripps Institute doctoral graduation, one should not assume that our understanding of the biomedical sciences is so profound that what is left for us is to fill in some gaps. He argued that much fundamental biomedical knowledge was still undiscovered and waiting to be illuminated. Among his many contributions to the pathogenesis of disease and application of therapy, his contributions to understanding the red cell and anemia were notable. These observations included a classic series of papers describing the effects of oxidant stress on individuals with red cell glucose-6-phosphate dehydrogenase deficiency and a life-long interest in the enzyme's variants and epidemiology. His monograph on methods for measuring red cell enzymes was an early contribution to enhancing the specificity of the diagnosis of hemolytic anemia. Published over five decades ago, it remains an unsurpassed source of methods for the assay of red cell enzymes. Beutler, also, used red cell enzyme measurement as a surrogate for diagnosis of systemic, until then difficult to diagnose diseases, such as galactosemia, glycogen storage disorders, and others. He found that red cell glucose-6-phosphate dehydrogenase deficiency was inherited as an X chromosome-linked disorder and described the mosaicism of normal and deficient red cells in heterozygous females. This finding of mosaicism provided the basis for an intellectual jump to the hypothesis of X chromosome inactivation in humans, coincident with Mary Lyon's description of the phenomenon in mice. He, also, made seminal contributions to understanding the effects of iron deficiency in non-anemic women and the expression of iron overload in those homozygous for the HFE mutation and the value of additives for prolonged storage of red cells, still in current use.

With no DNA or RNA synthesis, no mitochondria and their related enzymatic biochemical energy generating pathways, and with a relatively short life span, this amitotic cell is sustained at a normal concentration in the blood by a robust daily production of new cells in the marrow, the process of erythropoiesis. This process delivers two to three million new red cells to the blood per second. Although remarkable, it is also a vulnerability should red cell production be dampened by disease or substrate insufficiency: the latter, a principal cause of anemia.

In 1929, 3 years after obtaining his M.D. degree at the University of Manitoba, his family having immigrated to Canada from Austria, Maxwell Myer Wintrobe, obtained his Ph.D. at Tulane University, his doctoral thesis entitled "The Erythrocyte in Man." Wintrobe is considered the father of clinical hematology having published the first comprehensive text in the English language, Clinical Hematology, in 1942. He introduced the technique of the hematocrit device to measure the packed red cell volume at a time when hemoglobin and red cell count measurements were neither accurate nor reproducible. The word "hematocrit" was so appealing that it became a synonym for the packed red cell volume rather than the instrument of measurement as intended by Wintrobe. Initially, the "Wintrobe" tube, as it became known, was filled by pipette with blood to the 1 mL mark etched on the tube and the gradations on the tube allowed one to read the fraction of blood that was composed of red cells after centrifugation. Later, the microhematocrit centrifuge, which reached G-forces that removed plasma trapping as a significant consideration in the measurement in capillary tubes filled with blood, could be found on every ward and clinical laboratory as the principal means to measure the packed red cell volume and, thereby, identify anemia or erythrocytosis. A chart allowed the determination of the packed cell volume when the capillary tube, regardless of the volume of blood it contained, was placed against its scales. Wintrobe institutionalized the red cell indices, mean cell volume (MCV), mean cell hemoglobin (MCH), and mean cell hemoglobin concentration (MCHC) and showed in two classic paper in 1930 and 1934 that one could classify the anemias for diagnostic purposes by distinguishing among macrocytic, normocytic, simple microcytic, and hypochromic microcytic anemias, a method of differential diagnosis still used today. After moving to the University of Utah from Johns Hopkins University, Wintrobe established one of the most esteemed hematology clinical and research training programs in the world. He also described along with his colleague George Cartwright that the average hematocrit and hemoglobin concentration was higher in residents of Salt Lake City (elevation 4300 feet) than the value observed at Johns Hopkins in Baltimore (elevation 480 feet). He deduced from that prescient observation that hypoxia, in that instance from higher altitude, is a principal regulator of normal erythropoiesis.

In 1953, F. William Sunderman and colleagues enhanced the accuracy of blood hemoglobin measurement by introducing the cyanmethemoglobin method. In 1956, Wallace Coulter introduced his high-speed, automatic blood cell counter making blood cell counting accurate, reproducible, and capable of meeting the demands of a busy clinic and hospital environment. The "Coulter Principle" held that cells are poor conductors of electricity in a salt solution. Thus, when cells are diluted in saline and are drawn through a tiny aperture carrying a current, each cell produces a slight impedance to current flow as it passes through the narrow aperture. The pulse created by this impedance can be amplified and counted. Moreover, the size of the pulse is proportional to cell volume. Thus, the number and volume distribution of red cells in a measured volume of solution can be converted to red cell count and volume electronically. Their product, red cell count and red cell volume, provided the hematocrit, now a derived value. Thousands of cells can be counted per second. Since the red cells, leukocytes, and platelets are sufficiently different in size, they can be discriminated. The electronic particle counter's derivative technology of cell flow analysis, dependent on laser light, provided one of the most powerful diagnostic technologies in medicine, capable of measuring cell DNA content or the surface antigen array of a specific cell type. One could use the device to isolate purified, specific cell populations for analysis. The Coulter Principle and its derivative technologies revolutionized diagnostic medicine, biomedical, and industrial research and, more specifically, the diagnosis and management of red cell diseases.

A giant of studies of the red cell, perhaps little known to younger scientists, was Eric Ponder (d. 1970), an original member of the Red Cell Club (see further), whose treatise *Hemolysis and Related Phenomena* in 1948, reissued in 1971 by Grune and Stratton with a forward by Robert I. Weed, is an extraordinary compilation of his research on this cell. Many of his studies are still relevant. All scientist interested in the red cell should be familiar with this work. Weed, another gifted contributor to our understanding of the red cell, died prematurely in 1976, at the age of 48 years, of a glioblastoma. He was largely responsible for convincing the National Institutes of Health to expand the designation of the Heart and Lung Institute to the Heart, Lung and Blood Institute in 1976, facilitating research support for blood cells, especially red cell research. In 1976, in recognition of his leadership in that initiative and his contributions to research on the red cell, he was named the third recipient of the William Dameshek Award of the American Society of Hematology. At the time, the Society had two prizes, The Henry Stratton Lecture and The William Dameshek Prize. Stratton and Dameshek were very close friends. Dameshek was among the very top academic clinical hematologists in the United States and Stratton was the co-owner of Grune and Stratton Publishers. They were the prime movers of the establishment of the American Society of Hematology and started *Blood* in 1946. Dameshek was the founding editor and Grune and Stratton the publisher. Under Dameshek's editorship *Blood* became the most prestigious journal of clinical and research hematology in the world. In 1976, the journal became the official publication of the American Society of Hematology; however, the publisher still owned the title and, technically, editorial control, but some of it was ceded to the Society. In 1989, the American Society of Hematology bought the title to *Blood* from its then publisher Saunders, Inc. and it became *Blood, The Journal of the American Society of Hematology.* The purchase of title was an initiative led by H. Franklin Bunn, a distinguished hematologist at Harvard University and a world's authority on the structure and function of hemoglobin. The purchase of the Journal has provided the Society with an enormously successful economic engine to support its educational and research programs, full control of its editorial policies, and an outlet for the most impactful research in the field, including that of the red cell and its diseases.

Bob Weed's close colleagues at the University of Rochester, Claude Reed and Scott Swisher, were pioneers in forecasting the key role of a membrane protein abnormality as the primary lesion in hereditary spherocytosis, whereas others were distracted by epiphenomena, such as substrate transport. They showed that the membrane lipid composition of red cells in hereditary spherocytosis was normal but after 24 hours of incubation, lipids (cholesterol and phospholipids) were lost to the medium in their exact molar proportion as in the red cell membrane and this phenomenon could be decreased by adding glucose to the medium. This finding strongly suggested that the loss of surface area of the red cells and the disc to sphere transformation decreasing their surface area to volume ratio and moving toward their critical hemolytic volume was related to loss of pieces of membrane. This work published in 1966 was well before methods for membrane protein analysis were available. Later, the ability to characterize the protein composition of "pure" red cell membranes (ghosts) in cases of specific disorders of the red cell (eg, hereditary spherocytosis versus hereditary elliptocytosis) allowed the assignment of functional characteristics to the missing or mutant proteins. Red cell ghosts are a preparation of red cell membranes freed of their internal contents, notable hemoglobin and enzymes and substrates and colorless (ghostly pale) rather than red and are basically pure red cell membranes, a key specimen for study.

A longstanding focus on the red cell by basic and clinical investigators has been highlighted by the interactions of a group of scientists, referred to as "The Red Cell Club," which started in 1958 through the initiative of Joseph Hoffman and Daniel Tosteson, then young scientists at the National Institutes of Health. The spent their careers at Yale and Harvard, respectively. The meetings are small, informal, and an ideal milieu to focus on new science and the exchange of ideas. The Club, in its 63rd year in 2021, meets now once a year on the campus of a member to discuss new insights into the red cell and to share their current research. It is a collegial group with new "blood" being cycled in from laboratories throughout the United States and Canada as mentors introduce their acolytes to the red cell's charms. Usually, a preceding round of golf is held for those devotees of the game, weather permitting. Members, who for reasons of age or a change of interests leave the fold, are never dropped from the invitation list. Nonparticipants are tenderly referred to as "red cell ghosts." In the last several years, scientists from Europe and, occasionally Japan, have participated in these meetings. A European Red Cell Club has been established highlighting that the mysteries of the cell have not all been uncovered, confirming Beutler's admonition.

In this volume, we bring to the reader the most up-to-date consideration of the structure and function of the red cell. After two introductory chapters on the structure and biology of the red cell and erythropoiesis, the focus turns to the comprehensive set of diseases, either acquired or inherited, in which a quantitative (deficiency or excess) or qualitative (membrane, enzyme, hemoglobin) abnormality of the red cell results in disease. These chapters, also, may include important, relevant basic scientific aspects of the clinical problem under discussion. The role of certain plasma constituents, iron, folic acid, and cobalamin, critical to normal red cell production and hemoglobin synthesis, is described as well.

We believe the authors have brought to our reader an insightful exposition of the red cell and its disorders to enlighten the clinicians faced with their challenges and to the benefit of the care of their patients. In addition, we hope this text provides scientists a clear delineation of the remaining mysteries of the cell and provides them with new foundations for development of therapy of red cell diseases. We hope that this text will fill the vacuum that has existed since the monograph published in 1970 devoted to the red cell by John W. Harris, and Robert W. Kellermeyer: *The Red Cell: Production, Metabolism, Destruction: Normal and Abnormal.*

The authors acknowledge and thank Karen Edmonson, Senior Editor, formerly at McGraw-Hill, Education, for supporting the production of this text and convincing management of its merits, Susan Daley at the University of Rochester Medical Center for her administrative assistance, Harriet Lebowitz, Senior Project Development Editor at McGraw-Hill Education for stewarding the final preparation of the manuscript and Jason Malley, editor and Richard Ruzycka, production supervisor, each at McGraw-Hill Education, and Warishree Pant, the Project Manager at Knowledge Works Global, Ltd.

Marshall A. Lichtman, Rochester, NY
Josef T. Prchal, Salt Lake City, UT

Part I Structure and Physiology of the Red Cell

CHAPTER 1
STRUCTURE AND COMPOSITION OF THE ERYTHROCYTE*

Mohandas Narla

SUMMARY

Collectively, the erythroid progenitors, terminally differentiating erythroblasts (precursors), and adult red cells are termed the *erythron* to reinforce the idea that they function as an organ. The widely dispersed cells comprising this organ arise from pluripotential hematopoietic stem cells. Following commitment to the erythroid lineage (unipotential progenitor), further maturation gives rise to the erythroid progenitors, burst-forming unit–erythroid (BFU-E) and, subsequently, colony-forming unit–erythroid (CFU-E), that can be identified by their development into representative clonal colonies of red cells in vitro. The CFU-E then undergoes terminal differentiation, progressing through four to five morphologic stages, each having characteristic light microscopic and ultrastructural features. During terminal erythroid differentiation, there is an increasing amount of hemoglobin synthesis accompanied by nuclear chromatin condensation, and at the final stage of differentiation, there is nuclear extrusion to generate an anucleate polychromatophilic macrocyte (reticulocyte with supravital staining). The human polychromatophilic macrocyte (reticulocyte) matures over 2 to 3 days, first in the marrow and then in circulation into the discoid erythrocyte. During reticulocyte maturation, cytoplasmic inclusions, including residual mitochondria and ribosomes, are degraded, and the reticulocyte loses surface area to achieve the mean cell volume and surface area of a discoidal erythrocyte. Mature erythrocytes are approximately 7 to 8 μm in diameter and undergo extensive deformation to pass through 3-μm-diameter capillaries and the 1-μm-wide and 0.5-μm-thick endothelial slits in the red pulp of the spleen. The ability of the red cell to undergo extensive reversible deformation is essential for both its function and its survival. Red cell deformability is a function of its geometry, the viscosity

Acronyms and Abbreviations: BFU-E, burst-forming unit–erythroid; CFU-E, colony-forming unit–erythroid; cP, centipoise; DIC, disseminated intravascular coagulation; EMP, erythroblast macrophage protein; ICAM-4, intercellular adhesion molecule-4; IL, interleukin; MCH, mean cell hemoglobin content; MCHC, mean corpuscular hemoglobin concentration; MCV, mean cell volume; MDS, myelodysplastic syndrome; SA:V, surface area-to-volume ratio; TTP, thrombotic thrombocytopenic purpura.

*This chapter contains text written for previous editions of this book by Brian Bull, Paul Herrmann, and Ernest Beutler.

of the cytoplasm, largely determined by the concentration of hemoglobin. Decreased deformability is a feature of red cells in various pathologic states. The erythrocyte is unique among eukaryotic cells in that its principal physical structure is its cell membrane, which encloses a concentrated hemoglobin solution. Thus, all structural properties of this cell are in some way linked to the cell membrane. In contrast to other cells, the erythrocyte has no cytoplasmic structures or organelles. Among human cells, only red cells and platelets do not have a nucleus.

● ERYTHRON

The mass of circulating erythrocytes constitutes an organ responsible for the transport of oxygen to tissues and the removal of carbon dioxide from tissues for exhalation. Collectively, the progenitors, precursors, and adult red cells make up an organ termed the *erythron*, which arises from pluripotential hematopoietic stem cells. Following commitment to the erythroid lineage, unipotential progenitors mature into the erythroid progenitors, the burst-forming unit–erythroid (BFU-E) and, subsequently, the colony-forming unit–erythroid (CFU-E), which then undergoes further maturation to generate anucleate polychromatophilic macrocytes (reticulocytes on supravital staining). The BFU-E and CFU-E are identified by their development into morphologically identifiable clonal colonies of red cells in vitro. The reticulocyte further matures, first in the marrow for 2 to 3 days and, subsequently, in the circulation for approximately 1 day, to generate discoid erythrocytes.[1-5] The proerythroblast, the first morphologically recognizable erythroid precursor cell in the marrow, typically undergoes 5 mitoses (range 4-6) before maturation to an orthochromatic erythroblast, which then undergoes nuclear extrusion. A feature of erythropoiesis is that after each cell division, the daughter cells advance in their state of maturation with significant changes in gene and protein expression compared with the parent cell and, ultimately, become functional as mature erythrocytes.[4] In this process, they acquire the human blood group antigens, transport proteins, and all components of the erythrocyte membrane.[4,6]

In the adult stage of development, the total number of circulating erythrocytes is in a steady state, unless perturbed by a pathologic or environmental insult. This effect does not hold during growth of the individual in utero, particularly in the early stages of embryonic development and during neonatal development as the total blood volume increases markedly. Consequently, erythrocyte production in the embryo and fetus differs markedly from that in the adult.

THE EARLIEST ERYTHRON

In the very early stages of human growth and development, there are two forms of erythroid differentiation: primitive and definitive.[7-10] Chapters 2 and 17 provide detailed information of embryonic and fetal hematopoiesis. The primitive erythron supplies the embryo with oxygen during the phase of rapid growth before the definitive form of maturation has had a chance to develop and seed an appropriate niche. The hallmark of this primitive erythron is the release of nucleated erythroid precursors containing embryonic hemoglobin. Although primitive in the sense that the cells contain nuclei when released into the circulation, this form of maturation differs from avian and reptilian erythropoiesis in that the nucleus is eventually expelled from the mammalian cells as they circulate. The transient presence of a nucleus in the cells of the circulating primitive erythron can decrease the efficiency of gas exchange in the lungs and microvasculature because the nucleus prevents the red cell from behaving as a fluid droplet.[11] The definitive stage of maturation makes its appearance around week 5 of embryogenesis when multipotential stem cells develop and seed the liver, which maintains the erythron for most of fetal life. In later fetal life, skeletal development provides marrow niches to which erythropoiesis relocates, being sustained in the form of erythroblastic islands, a central macrophage with circumferential layers of developing erythroid cells.[12] The definitive stage of erythroid maturation predominates during the remainder of fetal development and is the only type of erythroid maturation present through childhood and adult life. All normal human erythropoiesis occurs in the marrow in the form of erythroblastic islands.[13]

ERYTHROID PROGENITORS

Burst-Forming Unit–Erythroid

The earliest identifiable progenitor committed to the erythroid lineage is the BFU-E (Chap. 2, Fig. 2-1). A BFU-E is defined in vitro by its ability to create a "burst" on semisolid medium, that is, a colony consisting of several hundred to thousands of cells by 10 to 14 days of growth, during which time smaller satellite clusters of cells form around a larger central group of erythroid cells, giving rise to the designation of a "burst." The generation of BFU-E from hematopoietic stem cells requires interleukin (IL)-3, stem cell factor, and erythropoietin for differentiation, proliferation, prevention of apoptosis, and maturation (Chap. 2).[5,13]

Colony-Forming Unit–Erythroid

As erythroid maturation progresses, a later progenitor, the CFU-E, derived from the BFU-E, can be defined in vitro. The CFU-E is dependent on erythropoietin for its development and can undergo only a few cell divisions.[5,14,15] Thus, the CFU-E forms a smaller colony of morphologically recognizable erythroid cells in 5 to 7 days (see Chap. 2, Fig. 2-1). Adhesion between erythroid cells and macrophages occurs at the CFU-E stage of maturation.

Using cell-surface markers, IL-3 receptor, CD34, and CD36, highly purified populations of BFU-E and CFU-E can be isolated from human marrow.[5] Gene expression profiling shows distinctive changes in gene expression profiles in hematopoietic stem cells, BFU-E, and CFU-E.[5] Some of the marrow failure syndromes are the result of defects in differentiation of stem cells into erythroid progenitors.

ERYTHROBLASTIC ISLAND

The anatomical unit of erythropoiesis in the normal adult is the erythroblastic island or islet.[13,16,17] The erythroblastic island consists of a centrally located macrophage surrounded by maturing terminally differentiating erythroid cells (Fig. 1-1A). Several binding proteins are implicated in the cell–cell adhesions important to this process. These include $\alpha_4\beta_1$ integrin, erythroblast macrophage protein (EMP), and intercellular adhesion molecule-4 (ICAM-4) on the erythroblasts and vascular cell adhesion molecule (VCAM-1) EMP, α_V integrin on macrophages.[16] Additional macrophage receptors include CD69 (sialoadhesin) and CD163, but the counterreceptors for these on erythroblasts remains to be defined.[16] Phase-contrast microcinematography reveals that the macrophage is far from passive or immobile. Evidence suggests that either the erythroblastic islands migrate or that erythroid precursors move from island to island, because islands near sinusoids are composed of more mature erythroblasts, whereas islands more distant from the sinusoids are composed of proerythroblasts.[18] The macrophage's pseudopodium-like cytoplasmic extensions move rapidly over cell surfaces of the surrounding wreath of erythroblasts. On phase-contrast micrographs, the central macrophage of the erythroblastic island appears spongelike, with surface invaginations in which the erythroblasts lie (Fig. 1-1B). As the erythroblast matures, it moves along a cytoplasmic extension of the macrophage away from the main body. When the erythroblast is sufficiently mature for nuclear expulsion, the erythroblast makes contact with an endothelial cell, passes through a pore in the cytoplasm of the endothelial cell, and enters the circulation as a polychromatophilic macrocyte (reticulocyte).[19-21] The nucleus is ejected before egress from the marrow, phagocytized, and degraded by marrow macrophages.[22] In addition to the unique cytologic features just described, the macrophage of the erythroblastic island is also molecularly distinct as demonstrated by a unique immunophenotypic signature.[23] In addition, the macrophage of the erythroblastic island appears to play a stimulatory role in erythropoiesis; independent of erythropoietin. The anemia of chronic inflammation and of the myelodysplastic syndrome (MDS) may result partly from inadequate stimulation of erythropoiesis by these macrophages (Chaps. 2 and 6).

Despite the central role of erythroid islands in erythropoiesis in vivo, morphologically normal development of erythroid cells can be

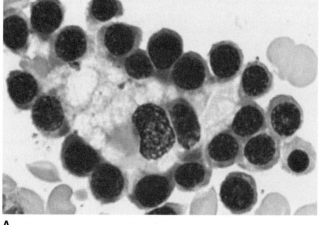

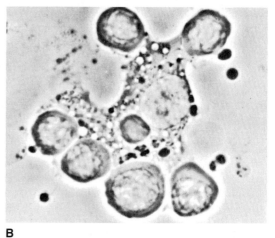

A   **B**

Figure 1–1. Erythroblastic island. **A.** Erythroblastic island as seen in Wright-Giemsa–stained marrow. Note central macrophage surrounded by a cohort of attached erythroblasts. **B.** Erythroblastic island in the living state examined by phase-contrast microscopy. The macrophage shows dynamic movement in relation to its surrounding erythroblasts. *(A, reproduced with permission from Lichtman MA, Shafer MS, Felgar RE, et al: Lichtman's Atlas of Hematology 2016. New York, NY: McGraw Hill; 2017.)*

recapitulated in vitro without these structures, assuming developing cells are provided with supraphysiologic concentrations of appropriate cytokines and growth factors. Such growth in vitro, however, is much less optimal than when erythroblasts form erythroblastic islands.[24] The erythroblastic island is a fragile structure. It is usually disrupted in the process of obtaining a marrow specimen by needle aspiration but can be seen in marrow biopsies.

Macrophages in erythroblastic islands not only affect erythroid differentiation and/or proliferation but also perform other functions, including rapid phagocytosis (<10 min) of extruded nuclei as a result of exposure of phosphatidylserine on the surface of the membrane surrounding the nucleus.[22] This phagocytosis is the reason for the inability to find extruded nuclei in marrow aspirates despite the fact that 2 million nuclei are extruded every second during steady-state erythropoiesis. A protective macrophage function linked to efficient phagocytosis has been described. In normal mice, DNase II in macrophages degrades the ingested nuclear DNA, but in DNase II-knockout mice, the inability to degrade DNA results in macrophage toxicity, with a resultant decrease in the number of marrow macrophages and in conjunction with severe anemia.[25] Macrophages can play both positive and negative regulatory roles in human erythropoiesis, but the mechanistic basis for these regulatory processes are not completely understood.[16,24] These processes may play a role in the ineffective erythropoiesis in disorders such as MDS, thalassemia, and malarial anemia.

Another potentially important role originally proposed for the central macrophage is direct transfer of iron to developing erythroblasts mediated by ferritin exchange between macrophages and erythroblasts

(Chap. 10).[13] This is an interesting evolving concept with identification of various transport proteins involved in this exchange.

ERYTHROID PROGENITORS AND PRECURSORS

Early Progenitors

A "progenitor" in the hematopoietic system is defined as a marrow cell that is a derivative of the pluripotent hematopoietic stem cell through the process of differentiation, and is antecedent to a "precursor" cell, the latter being identifiable by light microscopy by its morphologic characteristics. In erythropoiesis, the earliest precursor is the proerythroblast. Erythroid progenitor cells are identified as marrow cells capable of forming erythroid colonies in semisolid medium in vitro under conditions in which the appropriate growth factors are present. Progenitor cells also may be identified by characteristic profiles of surface CD antigens using flow cytometry. Numerically, erythroid progenitors, BFU-E, and CFU-E represent only a minute proportion of human marrow cells. BFU-E range from 300 to 1700 × 10^6 mononuclear cells and CFU-E range from 1500 to 5000 × 10^6 mononuclear cells.[5] In vitro cultures using CD34+ cells from blood, cord blood, and marrow as the starting material have identified the critical cytokines required for erythroid differentiation and maturation and have enabled the identification and isolation of pure cohorts of erythroid progenitors and erythroblasts at all stages of terminal erythroid maturation.[4,5]

Precursors

Figure 1-2 shows the sequence of precursors as seen in marrow films. Figure 1-3 shows the marrow precursors as isolated by flow cytometry.

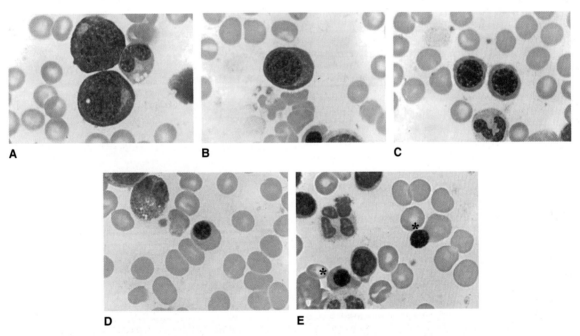

A   **B**   **C**

D   **E**

Figure 1–2. Human erythrocyte precursors. Light microscopic appearance. Marrow films stained with Wright stain. There are five stages of erythroblast development recognizable by light microscopy. **A.** Proerythroblasts. Two are present in this field. They are the largest red cell precursor, with a fine nuclear chromatin pattern, nucleoli, basophilic cytoplasm, and often a clear area at the site of the Golgi apparatus. **B.** Basophilic erythroblast. The cell is smaller than the proerythroblast, the nuclear chromatin is slightly more condensed, and cytoplasm is basophilic. **C.** Polychromatophilic erythroblasts. The cell is smaller on average than its precursors. The nuclear chromatin is more condensed, with a checkerboard pattern that develops. Nucleoli are usually not apparent. The cytoplasm is gray, reflecting the staining modulation induced by hemoglobin synthesis, which adds cytoplasmic content that takes an eosinophilic stain, admixed with the residual basophilia of the fading protein synthetic apparatus. **D.** Orthochromic normoblast. Smaller on average than its precursor, increased condensation of nuclear chromatin, with homogeneous cytoplasmic coloration approaching that of a red cell. **E.** Late orthochromatic erythroblasts *(asterisks)*. The orthochromatic erythroblast to the right is undergoing apparent enucleation. The other three mononuclear cells are lymphocytes. A degenerating four-lobed neutrophil is also present. *(Reproduced with permission from Lichtman MA, Shafer MS, Felgar RE, et al: Lichtman's Atlas of Hematology 2016. New York, NY: McGraw Hill; 2017.)*

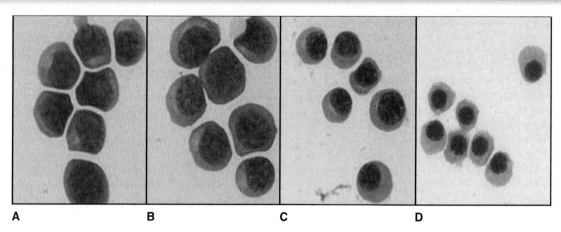

Figure 1–3. Human erythroblast precursors as isolated by cell flow cytometry. Images are of populations of human erythroblast precursors at stages of erythroid maturation when sorted from human marrow by flow cytometry. **A** and **B.** Proerythroblasts and early basophilic erythroblasts; **(C)** polychromatic erythroblasts; and **(D)** orthochromatic erythroblasts.

Proerythroblasts On stained films, the proerythroblast appears as a large cell, irregularly rounded or slightly oval.[13] The nucleus occupies approximately 80% of the cell area and contains fine chromatin delicately distributed in small clumps. One or several well-defined nucleoli are present. The high concentration of polyribosomes gives the cytoplasm of these cells its characteristic intense basophilia. At very high magnification, ferritin molecules are seen dispersed singly throughout the cytoplasm and lining the clathrin-coated pits on the cell membrane (Figs. 1-2 and 1-4). Diffuse cytoplasmic density on sections stained for peroxidase indicates that hemoglobin is already present. Dispersed glycogen particles are present in the cytoplasm.

Basophilic Erythroblasts Basophilic erythroblasts are smaller than proerythroblasts. The nucleus occupies three-fourths of the cell area and is composed of characteristic dark violet heterochromatin interspersed with pink-staining clumps of euchromatin linked by irregular strands.[13] The whole arrangement often resembles wheel spokes or a clock face. The cytoplasm stains deep blue, leaving a perinuclear halo that expands into a juxtanuclear clear zone around the Golgi apparatus. Cytoplasmic basophilia at this stage results from continued presence of polyribosomes (Figs. 1-2 and 1-5).

Polychromatophilic Erythroblasts After the mitotic division of the basophilic erythroblast, the cytoplasm changes from deep blue to gray as hemoglobin dilutes the polyribosome content. Cells at this stage are smaller than basophilic erythroblasts. The nucleus occupies less than half of the cell area. The heterochromatin is located in well-defined clumps spaced regularly about the nucleus, producing a checkerboard pattern. The nucleolus is lost, but the perinuclear halo persists.[13] It is at this point that erythroblasts lose their mitotic potential. Electron microscopy of the polychromatophilic erythroblast reveals increased aggregation of nuclear heterochromatin.[13] Active ferritin transport across the cell membrane is always evident, and siderosomes along with dispersed ferritin molecules can be identified within the cytoplasm (Figs. 1-2 and 1-6).

Orthochromic (syn. Orthochromatic) Erythroblasts After the final mitotic division of the erythropoietic series, the concentration of hemoglobin increases within the erythroblast. Under the light microscope, the nucleus appears almost completely dense and featureless. It is measurably decreased in size. This cell is the smallest of the erythroblastic series.[13] The nucleus occupies approximately one-fourth of the cell area and is eccentric. Cell movement can be appreciated under the phase-contrast microscope. Round projections appear suddenly in different parts of the cell periphery and are just as quickly retracted.[13] The movements probably are made in preparation for ejection of the nucleus. The cell ultrastructure is characterized by irregular borders, reflecting its motile state. The heterochromatin forms large masses. Mitochondria are reduced in number and size (see Figs. 1-2, 1-7, and 1-8).

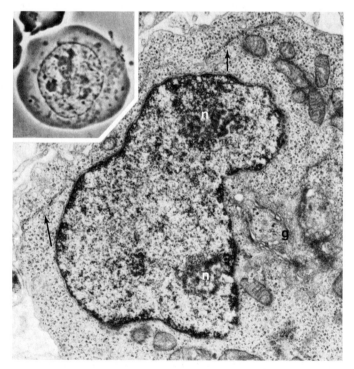

Figure 1–4. Proerythroblast. Phase-contrast micrograph *(inset)* of a proerythroblast showing the immature nucleus with nucleoli and finely dispersed nuclear chromatin. The centrosome (juxtanuclear clear zone) is apparent with its dense accumulation of mitochondria. Electron microscopic section of the proerythroblast shows nucleoli *(n)* in contact with the nuclear membrane. Chromatin is finely dispersed and forms small aggregates in the fixed nuclear membrane. The perinuclear canal is narrow but well defined. Polyribosome groups, many in helical configuration, are dispersed throughout the cytoplasm. The Golgi apparatus *(g)* is well developed, and regions of endoplasmic reticulum *(arrows)* are seen.

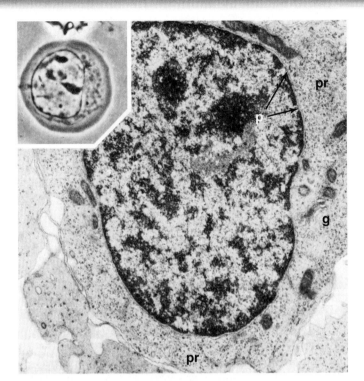

Figure 1–5. Basophilic erythroblast. Phase-contrast photomicrograph *(inset)* shows increased clumping of the nuclear chromatin and further rounding of the cell, with aggregation of the mitochondria and centrosome into the regions of nuclear indentation. The electron microscopic section shows clumping of the nuclear chromatin, nuclear pores *(p)*, organization of the nucleoli, increased density of polyribosomes *(pr)*, well-developed Golgi apparatus *(g)*, and a decrease in smooth endoplasmic reticulum.

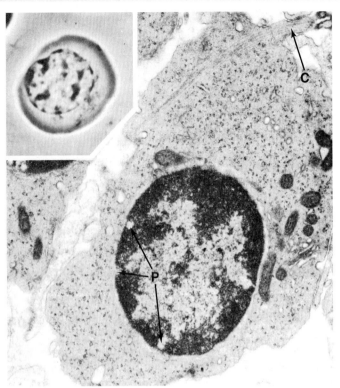

Figure 1–6. Polychromatophilic erythroblast. Phase-contrast micrograph *(inset)* demonstrates diminished size of this cell compared with its precursor. Further clumping of nuclear chromatin gives the nucleus a checkerboard appearance. The centrosome is condensed, and a perinuclear halo has developed. The electron microscopic section demonstrates relative reduction of the density of polyribosomes and dilution by the moderately osmiophilic hemoglobin in the cytoplasm. Nuclear chromatin shows a marked increase in clumping, and nuclear pores *(P)* are enlarged.

Normal Sideroblasts All normal erythroblasts are sideroblasts in that they contain iron in structures called *siderosomes*, as evident by transmission electron microscopy. These structures are essential for the transfer of iron for heme (hemoglobin) synthesis. By light microscopy, under the usual conditions of Prussian blue staining for iron, a minority of normal erythroblasts (approximately 15%-20%) can be identified as containing siderosomes, and those that can be so identified have very few (1-4) small Prussian blue–positive granules.

Pathologic Sideroblasts A heterogeneous group of erythrocyte disorders is accompanied by ineffective erythropoiesis, abnormal erythroblast morphology, and hyperferremia. These disorders include acquired megaloblastic anemia (Chap. 9), congenital dyserythropoietic anemias (Chap. 14), thalassemias (Chap. 17), the inherited and acquired sideroblastic anemias, pyridoxine-responsive anemia, alcohol-induced sideroblastic anemia, and lead intoxication (Chaps. 20 and 23). Some of these conditions are characterized by the presence of pathologic sideroblasts. Pathologic sideroblasts are of two types. The first is an erythroblast that has an increase in number and size of Prussian blue–stained siderotic granules throughout the cytoplasm. The second is the erythroblast that shows iron-containing granules that are arranged in an arc or a complete ring around the nucleus (Fig. 1-8). These pathologic sideroblasts are referred to as *ring* or *ringed sideroblasts*.[26,27] Electron microscopic studies show that granules in ringed sideroblasts are iron-loaded mitochondria. In cells with iron-loaded mitochondria, many ferritin molecules are deposited between adjacent erythroblast membranes.

RETICULOCYTE

Birth

Before enucleation at the late orthochromatic erythroblasts stage, intermediate filaments and the marginal band of microtubules disappear. Enucleation is a highly dynamic process that involves coordinated action of multiple mechanisms.[28-30] Tubulin and actin become concentrated at the point where the nucleus will exit. These changes, accompanied by microtubular rearrangements and actin polymerization, play a role in nuclear expulsion. Expulsion of the nucleus in vitro is not an instantaneous phenomenon; it requires a period of 6 to 8 minutes. The process begins with several vigorous contractions around the midportion of the cell, followed by a division of the cell into unequal portions. The smaller portion consists of the expelled nucleus surrounded by a thin ring of hemoglobin and plasma membrane (Fig. 1-9). In vivo, expulsion of the nucleus may occur while the erythroblast is still part of an erythroblastic island and the outer leaflet of the bilaminar membrane surrounding the expelled nucleus is high in phosphatidylserine, a signal for macrophage ingestion (Fig. 1-10).[22] Two hypotheses have been proposed to explain how the reticulocyte exits the marrow.[19-21] The reticulocyte may actively traverse the sinus epithelium to enter the lumen. More likely, however, the reticulocyte may be driven across by a pressure differential because it appears incapable of directed amoeboid motion. In vitro experimental evidence favors the hypothesis that pressure differential is likely the driver for reticulocyte release.[21]

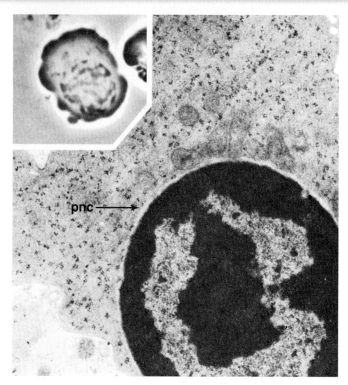

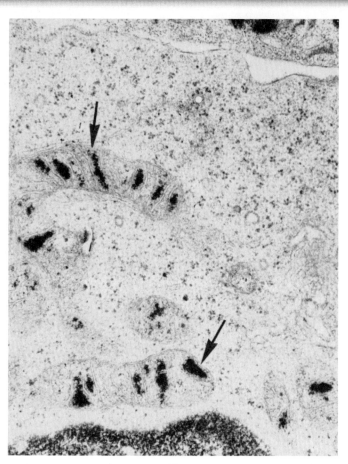

Figure 1–7. Orthochromic erythroblast. Phase-contrast appearance of this cell in the living state *(inset)* shows the irregular borders indicative of its characteristic motility, the eccentric nucleus making contact with the plasmalemma, further pyknosis of the nuclear chromatin, and condensation of the centrosome. The electron microscopic section shows further dilution of polyribosomes, some of which appear to be disintegrating into monoribosomes, by the increasing hemoglobin. The number of mitochondria is decreased, and some mitochondria are degenerating. Nuclear chromatin is clumped into large masses, and a perinuclear canal *(pnc)* is seen.

Figure 1–8. Pathologic sideroblast is an erythroblast characterized by the presence of mitochondrial deposits of iron-containing ferruginous micelles *(arrows)* between the cristae.

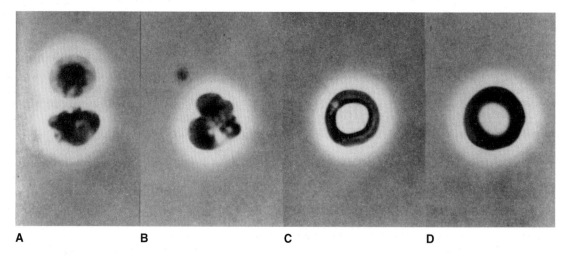

A   B   C   D

Figure 1–9. Morphology of cells during reticulocyte maturation. **A.** Orthochromatic erythroblast extruding its nucleus. **B.** Multilobular, motile reticulocyte generated after nuclear extrusion. **C.** The cup-shaped, nonmotile reticulocyte at a later stage of maturation. **D.** Mature discoid red cell.

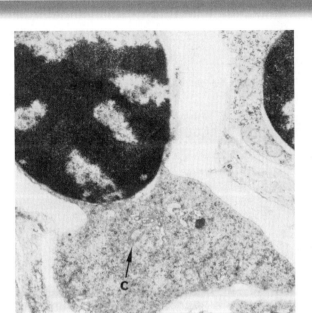

Figure 1–10. Orthochromic erythroblast ejecting its nucleus. A thin rim of cytoplasm surrounds the nucleus. In the cytoplasm, a single centriole (c) is partially encircled by some Golgi saccules.

Maturation

After nuclear extrusion, the reticulocyte retains mitochondria, small numbers of ribosomes, the centriole, and remnants of the Golgi apparatus. It contains no endoplasmic reticulum. Supravital staining with brilliant cresyl blue or new methylene blue produces aggregates of ribosomes, mitochondria, and other cytoplasmic organelles. These aggregates stain deep blue and, arranged in reticular strands, give the reticulocyte its name. Maturation of the reticulocyte requires 48 to 72 hours. During this period, approximately 20% of the membrane surface area is lost and cell volume decreases by 10% to 15%, and the final assembly of the membrane skeleton is completed.[31-33] Living reticulocytes observed by phase-contrast microscopy are irregularly shaped cells with a characteristically puckered exterior and a motile membrane. Examined by electron microscopy, reticulocytes are irregularly shaped and contain many remnant organelles.[13] The organelles, small smooth vesicles, and an occasional centriole are grouped in the region of the cell where the nucleus is expelled. In "young" reticulocytes, the majority of ribosomes dispersed throughout the cytoplasm are in the form of polyribosomes. As protein synthesis diminishes during maturation, the polyribosomes gradually transform into monoribosomes. During reticulocyte maturation, there is significant remodeling of the membrane, including loss of membrane proteins that include transferrin receptors, Na-K adenosine triphosphatase, and adhesion molecules, as well as loss of tubulin and cytoplasmic actin.[33] During the remodeling process, the membrane becomes more elastic and acquires increased membrane mechanical stability.[32]

Macroreticulocytes

"Stress" reticulocytes are released into the circulation during an intense erythropoietin response to acute anemia or experimentally in response to large doses of exogenously administered erythropoietin.[34] These cells may be twice the normal volume, with a corresponding increase in mean cell hemoglobin (MCH) content. Whether the increase results from one less mitotic division during maturation or from some other process such as changes in cell cycle is not clear. Mice do not have the ability to produce stress reticulocytes with increased mean cell volume

(MCV) and MCH. In contrast, even under moderate erythropoietic stress, some reticulocytes in the marrow pool shift to the circulating pool. These "shift" reticulocytes with normal MCH contain a higher-than-normal RNA content and can be quantified. Quantification is commonly performed by applying a fluorescent stain to tag RNA and then dividing reticulocytes into high-, medium-, and low-fluorescence categories using a fluorescence-sensitive flow cytometer. The "stress" reticulocytes of the older literature likely fall in the high- and medium-fluorescence categories. Currently, little attention is being paid to discriminate stress and shift reticulocytes.

Pathology of the Reticulocyte

The reticulocyte may show pathologic alterations in size or staining properties. The reticulocyte may contain inclusions visible by light microscopy or identifiable only from ultrastructural analysis. Most pathologic inclusions usually attributed to erythrocytes are found within reticulocytes and are nuclear or cytoplasmic remnants derived from late-stage erythroblasts. In patients who have undergone splenectomy, they may also be found in mature erythrocytes.

RED CELL INCLUSIONS

See Fig. 1-11 for images of red cell inclusions.

Howell-Jolly Bodies

Howell-Jolly bodies are small nuclear remnants that have the color of a pyknotic nucleus on Wright-stained films and show a positive Feulgen reaction for DNA.[35,36] They are spherically shaped, randomly distributed in the red cell, and usually no larger than 0.5 μm in diameter. Howell-Jolly bodies may be numerous, although only one is usually present. In pathologic situations, they appear to represent chromosomes that have separated from the mitotic spindle during abnormal mitosis, and they contain a high proportion of centromeric material along with heterochromatin. More commonly, during normal maturation they arise from nuclear fragmentation or incomplete expulsion of the nucleus. Howell-Jolly bodies are pitted from the reticulocytes during their transit through the interendothelial slits of the splenic sinus. They are characteristically present in the blood of persons who have undergone splenectomy and in patients with megaloblastic anemia, and hyposplenic states.

Pocked (or Pitted) Red Cells

When viewed by interference-phase microscopy, pocked red cells appear to have surface membrane "pits" or craters.[37-39] The vesicles or indentations characterizing these cells represent autophagic vacuoles adjacent to the cell membrane. The vacuoles appear to be instrumental in disposal of cellular debris as the erythrocyte passes through the microcirculation of the spleen. Within 1 week after splenectomy, a patient's pocked red cell counts begin to rise, reaching a plateau at 2 to 3 months. Pocked red blood cell counts are sometimes used as a surrogate test for splenic function.

Cabot Rings

The ring-like or figure-of-eight structures sometimes seen in megaloblastic anemia within reticulocytes and in an occasional, heavily stippled, late-intermediate megaloblast are designated *Cabot rings*.[40,41] Their composition is nuclear. Some investigators have suggested that Cabot rings originate from spindle material that was mishandled during abnormal mitosis. Others have found no indication of DNA or spindle filaments but have shown the rings are associated with adherent granular material containing arginine-rich histone and nonhemoglobin iron.

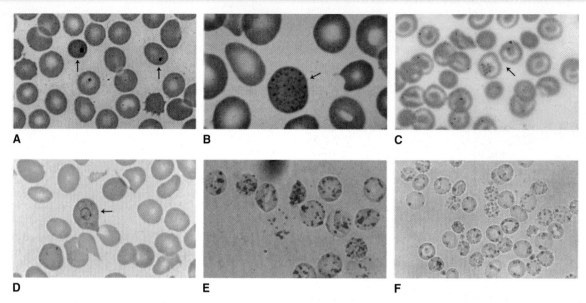

Figure 1–11. Red cell inclusions. Blood films. **A.** Red cells with Howell-Jolly bodies *(arrows)* postsplenectomy. The crisp circular border, dark blue color, and peripheral location are characteristics. **B.** Basophilic stippling. These basophilic inclusions may be fine or coarse. In this case, the cell contains coarse stippling seen in lead poisoning *(arrow)*. **C.** Siderocyte. These cells contain purple granules when stained with Wright stain (Pappenheimer bodies). Compared with basophilic stippling, siderotic granules are usually fewer in number and sometimes clustered. These Prussian blue–stained cells confirm that the granules contain iron (blue reaction product). The *arrow* points to two siderocytes. **D.** Cabot ring. Rare red cell inclusion *(arrow)*. See text for further description. **E.** Heinz bodies. These cells from a patient with glucose-6-phosphate dehydrogenase deficiency were incubated with a supravital dye, which stains the denatured globin precipitates. **F.** Red cells from a patient with hemoglobin H disease (α-thalassemia). The hemoglobin precipitates are stained with brilliant cresyl blue. *(Reproduced with permission from Lichtman MA, Shafer MS, Felgar RE, et al: Lichtman's Atlas of Hematology 2016. New York, NY: McGraw Hill; 2017.)*

Basophilic Stippling

Basophilic stippling consists of granulations of variable size and number that stain deep blue with Wright stain. Electron microscopic studies have shown that *punctate basophilia* represents aggregated ribosomes.[42] Clumps form during the course of drying and postvital staining of the cells, much as "reticulum" in reticulocytes precipitates from ribosomes during supravital staining. The clumped ribosomes may include degenerating mitochondria and siderosomes. In conditions such as lead intoxication (Chap. 23), pyrimidine 5'-nucleotidase deficiency (Chap. 16), and thalassemia (Chap. 17), the altered reticulocyte ribosomes have a greater propensity to aggregate. As a result, basophilic granulation appears larger and is referred to as *coarse basophilic stippling*.

Heinz Bodies

Heinz bodies are composed of denatured proteins, primarily hemoglobin, that form in red cells as a result of chemical insult; in hereditary defects of the hexose monophosphate shunt (Chap. 16); in the thalassemias (Chap. 17); and in unstable hemoglobin syndromes (Chap. 18).[43] Heinz bodies are not seen on ordinary Wright- or Giemsa-stained blood films. Heinz bodies are readily visible in red cells stained supravitally with brilliant cresyl blue or crystal violet and are eliminated as red cells traverse the endothelial slits of the splenic sinus.

Hemoglobin H Inclusions

Hemoglobin H is composed of β_4 tetramers, indicating that β chains are present in excess as a result of impaired α-chain production (Chap. 17). Exposure to redox dyes such as brilliant cresyl blue, methylene blue, or new methylene blue, results in denaturation and precipitation of abnormal hemoglobin.[44-46] Brilliant cresyl blue causes the formation of a large number of small membrane-bound inclusions, giving the cell a characteristic "golf ball–like" appearance when viewed by light microscopy.

Methylene blue and new methylene blue generate a smaller number of variably sized membrane-bound and floating inclusions. These changes are seen most frequently in α-thalassemia but can also be found in patients with unstable hemoglobin (Chap. 18) and in rare patients with primary myelofibrosis in whom acquired hemoglobin H disease has developed.

Siderosomes and Pappenheimer Bodies

Normal or pathologic red cells in blood containing siderosomes ("iron bodies") usually are reticulocytes. The iron granulations are larger and more numerous in the pathologic state. Electron microscopy shows that many of these bodies are mitochondria-containing ferruginous micelles rather than the ferritin aggregates characterizing normal siderocytes.[47] Siderosomes usually are found in the cell periphery, whereas basophilic stippling tends to be distributed homogeneously throughout the cell. Pappenheimer bodies are siderosomes that stain with Wright stain. Electron microscopy of Pappenheimer bodies shows that the iron often is contained within a lysosome, as confirmed by the presence of acid phosphatase. Siderosomes may contain degenerating mitochondria, ribosomes, and other cellular remnants.

STRUCTURE AND SHAPE OF ERYTHROCYTES

The normal resting shape of the erythrocyte is a biconcave disc (Fig. 1-12). Variations in the shape and dimensions of the red cell are useful in the differential diagnosis of anemias. Normal human red cells have a diameter of 7 to 8 μm, and the diameter decreases slightly with cell age. The decrease in size likely results from loss of membrane surface area during the erythrocyte life span by spleen-facilitated vesiculation. The cells have an average volume of approximately 90 fL and a surface area of approximately 140 μm². The membrane is present in sufficient excess to allow the cell to swell to a sphere of approximately 150 fL or to

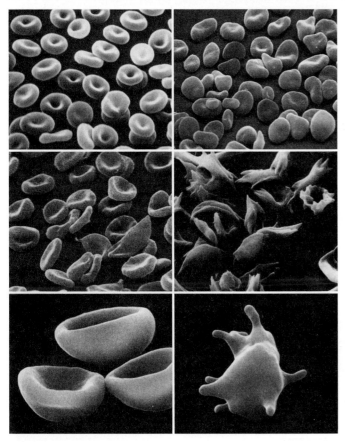

Figure 1–12. Scanning electron micrographs of distinct red cell morphologies. Discoid normal red cells *(top left panel)*. Elliptocytes and fragmented red cells *(top right panel)*. Oxygenated sickle red cells *(middle left panel)* and deoxygenated sickle red cells *(middle right panel)*. Stomatocytic red cells *(bottom left panel)*. Acanthocyte *(bottom right panel)*.

deform so as to enter a capillary with a diameter of 2.8 μm. The normal erythrocyte stains reddish-brown with Wright-stained blood films and pink with Giemsa stain. The central third of the cell appears relatively pale compared with the periphery, reflecting its biconcave shape. Many artifacts can be produced in the preparation of the blood film. They may result from contamination of the glass slide or coverslip with traces of fat, detergent, or other impurities. Friction and surface tension involved in the preparation of the blood film produce fragmentation, "doughnut cells" or anulocytes, and crescent-shaped cells. Observed under the phase-contrast or interference microscope, the red cell shows a characteristic internal scintillation known as red cell flicker.[48] The scintillation results from thermally excited undulations of the red cell membrane. Frequency analysis of the surface undulations has provided an estimate of the membrane curvature elastic constant and of changes in this constant resulting from alcohol, cholesterol loading, and exposure to cross-linking agents.

RED CELL SHAPE AND SURVIVAL IN CIRCULATION

The red cell spends most of its circulatory life within the capillary channels of the microcirculation. During its 100- to 120-day life span, the red cell travels approximately 250 km and loses approximately 15% to 20% of its cell surface area. The long survival of the red cell is at least partially a result of the unique capacity of its membrane to "tank tread,"

that is, to rotate around the red cell contents and thereby facilitate more efficient oxygen delivery. The physical arrangement of membrane skeletal proteins in a uniform shell of highly folded hexagonal spectrin lattice permits this unusual behavior.[49-51] The arrangement also is responsible for the characteristic biconcave shape of the resting cell. Red cells must also be able to withstand large shear forces and must be able to undergo extensive reversible deformation during transit through the microvasculature and in transiting from the splenic red cell pulp back into circulation. The resiliency and fluidity of the membrane to deformation is regulated by the spectrin-based membrane skeleton.[49] A deficiency in the amount of spectrin or the presence of mutant spectrin in the submembrane skeleton results in abnormally shaped cells in hereditary spherocytosis, elliptocytosis, and pyropoikilocytosis (Chap. 15).[49] In regions of circulatory standstill or very slow flow, red cells travel in aggregates of 2 to 12 cells, forming rouleaux. Within large vessels, increased shear forces disrupt this aggregation.

RED CELL COMPOSITION

The erythrocyte is a complex cell. The membrane is composed of lipids and proteins, and the interior of the cell contains metabolic machinery designed to sustain the cell through its 120-day life span and maintain the integrity of hemoglobin function. Each component of red blood cells may be expressed as a function of red cell volume, grams of hemoglobin, or square centimeters of cell surface. These expressions are usually interchangeable, but under certain circumstances each may have specific advantages. However, because disease may produce changes in the average red cell size, hemoglobin content, or surface area, the use of any of these measurements individually may, at times, be misleading. For convenience and uniformity, data in the accompanying tables (Tables 1-1 through 1-6)[52-125] are expressed in terms of cell constituent per milliliter of red cell and per gram of hemoglobin. In many instances, this process required recalculation of published data. These recalculations assume a hematocrit value of 45% and 33 g of hemoglobin per deciliter of red cells. To obtain concentration per gram of hemoglobin, the concentration per milliliter red blood cell can be multiplied by 3.03. The tables list only some of the most commonly referred to constituents of the erythrocyte. The reference on which each value is based is the first number presented in the last column of each table. Where applicable, additional confirmatory references are given. In some instances, only the percentage of the total of the type of constituent present is given. Chapter 15 discusses the detailed protein composition of the red cell membrane and its various protein constituents.

TABLE 1–1. Human Erythrocyte Protein and Water Content

Component	mg/mL RBC	Reference(s)
Water	721 ± 17.3	52
Total protein	371	52
Nonhemoglobin protein	9.2	52, 53
Insoluble stroma protein	6.3	53
Enzyme proteins	2.9	53
Extensive study by proteomic methods		54, 55

Abbreviation: RBC, red blood cell.

TABLE 1–2. Human Erythrocyte Phospholipids

Lipid	Amount	Reference
Total phospholipids	2.98 ± 0.20 mg/mL RBC	56
Cephalin	1.17 (0.38–1.91) mg/mL RBC	56
Ethanolamine phosphoglyceride	29% of total phospholipid	56
Mean plasmalogen content	67% of ethanolamine phosphoglyceride	56
Serine phosphoglyceride	10% of total phospholipid	56
Mean plasmalogen content	8% of serine phosphoglyceride	56
Lecithin	0.32 (0.03–0.95) mg/mL	57
Sphingomyelin	0.12–1.13 mg/mL	57
Lysolecithin	1.82% of total phospholipids	58

Abbreviation: RBC, red blood cell.

Some results are given as mean ± standard deviation.

ERYTHROCYTE DEFORMABILITY

During its 120-day life span, the erythrocyte must undergo extensive passive deformation and must be mechanically stable to resist fragmentation; cellular deformability is an important determinant of red cell survival in the circulation. Red cell deformability is influenced by three distinct cellular components: (1) cell shape or cell geometry, which determines the ratio of cell surface area to cell volume (SA:V; higher values of SA:V facilitate deformation); (2) cytoplasmic viscosity, which is primarily regulated by the mean corpuscular hemoglobin concentration (MCHC) and is therefore influenced by alterations in

TABLE 1–3. Human Erythrocyte Coenzyme and Vitamins

Compound	µmol/mL RBC	Reference
Ascorbic acid	0.02892 ± 0.00431	59
Choline free	Trace	60
Cocarboxylase	0.00021	61
Coenzyme A	0.0027	62
Nicotinic acid	0.105	63
Pantothenic acid	0.001 ± 0.00028	64
Pyridoxal phosphate	$20 \times 10^{-6} \pm 2 \times 10^{-6}$	65
Pyridoxal	$11 \times 10^{-6} \pm 3 \times 10^{-6}$	65
Total vitamin B_6 aldehydes	$30 \times 10^{-6} \pm 8 \times 10^{-6}$	65
Pyridoxamine phosphate	$8 \times 10^{-6} \pm 8 \times 10^{-6}$	65
4-Pyridoxic acid	$4 \times 10^{-6} \pm 4 \times 10^{-6}$	65
Riboflavin	0.00059 ± 0.00021	66
Flavin adenine dinucleotide	0.000398 ± 0.000042	67
Thiamine	0.00027	68

Abbreviation: RBC, red blood cell.

Some results are given as mean ± standard deviation.

TABLE 1–4. Nucleotides

Compound	µmol/mL RBC	Reference(s)
Adenosine monophosphate	0.021 ± 0.003	69-72
Adenosine diphosphate	0.216 ± 0.036	69-72
Adenosine triphosphate	1.35 ± 0.035	71-75
Cyclic adenosine monophosphate	0.015 ± 0.0024	76
Cyclic guanosine monophosphate	0.013 ± 0.0042	76
Guanosine diphosphate	0.018 ± 0.005	71
Guanosine triphosphate	0.052 ± 0.012	70, 71
Inosine monophosphate	0.031 ± 0.005	71-73
Nicotinamide adenine dinucleotide		77, 78
Reduced	0.0018 ± 0.001	77, 78
Oxidized	0.049 ± 0.006	
Nicotinamide adenine dinucleotide phosphate		77, 78
Reduced	0.032 ± 0.002	
Oxidized	0.0014 ± 0.0011	
S-adenosylmethionine	0.005	79
Total nucleotide	1.534 ± 0.033	80
Uridine diphosphoglucose	0.031 ± 0.005	71, 81
Uridine diphosphate N-acetyl glucosamine	0.018	81

Abbreviation: RBC, red blood cell.

Some results are given as mean ± standard deviation.

cell volume; and (3) membrane deformability and mechanical stability, which are regulated by multiple membrane properties, which include elastic shear modulus, bending modulus, and yield stress.[126-129] Either directly or indirectly, membrane components and their organization play an important role in regulating each of the factors that influence cellular deformability.

The biconcave disc shape of the normal red cell creates an advantageous SA:V relationship, allowing the red cell to undergo marked deformation while maintaining a constant surface area. The normal human adult red cell has a volume of 90 fL and a surface area of 140 µm². If the red cell were a sphere of identical volume, it would have a surface area of only 98 µm². Thus, the discoid shape provides approximately 40 µm² of excess surface area, or an extra 43%, which enables the red cell to undergo extensive deformation. Most deformations occurring in vivo and in vitro involve no increase in surface area. This is important because the normal red cell can undergo large linear extensions of up to 230% of its original dimension while maintaining its surface area, but an increase of even 3% to 4% in surface area results in cell lysis. Either membrane loss, leading to a reduction in surface area, or an increase in cell water content, leading to an increase in cell volume, will create a more spherical shape with less redundant surface area. This loss of surface area redundancy results in reduced cellular deformability, compromised red cell function, and diminished survival as a result of splenic sequestration of spherocytic red cells. A 17% reduction in surface area results in rapid removal of red cells by the human spleen.[130]

TABLE 1–5. Human Erythrocyte Carbohydrates, Organic Acids, and Metabolites

Compound	µmol/mL RBC	Reference(s)
Dihydroxyacetone phosphate	0.0094 ± 0.0028	69
2,3-Diphosphoglycerate	4.171 ± 0.636	69, 75
Fructose	0.000354 ± 0.0000191	82
Fructose 6-phosphate	0.0093 ± 0.002	69, 72, 75, 83
Fructose 3-phosphate	0.013 ± 0.001	84, 85
Fructose 2,6-diphosphate[a]	48 ± 13	86
Fructose 1,6-diphosphate	0.0019 ± 0.0006	69, 72, 75, 83
Glucuronic acid	Trace	87
Glucose	In equilibrium with plasma	88, 89
Glucose 6-phosphate	0.0278 ± 0.0075	69, 72, 75, 83
Glucose 1,6-diphosphate	0.18–0.30	72, 90
Glyceraldehyde 3-phosphate	Not detectable	69
Lactic acid	0.932 ± 0.211	53, 69, 91
Mannose 1,6-diphosphate	0.150	90
Octulose 1,8-diphosphate	Trace	92
Pyruvate	0.0533 ± 0.0215	69
3-Phosphoglycerate	0.0449 ± 0.0051	69, 75
2-Phosphoglycerate	0.0073 ± 0.0025	69, 75
Phosphoenol pyruvate	0.0122 ± 0.0022	69
Ribonucleic acid	1.355 mg	93
Ribose 1,5-diphosphate	<0.02	94, 95
Ribulose 5-phosphate	Trace	96
Sedoheptulose 7-phosphate	Trace	96
Sedoheptulose diphosphate	Trace	97
Sialic acid	0.825 ± 0.028	94
Sorbitol	31.1 ± 5.3	82, 84
Sorbitol 3-phosphate	0.013 ± 0.001	85

Abbreviation: RBC, red blood cell.

[a]Values are given in picomoles.

Some results are given as mean ± standard deviation.

TABLE 1–6. Human Erythrocyte Electrolytes

Electrolyte	µmol/mL RBC	Reference
Aluminum	0.0026	98
Bromide	0.1225	99, 100
Calcium	0.0089 ± 0.0030	100-102
Chloride	78	100, 103
Chromium	0.0004	104
Cobalt	0.0002	100, 105
Copper	0.018	104, 106, 107
Fluoride	0.0131	108
Iodine, protein-bound	0.0013	109
Lead	0.0082	98, 100, 106, 110
Magnesium	3.06	104, 111-113
Manganese	0.0034	98, 114
Nickel	0.0009	104
Phosphorus (acid soluble)		
Total P	13.2	115
Inorganic P	0.466	115
Lipid P	3.840	116
Unidentified P	0.955	115
Potassium	102.4 ± 3.9	111, 117-121
Rubidium	0.054	100
Silicon	0.036–0.060[a]	122
Silver	Trace	98
Sodium	6.2 ± 0.8	117-119
Sulfur	0.0044	123
Tin	0.0022	98
Zinc	0.153	104, 124, 125

Abbreviation: RBC, red blood cell.

[a]Obtained by subtracting plasma concentration from whole-blood concentration.

Some results are given as mean ± standard deviation.

Cytoplasmic viscosity, another regulatory component of red cell deformability, is largely determined by the MCHC, which is determined in large part by cell water content. As the hemoglobin concentration rises from 27 to 35 g/dL (the normal range for red blood cells), the viscosity of hemoglobin solution increases from 5 to 15 centipoise (cP), 5 to 15 times that of water. At these levels, the contribution of cytoplasmic viscosity to cellular deformability is negligible. However, viscosity increases exponentially at hemoglobin concentrations higher than 37 g/dL, reaching 45 cP at 40 g/dL, 170 cP at 45 g/dL, and 650 cP at 50 g/dL. At these levels, cytoplasmic viscosity may become the primary determinant of cellular deformability. Thus, cellular dehydration, usually caused by the failure of normal volume homeostasis mechanisms, can severely impair cellular deformability and thus decrease optimal oxygen delivery by impairing the ability of red cells to undergo rapid deformation necessary for passage through the microvasculature. As examples, cellular dehydration reduces red cell deformability in hereditary xerocytosis, sickle cell anemia, hemoglobin CC, and β-thalassemia.[129,131,132] However, changes in cellular dehydration by itself appear to have little influence on red cell survival.

The property of membrane deformability determines the extent of membrane deformation that can be induced by a defined level of applied force. The more deformable the membrane, the less the force required for the cell to pass through the capillaries and other narrow openings, such as fenestrations in the splenic cords. The property of membrane mechanical stability is defined as the maximum extent of deformation that a membrane can undergo, beyond which it cannot completely recover its initial shape. This is the point at which the membrane fails. Normal membrane stability allows human red cells to circulate for 100 to 120 days without fragmenting, whereas decreased stability leads to cell fragmentation under normal circulatory stresses. Both membrane deformability and membrane mechanical stability are regulated by structural organization of membrane proteins.[128] Although decreased membrane deformability can reduce effective tissue oxygen delivery, it appears to have little effect on red cell survival because Southeast Asian ovalocytes with marked reductions in membrane deformability have near-normal red cell survival. Loss of membrane mechanical stability leading to membrane fragmentation and consequent reduction in SA:V ratio, conversely, compromises red cell survival as in hemolytic hereditary elliptocytosis.[49]

RED CELL SENESCENCE

The reticulocyte loses membrane as it matures into a discocyte, and membrane loss by vesiculation continues throughout the erythrocyte's life span. The notion that erythrocyte aging is synonymous with membrane loss, increasing MCHC, and decreasing deformability largely results from studies on density-separated cells and the equating of dense cells with aged cells (Chap. 2). Although it is clear that loss of membrane surface area and decreased cell volume are the features of normal red cell senescence and that cell density increases with cell age, there is no direct relationship between cell age and cell density because there is a large heterogeneity in cell densities of reticulocytes as they enter circulation. What is clear is that the densest 1% of circulating red cells are the most aged—they have the highest levels of glycated hemoglobin, a very good marker of cell age. The loss of membrane surface area of the senescent red cells appears to be a result of membrane oxidation–induced band 3 clustering and consequent membrane vesiculation, and

the resultant critical decrease in SA:V ratio leads to their removal from circulation.[133,134]

PATHOPHYSIOLOGY OF ERYTHROCYTE SHAPES

Chapter 15 discusses erythrocytes in greater detail.

See Table 1-7 and Fig. 1-13 for scanning and blood film appearance of pathologically shaped red cells.

Spherocytes and Stomatocytes

Spherocytes represent red cells, with the most decreased SA:V ratio seen in hereditary spherocytosis (Chap. 15), immune hemolytic anemia (Chap. 26), stored blood (Chap. 30), Heinz body hemolytic anemia (Chap. 16), and caused by cell fragmentation (Chap. 22).[49,135] Stomatocytes are seen in hereditary stomatocytosis, as well as in hereditary spherocytosis, alcoholism, cirrhosis, obstructive liver disease, and erythrocyte sodium pump defects.[49,136,137] Red cells sensitized with antibodies, complement, or immune complexes lose cholesterol and surface area. As a result, they are less deformable and more osmotically fragile. Heinz body formation leads to membrane depletion by fragmentation, with spherocyte formation. A spherogenic mechanism common to Heinz body hemolytic anemias and immune hemolysis is partial phagocytosis of portions of the cell containing aggregates of denatured hemoglobin and portions of the sensitized membrane, respectively.

Stomatocytosis appear to be an intermediate form in the generation of spherocytosis with varying extents of decreased SA:V ratio as a

TABLE 1–7. Nomenclature of Red Cell Shapes and Associated Disease States

Terminology (Greek Meaning)	Old Terms, Synonyms	Description	Micrograph	Associated Disease States
Discocyte (disc)	Biconcave disc	Biconcave disc form of RBC		
Echinocyte (I-III) (sea urchin)	"Burr cell," crenated cell, "berry cell"	Spiculated RBC with short, equally spaced projections over entire surface; progressing from the "crenated disc" (echinocyte I) to the crenated sphere (echinocyte IV—not shown) with nearly complete loss of spicules		Uremia, liver disease Low-potassium red cells Immediately posttransfusion with aged or metabolically depleted blood Carcinoma of stomach and bleeding peptic ulcers
Acanthocyte (spike)	"Spur cell," acanthoid cell, acanthrocyte	Irregularly spiculated RBC with projections of varying length and position		Abetalipoproteinemia Alcoholic liver disease Postsplenectomy state Malabsorptive states
Stomatocyte (I-III) (mouth)	Mouth cell, cup form, mushroom cap, uniconcave disc, microspherocyte	Bowl-shaped RBC with single concavity; progressing from shallow bowl (I) to near sphere with small dimple (seen as mouth-shaped form in peripheral film)		Hereditary spherocytosis Hereditary stomatocytosis Alcoholism, cirrhosis, obstructive liver disease Erythrocyte sodium-pump defect

(continued)

TABLE 1–7. Nomenclature of Red Cell Shapes and Associated Disease States (Continued)

Terminology (Greek Meaning)	Old Terms, Synonyms	Description	Micrograph	Associated Disease States
Spherostomatocyte (sphere)	Spherocyte, prelytic sphere, microspherocyte	Spherical RBC with dense hemoglobin content; scanning electron microscopy shows a persistent minimal dimple		Hereditary spherocytosis (cells actually spherostomatocytes) Immune hemolytic anemia Posttransfusion Heinz body hemolytic anemia Water-dilution hemolysis Fragmentation hemolysis
Schizocyte (cut)	Schistocyte, helmet cell, fragmented cell	Split RBC, often showing half-disc shape with two or three pointed extremities; may be small, irregular fragment		Microangiopathic hemolytic anemia (TTP, DIC, vasculitis, glomerulonephritis, renal graft rejection) Carcinomatosis Heart-valve hemolysis (prosthetic or pathologic valves) Severe burns March hemoglobinuria
Elliptocyte (oval)	Ovalocyte	Oval to elongated ellipsoid RBC (with polarization of hemoglobin)		Hereditary elliptocytosis Thalassemia Iron deficiency Myelophthisic anemias Megaloblastic anemias
Drepanocyte (sickle)	Sickle cell	RBC containing polymerized hemoglobin S; showing varying shapes from bipolar, spiculated forms to holly-leaf and irregularly spiculated forms		Sickle cell disorders (SS, S trait, SC, SD, S thalassemia, etc.) Hemoglobin C-Harlem Hemoglobin Memphis/S
Codocyte (bell)	Target cell	Bell-shaped RBC that assumes a target shape on dried films of blood		Obstructive liver disease Hemoglobinopathies (S, C) Thalassemia Iron deficiency Postsplenectomy state Lecithin cholesterol acetyltransferase deficiency
Dacryocyte (tear)	Teardrop cell	RBC with a single elongated or pointed extremity		Primary myelofibrosis Myelophthisic anemias Thalassemia
Leptocyte (thin)	Thin cell, wafer cell	Thin, flat RBC with hemoglobin at periphery		Thalassemia Obstructive liver disease (± iron deficiency)
Keratocyte (horn)	Horn cell	RBC with spicules resulting from ruptured vacuole; cell appears half-moon shaped or spindle shaped		DIC or vascular prosthesis

Abbreviations: DIC, disseminated intravascular coagulation; RBC, red blood cell; TTP, thrombotic thrombocytopenic purpura.

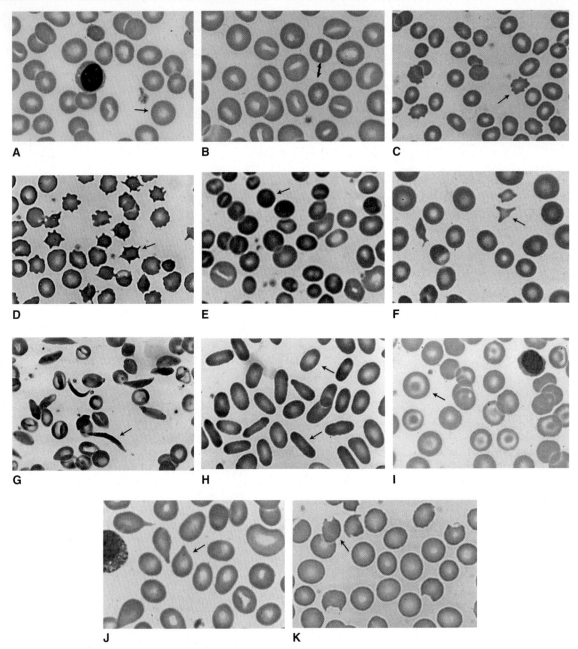

Figure 1–13. A. Normal blood. The *arrow* points to a normochromic-normocytic discocyte. **B.** Stomatocytes. The *double arrow* points to the two morphologic types of stomatocyte: upper cell with a slit-shaped pale area and lower cell with a small central circular pale area. **C.** Echinocytes. The field has several such cells. The *arrow* points to one example with evenly distributed, blunt, short, circumferentially positioned projections. **D.** Acanthocytes. The *arrow* points to one example with a few spike-shaped projections, unevenly distributed and of varying lengths. **E.** Spherocytes. Small, circular, densely-staining (hyperchromic) cells that, when fully developed, show no central pallor. **F.** Schizocytes (schistocytes, helmet cells, fragmented red cells). These microcytic cell fragments may assume varied shapes. The arrow points to a triangular shape, but two others of different shape are also present in the field. Despite being damaged and very small, they frequently maintain a biconcave appearance, as seen by their central pallor. **G.** Sickle cells (drepanocytes). Numerous sickle cells are shown. Two are in the classic shape of the blade on the agricultural sickle *(arrow)*. Many red cells that have undergone the transformation to a "sickle" cell take the slightly less extreme form of elliptical cells with a very narrow diameter with condensed hemoglobin in the center (para-crystallization). About eight such cells are in the field. **H.** Elliptocytes and ovalocytes. The *lower arrow* points to an elliptocyte (cigar-shaped). The *upper arrow* points to an ovalocyte (football-shaped). Because both forms may be seen together in a case of inherited disease (same gene mutation resulting in both shapes), as shown here, it has been proposed that all such shapes be called elliptocytes with a Roman numeral to designate the severity of the shape change toward the elliptical, that is, elliptocytes I, II, and III. **I.** Target cells (codocytes). The *arrow* points to one characteristic example among several in the field. The hemoglobin concentration corralled by membrane recurvature in the center of the cell gives it the appearance of an archery target. **J.** Tear-drop–shaped cells (dacryocytes). Three dacryocytes are in this field. One example is indicated by the *arrow*. **K.** Horn cell (keratocyte). Several examples are in the field. The *arrow* points to a typical such cell with two sharp projections. *(Reproduced with permission from Lichtman MA, Shafer MS, Felgar RE, et al: Lichtman's Atlas of Hematology 2016. New York, NY: McGraw Hill; 2017.)*

result of loss of membrane surface area or increased cell volume. Stomatocytosis is a feature of hereditary hydrocytosis caused by increased cell volume and consequent decrease in SA:V ratio. A spectrum of abnormal cells varying from normal discocytes to stomatocytes, spherostomatocytes, and dense microspherocytes is seen in hereditary spherocytosis.

Elliptocytes

Elliptocytes are seen in hereditary elliptocytosis (Chap. 15) as well as in thalassemia (Chap. 17), iron deficiency (Chap. 11), and megaloblastic anemia (Chap. 9).[49] In blood films of normal subjects, elliptical or oval cells usually constitute less than 1% of the erythrocytes. In various pathologic situations, with or without anemia (thalassemia trait, folate, and iron deficiency), the number of elliptocytes can increase to 10%. Exceptionally, as in dyserythropoiesis, the proportion can be as high as 50%. In hereditary elliptocytosis, the number of elliptical erythrocytes varies greatly, from 1% to 98%. Qualitative and quantitative anomalies of spectrin and protein 4.1, the major proteins of the membrane skeleton, are associated with hereditary elliptocytosis.[49,138] Severe hemolytic anemia is seen only in the homozygous or compound heterozygotes form of the disease (hereditary pyropoikilocytosis), in which extensive cell fragmentation produces *pyropoikilocytes* with marked decreases in SA:V ratio.

Acanthocytes

The acanthocyte (Chap. 15) is irregularly shaped, with 2 to 10 hemispherically tipped spicules of variable length and diameter. The bases of the spicules on the acanthocyte are of varying girth, unlike the spicules on echinocytes, which have remarkably uniform dimensions. Acanthocytes are seen in neuroacanthocytosis and in abetalipoproteinemia.[139] The lack of anemia in these conditions suggests that these cells have near normal life span in circulation.

Target Cells (Codocytes)

A relative excess of membrane surface area or decreased cell volume leading to increased SA:V ratio results in target cells.[140] Target cells may be seen in obstructive liver disease, hemoglobinopathies (S and C), thalassemia, iron deficiency, postsplenectomy, and lecithin cholesterol acetyltransferase deficiency. In patients with obstructive liver disease, lecithin cholesterol acetyltransferase activity is depressed. This increases the cholesterol-to-phospholipid ratio and produces an absolute increase in the surface area of the red cell membrane. In contrast, membrane excess is only relative in patients with iron-deficiency anemia and thalassemia because of the reduced cell volume. In contrast to spherocytes, which exhibit increased osmotic fragility, target red cells are osmotically resistant.

Sickle Cells (Drepanocytes)

The sickle cell displays a characteristic variation of form on stained blood films (Chap. 18). The fusiform cell in the crescent shape with two pointed extremities is encountered most commonly in deoxygenated blood samples as a result of polymerization of sickle hemoglobin. If sickle cell formation is observed by phase-contrast microscopy, the earliest change with deoxygenation is loss of flicker, followed by slight deformation at the discocyte border, with displacement of the hemoglobin to one region of the cell. The cell then elongates and becomes rigid as a result of polymerization of hemoglobin S. Upon reoxygenation, the sickle cell resumes the discocyte form and, in so doing, can lose membrane by microspherulation and fragmentation during retraction of long spicules.[141] Evidence suggests that the more typical sickle-shaped cells form under slow deoxygenation. With each sickling–unsickling cycle, membrane damage accumulates, resulting in the formation of irreversibly sickled cells.[142,143] These cells are incapable of reversion to the biconcave disc shape, even when fully oxygenated. They have an increased hemoglobin concentration, increased cation permeability, decreased potassium, and increased sodium.

Fragmented Cells (Schistocytes)

Schistocytes are seen in microangiopathic hemolytic anemias (thrombotic thrombocytopenic purpura [TTP], disseminated intravascular coagulation [DIC], vasculitis, glomerulonephritis, renal graft rejection), carcinomatosis, heart valve hemolysis (prosthetic or pathologic valves), severe burns, and march hemoglobinuria (Chap. 22). Fibrin strands in damaged blood vessels can be arrayed so that they sieve the passing red cells. If a passing red cell folds over or otherwise attaches to the strand, the bloodstream pulls on the arrested cell, stretches it, and eventually fragments it.[144] The spleen rapidly removes the schistocytes with a low relative SA:V ratio; the remainder may circulate for many days.

REFERENCES

1. Anstee DJ, Gampel A, Toye AM. Ex-vivo generation of human red cells for transfusion. *Curr Opin Hematol.* 2012;19:163.
2. Sato T, Maekawa T, Watanabe S, et al. Erythroid progenitors differentiate and mature in response to endogenous erythropoietin. *J Clin Invest.* 2000;106:263.
3. Giarratana MC, Kobari L, Lapillonne HC, et al. Ex vivo generation of fully mature human red blood cells from hematopoietic stem cells. *Nat Biotechnol.* 2005;23:69.
4. Hu J, Liu J, Xue F, et al. Isolation and functional characterization of human erythroblasts at distinct stages: implications for understanding of normal and disordered erythropoiesis in vivo. *Blood.* 2013;121:3246.
5. Li J, Hale J, Bhagia P, et al. Isolation and transcriptome analysis of human erythroid progenitors. *Blood.* 2014;124:3636.
6. Southcott MJG, Tanner MJA, Anstee DJ. The expression of human blood group antigens during erythropoiesis in a cell culture system. *Blood.* 1999;93:4425.
7. Palis J. Ontogeny of erythropoiesis. *Curr Opin Hematol.* 2008;15:155.
8. Palis J. Primitive and definitive erythropoiesis in mammals. *Front Physiol.* 2014;5:3.
9. Zambidis ET, Peault B, Park TS, et al. Hematopoietic differentiation of human embryonic stem cells progresses through sequential hematoendothelial, primitive, and definitive stages resembling human yolk sac development. *Blood.* 2005;106:860.
10. Pereda J, Niimi G. Embryonic erythropoiesis in human yolk sac: two different compartments for two different processes. *Microsc Res Tech.* 2008;71:856.
11. Schmid-Schonbein H, Wells R. Fluid drop-like transition of erythrocytes under shear. *Science.* 1969;165:288.
12. Sadahira Y, Mori M. Role of the macrophage in erythropoiesis. *Pathol Int.* 1999;49:841.
13. Bessis M. *Living Blood Cells and Their Ultrastructure.* Springer-Verlag; 1973.
14. Gregory CJ, Eaves AC. Three stages of erythropoietic progenitor cell differentiation distinguished by a number of physical and biologic properties. *Blood.* 1978;51:527.
15. McLeod DL, Shreeve MM, Axelrad AA. Improved plasma culture system for production of erythrocytic colonies in vitro: quantitative assay method for CFU-E. *Blood.* 1974;44:517.
16. Chasis JA, Mohandas N. Erythroblastic islands: niches for erythropoiesis. *Blood.* 2008;112:470.
17. Manwani D, Bieker JJ. The erythroblastic island. *Curr Top Dev Biol.* 2008;82:23.
18. Yokoyama T, Etoh T, Kitagawa H, et al. Migration of erythroblastic islands toward the sinusoid as erythroid maturation proceeds in rat bone marrow. *J Vet Med Sci.* 2003;65:449.
19. Lichtman MA, Santillo P. Red cell egress from the marrow—Vis-à-tergo. *Blood Cells.* 1986;12:11.
20. Chamberlain JK, Lichtman MA. Marrow cell egress: specificity of the site of penetration into the sinus. *Blood.* 1978;52:959.
21. Waugh RE, Sassi M. An in vitro model of erythroid egress in bone marrow. *Blood.* 1986;68:250.
22. Yoshida H, Kawane K, Koike M, et al. Phosphatidylserine-dependent engulfment by macrophages of nuclei from erythroid precursor cells. *Nature.* 2005;437:754.
23. Jacobsen RN, Forristal CE, Raggatt LJ, et al. Mobilization with granulocyte colony-stimulating factor blocks medullar erythropoiesis by depleting F4/80(+)VCAM1(+)CD169(+)ER-HR3(+)Ly6G(+) erythroid island macrophages in the mouse. *Exp Hematol.* 2014;42:547.
24. Rhodes MM, Kopsombut P, Bondurant MC, et al. Adherence to macrophages in erythroblastic islands enhances erythroblast proliferation and increases erythrocyte production by a different mechanism than erythropoietin. *Blood.* 2008;111:1700.
25. Kawane K, Fukuyama H, Kondoh G, et al. Requirement of DNase II for definitive erythropoiesis in the mouse fetal liver. *Science.* 2001;292:1546.
26. Bowman WD Jr. Abnormal ("ringed") sideroblasts in various hematologic and nonhematologic disorders. *Blood.* 1961;18:662.
27. Hines JD, Grasso JA. The sideroblastic anemias. *Semin Hematol.* 1970;7:86.
28. Konstantinidis DG, Pushkaran S, Johnson JF, et al. Signaling and cytoskeletal requirements in erythroblast enucleation. *Blood.* 2012;119:6118.

29. Ubukawa K, Guo YM, Takahashi M, et al. Enucleation of human erythroblasts involves non-muscle myosin IIB. *Blood.* 2012;119:1036.

30. Keerthivasan G, Small S, Liu H, et al. Vesicle trafficking plays a novel role in erythroblast enucleation. *Blood.* 2010;116:3331.

31. Nowak RB, Papoin J, Gokhin DS, et al. Tropomodulin 1 controls erythroblast enucleation via regulation of F-actin in the enucleosome. *Blood.* 2017;130:1144.

32. Chasis JA, Prenant M, Leung A, et al. Membrane assembly and remodeling during reticulocyte maturation. *Blood.* 1989;74:1112.

33. Liu J, Guo X, Mohandas N, et al. Membrane remodeling during reticulocyte maturation. *Blood.* 2010;115:2021.

34. Brecher G, Haley JE, Prenant M, Bessis M. Macronormoblasts, macroreticulocytes and macrocytes. *Blood Cells.* 1975;1:547.

35. Jolly JMJ. Recherches sur la formation des globules rouges des mammifères. *Arch Anat Microsc.* 1907;9:133.

36. Felka T, Lemke J, Lemke C, et al. DNA degradation during maturation of erythrocytes—molecular cytogenetic characterization of Howell-Jolly bodies. *Cytogenet Genome Res.* 2007;119:2.

37. Holroyde CP, Gardner FH. Acquisition of autophagic vacuoles by human erythrocytes. Physiological role of the spleen. *Blood.* 1970;36:566.

38. O'Grady JG, Harding B, Egan EL, et al. "Pitted" erythrocytes: impaired formation in splenectomized subjects with congenital spherocytosis. *Br J Haematol.* 1984;57:441.

39. Buchanan GR, Holtkamp CA, Horton JA. Formation and disappearance of pocked erythrocytes: studies in human subjects and laboratory animals. *Am J Hematol.* 1987;25:243.

40. Kass L. Origin and composition of Cabot rings in pernicious anemia. *Am J Clin Pathol.* 1975;64:53.

41. Kass L, Gray RH. Ultrastructural visualization of Cabot rings in pernicious anemia. *Experientia.* 1976;32:507.

42. Jensen WN, Moreno GD, Bessis MC. An electron microscopic description of basophilic stippling in red cells. *Blood.* 1965;25:933.

43. Heinz R. Uber Blutdegeneration und regeneration. *Beitr Pathol.* 1901;29:299.

44. Chinprasertsuk S, Piankijagum A, Wasi P. *In vivo* induction of intraerythrocytic inclusion bodies in hemoglobin H disease: an electron microscopic study. *Birth Defects Orig Artic Ser.* 1987;23:317.

45. Sansone G, Sciarratta GV, Ivaldi G, Chiappara G. Hb H-like inclusions in red cells of patients with unstable haemoglobin. *Haematologica.* 1987;72:481.

46. Wickramasinghe SN, Hughes M, Higgs DR, et al. Ultrastructure of red cells containing haemoglobin H inclusions induced by redox dyes. *Clin Lab Haematol.* 1981;3:51.

47. Bessis MC, Breton-Gorius J. Iron particles in normal erythroblasts and normal and pathological erythrocytes. *J Biophys Biochem Cytol.* 1957;3:503.

48. Evans J, Gratzer W, Mohandas N, et al. Fluctuations of the red cell membrane: relation to mechanical properties and lack of ATP-dependence. *Biophys J.* 2008;94:4134.

49. Mohandas N, Gallagher PG. Red cells: past, present and future. *Blood.* 2008;112:393.

50. Discher D, Mohandas N, Evans EA. Molecular maps of red cell deformation: hidden elasticity and in situ connectivity. *Science.* 1994;266:1032.

51. Liu SC, Derick LH, Palek J. Visualization of the hexagonal lattice in the erythrocyte membrane skeleton. *J Cell Biol.* 1987;104:527.

52. Ponder E. *Hemolysis and Related Phenomena.* Grune & Stratton; 1948.

53. Behrendt H. *Chemistry of Erythrocytes.* Charles C Thomas; 1957.

54. Tyan YC, Jong SB, Liao JD, et al. Proteomic profiling of erythrocyte proteins by proteolytic digestion chip and identification using two-dimensional electrospray ionization tandem mass spectrometry. *J Proteome Res.* 2005;4:748.

55. Pasini EM, Kirkegaard M, Mortensen P, et al. In-depth analysis of the membrane and cytosolic proteome of red blood cells. *Blood.* 2006;108:791.

56. Farquhar JW. Human erythrocytes phosphoglycerides. I. Quantification of plasmalogens, fatty acids and fatty aldehydes. *Biochim Biophys Acta.* 1962;60:80.

57. Kirk E. The concentration of lecithin, cephalin, ether-insoluble phosphatide, and cerebrosides in plasma and red blood cells of normal adults. *J Biol Chem.* 1938;123:637.

58. Phillips GB, Roome NS. Quantitative chromatographic analysis of the phospholipids of abnormal human red blood cells. *Proc Soc Exp Biol Med.* 1962;109:360.

59. Westerman MP, Zhang Y, McConnell JP, et al. Ascorbate levels in red blood cells and urine in patients with sickle cell anemia. *Am J Hematol.* 2000;65:174.

60. Luecke R, Pearson PB. The microbiological determination of free choline in plasma and urine. *J Biol Chem.* 1944;153:259.

61. Beerstecher E, Spangler S, Granick S, et al. Blood vitamins, hormones, enzymes. Blood coenzymes: vertebrates. In: Altman PL, Dittmer DS, eds: *Blood and Other Body Fluids.* Federation of American Societies for Experimental Biology; 1961:62.

62. Kaplan NO, Lipmann F. The assay of distribution of coenzyme A. *J Biol Chem.* 1948;174:37.

63. Klein JR, Perlzweig WA, Handler P. Determination of nicotinic acid in blood cells and plasma. *J Biol Chem.* 1942;145:27.

64. Pearson PB. The pantothenic acid content of the blood of mammalia. *J Biol Chem.* 1941;140:423.

65. Masse PG, Mahuren JD, Tranchant C, Dosy J. B-6, vitamers and 4-pyridoxic acid in the plasma, erythrocytes, and urine of postmenopausal women. *Am J Clin Nutr.* 2004;80:946.

66. Burch HB, Bessey OA, Lowry OH. Fluorometric measurements of riboflavin and its natural derivatives in small quantities of blood serum and cells. *J Biol Chem.* 1948;175:457.

67. Beutler E. Glutathione reductase: stimulation in normal subjects by riboflavin supplementation. *Science.* 1969;165:613.

68. Burch HB, Bessey OA, Love RH, Lowry OH. The determination of thiamine and thiamine phosphates in small quantities of blood and blood cells. *J Biol Chem.* 1952;198:477.

69. Beutler E. *Red Cell Metabolism: A Manual of Biochemical Methods.* Grune & Stratton; 1984.

70. Bishop C, Rankine D, Talbott JH. The nucleotides in normal human blood. *J Biol Chem.* 1959;234:1233.

71. Mandel P, Chambon P, Karon H, et al. Nucleotides libres des globules rouges et des reticulocytes. *Folia Haematol Int Mag Klin Morphol Blutforsch.* 1962;78:525.

72. Bartlett GR. Human red cell glycolytic intermediates. *J Biol Chem.* 1959;234:449.

73. Yoshikawa H, Nakano M, Miyamoto K, Tatibana M. Phosphorus metabolism in human erythrocyte. II. Separation of acid-soluble phosphorus compounds incorporating p32 by column chromatography with ion exchange resin. *J Biochem.* 1960;47:635.

74. Beutler E, Mathai CK. A comparison of normal red cell ATP levels as measured by the firefly system and the hexokinase system. *Blood.* 1967;30:311.

75. Minakami S, Suzuki C, Saito T, Yoshikawa H. Studies on erythrocyte glycolysis. I. Determination of the glycolytic intermediates in human erythrocytes. *J Biochem.* 1965;58:543.

76. Patterson WD, Hardman JG, Sutherland EW. A comparison of cyclic nucleotide levels in plasma and cells of rat and human blood. *Endocrinology.* 1974;95:325.

77. Canepa L, Ferraris AM, Miglino M, Gaetani GF. Bound and unbound pyridine dinucleotides in normal and glucose-6-phosphate dehydrogenase-deficient erythrocytes. *Biochim Biophys Acta.* 1991;1074:101.

78. Micheli V, Simmonds HA, Bari M, Pompucci G. HPLC determination of oxidized and reduced pyridine coenzymes in human erythrocytes. *Clin Chim Acta.* 1993;220:1.

79. Lagendijk J, Ubbink JB, Vermaak WJH. Quantification of erythrocyte S-adenosyl-L-methionine levels and its application in enzyme studies. *J Chromatogr B Biomed Appl.* 1992;576:95.

80. Overgard-Hansen K, Jorgensen S. Determination and concentration of adenine nucleotides in human blood. *Scand J Clin Lab Invest.* 1960;12:10.

81. Mills GC. Uridine diphosphate glucose and uridine diphosphate N-acetylglucosamine in erythrocytes. *Tex Rep Biol Med.* 1960;18:446.

82. Liang HR, Takagaki T, Foltz RL, Bennett P. Quantitative determination of endogenous sorbitol and fructose in human erythrocytes by atmospheric-pressure chemical ionization LC tandem mass spectrometry. *J Chromatogr B Analyt Technol Biomed Life Sci.* 2005;824:36.

83. Lionetti FJ, McLellan WL, Fortier NL, Foster JM. Phosphate esters produced from inosine in human erythrocyte ghosts. *Arch Biochem.* 1961;94:7.

84. Kawaguchi M, Fujii T, Kamiya Y, et al. Effects of fructose ingestion on sorbitol and fructose 3-phosphate contents of erythrocytes from healthy men. *Acta Diabetol.* 1996;33:100.

85. Petersen A, Szwergold BS, Kappler F, et al. Identification of sorbitol 3-phosphate and fructose 3-phosphate in normal and diabetic human erythrocytes. *J Biol Chem.* 1990;265:17424.

86. Colomer D, Pujades A, Carballo E, Vives Corrons JL. Erythrocyte fructose 2,6-bisphosphate content in congenital hemolytic anemias. *Hemoglobin.* 1991;15:517.

87. Deichmann WB, Dierker M. The spectrophotometric estimation of hexuronates (expressed as glucuronic acid) in plasma or serum. *J Biol Chem.* 1946;163:753.

88. Jung CY. Carrier-mediated glucose transport across human red cell membranes. In: Surgenor DM, ed. *The Red Blood Cell.* Academic Press; 1975:705.

89. Lacko L, Wittke B, Geck P. The temperature dependence of the exchange transport of glucose in human erythrocytes. *J Cell Physiol.* 1973;82:213.

90. Bartlett GR. Glucose and mannose diphosphates in the red blood cell. *Biochim Biophys Acta.* 1968;156:231.

91. Johnson RE, Edward HT, Dill DB, Wilson JW. Blood as a physicochemical system. XIII. The distribution of lactate. *J Biol Chem.* 1945;157:461.

92. Bartlett GR, Bucolo G. Octulose phosphates from the human red blood cell. *Biochem Biophys Res Commun.* 1960;3:474.

93. Mandel P, Métais P. Les acides nucléiques du plasma sanguin chez l'homme. *C R Seances Soc Biol Fil.* 1948;142:241.

94. Aminoff D, Anderson J, Dabich L, Gathmann WD. Sialic acid content of erythrocytes in normal individuals and patients with certain hematologic disorders. *Am J Hematol.* 1980;9:381.

95. Vanderheiden BS. Ribosediphosphate in the human erythrocyte. *Biochem Biophys Res Commun.* 1961;6:117.

96. Bruns FH, Noltmann E, Vahlhaus E. Über den Stoffwechsel von Ribose-5-phosphat in Hämolysaten. I. Aktivitäts-messung und Eigenschaften der Phosphoribose-isomerase. II. Der Pentosephosphate-Cyclus in roten Blutzellen. *Biochem Z.* 1958;330:483.

97. Bucolo G, Bartlett GR. Sedoheptulose diphosphate formation by the human red blood cell. *Biochem Biophys Res Commun.* 1960;3:620.

98. Kehoe RA, Cholak J, Story RV. A spectrochemical study of the normal ranges of concentration of certain trace metals in biological materials. *J Nutr.* 940;19:579.

99. Hunter G. Micro-determination of bromide in body fluids. *Biochem J.* 1955;60:261.

100. Ojo JO, Oluwole AF, Durosinmi MA, et al. Baseline levels of elemental concentrations in whole blood, plasma, and erythrocytes of Nigerian subjects. *Biol Trace Elem Res.* 1994;43-45:461.

101. Bernard J-F, Bournier O, Boivin P. Human erythrocytic calcium concentration in hemolytic anemia. *Biomedicine.* 1975;23:431.

102. Shoji S, Komiyama A, Nakamura M, Nomoto S. Calcium content of healthy human erythrocytes. *Clin Chem.* 1989;35:1264.

103. Bernstein RE. Potassium and sodium balance in mammalian red cells. *Science.* 1954;120:459.

104. Herring WB, Leavell BS, Paizao LM, Yoe JH. Trace metals in human plasma and red blood cells: a study of magnesium, chromium, nickel, copper, and zinc. I. Observations of normal subjects. *Am J Clin Nutr.* 1960;8:846.

105. Heyrovsky A. The biochemistry of cobalt. III. Amounts of cobalt in plasma, erythrocytes, urine, and feces of normal subjects. *Cas Lek Cesk.* 1952;91:680.

106. Mahalingam TR, Vijayalakshmi S, Prabhu RK, et al. Studies on some trace and minor elements in blood—a survey of the Kalpakkam (India) population. 2. Reference values for plasma and red cells, and correlation with coronary risk index. *Biol Trace Elem Res.* 1997;57:207.

107. Lahey ME, Gubler CJ, Cartwright GE, Wintrobe MM. Studies on copper metabolism. VI. Blood copper in normal human subjects. *J Clin Invest.* 1953;32:322.

108. Largent EJ, Cholak J. Blood electrolytes. Man. In: Altman PL, Dittmer DS, eds. *Blood and Other Body Fluids.* Federation of American Societies for Experimental Biology; 1961:21.

109. McClendon JF, Foster WC. Protein-bound iodine in erythrocytes and plasma and elsewhere. *Am J Med Sci.* 1944;207:549.

110. Jensovsky L, Roth Z. Der normale Bleigehalt im menschlichen Blute. *Naturwissenschaften.* 1961;48:382.

111. McCance R, Widdowson EM. The effect of development, anaemia, and undernutrition on the composition of the erythrocyte. *Clin Sci.* 1956;15:409.

112. Huijgen HJ, Sanders R, van Olden RW, et al. Intracellular and extracellular blood magnesium fractions in hemodialysis patients: is the ionized fraction a measure of magnesium excess? *Clin Chem.* 1998;44:639.

113. Martin BJ, Lyon TD, Fell GS, McKay P. Erythrocyte magnesium in elderly patients: not a reliable guide to magnesium status. *J Trace Elem Med Biol.* 1997;11:44.

114. Miller DO, Yoe JH. Spectrophotometric determination of manganese in human plasma and red cells with benzohydroxamic acid. *Anal Chim Acta.* 1962;26:224.

115. Bartlett GR, Savage E, Hughes L, Marlow AA. Carbohydrate intermediates and related cofactors with benzohydroxamic acid. *J Appl Physiol.* 953;6:51.

116. Ferranti F, Giannetti O. The microdetermination of phosphorus (inorganic, acid-soluble, lipoid and total) in the blood and excretions. *Diagn Tec Lab Napoli Riv Mens.* 1933;4:664.

117. Overman RR, Davis AK. The application of flame photometry to sodium and potassium determinations in biological fluids. *J Biol Chem.* 1947;168:641.

118. Mayer KDF, Starkey BJ. Simpler flame photometric determination of erythrocyte sodium and potassium: the reference range for apparently healthy adults. *Clin Chem.* 1977;23:275.

119. Bernard JF, Bournier O, Renoux M, et al. Unclassified haemolytic anaemia with splenomegaly and erythrocyte cation abnormalities—a disease of the spleen? *Scand J Haematol.* 1976;17:231.

120. Hald PM. Notes on the determination and distribution of sodium and potassium in cells and serum of normal human blood. *J Biol Chem.* 1946;163:429.

121. Streef GM. Sodium and calcium content of erythrocytes. *J Biol Chem.* 1939;129:661.

122. Tamada T. An indirect spectrophotometric method for the determination of silicon in serum, whole blood and erythrocytes. *Anal Sci.* 2003;19:1291.

123. Reed L, Denis W. On the distribution of the non-protein sulfur of the blood between serum and corpuscles. *J Biol Chem.* 1927;73:623.

124. Vallee BL, Gibson JG. The zinc content of normal human whole blood, plasma, leucocytes, and erythrocytes. *J Biol Chem.* 1948;176:445.

125. Zak B, Nalbandian RM, Williams LA, Cohen J. Determination of human erythrocyte zinc: hemoglobin ratios. *Clin Chim Acta.* 1962;7:634.

126. Mohandas N, Clark MR, Jacobs MS, Shohet SB. Analysis of factors regulating erythrocyte deformability. *J Clin Invest.* 1980;66:563.

127. Mohandas N, Chasis JA, Shohet SB. The influence of membrane skeleton on red cell deformability, membrane material properties and shape. *Semin Hematol.* 1983;20:225.

128. Chasis JA, Mohandas N. Erythrocyte membrane deformability and stability. Two distinct membrane properties which are independently regulated by skeletal protein associations. *J Cell Biol.* 1986;103:343.

129. Mohandas N, Chasis JA. Red cell deformability, membrane material properties and shape: regulation by transmembrane, skeletal and cytosolic proteins and lipids. *Semin Hematol.* 1993;30:171.

130. Safeukui I, Buffet P, Delpaine G, et al. Quantitative assessment of sensing and sequestration of spherocytic erythrocytes by human spleen: implications for understanding clinical variability of membrane disorders. *Blood.* 2012;120:424.

131. Clark MR, Mohandas N, Caggiano V, Shohet SB. Effects of abnormal cation transport on deformability of desiccytes. *J Supramol Struct.* 1978;8:521.

132. Evans E, Mohandas N, Leung A. Static and dynamic rigidities of normal and sickle erythrocytes: major influence of cell hemoglobin concentration. *J Clin Invest.* 1984;73:477.

133. Pantaleo A, Giribaldi G, Mannu F, et al. Naturally occurring anti-band 3 antibodies and red cell removal under physiological and pathological conditions. *Autoimmun Rev.* 2008;7:457.

134. Arashiki N, Kimata N, Manno S, et al. Membrane peroxidation and methemoglobin formation are both necessary for band 3 clustering: mechanistic insights into erythrocyte senescence. *Biochemistry.* 2013;52:5760.

135. Cooper RA. Loss of membrane components in pathogenesis of antibody-induced spherocytosis. *J Clin Invest.* 1972;51:16.

136. Lock SP, Smith RS, Hardisty RM. Stomatocytosis: a hereditary red cell anomaly associated with haemolytic anaemia. *Br J Haematol.* 1961;7:303.

137. Delaunay J, Stewart G, Iolascon A. Hereditary dehydrated and overhydrated stomatocytosis: recent advances. *Curr Opin Hematol.* 1999;6:110.

138. Delaunay J. The molecular basis of hereditary red cell membrane disorders. *Blood Rev.* 2007;21:1.

139. De Franceschi L, Bosman GJ, Mohandas N. Abnormal red cell features associated with hereditary neurodegenerative disorders: the neuroacanthocytosis syndromes. *Curr Opin Hematol.* 2014;21:201.

140. Cooper RA, Jandl JH. Bile salts and cholesterol in the pathogenesis of target cells in obstructive jaundice. *J Clin Invest.* 1968;47:809.

141. Padilla F, Bromberg PA, Jensen WN. Sickle–unsickle cycle—cause of cell fragmentation leading to permanently deformed cells. *Blood.* 1973;41:653.

142. Horiuchi K, Ballas SK, Asakura T. The effect of deoxygenation rate on the formation of irreversibly sickled cells. *Blood.* 1988;71:46.

143. Bertles JF, Milner PF. Irreversibly sickled erythrocytes: a consequence of the heterogeneous distribution of hemoglobin types in sickle-cell anemia. *J Clin Invest.* 1968;47:1731.

144. Bull BS, Kuhn IN. Production of schistocytes by fibrin strands (a scanning electron microscope study). *Blood.* 1970;35:104.

CHAPTER 2
ERYTHROPOIESIS AND RED CELL TURNOVER

Josef T. Prchal and Perumal Thiagarajan

SUMMARY

Production of red cells, or *erythropoiesis*, is a tightly regulated process by which hematopoietic stem cells (HSCs) differentiate into erythroid progenitors and then mature into red cells. Erythropoiesis generates ~2×10^{11} new

Acronyms and Abbreviations: ACEIs, angiotensin converting enzyme inhibitors; AMP, adenosine monophosphate; ASXL1, a polycomb group protein-epigenetic modifier; ATP, adenosine triphosphate; BCL11A, a critical switching factor for silencing gamma globin; Bcl-x_L, an antiapoptotic factor; BFU-E, burst-forming units—erythroid; BNIP3L, an hypoxic regulated gene that facilitates mitochondrial autophagy; C_3, third component of complement; ^{14}C, radioactive carbon; CBP, a coactivator of a transcription factor; CD 44, cell differentiation antigen; CDA, congenital dyserythropoietic anemia; CFU-E, colony-forming units—erythroid; CIS, a signal transduction protein that downregulates activity of erythropoietin receptor; CO, carbon monoxide; COHb, carboxyhemoglobin; CPM, counts per minute; ^{51}Cr, chromium-51; ^{50}Cr, chromium-50; DFP, diisopropylfluorophosphate; E2A, transcription factor import for early erythropoiesis; E2F-2, a transcription factor that plays a crucial role in the control of cell cycle and also act as a tumor suppressor protein; EKLF, erythroid Krüppel-like factor—encoded by *KLF1* gene; Emp, erythroblast-macrophage protein; EPO, erythropoietin; EPOR, EPO receptor; ETCO, end-tidal CO; ^{55}Fe or ^{59}Fe, radioactive iron; FOG, "friend of GATA," a GATA-1 interacting protein; Fox03, a member of the forkhead family of transcription factors; G-6-PD, glucose-6-phosphate dehydrogenase; Gas6, growth arrest-specific 6; GATA-1 transcription factor 1 binding to the DNA sequence GATA; Gfi-1B, growth factor independence-1B; HbF, fetal hemoglobin; Hct, hematocrit; HCP, hematopoietic cell phosphatase; HIF, hypoxia-inducible transcription factor; HO, heme oxygenase; HRE, hypoxia-responsive element; HSC, hematopoietic stem cell; ICSH, International Committee on Standardization in Hematology; Ig, immunoglobulin; IGF-1, insulin-like growth factor-1; ^{111}In, indium-111; IRP, iron regulatory protein; JAK2, a tyrosine kinase that interacts with erythropoietin receptor; KAP1, KRAB-associated protein-1 is a transcriptional cofactor; KRAB-ZFP, 1 of the 400 human zinc finger protein-based transcription factors; MCV, mean cell volume; mRNA, messenger RNA; mDia2, a protein that regulates actin and focal adhesion dynamics; miRs, microRNAs are small non-coding RNA molecules; ^{15}N, nitrogen; Nix, a protein that is expressed during erythropoiesis and regulates mitochondrial apoptosis (autophagy); PHD, proline hydroxylase; PK, pyruvate kinase; PU.1, transcription factor; RACK1, receptor of activated protein kinase C; RAS, the renin–angiotensin system; Rb, tumor suppressor retinoblastoma (protein); RCM, red cell mass; SCL/TAL1, stem cell leukemia/t-cell acute lymphoblastic leukemia 1 factor; SCL/tal-1, basic helix-loop-helix transcription factor; SNPs, single-nucleotide polymorphisms; SOCS3, a signal transduction protein (also known as CIS3) that downregulates activity of erythropoietin receptor; ^{99m}Tc, technetium-99; VHL, von Hippel-Lindau protein.

erythrocytes to replace the 2×10^{11} red cells (approximately 1% of the total red cell mass [RCM]) removed from the circulation each day. Red cell production increases several-fold after blood loss or hemolysis. When one of the progeny of an HSC becomes committed to the erythroid lineage, this early erythroid progenitor undergoes a series of divisions and concurrent maturation that eventually result in morphologically recognizable erythroblasts. After expulsion of the nucleus, a macrocyte (polychromatophilic when Wright-stained, or a reticulocyte if new methylene blue–stained) leaves the marrow. During the first 24 to 48 hours in the circulation, reticulocytes lose their residual organelles (mitochondria and ribosomes) through an autophagic process (Chap. 1) and undergo reconditioning of the membrane to become mature red cells with a biconcave disc shape. Erythropoiesis is controlled by transcription factors and cytokines, the principal ones being GATA 1 and erythropoietin (EPO), respectively, which influence lineage commitment, proliferation, apoptosis, differentiation, and number of divisions, from the earliest progenitor to late erythroblasts. The number of red cells produced varies in response to tissue oxygenation, which determines the level of the transcription factors, hypoxia-inducible factors (HIFs)—HIF-1 and HIF-2—the principal regulators of the response to hypoxia. HIFs modulate erythropoiesis by regulation of EPO production by direct EPO-independent mechanism(s) and by facilitating iron availability.

The survival of red cells in the circulation can be measured in a variety of ways: (1) by labeling with radioactive isotopes, particularly ^{51}Cr, and assessing the disappearance of the radioactive tag from the circulation over time; (2) by labeling the erythrocytes with biotin or a fluorescent dye and measuring this marker over time; (3) by determining the disappearance of transfused antigen-matched allogeneic erythrocytes using immunologic markers; and (4) by measuring the excretion of carbon monoxide (CO), a product of heme catabolism.

Such studies show that normal human red cells have a finite life span averaging 120 days, with some component of random destruction. The mitochondrial and ribosomal removal highlighting maturation of the reticulocyte is accompanied by increasing cell density, but after a few days of intravascular life span, there is little further increase in density or other changes in the physical property of the red cells. Thus, cell density is not a good marker for aged red cells. This has made study of the senescent changes in the red cell that mark it for destruction difficult. Candidates for such changes include changes in membrane AE-1 (anion exchanger-1; also known as band 3) and exposure of phosphatidylserine on the membrane, which may be of major importance.

● HISTORY

Erythrocytes evolved largely for the purpose of transporting oxygen to tissues and carbon dioxide from tissues. Thus, the size of the red cell mass (RCM) and the rate of red cell production must be closely related to supply and demand for oxygen in the tissues. French mountaineers and physiologists at the end of the 19th century established that a low tissue tension of oxygen stimulates red cell production.[1] In 1906, Paul Carnot, a professor at the Sorbonne, and Mademoiselle DeFlandre, his associate, suggested that hypoxia generates a humoral factor capable of stimulating red cell production.[2] In 1950, Kurt Reissmann[3] provided evidence for the existence of an indirect humoral mechanism using parabiotic rats. The work of Erslev and colleagues,[4,5] demonstrated that the plasma from anemic rabbits and primates contains an erythrocyte stimulating factor, appropriately named erythropoietin (EPO). Then, EPO was shown to be produced by the kidney,[6] a finding that raised the possibility that EPO might be of therapeutic benefit to anemic uremic patients. After cloning the *EPO* gene and production of recombinant EPO in therapeutic quantities, EPO has proved invaluable for the therapy of many forms of anemia.

PHYLOGENY OF RED CELL PRODUCTION

HEMOGLOBIN AND RED CELLS

The existence of hemoglobin in virtually all animals is a testimony to the ancient origin of the molecule.[7] Hemoglobin is present in the most primitive animal forms, such as *Paramecium* and *Tetrahymena*, although very primitive organisms, such as *Daphnia* (a small planktonic crustacean), are capable of developing an oxygen transport system without circulating red cells.[8] They accommodate their oxygen need by modulating hemoglobin synthesis.[9] One interesting exception is the Antarctic ice fish (*Chaenocephalus aceratus*) lacking hemoglobin.[10] These ice fish compensate for the absence of hemoglobin by their unusual nitric oxide metabolism.[11-13] They have very large hearts and unusually large diameter capillaries. This permits a large volume of blood to circulate at high flow rate and at low vascular pressure because of decreased peripheral resistance. This permits their survival in the very high oxygen content of Antarctic waters.[13]

An erythroid cell that can synthesize, carry, package, and protect hemoglobin from oxidation developed along with the evolution of a body cavity and with the development of a circulatory system.[14] Circulating nucleated erythrocytes first appear in worms (the phylum *Nemertina*) and in the immobile marine phylum *Phoronida*. In these primitive invertebrates, erythropoiesis is derived from endothelial cells on the peritoneal surface.[15] Nucleated red cells still exist in more advanced reptiles and birds.[16] All mammalian erythrocytes are non-nucleated; in most species they are disc-shaped, but are oval in others.[17] Enucleation decreases the workload of the heart as it reduces one-third of the cell weight, facilitates the passage of red cells through the microvasculature by preventing possible blockage of small capillaries by nondeformable red cells, and provides additional intracellular space for carrying hemoglobin.

In nonmammalian species, the spleen is the erythropoietic organ; however, in some fish, the kidneys are also involved in red cell production.[18,19] In vertebrates, an evolutionary shift occurred from the spleen to the liver and from the liver to the marrow.[20] In higher animals, erythropoiesis is controlled by EPO, which adjusts red cell production to tissue oxygen demand. EPO of mammals has considerable biologic similarity and genetic homology.[21]

ONTOGENY OF RED CELL PRODUCTION

EMBRYONIC AND FETAL ERYTHROPOIESIS

The environment within the marrow appears optimal for cellular proliferation and maturation. However, bone cavities do not develop until the fifth fetal month in humans. Other sites are responsible for red cell production during early embryonic life.[22] The large nucleated blood cells are first formed in the human yolk sac[23] and some enucleate.[24] They cluster in blood islands that become enveloped by endothelial cells forming the vascular plexus of the yolk sac.[25] This is referred to as *primitive erythropoiesis* and is contrasted with *definitive erythropoiesis*, which occurs in the context of a fully formed and functional vascular

system. Hematopoietic stem cells (HSCs) that provide differentiated cells essential for oxygen transport, hemostasis, and protection from infection throughout adult life arise from a specialized population of cells termed *hemogenic endothelium* located on the ventral floor of the dorsal aorta (Chap. 1). In a process known as *endothelial-to-hematopoietic transition*, endothelial cells in the ventral floor of the aorta bud into the extravascular space, followed by reentry into the circulation.[26] These are the first definitive HSCs produced in humans, and they proceed to seed hematopoietic niches throughout development.[27] One of the microenvironmental clues appears to be the circumferential strain in the ventral wall transmitted by the pulsating heart, which activates mechanosensitive ion channel Piezo-1, which promotes the endothelial-to-hematopoietic transition.[28] During the neonatal period, the volume of available marrow space is almost the same as the total volume of hematopoietic cells and marrow vasculature.[29] This process continues for a few years until the growth of bones and bone cavities exceeds the growth of (need for) hematopoietic mass. However, when the demand on erythropoiesis increases (eg, blood loss, hypoxia, ineffective erythropoiesis, or hemolysis), the proportion of hematopoiesis-bearing marrow space increases in adults, but the lack of reserve space in neonates and small children reactivates extramedullary erythropoiesis in the liver and spleen.[30] In adults, expansion of marrow space continues with aging, and the amount of fatty tissue gradually increases in all bone cavities. Because of the abundant marrow space, compensatory reactivation of extramedullary sites rarely occurs in later life. Extramedullary hematopoiesis during adult years indicates pathologic rather than compensatory blood formation, such as is seen in patients with primary myelofibrosis (Chap. 1) wherein the stem cells have abnormal interaction with the extracellular matrix.[31] During fetal life, EPO production is primarily hepatic.[32] At birth, a gradual switch to renal production of EPO occurs. In the adult, the kidney is responsible for approximately 85% of total production.[33,34]

In the yolk sac prior to week 8 of intrauterine life, normoblasts produce three embryonic hemoglobins—Gower 1 ($\xi2\epsilon2$), Gower 2 ($\alpha2\epsilon2$), and Portland ($\xi2 \gamma2$). The ξ- and ϵ-globin chains are the embryonic counterparts of the adult α- and β-, γ- and δ-globin chains, respectively. As erythropoiesis moves to the liver and spleen, and there is an orderly switch from ξ- to α-globin chain and from ϵ- to γ-globin chain production, and the predominant hemoglobin is in the fetus is fetal hemoglobin (HbF) ($\alpha2\gamma2$). Postnatally, γ-globin chain production (HbF) is replaced by β-globin chain production. This is commonly referred to as hemoglobin switching, such that between 6 and 12 months of age, Hb A ($\alpha2\beta2$) becomes the predominant hemoglobin.

CELLULAR COMPONENTS OF ERYTHROPOIESIS AND ITS REGULATION

PROGENITOR CELLS

Self-renewing HSCs progressively differentiate into multilineage blood progenitors that diversify into each of the lineage-restricted progenitors, in an evolutionarily conserved hierarchical processes. The precise mechanisms that underlie lineage commitment are not fully understood. Two competing hypotheses have been proposed to explain commitment and differentiation of multipotential progenitors toward the erythroid lineage: a deterministic model and a stochastic model.[35] In both models, a set of transcription factors uniquely induces and regulates the transcriptional program for each lineage. According to the deterministic model, extrinsic factors such as cytokines play an instructive role in lineage specification, by inducing the expression of lineage-specific transcription factors. In contrast, the stochastic model proposes that the transcription factors encoding any specific lineage are expressed stochastically, in an autonomous, temporally regulated process, independent of extrinsic signals. These transcription factors activate a unique set of genes for a particular lineage and repress the action of alternative transcription factors. The role of cytokines is permissive rather than instructive, supporting functions such as cell survival or proliferation. Both in vitro and in vivo studies support a permissive, rather than instructive, role for cytokine receptors in lineage commitment and differentiation.[36] However, this does not exclude the possibility that other types of extrinsic signals might influence lineage commitment in early stem and progenitor cells.

Advances in sequencing technologies and mass spectrometry allow identification of gene and protein expression patterns simultaneously in thousands of single cells in an unprecedented detail. Furthermore, chromatin immunoprecipitation techniques and assays for transposase-accessible chromatin identify actively transcribed genes. These recent single-cell approaches suggest an unexpected model of hematopoietic development. The classical model viewed the hematopoietic hierarchy as deterministic, with the paths from stem cells to each blood lineage consisting of sequential transitions between well-defined and discrete developmental stages. This view has now been modified based on single-cell studies from several laboratories.[37-40] They show that single-cell transcriptomes of early hematopoietic progenitors fall into a continuum, rather than into discrete clusters (as may have been expected if developmental stages were discrete). The hematopoietic structure is nevertheless hierarchical, but developmental paths from multipotential progenitors to committed unipotential progenitor are both continuous and somewhat variable, though not random: certain types of oligopotential progenitors are found more than expected by chance, suggesting that specific developmental paths are preferred over others. Some previously unexpected pathways have been identified, including a previously unknown coupling between the erythroid and basophil/mast cell fates.[40,41] A number of studies indicate that the transcription factors GATA-1, FOG1, erythroid Krüppel-like factor–encoded by *KLF1* gene (EKLF), PU.1, and SCL/tal-1 are critical regulators of erythroid differentiation. Moreover, studies have shown a surprising hierarchical branching structure, in which the erythroid and basophil/mast cell fates are unexpectedly coupled.[38]

GATA Family of Transcription Factors

The GATA family of zinc-finger transcription factors was first identified as the nuclear factors that bind to the tetra-nucleotide G-A-T-A sequence in the enhancer region of the globin genes.[42,43] GATA-1 protein is expressed during erythroid differentiation, with highest expression in colony-forming units–erythroid (CFU-Es) and pronormoblasts. GATA-1 promotes erythroid differentiation by activating several erythroid-specific genes and represses transcription of KIT receptor and GATA-2. GATA-1–deficient mice die at embryonic day 10.5 with severe anemia as a result of maturation arrest at the stage of pronormoblasts.[44] In vitro, GATA-1 null embryonic stem cells fail to mature beyond pronormoblast and undergo apoptosis. GATA-1 and its cofactor CBP are essential for the formation of an erythroid-specific histone acetylation pattern of histones at the active globin genes and the β-globin locus control region.[45] GATA-1, along with EPO, induces expression of the antiapoptotic protein Bcl-x$_L$[46] and interacts with multiple proteins, including friends of GATA (FOG)-1 and transcription factor (PU.1)[47]; FOG-1 acts as a cofactor for GATA-1.[48] GATA-1 interaction with PU.1 appears to counteract erythropoiesis by inducing differentiation of pluripotent stem cell to myeloid and B lymphopoiesis and inhibition of erythropoiesis.[47,49,50] Whereas PU.1 absence appears to be required for completion of terminal erythroid differentiation, low levels of PU.1 expression are essential for fetal erythropoiesis and for proper augmentation of adult erythropoiesis at times of stress.[51] The pivotal role of GATA-1 in erythropoiesis is further demonstrated in patients with Diamond-Blackfan syndrome, an inherited marrow failure syndrome with selective deficiency of erythroid precursors in the marrow. In most instances the disease is caused by haploinsufficiency of ribosomal protein genes.[52] The erythroid defects are caused by reduced translation of *GATA1* messenger RNA (mRNA).[53] Moreover, rare instances of Diamond-Blackfan syndrome are caused by point mutations in GATA-1 (Chap. 5).[54]

Friends of GATA

FOG-1, a member of the friend of GATA family of zinc-finger proteins, acts as a cofactor for GATA-1. The gene was first identified in a yeast two-hybrid screen for GATA-1 interacting proteins.[48] FOG-1 binds to the amino zinc finger of GATA-1. Mice deficient in FOG-1$^{-/-}$ die during embryonic days 10.5 to 11.5 because of severe anemia with arrest in erythroid maturation at a stage similar to that observed in the GATA1- mice.[55] FOG-1 physically interacts with GATA-1 to augment or inhibit its transcriptional activity depending on the promoter context.

GATA-2 was initially cloned as a GATA motif-binding factor and is present in all erythroid cells. Targeted deletion of GATA2 results in embryonic lethality at day 10.5 as a result of ablation of blood cell development.[56] *GATA1* and *GATA2* directly regulate GATA2 transcription in a reciprocal fashion during erythroid differentiation.[57,58] *GATA2* autoregulates its transcription by binding to its own regulatory elements in the promoter region. This autoregulation is abolished by the displacement of GATA2 by GATA-1 (GATA2/GATA-1 switch), an interaction facilitated by FOG-1.[59] Chromatin immunoprecipitation studies indicate that FOG-1 facilitates occupancy by GATA-1 at selected cis-regulatory chromatin elements. Double knockout of *GATA1* and *GATA2* results in embryonic lethality with complete absence of primitive erythropoiesis.[60] The severity of this phenotype compared with either single *GATA1* or *GATA2* knockout suggests overlapping functions of these two transcription factors in primitive erythropoiesis.

Krüppel-Like Factor

Erythroid Krüppel-like factor (EKLF encoded by *KLF1* gene) is a zinc-finger protein identified by subtractive hybridization of the mRNA of erythroid cells, with common messages in a myeloid cell line.[61] It interacts with CACCC sequence in the β-globin promoter, where it modifies chromatin structure permitting β-globin gene transcription. EKLF-deficient mice die at embryonic day 14.5 to 15 from severe anemia caused by defective definitive erythropoiesis.[62] There is a marked decrease in β-globin mRNA and protein levels in EKLF-deficient erythroid cells. Large amounts of iron accumulate in the mononuclear phagocyte system of EKLF-deficient mice, consistent with the ineffective erythropoiesis in these animals. Despite the embryonic lethality of *Klf1*$^{-/-}$ mice, *KLF1*-null humans survive to birth with severe nonspherocytic hemolytic anemia and kernicterus.[63] HbF expression is very high in such children, consistent with a key role for EKLF1 in adult hemoglobin switching. Loss-of-function mutation in one allele of *KLF1* causes asymptomatic blood type called In(Lu), reduced levels of the red-cell membrane glycoproteins BCAM and CD44, and elevated levels of HbF.[64] Mutations within the second zinc-finger domain of the *KLF1* gene have been shown to cause a congenital dyserythropoietic anemia (CDA) now labeled as CDA type IV.[65]

Stem Cell Leukemia/T-Cell Acute Lymphoblastic Leukemia 1 Factor

Stem cell leukemia/t-cell acute lymphoblastic leukemia 1 (SCL/tal-1) is a member of basic helix-loop-helix transcription factors essential for maturation of the erythroid and megakaryocytic lineages.[66] Knockout of SCL/tal-1 leads to failure of hematopoiesis.[67] Selective rescue of SCL/

tal-1 null embryonic stem cells under the control of stem cell enhancer revealed differentiation blocks in erythroid and megakaryocytic maturation.[68] Conditional knockout studies have revealed that erythroid and megakaryocytic precursors do not develop in the marrow of mice upon deletion of SCL/tal-1.[69] Heterodimerization of SCL with other transcription factors, such as transcription factor import for early erythropoiesis (E2A), is a prerequisite for its functions.[70]

Growth Factor Independence-1B

Growth factor independence-1B (Gfi-1B) is a transcription factor with highly conserved transcriptional repressor domains. Gfi-1B–deficient mouse embryos die by E15 failing to produce definitive enucleated red blood cells; tissue examination revealed developmental arrest of splenic erythroid and megakaryocytic precursors.[71] In contrast, overexpression of Gfi-1B in early erythroid progenitors leads to their drastic expansion.[72] The homologous protein Gfi-1 plays a major role during myeloid differentiation, and its deficiency is a rare cause of human neutropenia.[73]

BCL11A

A critical switching factor for silencing gamma globin (BCL11A), a transcription factor initially identified in lymphoid cells, has been shown to regulate erythroid differentiation, especially during the switch from fetal to adult hemoglobin.[70] HbF levels decline after birth and are simultaneously replaced by adult hemoglobin A. Genome-wide association studies have identified the stage-specific repressor BCL11A as regulating the expression of HbF.[74,75]

An inverse relationship exists between BCL11A and HbF expression in erythroid cells. BCL11A binds to the β-globin enhancer and also to an intergenic region between the γ-globin genes and delta-lobin gene, a region often deleted in individuals with hereditary persistence of HbF. Further, single-nucleotide polymorphisms (SNPs) in these loci increase HbF levels.[76] The precise mechanism of action of BCL11A in silencing HbF is unclear and may involve direct modification of chromatin and/or alteration in long-range interactions.[77] In aggregate, these studies suggest that manipulation of BCL11A levels could enhance expression of HbF in adult cells, potentially ameliorating the severity of β thalassemia and sickle cell disease. CRISPR-mediated editing of the BCL11A enhancer sequence in hemoglobin locus induces HbF production, validating BCL11A as therapeutic target.[78] For results of ongoing clinical trials refer to Chap. 17.

Growth Arrest-Specific 6 Protein

Growth arrest-specific 6 (Gas6) protein is a secreted vitamin K–dependent protein that interacts with cell membranes and leads to intracellular signaling (via its receptor's tyrosine kinases). Gas6 receptors are expressed on megakaryocytes, myelomonocytic precursors, and marrow stromal cells. Gas6 has been shown to amplify the erythropoietic response to EPO using a mouse model of Gas6 knockout.[79] Gas6 is known to downregulate the expression of inflammatory cytokines such as tumor necrosis factor-α by macrophages.[80]

Pleckstrin-2

Pleckstrin-2 is involved in actin dynamics and plays important roles in erythroblast survival and enucleation in the early and late stages of terminal erythropoiesis.[81] In mice, *Pleckstrin-2* transcription is a downstream target of EPO-EPOR–induced JAK2/STAT5 signaling.[82]

Other Regulators of Lineage-Specific Differentiation The molecular mechanisms that regulate lineage-specific differentiation and commitment must account for the existence of separate megakaryocytic/erythroid, myeloid, and lymphoid lineage progenitors[83] (see **Erythropoietin, oxygen sensing, and hypoxia-inducible factor,** *Erythropoietin receptor* **and accompanying Fig. 2-6**).

Hormones

Several hormones that activate nuclear receptor transcription factors also regulate erythropoiesis. Glucocorticoids promote the self-renewal of burst-forming unit–erythroid (BFU-E) and prevent their differentiation to the more mature colony-forming units–erythroid (CFU-E).[84] They play an important role during stress erythropoiesis[85]; synthetic glucocorticoids have been used to treat anemia in Diamond-Blackfan syndrome.[86] Anemia is often observed in patients with hypothyroidism,[87] and thyroid hormones play an essential role during terminal human erythroid cell differentiation by promoting nuclear receptor coactivator 4 recruitment to chromatin regions that are in proximity to RNA polymerase II.[88]

PROGENITOR CELLS

Early erythropoiesis can be evaluated by functional assays and morphologic studies of hematopoietic colonies formed on semisolid media. The developmentally earliest unipotential progenitor committed to the erythroid lineage is the BFU-E. It was initially termed a "burst" because it contains cells still capable of migration, resulting in satellite accumulations of cells. Thus, these cells form smaller clusters around a larger central colony, composed of 2000 to 3000 cells, giving the appearance of a sunburst with satellite colonies (Fig. 2-1). However, all the cells in the colony and its satellites are derived from a single BFU-E cell and, thus, are clonal. BFU-Es take longer than more mature erythroid progenitors to form a colony of erythroblasts, the progenitor of which is termed a CFU-E. BFU-Es express low levels of EPO receptors (EPORs) and transferrin receptors (CD71).[89] BFU-Es mature into CFU-Es—the latter with higher-level expression of EPOR and transferrin receptor density and higher EPO dependency—and form smaller colonies (50-200 cells) that mature in 3 to 5 days.[35,36] Individual BFU-E and CFU-E cells cannot be identified by microscopy (Chap. 1), but they can be studied in vitro by their ability to generate microscopically recognizable hemoglobinized precursors (ie, erythroblasts) using clonogenic assays on semisolid media. The ability to isolate highly pure human BFU-E and CFU-E progenitors revealed unique transcriptomes for BFU-E and CFU-E.[89] The BFU-E gives rise to (EPO)-dependent CFU-E, and these mature into reticulocytes and mature erythrocytes.

PRECURSOR CELLS

In contrast to BFU-E and CFU-E, precursor cells that constitute the latter stages of erythropoiesis can be identified by light microscopy (Chap. 1). The earliest morphologically recognizable erythroid precursor in the adult marrow is the proerythroblasts. Proerythroblasts are large cells and have large uncondensed nuclei and deep basophilic cytoplasm caused by numerous RNA-containing polyribosomes. The proerythroblast has a volume of 900 fL, 10 times the volume of the mature red blood cell. With each successive division, the precursor cells give rise to daughter cells of about half the preceding cell volume. Furthermore, with each division there is an increase in hemoglobin synthesis and condensation of the nucleus. Thus, when the proerythroblasts divide to become basophilic erythroblasts, the daughter cells have less deep-blue cytoplasm because of the admixture of the coloration of hemoglobin being synthesized, and also a more condensed nucleus. When the basophilic erythroblasts divide further, they give rise to mature cells, with more cytoplasmic hemoglobin that is stainable with both acid and basic dyes, resulting in light gray–colored cytoplasm. These cells are termed *polychromatophilic erythroblasts*, whereas the offspring of polychromatophilic erythroblasts are termed *orthochromic erythroblasts*. Their nuclear chromatin is completely condensed and its cytoplasm is pink as a result of complete hemoglobinization. These erythroid cells

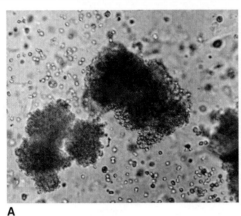
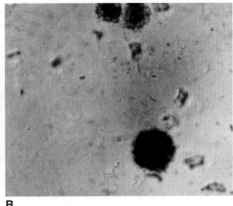

A   **B**

Figure 2–1. BFU-E and CFU-E. Erythroid colony growth in methylcellulose medium in the presence of erythropoietin. Normal human marrow. The colonies are stained for hemoglobin. **A.** Burst-forming unit–erythroid (BFU-E). This colony grows from a single-marrow erythroid progenitor cell (BFU-E). It was photographed at 14 days in culture. The BFU-E is a differentiated cell, committed to the erythroid lineage. The BFU-E is a more primitive progenitor in the erythroid maturation pathway than the colony-forming unit–erythroid (CFU-E). The colony it forms is large, compared with the CFU-E, has spreading margins, and often satellite colonies. **B.** CFU-E. This colony was photographed at day 7 in culture. The CFU-E originates from a more mature single progenitor cell than the BFU-E. The CFU-E is smaller and grows typically in a tight, dense colony, compared with the BFU-E. The sequence established in the erythroid lineage is BFU-E, CFU-E, erythrocyte precursors (proerythroblast, etc). *(Reproduced with permission from Lichtman MA, Shafer MS, Felgar RE, et al: Lichtman's Atlas of Hematology 2016. New York, NY: McGraw Hill; 2017.)*

cannot divide further. After extrusion of the nucleus, the enucleated cells derived from orthochromic erythroblasts are termed *polychromatophilic erythrocytes*, reticulocytes when stained supravitally and so named after the cytoplasmic remnants of the endoplasmic reticulum and the persistence of a few mitochondria and strings of ribosomes they contain. These anucleate cells (ie, reticulocytes) remain in the marrow for 48 to 72 hours before being released into the blood. The polychromatophilic erythrocytes (reticulocytes) have an irregular, polylobated shape and various membrane-bound organelles.[90] In the blood, these newly released polychromatophilic macrocytes (reticulocytes) undergo further maturation with the removal of vestiges of organelles and reconditioning of the membrane and a decrease in cell volume from circa 140fL to 90fL to become mature red blood cells with the morphology of a biconcave disk.[91]

The number of erythroid precursor cells determines to a great extent the number of red cells produced. The proerythroblasts also contain EPORs that, in the presence of higher-than-normal levels of EPO, may accelerate their entry into their first mitotic division. This process may lead to a shortened marrow transit time of erythroblasts[92] and result in release of still-immature erythrocytes (polychromatophilic macrocytes), so-called *stress* or *shift* reticulocytes (larger, gray-blue–stained and often showing some folding on the blood film) (Fig. 2-2).[93] These stress reticulocytes may be up to twice the size of normal mature red cells, and their presence in the blood film is an indication of the marrow's response to anemia. Creation of normalized and-shaped red cells, devoid of organelles and discoid round-shaped red cells, is the end result of an orderly transformation of a proerythroblast with a large nucleus and a volume of approximately 900 fL to a hemoglobinized anucleate disc-shaped cell with a volume of approximately 90 fL, and takes about 5 days to occur. Although cytoplasmic maturation is continuous, the interposed mitotic divisions cause a stepwise reduction in cytoplasmic and nuclear volumes, enabling recognition of proerythroblasts, erythroblasts, and polychromatophilic macrocytes (reticulocytes) with light microscopy (Chap. 1). Direct measurements of the number of marrow erythroblasts and reticulocytes have shown approximately 50 erythroblasts and approximately 124 reticulocytes for each proerythroblast (Table 2-1).[94,95] This distribution conforms to the number of cells in a theoretic erythroid pyramid (Table 2-1, Fig. 2-3). In the

pyramid, each erythroblast undergoes five mitotic divisions over 5 days before the orthochromatic erythroblast loses its nucleus and as an immature erythrocyte enters a 2- to 3-day period of maturation before its release from the marrow. The size and shape of these erythroid pyramids undoubtedly vary, but such variations play a role in the physiologic control of red cell production. When production is suppressed, as in the circumstance of low EPO secretion seen in anemia of chronic renal disease, the distribution of erythroblasts appears normal, with no morphologic or ferrokinetic evidence of ineffective erythropoiesis, but the number of erythroid progenitors is decreased.[92] When production is increased, as in severe hemolytic anemia, the pyramid of erythroid precursors also appears normal, with no evidence of additional mitotic divisions, but the number of erythroid progenitors is increased. Consequently, the rate of red cell production largely depends on the number of erythroid progenitors formed.

As the erythroblast matures, its synthetic activities increase rapidly, producing all proteins characteristic of mature red blood cells, particularly globin chain synthesis. Eventually, 95% of all protein in the red cell is hemoglobin, almost all hemoglobin A ($\alpha_2\beta_2$) in adults, with only small amounts of hemoglobin F ($\alpha_2\gamma_2$) and hemoglobin A^2 ($\alpha_2\delta_2$). Hemoglobin F is unequally distributed and is present only in some erythrocytes, designated as *F cells* (Chaps. 17 and 18).

EPOR density declines sharply on early erythroblasts, and EPORs are absent from the more mature erythroblast forms, whereas the number of receptors for transferrin increases, reflecting the increased demands for iron for heme synthesis.

ERYTHROBLAST ENUCLEATION

The microenvironment may be important for proliferation and maturation of erythroblasts. However, in situ secreted or circulating growth factors and cytokines appear to be less important for precursor cells than for progenitor cells. Intercellular adhesion molecules secure the structural integrity of the marrow, and fibronectin is of special importance for erythroblasts.[96] Loss of fibronectin receptors heralds the translocation of polychromatophilic macrocytes (reticulocytes) into blood, but some newly emerging erythrocytes remain adherent, even

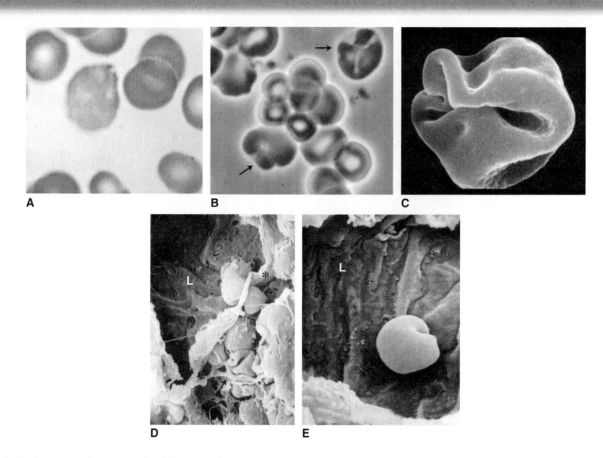

Figure 2–2. Stress reticulocytes. **A.** Blood film. Hemolytic anemia. The polychromatophilic macrocyte with puckering evident by the clover-leaf-shaped clear areas (folds) is a characteristic stress erythrocyte, so named because they are prematurely released from the marrow by high levels of erythropoietin, usually as a result of a hemolytic anemia. They are large, intensely polychromatophilic, and often have evidence of excess surface area as evident by the folds. **B.** Phase-contrast microscopy of the blood cells in suspension from a case of hemolytic anemia. The *arrows* point to two macrocytes with puckered (folded) surfaces, characteristic of stress reticulocytes. **C.** A scanning electron micrograph of a stress reticulocyte. Note the markedly increased surface area-to-volume relationship for a red cell. **D.** Scanning electron micrograph of a marrow sinus of a mouse. *L* denotes the sinus lumen. The *asterisk* is the edge of the endothelial lining of the sinus, torn in preparation for microscopy. The *arrow* points to two anuclate red cells folded amidst the reticular cell extensions that make up the stroma of marrow. Note the severe folding of reticulocytes in situ. Note similarity between folds of the cell to the scanning image in (*C*). Just below the *asterisk* is an enucleated red cell (reticulocyte), half in the hematopoietic space and half in the lumen, presumptively in egress. Note the surface folding required when traversing the narrow pore in endothelium. **E.** A marrow sinus with an anuclate red cell emerging into the lumen. Note the folding required to negotiate the narrow pore through which the cell is exiting. (See Chap. 1 for details of erythrocyte egress.) *(Reproduced with permission from Lichtman MA, Shafer MS, Felgar RE, et al: Lichtman's Atlas of Hematology 2016. New York, NY: McGraw Hill; 2017.)*

TABLE 2–1. Erythroid Pools		
Cell Number × 10⁸ per kg/Body Weight		
Cell Type	**Observed**	**Theoretic Model (Fig. 2-3)**
Proerythroblasts	1	1
Erythroblasts	49	58
Marrow reticulocytes	82	64
Blood reticulocytes	31	32
Mature red cells	3300	3800

Data from Donohue DM, Reiff RH, Hanson ML, et al. Quantitative measurement of the erythrocytic and granulocytic cells of the marrow and blood. *J Clin Invest*. 1958;37(11):1571-1576; and Finch CA, Harker LA, Cook JD. Kinetics of the formed elements of human blood. *Blood*. 1977;50(4):699-707.

after release, and are temporarily sequestered by the spleen (Chaps. 1 and 25). Because erythroid colonies developed in vitro consist principally of nucleated red cells, enucleation may primarily be induced by marrow stromal cells (Chap. 1).

The extrusion process is an active process involving cytokinetic machinery of the actin cytoskeleton and microtubules. The nucleus is displaced to one side of the cytoplasm by cytokinesis.[97] Morphologic examination, time-lapse live-cell imaging, and electron microscopic studies have shown F-actin bundles concentrate at the furrow behind the extruding nucleus, and a contractile actin ring forms at the boundary between the cytoplasm and the nucleus of enucleating cells. Inhibitors of actin polymerization[98] and microtubule disrupting agents[99] inhibit contractile ring formation. Rac1 GTPase, a pleiotropic regulator of multiple cellular processes, and its effector mDia2 are essential because downregulation of these two proteins disrupts the contractile ring formation and erythroblast enucleation.[100] During enucleation, major plasma membrane proteins partition to the developing reticulocyte via the cytoskeleton and are excluded from the plasma membrane

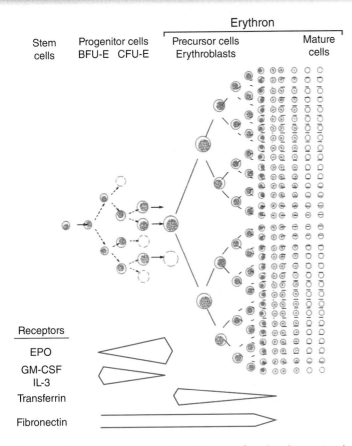

Figure 2–3. Theoretical model of proliferation of erythroid-committed marrow cells, including their most important receptors. BFU-E, burst-forming unit–erythroid; CFU-E, colony-forming unit–erythroid; EPO, erythropoietin; GM-CSF, granulocyte-macrophage colony-stimulating factor; IL, interleukin.

surrounding the extruded nucleus.[101] Extrusion results in a polychromatophilic macrocyte (reticulocyte) and a nucleus enveloped with a thin layer of cytoplasm and the plasma membrane is called *pyrenocyte*. Pyrenocytes are then rapidly eliminated by marrow macrophages by phosphatidylserine-dependent phagocytosis.[102]

The enucleation process is orchestrated by transcription factors, including KFL1, which is required for enucleation through its regulation of the expression of cell cycle proteins, deacetylases, caspases, and nuclear membrane proteins. In addition, a polycomb group protein-epigenetic modifier (ASXL1)[103] and FoxO3,[104] a transcription factor that plays a crucial role in the control of cell cycle and also act as a tumor suppressor protein (E2F-2),[105] and micro-RNAs (miRs) also play critical roles by modulating the expression activity of adhesion proteins, cytoskeletal components, and the acetylation status of histones. The erythroblasts in culture do not enucleate as they do in the marrow, revealing the important role for the marrow microenvironment in the process.[106] Consistent with this conclusion, erythroid colonies developed in vitro consist principally of nucleated red cells (Chap. 1). Erythroblast macrophage protein (Emp) appears to be particularly important for erythroblast-macrophage interaction during enucleation.[107,108] Genetic ablation of *Emp* in the mouse leads to a dramatic increase of nucleated red cells in the blood, and no fetal liver erythroblastic islands are observed in Emp-deficient mice. *Emp*[null] mice do not extrude their nuclei from erythroid cells, and actin localization during terminal erythroblast differentiation is disrupted.

Other proteins that are involved in the macrophage-erythroblast interaction include the tumor suppressor retinoblastoma (Rb) protein. Rb deficiency in murine fetal liver prevents interactions between macrophages and erythroblasts and blocks erythroblast enucleation.[109] Rb also promotes erythropoiesis by coupling cell-cycle exit with mitochondrial biogenesis.[110]

Microscopic determination of marrow cellularity and the proportion of erythroblasts permits semiquantitative evaluation of erythropoiesis. However, the presence of ineffective erythropoiesis in disease states, such as iron deficiency, anemia of inflammation, megaloblastic anemias, and thalassemias, often makes a morphologic approach misleading (Chaps. 6, 9, 11, 14, and 17). Red cell production can be accurately estimated by ferrokinetic studies using ^{59}Fe. Similarly, the amount of the final product of erythropoiesis, the RCM, can also be accurately measured. Unfortunately, the ever-increasing regulation of even minute amounts of radioisotopes used in vivo makes these methods virtually unavailable. Methods based on inhalation of minute amounts of CO allowing measurement of changes of blood carboxyhemoglobin (COHb) levels are useful and are available in some centers, see section *Nonradioactive Methods*.

Chapters 1, 16, and 17 discuss developmental control of erythropoiesis, differential use of enzyme and globin genes, and the crucial differences between embryonic yolk sac and fetal/adult definite erythropoiesis. This chapter focuses mainly on adult erythropoiesis.

ERYTHROPOIETIN, OXYGEN SENSING, AND HYPOXIA-INDUCIBLE FACTOR

Erythropoietin

The principal hormone regulating erythropoiesis is EPO, which is produced in adult life principally in the kidney[6] (Figs. 2-4a and b). Erythroid progenitors express their own EPO at very low levels.[111] Different levels of kidney-produced EPO are optimal for various stages of erythroid maturation.[112] EPO and its recombinant form are heavily glycosylated α-globulins with a molecular mass of 34,000 Da and a specific activity of approximately 200,000 IU/mg.[113,114] Sixty percent of the molecular weight of the recombinant protein is contributed by amino acids; the remaining 40% is composed of carbohydrate. Using molecular probes for *EPO*, mRNA enabled the localization of the synthesis of EPO to renal interstitial fibroblasts.[115,116] The cells appear to function in an all-or-none fashion, with the overall production of mRNA dependent on the number of cells activated.[117]

Certain 5′ sequences located 6000 to 12,000 bp upstream regulate *EPO* gene transcription.[118] These sequences are not hypoxia-sensitive but appear necessary for tissue and cellular specificity. Hepatic production is contributed primarily by hepatocytes but is a much less important source than is the kidney in adults.[119] During fetal life, however, hepatic EPO production is of major importance for red cell production (Chap. 1).[120,121] EPO production is regulated exclusively at the level of its transcription by hypoxia. The transcriptional activation of the *EPO* gene is controlled by a specific sequence located in the 3′ flanking *EPO* noncoding region termed *hypoxia-responsive element* (HRE).[122-124] The core of the enhancer is constituted by the sequence CACGTGCT, and mutations in this core sequence abolish hypoxia responsiveness.

EPO is not stored but secreted immediately.[115-117] Circulating recombinant EPO and presumably native EPO have a half-life (T$_{1/2}$) of 4 to 12 hours; EPO is eliminated after it binds to EPOR (see "Erythropoietin Receptor,") by internalization and degradation.[125]

Erythropoietin Receptor

Interaction of EPO with its receptor EPOR results in (1) stimulation of erythroid cell division, (2) erythroid differentiation by induction of

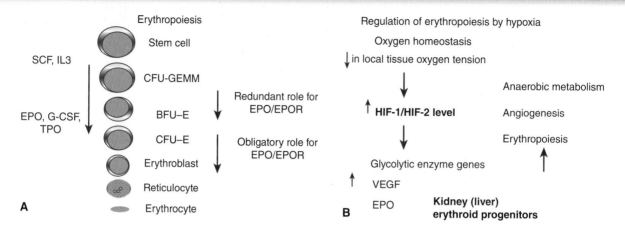

Figure 2–4. A. Cytokine influence on hematopoiesis. CFU-GEMM, colony-forming unit–growing granulocyte, erythrocyte, megakaryocyte, and macrophage precursors; EPO, erythropoietin; EPOR, erythropoietin receptor; G-CSF, granulocyte colony-stimulating factor; IL3, interleukin-3; SCF, stem cell factor; TPO, thrombopoietin. **B.** Regulation of erythropoiesis by hypoxia. HIF-1/HIF-2, hypoxia inducible factors-1 and -2; VEGF, vascular endothelial growth factor-I.

erythroid-specific protein expression, and (3) prevention of erythroid progenitor apoptosis.[126] Several lines of evidence suggest that EPOR is a preformed homodimer that undergoes a major conformational change upon ligand binding,[127] which initiates the EPO-specific erythroid signal transduction cascade (Fig. 2-5). The cytoplasmic portion of EPOR contains a positive regulatory domain that interacts with Janus kinase 2 (JAK2).[129] Immediately after EPO binding, JAK2 cross-phosphorylates the EPOR itself and other proteins such as STAT5, thus initiating a cascade of erythroid-specific signaling.[130] JAK2/STAT5 signaling plays an essential role in EPO–EPOR-mediated regulation of erythropoiesis (see Fig. 2-5).[131] Deficiency of EPO–EPOR is lethal by abrogating fetal liver erythropoiesis (but not the "primitive" yolk sac erythropoiesis). However, in these *EPO* or *EPOR*-knockout mice, differentiation of pluripotential stem cells to BFU-E occurs, but does not fully complete erythroid differentiation. These observations demonstrate the crucial role of EPO in terminal erythroid maturation.[132-134] The C-terminal cytoplasmic portion of EPOR also possesses a domain essential for the prevention of apoptosis (see Fig. 2-5) by inducing expression of Bcl-x$_L$ via phosphoinositide 3 kinase.[46] Moreover, the cytoplasmic portion of EPOR also contains a negative regulatory domain[135] that interacts with hematopoietic cell phosphatase (HCP, also known as SHP1) and downmodulates signal transduction.[136] Once recruited by EPOR tyrosine (Y)429, HCP attaches to the cytoplasmic EPOR domain and dephosphorylates JAK2 (Fig. 2-6). Deletion of the HCP binding site leads to prolonged phosphorylation of JAK2/STAT5 (see Chaps. 3 and 27).[136,137] CIS3 (also known as SOCS3), another negative regulator of erythropoiesis, binds to the cytoplasmic portion of the EPOR Y401 and suppresses EPO-dependent JAK2/ STAT5 signaling.[138,139] Thus, deletion of the distal C-terminal cytoplasmic portion of EPOR abolishes negative regulatory elements and results in increased proliferation of erythroid progenitor cells (Chap. 27), and is found in the individuals with primary familial and congenital erythrocytosis (also referred to as polycythemia), are rarely found in erythroleukemia.[140] The rearranged EPOR has also been identified in a subtype of high-risk B-progenitor acute lymphoblastic leukemia.[141]

As the activation signal after EPO binding to its receptor is rapidly downregulated and EPO briskly disappears after binding to EPOR, EPO–EPOR internalization is one mechanism of downregulation of EPO signaling.[125] After EPO binds to its receptor, EPO–EPOR complexes are ubiquinated, rapidly internalized, and targeted for degradation. This process involves two proteolytic systems, the proteosomes

that remove part of the intracellular domain of EPOR at the cell surface and the lysosomes that degrade the EPO–EPOR complex in the cytoplasm.[142]

Another incompletely understood mechanism of erythropoiesis regulation is the presence of several EPOR isoforms, some of which may have an inhibitory function on erythropoiesis.[143-145]

Nonerythroid Effect of Erythropoietin Signaling

Soon after the erythroid effects of recombinant EPO were described, nonerythroid effects of EPO were identified.[146] Some of these effects are beneficial, including roles in neural, cardiovascular, and retinal tissues; immune function; and tissue repair. It has been claimed that EPO also exerts beneficial effects on athletic performance and improved neurocognition, but these are not substantiated. The effects of EPO in nonerythroid tissues are the result of EPO binding to EPOR and, as in erythroid cells, the EPO–EPOR interaction initiates a signal transduction process that regulates the survival, growth, and differentiation of the involved tissue.[147] EPO and EPOR have been shown to play a physiologic role in many nonerythroid cells including endothelial cells,[148] megakaryocytes, and cells of the brain,[149] heart, uterus, breast, and testis. However, in some tissues (eg, brain, heart, kidney), the signaling mechanism may be different because EPO can interact with heterodimers composed of EPOR and CD131.[150,151]

Detrimental EPO effects include a poorly understood increased cancer mortality,[129,152,153] increased blood pressure, and thrombosis.[150,154]

Hypoxia-Inducible Factors

EPO production is mediated by hypoxemia.[112] Hypoxia plays an important role in development, energy metabolism, vasculogenesis, iron metabolism, and tumor promotion, and is the principal regulator of erythropoiesis. The response to hypoxia is controlled by transcriptional factors termed hypoxia-inducible factors (HIFs).[155,156] Adaptive physiologic responses to hypoxia serve to (1) increase O$_2$ delivery to tissue cells, (2) allow cells to survive under reduced O$_2$ by activating glycolysis, and (3) reduce the formation of reactive oxygen species.[157] HIFs are heterodimeric transcription factors composed of a highly regulated α subunit and a constitutively expressed β subunit that belongs to the basic helix-loop-helix containing the PER-ARNTSIM (PAS)-domain family of transcription factors. The first HIF to be discovered, HIF-1, is induced in hypoxic cells and binds to a cis-acting nucleotide sequence of HRE, first identified in the 3′-flanking region of the

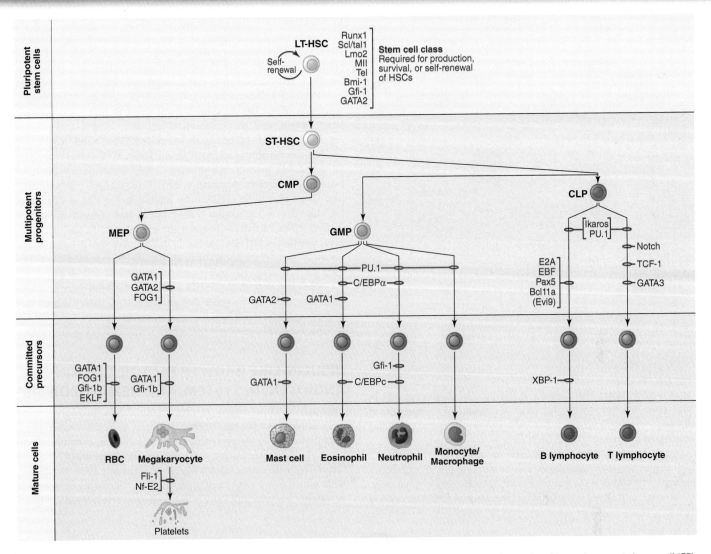

Figure 2–5. Schematic outline of emerging hierarchy of hematopoiesis outlining a separate progenitor for erythroid/megakaryocytic lineage (MEP). RUNX-1, Scl1/Tal1, Lmo1, MllTel, PU.1, GATA1, GATA2, gf-1,C/EBPα, FOG1, EKLF, Ikaros, E2A, EBF, PAX-5, BCL 11A, NOTCH, TCF-1 are transcription factors. CLP, common lymphoid progenitor; CMP, common myeloid progenitor; GMP, granulocyte/macrophage progenitor; LT-HSC, long-term hematopoietic stem cell; MEP, megakaryocyte/erythroid progenitor; RBCs, red blood cells; ST-HSC, short-term hematopoietic stem cell. *(Reproduced with permission from Orkin SH, Zon LI: Hematopoiesis: an evolving paradigm for stem cell biology. Cell. 2008 Feb 22;132[4]:631-644.)*

human *EPO* gene.[122-124] Two other HIF homologues, HIF-2 and HIF-3, have been identified. HIF-1α is expressed ubiquitously, whereas HIF-2α expression is restricted to certain tissues.[155,165] HIF-2 is the principal regulator of EPO expression.[121,158] Approximately 3% of all genes expressed in endothelial tissue are HIF-1–regulated.[159] The mechanism of HIF regulation is complex. The half-life of HIF-1α in the cell is about a minute under normoxic conditions. In normoxia, HIF-1 and HIF-2 α subunits are rapidly degraded in a protein-ubiquitin proteasome pathway[160-162] and thus have extremely short half-life.[163] This degradation of HIFs α subunits is initiated by a posttranslational hydroxylation of proline 564 (P564) by one of several iron-containing proline hydroxylases (PHDs) whose activity is dependent on oxygen and requires a substrate. Thus, under normoxic conditions, HIFs α subunits are hydroxylated at the conserved proline, binds to the von Hippel-Lindau (VHL) followed by subsequent ubiquitination and proteasomal degradation. This targeting and subsequent polyubiquitination and destruction of HIFs α subunits requires PHD activity, VHL, iron, O_2, and this complex constitutes the oxygen sensor (Fig. 2-7).[161,164]

Under hypoxic conditions, HIF-1 and HIF-2 α proteins are not degraded and are translocated to the cell nucleus, where they dimerize with constitutively expressed HIF-β to form the HIF heterodimer that activates transcription through binding to specific HREs on target genes. Another regulatory step involves O_2-dependent asparaginyl-hydroxylation of asparagine (N) 803 in HIF-1α that requires the enzyme HIF-3, also known as FIH-1 (factor inhibiting HIF-1). Hydroxylation of N803 during normoxia blocks the binding of transcription factors p300 and CBP to HIF-1, resulting in inhibition of HIF-1–mediated gene transcription. Under hypoxic conditions, HIFs α subunits are not hydroxylated. The unmodified protein escapes VHL-binding, ubiquitination, and degradation (see Fig. 2-7), allowing it to form the requisite heterodimer, enter the nucleus, and activate transcription of HIF-1 target genes. Iron metabolism and erythropoiesis closely interact and iron availability is central to productive erythropoiesis via hepcidin and erythroferrone (see Chap. 10). In addition to indirect regulation of HIFs by iron regulation of principal negative regulator of HIFs—PHD2—there is also direct regulation of HIF-2 by iron. The 5' untranslated region of

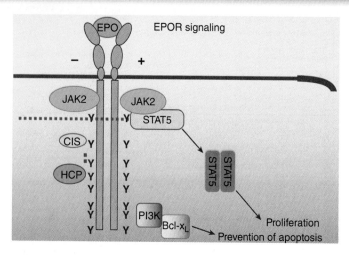

Figure 2–6. Outline of erythropoietin–erythropoietin receptor (EPO–EPOR) signaling. Activation of JAK2 and STAT5 represents erythropoiesis-promoting signals. Interaction of CIS and HCP inhibit erythropoiesis. PI3 kinase (PI3K) activation of Bcl-x$_L$ inhibits apoptosis of erythroid progenitors. HCP, hematopoietic cell phosphatase.

EPAS1 gene encoding HIF-2α contains the iron-responsive element that represses the translation of *EPAS1*.[165] The iron regulatory protein (IRP-1) binds to this 5'untranslated region of HIF-2α. The deletion of *Irp1* in mice results in erythrocytosis, attributable to translational de-repression of Hif-2α.[166] Four families from Iceland with erythrocytosis and mutations in IRP1 are described in Chap. 28.[167]

HIF Transcription Factors HIF-1α and HIF-2α exhibit a high-degree sequence homology but have differing mRNA expression patterns. The kidney is the main site of EPO production (ie, renal interstitial cells), and HIF-2 is the principal regulator of *EPO* transcription in the kidney.[155,168] The importance of HIF-2α in regulation[164] of the *EPO* gene was demonstrated by a gain-of-function *EPAS1* encoding HIF-2α mutation, causing erythrocytosis.[169] In other tissues, such as the brain[149,170] and liver[121] (which generates approximately 15% of circulating EPO), HIF-1α appears to play an important role.

Hypoxia-Independent Regulation of HIF Although O$_2$-dependent regulation of the HIF-1α subunit is mediated by prolyl hydroxylases, VHL protein, and the proteasomal complex, hypoxia-independent regulation of HIF-1α has been uncovered. This novel mechanism involves the receptor of activated protein kinase C (RACK1) as an HIF-1α–interacting protein that promotes prolyl hydroxylase/VHL-independent proteasomal degradation of HIF-1α. RACK1 competes with heat shock protein 90 (HSP90) for binding to the PAS-A domain of HIF-1α. HIF-1α degradation is abolished by loss-of-function RACK1. RACK1 binds to the proteasomal subunit, elongin-C, and promotes ubiquitination of HIF-1α (see Fig. 2-7). Therefore, RACK1 and HSP90 are the essential components of an O$_2$/PHD/VHL-independent mechanism for regulating HIF-1α.[171]

The rapid degradation of HIF is complex and tightly regulated, and mutations affecting the genes that encode the regulatory factors may underlie some yet unexplained congenital erythrocytoses. This complex (Chaps. 3 and 28) constitutes the oxygen sensor (see Fig. 2-7).[161,164,172]

INSULIN-LIKE GROWTH FACTOR-1, RENIN–ANGIOTENSIN SYSTEM, AND HEMATOPOIESIS

Although in vitro studies of erythropoiesis have provided crucial information about the regulation of erythropoiesis, many experiments were performed in the presence of serum and serum-component proteins capable of stimulating and inhibiting erythropoiesis.[173,174] Using serum-free conditions, insulin-like growth factor-1 (IGF-1) can partially substitute for EPO in cultures of BFU-E. Furthermore, anephric, nonanemic patients with low EPO have elevated levels of IGF-1.[175]

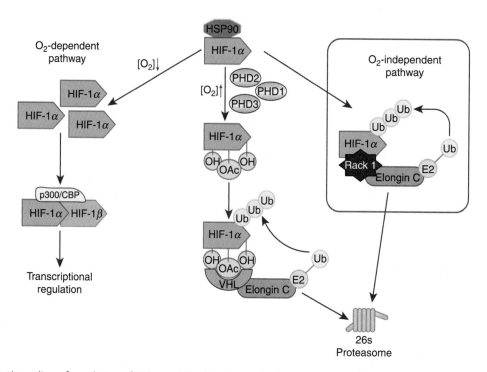

Figure 2–7. Schematic outline of regulation of HIF-2 and HIF-2α subunits by hypoxic and nonhypoxic pathways. HIF, hypoxiainducible factor; HSP90, heat shock protein 90; PHDs, proline hydroxylases; p300 and CBP, cofactors of hypoxia response transcription with HIF-1; RACK1, receptor of activated protein kinase C; ub, ubiquitin residues; VHL, von Hippel–Lindau protein.

RED CELL LIFE SPAN

Normal human red cells have a life span of about 120 days, after which they are engulfed by macrophages. This is an extremely efficient process because macrophages phagocytose about 5 million erythrocytes every second without a significant release of hemoglobin into the circulation. The precise molecular mechanism(s) by which macrophages recognize senescent red blood cells for phagocytosis is (are) still not fully understood. As red blood cells age, several physiologic changes occur that may serve as signals for recognition by macrophages.[176,177] These include (1) a decrease in the activity of enzymes[178]; (2) a progressive decrease of adensine triphosphate (ATP) content[179]; (3) a loss of lipid asymmetry with exposure of phosphatidylserine[180]; (4) an accumulation of lipid peroxidation products[181]; (5) a desialylation of membrane glycoprotein[182]; (6) an exposure of cryptic senescent antigens[183] and aggregation of AE-1 (band 3) protein (Chap. 15)[184]; (7) a decrease in deformability caused by increased oxidative stress[185]; and (8) an increase in cell surface–bound immunoglobulins and complement components (Chap. 26).[186,187] All of these changes have been investigated as signals for recognition by the macrophages. Further, hypoxia may ameliorate red cell destruction and increase red cell survival, constituting an independent mechanism for expansion of RCM.[188]

REMOVAL OF ERYTHROCYTE ORGANELLES

DOWNREGULATION OF CELL SURFACE PROTEINS AND OTHER ORGANELLES

During erythroid maturation, reticulocytes release small vesicles containing cellular proteins. These vesicles are exosomes that are involved in the clearance of cell surface proteins, such as acetyl cholinesterase, CD71 transferrin receptor, and integrin α4β1.[189,190] The enrichment of these surface molecules in exosomes suggests that the exosomal pathway plays a major role in the clearance of these surface molecules. Other cellular components, such as nuclei, mitochondria, ribosomes, lysosomes, endoplasmic reticulum, Golgi apparatus, ribosomes, and RNA, are also cleared during erythroid maturation. The precise mechanisms for the removal of these components are unclear. In Nix-deficient mice (a proapoptotic Bcl-2–related protein, important in mitochondrial elimination), the loss of CD71 and ribosomes are normal during erythroid maturation, suggesting that exosomal pathways play a major role in the clearance of CD71 or ribosomes.[191]

Erythroblast Enucleation

Erythroblast enucleation is accompanied by chromatin condensation and by a rearrangement of actin cytoskeleton involving interaction between the erythroblasts and macrophages at the erythroblastic island, and is described in an early paragraph of this chapter. It occurs in orthochromatic erythroblasts, producing two kinds of cells, the reticulocyte and the pyrenocyte (the nucleus surrounded by a tiny layer of cytoplasm and the plasma membrane). Pyrenocytes are rapidly eliminated by the macrophages of the erythroblastic island.[90]

Clearance of Mitochondria by Autophagy

During terminal erythroid differentiation, erythroid cells discard all their internal organelles including mitochondria. Autophagy (Chap. 1) plays an important role in this process based on early morphologic studies.[192,193] This role is confirmed by studies using chemical inhibitors of autophagy and siRNA knockdown of essential autophagy-associated genes.[191,194] At the initial stage of autophagy, a double-membrane structure is formed to sequester cytoplasmic components in autophagosomes. Autophagosomes then fuse with lysosomes and become autophagolysosomes to degrade the sequestered components. Nixdeficient mice display defects in the clearance of mitochondria. The formation of autophagosomes in reticulocytes is normal in the absence of Nix, suggesting that Nix is not required for the initiation of autophagy or the formation of autophagosomes. Instead, mitochondria remain clustered outside of autophagosomes in Nix[-/-] reticulocytes.[191] This finding indicates that Nix is required for the sequestration of mitochondria by autophagosomes. Another study using virally transformed Nix[-/-] erythroid cells also described defective inclusion of mitochondria by autophagosomes.[195] Therefore, Nix deficiency leads to a specific defect in mitochondrial removal without causing a general block in autophagy or erythroid maturation. Nix[-/-] reticulocytes are defective in the loss of mitochondrial membrane potential during in vitro maturation.[191] The role of other genes in mitophagy has also been described; when the *Atg7* gene was deleted in mice, mitophagy was impaired.[106] However, some differences of murine and human hematopoietic lineages have been described.[196,197]

Removal of Ribosomes in Reticulocytes

Removal of erythrocyte ribosomes is incompletely understood, although it is clear that the *Ulk1* gene (an autophagy-activating Ser/Thr protein kinase) is involved in both ribosome and mitochondria degradation.[194] However, the impaired clearance of ribosomes is highly detrimental, as seen in hemolytic anemia associated with congenital defect of erythrocyte 5′ nucleotidase (Chap. 16).[198]

MICRORNAS (miRNAS) IN ERYTHROPOIESIS

miRNAs are small 18- to -22–nucleotide noncoding RNAs that regulate gene expression by inhibiting protein translation or by destabilizing target mRNAs; they are important regulators of hematopoiesis. The role of miRNAs in regulation of erythropoiesis is being actively defined. Some miRNAs are mainly expressed in the early stages of erythropoiesis, others in late stages, and some have biphasic expression during erythroid differentiation. Some appear to have erythroid-specific expression.[199] The critical role of miRNAs and their relationship to the essential transcription factors regulating erythropoiesis is outlined by the report that the pivotal transcription factors for erythropoiesis, GATA-1 and NF-E2, directly regulate and control differentiation via miR-199b-5p. This miRNA then targets c-Kit, an important receptor for early erythroid cells.[200] Some miRNAs likely play a role in the commitment to erythroid versus megakaryocytic differentiation. Thus, miR-18a was reported to be upregulated during erythropoiesis and downregulated during megakaryopoiesis, whereas miR-145 was upregulated in megakaryopoiesis and downregulated in erythropoiesis. Their mRNA targets and their functional significance are being defined.[201] LIN28B and its targeted let-7 have regulated expression during the fetal-to-adult erythroid cell transition.[202] Another important phase of erythroid development and function is regulated by miR-351. A complex regulatory transcriptional repressor system controlling heterochromatin formation exists, composed of one of the 400 human zinc finger protein-based transcription factors (KRAB-ZFP)–mediated repression that includes cofactor KAP1. Deletion of KAP1 in mice upregulates miR-351 and several other miRs, which then downregulate Nix and mitochondrial autophagy. MiR21 is hypoxia-induced and downregulates catalase after rapid normoxic return from hypoxia (see "Neocytolysis" in the next section), resulting in expansion of mitochondria in erythroid progenitors and transient hypoproliferative anemia phenotype.[203]

MEASUREMENTS OF RED CELL MASS

The RCM is maintained and regulated by the kidney and marrow, which, under steady-state conditions, precisely replaces cells lost by senescence. RCM defines anemia and erythrocytosis. The kinetics of red cell production and destruction help establish their pathogenesis. A number of tests have been developed to measure the three main components of red cell kinetics: RCM, rate of red cell production, and rate of red cell destruction. Some of these tests are simple but indirect and only semiquantitative, such as hematocrit (Hct), reticulocyte count, haptoglobin, lactate dehydrogenase, unconjugated bilirubin concentration, and CO formation. Examination of the marrow allows assessment of total cellularity and relative erythroid contribution but is limited in that the kinetics of cell production cannot be inferred from a single static image obtained from a very small fraction of the whole marrow. These tests are very useful in the aggregate but can be supplemented by more complex but direct quantitation; however, most require use of radioisotopes.

PACKED RED CELL VOLUME OR HEMATOCRIT

Packed red cell volume is commonly referred to as the *hematocrit*. It is measured as the percentage of the volume of whole blood that is made up by red cells. Historically it was measured by high speed centrifugation of blood and determination of the fraction of the total blood column composed of tightly packed red cells. Modern electronic particle counters calculate the Hct from the product of the red cell count and the mean cell volume (MCV) (Chap. 1). Total body Hct is the RCM in the circulation divided by the total blood volume. Blood Hct is the simplest and most widely used test for estimating the size of RCM. In most anemic patients, blood Hct gives an excellent approximation of total RCM and a functional estimation of the oxygen-carrying capacity and of blood viscosity. Its main drawback is that it is a measure that is influenced by changes in plasma volume and may not reflect the size of the RCM in dehydrated or overhydrated patients. Dehydration usually is clinically apparent and, in most cases, can be taken into account when evaluating the significance of a specific Hct determination. Only direct measurement of RCM can differentiate between relative and absolute erythrocytosis. Thus, although Tibetans have lower Hct than sojourners to high altitude or other non-Tibetan high-altitude residents, the direct measurements of the Tibetan subgroup Sherpas showed they have increased RCM as well as increased plasma volume.[204] However, when the Hct is greater than 60%, almost all patients have an increase in total RCM.[205]

Isotopic Methods

A more direct and accurate estimate of the size of the RCM is obtained from labeling a known quantity of red cells and determining the dilution of this label in the blood. Many of these time-honored methods used radioactive labels and led to our current knowledge of red cell production and destruction. These methods are usually unavailable, largely because of poorly justified apprehension of the insignificant risk of this degree of radiation exposure. Moreover, because differentiation of secondary causes of modest increases in hemoglobin concentration from normal and from polycythemia vera is the principal use of the RCM, with the discovery that nearly every patient with polycythemia vera bears the JAK2V617F mutation (Chap. 28), the need for determining RCM has diminished. Nevertheless, the knowledge acquired from formal determination of RCM will be briefly outlined here. Radioactive iron is an excellent label of red cells because it is biosynthetically incorporated into hemoglobin in vivo and permits assessment of effective and ineffective erythropoiesis, RCM, and the site of red cell destruction[206]

and is described in detail in section "Ferrokinetics." However, the radiation exposure to the donor virtually precludes its use in humans but it is still being used in experimental animals.

Almost all current clinical methods use labeling of autologous red cells in vitro by any one of a number of isotopes or biotin.[207] Among the isotopes, chromium-51 (^{51}Cr) was the most widely used label for measurement of RCM, survival, and the site of destruction, although technetium-99m (^{99m}Tc) use is also convenient and accurate.[208] Chromium in the form of the chromate ion (CrO_2^-) readily enters the red cell and binds to globin chains. Excess isotope in the incubation mixture can be removed by washing or by using ascorbic acid to reduce the chromate ion to a non-permeable chromic ion. Approximately 15 minutes after injection of a known amount of labeled cells, a sample of blood is obtained; its volume, Hct, and radioactivity are determined; and the total red cell volume is calculated from the equation:

$$RCM\,(mL) = \frac{CPM\ of\ isotope\ injected}{CPM\ of\ red\ cells\ in\ sample}$$

where CPM = counts per minute. Sampling time is usually 15 minutes. The replicate determination can be made with a coefficient of variation of approximately 1.5%.[209] The principal problem lies in reporting the measured RCM. The total RCM can be expressed as a volume related to body surface (mL/m^2) or as a volume related to body weight (mL/kg). A committee of the International Committee on Standardization in Hematology (ICSH) has extensively examined existing data and concluded that the most reproducible expressions of RCM are related to body surface area estimated from height and weight[210]:

$$RCM_{Males} = (1486 \times S) - 285$$
$$RCM_{Females} = (822 \times S) + (1.06 \times Age)$$

where RCM = red cell mass, S = body surface area in square meters, and Age = age in years. The calculated values ± 25% included 98% of the measured male values and 99% of the measured female values.[15]

Despite the ICSH recommendation, the most common method is to report RCM values in terms of milliliters per kilogram. However, this method of expression gives erroneously low values in obese individuals because adipose tissue is hypovascular. A better method might be to express the RCM in terms of lean weight. In general, lean weight is 20% less than actual weight in normal males and 25% less in normal females.[208] However, estimation of lean weight in obese individuals is inaccurate. From a practical point of view, RCM probably is best reported in terms of actual weight, with clinical inferences made based on body configuration. In general, the RCM of normal females ranges from 23 to 29 mL/kg body weight and of normal males ranges from 26 to 32 mL/kg.[210]

Nonradioactive Methods

Whereas biotin labelling for RCM is being used in experimental animals[211] and also in humans,[212] currently no FDA-approved biotin preparation for human administration is available. CO binds with high affinity to hemoglobin, generating COHb, as discussed in Chap. 19, and the CO inhalation and rebreathing has been used for decades by physiologists as a nonradioactive method to determine directly RCM and indirectly plasma volume.[213] With CO rebreathing, COHb levels increase and using the *dilution principle*, hemoglobin content and, indirectly, red cell and plasma volumes can be calculated.[214] The commercial equipment (Detalo Instruments APS) has been used in Europe; this procedure takes 10 minutes, and thus exposure time to CO is short and equivalent to that of smoking a cigarette.

PLASMA LABELS

RCM also can be estimated from plasma volume. Radioactive iodine (^{125}I) is used to label albumin and measure its distribution volume.[215] Other radioactive isotopes such as ^{99m}Tc have been used. Albumin labeled with radioactive iodine was readily commercially available in the past, and a known amount was injected intravenously. Several blood samples are obtained within the first 15 minutes and centrifuged. CPM per milliliter of plasma is measured, plotted on semilogarithmic paper, and extrapolated to zero time. This procedure is necessary because, in contradistinction to labeled red cells, labeled albumin is removed gradually, beginning immediately after injection. Plasma volume is calculated according to the equation:

$$\text{Plasma volume (mL)} = \frac{\text{CPM of labeled albumin injected}}{\text{CPM/mL Plasma at 0 hour}}$$

The continuous exchange of intravascular with extravascular albumin is the major problem encountered when plasma volume is measured with labeled albumin. Even with extrapolation to 0 hour, plasma volume is larger than that measured with a strictly intravascular protein such as fibrinogen.[216] Consequently, if measurement of the plasma volume is used to calculate the size of the total RCM, it is a less reliable measure than determining RCM directly with tagged red cells. This inaccuracy is further augmented by the fact that the venous Hct used to calculate RCM from measured plasma volume does not accurately reflect the distribution of plasma and red cells in the body. However, from a practical point of view, the results of estimating RCM from plasma volume are reasonably accurate and have been advocated based on simplicity.[215]

TOTAL BODY HEMATOCRIT

When total RCM is measured with labeled red cells, the value is approximately 10% lower than that calculated from plasma volume and the Hct of blood. In fact, the mean Hct of blood in all of the vessels (total body Hct) clearly is somewhat lower than the Hct measured from blood obtained from large vessels; these differences are a result of varying proportions of plasma in different-sized vessels.

In general, the ratio of total body Hct as estimated by direct measurements of red cell volume and plasma volume to the large-vessel Hct ranges from 0.89 to 0.92 mL.[217] Consequently, when using the determined plasma volume to calculate RCM and total blood volume, a correction factor is necessary, and a value of 0.90 is generally used:

$$\text{Corrected RCM} = \frac{\text{Hct plasma volume} \times 0.90}{100\,\text{Hct}}$$

where Hct = hematocrit.

Recommended procedures for determination and evaluation of blood volume are outlined by the ICSH.[218]

● MEASUREMENTS OF RED CELL PRODUCTION

Under certain conditions, a fraction of red cell production is ineffective, with destruction of nonviable red cells within either the marrow or shortly after the cells reach the blood.[92]

EFFECTIVE RED CELL PRODUCTION

Effective erythropoiesis is most simply estimated by determining the reticulocyte count. Most modern automated counters measure reticulocytes by nucleic acid–binding dyes such as thioazole orange using flow cytometry. These are fast and reliable assays. This count usually is expressed as the percentage of red cells that are reticulocytes, but it can also be expressed as the total number of circulating reticulocytes per unit of blood (absolute reticulocyte count and corrected reticulocyte counts):

$$\text{Absolute reticulocyte count} = \frac{\%\text{reticulocytes} \times \text{red cell count}}{100}$$

A simple clinical method to estimate effective erythropoiesis uses the reticulocyte count to calculate the reticulocyte index (see the equation below).[219] This measurement depends on several assumptions: (1) the human red cell life span is approximately 100 days (actual, 120 days); (2) the life span is finite and, thus, the oldest 1 of 100 or 1% of red cells is removed (and replaced) each day; (3) the reticulocyte is identifiable as such in the blood for 1 day using supravital stain; and (4) the reticulocyte count of 1% in a person with a normal Hct represents normal red cell production and thus "1" is the basal reticulocyte index. However, although these assumptions are useful in clinical practice, a certain component of red cell destruction is random.

In anemic patients, two calculations are needed to measure the reticulocyte index and compare it with the normal of 1 in the basal state. To correct the reticulocyte percentage for the lower red cell count in anemic subjects, the reticulocyte percent is multiplied by the ratio of the patient's Hct over the normal mean Hct (45 is typically used), providing a corrected reticulocyte percent. Because modern counters provide a measured red blood cell count, it is appropriate with red cell count rather than Hct, which is a derived value. With conversion of the reticulocyte count (see the previous equation), the reticulocyte index (see equation below) is achieved by taking into account the estimated life span of reticulocytes. The life span of reticulocytes in blood in a normal individual is approximately 1 day. However, when red cell production is increased under conditions of erythropoietic stress (eg, in severe anemia), reticulocytes are released prematurely and circulate as reticulocytes for 2 to 4 days, except in situations with low EPO levels, as in renal insufficiency. These prematurely released reticulocytes appear as large polychromatophilic erythrocytes on Wright-stained blood smear and are called *stress* or *shift reticulocytes*.

$$\text{Reticulocyte index} = \frac{\text{absolute reticulocyte count}}{\text{correction factor (usually 2)}}$$

Accordingly, the elevated reticulocyte count may give an erroneous impression of the actual rate of daily red cell production. To take this situation into account when estimating the rate of red cell production in anemic patients with high reticulocyte counts, dividing the absolute reticulocyte count by a factor may provide a more accurate estimate of red cell production.[219] For simplicity, an average factor of 2 often is used; however, the factor depends on the degree of anemia: 1.5 in mild cases, 2.5 in moderate cases, and 3.0 in severe cases. An example follows:

A patient with autoimmune hemolytic anemia has a Hct of 10 and reticulocyte count of 70%. The marrow cannot increase production by 70-fold, illustrating the need for corrections. To measure the approximate true increase, we calculate the reticulocyte index as follows:

$$\text{Corrected reticulocyte count} = 70 \times 10/45 = 15\text{, and}$$
$$\text{Reticulocyte index} = 15/3 = 5 \times \text{Basal erythroid production}$$

Thus, marrow erythroid production in response to this severe anemia has increased fivefold, a plausible response to this severity of hemolytic anemia. If the laboratory reports the absolute reticulocyte count per liter of blood rather than the percent of reticulocytes, only the second correction is required.

INEFFECTIVE RED CELL PRODUCTION

Ineffective erythropoiesis is suspected when the reticulocyte count is normal or only slightly increased despite erythroid hyperplasia of the marrow. Ineffective erythropoiesis was first recognized as an entity from the study of isotope incorporation into fecal stercobilin after administration of labeled glycine, a precursor of heme.[220] Two peaks were observed: an early peak at 3 to 5 days and a late peak at 100 to 120 days. One of the sources of the early labeled peak was suggested to be the hemoglobin of red cells that had never completed their development, having been destroyed either in the marrow or shortly after reaching the blood. Subsequent studies revealed that in certain disorders, such as pernicious anemia, thalassemia, and sideroblastic anemia, ineffective erythropoiesis is a major component of total erythropoiesis. This component can be quantitated by measuring ^{15}N-labeled glycine incorporation into the early bilirubin peaks[220] or ferrokinetics.[92,206] Calculated from bilirubin peaks and turnover, ineffective erythropoiesis under normal conditions amounts to approximately 4% to 12% of total erythropoiesis. Using ferrokinetic methods, ineffective erythropoiesis is calculated as the difference between total plasma iron turnover and erythrocyte iron turnover plus storage iron turnover (see "Ferrokinetics"). The values estimated from such studies in normal subjects are higher, ranging from 14% to 34%.[92] However, the results, both high and low, probably are misleading because none of the methods actually measures cell death, only the turnover of heme and iron. The premature death of cells (apoptosis) occurs in normal subjects, but much of the early release of bilirubin and iron is derived from the rim of hemoglobin extruded during enucleation of erythroblasts (Chap. 1).

TOTAL ERYTHROPOIESIS

Total erythropoiesis, which is the sum of effective and ineffective red cell production, can be estimated from a marrow examination. Films or sections from marrow aspirates and biopsies are first examined for relative content of fat and hematopoietic tissue. This examination gives an estimate of overall hematopoietic activity within the marrow space. A differential count then is performed, determining the ratio between granulocytic and erythroid precursors (M:E ratio). In a normal adult, the ratio is approximately 3:1 to 5:1. The ratio can be used to estimate whether erythropoiesis is normal, increased, or decreased (Chap. 1). The ratio is only an approximation of total erythroid activity because the ratio can be altered by changing the myeloid and erythroid components, and an aspirate or biopsy of a small segment of the marrow may not always reflect total marrow activity. These assumptions are valid as long as the marrow reflects the steady state. However, when used in conjunction with determination of red blood cell count and reticulocyte count, under most circumstances the ratio provides qualitative information about the rate and effectiveness of red blood cell production. A more accurate quantitation of total erythropoiesis can be made by measuring the rate of production of red cells (ferrokinetics) or, in steady-state conditions, the rate of destruction of red cells (red cell life span, bilirubin production, CO excretion).

FERROKINETICS

In 1950, Huff and associates[221] described a method for measuring the rate of red cell production using a simple model of iron metabolism (Figs. 2-8 and 2-9) (Chap. 10). In this method, radioactive iron is complexed to transferrin in vitro and injected intravenously. Alternatively, ^{59}Fe can be injected directly intravenously as the gluconate without preincubation with the patient's own plasma, providing enough unbound transferrin is available, because binding is almost instantaneous. The rate of clearance of the transferrin-bound iron from the plasma

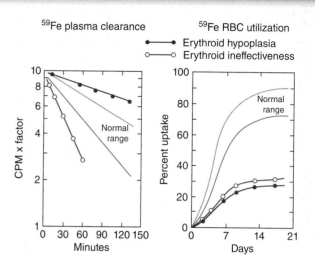

Figure 2–8. Iron clearance and iron utilization in normal subjects, patients with decreased effective red cell production (erythroid hypoplasia), and patients with ineffective red cell production. CPM, counts per minute; RBC, red blood cell.

(^{59}Fe plasma $T_{1/2}$) and the subsequent uptake in the red cells are measured. From these two values and from determinations of plasma iron concentration and plasma volume, the rate of formation of red cells can be calculated.[92,206]

The initial clearance of iron is exponential, and sampling during this period can be used to calculate $T_{1/2}$. In normal individuals, initial clearance averages approximately 90 minutes. Initial clearance is shorter in patients with hyperplasia of the erythropoietic tissue and longer in patients with marrow hypoplasia (see Fig. 2-9). However, the clearance rate is not a direct measurement of erythropoietic activity because it depends on the size of the pool of unlabeled, circulating iron. Consequently, calculation of the plasma iron turnover rate must include the plasma iron concentration. Clearance is expressed in milligrams of iron. The point of reference can be hemoglobin mass, blood volume,

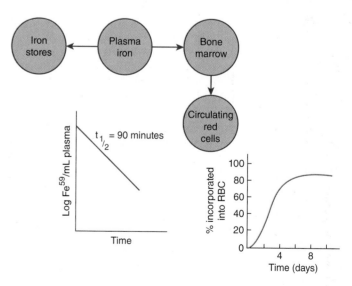

Figure 2–9. Single dynamic pool model of iron metabolism. Radioactive iron injected into the plasma iron pool is cleared from the plasma as a single exponential, and approximately 80% is incorporated into circulating blood cells.

or weight, but a commonly used expression is micrograms of iron per deciliters of whole blood per day:

$$\text{Plasma iron turnover rate (mg iron/dL blood/24 h)}$$
$$= \frac{\text{plasma iron (mg/dL)} \times (100\,\text{Hct})}{T_{1/2}(\text{min}) \times 100}$$

Under normal conditions, radioactive iron is incorporated into newly formed red cells after a few days and reaches a maximum approximately 10 to 14 days after injection (see Fig. 2-9). Normal utilization is 70% to 90% on days 10 to 14, a value so high that further increases have little significance. However, decreased utilization is an important finding and suggests immature red cells are destroyed in the marrow before they are released to the circulation (ineffective erythropoiesis) or that serum iron is diverted to nonerythropoietic tissues (marrow hypoplasia). The shape of the red cell utilization curve is also important. An early and steep rise (rapid marrow transit time) suggests a high EPO level. Finally, an early rise in utilization with a subsequent fall-off suggests hemolysis.

When calculating utilization, the blood volume must be known:

$$\text{Red cell iron utilization (\%)}$$
$$= \frac{\text{CPM of 1 mL blood} \times \text{blood volume} \times 100}{\text{CPM of } ^{59}\text{Fe injected}}$$

Using the plasma iron clearance and utilization of iron, the red cell turnover in milligrams per deciliter of blood for 24 hours is calculated as follows:

$$\text{Red cell iron turnover (mg iron/dL blood/24 h)}$$
$$= \text{plasma iron turnover maximal red cell iron utilization}$$

The normal value of red cell iron turnover is 0.30 to 0.70 mg/dL blood per 24 hours.[92] This range fits very well with a crude estimation of the iron used for maintaining the RCM in 1 dL of blood or 45 mL of packed red cells. The daily red cell production must equal the daily red cell destruction (45 mL/120 = 0.38 mL), assuming a red cell life span of 120 days. Because 1 mL of packed red cells contains approximately 1 mg of iron, a daily plasma iron turnover of 0.38 mg is needed by 1 dL of blood to maintain homeostasis.

Calculating red cell iron turnover has provided useful information about the total volume and effectiveness of erythroid tissue (Table 2-2). However, an elevated serum iron concentration gives erroneous impressions of the state of erythropoiesis. Moreover, prolonged sampling of plasma after an intravenous injection of ^{59}Fe has shown that clearance is

TABLE 2–2. Plasma Radioactive Iron Clearance and Red Blood Cell Uptake

Condition	Plasma ^{59}FE T$_{1/2}$	Red Blood Cell Uptake (%)
Normal	90 min	80-90
Increased erythropoiesis	Rapid (10-40 min)	80-90
Hemolytic anemia	Rapid	20-90[a]
Ineffective erythropoiesis	Normal to rapid	10-30
Iron-deficiency anemia	Normal to rapid	100
Decreased erythropoiesis	Slow (≥180 min)	0-20

[a]Variability a result of variability in intensity of hemolysis and size of iron stores.

not a single exponential but must be represented by several exponential components.[222] This finding has led to the introduction of more complex models of iron kinetics with a single pool of plasma iron exchanging with a number of extravascular erythroid and nonerythroid pools. Careful analysis of such models has generated computer-supported methods calculating the degree and effectiveness of erythroid activity.[223] Although possibly more accurate than the conventional method of calculating iron turnover, the models appear to be too cumbersome for clinical use. Moreover, even these sophisticated methods may not give an accurate account of the state of erythropoiesis. Despite a constant rate of red cell production, the plasma iron turnover was found to increase with increasing plasma iron and transferrin saturation. This finding was first thought to result from increased nonerythroid iron uptake and led to the introduction of various correction factors in the calculation of red cell iron turnover.[223] However, the iron in plasma is present in two pools, a diferric and a monoferric transferrin pool (Chap. 10), and the erythroid and nonerythroid receptors have a four times greater avidity for diferric transferrin than for monoferric transferrin. Consequently, total plasma iron turnover depends on the degree of saturation and does not necessarily reflect the number of transferrin receptors, presumably a critical measure of erythropoietic capacity.[224] To measure the number of transferrin receptors, adjusting the plasma iron turnover equations for both nonerythroid uptake and degree of transferrin saturation, and expressing the plasma turnover in terms of transferrin rather than iron, have been proposed.[225] Normal erythroid uptake of transferrin is 60 ± 12 μmol/L of blood per day, a value that has appropriately decreased and increased in patients with hypoplastic and hyperplastic marrow.

MEASUREMENT OF RED CELL DESTRUCTION

The original method for the measurement of the red cell life span consisted in the transfusion of cells that were compatible but identifiable immunologically—the Ashby technique; type O red cells were infused into individuals with type A or B cells. The differential agglutination technique used anti-A or anti-B antiserum to measure the life span of type O red cells that were transfused to type A or type B recipients, and the recipients' own cells were removed using anti-A or anti-B serum.[226] During World War II and shortly after, this method was used extensively, but in recent years, because of the hazards associated with the administration of allogeneic erythrocytes, it has been replaced by techniques based on labeling of autologous blood.

In 1946, Shemin and Rittenberg demonstrated that the incorporation of nitrogen (^{15}N)-labeled glycine into heme could be used to measure the life span of the red cells.[227] Since then, a number of other isotopic methods have been developed. These can be divided into three groups: (1) those that label a cohort of cells, (2) those that label cells randomly, and (3) those that use indirect measurements such as the rate of production of red cells or the rate of heme breakdown. The first two methodologic approaches yield information about the nature of the shortening of the red cell life span, age-dependent or random. The third methodology yields only mean life span.

COHORT METHODS

Cohort methods depend on the biosynthetic incorporation of the label into the developing red cells. In these methods a group of cells of approximately the same age is labeled. The labels used are glycine-containing labeled ^{15}N,[227] radioactive carbon (^{14}C),[228] or radioactive iron (either ^{55}Fe or ^{59}Fe).[229-231] The main disadvantage of cohort labeling is the need for prolonged periods of sampling, especially if the life span is only moderately reduced (Figs. 2-10 and 2-11). In addition, radioiron from destroyed red cells may be reused, making it difficult to interpret

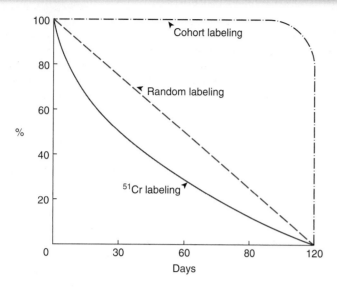

Figure 2–10. Red cell life span measured by cohort labeling or random labeling. When red cells are labeled randomly with chromium-51 (^{51}Cr), there is a daily 1% elution that needs to be corrected for in the calculation of total red cell life span.

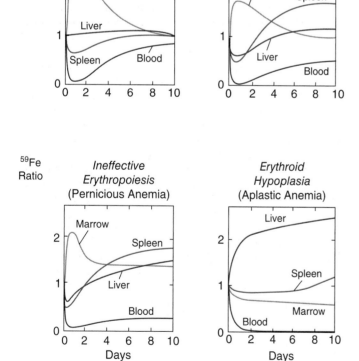

Figure 2–11. Tissue distribution of ^{59}Fe in normal subjects, hypersplenic patients, and anemic patients with ineffective and effective erythropoiesis. The radioactivity is expressed on the ordinate as a ratio relative to the radioactivity measured in the same organ 15 minutes after the intravenous administration of the isotope. *(Reproduced with permission from Finch CA, Deubelbeiss K, Cook JD, et al. Ferrokinetics in man, Medicine 1970 Jan;49(1):17-53.)*

results. Further, the increasing restrictions on use of radiochemicals has drastically decreased availability of these two previously widely used nuclear medicine tests.

A simple double-labeling technique that allows nonradioactive cohort labeling was described using two distinct labeling steps separated by a defined time interval. Cells are subsequently evaluated by the relative proportions of these labels. The initial labeling step uses biotin that binds to all circulating cells (the red blood cells accounting for most of the label), the second administered labeling substance at a later time, digoxygenin, then distinguishes erythrocyte subpopulation of known age.[232]

RANDOM-LABEL METHODS

The random-label methods are the Ashby differential agglutination technique,[226] which uses an immunologic marker, and the use of various red cell labels such as chromium (^{50}Cr, ^{51}Cr, or^{53}Cr),[233-235] diisopropylfluorophosphate (DFP) labeled with ^{32}P, ^{103}H,[236] or ^{14}C,[237] ^{14}C cyanate,[238] a lipophilic dye,[239,240] or biotin.[241,242]

Chromium-51 Method

The most widely used radioactive isotope for the measurement of the red cell life span is ^{51}Cr. As the chromate ion penetrates the red cell membrane, it binds to the α and β chains of globin. Unfortunately, these bonds are not covalent and there is a continuous elution of the isotope, varying from 0.5% to 2.9% per day.[243]

DF^{32}P Method

DFP, on the other hand, is irreversibly bound to red cell cholinesterase. There is some elution of unbound DFP during the first 2 to 3 days of study, but after that, DFP disappearance closely matches red cell destruction.[236,244] Nevertheless, because sample preparation is somewhat complicated, this label is not commonly used.

The life span is estimated by measuring the survival of randomly labeled red cells. Immediately after transfusion, the labeled erythrocytes equilibrate with unlabeled red cells. This normally takes about 5 minutes[245] but may be longer in patients with splenomegaly. After equilibration, during the next 24 hours the cells damaged by the labeling process will be removed from the circulation. Red blood cells that survive this period are assumed to have their expected long-term survival.[246]

To accurately calculate red cell life span using a random-label method requires steady-state conditions or that correction can be made for concurrent blood loss or blood transfusion. However, it is usually possible to gain an accurate estimate of red cell half-life by sampling three times a week for 1 to 2 weeks.

In the normal human the red cell lifes pan is finite with an average of about 120 days, with some random destruction (ie, 0.06%-0.4% per day). In some mammalian species, the amount of random destruction is much greater.[247] The survival curve of randomly labeled human red cells should consequently be nearly linear from day 0 to 120, with a half-life of 60 days. When ^{51}Cr is used as the label, approximately 1% of label elutes per day and the survival curve becomes exponential with a half-life of approximately 30 days (see Fig. 2-10).

Because merely expressing the red cell life span measured by chromium will not give information about the character of destruction, senescence versus random, it has been recommended that in addition, a correction factor for chromium elution be used and the data recorded using linear coordinates.[248] If the data lie on a straight line, the destruction is by senescence and the life span can be calculated as twice the half-life. If the data indicate exponential disappearance and it is necessary to use a semilogarithmic plot to depict the data on a straight line, the destruction is random and the life span is 1.44 times the half-life.

One objection to this method is that the degree of chromium elution is not a constant but varies from day to day and is influenced by various disease states.[243] Furthermore, the best fit of data is rarely linear or exponential, but somewhere between. Although computer-assisted methods can resolve ambiguities, the inherent biologic and technical variations in measuring red cell life span are such that it is better to rely on chromium $T_{1/2}$ with intuitive adjustments based on clinical findings.

Biotin Method

A nonradioactive label has also been developed to label the red blood cells in humans by covalent attachment of biotin to red cell membrane proteins and enumerating the survival by flow cytometry.[207] Biotin labeling estimates red cell survival comparable with that obtained with a concurrent ^{51}Cr label for both normal volunteers and patients with sickle cell disease. In addition to being a nonradioactive probe, biotin labeling has other advantages. The transfused cells can be isolated from the patients on avidin substrates for further characterization. Biotin labeling has been used to demonstrate that sickle cells without HbF have a shorter in vivo survival compared with those with HbF,[249] and has also been instrumental in showing a role for phosphatidylserine exposure in the clearance of sickle cells (Chap. 18).[250] Recently, a rapid and robust method was developed to manufacture biotin-labeled red blood cells for clinical research compliant to good practice guidelines for blood establishments.

INDIRECT METHODS

There are two approaches to the calculation of the red cell life span by indirect methods: (1) from a measurement of the rate of production of red cells using radioactive iron and (2) from a measurement of the rate of breakdown of heme to bilirubin,[251] that is, the release of CO from catabolized heme.[252] Both of these compounds are derived almost exclusively from catabolized hemoglobin, and measurements of their rate of production have provided useful information about the red cell life span. There are too many variables that affect the serum bilirubin level to make it a reliable, quantitative measurement of red cell destruction. The measurement of CO production was formerly very tedious, requiring elaborate rebreathing apparatus. With the development of newer technologies,[253,254] measuring CO levels as an exhaled CO (endtidal CO; ie, ETCO) has become more practical. An advantage of the measurement of ETCO as an indication of the rate of red cell destruction is that it gives the rate of destruction at a single point in time. An instrument by CoSense (Capnia Inc) obtained FDA 510(k) clearance in December 2013, and provides a substitute for the previously approved instruments that are no longer available. This device is compact and portable, and uses a sterile single-use nasal cannula for quantifying ETCO quantification and also samples ambient CO, which is subtracted from the value in exhaled breath and is suitable for use in neonates. This device also counts the breath rate, analyzed CO in individual breaths, and provides CO measurements in parts per million in a matter of minutes. However, major shortcomings of the current version of this instrument is that the baseline level of ETCO is set up too high, thus allowing detection of only moderate to severe hemolysis, but not mild hemolysis.[255]

SENESCENCE OF NORMAL ERYTHROCYTES

Methodologic Considerations

Labeling a cohort of human erythrocytes with ^{59}Fe and centrifuging the cells in a density gradient demonstrates that reticulocytes and young red cells are less dense than mature red cells.[256,257] However, at the end of the life span of the labeled cohort, radioactivity is fairly evenly distributed throughout red cells of all densities, with only a slight tendency of the radioactivity to be concentrated in the denser cells. Unfortunately, many studies of the properties of senescent cells in the past have been done based on the characteristics of the densest fraction of erythrocytes, using various fractionating techniques. In fact, the densest fraction of red cells is only slightly enriched with old erythrocytes.[258,259] A combination of density separation and elutriation (a process for separating particles based on their size, shape, and density) seemed to provide results superior to density separation alone using hemoglobin A_{1C} content as a marker. However, none of the current methods provides perfect identification of senescent red cells.[260]

In two animal models and one human disease model, the cells that are truly aged provide some insight into the senescence. In mice, in vivo aged erythrocytes have been produced by serially transfusing mice, maintaining an increased RCM to suppress virtually all erythropoiesis.[261] In the rabbit, red cells have been labeled with traces of biotin, which allows them to be recovered from the circulation.[262] In the human disease *transient erythroblastopenia of childhood* (Chaps. 5 and 27), a disorder in which there is cessation of all erythropoiesis for several months, the density and deformability of the aged cells in erythroblastopenia of childhood remains surprisingly normal.[258] The use of the latter model has been criticized because this disorder is not fully understood and the red cells in the circulation may not be entirely normal.[263]

PROPERTIES OF AGED CELLS

Although the activities of a large number of enzymes, including hexokinase, glucose-6-phosphate dehydrogenase (G-6-PD), and pyruvate kinase (PK), are higher in reticulocytes than in mature erythrocytes, the activities of these enzymes do not normally continue to decline during the aging of the erythrocyte.[262,264] Pyrimidine-5′-nucleotidase[265,266] and adenosine monophosphate (AMP)-deaminase[267-269] appear to be exceptions to this rule because there is a continuing decline of enzyme activity throughout the life span of the red cell. The decrease in the activity of these enzymes is not linear with age, but exponential.[178] This stability of many of the red cell enzymes during the aging of normal erythrocytes contrasts to the circumstances that are brought about by mutations in enzymes such as G-6-PD and PK, where instability of the abnormal enzyme leads to accelerated decay in the amount of enzyme protein, a factor that surely plays an important role in the ultimate, premature demise of the cell (Chap. 16). Fluorescent sorting of blood type NN erythrocytes transfused into humans shows that the densest fractions are only minimally enriched with old cells,[270] and biotinylated aged cells of rabbits have been found to have only a modestly decreased surface area, volume, cell water, and density, and therefore slightly decreased deformability.[259,271]

As they circulate, red cells lose a substantial portion of their membrane and hemoglobin in the form of vesicles.[272] Thus, the loss of membrane material in hemoglobin vesicles may play a role in the aging process.[273] In normal blood, a small number of red cell vesicles, approximately 190 per microliter blood, can be harvested. During storage of red blood cells, the aggregates of vesicles are formed and may contribute to acute lung injury by interacting with neutrophils.[274]

MECHANISM OF DESTRUCTION OF NORMAL, AGED CELLS

Several different mechanisms of senescent red cell destruction have been proposed. Determining the actual mechanism(s) is especially difficult because the cells that are marked for removal are bound to be present at very low concentrations or not at all in the circulating blood—they have been removed. Many of the earlier data are predicated upon the isolation of dense cells, and the consideration that they are "old" has been erroneous (see "Methodologic Considerations," previously in the chapter). Moreover, it is likely that there is more than one mechanism that serves to remove effete red cells from the circulation; there is no known mutation that lengthens red cell life span.

Loss of deformability

During its life span the red cells must pass innumerable times without rupturing through capillaries with diameters of approximately 2 to 4 μm. Physical stress encountered by red cells is especially severe when they traverse interendothelial slits of ~2 μm in the venous sinus. The deformability of the membrane allows the red cell to distort sufficiently to complete its journey through the microcirculation and regain its efficient biconcave disc shape again in the peripheral blood. The principal determinants of the red blood cell deformability are the ratio of cell surface area to volume that also may determine some erythrocyte pathological shaped such a spherocytes (see Chap. 15), intracellular viscosity (determined the physical properties of hemoglobin), and membrane elasticity (determined by rheological properties of the membrane). Repeated physical stress encountered in the microcirculation results in accumulated loss of deformability that adversely may affect its life span.[275] Even though the loss of red cell membrane is postulated in senescence, studies of biotinylated rabbit red cells showed that old cells had both decreased surface area (10.5%) and volume (8.4%), resulting in little change in surface-to-volume ratio during aging. The aged cells were found to have normal membrane elasticity with only a minority of the cells being recovered from denser fractions following centrifugation.[276] However, loss of membrane plays a role in many types of pathologic hemolysis, including hereditary spherocytosis, and in autoimmune hemolytic anemia (see Chaps. 15 and 26). In sickle cell disease and hemoglobin C disease the internal viscosity of the cell is increased (see Chap. 18). Loss of water from the red cell, as may occur when the membrane is damaged and leaks potassium as in hereditary xerocytosis, also markedly impairs the deformability of the cell (see Chap. 15). In southeast Asian ovalocytosis, despite an increased rigidity of red blood cell membrane there is no increase in hemolysis or anemia calling into question importance of rigidity as a sole determinant of red cell clearance.[277]

AE-1 (Band 3) Clustering Models

It has been proposed that an altered membrane AE-1 serves as a receptor for antibodies directed against a neoantigen, designated senescent cell antigen, and that, possibly, after-binding complement marks the senescent cell for destruction. It is not known how clustering of AE-1 occurs in vivo, and recent work suggests peroxidation of cytoplasmic aspect of the protein results in carbonylation. Methemoglobin binds to the cytoplasmic peroxidized domain of AE-1 and induces cluster formation.[278] But much, if not all, of the evidence for these models depends on the assumptions that dense cells are old, and the uptake of cells by monocytes is a surrogate for their being marked for destruction.[279] However, immunoglobulin levels on aged, biotinylated rabbit cells are not increased,[280] and the fact that red cell life span has never been demonstrated to be prolonged in agammaglobulinemic patients casts serious doubt on the concept that immunoglobulins mediate removal of senescent red cells.

Phosphatidylserine Exposure Models

In red blood cells, as in most other cells, the anionic phospholipid phosphatidylserine is present exclusively in the inner cytoplasmic leaflet of the membrane bilayer.[281] The exposure of phosphatidylserine on the outer leaflet of the cell membrane is one of the signals that allows macrophages to recognize apoptotic cells. It is thus likely that surface expression of phosphatidylserine is at least one of the signals by which macrophages recognize senescent erythrocytes.[180,282,283] Data from a biotinylated rabbit erythrocyte model suggest that the average time during which phosphatidylserine is exposed is only 0.3 to 0.5 days, so that few cells with increased exposure of the phospholipid are in the circulation at any time.[282] An increase of phosphatidylserine exposure has also been documented in humans descending from high altitudes[284] that may be relevant with decreased red cell survival documented in *neocytolysis* (discussed in the next section). The exposure of phosphatidylserine on the outer leaflet of the cell membrane is one of the signals. A proposed model for the destruction of newly formed cells was that endothelial cells might respond to changes in circulating erythropoietin by influencing the interaction of phagocytes with young red cells, targeting the cells by surface adhesion molecules.[285] A study in mice, using somewhat different methods, suggested that phosphatidylserine exposure is greatest in young erythrocytes, and does not increase with aging.[286] It is not yet clear whether phosphatidylserine exposure is the only or even the primary signal that indicates that a cell has reached the end of its life span, but it is the only major difference between senescent and nonsenescent erythrocytes that has been clearly documented.[283]

Several proteins were described that bind to phosphatidylserine-expressing apoptotic cells including lactadherin,[287] gas-6,[288] Del-1,[289] and several complement components.[290] These proteins act as opsonins in promoting the clearance of phosphatidylserine-expressing cells by macrophages. Angiogenic endothelial cells also express several integrins associated with phagocytosis in macrophages and can engulf phosphatidylserine-expressing "aged" erythrocytes and may play a role in clearance of senescent cells.[291]

Eryptosis is defined as cell shrinkage and exposure of phosphatidylserine caused by entry of calcium ions followed by activation of a scramblase, an enzyme capable of randomizing the distribution of phospholipid in both membrane bilayers.[281] It may contribute to red cell clearance in diseased states,[292] but its role in senescence-associated clearance is not clear.[293] Eryptosis in chronic hypobaric hypoxic rats is decreased. They reported that the decreased eryptosis was due to reduction of phosphatidylserine and cytosolic Ca^{2+} and the increase of integrin-associated protein CD47. Using biotin labeling, they showed that red cells produced in hypoxia had a longer life span than controls, further proving the relevance of the decreased eryptosis and the increased red cell survival with hypoxia.[294] This may be the first evidence suggesting that hypoxia-induced erythrocytosis (Chap. 28) may be contributed to by prolonged red cell survival.[188]

Another model that has been proposed for normal red cell clearance is based on a slight increase in green autofluorescence, believed to represent the result of oxidative damage, which has been observed in aging murine erythrocytes.[295] The interaction of erythrocyte cell-surface antigen cell differentiation antigen (CD 44) with hyaluronic acid may play a role in the clearance of aged erythrocytes from the circulation, but such clearance seems limited to primates, with an exception of a patient with CD 44 deficiency that manifested as congenital dyserythropoietic anemia (Chap. 14).[296]

NEOCYTOLYSIS

Hypoxia increases red cells by enhancing HIFs with subsequent EPO-stimulated erythropoiesis. Upon return to normoxia, the secondary erythrocytosis (Chap. 28) is overcorrected, as the accumulated, newly formed red cells undergo preferential destruction, a process termed *neocytolysis*.[285] Neocytolysis was originally observed during space travel at zero gravity, wherein the mechanism is not clear. On return to normoxia, there is excessive generation of reactive oxygen species from increased mitochondrial mass correlating with decreased hypoxia-controlled gene Bnip3L transcripts.[191,297] Bnip3L mediates removal of reticulocyte mitochondria that generate increased reactive oxygen species accompanied by reduced catalase activity mediated by hypoxia-regulated miR21.[298] Rapid changes in Hct in human newborns also suggest that neocytolysis also occurs after birth when a hypoxic fetus has an exaggerated increase in hemoglobin concentration at birth, but the neonate rapidly overcorrects its increased RCM and becomes anemic in the first 2 weeks of life.[299,300]

MECHANISMS OF DESTRUCTION OF ABNORMAL RED BLOOD CELLS

The previous section, "Senescence of Normal Erythrocytes" enumerated some mechanisms that may be involved in normally terminating the life of the effete erythrocyte. It has sometimes been assumed that the mechanisms by which red cells are destroyed prematurely in disease states reflect these normal mechanisms. Although there may well be some overlap, the mechanisms of red cell destruction in disease states are likely different. The assumption that the mechanisms responsible for hemolytic anemia represent premature aging of the erythrocyte is no more logical than to suggest that an animal's death through pneumonia, renal failure, or cancer represents premature aging. Classically, the destruction of red blood cells is considered intravascular when hemoglobin is released into the plasma, and extravascular, when the macrophages in the spleen and liver engulf the red cells with little release of hemoglobin.

INTRAVASCULAR DESTRUCTION

If the red cell membrane is breached in the circulation, the red cell is destroyed. This mode of erythrocyte demise occurs at a low frequency, but may be the predominant mode of destruction in some hemolytic disorders—for example, ABO-incompatible transfusions (Chap. 29) and paroxysmal nocturnal hemoglobinuria (Chap. 8), where the surface complement complex creates pores in the red cell membrane; and in cardiac valve-induced hemolysis (Chap. 22) and microangiopathic hemolytic anemia (Chap. 22), where the shear stress may be so strong as to break open the membrane.

Antibody-mediated intravascular hemolysis occurs due to complement activation by the classical pathway (Chap. 26). Immune complexes activate the classical complement pathway by binding the C1q portion of the C1 complex. IgM (Immunoglobulin M) antibodies fix complement more avidly than IgG antibodies because they are pentameric and has multiple binding sites for C1q. However, two IgG molecules in close proximity on the red blood cell surface can also activate complement. Hence, the antigen density is a critical determinate of complement activation in IgG-mediated immune hemolytic anemia.[301] As the macrophages do not express IgM Fc receptors.[302] IgM-mediated red cell destruction is mediated directly through complement-induced damage and indirectly through macrophage clearance of complement opsonized cells. Exposure of the collagen-like regions of C1q makes it recognizable by macrophage complement receptor 1 (CR1),[303] however, C1q opsonization does not contribute significantly to the pathophysiology of immune-mediated hemolytic anemia. Rather, during complement activation, the third component of complement (C3) is cleaved to C3b, which can bind covalently to cell surface carbohydrate and peptide moieties. Bound C3b is rapidly cleaved to an inactivated form, iC3b. Macrophages have receptors for C3b (CR1) and iC3b (CR3). Unlike FcγRs, which are constitutively active, the phagocytic function of CR3 requires activation through a distinct pathway.[304] Cell-bound iC3b is rapidly degraded enzymatically to C3dg and C3d. C3d/C3dg binds to CR2 with low affinity expressed primarily by B lymphocytes.

Therefore, clearance of C3d/C3dg opsonized red cells is inefficient, and red cells opsonized by C3d/C3dg can be found circulating in the peripheral blood of patients with immune hemolytic anemia, particularly in patients with cold agglutinin disease.[305]

EXTRAVASCULAR DESTRUCTION

Extravascular hemolysis is mediated by macrophages mostly in the spleen and liver.[306] The spleen plays a central role especially in pathological destruction. The spleen is a lymphoid organ that functions primarily as a filter for the blood.[307] Splenic blood flow is unique consisting of both an open and circulation. Most splenic arterioles empty into red pulp, a reticular meshwork-rich in macrophages and they are not lined by endothelial cells. Red cells traverse the red pulp slowly under low shear stress to reach the splenic sinuses (see Chap. 25). The high density of macrophages in the red pulp results in close contact with the red cells. Macrophages recognize damaged and deformed red cell and remove them by phagocytosis. In addition, without damaging the red cell, macrophages remodel the cell by removing nuclear remnants (Howell-Jolly bodies) and other inclusions such as Heinz bodies (denatured hemoglobin caused by oxidative damage) and Pappenheimer bodies (phagosomes containing excess iron). The red pulp is separated from splenic sinuses by interendothelial fenestrations $\sim$2 μM in diameter. The red cells have to traverse these tight spaces to reach the splenic sinuses. Phagocytosis of defective or antibody-coated red cells readily occur. IgG antibodies bind red cell antigens, and the Fc portion of the bound immunoglobulin is recognized by specific macrophage receptors that mediate phagocytosis. There are three types of Fcγ receptors that activate phagocytosis, FcγRI (CD64), FcγRIIA (CD32a), and FcγRIII (CD16). Phagocytosed red cells are targeted to phagolysosomes. There are four subtypes of IgG—IgG1, IgG2, IgG3, and IgG4 with varying affinities for FcγRs.[308] They transduce signals that induce efficient erythrophagocytosis via immunoreceptor tyrosine-based activating motifs (ITAMs) with little free hemoglobin is released into the circulation.[309] PMacrophages also contain FcγRIIB, which is an inhibitory receptor that transmits signals through an immunoreceptor tyrosine-based inhibitory motif (ITIM). Intravenous immunoglobulin (IVIG) is a modestly effective treatment for autoimmune hemolytic anemia (see Chap. 26).[310] Although other mechanisms contribute, the therapeutic activity of IVIgG appears to be mediated in part through binding to FcγRIIB.

FATE OF HEMOGLOBIN IN INTRAVASCULAR DESTRUCTION

Hemoglobin

When red cells are destroyed in the vascular compartment, the hemoglobin escaping into the plasma is bound to haptoglobin. A dimeric glycoprotein, each molecule of haptoglobin can bind two hemoglobin dimers. The binding of hemoglobin not only obviates its potential toxicity, it also triggers the second step of the scavenging process, that is, recognition by macrophage receptor CD163, and subsequent clearance of the entire complex by receptor-mediated endocytosis.[317] CD163 belongs to the scavenger receptor cysteine-rich family of proteins and the haptoglobin–hemoglobin complex is cleared from the plasma with a $T_{1/2}$ of 10 to 30 minutes. The heme of the hemoglobin is converted to iron, CO, and biliverdin by heme oxygenase (HO) and the biliverdin is further catabolized to bilirubin. CO is released (see section "Indirect Methods" on measuring red cell life span) in the course of cleavage of heme-by-heme oxygenase.[318] Bilirubin, initially thought to have no physiologic role, has now been shown to have potent antioxidant effect by being oxidized to biliverdin and then recycled by biliverdin reductase back to bilirubin.[319]

Haptoglobin

Free haptoglobin, in contrast to the hemoglobin–haptoglobin complex, has a $T_{1/2}$ of 5 days, and when large amounts of the rapidly turned-over haptoglobin–hemoglobin complex are formed, the haptoglobin content of the plasma is depleted. The haptoglobin content of the plasma is diminished not only in the plasma of patients undergoing frank intravascular hemolysis, but also from the plasma of patients who, like those with sickle cell disease, have accelerated red cell destruction occurring primarily within macrophages. Presumably there is either enough intravascular hemolysis in such hemolytic disorders to lower the plasma haptoglobin level or sufficient leakage from the phagocytic cells into the plasma to bind to haptoglobin. Thus, the measurement of plasma haptoglobin levels is useful in diagnosing hemolysis, although it cannot, as previously suggested, serve to clearly distinguish extravascular from intravascular hemolysis.

Heme

Free heme that is released into the circulation is bound in a 1:1 ratio to the plasma glycoprotein hemopexin,[320] which is cleared from the plasma with a $T_{1/2}$ of 7 to 8 hours.[321,322] The heme–hemopexin complex is taken up by a low-density-lipoprotein–related receptor, CD91.[323] Figure 2-12 illustrates the parallel functions of hemopexin and haptoglobin. When the capacity of hemopexin to bind heme is saturated, excess heme may bind to albumin to form methemalbumin.[324] Excess heme is toxic to cells because of the ability of heme to catalyze the so-called Fenton reaction, generating hydroxyl radicals, a highly reactive oxygen species. To avoid the phenomenon and complement the negative feedback regulation of heme synthesis, the expression of HO-1 is induced in response to an increased level of heme, which subsequently results in the degradation of excess heme not bound to proteins. In contrast to HO-1, HO-2 is constitutively expressed and participates in the regulation of a basal heme level. HO-1 deficiency in humans showed severe inflammatory complications, persistent hemolytic anemia characterized by marked erythrocyte fragmentation and intravascular hemolysis, with paradoxic increase of serum haptoglobin and very low bilirubin and an early death.[325]

FATE OF HEMOGLOBIN IN EXTRAVASCULAR DESTRUCTION

Red cells that are engulfed by phagocytic cells are degraded within lysosomes into lipids, protein, and heme. The proteins and lipids are reprocessed in their respective catabolic pathways and the heme is cleaved by

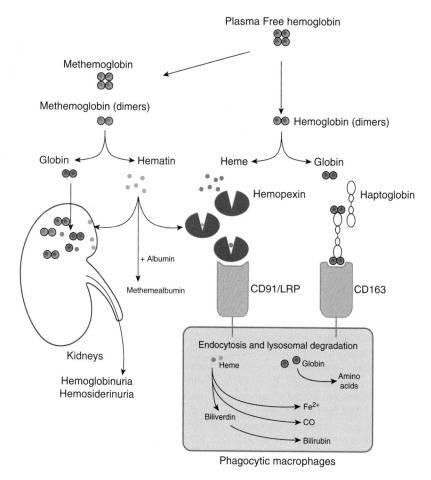

Figure 2–12. Overview of extracellular hemoglobin catabolism. LRP/CD91 and CD163 internalize of extracellular heme and hemoglobin in complex with hemopexin and haptoglobin by receptor-mediated endocytosis. Both receptors are highly expressed in phagocytic macrophages, which are known to metabolize heme into bilirubin, Fe, and CO. In addition to the expression in macrophages, LRP/CD91 is highly expressed in several other cell types including hepatocytes, neurons, and syncytiotrophoblasts. Globin chains and heme (or hematin) are filtered in the glomerulus and engulfed by the tubular cells. When their capacities are exceeded, they appear in the urine.

a microsomal HO.[326] HO catalyzes the oxygen-dependent degradation of heme to biliverdin with the release of CO (forming rapidly COHb, and then partially excreted by ETCO) and "free" iron. Biliverdin is converted into bilirubin by biliverdin reductase α, which is expressed ubiquitously in all tissues under basal conditions with high levels in macrophages in the spleen and liver.[327] The overall reduction of biliverdin to bilirubin is very efficient, and under physiologic circumstances the concentration of serum biliverdin is low.

Bilirubin Excretion

Regardless of the site of destruction of hemoglobin, one of the final products is bilirubin. Bilirubin is very insoluble and transported in plasma bound to albumin. Unconjugated bilirubin (ie, before conjugation to glucuronic acid) is taken up into hepatocytes by transporters of the organic anion-transporting polypeptide family, followed by conjugation with glucuronic acid in the microsomes, yielding bilirubin glucuronosyl isoforms, which are then transported into the bile ducts in an ATP-dependent fashion. This efflux across the canalicular membrane is mediated by multidrug-resistance protein 2, which has high affinity for monoglucuronosyl bilirubin and bisglucuronosyl bilirubin.[328] In the gastrointestinal tract, the bilirubin is converted to urobilinogens by bacterial reduction.[329] A small fraction of urobilinogen is reabsorbed and excreted into the urine. Thus, the fecal and urinary urobilinogen excretion have been used as an indicator of the rate of hemolysis, but are only uncommonly used for this purpose in modern practice because the collections are cumbersome and because alternative degradative pathways detract from the accuracy of the estimates of the rate of heme catabolism.

REFERENCES

1. Erslev AJ. Blood and mountains. In: Wintrobe MM, ed. *Blood, Pure and Eloquent*. McGraw Hill; 1980:257.
2. Carnot P, Deflandre C. Sur l'activité hématopoïétique des serum au cours de la régénération du sang. *Acad Sci Med*. 1906;3.
3. Reissmann KR. Studies on the mechanism of erythropoietic stimulation in parabiotic rats during hypoxia. *Blood*. 1950;5:372.
4. Erslev A. Humoral regulation of red cell production. *Blood*. 1953;8:349.
5. Erslev A, Lavietes PH, Van Wagenen G. Erythropoietic stimulation induced by anemic serum. *Proc Soc Exp Biol Med*. 1953;83:548.
6. Jacobson LO, Goldwasser E, Fried W, et al. Role of the kidney in erythropoiesis. *Nature*. 1957;179:633.
7. Hardison R. Hemoglobins from bacteria to man: evolution of different patterns of gene expression. *J Exp Biol*. 1998;201:1099.
8. Fox H. The hemoglobin of *Daphnia*. *Proc R Soc Lond (Biol)*. 1948;135.
9. Zeis B, Becher B, Lamkemeyer T, et al. The process of hypoxic induction of *Daphnia magna* hemoglobin: subunit composition and functional properties. *Comp Biochem Physiol B Biochem Mol Biol*. 2003;134:243.
10. Hemmingsen EA, Douglas EL. Respiratory characteristics of the hemoglobin-free fish *Chaenocephalus aceratus*. *Comp Biochem Physiol*. 1970;33:733.
11. Garofalo F, Amelio D, Cerra MC, et al. Morphological and physiological study of the cardiac NOS/NO system in the Antarctic (Hb-/Mb-) icefish *Chaenocephalus aceratus* and in the red-blooded *Trematomus bernacchii*. *Nitric Oxide*. 2009;20:69.
12. Garofalo F, Pellegrino D, Amelio D, Tota B. The Antarctic hemoglobinless icefish, fifty five years later: a unique cardiocirculatory interplay of disaptation and phenotypic plasticity. *Comp Biochem Physiol A Mol Integr Physiol*. 2009;154:10-28.
13. Sidell BD, O'Brien KM. When bad things happen to good fish: the loss of hemoglobin and myoglobin expression in Antarctic icefishes. *J Exp Biol*. 2006;209:1791.
14. Cooper EL. Evolution of blood cells. *Ann Immunol (Paris)*. 1976;127:817.
15. Scott RB. Comparative hematology: the phylogeny of the erythrocyte. *Blut*. 1966;12:340.
16. Andrew W. *Comparative Hematology*. Grune & Stratton; 1965.
17. Bolliger A. Observations on the blood of a monotreme *Tachyglossus aculeatus*. *Aust J Sci*. 1959;22.
18. Iorio RJ. Some morphologic and kinetic studies of the developing erythroid cells of the common gold fish *Carassius auratus*. *Cell Tissue Kinet*. 1969;2.
19. Jordan HE. Comparative hematology. In: Downy H, ed. *Handbook of Hematology*. Hoeber-Harper; 1938:703.
20. Robb-Smith AHT. *The Growth of Knowledge of the Functions of the Blood*. Macfarlane R, ed. Academic Press; 1961.
21. Shoemaker CB, Mitsock LD. Murine erythropoietin gene: cloning, expression, and human gene homology. *Mol Cell Biol*. 1986;6:849.
22. Palis J, Segel G. Hematology of the fetus and newborn. In: Kaushansky K, Lichtman MA, Prchal JT, Levi M, Burns LJ, Linch DC, eds. *Williams Hematology*. 10th ed. New York, NY; McGraw Hill; 2021.
23. Le Douarin NM. Cell migrations in embryos. *Cell*. 1984;38:353.
24. Kingsley PD, Malik J, Emerson RL, et al. "Maturational" globin switching in primary primitive erythroid cells. *Blood*. 2006;107:1665.
25. Ferkowicz MJ, Yoder MC. Blood island formation: longstanding observations and modern interpretations. *Exp Hematol*. 2005;33:1041.
26. Kissa K, Herbomel P. Blood stem cells emerge from aortic endothelium by a novel type of cell transition. *Nature*. 2010;464:112.
27. Chen AT, Zon LI. Zebrafish blood stem cells. *J Cell Biochem*. 2009;108:35.
28. Scapin G, Shah DI. Pulsation activates Mechanosensitive Piezo1 to form long-term hematopoietic stem cells. Abstract presented at: 61st ASH Annual Meeting & Exposition; 2019; Orlando, FL. Session 445.
29. Hudson G. Bone-marrow volume in the human foetus and newborn. *Br J Haematol*. 1965;11:446.
30. Brannon D. Extramedullary hematopoiesis in anemia. *Bull Johns Hopkins Hosp*. 1927;41.
31. Erslev AJ. Medullary and extramedullary blood formation. *Clin Orthopaed Rel Res*. 1967;52:25.
32. Zanjani ED, Poster J, Burlington H, et al. Liver as the primary site of erythropoietin formation in the fetus. *J Lab Clin Med*. 1977;89:640.
33. Flake AW, Harrison MR, Adzick NS, et al. Erythropoietin production by the fetal liver in an adult environment. *Blood*. 1987;70:542.
34. Zanjani ED, Ascensao JL, McGlave PB, et al. Studies on the liver to kidney switch of erythropoietin production. *J Clin Invest*. 1981;67:1183.
35. Till JE, McCulloch EA, Siminovitch L. A stochastic model of stem cell proliferation, based on the growth of spleen colony-forming cells. *Proc Natl Acad Sci U S A*. 1964;51:29.
36. Socolovsky M, Lodish HF, Daley GQ. Control of hematopoietic differentiation: lack of specificity in signaling by cytokine receptors. *Proc Natl Acad Sci U S A*. 1998;95:6573.
37. Velten L, Haas SF, Raffel S, et al. Human haematopoietic stem cell lineage commitment is a continuous process. *Nat Cell Biol*. 2017;19:271.
38. Tusi BK, Wolock SL, Weinreb C, et al. Population snapshots predict early haematopoietic and erythroid hierarchies. *Nature*. 2018;555:54.
39. Dahlin JS, Hamey FK, Pijuan-Sala B, et al. A single-cell hematopoietic landscape resolves 8 lineage trajectories and defects in Kit mutant mice. *Blood*. 2018;131:e1.
40. Pellin D, Loperfido M, Baricordi C, et al. A comprehensive single cell transcriptional landscape of human hematopoietic progenitors. *Nat Commun*. 2019;10:2395.
41. Psaila B, Mead AJ. Single-cell approaches reveal novel cellular pathways for megakaryocyte and erythroid differentiation. *Blood*. 2019;133:1427.
42. Evans T, Felsenfeld G. The erythroid-specific transcription factor Eryf1: a new finger protein. *Cell*. 1989;58:877.
43. Tsai SF, Martin DI, Zon LI, et al. Cloning of cDNA for the major DNA-binding protein of the erythroid lineage through expression in mammalian cells. *Nature*. 1989;339:446.
44. Pevny L, Lin CS, D'Agati V, et al. Development of hematopoietic cells lacking transcription factor GATA1. *Development*. 1995;121:163.
45. Letting DL, Chen YY, Rakowski C, et al. Context-dependent regulation of GATA1 by friend of GATA1. *Proc Natl Acad Sci U S A*. 2004;101:476.
46. Gregory T, Yu C, Ma A, et al. GATA1 and erythropoietin cooperate to promote erythroid cell survival by regulating bcl-xL expression. *Blood*. 1999;94:87.
47. Nerlov C, Querfurth E, Kulessa H, et al. GATA1 interacts with the myeloid PU.1 transcription factor and represses PU.1-dependent transcription. *Blood*. 2000;95:2543.
48. Tsang AP, Visvader JE, Turner CA, et al. FOG, a multitype zinc finger protein, acts as a cofactor for transcription factor GATA1 in erythroid and megakaryocytic differentiation. *Cell*. 1997;90:109.
49. Cantor AB, Orkin SH. Transcriptional regulation of erythropoiesis: an affair involving multiple partners. *Oncogene*. 2002;21:3368.
50. Xie H, Ye M, Feng R, et al. Stepwise reprogramming of B cells into macrophages. *Cell*. 2004;117:663.
51. Back J, Dierich A, Bronn C, et al. PU.1 determines the self-renewal capacity of erythroid progenitor cells. *Blood*. 2004;103:3615.
52. Mirabello L, Khincha PP, Ellis SR, et al. Novel and known ribosomal causes of Diamond-Blackfan anaemia identified through comprehensive genomic characterisation. *J Med Genet*. 2017;54:417.
53. Ludwig LS, Gazda HT, Eng JC, et al. Altered translation of GATA1 in Diamond-Blackfan anemia. *Nat Med*. 2014;20:748.
54. Sankaran VG, Ghazvinian R, Do R, et al. Exome sequencing identifies GATA1 mutations resulting in Diamond-Blackfan anemia. *J Clin Invest*. 2012;122:2439.
55. Tsang AP, Fujiwara Y, Hom DB, et al. Failure of megakaryopoiesis and arrested erythropoiesis in mice lacking the GATA1 transcriptional cofactor FOG. *Genes Dev*. 1998;12:1176.
56. Tsai FY, Keller G, Kuo FC, et al. An early haematopoietic defect in mice lacking the transcription factor GATA2. *Nature*. 1994;371:221.
57. Leonard M, Brice M, Engel JD, et al. Dynamics of GATA transcription factor expression during erythroid differentiation. *Blood*. 1993;82:1071.
58. Mouthon MA, Bernard O, Mitjavila MT, et al. Expression of tal-1 and GATA-binding proteins during human hematopoiesis. *Blood*. 1993;81:647.
59. Pal S, Cantor AB, Johnson KD, et al. Coregulator-dependent facilitation of chromatin occupancy by GATA1. *Proc Natl Acad Sci U S A*. 2004;101:980.

60. Fujiwara Y, Chang AN, Williams AM, et al. Functional overlap of GATA1 and GATA2 in primitive hematopoietic development. *Blood.* 2004;103:583.

61. Miller IJ, Bieker JJ. A novel, erythroid cell-specific murine transcription factor that binds to the CACCC element and is related to the Kruppel family of nuclear proteins. *Mol Cell Biol.* 1993;13:2776.

62. Nuez B, Michalovich D, Bygrave A, et al. Defective haematopoiesis in fetal liver resulting from inactivation of the EKLF gene. *Nature.* 1995;375:316.

63. Magor GW, Tallack MR, Gillinder KR, et al. KLF1-null neonates display hydrops fetalis and a deranged erythroid transcriptome. *Blood.* 2015;125:2405.

64. Helias V, Saison C, Peyrard T, et al. Molecular analysis of the rare in(Lu) blood type: toward decoding the phenotypic outcome of haploinsufficiency for the transcription factor KLF1. *Hum Mutat.* 2013;34:221.

65. Jaffray JA, Mitchell WB, Gnanapragasam MN, et al. Erythroid transcription factor EKLF/KLF1 mutation causing congenital dyserythropoietic anemia type IV in a patient of Taiwanese origin: review of all reported cases and development of a clinical diagnostic paradigm. *Blood Cells Mol Dis.* 2013;51:71.

66. Aplan PD, Nakahara K, Orkin SH, et al. The SCL gene product: a positive regulator of erythroid differentiation. *EMBO J.* 1992;11:4073.

67. Robb L, Lyons I, Li R, et al. Absence of yolk sac hematopoiesis from mice with a targeted disruption of the scl gene. *Proc Natl Acad Sci U S A.* 1995;92:7075.

68. Sanchez MJ, Bockamp EO, Miller J, et al. Selective rescue of early haematopoietic progenitors in Scl(-/-) mice by expressing Scl under the control of a stem cell enhancer. *Development.* 2001;128:4815.

69. Mikkola HK, Klintman J, Yang H, et al. Haematopoietic stem cells retain long-term repopulating activity and multipotency in the absence of stem-cell leukaemia SCL/tal-1 gene. *Nature.* 2003;421:547.

70. Zaitseva MP. Effect of labor conditions on the development and course of rheumatism. *Voprosy revmatizma.* 1970;10:59.

71. Saleque S, Cameron S, Orkin SH. The zinc-finger proto-oncogene Gfi-1b is essential for development of the erythroid and megakaryocytic lineages. *Genes Dev.* 2002;16:301.

72. Garcon L, Lacout C, Svinartchouk F, et al. Gfi-1B plays a critical role in terminal differentiation of normal and transformed erythroid progenitor cells. *Blood.* 2005;105:1448.

73. Person RE, Li FQ, Duan Z, et al. Mutations in proto-oncogene GFI1 cause human neutropenia and target ELA2. *Nat Genet.* 2003;34:308.

74. Sankaran VG, Menne TF, Xu J, et al. Human fetal hemoglobin expression is regulated by the developmental stage-specific repressor BCL11A. *Science.* 2008;322:1839.

75. Menzel S, Garner C, Gut I, et al. A QTL influencing F cell production maps to a gene encoding a zinc-finger protein on chromosome 2p15. *Nat Genet.* 2007;39:1197.

76. Lettre G, Sankaran VG, Bezerra MA, et al. DNA polymorphisms at the BCL11A, HBS1L-MYB, and beta-globin loci associate with fetal hemoglobin levels and pain crises in sickle cell disease. *Proc Natl Acad Sci U S A.* 2008;105:11869.

77. Bao EL, Cheng AN, Sankaran VG. The genetics of human hematopoiesis and its disruption in disease. *EMBO Mol Med.* 2019;11:e10316.

78. Wu Y, Jing Zeng J, Roscoe BP et al. Highly efficient therapeutic gene editing of human hematopoietic stem cells. *Nat Med.* 2019;May;25(5):776.

79. Angelillo-Scherrer A, Burnier L, Lambrechts D, et al. Role of Gas6 in erythropoiesis and anemia in mice. *J Clin Invest.* 2008;118:583.

80. Lemke G, Lu Q. Macrophage regulation by Tyro 3 family receptors. *Curr Opin Immunol.* 2003;15:31.

81. Zhao B, Keerthivasan G, Mei Y, et al. Targeted shRNA screening identified critical roles of pleckstrin-2 in erythropoiesis. *Haematologica.* 2014;99:1157.

82. Zhao B, Mei Y, Cao L, et al. Loss of pleckstrin-2 reverts lethality and vascular occlusions in JAK2V617F-positive myeloproliferative neoplasms. *J Clin Invest.* 2018;128:125.

83. Orkin SH, Zon LI. Hematopoiesis: an evolving paradigm for stem cell biology. *Cell.* 2018;132:631.

84. Flygare J, Rayon Estrada V, Shin C, et al. HIF1alpha synergizes with glucocorticoids to promote BFU-E progenitor self-renewal. *Blood.* 2011;117:3435.

85. Bauer A, Tronche F, Wessely O, et al. The glucocorticoid receptor is required for stress erythropoiesis. *Genes Dev.* 1999;13:2996.

86. Li H, Lodish HF, Sieff CA. Critical issues in Diamond-Blackfan anemia and prospects for novel treatment. *Hematol Oncol Clin North Am.* 2018;32:701.

87. Dainiak N, Hoffman R, Maffei LA, et al. Potentiation of human erythropoiesis in vitro by thyroid hormone. *Nature.* 1978;272:260.

88. Gao X, Lee HY, Li W, et al. Thyroid hormone receptor beta and NCOA4 regulate terminal erythrocyte differentiation. *Proc Natl Acad Sci U S A.* 2017;114:10107.

89. Li J, Hale J, Bhagia P, et al. Isolation and transcriptome analyses of human erythroid progenitors: BFU-E and CFU-E. *Blood.* 2014;124:3636.

90. Bessis M, Breton-Gorius J. [The reticulocyte. vital staining and electron microscopy]. *Nouv Rev Fr Hematol.* 1964;4:77.

91. Gronowicz G, Swift H, Steck TL. Maturation of the reticulocyte in vitro. *J Cell Sci.* 1984;71:177.

92. Finch CA, Deubelbeiss K, Cook JD, et al. Ferrokinetics in man. *Medicine.* 1970;49:17.

93. Noble NA, Xu QP, Hoge LL. Reticulocytes II: reexamination of the in vivo survival of stress reticulocytes. *Blood.* 1990;75:1877.

94. Donohue DM, Reiff RH, Hanson ML, et al. Quantitative measurement of the erythrocytic and granulocytic cells of the marrow and blood. *J Clin Invest.* 1958;37:1571.

95. Finch CA, Harker LA, Cook JD. Kinetics of the formed elements of human blood. *Blood.* 1977;50:699.

96. Goltry KL, Patel VP. Specific domains of fibronectin mediate adhesion and migration of early murine erythroid progenitors. *Blood.* 1997;90:138.

97. Ji P, Murata-Hori M, Lodish HF. Formation of mammalian erythrocytes: chromatin condensation and enucleation. *Trends Cell Biol.* 2011;21:409.

98. Koury ST, Koury MJ, Bondurant MC. Cytoskeletal distribution and function during the maturation and enucleation of mammalian erythroblasts. *J Cell Biol.* 1989;109:3005.

99. Chasis JA, Prenant M, Leung A, et al. Membrane assembly and remodeling during reticulocyte maturation. *Blood.* 1989;74:1112.

100. Ji P, Jayapal SR, Lodish HF. Enucleation of cultured mouse fetal erythroblasts requires Rac GTPases and mDia2. *Nat Cell Biol.* 2008;10:314.

101. Lee JC, Gimm JA, Lo AJ, et al. Mechanism of protein sorting during erythroblast enucleation: role of cytoskeletal connectivity. *Blood.* 2004;103:1912.

102. Yoshida H, Kawane K, Koike M, et al. Phosphatidylserine-dependent engulfment by macrophages of nuclei from erythroid precursor cells. *Nature.* 2005;437:754.

103. Shi H, Yamamoto S, Sheng M, et al. ASXL1 plays an important role in erythropoiesis. *Sci Rep.* 2016;6:28789.

104. Liang R, Camprecios G, Kou Y, et al. A systems approach identifies essential FOXO3 functions at key steps of terminal erythropoiesis. *PLoS Genet.* 2015;11:e1005526.

105. Swartz KL, Wood SN, Murthy T, et al. E2F-2 promotes nuclear condensation and enucleation of terminally differentiated erythroblasts. *Mol Cell Biol.* 2017;37.

106. Moras M, Lefevre SD, Ostuni MA. From erythroblasts to mature red blood cells: organelle clearance in mammals. *Front Physiol.* 2017;8:1076.

107. Hanspal M, Smockova Y, Uong Q. Molecular identification and functional characterization of a novel protein that mediates the attachment of erythroblasts to macrophages. *Blood.* 1998;92:2940.

108. Soni S, Bala S, Gwynn B, et al. Absence of erythroblast macrophage protein (Emp) leads to failure of erythroblast nuclear extrusion. *J Biol Chem.* 2006;281:20181.

109. Iavarone A, King ER, Dai XM, et al. Retinoblastoma promotes definitive erythropoiesis by repressing Id2 in fetal liver macrophages. *Nature.* 2004;432:1040.

110. Sankaran VG, Orkin SH, Walkley CR. Rb intrinsically promotes erythropoiesis by coupling cell cycle exit with mitochondrial biogenesis. *Genes Dev.* 2008;22:463.

111. Stopka T, Zivny JH, Stopkova P, et al. Human hematopoietic progenitors express erythropoietin. *Blood.* 1998;91:3766.

112. Krantz SB. Erythropoietin. *Blood.* 1991;77:419.

113. Jelkmann W. Erythropoietin: structure, control of production, and function. *Physiol Rev.* 1992;72:449.

114. Jelkmann W, Metzen E. Erythropoietin in the control of red cell production. *Ann Anat.* 1996;178:391.

115. Koury ST, Bondurant MC, Koury MJ. Localization of erythropoietin synthesizing cells in murine kidneys by in situ hybridization. *Blood.* 1988;71:524.

116. Lacombe C, Da Silva JL, Bruneval P, et al. Peritubular cells are the site of erythropoietin synthesis in the murine hypoxic kidney. *J Clin Invest.* 1988;81:620.

117. Koury ST, Koury MJ, Bondurant MC, et al. Quantitation of erythropoietin-producing cells in kidneys of mice by in situ hybridization: correlation with hematocrit, renal erythropoietin mRNA, and serum erythropoietin concentration. *Blood.* 1989;74:645.

118. Semenza GL, Dureza RC, Traystman MD, et al. Human erythropoietin gene expression in transgenic mice: multiple transcription initiation sites and cis-acting regulatory elements. *Mol Cell Biol.* 1990;10:930.

119. Schuster SJ, Koury ST, Bohrer M, et al. Cellular sites of extrarenal and renal erythropoietin production in anaemic rats. *Br J Haemotol.* 1992;81:153.

120. Mole DR, Radcliffe PJ. Regulation of endogenous erythropoietin production. In: Molineux G, Foote MA, Elliot SG, eds. *Erythropoietins and Erythropoiesis.* 2nd ed. Birkhäuser-Verlag AG; 2009:19.

121. Rankin EB, Biju MP, Liu Q, et al. Hypoxia-inducible factor-2 (HIF-2) regulates hepatic erythropoietin in vivo. *J Clin Invest.* 2007;117:1068.

122. Semenza GL, Nejfelt MK, Chi SM, et al. Hypoxia-inducible nuclear factors bind to an enhancer element located 3′ to the human erythropoietin gene. *Proc Natl Acad Sci U S A.* 1991;88:5680.

123. Beck I, Ramirez S, Weinmann R, et al. Enhancer element at the 3′-flanking region controls transcriptional response to hypoxia in the human erythropoietin gene. *J Biol Chem.* 1991;266:15563.

124. Pugh CW, Tan CC, Jones RW, et al. Functional analysis of an oxygen-regulated transcriptional enhancer lying 3′ to the mouse erythropoietin gene. *Proc Natl Acad Sci U S A.* 1991;88:10553.

125. Sawyer ST, Krantz SB, Goldwasser E. Binding and receptor-mediated endocytosis of erythropoietin in friend virus-infected erythroid cells. *J Biol Chem.* 1987;262:5554.

126. Ebert BL, Bunn HF. Regulation of the erythropoietin gene. *Blood.* 1999;94:1864.

127. Constantinescu SN, Keren T, Socolovsky M, et al. Ligand-independent oligomerization of cell-surface erythropoietin receptor is mediated by the transmembrane domain. *Proc Natl Acad Sci U S A.* 2001;98:4379.

128. Wilmes S, Hafer M, Vuorio J, et al. Mechanism of homodimeric cytokine receptor activation and dysregulation by oncogenic mutations. *Science.* 2020;367:643.

129. Witthuhn BA, Quelle FW, Silvennoinen O, et al. JAK2 associates with the erythropoietin receptor and is tyrosine phosphorylated and activated following stimulation with erythropoietin. *Cell.* 1993;74:227.

130. Damen JE, Wakao H, Miyajima A, et al. Tyrosine 343 in the erythropoietin receptor positively regulates erythropoietin-induced cell proliferation and Stat5 activation. *EMBO J.* 1995;14:5557.

131. Parganas E, Wang D, Stravopodis D, et al. Jak2 is essential for signaling through a variety of cytokine receptors. *Cell.* 1998;93:385.

132. Divoky V, Prchal JT. Mouse surviving solely on human erythropoietin receptor (EpoR): model of human EpoR-linked disease. *Blood.* 2002;99:3873.

133. Lin CS, Lim SK, D'Agati V, et al. Differential effects of an erythropoietin receptor gene disruption on primitive and definitive erythropoiesis. *Genes Dev.* 1996;10:154.

134. Wu H, Liu X, Jaenisch R, et al. Generation of committed erythroid BFU-E and CFU-E progenitors does not require erythropoietin or the erythropoietin receptor. *Cell.* 1995;83:59.

135. D'Andrea AD, Yoshimura A, Youssoufian H, et al. The cytoplasmic region of the erythropoietin receptor contains nonoverlapping positive and negative growth-regulatory domains. *Mol Cell Biol.* 1991;11:1980.

136. Klingmuller U, Lorenz U, Cantley LC, et al. Specific recruitment of SH-PTP1 to the erythropoietin receptor causes inactivation of JAK2 and termination of proliferative signals. *Cell.* 1995;80:729.

137. Arcasoy MO, Harris KW, Forget BG. A human erythropoietin receptor gene mutant causing familial erythrocytosis is associated with deregulation of the rates of Jak2 and Stat5 inactivation. *Exp Immunol.* 1999;27:63.

138. Marine JC, McKay C, Wang D, et al. SOCS3 is essential in the regulation of fetal liver erythropoiesis. *Cell.* 1999;98:617.

139. Sasaki A, Yasukawa H, Shouda T, et al. CIS3/SOCS-3 suppresses erythropoietin (EPO) signaling by binding the EPO receptor and JAK2. *J Biol Chem.* 2000;275:29338.

140. Prchal JT, Gregg XT. Erythropoiesis. Genetic abnormalities. In: Molineux G, Foote MA, Elliot SG, eds. *Erythropoietins and Erythropoiesis.* 2nd ed. Birkhäuser-Verlag AG; 2009:61.

141. Roberts KG, Morin RD, Zhang J, et al. Genetic alterations activating kinase and cytokine receptor signaling in high-risk acute lymphoblastic leukemia. *Cancer Cell.* 2012;22:153.

142. Walrafen P, Verdier F, Kadri Z, et al. Both proteasomes and lysosomes degrade the activated erythropoietin receptor. *Blood.* 2005;105:600.

143. Arcasoy MO, Jiang X, Haroon ZA. Expression of erythropoietin receptor splice variants in human cancer. *Biochem Biophys Res Commun.* 2003;307:999.

144. Barron C, Migliaccio AR, Migliaccio G, et al. Alternatively spliced mRNAs encoding soluble isoforms of the erythropoietin receptor in murine cell lines and bone marrow. *Gene.* 1994;147:263.

145. Nakamura Y, Nakauchi H. A truncated erythropoietin receptor and cell death: a reanalysis. *Science.* 1994;264:588.

146. Prchal JT, Semenza GL, Prchal J, et al. Familial polycythemia. *Science.* 1995;268:1831.

147. Noguchi CT, Wang L, Rogers HM, et al. Survival and proliferative roles of erythropoietin beyond the erythroid lineage. *Exp Rev Mol Med.* 2008;10:e36.

148. Anagnostou A, Lee ES, Kessimian N, et al. Erythropoietin has a mitogenic and positive chemotactic effect on endothelial cells. *Proc Natl Acad Sci U S A.* 1990;87:5978.

149. Chen ZY, Asavaritikrai P, Prchal JT, et al. Endogenous erythropoietin signaling is required for normal neural progenitor cell proliferation. *J Biol Chem.* 2007;282:25875.

150. Arcasoy MO. The non-haematopoietic biological effects of erythropoietin. *Br J Haematol.* 2008;141:14.

151. Brines M, Cerami A. Discovering erythropoietin's extra-hematopoietic functions: biology and clinical promise. *Kidney Int.* 2006;70:246.

152. Agarwal N, Gordeuk VR, Prchal JT. Are erythropoietin receptors expressed in tumors? Facts and fiction—more careful studies are needed. *J Clin Oncol.* 2007;25:1813.

153. Hardee ME, Cao Y, Fu P, et al. Erythropoietin blockade inhibits the induction of tumor angiogenesis and progression. *PLoS ONE.* 2007;2:e549.

154. Biggar P, Kim GH. Treatment of renal anemia: erythropoiesis stimulating agents and beyond. *Kidney Res Clin Pract.* 2017;36:209.

155. Hirota K, Semenza GL. Regulation of angiogenesis by hypoxia-inducible factor 1. *Crit Rev Oncol Hematol.* 2006;59:15.

156. Yoon D, Pastore YD, Divoky V, et al. Hypoxia-inducible factor-1 deficiency results in dysregulated erythropoiesis signaling and iron homeostasis in mouse development. *J Biol Chem.* 2006;281:25703.

157. Fukuda R, Zhang H, Kim JW, et al. HIF-1 regulates cytochrome oxidase subunits to optimize efficiency of respiration in hypoxic cells. *Cell.* 2007;129:111.

158. Pugh CW. Modulation of the hypoxic response. *Adv Exp Med Biol.* 2016;903:259.

159. Manalo DJ, Rowan A, Lavoie T, et al. Transcriptional regulation of vascular endothelial cell responses to hypoxia by HIF-1. *Blood.* 2005;105:659.

160. Maxwell PH, Wiesener MS, Chang GW, et al. The tumour suppressor protein VHL targets hypoxia-inducible factors for oxygen-dependent proteolysis. *Nature.* 1999;399:271.

161. Ivan M, Kondo K, Yang H, et al. HIFalpha targeted for VHL-mediated destruction by proline hydroxylation: implications for O_2 sensing. *Science.* 2001;292:464.

162. Jaakkola P, Mole DR, Tian YM, et al. Targeting of HIF-alpha to the von Hippel-Lindau ubiquitylation complex by O_2-regulated prolyl hydroxylation. *Science.* 2001;292:468.

163. Jewell UR, Kvietikova I, Scheid A, et al. Induction of HIF-1alpha in response to hypoxia is instantaneous. *FASEB J.* 2001;15:1312.

164. Jaakkola P, Mole DR, Tian YM, et al. Targeting of HIF-alpha to the von Hippel-Lindau ubiquitylation complex by O_2-regulated prolyl hydroxylation. *Science.* 2001;292:468.

165. Sanchez M, Galy B, Muckenthaler MU, Hentze MW. Iron-regulatory proteins limit hypoxia-inducible factor-2alpha expression in iron deficiency. *Nat Struct Mol Biol.* 2007, 14:420.

166. Ghosh MC, Zhang DL, Jeong SY, et al. Deletion of iron regulatory protein 1 causes polycythemia and pulmonary hypertension in mice through translational derepression of HIF2alpha. Cell Metab. 2013;17(2):271

167. Oskarsson GR, Oddsson A, Magnusson MK, et al. Predicted loss and gain of function mutations in ACO1 are associated with erythropoiesis. Commun Biol. 2020;3:189

168. Percy MJ, Furlow PW, Lucas GS, et al. A gain-of-function mutation in the HIF2A gene in familial erythrocytosis. *N Engl J Med.* 2008;358:162.

169. Gruber M, Hu CJ, Johnson RS, et al. Acute postnatal ablation of Hif-2alpha results in anemia. *Proc Natl Acad Sci U S A.* 2007;104:2301.

170. Chavez JC, Baranova O, Lin J, et al. The transcriptional activator hypoxia inducible factor 2 (HIF-2/EPAS-1) regulates the oxygen-dependent expression of erythropoietin in cortical astrocytes. *J Neurosci.* 2006;26:9471.

171. Liu YV, Baek JH, Zhang H, et al. RACK1 competes with HSP90 for binding to HIF-1alpha and is required for O_2-independent and HSP90 inhibitor-induced degradation of HIF-1alpha. *Mol Cell.* 2007;25:207.

172. Epstein AC, Gleadle JM, McNeill LA, et al. C. elegans EGL-9 and mammalian homologs define a family of dioxygenases that regulate HIF by prolyl hydroxylation. *Cell.* 2001;107:43.

173. Correa PN, Eskinazi D, Axelrad AA. Circulating erythroid progenitors in polycythemia vera are hypersensitive to insulin-like growth factor-1 in vitro: studies in an improved serum-free medium. *Blood.* 1994;83:99.

174. Mirza AM, Ezzat S, Axelrad AA. Insulin-like growth factor binding protein-1 is elevated in patients with polycythemia vera and stimulates erythroid burst formation in vitro. *Blood.* 1997;89:1862.

175. Brox AG, Congote LF, Fafard J, et al. Identification and characterization of an 8-kd peptide stimulating late erythropoiesis. *Exp Hematol.* 1989;17:769.

176. Bratosin D, Mazurier J, Tissier JP, et al. Cellular and molecular mechanisms of senescent erythrocyte phagocytosis by macrophages. A review. *Biochimie.* 1998;80:173.

177. Lutz HU, Bogdanova A. Mechanisms tagging senescent red blood cells for clearance in healthy humans. *Front Physiol.* 2013;4:387.

178. Clark MR. Senescence of red blood cells: progress and problems. *Physiol Rev.* 1988;68:503.

179. Lichtman MA. Does ATP decrease exponentially during red cell aging? *Nouv Rev Fr Hematol.* 1975;15:625.

180. Connor J, Pak CC, Schroit AJ. Exposure of phosphatidylserine in the outer leaflet of human red blood cells. Relationship to cell density, cell age, and clearance by mononuclear cells. *J Biol Chem.* 1994;269:2399.

181. Ando K, Beppu M, Kikugawa K. Evidence for accumulation of lipid hydroperoxides during the aging of human red blood cells in the circulation. *Biol Pharm Bull.* 1995;18:659.

182. Shinozuka T. Changes in human red blood cells during aging in vivo. *Keio J Med.* 1994;43:155.

183. Kay MM. Generation of senescent cell antigen on old cells initiates IgG binding to a neoantigen. *Cell Mol Biol (Noisy-le-Grand).* 1993;39:131.

184. Low PS, Waugh SM, Zinke K, et al. The role of hemoglobin denaturation and band 3 clustering in red blood cell aging. *Science.* 1985;227:531.

185. Mohanty JG, Nagababu E, Rifkind JM. Red blood cell oxidative stress impairs oxygen delivery and induces red blood cell aging. *Front Physiol.* 2014;5:84.

186. Lutz HU, Gianora O, Nater M, et al. Naturally occurring anti-band 3 antibodies bind to protein rather than to carbohydrate on band 3. *J Biol Chem.* 1993;268:23562.

187. Gattegno L, Bladier D, Vaysse J, et al. Inhibition by carbohydrates and monoclonal anticomplement receptor type 1, on interactions between senescent human red blood cells and monocytic macrophagic cells. *Adv Exp Med Biol.* 1991;307:329.

188. Song J, Tashi T, Prchal JT. Editorial comment on: inhibition of suicidal erythrocyte death by chronic hypoxia by Tang et al. (From: Tang F, Feng L, Li R, et al. High Alt Med Biol 2019;20:112-119. High Alt Med Biol. 2019;20:120).

189. Hong CI, De NC, Tritsch GL, et al. Synthesis and biological activities of some N4-substituted 4-aminopyrazolo(3,4-d)pyrimidines. *J Med Chem.* 1976;19:555.

190. Eshghi S, Vogelezang MG, Hynes RO, et al. Alpha4beta1 integrin and erythropoietin mediate temporally distinct steps in erythropoiesis: integrins in red cell development. *J Cell Biol.* 2007;177:871.

191. Sandoval H, Thiagarajan P, Dasgupta SK, et al. Essential role for Nix in autophagic maturation of erythroid cells. *Nature.* 2008;454:232.

192. Kent G, Minick OT, Volini FI, et al. Autophagic vacuoles in human red cells. *J Am Pathol.* 1966;48:831.

193. Heynen MJ, Tricot G, Verwilghen RL. Autophagy of mitochondria in rat bone marrow erythroid cells. Relation to nuclear extrusion. *Cell Tissue Res.* 1985;239:235.

194. Kundu M, Lindsten T, Yang CY, et al. Ulk1 plays a critical role in the autophagic clearance of mitochondria and ribosomes during reticulocyte maturation. *Blood.* 2008;112:1493.

195. Schweers RL, Zhang J, Randall MS, et al. NIX is required for programmed mitochondrial clearance during reticulocyte maturation. *Proc Natl Acad Sci U S A.* 2007;104:19500.

196. Mortensen M, Ferguson DJ, Edelmann M, et al. Loss of autophagy in erythroid cells leads to defective removal of mitochondria and severe anemia in vivo. *Proc Natl Acad Sci U S A.* 2010;107:832.

197. Notta F, Zandi S, Takayama N, et al. Distinct routes of lineage development reshape the human blood hierarchy across ontogeny. *Science.* 2016;351:aab2116.

198. Gregg XT, Prchal JT. Red blood cell enzymopathies. In: Hoffman R, Benz E, et al, eds. *Hematology: Basic Principles and Practice.* 7th ed. Elsevier; 2018.

199. Bruchova H, Yoon D, Agarwal AM, et al. Regulated expression of microRNAs in normal and polycythemia vera erythropoiesis. *Exp Hematol.* 2007;35:1657.

200. Li Y, Bai H, Zhang Z, et al. The up-regulation of miR-199b-5p in erythroid differentiation is associated with GATA1 and NF-E2. *Mol Cell.* 2014;37:213.

201. Raghavachari N, Liu P, Barb JJ, et al. Integrated analysis of miRNA and mRNA during differentiation of human CD34+ cells delineates the regulatory roles of microRNA in hematopoiesis. *Exp Hematol.* 2014;42:14.

202. Lee YT, de Vasconcellos JF, Yuan J, et al. LIN28B-mediated expression of fetal hemoglobin and production of fetal-like erythrocytes from adult human erythroblasts ex vivo. *Blood.* 2013;122:1034.

203. Barde I, Rauwel B, Marin-Florez RM, et al. A KRAB/KAP1-miRNA cascade regulates erythropoiesis through stage-specific control of mitophagy. *Science.* 2013;340:350.

204. Stembridge M, Williams AM, Gasho C, et al. The overlooked significance of plasma volume for successful adaptation to high altitude in Sherpa and Andean natives. *Proc Natl Acad Sci U S A.* 2019;116:16177.

205. Pearson TC, Botterill CA, Glass UH, et al. Interpretation of measured red cell mass and plasma volume in males with elevated venous PCV values. *Scand J Haemotol.* 1984;33:68.

206. Ersley A. Erythrokinetics. In: *Hematology.* 3rd ed. McGraw Hill; 1983:1638.

207. Cavill I, Trevett D, Fisher J, et al. The measurement of the total volume of red cells in man: a non-radioactive approach using biotin. *Br J Haemotol.* 1988;70:491.

208. Jones J, Mollison PL. A simple and efficient method of labelling red cells with 99mTc for determination of red cell volume. *Br J Haemotol.* 1978;38:141.

209. Baek JH, Liu YV, McDonald KR, et al. Spermidine/spermine N1-acetyltransferase-1 binds to hypoxia-inducible factor-1alpha (HIF-1alpha) and RACK1 and promotes ubiquitination and degradation of HIF-1alpha. *J Biol Chem.* 2007;282:33358.

210. Pearson TC, Guthrie DL, Simpson J, et al. Interpretation of measured red cell mass and plasma volume in adults: Expert Panel on Radionuclides of the International Council for Standardization in Haematology. *Br J Haemotol.* 1995;89:748.

211. Mock DM, Lankford GL, Widness JA, et al. Measurement of red cell survival using biotin-labeled red cells: validation against 51Cr-labeled red cells. *Transfusion.* 1999;39:156.

212. Mock DM, Nalbant D, Kyosseva SV, et al. Development, validation, and potential applications of biotinylated red blood cells for posttransfusion kinetics and other physiological studies: evidenced-based analysis and recommendations. *Transfusion.* 2018;58:2068.

213. Haldane J, Smith JL. The mass and oxygen capacity of the blood in man. *J Physiol.* 1900;331.

214. Ahlgrim C, Birkner P, Seiler F, et al. Applying the optimized CO rebreathing method for measuring blood volumes and hemoglobin mass in heart failure patients. *Front Physiol.* 2018;9:1603.

215. Fairbanks VF, Klee GG, Wiseman GA, et al. Measurement of blood volume and red cell mass: re-examination of 51Cr and 125I methods. *Blood Cells Mol Dis.* 1996;22:169.

216. Larson RA. Studies of the body hematocrit phenomenon: dynamic hematocrit of large vessel and initial distribution space of albumin and fibrinogen in the whole body. *Scand J Clin Lab Invest.* 1998;22.

217. Button LN, Gibson JG 2nd, Walter CW. Simultaneous determination of the volume of red cells and plasma for survival studies of stored blood. *Transfusion.* 1965;5:143.

218. Recommended methods for measurement of red-cell and plasma volume: International Committee for Standardization in Haematology. *J Nucl Med.* 1980;21:793.

219. Hillman RS, Finch CA. Erythropoiesis: normal and abnormal. *Semin Hematol.* 1967;4:327.

220. Samson D, Halliday D, Nicholson DC, et al. Quantitation of ineffective erythropoiesis from the incorporation of [15N] delta-aminolaevulinic acid and [15N] glycine into early labelled bilirubin. I. Normal subjects. *Br J Haemotol.* 1976;34:33.

221. Huff RL, Hennessy TG, Austin RE, et al. Plasma and red cell iron turnover in normal subjects and in patients having various hematopoietic disorders. *J Clin Invest.* 1950;29:1041.

222. Cook JD, Marsaglia G, Eschbach JW, et al. Ferrokinetics: a biologic model for plasma iron exchange in man. *J Clin Invest.* 1970;49:197.

223. Ricketts C, Cavill I, Napier JA, et al. Ferrokinetics and erythropoiesis in man: an evaluation of ferrokinetic measurements. *Br J Haemotol.* 1977;35:41.

224. Bauer W, Stray S, Huebers H, et al. The relationship between plasma iron and plasma iron turnover in the rat. *Blood.* 1981;57:239.

225. Beguin Y. The soluble transferrin receptor: biological aspects and clinical usefulness as quantitative measure of erythropoiesis. *Haematologica.* 1992;77:1.

226. Ashby W. The determination of the length of life of transfused blood corpuscles in man. *J Exp Med.* 1919;29:267.

227. Shemin D, Rittenberg D. The life span of the human red blood cell. *J Biol Chem.* 1946;166:627.

228. Berlin NI, Meyer LM, Lazarus M. Life span of the rat red blood cell as determined by glycine-2-C14. *Am J Physiol.* 1951;165:465.

229. Beutler E, Dern RJ, Alving AS. The hemolytic effect of primaquine. IV. The relationship of cell age to hemolysis. *J Lab Clin Med.* 1954;44:439.

230. Birgens HS, Hansen OP, Henriksen JH, et al. Quantitation of erythropoiesis in myelomatosis. *Scand J Haemotol.* 1979;22:357.

231. Weinstein IM, Beutler E. The use of Cr51 and Fe59 in a combined procedure to study erythrocyte production and destruction in normal human subjects and in patients with hemolytic or aplastic anemia. *J Lab Clin Med.* 1955;45:616.

232. Gifford SC, Yoshida T, Shevkoplyas SS, et al. A high-resolution, double-labeling method for the study of in vivo red blood cell aging. *Transfusion.* 2006;46:578.

233. Beutler E, West C. Measurement of the viability of stored red cells by the single-isotope technique using 51Cr. Analysis of validity. *Transfusion.* 1984;24:100.

234. Lindsell CJ, Franco RS, Smith EP, et al. A method for the continuous calculation of the age of labeled red blood cells. *Am J Hematol.* 2008;83:454.

235. Silver HM, Seebeck MA, Cowett RM, et al. Red cell volume determination using a stable isotope of chromium. *J Soc Gynecol Invest.* 1997;4:254.

236. Cline MJ, Berlin NI. Measurement of red cell survival with tritiated diisopropylfluorophosphate. *J Lab Clin Med.* 1962;60:826.

237. Milner PF, Charache S. Life span of carbamylated red cells in sickle cell anemia. *J Lab Clin Med.* 1973;52:3161.

238. Eschbach JW, Korn D, Finch CA. 14C cyanate as a tag for red cell survival in normal and uremic man. *J Lab Clin Med.* 1977;89:823.

239. Horan PK, Slezak SE. Stable cell membrane labelling. *Nature.* 1989;340:167.

240. Slezak SE, Horan PK. Fluorescent in vivo tracking of hematopoietic cells. Part I. Technical considerations. *Blood.* 1989;74:2172.

241. Strauss RG, Mock DM, Widness JA, et al. Posttransfusion 24-hour recovery and subsequent survival of allogeneic red blood cells in the bloodstream of newborn infants. *Transfusion.* 2004;44:871.

242. Suzuki T, Dale GL. Biotinylated erythrocytes: in vivo survival and in vitro recovery. *Blood.* 1987;70:791.

243. Bentley SA, Glass HI, Lewis SM, et al. Elution correction in 51Cr red cell survival studies. *Br J Haemotol.* 1974;26:179.

244. McCurdy PR, Sherman AS. Irreversibly sickled cells and red cell survival in sickle cell anemia: a study with both DF32P and 51CR. *Am J Med.* 1978;64:253.

245. Franco RS. Measurement of red cell lifespan and aging. *Transfus Med Hemother.* 2012;39:302.

246. Mollison PEC, Contreras M. The transfusion of red cells. In: *Blood Transfusion in Clinical Medicine.* Blackwell; 1987:95.

247. Eadie GS, Brown IW Jr. Red blood cell survival studies. *Blood.* 1953;8:1110.

248. Recommended method for radioisotope red-cell survival studies. International Committee for Standardization in Haematology. *Br J Haemotol.* 1980;45:659.

249. Franco RS, Yasin Z, Palascak MB, et al. The effect of fetal hemoglobin on the survival characteristics of sickle cells. *Blood.* 2006;108:1073.

250. Yasin Z, Witting S, Palascak MB, et al. Phosphatidylserine externalization in sickle red blood cells: associations with cell age, density, and hemoglobin F. *Blood.* 2003;102:365.

251. Berlin NI, Berk PD. Quantitative aspects of bilirubin metabolism for hematologists. *Blood.* 1981;57:983.

252. Doyle J, Vreman HJ, Stevenson DK, et al. Does vitamin C cause hemolysis in premature newborn infants? Results of a multicenter double-blind, randomized, controlled trial. *J Pediatr.* 1997;130:103.

253. Furne JK, Springfield JR, Ho SB, et al. Simplification of the end-alveolar carbon monoxide technique to assess erythrocyte survival. *J Lab Clin Med.* 2003;142:52.

254. Vreman HJ, Stevenson DK. Carboxyhemoglobin determined in neonatal blood with a CO-oximeter unaffected by fetal oxyhemoglobin. *Clin Chem.* 1994;40:1522.

255. Christensen RD, Malleske DT, Lambert DK, et al. Measuring end-tidal carbon monoxide of jaundiced neonates in the birth hospital to identify those with hemolysis. *Neonatology.* 2016;109:1.

256. Borun ER, Figueroa WG, Perry SM. The distribution of Fe59 tagged human erythrocytes in centrifuged specimens as a function of cell age. *J Clin Invest.* 1957;36:676.

257. Luthra MG, Friedman JM, Sears DA. Studies of density fractions of normal human erythrocytes labeled with iron-59 in vivo. *J Lab Clin Med.* 1979;94:879.

258. Linderkamp O, Friederichs E, Boehler T, et al. Age dependency of red blood cell deformability and density: studies in transient erythroblastopenia of childhood. *Br J Haemotol.* 1993;83:125.

259. Dale GL, Norenberg SL. Density fractionation of erythrocytes by Percoll/ hypaque results in only a slight enrichment for aged cells. *Biochim Biophys Acta.* 1990;1036:183.

260. Bosch FH, Werre JM, Roerdinkholder-Stoelwinder B, et al. Characteristics of red cell populations fractionated with a combination of counterflow centrifugation and Percoll separation. *Blood.* 1992;79:254.

261. Ganzoni AM, Oakes R, Hillman RS. Red cell aging in vivo. *J Clin Invest.* 1971;50:1373.

262. Suzuki T, Dale GL. Senescent erythrocytes: isolation of in vivo aged cells and their biochemical characteristics. *Proc Natl Acad Sci U S A.* 1988;85:1647.

263. Haram S, Carriero D, Seaman C, et al. The mechanism of decline of age-dependent enzymes in the red blood cell. *Enzyme.* 1991;45:47.

264. Zimran A, Forman L, Suzuki T, et al. In vivo aging of red cell enzymes: study of biotinylated red blood cells in rabbits. *Am J Hematol.* 1990;33:249.

265. Beutler E, Hartman G. Age-related red cell enzymes in children with transient erythroblastopenia of childhood and with hemolytic anemia. *Pediatr Res.* 1985;19:44.

266. Beutler E. The relationship of red cell enzymes to red cell life-span. *Blood Cells.* 1988;14:69.

267. Dale GL, Norenberg SL. Time-dependent loss of adenosine 5'-monophosphate deaminase activity may explain elevated adenosine 5'-triphosphate levels in senescent erythrocytes. *Blood.* 1989;74:2157.

268. Paglia DE, Valentine WN, Nakatani M, et al. AMP deaminase as a cell-age marker in transient erythroblastopenia of childhood and its role in the adenylate economy of erythrocytes. *Blood.* 1989;74:2161.

269. Dale GL, Norenberg SL, Suzuki T, et al. Altered adenine nucleotide metabolism in senescent erythrocytes from the rabbit. *Prog Clin Biol Res.* 1989;319:259.

270. Clark MR CL, Jensen RH. Density distribution of aging, transfused human red cells. *Blood.* 1989;74(Suppl 1):217a.

271. Waugh RE, Narla M, Jackson CW, et al. Rheologic properties of senescent erythrocytes: loss of surface area and volume with red blood cell age. *Blood.* 1992;79:1351.

272. Tissot JD, Rubin O, Canellini G. Analysis and clinical relevance of microparticles from red blood cells. *Curr Opin Hematol.* 2010;17:571.

273. Willekens FL, Werre JM, Groenen-Dopp YA, et al. Erythrocyte vesiculation: a self-protective mechanism? *Br J Haemotol.* 2008;141:549.

274. Jank H, Salzer U. Vesicles generated during storage of red blood cells enhance the generation of radical oxygen species in activated neutrophils. *Sci World J.* 2011;11:173.

275. Waugh RE, Narla M, Jackson CW, et al. Rheologic properties of senescent erythrocytes: loss of surface area and volume with red blood cell age. *Blood.* 1992;79(5):1351.

276. Dale GL, Daniels RB, Beckman J, Norenberg SL. Characterization of senescent red cells from the rabbit. *Adv Exp Med Biol.* 1991;307:93.

277. Safeukui I, Buffet PA, Deplaine G Sensing of red blood cells with decreased membrane deformability by the human spleen. *Blood Adv.* 2018;2(20):2581.

278. Arashiki N, Kimata N, Manno S, et al. Membrane peroxidation and methemoglobin formation are both necessary for band 3 clustering: mechanistic insights into human erythrocyte senescence. *Biochemistry.* 2013;52:5760.

279. Arese P, Turrini F, Schwarzer E. Band 3/complement-mediated recognition and removal of normally senescent and pathological human erythrocytes. *Cell Physiol Biochem.* 2005;16:133.

280. GL D. Does surface bound immunoglobulin mediate erythrocyte death? Commentary. *Blood Cells.* 1988;14:36.

281. Zwaal RF, Comfurius P, Bevers EM. Surface exposure of phosphatidylserine in pathological cells. *Cell Mol Life Sci.* 2005;62:971.

282. Boas FE, Forman L, Beutler E. Phosphatidylserine exposure and red cell viability in red cell aging and in hemolytic anemia. *Proc Natl Acad Sci U S A.* 1998;95:3077.

283. Kuypers FA, de Jong K. The role of phosphatidylserine in recognition and removal of erythrocytes. *Cell Mol Biol (Noisy-le-Grand).* 2004;50:147.

284. Risso A, Turello M, Biffoni F, et al. Red blood cell senescence and neocytolysis in humans after high altitude acclimatization. *Blood Cells Mol Dis.* 2007;38:83.

285. Rice L, Alfrey CP. The negative regulation of red cell mass by neocytolysis: physiologic and pathophysiologic manifestations. *Cell Physiol Biochem.* 2005;15:245.

286. Khandelwal S, Saxena RK. A role of phosphatidylserine externalization in clearance of erythrocytes exposed to stress but not in eliminating aging populations of erythrocyte in mice. *Exp Gerontol.* 2008;43:764.

287. Dasgupta SK, Abdel-Monem H, Guchhait P, et al. Role of lactadherin in the clearance of phosphatidylserine-expressing red blood cells. *Transfusion.* 2008;48:2370.

288. Ishimoto Y, Ohashi K, Mizuno K, et al. Promotion of the uptake of PS liposomes and apoptotic cells by a product of growth arrest-specific gene, gas6. *J Biochem.* 2000;127:411.

289. Hanayama R, Tanaka M, Miwa K, et al. Expression of developmental endothelial locus-1 in a subset of macrophages for engulfment of apoptotic cells. *J Immunol.* 2004;172:3876.

290. Wang RH, Phillips G, Jr., Medof ME, et al. Activation of the alternative complement pathway by exposure of phosphatidylethanolamine and phosphatidylserine on erythrocytes from sickle cell disease patients. *J Clin Invest.* 1993;92:1326.

291. Fens MH, Storm G, Pelgrim RC, et al. Erythrophagocytosis by angiogenic endothelial cells is enhanced by loss of erythrocyte deformability. *Exp Hematol.* 2010;38:282.

292. Lang F, Gulbins E, Lerche H, et al. Eryptosis, a window to systemic disease. *Cell Physiol Biochem.* 2008;22:373.

293. Franco RS, Puchulu-Campanella ME, Barber LA, et al. Changes in the properties of normal human red blood cells during in vivo aging. *Am J Hematol.* 2013;88:44.

294. Tang F, Feng L, Li R, et al. Inhibition of suicidal erythrocyte death by chronic hypoxia. *High Alt Med Biol.* 2019;20:112.

295. Khandelwal S, Saxena RK. Age-dependent increase in green autofluorescence of blood erythrocytes. *J Biosci.* 2007;32:1139.

296. Kerfoot SM, McRae K, Lam F, et al. A novel mechanism of erythrocyte capture from circulation in humans. *Exp Hematol.* 2008;36:111.

297. Fei P, Wang W, Kim SH, et al. Bnip3L is induced by p53 under hypoxia, and its knockdown promotes tumor growth. *Cancer Cell.* 2004;6:597.

298. Song J, Yoon J, Christensen RD, et al. HIF-mediated increased ROS from reduced mitophagy and decreased catalase causes neocytolysis. *J Mol Med (Berl).* 2015;93:857.

299. Javier MC, Krauss A, Nesin M. Corrected end-tidal carbon monoxide closely correlates with the corrected reticulocyte count in Coombs' test-positive term neonates. *Pediatrics.* 2003;112:1333.

300. Christensen RD, Lambert DK, Henry E, et al. Unexplained extreme hyperbilirubinemia among neonates in a multihospital healthcare system. *Blood Cells Mol Dis.* 2013;50:105.

301. Garratty G. The James Blundell Award Lecture 2007: do we really understand immune red cell destruction? *Transfus Med.* 2008;18(6):321.

302. Kubagawa H, Oka S, Kubagawa Y, et al. Identity of the elusive IgM Fc receptor (FcmuR) in humans. *J Exp Med.* 2009;206(12):2779.

303. Eggleton P, Tenner AJ, Reid KB. C1q receptors. *Clin Exp Immunol.* 2000;120(3):406.

304. Kubagawa H, Oka S, Kubagawa Y, et al. Identity of the elusive IgM Fc receptor (FcmuR) in humans. *J Exp Med.* 2009;206(12):2779.

305. Aderem A, Underhill DM. Mechanisms of phagocytosis in macrophages. *Annu Rev Immunol.* 1999;7:593.

306. Eggleton P, Tenner AJ, Reid KB. C1q receptors. *Clin Exp Immunol.* 2000;Aug 5(8):606.

307. Mebius RE, Kraal G. Structure and function of the spleen. 2005;Aug 5 (8):606-16.

308. Vidarsson G, Dekkers G, Rispen T. IgG subclasses and allotypes: from structure to effector functions. *Front Immunol.* 2014;Oct 20;5:520.

309. Bournazos S, Wang TT, Ravetch JV. The Role and Function of Fcγ Receptors on Myeloid Cells. *Microbiol Spectr.* 2016;Dec;4(6):0045.

310. Flores G, Cunningham-Rundles C, Newland AC, Bussel JB. Efficacy of intravenous immunoglobulin in the treatment of autoimmune hemolytic anemia: results in 73 patients. *Am J Hematol.* 1993 Dec;44(4):237.

311. Rigal CS. The place of instruments in the scientific work of Marcel Bessis (1917-1994): the electron microscope and the ektacytometer. *Hematol Cell Ther.* 2000;42:250.

312. Shin S, Hou JX, Suh JS, et al. Validation and application of a microfluidic ektacytometer (RheoScan-D) in measuring erythrocyte deformability. *Clin Hemorheol Microcirc.* 2007;37:319.

313. LoBuglio AF, Cotran RS, Jandl JH. Red cells coated with immunoglobulin G: binding and sphering by mononuclear cells in man. *Science.* 1967;158:1582.

314. Jandl JH, Tomlinson AS. The destruction of red cells by antibodies in man. II. Pyrogenic, leukocytic and dermal responses to immune hemolysis. *J Clin Invest.* 1958;37:1202.

315. Lutz HU SP, Kock D, Taylor RP. Opsonic potential of C3b-anti-band 3 complexes when generated on senescent and oxidatively stressed red cells or in fluid phase. In: Magnani M, et al, eds. *Red Blood Cell Aging.* Plenum Press; 1991.

316. Beppu M, Mizukami A, Nagoya M, et al. Binding of anti-band 3 autoantibody to oxidatively damaged erythrocytes. Formation of senescent antigen on erythrocyte surface by an oxidative mechanism. *J Biol Chem.* 1990;265:3226.

317. Nielsen MJ, Andersen CB, Moestrup SK. CD163 binding to haptoglobin-hemoglobin complexes involves a dual-point electrostatic receptor-ligand pairing. *J Biol Chem.* 2013;288:18834.

318. Carter K, Worwood M. Haptoglobin: a review of the major allele frequencies worldwide and their association with diseases. *Int J Lab Hematol.* 2007;29:92.

319. Baranano DE, Rao M, Ferris CD, et al. Biliverdin reductase: a major physiologic cytoprotectant. *Proc Natl Acad Sci U S A.* 2002;99:16093.

320. Piccard H, Van den Steen PE, Opdenakker G. Hemopexin domains as multifunctional liganding modules in matrix metalloproteinases and other proteins. *J Leukoc Biol.* 2007;81:870.

321. Sears DA. Disposal of plasma heme in normal man and patients with intravascular hemolysis. *J Clin Invest.* 1970;49:5.

322. Wochner RD, Spilberg I, Iio A, et al. Hemopexin metabolism in sickle-cell disease, porphyrias and control subjects–effects of heme injection. *N Engl J Med.* 1974;290:822.

323. Hvidberg V, Maniecki MB, Jacobsen C, et al. Identification of the receptor scavenging hemopexin-heme complexes. *Blood.* 2005;106:2572.

324. Rosen H, Sears DA, Meisenzahl D. Spectral properties of hemospexin-heme. The Schumm test. *J Lab Clin Med.* 1969;74:941.

325. Yachie A, Niida Y, Wada T, et al. Oxidative stress causes enhanced endothelial cell injury in human heme oxygenase-1 deficiency. *J Clin Invest.* 1999;103:129.

326. Maines MD. The heme oxygenase system: a regulator of second messenger gases. *Ann Rev Pharmacol Toxicol.* 1997;37:517.

327. Komuro A, Tobe T, Nakano Y, et al. Cloning and characterization of the cDNA encoding human biliverdin-IX alpha reductase. *Biochim Biophys Acta.* 1996;1309:89.

328. Erlinger S, Arias IM, Dhumeaux D. Inherited disorders of bilirubin transport and conjugation: new insights into molecular mechanisms and consequences. *Gastroenterology.* 2014;146(7):1625-1638.

329. Elder G, Gray CH, Nicholson DC. Bile pigment fate in gastrointestinal tract. *Semin Hematol.* 1972;9:71.

Part II **Classification of Red Cell Diseases**

CHAPTER 3
CLINICAL MANIFESTATIONS AND CLASSIFICATION OF ERYTHROCYTE DISORDERS

Josef T. Prchal

SUMMARY

Anemias are characterized by a decrease and erythrocytoses by an increase of the red cell mass. In most clinical situations, changes in red cell mass are inferred from the hemoglobin concentration or hematocrit. Some red cell disorders are associated with compensated hemolysis without or with only slight anemia. Their clinical manifestations are evident not by the effects of anemia but by changes associated with catabolism of hemoglobin such as an increase in serum bilirubin and, if sustained, cholelithiasis, decreased haptoglobin, and usually chronic reticulocytosis. Some red cell disorders are only showcased by morphologic abnormalities as exemplified by hereditary elliptocytosis unaccompanied by hemolysis or anemia, or by cyanosis such as that seen with methemoglobinemia and sulfhemoglobinemia.

The anemias have their principal effect by decreasing the oxygen-carrying capacity of blood and their severity is most conveniently considered in terms of blood hemoglobin concentration; however, oxygen-carrying capacity of blood is also influenced by red cell and plasma volumes. Anemia may cause symptoms because of tissue hypoxia (eg, fatigue, dyspnea on exertion). Some manifestations are also caused by compensatory attempts to ameliorate hypoxia (eg, hyperventilation, tachycardia, and increased cardiac output). These manifestations are a function of the severity and rapidity of onset of the anemia. Tissue hypoxia sensing is ubiquitous and is signaled by an increased level of hypoxia-inducible transcription factors (HIFs), HIF-1 and HIF-2. HIFs upregulate transcription of many genes, in addition to the principal erythropoietic factor erythropoietin (EPO), that are involved in erythropoiesis, but also in angiogenesis, energy metabolism, and iron balance. The classification of anemia distinguishes whether the anemia is inherited or acquired and considers new kinetic and molecular findings. Some anemic disorders can be accompanied by nonerythroid pathologic indicators, such as mutated red cell enzyme aldolase, which is also associated with glycogen storage disease and developmental disability in addition to hemolytic anemia.

Acronyms and abbreviations: *EGLN1*, a gene encoding PHD2 protein; *EPAS1*, a gene encoding hypoxia-inducible factor-2alpha; EPO, erythropoietin; EPOR, erythropoietin receptor; HIF, hypoxia-inducible factor; IRP-1, iron regulatory protein; MCHC, mean corpuscular hemoglobin concentration; MCV, mean corpuscular volume, PFCP, primary familial and congenital polycythemia; PHD2, prolyl hydroxylase domain-containing protein 2; *VHL*, a gene encoding von Hippel–Lindau tumor suppressor.

The erythrocytoses are most conveniently expressed in terms of the packed red cell volume (hematocrit), because their clinical manifestations are primarily related to the expanded red cell mass and resulting increased viscosity of blood, and other specific features related to the pathophysiology stemming from a molecular causative defect (eg, thrombosis in polycythemia vera and Chuvash erythrocytosis [also Chuvash polycythemia], cyanosis in congenital methemoglobinemia). However, normal hematocrit levels associated with increased plasma volume may mask an increase in red cell mass and, in turn, elevated hematocrit levels with decreased plasma volume may falsely lead to a diagnosis of erythrocytosis (spurious erythrocytosis). The erythrocytoses may be primary, caused by acquired somatic or inherited germline mutation(s) dysregulating expansion of erythroid progenitors and, thus, red cell production (eg, clonal expansion of a multipotential hematopoietic cell [polycythemia vera]); or it may be caused by germline gain-of-function mutations of the EPO receptor (*EPOR*), resulting in polyclonal hematopoiesis; both are associated with low EPO. Secondary erythrocytoses may be acquired, caused by increased levels of circulating erythropoiesis-stimulating factors, usually EPO, as a result of tissue hypoxia (eg, chronic pulmonary disease, exposure to high-altitude hypoxia), or occurring post renal transplant, aberrant EPO expression, and EPO doping, induced by testosterone and other androgen medications, high cobalt, and manganese. Secondary erythrocytoses may also be inherited (eg, high oxygen affinity hemoglobins or decreased 2,3BPG), and from congenital disorders of hypoxia sensing (mutations of genes in the HIFs' pathway), resulting in the augmentation of HIF-2 and HIF-1. Some secondary erythrocytoses have hypersensitive erythroid progenitors and increased levels of EPO and so share features of both primary and secondary erythrocytosis, exemplified by Chuvash erythrocytosis (also known as Chuvash polycythemia). Some erythrocytoses are associated with phenotypes that extend beyond the erythroid system, such as polycythemia vera, a stem cell disorder, with thrombotic complications. Erythrocytosis with *VHL* mutations and some HIF2a (*EPAS1*) mutations have thrombotic complications as a major cause of morbidity even when red cell mass is controlled with phlebotomy. Also, in type II congenital methemoglobinemia, the latter is accompanied by developmental failure and moderate erythrocytosis.

● ANEMIA

PATHOPHYSIOLOGY AND MANIFESTATIONS

Effects on Oxygen Transport

The clinical manifestations of anemia are a function of the degree of tissue hypoxia and the etiology and pathogenesis of the specific anemia (eg, splenomegaly characteristic of hereditary spherocytosis, neurologic defects, and gastric atrophy of pernicious anemia). Decreased oxygen-carrying capacity mobilizes compensatory mechanisms designed to prevent or ameliorate tissue hypoxia. Red cells also transport carbon dioxide from tissues to the lungs and help distribute nitric oxide throughout the body (Chap. 19), but transport of these gases does not appear to be dependent on the concentration of red cells in the blood and is normal in anemic patients. Tissue hypoxia occurs when the pressure of oxygen in the capillaries is too low to provide cells with enough oxygen for their metabolic needs. In an average person, the red cell mass must provide the total body tissues with approximately 0.25 L/min of oxygen to support life. The oxygen-carrying capacity of normal blood is 1.34 mL/g of hemoglobin (approximately 0.2 L/L of normal blood), and cardiac output is approximately 5 L/min; thus, 1 L/min of oxygen is available at the tissue level. Extraction of one-fourth of this amount reduces the oxygen tension of 100 torr in the arterial end of the capillary to 40 torr in the venous end. This partial extraction ensures the presence of sufficient diffusion pressure throughout the capillaries to provide all cells with enough oxygen for the cell's metabolic needs (Fig. 3-1). In anemia, extraction of the same amount of oxygen leads to greater hemoglobin desaturation and lower oxygen tension at the venous end of the capillary. The resulting hypoxia in the immediate vicinity initiates several compensatory, and frequently symptomatic, adjustments in the supply of blood and oxygen.

Hypoxia-Inducible Transcription Factors

Hypoxia-inducible factor (HIF)-1 and its homologue with tissue-restricted expression, HIF-2, play a central role in the body's response to hypoxia (Chaps. 2 and 28). HIF-1 was first identified as a factor regulating the transcriptional activity of the *erythropoietin (EPO)* gene (Chap. 2).[1] The essential role of this transcriptional factor in global regulation of protection against hypoxia soon became clear. Its actions include respiratory control, transcriptional regulation of glycolytic enzyme genes, angiogenesis, and energy metabolism.[2-4] The degradation of the hypoxia-regulated α subunits of HIFs is controlled by enzymes sensitive to the presence or absence of oxygen.[5] Thus, HIFs' downregulation is mediated by two principal negative regulators, von Hippel–Lindau tumor suppressor (VHL) and prolyl hydroxylase domain-containing proteins (PHD), PHD2 (encoded by *EGLN1*) being the principal PHD for regulation of erythropoiesis. Chapter 2 describes the current knowledge of hypoxia sensing in greater detail; however, HIF-2 is the major regulator of EPO production. Tissue-specific factors are responsible for tissue-specific mobilization of the compensatory mechanisms listed in the next section permit survival under hypoxic conditions. Figure 3-2 outlines the regulation of some physiologic processes by hypoxia.

Decreased Oxygen Consumption

Energy metabolism at the optimal oxygen supply is sustained by energy-efficient oxidative phosphorylation. In hypoxia, energy is produced by less efficient glycolysis accomplished by upregulation of transcription of glycolytic enzyme genes[4] and increased glucose transport, a process known as the *Pasteur effect*. The Pasteur effect and its exception in the metabolism observed in malignant tissue, referred to as the *Warburg effect*, are both explained at the molecular level by changes in HIF-1 levels.[4,6–8]

Decreased Oxygen Affinity

Efficient increase in tissue oxygen delivery is accomplished by decreasing the affinity of hemoglobin for oxygen (right-shifted hemoglobin oxygen dissociation curve). This action permits increased oxygen extraction from the same amount of hemoglobin (Chaps. 18 and 19).[9] Acutely, a very small shift in pH produces a large effect on the dissociation curve because of the Bohr effect (described by Danish physician Christian Bohr in 1904: *Hemoglobin's oxygen binding affinity is inversely related both to acidity and to the concentration of carbon dioxide*).[10] In chronic anemia, increased oxygen tissue delivery is accomplished by increased amounts of 2,3-bisphosphoglycerate (Chaps. 16 and 18).[9] The increased synthesis of 2,3-bisphosphoglycerate in anemia is accomplished by increasing the intracellular pH of red cells (Chap. 1) by respiratory alkalosis resulting from increased respiration. This effect is clearly demonstrated in individuals with high-altitude hypoxemia.[11]

Increased Tissue Perfusion

The effect of decreased oxygen-carrying capacity on the tissue tension of oxygen can be compensated acutely by increasing tissue perfusion locally via changing vasomotor activity and, in the long term, by enhanced tissue angiogenesis.[2] Because in chronic anemia the blood volume is not changed (Fig. 3-3),[12] increased tissue perfusion is organ-selective, accomplished by shunting the blood from nonvital donor-tissue areas to oxygen-sensitive essential recipient organs. In acute anemia, the major donor areas for redistribution of blood are the mesenteric and iliac beds.[13] In chronic anemia in humans, the donor areas are the cutaneous tissue[14] and the kidneys.[15] Vasoconstriction and oxygen deprivation in the skin cause the characteristic pallor of anemia. In the kidneys, the oxygen supply under normal conditions exceeds oxygen demands. The arteriovenous oxygen difference in the kidney is as low as 14 mL/L (compared with the myocardium, where the difference can be as high as 200 mL/L), indicating that even a severe reduction in kidney blood perfusion can be tolerated. Nevertheless, enough renal hypoxia must be present to activate HIF-2 and stimulate increased EPO production and erythropoiesis (Chap. 2). The effect on renal excretory mechanisms is slight because the reduction in renal blood flow is offset by a high plasmacrit. Thus, organs with the most pressing need for oxygen, such as the myocardium and brain, are largely unimpeded by a moderate reduction in oxygen-carrying capacity, whereas in other tissues, severe anemia leads to tissue hypoxia, with some tissue-specific consequences such as retinal hemorrhages.[16]

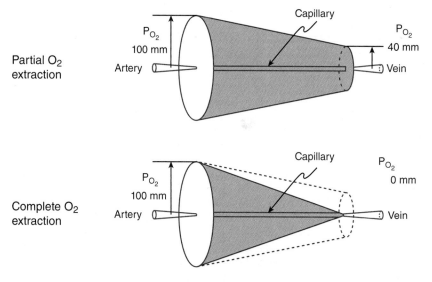

Figure 3–1. Theoretical tissue segment provided with oxygen from one capillary. With an arterial diffusion pressure of oxygen of 100 torr and partial oxygen extraction resulting in a venous oxygen pressure of 40 torr, one capillary can provide oxygen to cells within a truncated cone segment. With complete oxygen extraction, however, oxygen cannot be supplied to cells within a rim of tissue around the apex of the cone.

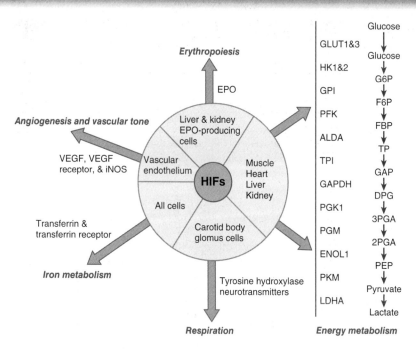

Figure 3–2. Regulation of erythropoiesis, angiogenesis, iron metabolism, respiration, and energy metabolism by HIF-1 are examples of physiologic processes regulated by hypoxia. iNOS, inducible nitrous oxide synthase; VEGF, vascular endothelial growth factor. *Right panel, left column, in order:* GLUT1&3, glucose transporters 1 and 3; glycolytic enzymes: HK1&2, hexokinase 1 and 2; GPI, glucose phosphate isomerase; PFK, phosphofructokinase; ALDA, aldolase A; TPI, triosephosphate isomerase; GAPDH, glycerol phosphate dehydrogenase; PGK1, phosphoglycerate kinase; PGM, phosphoglycerate mutase; ENOL1, enolase 1; PKM, pyruvate kinase M isoform; LDHA, lactic dehydrogenase A isoform. *Right column:* Metabolic intermediates generated by the depicted enzymes.

Increased Cardiac Output

Increased cardiac output is a metabolically expensive compensatory device.[17] It decreases the fraction of oxygen that must be extracted during each circulation, thereby maintaining higher oxygen pressure. Because the viscosity of blood in anemia is decreased and selective vascular dilatation decreases peripheral resistance, high cardiac output can be maintained without any increase in blood pressure.[18] In an otherwise healthy person, a measurable increase in resting cardiac output does not occur until hemoglobin concentration is less than 70 g/L, and clinical signs of cardiac hyperactivity usually are not present until hemoglobin concentration reaches even lower levels.[19]

Signs of cardiac hyperactivity include tachycardia, increased arterial and capillary pulsation, and hemodynamic "flow" murmurs.[20]

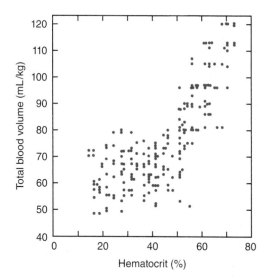

Figure 3–3. Relationship between hematocrit and total blood volume in normal individuals and in patients with anemia and erythrocytosis. *(Reproduced with permission from Huber H, Lewis SM, Szur L. The Influence of Anaemia, Polycythaemia and Splenomegaly on the Relationship between Venous Haematocrit and Red-Cell Volume. Br J Haematol. 1964 Oct;10:567-575.)*

Murmurs usually are heard during systole. Murmurs and bruits have been described in many regions, such as over the jugular vein, the closed eye, and the parietal region of the skull, and may be sensed by the patient as roaring in the ears (tinnitus), especially at night. They disappear promptly after the hemoglobin concentration returns to normal.[20] The myocardium tolerates a prolonged period of sustained hyperactivity. However, angina pectoris and high-output failure may supervene if anemia is severe that it does not fulfill myocardial oxygen demands, or if the patient has coronary artery disease. Cardiomegaly, pulmonary congestion, ascites, and edema have been observed, and they require prompt treatment with oxygen and transfusion of packed red cells.

Increased Pulmonary Function

Significant anemia leads to a compensatory increase in respiratory rate that decreases the oxygen gradient from ambient air to alveolar air and increases the amount of oxygen available to oxygenate a greater than normal cardiac output. Consequently, exertional dyspnea and orthopnea are characteristic clinical manifestations of moderate to severe anemia.[19-22]

Increased Red Cell Production

The most appropriate response to anemia is a compensatory increase of red cell production, which may increase about two- to threefold acutely and four- to sixfold chronically, and 10-fold in the most extreme case. The increase is mediated by increased production of EPO. The rate of EPO synthesis is inversely and logarithmically related to hemoglobin concentration (Chap. 2). EPO concentration can increase from approximately 10 U/L at normal hemoglobin concentrations to 10,000 U/L in severe anemia (Fig. 3-4).[23,24] The change in EPO levels ensures that red cell production increases in response to hemolytic and other anemias or subacute blood loss. If the former is mild, the anemia may be compensated and, if iron is available, the blood loss will be repaired after it ceases. Augmented erythroid activity expands marrow space, which, if intense, can cause sternal tenderness and diffuse bone pains. The proportion and number of reticulocytes increase. Because erythroid transit time through the marrow is shortened, "stress reticulocytes" have increased cell volume and surface area (see Chap. 2, Fig. 2-2). They develop characteristic surface folds as a result of the

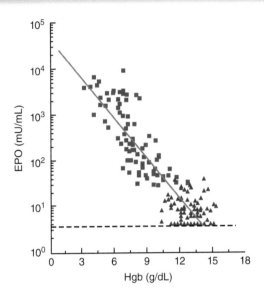

Figure 3–4. Erythropoietin (EPO) levels in plasma of normal individuals and patients with anemia uncomplicated by renal or inflammatory disease. The lower limit of accuracy of the erythropoietin assay is 3 mU/mL and is indicated by the broken line. ■, Anemias; ▲, normals.

increased surface-area-to-volume ratio that can be identified in the blood film. Nucleated red cells may be observed in the blood in severe anemia.[25]

Administration of human recombinant EPO augments or replaces endogenous synthesis. In pharmacologic amounts, the effect on hemoglobin concentration is most noticeable if endogenous production is subnormal as a result of renal failure or systemic illnesses (Chap. 6). In severe anemia where endogenous EPO production (providing production is not impaired) has already increased red cell production maximally, administration of EPO may not help, and the patients require transfusion.[24]

Uncorrected Tissue Hypoxia

A certain residual degree of tissue hypoxia remains despite mobilization of compensatory mechanisms. Hypoxia is essential for initiation of adequate cardiovascular and erythropoietic compensation mechanisms, but severe tissue hypoxia can cause the following symptoms: dyspnea on exertion or even at rest; angina; intermittent claudication; muscle cramps, typically at night; headache; light-headedness; and fatigue. Some diffuse gastrointestinal and genitourinary symptoms are associated with anemia (eg, abdominal cramps, nausea), but whether the symptoms should be attributed to tissue hypoxia, compensatory redistribution of blood, or the underlying cause of anemia is uncertain.

CLASSIFICATION

Anemia can be classified, based on determination of the red cell mass, as (1) *relative* or (2) *absolute*. Relative anemia is characterized by a normal total red cell mass in an increased plasma volume, resulting in a dilution anemia, a disturbance in plasma volume regulation.

Classification of the *absolute anemias* with decreased red cell mass may be challenging because the classification must consider kinetic, morphologic, and pathophysiologic interacting criteria. Anemia of acute hemorrhage is not a diagnostic problem and is usually a genitourinary or gastrointestinal matter, not a hematologic consideration. Initially, all anemias should be divided into anemias caused by decreased production and anemias caused by increased destruction of red cells.

The differentiation is based largely on the reticulocyte count. Subsequent diagnostic breakdown can be based on either morphologic or pathophysiologic criteria.

Morphologic classification subdivides anemia into (1) macrocytic anemia, (2) normocytic anemia, and (3) microcytic hypochromic anemia. The main advantages of this classification are that the classification is simple, is based on readily available red cell indices (eg, mean cell volume [MCV] and mean cell hemoglobin concentration [MCHC]), and forces the physician to consider the most important types of curable anemia: vitamin B_{12}, folic acid, and iron-deficiency anemias. Such practical considerations have led to wide acceptance of this classification.

Pathophysiologic classification (Table 3-1) is best suited for relating disease processes to potential treatment. In addition, anemia resulting from vitamin or iron-deficiency states occurs in a significant proportion of patients with normal red cell indices.

This chapter presents a classification based on our present concepts of normal red cell production and red cell destruction. Figure 3-5 outlines the cascade of proliferation, differentiation, and maturation underlying the transformation of a multipotential stem cell, first to erythroid progenitor cells, then to erythroid precursor cells, and finally to mature red cells. Each of these steps can become impaired and cause anemia. Therapeutic intervention depends on identifying the defective step and instituting the specific therapy. The limitation of such a classification is that in most anemias, the pathogenesis involves several steps. For example, a decreased rate of production most often results in production of defective red cells with a shortened life span. Thus, the outline provided is a conceptual guide to our present understanding of the processes underlying the production and destruction of red cells.

● ERYTHROCYTOSIS

Erythrocytosis is also known as polycythemia.

TERMINOLOGY

Increased red cell mass has been variably termed either *erythrocytosis* or *polycythemia*; no clear consensus for either term has been achieved. In this and related chapters, we have chosen to use the term "polycythemia" only for polycythemia vera and refer to other primary and secondary increases in red cell mass as "erythrocytosis". Here, we and many others interpret the meaning of polycythemia to imply that several hematopoietic lineages are increased, that is, erythrocytosis, neutrophilia, and thrombocytosis. In that case the only form of polycythemia is polycythemia vera. In contrast, an editor of earlier editions of *Williams Hematology*, the late Allan Erslev as well as other red cell experts, argued that the proper meaning of polycythemia is "too many cells in the blood". In that case, other primary and secondary increases in red cell mass also have been termed polycythemias. However, this chapter will reserve the term polycythemia for polycythemia vera.

PATHOPHYSIOLOGY

The production and presence of an increased number of red cells are associated with general and specific effects generated by changes in blood viscosity and blood volume.

The viscosity of blood increases logarithmically with an increase in hematocrit (Fig. 3-6). At hematocrits above the normal range, the increase in blood viscosity impairs blood flow and increases cardiac workload. The resulting decrease in blood flow reduces the transport of oxygen, with average optimal values at hematocrit readings between 40% and 45%.[26,27] In a study of red cells from a number of animal species, the optimal value of oxygen transport corresponded closely to their normal hematocrit levels,[28] which may explain the evolutionary

TABLE 3–1. Classification of Anemia

I. Absolute anemia (decreased red cell volume)

  A. Decreased red cell production

    1. Acquired

      a. Pluripotential hematopoietic stem cell failure

        (1) Autoimmune (aplastic anemia) (Chap. 4)

          (a) Radiation-induced

          (b) Drugs and chemicals (chloramphenicol, benzene, etc)

          (c) Viruses (non-A-G, H hepatitis, Epstein-Barr virus, etc)

          (d) Idiopathic

        (2) Anemia of leukemia and of myelodysplastic syndromes

        (3) Anemia associated with marrow infiltration (Chap. 13)

        (4) Postchemotherapy

      b. Erythroid progenitor cell failure

        (1) Pure red cell aplasia (parvovirus B19 infection, drugs, associated with thymoma, autoantibodies, etc [Chap. 5])

        (2) Endocrine disorders (Chap. 7)

        (3) Acquired sideroblastic anemia (drugs, copper deficiency, etc [Chap. 20])

      c. Functional impairment of erythroid and other progenitors from nutritional and other causes

        (1) Megaloblastic anemias (Chap. 9)

          (a) Vitamin B_{12} deficiency

          (b) Folate deficiency

          (c) Acute megaloblastic anemia because of nitrous oxide (N_2O)

          (d) Drug-induced megaloblastic anemia (pemetrexed, methotrexate, phenytoin toxicity, etc)

        (2) Iron-deficiency anemia (Chap. 11)

        (3) Anemia resulting from other nutritional deficiencies (Chap. 12)

        (4) Anemia of chronic disease and inflammation (Chap. 6)

        (5) Anemia of renal failure (Chap. 2)

        (6) Anemia caused by chemical agents (lead toxicity [Chap. 23])

        (7) Acquired thalassemias (seen in some clonal hematopoietic disorders [Chaps. 17 and 20])

        (8) Erythropoietin antibodies (Chap. 2)

    2. Hereditary

      a. Pluripotential hematopoietic stem-cell failure (Chap. 4)

        (1) Fanconi anemia

        (2) Shwachman syndrome

        (3) Dyskeratosis congenita

      b. Erythroid progenitor cell failure

        (1) Diamond-Blackfan syndrome (Chap. 5)

        (2) Congenital dyserythropoietic syndromes (Chap. 14)

      c. Functional impairment of erythroid and other progenitors from nutritional and other causes

        (1) Megaloblastic anemias (Chap. 9)

          (a) Selective malabsorption of vitamin B_{12} (Imerslund-Gräsbeck disease)

          (b) Congenital intrinsic factor deficiency

          (c) Transcobalamin II deficiency

          (d) Inborn errors of cobalamin metabolism (methylmalonic aciduria, homocystinuria, etc)

          (e) Inborn errors of folate metabolism (congenital folate malabsorption, dihydrofolate deficiency, methyltransferase deficiency, etc)

        (2) Inborn purine and pyrimidine metabolism defects (Lesch-Nyhan syndrome, hereditary orotic aciduria, etc)

        (3) Disorders of iron metabolism (Chap. 11)

          (a) Hereditary atransferrinemia

          (b) Hypochromic anemia caused by divalent metal transporter (DMT)-1 mutation

        (4) Hereditary sideroblastic anemia (Chap. 20)

        (5) Thalassemias (Chap. 17)

(continued)

TABLE 3–1. Classification of Anemia (Coninued)

B. Increased red cell destruction
  1. Acquired
     a. Mechanical
        (1) Macroangiopathic (march hemoglobinuria, artificial heart valves [Chap. 22])
        (2) Microangiopathic (disseminated intravascular coagulation [DIC]; thrombotic thrombocytopenic purpura [TTP]; vasculitis [Chaps. 22])
        (3) Parasites and microorganisms (malaria, bartonellosis, babesiosis, *Clostridium perfringens*, etc (Chap. 24)
     b. Antibody and complement mediated
        (1) Warm-type autoimmune hemolytic anemia (Chap. 26)
        (2) Cryopathic syndromes (cold agglutinin disease, paroxysmal cold hemoglobinuria, cryoglobulinemia (Chaps. 26 and 29)
        (3) Transfusion reactions (immediate and delayed [Chap. 30])
        (4) Paroxysmal nocturnal hemoglobinuria (Chap. 8)
     c. Hypersplenism (Chap. 25)
     d. Red cell membrane disorders (Chap. 15)
        (1) Spur cell hemolysis
        (2) Acquired acanthocytosis and acquired stomatocytosis, etc
     e. Chemical injury and complex chemicals (arsenic; copper; chlorate; spider, scorpion, and snake venoms, etc [Chap. 23])
     f. Physical injury (heat, oxygen, radiation [Chap. 23])
  2. Hereditary
     a. Hemoglobinopathies (Chap. 18)
        (1) Sickle cell disease
        (2) Unstable hemoglobins
     b. Red cell membrane disorders (Chap. 15)
        (1) Cytoskeletal membrane disorders (hereditary spherocytosis, elliptocytosis, pyropoikilocytosis)
        (2) Lipid membrane disorders (hereditary abetalipoproteinemia, hereditary stomatocytosis, etc)
        (3) Membrane disorders associated with abnormalities of erythrocyte antigens (McLeod syndrome, Rh deficiency syndromes, etc)
        (4) Membrane disorders associated with abnormal transport (hereditary xerocytosis)
     c. Red cell enzyme defects (pyruvate kinase, 5'-nucleotidase, glucose-6-phosphate dehydrogenase deficiencies, other red cell enzyme disorders [Chap. 16]
     d. Porphyrias (congenital erythropoietic and hepatoerythropoietic porphyrias, rarely congenital erythropoietic protoporphyria [Chap. 21])
C. Blood loss and blood redistribution
  1. Acute blood loss
  2. Splenic sequestration crisis (Chap. 25)
II Relative (increased plasma volume)
  A. Macroglobulinemia
  B. Pregnancy
  C. Athletes (Chap. 2)
  D. Postflight astronauts (Chap. 2)
  E. Rapid descent from high to low altitude, ie, neocytolysis (Chap. 2)

determination of optimal hematocrit levels.[29] However, before concluding that an elevated red cell mass is always a suboptimal condition, it is inappropriate to correlate viscosity readings, derived from blood tested in a rigid glass viscometer (Ostwald) or even in a cone-plate viscometer, with those in flowing blood through tiny distensible vessels in vivo.[30] First, the flow through these narrow channels is rapid (high shear rate), which in a non-Newtonian fluid such as blood causes a marked decrease in viscosity. Second, blood flowing through narrow channels in vivo is axial, with a central core of packed red cells sliding over a peripheral layer of lubricating low-viscosity plasma. Finally, and most importantly, absolute erythrocytosis is not normovolemic but is accompanied by increased blood volume, which in turn enlarges the vascular bed and decreases peripheral resistance. Because blood pressure remains stable,

the increased blood volume must be associated with increased cardiac output and increased oxygen transport (cardiac output × hemoglobin concentration). Using measurements of cardiac output in dogs[31] and tissue oxygen tension in rats and mice,[30] construction of curves (Fig. 3-7) that relates oxygen transport to hematocrit in normovolemic and hypervolemic states is possible. These curves show that hypervolemia per se increases oxygen transport and that the optimum oxygen transport in these conditions occurs at higher hematocrit values than in normovolemic states. Consequently, despite the increased viscosity, a moderate increase in hematocrit is beneficial. The same may not be true of a more pronounced increase in hematocrit. Observations in humans[32] and experimental animals[31] indicate that high viscosity causes reduced blood flow to most tissues and may be responsible for the cerebral and

ERYTHROPOIESIS

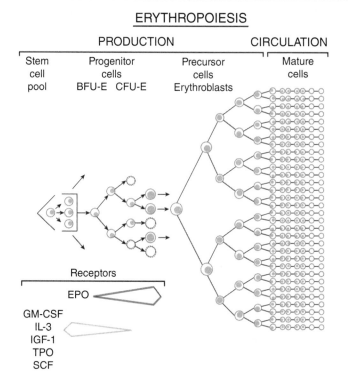

Figure 3–5. Outline of the process of differentiation, proliferation, and maturation underlying the production and destruction of red blood cells. Multipotential stem cells responding to a number of growth factors, including granulocyte-monocyte colony-stimulating factor (GM-CSF), interleukin 3 (IL-3), insulin growth factor 1 (IGF-1), thrombopoietin (TPO), and stem cell factor (SCF), differentiate to progenitor cells committed to erythroid development. Progenitor cells, burst-forming unit–erythroid (BFU-E), and colony-forming unit–erythroid (CFU-E) proliferate under the control of erythropoietin (EPO) and finally differentiate to precursor cells (erythroblasts). In the presence of adequate amounts of nutrients, such as vitamin B_{12}, folic acid, and iron, precursor cells proliferate and mature into nucleated red cells, reticulocytes, and mature red blood cells. After 120-day life span in the circulation, the red cell has undergone age-related changes at which they are removed by the mononuclear phagocyte system with a small residual component of random destruction.

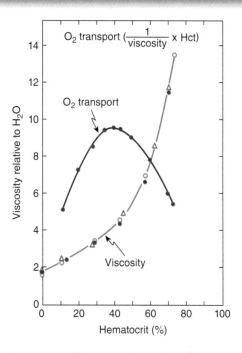

Figure 3–6. Viscosity of heparinized normal human blood related to hematocrit (Hct). Viscosity is measured with an Ostwald viscosimeter at 37°C (98.6°F) and expressed in relation to viscosity of saline solution. Oxygen transport is computed from Hct and O_2 flow (1/*Viscosity*) and is recorded in arbitrary units.

cardiovascular impairment experienced occasionally by high-altitude dwellers,[33] patients with severe erythrocytosis or polycythemia vera,[34,35] and athletes self-administering overdoses of EPO (Chap. 28). Although it has been long argued that the Tibetan evolutionary adaptation to high altitude–associated hypoxia is associated with lower than expected hemoglobin/hematocrit levels similar to low-altitude dwellers,[36] perhaps to protect them from high blood viscosity, the direct measurements of Tibetan subgroup Sherpas in fact showed they have increased red cell volume as well as increased plasma volume, providing not only increased oxygen-binding capacity but also increased tissue oxygen delivery from the increased blood volume.[37]

MANIFESTATIONS

The rate of red cell production is increased in true erythrocytosis, but changes in erythroid marrow cellularity can be difficult to assess by microscopy, although the marrow is hypercellular in a typical patient with polycythemia vera. Under normal conditions, the rate of red cell production is adjusted to maintain the red cell mass at about 30 mL/kg of body weight. Because the life span of red cells in erythrocytosis is

normal, a doubling of the daily rate of red cell production is adequate to maintain a polycythemic red cell mass of 60 mL/kg. Consequently, the morphology and volume of the marrow are only moderately altered in erythrocytosis compared with the changes observed in some types of hemolytic anemia, in which the rate of red cell production can be four to six times normal. In erythrocytosis, the number of red cells destroyed daily merely causes a slight increase in bilirubin levels. The presence of secondary gout and splenomegaly are usually signs of a myeloproliferative neoplasm rather than of erythrocytosis alone. Although considerable homology exists between EPO and thrombopoietin,[38] there is no evidence that the two molecules cross-react at the level of their respective receptors, as discussed in Chap. 28.[39] EPO-driven erythrocytosis is generally not associated with increased platelet production.

The increased viscosity and vascular space are responsible for many of the signs and symptoms of polycythemia vera. The characteristic *rubor* in patients with polycythemia vera is caused by excessive deoxygenation of blood flowing sluggishly through dilated cutaneous vessels. Nonspecific symptoms such as headaches, dizziness, tinnitus, and a reported feeling of fullness of the face and head are probably caused by a combination of increased viscosity and vascular dilatation. In cases of extreme increases in red cell mass and some specific types of erythrocytosis (eg, methemoglobinemia; Chap. 19), cyanosis can result from greater than 40 to 50 g/L of deoxygenated hemoglobin (accomplished more easily at higher hemoglobin concentrations [see "blue bloaters" and "pink puffers" in Chap. 28]) or greater than 15 g/L of methemoglobin and 5 g/L of sulfhemoglobin (Chap. 19).

Hemorrhage from the nose or stomach in patients with normal platelets and coagulation proteins can be attributed to capillary distention; however, circulatory stagnation causing ischemia and necrosis may contribute. Thromboses are common in polycythemia vera but are not seen at similar frequencies in other types of erythrocytoses (Chap. 28). Coronary blood flow is assumed to be decreased in patients

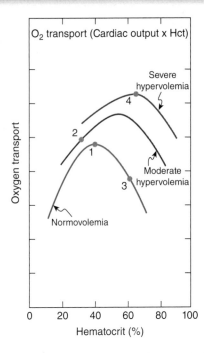

Figure 3–7. Oxygen transport at various hematocrit (Hct) levels in normovolemia, mild hypervolemia, and severe hypervolemia. Oxygen transport is estimated by multiplying Hct by cardiac output. (1) Optimal oxygen transport for normovolemic subjects is at a Hct of approximately 45%, with a progressive increase in optimal Hct as blood volume increases. (2) Suboptimal Hct in a hypervolemic person (anemia of pregnancy) may be associated with higher oxygen transport than in a normovolemic person with normal Hct. (3) High Hct without an increase in blood volume may be associated with an absolute reduction in oxygen transport and tissue hypoxia. (4) Only high Hct coupled with high blood volume enhances oxygen transport to the tissues. *(Data from Murray JF, Gold P, Johnson BL, Jr. The circulatory effects of hematocrit variations in normovolemic and hypervolemic dogs. J Clin Invest. 1963;42:1150; and Thorling EB, Erslev AJ. The "tissue" tension of oxygen and its relation to hematocrit and erythropoiesis. Blood. 1968;31:332.)*

with an increased red cell mass,[34] so the risk of coronary thrombosis in patients with a high hematocrit reading is assumed to be increased; however, statistical analyses have yielded equivocal evidence of such a relationship.[35,40,41] The relationship of the hematocrit to thrombosis has been critically reviewed, indicating that hematocrit does not on its own increase thrombotic risk unless the somatic or germline mutations causing polycythemia and erythrocytosis, respectively, also promote thrombosis (Chap. 28).[42] Erythrocytosis does not pose a risk in surgical patients.[43] Although cerebral blood flow is materially reduced in patients with moderately elevated hematocrit,[32,44] such reductions may have little practical significance. Moreover, in normovolemic individuals, cerebral blood flow decreases after a certain point of hematocrit elevation.[44] However, blood flow is also influenced by the oxygen demand of tissues through incompletely understood mechanisms,[45] and cerebral blood flow remains high at increased hematocrit levels when oxygen delivery is impaired. Thus, patients with high hemoglobin oxygen-affinity variants (Chap. 18) had cerebral blood flow higher than the subjects of comparable age, matched for hematocrit and viscosity, but without the hemoglobin variant.[46] In polycythemia vera, however, it has been advocated that normalization of red cell mass should be accomplished before surgery, but firm data supporting this practice are lacking.

CLASSIFICATION

Erythrocytosis is a condition in which the hematocrit percentage is above the upper limits of normal: higher than 51% in men and 48% in women. Erythrocytosis can be classified as: (1) relative, in which the red cell mass is normal but the plasma volume is decreased, or (2) absolute, in which the red cell mass is increased above normal (Chap. 28). Table 3-2 outlines the types of erythrocytosis.

Differentiation of absolute from relative erythrocytosis can be difficult at hematocrit levels lower than 60%. Designation of a measured red cell mass as normal is imprecise because the red cell mass depends on the patient's age, sex, weight, height, and body frame, and because only increases above the mean of more than 25% of red cell mass are considered abnormal.

Primary Erythrocytosis and Polycythemia

Primary polycythemias are caused by either acquired somatic (polycythemia vera) or inherited germline mutations (such as gain-of-function *EPOR* mutations expressed within hematopoietic progenitors), leading to increased production of red cells causing primary familial and congenital polycythemia (PFCP), also referred to as erythrocytosis.

Secondary Erythrocytosis

Secondary erythrocytosis is caused by augmentation of erythropoiesis by circulating stimulatory factors such as EPO that is hypoxia-induced (eg, high altitude, lung disease), EPO-producing tumors, or cobalt and manganese toxicity (see Table 3-2 for a full list of causes of secondary erythrocytosis and Chap. 28 for a more extensive discussion of the causes of secondary erythrocytosis).

Disorders of Hypoxia Sensing

Erythrocytosis from *VHL* Gene Mutation Chuvash erythrocytosis and some other disorders of hypoxia sensing, including several recessively inherited mutations of the *VHL* gene, have elevated or inappropriately normal EPO levels in relation to elevated hematocrit. This phenotype is different from other, more common *VHL* mutations encompassing VHL tumor predisposition syndrome, wherein dominantly inherited germline *VHL* mutations precede the acquired somatic mutations that eventually result in tumorigenesis (hemangioblastoma, renal cell carcinoma, pheochromocytoma, pancreatic endocrine tumors, and endolymphatic sac tumors). Following the description of Chuvash erythrocytosis (aka Chuvash polycythemia), other homozygous and compound heterozygous inherited *VHL* mutations causing erythrocytosis, but not tumors, have been described (Chap. 28). Some patients with tumor predisposition VHL syndrome also develop acquired erythrocytosis caused by EPO production in tumor tissue.[47]

Clinically, patients with Chuvash erythrocytosis are prone to develop thrombosis, have elevated pulmonary pressure, and have increased mortality independent of the increase in hematocrit.[42]

Erythrocytosis from HIF2α (*EPAS1*) and PHD2 (*EGLN1*) Mutations Dominantly inherited gain-of-function HIF2α (encoded by *EPAS1*) gene mutations have elevated or inappropriately normal EPO levels in relation to elevated hematocrit. All reported polycythemic heterozygotes for loss-of-function PHD2 variants (encoded by the *EGLN1* gene) have normal EPO levels.

The iron availability is needed for the enzyme activity of the principal negative regulator of HIFs—PHD2 and thus iron deficiency increases HIF-1 and HIF-2 levels; these augment erythropoiesis. Further, there is also direct regulation of HIF-2 by iron. The 5′-untranslated region of HIF-2α contains the iron-responsive element that represses the translation of HIF-2. The iron regulatory protein (IRP-1) binds to this 5′-untranslated region of HIF-2α. The deletion of *Irp-1* causes

TABLE 3–2. Classification of Erythrocytosis and Poly

I. Absolute (true) polycythemia (increased red cell volume) (Chap. 28)

  A. Primary erythrocytosis

    1. Acquired

      a. Polycythemia vera

    2. Hereditary (Chap. 28)

      a. Primary familial and congenital erythrocytosis (or polycythemia) (PFCP)

        (1) Erythropoietin receptor mutations

        (2) Unknown gene mutations

  B. Secondary erythrocytosis

    1. Acquired (Chap. 28)

      a. Hypoxemia

        (1) Chronic lung disease

        (2) Right-to-left cardiac shunts

        (3) High altitude

        (4) Smoking

      b. Carboxyhemoglobinemia (Chap. 19)

        (1) Smoking

        (2) Carbon monoxide poisoning

      c. Autonomous erythropoietin production (Chap. 28)

        (1) Hepatocellular carcinoma

        (2) Renal cell carcinoma

        (3) Cerebellar hemangioblastoma

        (4) Pheochromocytoma

        (5) Parathyroid carcinoma

        (6) Meningioma

        (7) Uterine leiomyoma

        (8) Polycystic kidney disease

        (9) Cobalt toxicity

        (10) Manganese toxicity

      d. Exogenous erythropoietin administration ("EPO doping") (Chap. 28)

      e. Complex or uncertain etiology

        (1) Postrenal transplant (probable abnormal angiotensin II signaling) (Chap. 28)

        (2) Androgen/anabolic steroids (Chap. 28)

    2. Hereditary

      a. High-oxygen affinity hemoglobins (Chap. 18)

      b. 2,3-Bisphosphoglycerate deficiency (Chap. 16)

      c. Congenital methemoglobinemias (recessive, ie, cytochrome b5 reductase deficiency, dominant globin mutations [Chap. 19])

  C. Disorders of hypoxia sensing (Chap. 28)

    1. Proven or suspected congenital disorders of hypoxia sensing

      a. Chuvash erythrocytosis (aka Chuvash polycythemia)

      b. High erythropoietin polycythemias caused by mutations of von Hippel–Lindau (*VHL*) gene other than Chuvash mutation

      c. HIF2α (*EPAS1*) mutations

      d. PHD2 (*EGLN1*) mutations

II. Relative (spurious) erythrocytosis (normal red cell volume) (Chap. 28)

  A. Dehydration

  B. Diuretics

  C. Smoking

  D. Gaisböck syndrome

erythrocytoses in mice and incompletely defined inherited polymorphisms of *IRP-1* in several Northern European families and correlate with erythrocytoses and anemia. For more details refer to Chaps. 2 and 28.

Because of the rarity of *EPAS1* and *EGLN1* mutations (Chap. 28), their nonerythroid phenotype is not well-defined; however, some *EPAS1* (HIF2α) mutations, also have a propensity to thrombosis, independent of whether their hematocrit is controlled by phlebotomies.[48] Some *EPAS1* (HIF2α) mutations, associated with genetic mosaicism, have been associated with congenital erythrocytosis and later development of pheochromocytoma/paraganglioma and somatostatinoma tumors. In these instances, in most patients, the *EPAS1* mutation is present in the tumors, which frequently recur, but is difficult to detect in peripheral blood (see Chap. 28).[49,50]

REFERENCES

1. Semenza GL, Nejfelt MK, Chi SM, et al. Hypoxia-inducible nuclear factors bind to an enhancer element located 3′ to the human erythropoietin gene. *Proc Natl Acad Sci U S A.* 991;88:5680.
2. Guillemin K, Krasnow MA. The hypoxic response: huffing and HIFing. *Cell.* 1997;89:9.
3. Hochachka PW, Buck LT, Doll CJ, et al. Unifying theory of hypoxia tolerance: molecular/metabolic defense and rescue mechanisms for surviving oxygen lack. *Proc Natl Acad Sci U S A.* 1996;93:9493.
4. Semenza GL. O2-regulated gene expression: transcriptional control of cardiorespiratory physiology by HIF-1. *J Appl Physiol (1985).* 2004;96:1173.
5. Srinivas V, Zhu X, Salceda S, et al. Hypoxia-inducible factor 1alpha (HIF-1alpha) is a non-heme iron protein. Implications for oxygen sensing. *J Biol Chem.* 1998;273:18019.
6. Ivan M, Kondo K, Yang H, et al. HIFalpha targeted for VHL-mediated destruction by proline hydroxylation: implications for O2 sensing. *Science.* 2001;292:464.
7. Jaakkola P, Mole DR, Tian YM, et al. Targeting of HIF-alpha to the von Hippel-Lindau ubiquitylation complex by O2-regulated prolyl hydroxylation. *Science.* 2001;292:468.
8. Epstein AC, Gleadle JM, McNeill LA, et al. *C. elegans* EGL-9 and mammalian homologs define a family of dioxygenases that regulate HIF by prolyl hydroxylation. *Cell.* 2001;107:43.
9. Edwards MJ, Novy MJ, Walters CL, et al. Improved oxygen release: an adaptation of mature red cells to hypoxia. *J Clin Invest.* 1968;47:1851.
10. Bohr C, Hasselbalch K, Krogh A. Concerning a biologically important relationship: the influence of the carbon dioxide content of blood on its oxygen binding. *Skan Arch Physiol.* 1904;16:401.
11. Moore LG, Brewer GJ. Beneficial effect of rightward hemoglobin-oxygen dissociation curve shift for short-term high-altitude adaptation. *J Lab Clin Med.* 1981;98:145.
12. Huber H, Lewis SM, Szur L. The influence of anaemia, polycythaemia and splenomegaly on the relationship between venous haematocrit and red-cell volume. *Br J Haematol.* 1964;10:567.
13. Vatner SF. Effects of hemorrhage on regional blood flow distribution in dogs and primates. *J Clin Invest.* 1974;54:225.
14. Abramson D, Fierst SM, Flachs K. Resting peripheral blood flow in the anemia state. *Am Heart J.* 1954;25.
15. Bradley SE, Bradley GP. Renal function during chronic anemia in man. *Blood.* 1947;2:192.
16. Merin S, Freund M. Retinopathy in severe anemia. *Am J Ophthalmol.* 1968;66:1102.
17. Duke M, Abelmann WH. The hemodynamic response to chronic anemia. *Circulation.* 1969;39:503.
18. Sharpey-Schafer EP. Cardiac output in severe anemia. *Clin Sci.* 1944;5.
19. Wintrobe MM. The cardiovascular system in anemia; with a note on the particular abnormalities in sickle cell anemia. *Blood.* 1946;1:121.
20. Wales RT, Martin EA. Arterial bruits in anaemia. *Br Med J.* 1963;2:1444.
21. Blumgart HL, Altschule MD. Clinical significance of cardiac and respiratory adjustments in chronic anemia. *Blood.* 1948;3:329.
22. Fatemian M, Gamboa A, Leon-Velarde F, et al. Selected contribution: ventilatory response to CO2 in high-altitude natives and patients with chronic mountain sickness. *J Appl Physiol (1985).* 2003;94:1279.
23. Adamson JW. The erythropoietin-hematocrit relationship in normal and polycythemic man: implications of marrow regulation. *Blood.* 1968;32:597.
24. Erslev AJ. Erythropoietin. *N Engl J Med.* 1991;324:1339.
25. Ward HP, Holman J. The association of nucleated red cells in the peripheral smear with hypoxemia. *Ann Intern Med.* 1967;67:1190.
26. Dintenfass L. A preliminary outline of the blood high viscosity syndromes. *Arch Intern Med.* 1966;118:427.
27. Stone HO, Thompson HK Jr, Schmidt-Nielsen K. Influence of erythrocytes on blood viscosity. *Am J Physiol.* 1968;214:913.
28. Erslev AJ, Caro J, Schuster SJ. Is there an optimal hemoglobin level? *Transfus Med Rev* 1989;3:237.
29. Murray JF, Gold P, Johnson BL Jr. The circulatory effects of hematocrit variations in normovolemic and hypervolemic dogs. *J Clin Invest.* 1963;42:1150.
30. Thorling EB, Erslev AJ. The "tissue" tension of oxygen and its relation to hematocrit and erythropoiesis. *Blood.* 1968;31:332.
31. Fan FC, Chen RY, Schuessler GB, et al. Effects of hematocrit variations on regional hemodynamics and oxygen transport in the dog. *Am J Physiol.* 1980;238:H545.
32. Pearson TC, Humphrey PRD, Thomas DJ, et al. hematocrit, blood viscosity, cerebral blood flow, and vascular occlusion. In: Lowe GDO, ed. *Clinical Aspects of Blood Viscosity and Cell Deformability.* Springer-Verlag; 1981.
33. Monge CM, Monge CC. *High-Altitude Diseases: Mechanism and Management.* Chas. C. Thomas; 1966.
34. Kershenovich S, Modiano M, Ewy GA. Markedly decreased coronary blood flow in secondary polycythemia. *Am Heart J.* 1992;123:521.
35. Conley CL, Russell RP, Thomas CB, et al. Hematocrit values in coronary artery disease. *Arch Intern Med.* 1964;113:170.
36. Beall CM. Two routes to functional adaptation: Tibetan and Andean high-altitude natives. *Proc Natl Acad Sci U S A.* 2007;104(Suppl 1):8655.
37. Stembridge M, Williams AM, Gasho C, et al. The overlooked significance of plasma volume for successful adaptation to high altitude in Sherpa and Andean natives. *Proc Natl Acad Sci U S A.* 2019;116:16177.
38. Kaushansky K. Thrombopoietin. *N Engl J Med.* 1998;339:746.
39. Geddis AE, Kaushansky K. Cross-reactivity between erythropoietin and thrombopoietin at the level of Mpl does not account for the thrombocytosis seen in iron deficiency. *J Pediatr Hematol Oncol.* 2003;25:919.
40. Mayer GA. Hematocrit and coronary heart disease. *Can Med Assoc J.* 1965;93:1151.
41. Hershberg PI, Wells RE, McGandy RB. Hematocrit and prognosis in patients with acute myocardial infarction. *JAMA.* 1972;219:855.
42. Gordeuk VR, Key NS, Prchal JT. Re-evaluation of hematocrit as a determinant of thrombotic risk in erythrocytosis. *Haematologica.* 2019;104:653.
43. Lubarsky DA, Gallagher CJ, Berend JL. Secondary polycythemia does not increase the risk of perioperative hemorrhagic or thrombotic complications. *J Clin Anesth.* 1991;3:99.
44. Thomas DJ, du Boulay GH, Marshall J, et al. Cerebral blood-flow in polycythaemia. *Lancet.* 1977;2:161.
45. Borzage MT, Bush AM, Choi S, et al. Predictors of cerebral blood flow in patients with and without anemia. *J Appl Physiol (1985).* 2016;120:976.
46. Wade JP, du Boulay GH, Marshall J, et al. Cerebral blood flow, haematocrit and viscosity in subjects with a high oxygen affinity haemoglobin variant. *Acta Neurol Scand.* 1980;61:210.
47. Friedrich CA. Genotype-phenotype correlation in von Hippel-Lindau syndrome. *Hum Mol Genet.* 2001;10:763.
48. Gordeuk VR, Miasnikova GY, Sergueeva AI, et al. Thrombotic risk in congenital erythrocytosis due to up-regulated hypoxia sensing is not associated with elevated hematocrit. *Haematologica.* 2020;105(3):e87-e90.
49. Zhuang Z, Yang C, Lorenzo F, et al. Somatic HIF2A gain-of-function mutations in paraganglioma with polycythemia. *N Engl J Med.* 2012;367:922.
50. Lorenzo FR, Yang C, Ng Tang Fui M, et al. A novel EPAS1/HIF2A germline mutation in a congenital polycythemia with paraganglioma. *J Mol Med (Berl).* 2013;91:507.

PART III Diseases of Red Cell Production

CHAPTER 4
APLASTIC ANEMIA: ACQUIRED AND INHERITED

George B. Segel and Marshall A. Lichtman

SUMMARY

Acquired aplastic anemia is a clinical syndrome in which there is a deficiency of red cells, neutrophils, monocytes, and platelets in the blood, and fatty replacement of the marrow with a near absence of hematopoietic precursor cells. Reticulocytopenia is a constant feature. Neutropenia, monocytopenia, and thrombocytopenia, when severe, are life-threatening because of the risk of infection and bleeding, complicated by severe anemia. Most cases occur without an evident precipitating cause and are the result of autoreactive cytotoxic T lymphocytes that suppress or destroy primitive CD34+ multipotential hematopoietic cells. The disorder also can occur after (1) prolonged high-dose exposure to certain toxic chemicals (eg, benzene); (2) after specific viral infections (eg, Epstein-Barr virus [EBV]); (3) as an idiosyncratic response to certain pharmaceuticals (eg, ticlopidine, chloramphenicol); (4) as a feature of an autoimmune disorder (eg, lupus erythematosus); or, rarely, (5) in association with pregnancy. The final common pathway is through cytotoxic T-cell autoreactivity, whether idiopathic or associated with an inciting agent, because they all respond in a similar fashion to immunosuppressive therapy. The differential diagnosis of acquired aplastic anemia includes a hypoplastic marrow that can accompany paroxysmal nocturnal hemoglobinuria (PNH) or hypoplastic oligoblastic (myelodysplastic syndrome [MDS]) or polyblastic (acute) myelogenous leukemia. Allogeneic hematopoietic cell transplantation is curative in approximately 80% of younger patients with high-resolution human leukocyte antigen (HLA)–matched sibling donors, although the posttransplant period may be complicated by severe graft-versus-host disease. The disease may be significantly ameliorated or sometimes cured by immunotherapy, especially a regimen coupling antithymocyte globulin (ATG) with cyclosporine. However, after successful treatment with immunosuppressive agents, the disease may relapse or evolve into a clonal myeloid disorder, such as PNH, a clonal cytopenia, or oligoblastic or polyblastic myelogenous leukemia. The addition of eltrombopag (EPAG) to immunotherapy has increased the response rate and the quality of the response. Several uncommon inherited disorders, including Fanconi anemia (FA), Shwachman-Diamond syndrome, dyskeratosis congenita, and others have aplastic hematopoiesis as a primary manifestation.

INTRODUCTION
ACQUIRED APLASTIC ANEMIA

DEFINITION AND HISTORY

Aplastic anemia is a clinical syndrome that results from a marked diminution of marrow blood cell production. The decrease in hematopoiesis results in reticulocytopenia, anemia, granulocytopenia, monocytopenia, and thrombocytopenia. The diagnosis usually requires the presence of pancytopenia with a neutrophil count fewer than 1.5×10^9/L, a platelet count fewer than 50×10^9/L, a hemoglobin concentration less than 100 g/L, and an absolute reticulocyte count fewer than 40×10^9/L, accompanied by a hypocellular marrow without abnormal or malignant cells or fibrosis.[1] For the purpose of therapeutic decision making, comparative clinical trials, and international sharing of data, the disease has been stratified into moderately severe, severe, and very severe acquired aplastic anemia based on the blood counts (especially the neutrophil count) and the degree of marrow hypocellularity (Table 4-1). Most cases of aplastic anemia are acquired; many fewer cases are the result of an inherited disorder, such as Fanconi anemia (FA), Shwachman-Diamond syndrome, and others (see "Hereditary Aplastic Anemia" fruther).

Aplastic anemia was first recognized by Paul Ehrlich in 1888.[2] He described a young, pregnant woman who died of severe anemia and neutropenia. Thrombocytopenia was difficult to measure and the role of blood dust (platelets) was controversial at that time. Autopsy examination revealed a fatty marrow with essentially no hematopoiesis. The name *anémie pernicieuse aplastique* was subsequently applied to this disease by Chauffard, a French hematologist, in 1904,[3] and although an anachronistic term because the morbidity is the result of pancytopenia, especially neutropenia and thrombocytopenia, the designation "aplastic anemia" is entrenched in medical usage. For the next 40 years, many conditions that caused pancytopenia were confused with aplastic anemia based on incomplete or inadequate histologic study of the patient's marrow.[4] The development of improved instruments for percutaneous marrow biopsy in the last half of the 20th century improved diagnostic precision. In 1972, Thomas and his colleagues established that marrow transplantation from a histocompatible sibling donor could cure the disease.[5] The disease initially was thought to result from an atrophy or chemical injury of primitive marrow hematopoietic cells. The unexpected recovery of marrow recipients who were given immunosuppressive conditioning therapy, but who did not engraft with donor stem cells raised the possibility that the disease may not be intrinsic to primitive hematopoietic cells but the result of a suppression of hematopoietic cells by immune cells, notably T lymphocytes.[6] The requirement to treat the recipient of a marrow transplant from an identical twin with immunosuppressive conditioning therapy for optimal results of transplant, buttressed this concept.[7] This supposition was confirmed by a clinical trial that established antilymphocyte globulin (ALG) capable of ameliorating the disease in the majority of patients.[8] Since that time, compelling

Acronyms and Abbreviations: A, adenine; ALG, antilymphocyte globulin; ALL, acute lymphocytic leukemia; AML, acute myelogenous leukemia; ATG, antithymocyte globulin; ATR, ataxia-telangiectasia mutated and rad3-related kinase; BFU-E, burst-forming unit–erythroid; CAMT, congenital (hereditary) amegakaryocytic thrombocytopenia; CD, cluster of differentiation; CFU-GM, colony-forming unit–granulocyte-macrophage; cMpl, thrombopoietin receptor; CMV, cytomegalovirus; DDT, dichlorodiphenyltrichloroethane; EBV, Epstein-Barr virus; EPAG, eltrombopag; ELF6, eukaryotic initiation factor 6; EPO, erythropoietin; G, guanine; G-CSF, granulocyte colony-stimulating factor; HIV, human immunodeficiency virus; HLA, human leukocyte antigen; IL, interleukin; JAK, Janus kinase; MDS, myelodysplastic syndrome; MRI, magnetic resonance imaging; NIH, National Institutes of Health; PCP, pentachlorophenol; PNH, paroxysmal nocturnal hemoglobinuria; ppm, parts per million; SCF, stem cell factor; TERC, telomerase RNA component; TERT, telomerase reverse transcriptase; Th1, T-cell helper type 1; TNF, tumor necrosis factor; TNT, trinitrotoluene; TPO, thrombopoietin.

TABLE 4–1. Degree of Severity of Acquired Aplastic Anemia

Diagnostic Categories	Hemoglobin	Reticulocyte Concentration	Neutrophil Count	Platelet Count	Marrow Biopsy	Comments
Moderately severe	<100 g/L	$<40.0 \times 10^9$/L	$<1.5 \times 10^9$/L	$<50.0 \times 10^9$/L	Marked decrease of hematopoietic cells	At the time of diagnosis at least 2 of 3 blood counts should meet these criteria
Severe	<90 g/L	$<30.0 \times 10^9$/L	$<0.5 \times 10^9$/L	$<30.0 \times 10^9$/L	Marked decrease or absence of hemato-poietic cells	Search for a histocompatible donor should be made if age permits
Very severe	<80 g/L	$<20.0 \times 10^9$/L	$<0.2 \times 10^9$/L	$<20.0 \times 10^9$/L	Marked decrease or absence of hemato-poietic cells	Search for a histocompatible donor should be made if age permits

These values are approximations and must be considered in the context of an individual patient's situation. In some clinical trials, the blood count thresholds for moderately severe aplastic anemia are higher (eg, platelet count $<100 \times 10^9$/L and absolute reticulocyte count $<60 \times 10^9$/L.) The marrow biopsy may contain the usual number of lymphocytes and plasma cells; "hot spots," infrequent focal areas of erythroid cells, may be seen. No fibrosis, abnormal cells, or malignant cells should be evident in the marrow. Dysmorphic features of blood or marrow cells are not features of acquired aplastic anemia. Ethnic differences in the lower limit of the absolute neutrophil count should be considered.

evidence for a cellular autoimmune mechanism has accumulated (see "Etiology and Pathogenesis" further).

EPIDEMIOLOGY

The International Aplastic Anemia and Agranulocytosis Study and a French study found the incidence of acquired aplastic anemia to be approximately 2 per 1,000,000 persons per year.[1,9] This annual incidence has been confirmed by studies in Spain (Barcelona),[10] Brazil (State of Parana),[11] and Canada (British Columbia).[12] The highest frequency of aplastic anemia occurs in persons between the ages of 15 and 25 years; a second peak occurs between the ages of 65 and 69 years.[1] Aplastic anemia is more prevalent in the Far East, where the incidence is approximately 7 per 1,000,000 in parts of China,[13] approximately 4 per 1,000,000 in sections of Thailand,[14] approximately 5 per 1,000,000 in areas of Malaysia,[15] and approximately 7 per 1,000,000 among children of Asian descent living in Canada.[12] The explanation for a twofold or greater incidence in the Orient compared to the Occident may be multifactorial,[16] but a predisposition gene or genes is a likely component.[12,17] Studies have not established the use of chloramphenicol in Asia as a cause. Poorly regulated exposure of workers to benzene is a factor,[18] but the attributable risk from benzene and other toxic exposures does not explain the magnitude of the difference in the incidence in Asia compared with that in Europe and South America.[16,17] A relationship to impure water use in Thailand has led to speculation of an infectious etiology, although no agent, including seronegative hepatitis, a known association with the onset of acquired aplastic anemia,[16] has been identified. Seronegative viral hepatitis is a forerunner of approximately 7% of cases of acquired aplastic anemia.[17,19] The male-to-female incidence ratio of aplastic anemia in most studies is approximately one.[17] A high incidence of acquired aplastic anemia (23%-33%) also has been documented in patients after receiving liver transplant for seronegative hepatitis.[20]

● ETIOLOGY AND PATHOGENESIS

Table 4-2 lists the conditions associated with aplastic anemia.

The final common pathway to the clinical disease is a decrease in blood cell formation in the marrow. The number of marrow CD34+ cells (multipotential hematopoietic progenitors) and their derivative colony-forming unit–granulocyte-macrophage (CFU-GM) and burst-forming unit–erythroid (BFU-E) are reduced markedly in patients

with aplastic anemia,[21-24] as are colony-forming unit-megakaryocytes (CFU-Mk). Long-term culture-initiating cells, an in vitro surrogate assay for hematopoietic stem cells, also are reduced to approximately 1% of normal values.[24] Potential mechanisms responsible for acquired marrow cell failure include (1) cellular or humoral immune suppression of the marrow multipotential or stem cells, (2) progressive erosion of chromosome telomeres, (3) direct toxicity to hematopoietic multipotential or stem cells, (4) a defect in the stromal microenvironment of the marrow required for hematopoietic cell development, and (5) impaired production or release of essential multilineage hematopoietic growth factors. There is little experimental evidence for a stromal microenvironmental defect or a deficit of critical hematopoietic growth factors or their receptors. Telomerase mutations with consequent telomere shortening may be involved in as many as 40% of patients.[25] A susceptibility to the development of aplastic anemia is present in persons with certain human leukocyte antigen (HLA) types, such as HLA-DR15.[25]

Deficiencies in telomere repair could predispose to aplastic anemia by affecting the size of the multipotential hematopoietic cell compartment and by decreasing the multipotential cell's response to marrow injury, and could play a role in the evolution of aplastic anemia to a clonal myeloid disease by contributing to genomic instability.[26] Reduced hematopoiesis in most cases of aplastic anemia results from cytotoxic T-cell–mediated immune suppression of very early CD34+ hematopoietic multipotential progenitor or stem cells.[27] A small fraction of cases is initiated by a toxic exposure, drug exposure, or viral infection, and in these cases the pathogenesis also may relate to autoimmunity because there is evidence of immune dysfunction in seronegative hepatitis after benzene exposure, and many such patients respond to anti–T-cell therapy.[27]

Autoreactive Cytotoxic T Lymphocytes

In vitro and clinical observations have resulted in the identification of a cytotoxic T-cell–mediated attack on multipotential hematopoietic cells in the CD34+ cellular compartment as the basis for most cases of acquired aplastic anemia.[28] Cellular immune injury to the marrow after drug-, viral-, or toxin-initiated marrow aplasia could result from the induction of neoantigens that provoke a secondary T-cell–mediated attack on hematopoietic cells. This mechanism could explain the response to immunosuppressive treatment in cases that follow exposure to an exogenous agent.

Spontaneous or mitogen-induced increases in mononuclear cell production of interferon-γ,[29,30] interleukin (IL)-2,[30] and tumor necrosis

TABLE 4–2. Etiologic Classification of Aplastic Anemia

Acquired

Autoimmune

Drugs

   See Table 4-3

Toxins

   Benzene

   Chlorinated hydrocarbons

   Organophosphates

Viruses

   Epstein-Barr virus

  Non-A, -B, -C, -D, -E, or -G hepatitis virus

   HIV

Paroxysmal nocturnal hemoglobinuria

Autoimmune/connective tissue disorders

   Eosinophilic fasciitis

   Immune thyroid disease (Graves disease, Hashimoto thyroiditis)

   Rheumatoid arthritis

   Systemic lupus erythematosus

Thymoma

Pregnancy

Iatrogenic

   Radiation

   Cytotoxic drug therapy

Inherited

Fanconi anemia

Dyskeratosis congenita

Shwachman-Diamond syndrome

Other rare syndromes (see Table 4-12)

factor-α (TNF-α)[31,32] occur. These factors are inhibitory to hematopoietic cell development. Elevated serum levels of interferon-γ are present in 30% of patients with aplastic anemia, and interferon-γ expression has been detected in the marrow of most patients with acquired aplastic anemia.[33] Addition of antibodies to interferon-γ enhances in vitro colony growth of marrow cells from affected patients.[34] Long-term marrow cultures manipulated to elaborate exaggerated amounts of interferon-γ, markedly reduced the frequency of long-term culture-initiating cells.[27] These observations indicate that acquired aplastic anemia is the result of cellular immune-induced apoptosis of primitive CD34+ multipotential hematopoietic progenitors, mediated by cytotoxic T lymphocytes, in part, through the expression of T-helper type 1 (Th1) inhibitory cytokines, interferon-γ, and TNF-α (Fig. 4-1).[35] The secretion of interferon-γ is a result of the upregulation of the regulatory transcription factor T-bet,[36] and apoptosis of CD34+ cells is, in part, mediated through a FAS-dependent pathway.[27] Because HLA-DR2 is more prevalent in patients with aplastic anemia, antigen recognition may be a factor in those patients.

A variety of other potential factors have been found in some patients, including nucleotide polymorphisms in cytokine genes, overexpression of perforin in marrow cells, and decreased expression of SLAM-associated protein (SAP), a modulator protein that inhibits interferon-γ secretion.[27]

A decrease in regulatory T cells (CD4+CD25+FoxP3+) contributes to the expansion of an autoreactive CD8+CD28− T-cell population

and results in altered expression of T-cell receptor signaling molecules, which induces apoptosis of autologous hematopoietic multipotential hematopoietic cells.[37-40] T-regulatory cells are a component of the immune system that suppress immune responses of other cells. They provide a "stop" for immune reactions that have achieved their purpose. They also play a role in preventing autoimmune reactions. One mouse model of immune-related marrow failure, induced by infusion of parental lymph node cells into F1 hybrid recipients, caused a fatal aplastic anemia. The aplasia could be prevented by immunotherapy or with monoclonal antibodies to interferon-γ and TNF-α.[27] Another mouse model of aplastic anemia induced by the infusion of lymph node cells histoincompatible for the minor H antigen, H60, resulted from the expansion of H60-specific CD8 T cells in recipient mice. The result was severe marrow aplasia. The effect of the CD8 T cells could be abrogated by either immunosuppressive agents or administration of CD4+CD25+ regulatory T cells,[41] providing additional experimental evidence for the role of regulatory T cells in the prevention of aplastic anemia. There are two subsets of regulatory T cells, Treg A and Treg B, with distinct phenotypes.[42] Treg B cells have a greater expression of CD95, CCR4, and CD45RO antigens than do Treg A cells. Patients with aplastic anemia who respond to immunotherapy have a predominance of Treg B cells.

Several putative target antigens on affected hematopoietic cells have been identified. Autoantibodies to one putative antigen, kinectin, have been found in patients with aplastic anemia. T cells, responsive to kinectin-derived peptides, suppress granulocyte-monocyte colony growth in vitro. However, in these studies, cytotoxic T lymphocytes with that specificity were not isolated from patients.[43] Thus, the putative antigen(s) that is (are) the target of the autoreactive T cells has (have) not been identified.

Telomere Shortening

A relationship between acquired aplastic anemia and hereditary aplastic anemia (FA or dyskeratosis congenita) has been suggested because the defects in telomerase and telomere repair, characteristic of FA and dyskeratosis congenital, are shared in some adult patients with aplastic anemia, but in these cases there is no family history of such a disorder and no phenotypic abnormalities that characterize the hereditary disorders (see "Fanconi Anemia" and "Dyskeratosis Congenita" further). Telomeres shorten physiologically with age as telomerase becomes less active. T-cell–mediated acquired aplastic anemia is associated with telomere shortening, which could reflect an inherited defect in telomerase or a senescent erosion of activity. The telomerase mechanism consists of a telomerase reverse transcriptase (TERT), an RNA template for TERT, the telomerase RNA component (TERC), and other stabilizing proteins.[44,45] Cells with shortened telomeres normally undergo apoptosis unless DNA repair mechanisms are impaired, allowing the development of aneuploidy and neoplastic transformation.

Drugs

Chloramphenicol is the most notorious drug documented to cause aplastic anemia. Although this drug is directly myelosuppressive at very high doses because of its effect on mitochondrial DNA, the occurrence of aplastic anemia appears to be idiosyncratic; perhaps related to an inherited sensitivity to the nitroso-containing toxic intermediates.[46] This sensitivity may produce immunologic marrow suppression, because a substantial proportion of affected patients respond to treatment with immunosuppressive therapy.[47] The risk of developing aplastic anemia in patients treated with chloramphenicol is approximately 1 in 20,000, or 25 times that of the general population.[48] Although its use as an antibiotic has been largely abandoned in industrialized countries, global reports of fatal aplastic anemia continue to appear with topical or systemic use of the drug.

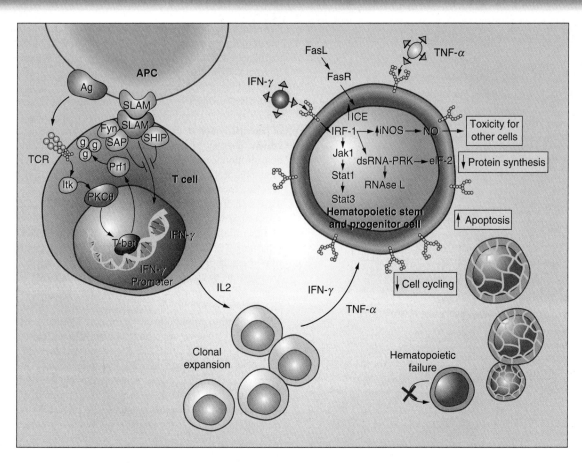

Figure 4–1. Immune pathogenesis of apoptosis of CD34 multipotential hematopoietic cells in acquired aplastic anemia. Antigens are presented to T lymphocytes by antigen-presenting cells (APCs). This triggers T cells to activate and proliferate. T-bet, a transcription factor, binds to the interferon-γ (IFN-γ) promoter region and induces gene expression. SLAM-associated protein (SAP) binds to Fyn and modulates the signaling lymphocyte activation molecule (SLAM) activity on IFN-γ expression, diminishing gene transcription. Patients with aplastic anemia show constitutive T-bet expression and low SAP levels. IFN-γ and tumor necrosis factor-α (TNF-α) upregulate both the T cell's cellular receptors and the Fas receptor. Increased production of interleukin-2 leads to polyclonal expansion of T cells. Activation of the Fas receptor by the Fas ligand leads to apoptosis of target cells. Some effects of IFN-γ are mediated through interferon regulatory factor 1 (IRF-1), which inhibits the transcription of cellular genes and entry into the cell cycle. IFN-γ is a potent inducer of many cellular genes, including inducible nitric oxide synthase (iNOS), and production of the toxic gas, nitric oxide (NO), may further diffuse the toxic effects. These events ultimately lead to reduced cell cycling and cell death by apoptosis. *(Reproduced with permission from Young NS, Calado RT, Scheinberg P: Current concepts in the pathophysiology and treatment of aplastic anemia,* Blood *2006 Oct 15;108[8]:2509-2519.)*

Epidemiologic evidence established that quinacrine (Atabrine) increased the risk of aplastic anemia.[49] This drug was administered to all US troops in the South Pacific and Asiatic theaters of operations as prophylaxis for malaria during 1943 and 1944. The incidence of aplastic anemia was 7 to 28 cases per 1,000,000 personnel per year in the prophylaxis zones, whereas untreated soldiers had 1 to 2 cases per 1,000,000 personnel per year. The aplasia occurred during administration of the offending agent and was preceded by a characteristic rash in nearly half the cases. Many other drugs have been reported to increase the risk of aplastic anemia but, owing to incomplete reporting of information and the infrequency of the association, the spectrum of drug-induced aplastic anemia may not be fully appreciated. Table 4-3 is a partial list of drugs that have been implicated.[50-58]

Many of these drugs are known to also induce selective cytopenias, such as agranulocytosis, which usually are reversible after discontinuation of the offending agent. These reversible reactions are not correlated with the risk of aplastic anemia, casting doubt on the effectiveness of routine monitoring of blood counts as a strategy to avoid aplastic anemia.

Because aplastic anemia is a rare event with drug use, it may occur because of an underlying metabolic or immunologic predisposition (gene polymorphism) in susceptible individuals. In the case of phenylbutazone-associated marrow aplasia, there is delayed oxidation and clearance of a related compound, acetanilide, compared with either normal controls or those with aplastic anemia from other causes. This finding suggests excess accumulation of the drug as a potential mechanism for the aplasia. In some cases, drug interactions or synergy may be required to induce marrow aplasia. Cimetidine, a histamine H_2-receptor antagonist, is occasionally implicated in the onset of cytopenias and aplastic anemia, perhaps owing to a direct effect on early hematopoietic progenitor cells.[59] This drug accentuates the marrow-suppressive effects of the chemotherapy drug carmustine.[60] In several instances, it has been reported as a possible cause of marrow aplasia when given with chloramphenicol. An association of the immune check-point inhibitor, nivolumab, with marrow aplasia was described in a patient treated for a glioblastoma.[61]

There appears to be little difference in the age distribution, gender, response to immunotherapy or hematopoietic cell transplantation, or

TABLE 4–3. Drugs Associated with Aplastic Anemia

Category	High Risk	Intermediate Risk	Low Risk
Analgesic			Phenacetin, aspirin, salicylamide
Antiarrhythmic			Quinidine, tocainide
Antiarthritic		Gold salts	Colchicine
Anticonvulsant		Carbamazepine, hydantoins, felbamate	Ethosuximide, phenacemide, primidone, trimethadione, sodium valproate
Antihistamine			Chlorpheniramine, pyrilamine, tripelennamine
Antihypertensive			Captopril, methyldopa
Anti-inflammatory		Penicillamine, phenylbutazone, oxyphenbutazone	Diclofenac, ibuprofen, indomethacin, naproxen, sulindac
Antimicrobial			
Antibacterial		Chloramphenicol	Dapsone, methicillin, penicillin, streptomy-cin, β-lactam antibiotics
Antifungal			Amphotericin, flucytosine
Antiprotozoal		Quinacrine	Chloroquine, mepacrine, pyrimethamine
Antineoplastic drugs			
Alkylating agent	Busulfan, cyclophosphamide, melphalan, nitrogen mustard		
Antimetabolite	Fluorouracil, mercaptopurine, methotrexate		
Cytotoxic antibiotic	Daunorubicin, doxorubicin, mitoxantrone		
Antiplatelet			Ticlopidine
Antithyroid			Carbimazole, methimazole, methylthiouracil, potassium perchlorate, propylthiouracil, sodium thiocyanate
Sedative and tranquilizer			Chlordiazepoxide, chlorpromazine (and other phenothiazines), lithium, meprobam-ate, methyprylon
Sulfa derivative		Sulfonamides	
Antibacterial			Numerous sulfonamides
Diuretic		Acetazolamide	Chlorothiazide, furosemide
Hypoglycemic			Chlorpropamide, tolbutamide
Miscellaneous			Allopurinol, interferon, pentoxifylline, penicillamine

Drugs that invariably cause marrow aplasia with high doses are considered high risk; drugs with 30 or more reported cases are listed as moderate risk; others are less often associated with aplastic anemia (low risk).[50]

This list was compiled from the AMA Registry, publications of the International Agranulocytosis and Aplastic Anemia Study, and other reviews and studies.

survival, related to whether a drug exposure preceded the onset of the marrow aplasia.

Toxic Chemicals

Benzene was the first chemical linked to aplastic anemia, based on studies in factory workers before the 20th century.[62-64] Benzene is used as a solvent and is employed in the manufacture of chemicals, drugs, dyes, and explosives. It has been a vital chemical in the manufacture of rubber and leather goods and has been used widely in the shoe industry, leading to an increased risk for aplastic anemia (and acute myelogenous leukemia [AML]) in workers exposed to a poorly regulated environment.[64] In studies in China, aplastic anemia among workers was sixfold higher than in the general population.[18]

The United States Occupational Safety and Health Administration has lowered the permissible atmospheric exposure limit of benzene to 1 part per million (ppm) (8-hour time-weighted average) and short-term exposure to 5 ppm (15-minute time-weighted average). The National Institute for Occupational Safety and Health recommends limits of exposure of 0.1 ppm as the 8-hour weighted average and 1 ppm for 15-minute short-term exposure. Before that regulatory change, the frequency of aplastic anemia in workers exposed to greater than 100 ppm benzene was approximately 1 in 100 workers, which decreased to 1 in 1000 workers at 10 to 20 ppm exposure.[63]

Organochlorine and organophosphate pesticide compounds have been suspected in the onset of aplastic anemia,[65,66] and several studies have indicated an increased relative risk, especially for agricultural exposures[11,16,67,68] and household[11,68] exposures. These relationships are suspect because dose–disease relationships and other important factors have not been delineated, and several studies have not found an association with environmental exposures.[12,69] Dichlorodiphenyl-trichloroethane (commonly known as DDT), lindane, and chlordane are insecticides that also have been associated with cases of aplastic anemia.[16,66] Occasional cases still occur after heavy exposure at industrial plants or after its use as a pesticide.[70] Lindane is metabolized in part to pentachlorophenol (PCP), another potentially toxic chlorinated hydrocarbon that is manufactured for use as a wood preservative. Cases of aplastic anemia and related blood disorders have been attributed to PCP over the past 25 years.[66,71] Prolonged exposures to petroleum distillates in the form of Stoddard solvent[72] and acute exposure to toluene through the practice of glue sniffing[73,74] also have been reported to cause marrow aplasia. Trinitrotoluene (commonly known as TNT), an explosive used extensively during World Wars I and II, is absorbed readily by inhalation and through the skin.[75] Fatal cases of aplastic anemia were observed in munitions workers exposed to TNT in Great Britain[76] from 1940 to 1946. In most cases, these conclusions have not been derived from specific studies but from accumulation of case reports or from patient histories, making conclusions provisional, although the argument for minimizing exposures to potential toxins is logical in any case.

Viruses

Non-A, -B, -C, -D, -E, -G Hepatitis Virus A relationship between hepatitis and the subsequent development of aplastic anemia has been the subject of a number of case reports, and this association was emphasized by two major reviews in the 1970s.[77,78] In the aggregate, these reports summarized findings in more than 200 cases. In many instances, the hepatitis was improving or had resolved when the aplastic anemia was noted 4 to 12 weeks later. Approximately 10% of cases occurred more than 1 year after the initial diagnosis of hepatitis. Most patients were young (18-20 years); two-thirds were male, and their survival was short (10 weeks). Although hepatitides A and B have been implicated in aplastic anemia in a small number of cases, most cases are related to non-A, non-B, non-C hepatitis.[79-81] Severe aplastic anemia developed in 9 of 31 patients who underwent liver transplantation for non-A, non-B, non-C hepatitis, but in none of 1463 patients who received transplants for other indications.[82] Several lines of evidence indicate there is no causal association with hepatitis C virus, suggesting that an unknown viral agent is involved.[16,83,84] Hepatitis virus B or C can be a secondary infection if carefully screened blood products are not used for transfusion. In 15 patients with posthepatitic aplastic anemia, no evidence was found for hepatitis A, B, C, D, E, or G, transfusion-transmitted virus, or parvovirus B19.[85] Several reports have suggested a relationship of parvovirus B19 to aplastic anemia,[86,87] whereas others have not.[82] This relationship has not been established (Chap. 5). The effect of seronegative hepatitis may be mediated through an autoimmune T-cell effect because of evidence of T-cell activation and cytokine elaboration.[27] These patients also have a similar response to hematopoietic cell transplantation[88] and to combined immunotherapy as do those with idiopathic aplastic anemia[89-91] (see "Treatment: Combination Immunotherapy" further).

Epstein-Barr Virus Epstein-Barr virus (EBV) has been implicated in the pathogenesis of aplastic anemia.[92,93] The onset usually occurs within 4 to 6 weeks of infection. In some cases, infectious mononucleosis is subclinical, with a finding of reactive lymphocytes in the blood film and serologic results consistent with a recent infection. EBV has been detected in marrow cells,[93] but it is uncertain whether marrow aplasia results from a direct effect or an immunologic response by the host. Patients have recovered after therapy with antithymocyte globulin (ATG).[93]

Other Viruses Human immunodeficiency virus (HIV) infection frequently is associated with varying degrees of cytopenia. The marrow is often cellular, but occasional cases of aplastic anemia have been noted.[94-96] Marrow hypoplasia may result from viral suppression and from the drugs used to control viral replication in this disorder. Human herpesvirus-6 has caused severe marrow aplasia subsequent to hematopoietic cell transplantation for other disorders.[97]

Autoimmune Diseases

The incidence of severe aplastic anemia was sevenfold greater than expected in patients with rheumatoid arthritis.[56] It is uncertain whether the aplastic anemia is related directly to rheumatoid arthritis or to the various drugs used to treat the condition (gold salts, d-penicillamine, and nonsteroidal anti-inflammatory agents). Occasional cases of aplastic anemia are seen in conjunction with systemic lupus erythematosus.[98] In vitro studies found either the presence of an antibody[99] or suppressor cell[100,101] directed against hematopoietic progenitor cells. Patients have recovered after plasmapheresis,[98] glucocorticoids,[100] or cyclophosphamide therapy,[99,101,102] which is compatible with an immune etiology.

Eosinophilic fasciitis, an uncommon connective tissue disorder with painful swelling and induration of the skin and subcutaneous tissue, has been associated with aplastic anemia.[103,104] Although it may be antibody-mediated in some cases, it has been largely unresponsive to therapy.[103] Nevertheless, (1) hematopoietic cell transplantation, (2) immunosuppressive therapy using cyclosporine, (3) immunosuppressive therapy using ATG, or (4) immunosuppressive therapy with ATG and cyclosporine has cured or significantly ameliorated the disease in a few patients.[103,104]

Severe aplastic anemia also has been reported coincident with immune thyroid disease (Graves disease)[105-109] and the aplasia has been reversed with treatment of the hyperthyroidism. Aplastic anemia has occurred in association with thymoma.[110-115] Autoimmune renal disease and aplastic anemia have occurred concurrently. The underlying relationship may be the role of cytotoxic T lymphocytes in the pathogenesis of several autoimmune diseases and in aplastic anemia.[116]

Pregnancy

There are a number of reports of pregnancy-associated aplastic anemia, but the relationship between the two conditions is not always clear.[117-122] In some patients, preexisting aplastic anemia is exacerbated with pregnancy, only to improve after termination of the pregnancy.[117,118] In other cases, the aplasia develops during pregnancy with recurrences during subsequent pregnancies.[118-121] Termination of pregnancy or delivery may improve the marrow function, but the disease may progress to a fatal outcome even after delivery.[117-119] Therapy may include elective termination of early pregnancy, supportive care, immunosuppressive therapy, or hematopoietic cell transplantation after delivery. Pregnancy in women previously treated with immunosuppression for aplastic anemia can result in the birth of a normal newborn.[122] In this latter study of 36 pregnancies, 22 were uncomplicated, 7 were complicated by a relapse of the marrow aplasia, and 5 without marrow aplasia required red cell transfusion during delivery.[119] One death occurred from cerebral thrombosis in a patient with paroxysmal nocturnal hemoglobinuria (PNH) and marrow aplasia.

Iatrogenic Causes

Although marrow toxicity from cytotoxic chemotherapy or radiation produces direct damage to stem cells and more mature cells, resulting in marrow aplasia, most patients with acquired aplastic anemia cannot relate an exposure that would be responsible for marrow damage.

Chronic exposure to low doses of radiation or use of spinal radiation for ankylosing spondylitis is associated with an increased, but delayed, risk of developing aplastic anemia and acute leukemia.[123,124] Patients who were given thorium dioxide (Thorotrast) as an intravenous contrast medium had numerous late complications, including malignant liver tumors, acute leukemia, and aplastic anemia.[125] Chronic radium poisoning, with osteitis of the jaw, osteogenic sarcoma, and aplastic anemia, was seen in workers who painted watch dials with luminous paint when they moistened the brushes orally.[126]

Acute exposures to large doses of radiation are associated with the development of marrow aplasia and a gastrointestinal syndrome.[127-130] Total-body exposure to between 1 and 2.5 Gy leads to gastrointestinal symptoms and depression of leukocyte counts, but most patients recover. A dose of 4.5 Gy leads to death in half the individuals (LD_{50}) owing to marrow failure. Higher doses in the range of 10 Gy are universally fatal unless the patient receives extensive supportive care followed by hematopoietic cell transplantation. Aplastic anemia associated with nuclear accidents was seen after the disaster that occurred at the Chernobyl nuclear power station in the Ukraine in 1986.[129]

Antineoplastic drugs such as alkylating agents, antimetabolites, and certain cytotoxic antibiotics have the potential for producing marrow aplasia. In general, this is transient, is an extension of their pharmacologic action, and resolves within several weeks of completing chemotherapy. Although unusual, severe marrow aplasia can follow use of the alkylating agent, busulfan, and may persist indefinitely. Marrow aplasia may develop in patients 2 to 5 years after discontinuation of alkylating agent therapy. These cases often evolve into hypoplastic myelodysplastic syndromes (MDS).

Stromal Microenvironment and Growth Factors

Short-term clonal assays for marrow stromal cells have shown variable defects in stromal cell function in patients with aplastic anemia. Serum levels of stem cell factor (SCF) have been either moderately low or normal in several studies of aplastic anemia.[131,132] Although SCF augments the growth of hematopoietic colonies from aplastic anemia patients' marrows, its use in patients has not led to clinical remissions. Another early-acting growth factor, FLT-3 ligand, is 30- to 100-fold elevated in the serum of patients with aplastic anemia; although the pathobiologic effect of this change is unclear.[133] Fibroblasts grown from patients with severe aplastic anemia have subnormal cytokine production. However, serum levels of granulocyte colony-stimulating factor (G-CSF),[134] erythropoietin (EPO),[135] and thrombopoietin (TPO)[136] are usually high. Synthesis of IL-1, an early stimulator of hematopoiesis, is decreased in mononuclear cells from patients with aplastic anemia.[137] Studies of the microenvironment have shown relatively normal stromal cell proliferation and growth factor production.[138] These findings, coupled with the limited response of patients with aplastic anemia to growth factors, suggest that cytokine deficiency is not the etiologic problem in most cases. The marrow stem cell niche may be altered by the immune disorder in aplastic anemia, but conclusive evidence of such a contributing factor is still being explored.[139] Because most patients transplanted for aplastic anemia are cured with allogeneic donor stem cells and, presumably, autologous stroma, the primary etiology appears to be the cytoxic T-cell effect.[140]

A rare exception to the negligible pathogenetic role of hematopoietic growth factors in the etiology of aplastic anemia is the homozygous or mixed heterozygous mutation of the TPO receptor gene, *MPL*, which can cause amegakaryocytic thrombocytopenia that evolves later into aplastic anemia. Furthermore, eltrombopag (EPAG), a TPO receptor agonist, can stimulate mono- or, in some patients, bilineage or trilineage recovery of blood counts that may be sustained off therapy (see "Treatment: Eltrombopag" further).

CLINICAL FEATURES

The onset of symptoms of aplastic anemia may be gradual with pallor, weakness, dyspnea, and fatigue as a result of the anemia. Dependent petechiae, bruising, epistaxis, vaginal bleeding, and unexpected bleeding at other sites secondary to thrombocytopenia are frequent presenting signs of the underlying marrow disorder. Rarely, it may be more dramatic with fever, chills, and pharyngitis or other sites of infection resulting from severe neutropenia and monocytopenia. Physical examination generally is unrevealing except for evidence of anemia (eg, conjunctival and cutaneous pallor, resting tachycardia) or cutaneous bleeding (eg, ecchymoses and petechiae), gingival bleeding, and intraoral purpura. Lymphadenopathy and splenomegaly are not features of aplastic anemia; such findings suggest an alternative diagnosis such as a clonal myeloid or lymphoid disease.

LABORATORY FEATURES

Blood Findings

Patients with aplastic anemia have varying degrees of pancytopenia. Anemia is associated with a low reticulocyte index. The reticulocyte count is usually less than 1% and may be zero despite the high levels of EPO. Absolute reticulocyte counts are usually fewer than 40×10^9/L. Macrocytes may be present in the blood film and the mean cell volume increased. The absolute neutrophil and monocyte count are low. An absolute neutrophil count fewer than 0.5×10^9/L along with a platelet count fewer than 30×10^9/L is indicative of severe disease, and a neutrophil count below 0.2×10^9/L denotes very severe disease (see Table 4-1). Lymphocyte production is thought to be normal, but patients may have mild lymphopenia. Platelets function normally. Significant qualitative changes of red cell, leukocyte, or platelet morphology on the blood film are not features of classical acquired aplastic anemia. Occasionally only one cell line is depressed initially, which may lead to an early diagnosis of pure red cell aplasia or amegakaryocytic thrombocytopenia. In such patients, other cell lines will fail shortly thereafter (days to weeks) and permit a definitive diagnosis. Table 4-4 is a plan for the initial laboratory investigation.

Plasma Findings

The plasma contains high levels of hematopoietic growth factors, including EPO, TPO, and myeloid colony-stimulating factors. Growth factor levels need not be measured, however, for clinical care. Plasma iron values are usually high, and ^{59}Fe clearance is prolonged, with decreased incorporation into red cells.

Marrow Findings

Morphology The marrow aspirate typically contains numerous spicules with empty, fat-filled spaces, and relatively few hematopoietic cells. Lymphocytes, plasma cells, macrophages, and mast cells may be present. Occasional spicules are cellular or even hypercellular ("hot spots"), but megakaryocytes usually are reduced. These focal areas of residual hematopoiesis do not appear to be of prognostic significance. Residual granulocytic cells generally appear normal, but it is not unusual to see mild macronormoblastic erythropoiesis, presumably as a result of the high levels of EPO. Marrow biopsy is essential to confirm the overall hypocellularity (Fig. 4-2), because a poor yield of spicules

TABLE 4–4. Approach to Diagnosis

- History and physical examination
- Complete blood counts, reticulocyte count, and examination of the blood film
- Marrow aspiration and biopsy
- Marrow cell cytogenetics to evaluate clonal myeloid disease
- DNA stability test as an initial marker of FA (may occur in early adulthood without phenotypic changes)
- Telomerase length as initial marker for dyskeratosis congenita (may occur in adulthood without phenotypic changes)
- Immunophenotyping of red and white cells, especially for CD55, CD59 to exclude PNH
- Direct and indirect antiglobulin (Coombs) test to rule out immune cytopenia
- Serum lactate dehydrogenase and uric acid, which if increased may reflect neoplastic cell turnover
- Liver function tests to assess for evidence of any recent viral hepatitis
- Screening tests for hepatitis viruses A, B, and C
- Screening tests for EBV, CMV, and HIV
- Serum B_{12} and red cell folic acid levels to rule out cryptic megaloblastic pancytopenia
- Serum iron, iron-binding capacity, and ferritin as a baseline before chronic transfusion therapy

Abbreviations: CMV, cytomegalovirus; EBV, Epstein-Barr virus; FA, Fanconi anemia; HIV, human immunodeficiency virus; PNH, paroxysmal nocturnal hemoglobinuria.

and cells occurs in marrow aspirates in other disorders, especially if fibrosis is present.

In severe aplastic anemia, as defined by the International Aplastic Anemia Study Group, less than 25% cellularity or less than 50% cellularity with less than 30% hematopoietic cells is seen in the marrow.

Progenitor Cell Growth In vitro CFU-GM and BFU-E CFU-Mk colony assays reveal a marked reduction in progenitor cells.[22-24]

Cytogenetic and Genetic Studies Cytogenetic analysis may be difficult to perform owing to low cellularity; thus, multiple aspirates may be required to provide enough cells for study. The results are normal in aplastic anemia. Clonal cytogenetic abnormalities in otherwise apparent aplastic anemia are indicative of an underlying hypoplastic clonal myeloid disease.[141] The move to newer techniques such as microarray-based comparative genomic hybridization permits detection of aneuploidies, deletions, duplications, and/or amplifications of any locus represented on an array. In addition, microarray-based comparative genomic hybridization is an effective tool for the detection of submicroscopic chromosomal abnormalities. This approach would increase the sensitivity to detect chromosome abnormalities in very hypocellular marrow samples, compared with standard G-banding, despite dilution of scant hematopoietic cells with nonhematopoietic stromal cells (eg, fibroblasts). Next-generation sequencing of targeted exons has uncovered 32 mutations associated with myeloid malignancies. These mutations occurred in nearly 20% (29 of 150 patients) of cases of aplastic anemia. These mutations include the genes *ASXL1*, *DNMT3A*, and *BCOR*, which are considered driver mutations in MDS and AML. Seventeen of the 29 patients with one of these three mutations had progression to overt myelodysplasia.[142]

Imaging Studies Magnetic resonance imaging (MRI) can be used to distinguish between marrow fat and hematopoietic cells.[143] This approach may be a more useful overall estimate of marrow hematopoietic cell density than morphologic techniques and may help differentiate hypoplastic myelogenous leukemia from aplastic anemia.

DIFFERENTIAL DIAGNOSIS

Any disease that can present with pancytopenia may mimic aplastic anemia if only the blood counts are considered. Measurement of the reticulocyte count and an examination of the blood film and marrow biopsy are essential early steps to arrive at a diagnosis. A reticulocyte percentage of less than 0.5% is strongly indicative of aplastic erythropoiesis and, when coupled with leukopenia and thrombocytopenia, points to aplastic anemia. Absence of qualitative abnormalities of cells on the blood film and a markedly hypocellular marrow are characteristics of acquired aplastic anemia. The disorders most commonly confused with severe aplastic anemia include approximately 5% to 10%

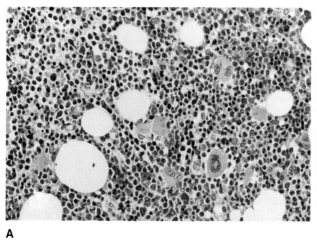
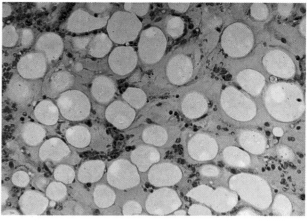

A

B

Figure 4–2. Marrow biopsy in aplastic anemia. **A.** A normal marrow biopsy section of a young adult. **B.** The marrow biopsy section of a young adult with very severe aplastic anemia. The specimen is devoid of hematopoietic cells and contains only scattered lymphocytes and stromal cells. The hematopoietic space is replaced by reticular cells (pre-adipocytic fibroblasts) converted to adipocytes.

of patients with MDS who present with a hypoplastic rather than a hypercellular marrow. Myelodysplasia should be considered if there is abnormal blood film morphology consistent with myelodysplasia (eg, poikilocytosis, basophilic stippling, neutrophils with hypogranulation, or the pseudo–Pelger-Hüet anomaly). Marrow erythroid precursors in myelodysplasia may have dysmorphic features. Pathologic sideroblasts are inconsistent with aplastic anemia and a frequent feature of myelodysplasia. Granulocyte precursors may have reduced or abnormal granulation. Megakaryocytes may have abnormal nuclear lobulation (eg, unilobular micromegakaryocytes). If clonal cytogenetic abnormalities are found, a clonal myeloid disorder, especially MDS or hypocellular myelogenous leukemia is likely. MRI studies of bone may be useful in differentiating severe aplastic anemia from clonal myeloid syndromes. The former gives a fatty signal and the latter a diffuse cellular pattern.

A hypocellular marrow frequently is associated with PNH. PNH is characterized by an acquired mutation in the *PIG-A* gene that encodes an enzyme that is required to synthesize mannolipids. The gene mutation prevents the synthesis of the glycosylphosphatidylinositol anchor precursor. This moiety anchors several proteins, including inhibitors of the complement pathway to blood cell membranes, and its absence accounts for the complement-mediated hemolysis in PNH. As many as 50% of patients with otherwise typical aplastic anemia have evidence of glycosylphosphatidylinositol molecule defects and diminished phosphatidylinositol-anchored protein on leukocytes and red cells as judged by flow cytometry, analogous to that seen in PNH.[144] The decrease or absence of these membrane proteins may make the PNH clone of cells resistant to the acquired immune attack on normal marrow components, or the phosphatidylinositol-anchored protein(s) on normal cells provides an epitope that initiates an aberrant T-cell attack, leaving the PNH clone relatively resistant (Chap. 8).[27]

Occasionally, apparent aplastic anemia may be the prodrome to childhood[145] or, less commonly, adult[146] acute lymphoblastic leukemia. Sometimes, careful examination of marrow cells by light microscopy or flow cytometry will uncover a population of leukemic lymphoblasts. In other cases, the acute leukemia may appear later. Hairy-cell leukemia, Hodgkin lymphoma, or another lymphoma subtype, rarely, may be preceded by a period of marrow hypoplasia. Immunophenotyping of marrow and blood cells by flow cytometry for CD25 may uncover the presence of hairy cells. Other clinical features may be distinctive. Organomegaly such as lymphadenopathy, hepatomegaly, or splenomegaly are inconsistent with the atrophic (hypoproliferative) features of aplastic anemia. Large granular lymphocytic leukemia also has been associated with aplastic anemia. Rare cases of typical acquired aplastic anemia have been followed by t(9;22)-positive acute lymphocytic leukemia or chronic myelogenous leukemia.[146]

RELATIONSHIP AMONG APLASTIC ANEMIA, PAROXYSMAL NOCTURNAL HEMOGLOBINURIA, AND CLONAL MYELOID DISEASES

In addition to the diagnostic difficulties occasionally presented by patients with hypoplastic MDS, hypoplastic AML, or PNH with hypocellular marrows, there may be a more fundamental relationship among these three diseases and aplastic anemia. The development of clonal cytogenetic abnormalities such as monosomy 7 or trisomy 8 in a patient with aplastic anemia portends the evolution of a MDS or acute leukemia. Occasionally, these cytogenetic markers have been transient, and in cases with disappearance of monosomy 7, hematologic improvement has occurred as well.[147] Persistent monosomy 7 carries a poor prognosis compared with trisomy 8.[148,149]

As many as 20% of patients with aplastic anemia have a 5-year probability of myelodysplasia developing.[147] If one excludes any transformation to a clonal myeloid disorder that occurs up to 6 months after treatment to avoid misdiagnosis among the hypoplastic clonal myeloid diseases, the frequency of a clonal myeloid disorder was nearly 15 times greater in patients treated with immunosuppression compared with those treated with hematopoietic cell transplantation after 39 months of observation.[150] This finding suggests that either immune suppression by anti–T-cell therapy enhances the evolution of a neoplastic clone or that it does not suppress the intrinsic tendency of aplastic anemia to evolve to a clonal disease, but provides the increased longevity of the patient required to express that potential. The latter interpretation is more likely because patients successfully treated solely with androgens developed clonal disease as frequently as those treated with immunosuppression.[151] Transplantation may reduce the potential to clonal evolution in patients with aplastic anemia by reestablishing robust lymphohematopoiesis.

Telomere shortening also may play a pathogenetic role in the evolution of aplastic anemia into myelodysplasia. Patients with aplastic anemia have shorter telomere lengths than matched controls, and patients with aplastic anemia with persistent cytopenias had greater telomere shortening over time than matched controls. Clonal cytogenetic changes developed in 3 of 5 patients with telomere lengths less than 5 kb, whereas such diseases did not develop in patients with longer telomeres.[24,152]

The findings of mutated genes considered driver mutations in MDS or AML (see "Marrow Findings: Cytogenetic and Genetic Studies" earlier) in nearly 20% of a population of patients with clinical aplastic anemia indicate that clonal hematopoiesis may develop or be present surreptitiously. The precise relationships to aplastic anemia are uncertain but could be the result of the outgrowth of a clone of cells in the background of severally suppressed polyclonal hematopoietic stem cells. These findings are more common in patients with a long duration of disease and with shorter telomeres.[142]

The relationship of PNH to aplastic anemia remains enigmatic. Because hematopoietic stem cells lacking the phosphatidylinositol-anchored proteins are present in many or all normal persons in very small numbers,[153] it is not surprising that more than 50% of patients with aplastic anemia may have a PNH cell population detected by immunophenotyping.[144] The probability of patients with aplastic anemia developing a clinical syndrome consistent with PNH is 10% to 20%, and this is not a consequence of immunosuppressive treatment.[147] Patients also may present with the hemolytic anemia of PNH, and progressive marrow failure may later develop, so that any pathogenetic explanation should consider both types of development of aplastic marrows in PNH, one preceding the diagnosis of PNH and one following the diagnosis of PNH. The *PIG-A* mutation may confer either a proliferative or survival advantage to PNH cells.[154,155] A survival advantage could result if the anchor protein or one of its ligands served as an epitope for the T-lymphocyte cytotoxicity, which induces the marrow aplasia. In this case, the presenting event could either reflect cytopenias or the sensitivity of red cells to complement lysis and hemolysis, depending on the intrinsic proliferative potential of the PNH clone.

Within our current state of knowledge, aplastic anemia is an autoimmune process, and any residual hematopoiesis is presumably polyclonal. This concept is a critical distinction from de novo hypoplastic leukemia and PNH, which are clonal (neoplastic) diseases. However, many patients with aplastic anemia develop somatic mutations in *BCOR*, *BCORL1*, *ASXL1*, and *DNMT3A* genes in addition to the clonal expansion of the PNH clone (*PIGA* gene). *ASXL1* and *DNMT3A* mutations increased in prevalence with patient age, whereas *BCOR*, *BCORL1*, and *PIGA* mutations were of similar frequency in all age groups. Mutations in

BCOR1/BCORL1 portend a favorable outcome of therapy, but the significance of other mutations is as yet unclear.[156] The environment of the aplastic marrow, however, may favor the eventual evolution of a mutant (malignant) clone, especially if immunotherapy is used, whereas hematopoietic cell transplantation may either ablate threatening minor clones or establish more robust hematopoiesis, an environment less conducive to clonal evolution.

TREATMENT

Approach to Therapy

Severe anemia, bleeding from thrombocytopenia, and, uncommonly at the time of diagnosis, infection secondary to granulocytopenia and monocytopenia requires prompt attention to remove potential life-threatening conditions and improve patient comfort (Table 4-5). More specific treatment of the marrow aplasia involves three principal options: (1) syngeneic or allogeneic hematopoietic cell transplantation or (2) combination immunosuppressive therapy with ATG and cyclosporine, and, since 2014, (3) EPAG, a cytokine shown to improve hematopoiesis in a significant proportion of patients with aplastic anemia. The latter has been used alone to rescue refractory or relapsed patients after immunotherapy or, now, as part of a triple-drug treatment combined with ATG and cyclosporine. The selection of the specific mode of treatment depends on several factors, including the patient's age and condition and the availability of a suitable allele-level HLA-matched hematopoietic stem cell donor. In general, transplantation is the preferred treatment for children and most otherwise healthy younger adults. Early histocompatibility testing of siblings or of unrelated donors is of particular importance because it establishes whether there is an optimal donor available to the patient for transplantation. The preferred stem cell source is a histocompatible sibling matched at the HLA-A, -B, -C, and -DR loci, but an allele-level HLA-matched unrelated donor can be used in younger patients.

Supportive Care

The Use of Blood Products   Although it has been recommended that red cell and platelet transfusions be used sparingly in potential transplant recipients to minimize sensitization to histocompatibility antigens, this has become less important since ATG and cyclophosphamide

---

TABLE 4–5. Initial Management of Aplastic Anemia

- Discontinue any potential offending drug and use an alternative class of agents if essential.
- Anemia: Transfusion of leukocyte-depleted, irradiated red cells as required for very severe anemia.
- Very severe thrombocytopenia or thrombocytopenic bleeding: Consider ε-aminocaproic acid; transfusion of CMV-negative, leukocyte-reduced, and irradiated platelets as required.
- Severe neutropenia; use infection precautions
- Fever (suspected infection): Microbial cultures; broad-spectrum antibiotics if specific organism not identified, G-CSF in dire cases. If child or small adult with profound infection (eg, gram-negative bacteria, fungus, persistent positive blood cultures) can consider granulocyte transfusion from a G-CSF pretreated donor.
- Immediate assessment for allogeneic hematopoietic cell transplantation: Histocompatibility testing of patient, parents, and siblings. Search databases for unrelated donor, if appropriate.

Abbreviations: CMV, cytomegalovirus; G-CSF, granulocyte colony-stimulating factor.

---

have been used as the preparative regimen for transplantation in aplastic anemia, because their use has markedly reduced the problem of graft rejection.[157]

Cytomegalovirus (CMV)-reduced-risk red cells and platelets should be given to a potential transplant recipient to minimize problems with CMV infections after transplantation. Once a patient is shown to be CMV-positive, this restriction is no longer necessary. Leukocyte-depletion filters or CMV serotesting are equivalent methods of decreasing the risk of transmitting CMV.

Red Cell Transfusion   Packed red cells to alleviate symptoms of anemia usually are indicated at hemoglobin values below 80 g/L, unless comorbid medical conditions require a higher hemoglobin concentration. These products should be leukocyte-depleted to lessen leukocyte and platelet sensitization and to reduce subsequent transfusion reactions and radiated to reduce the potential for a transfusion-related graft-versus-host reaction. It is important not to transfuse patients with red cells (or platelets) from family members if transplantation within the family is remotely possible, because this approach may sensitize patients to minor histocompatibility antigens, increasing the risk of graft rejection after hematopoietic cell transplantation. After a transplant, or in those individuals in whom transplantation is not a consideration, family members may be ideal donors for platelet products. Because each unit of red cells adds approximately 200 mg of iron to the total-body iron, over the long-term, transfusion-induced iron overload may occur. This is not a major problem in patients who respond to transplantation or immunosuppressive therapy, but it is an issue in nonresponders who require continued transfusion support. In the latter case, consideration should be given to iron-chelation therapy. Newer oral agents make this procedure easier to effect (Chap. 17).[158]

Platelet Transfusion   It is important to assess the risk of bleeding in each patient. Most patients tolerate platelet counts of $10 \times 10^9/L$ without undue bruising or bleeding, unless a systemic infection is present or vascular integrity is impaired.[159,160] A traumatic injury or surgery requires transfusion to greater than $50 \times 10^9/L$ platelets or greater than $100 \times 10^9/L$, respectively. Administration of ε-aminocaproic acid, 50 mg/kg per dose every 4 hours orally or intravenously, may reduce the bleeding tendency.[161] Pooled random-donor platelets may be used until sensitization ensues, although it is preferable to use leukocyte-reduced and irradiated single-donor platelets from the onset to minimize sensitization to HLA or platelet antigens. Subsequently, single-donor apheresis products or HLA-matched platelets may be required.

Platelet refractoriness is a major problem with long-term transfusion support.[162] This event may occur transiently, with fever or infection, or as a chronic problem secondary to HLA sensitization. In the past, this occurred in approximately 50% of patients after 8 to 10 weeks of transfusion support. Filtration of blood and platelet concentrates to remove leukocytes reduces this problem to approximately 15% of patients receiving chronic transfusions.[162,163] Patients should also receive ABO-identical platelets because this enhances platelet survival and further decreases refractoriness to platelet transfusion. Single-donor HLA-matched apheresis-harvested platelets may be necessary in previously pregnant or transfused patients who are already allosensitized or who become so after treatment with leukoreduced platelets. The frequency of either of these events is less than 10%.

Management of Neutropenia   Neutropenic precautions should be applied to hospitalized patients with a severe depression of the neutrophil count. The level of neutrophils requiring precautions is fewer than $0.5 \times 10^9/L$. One approach is to use private rooms, with requirements for face masks and handwashing with antiseptic soap. Unwashed fresh fruits and vegetables should be avoided because they are sources of bacterial contamination. It is uncommon for patients with aplastic anemia to present with a significant infection. When patients with aplastic anemia become febrile, cultures should be obtained from the throat, sputum (if any), blood, urine, stool, and any suspicious lesions. Broad-spectrum bactericidal antibiotics should be initiated promptly, without awaiting culture results. The choice of antibiotics depends on the prevalence of organisms and their antibiotic sensitivity in the local setting. Organisms of concern usually include *Staphylococcus aureus* (notably methicillin- and oxacillin-resistant strains), *S. epidermidis* (in patients with venous access devices), and gram-negative organisms. Patients with persistent culture-negative fevers should be considered for antifungal treatment.

Documented invasive aspergillosis unresponsive to amphotericin (particularly in the posttransplant setting), infections with organisms resistant to all-known antibiotics, and blood cultures that remain positive despite antibiotic treatment may require leukocyte transfusions from G-CSF–treated donors.[164] Granulocyte transfusion is more effective in children and adults with smaller body size, because transfused leukocytes have a smaller distribution space, which results in higher blood and tissue concentrations.

Specific Treatment

Hematopoietic Cell Transplantation as Primary Treatment Prompt therapy usually is indicated for patients with severe aplastic anemia. The major curative approach is hematopoietic cell transplantation from a histocompatible sibling (Table 4-6).[165-167] Only 20% to 30% of patients in the United States have compatible sibling donors (related to average family size). Haploidentical transplants are feasible when combined with intensive graft-versus-host disease prophylaxis.[168] In the unusual case of an identical twin donor, conditioning is required to obliterate the immune disease in the recipient, but it can be limited to cyclophosphamide. In this setting, an 80% to 90% 10-year survival rate is expected. Marrow stem cells perform better than blood stem cells when used as a source for patients with aplastic anemia, although this is under continued study. The results of transplantation are best in patients younger than 20 years (80%-90% long-term survival), but decrease every decade of increasing age thereafter. Posttransplant mortality is increased and survival decreased with increasing age. In patients older than 40 years, survival in matched-sibling transplant is reduced to approximately 50%.[169] There are still uncertainties about the optimal conditioning program in younger and older patients. ATG, cyclophosphamide, total-body radiation, fludarabine, and alemtuzumab are among the agents being studied.[165,167-170] Alemtuzumab-containing regimens appear to improve outcome by decreasing the frequency of chronic graft-versus-host disease, which could make it useful in treating older patients.[170-172]

Table 4-6 displays results of hematopoietic cell transplantation for aplastic anemia in children and adults compiled by the Center for International Blood & Marrow Transplant Research.

The longer the delay between diagnosis and transplantation, the less likely is a salutary outcome, probably as a result of a greater number of transfusions and a higher likelihood of pretransplantation infection. Acute and chronic graft-versus-host disease are serious complications, and therapy to prevent or ameliorate them is a standard part of post-transplantation treatment.[165,169] Transplantations have been performed using stem cells from partially matched siblings or unrelated, histocompatible donors recruited through the National Marrow Donor Program or similar organizations in other countries.[173,174] Umbilical cord blood is an effective alternative source of stem cells from unrelated donors (or, rarely, siblings) for transplantation in children or young adults,[171] but the results are optimal with HLA-matched sibling transplantation. Alternatively, the use of high-resolution, HLA typing of a matched, unrelated donor markedly improves the prognosis for transplantation.[175] High-resolution DNA donor-recipient matching at HLA-A, -B, -C, and -DRB1 (8 of 8 alleles) is considered the lowest level of matching consistent with the highest level of survival. If there is an HLA mismatch at one or more loci, especially HLA-A or -DRB1, the outcome is compromised,[175] and immunosuppression with combined therapy may be preferred initially, depending on patient age, CMV status, and disease severity. Older patients have a much less frequent favorable response with alternative, non–matched-sibling donor transplantations. The use of hematopoietic cell transplantation can be considered for patients who do not or no longer respond to immunotherapy.[168] If the patient in question is a candidate for hematopoietic cell transplantation based on all relevant factors, transplantation could be considered at any age for a patient with a syngeneic donor; transplantation could be considered a first-choice therapy up to 50 years of age for a patient with an HLA allele-level–matched sibling donor; and transplantation could be considered a first-choice therapy if an allele-level HLA-matched unrelated donor is available for patients younger than 20 years, especially if the transplant can be initiated within 3 months from diagnosis.[168,176] These guidelines are subject to the special circumstances of an individual case. For example, if patients with aplastic anemia undergo gene sequencing and a mutation known to be a driver mutation for myelodysplasia or AML is found, allogeneic hematopoietic cell transplantation may be a preferred treatment approach.

Components of Immunosuppressive Therapy

Antilymphocyte and Antithymocyte Globulin ATG and ALG act principally by reducing cytotoxic T cells. This involves ATG-induced apoptosis through both FAS and TNF pathways.[177] Cathepsin B also plays a role in T-cell cytotoxicity at clinical concentrations of ATG, but may involve an independent apoptosis pathway.[178] ATG and ALG also release hematopoietic growth factors from T cells.[179,180] Horse and rabbit ATG are licensed in the United States. Skin tests against horse serum should be performed before administration.[181] If found to be positive, the patient may be desensitized. For example, ATG therapy, 40 mg/kg, can be given intravenously, over 4 hours daily for 4 days. Several studies have compared equine with rabbit ATG in the immunotherapy of aplastic anemia, contemporaneously or using historical comparisons.

TABLE 4–6. Allogeneic Marrow Transplantation for Severe Aplastic Anemia (Percent Survival)

		Years of Observation					
		1	2	3	4	5	6
HLA-matched related	Pediatric <18 y, N = 1044	92	91	90	90	90	90
HLA-matched related	Adult ≥18 y, N = 1427	81	79	78	78	78	77
HLA-matched unrelated	Pediatric <18 y, N = 727	81	80	79	79	79	78
HLA-matched unrelated	Adult ≥18 y, N = 1024	72	69	68	67	65	64

Abbreviation: HLA, human leukocyte antigen.

The consensus is that equine ATG is superior to rabbit and, if available, is recommended as the first line of therapy (Table 4-7).[182-190] Nevertheless, rabbit ATG is effective and should be considered if equine ATG does not result in a satisfactory outcome (Fig. 4-3).

ATG treatment may accelerate platelet destruction, reduce the absolute neutrophil count, and cause a positive direct antiglobulin (Coombs') test. This effect may lead to an increase in transfusion requirements during the period of treatment. Serum sickness, characterized by spiking fevers, skin rashes, and arthralgia, commonly occurs 7 to 10 days from the first dose. The clinical manifestations of serum sickness can be diminished by administering a glucocorticoid (eg, prednisone 1 mg/kg) from day 1 of ATG treatment and for 2 weeks thereafter. Fever, rigors, rash, hypotention, and hypoxia can be minimized by administration of acetaminophen and diphenhydramine before each dose of ATG. This approach may require supplementation with intravenous hydration for hypotension and oxygen administration for hypoxia. Occasionally, a patient may require continuation of therapy in an intensive care unit. In cases of severe reactions, the administration of ATG can be slowed or temporarily discontinued until improvement occurs, and then reinstituted at a slower rate of infusion if necessary. With these adaptions, the course of ATG can be completed in most patients.[191] Approximately one-third of patients no longer require transfusion support after treatment with ATG alone.[192-194]

Of 358 patients responding to immunosuppressive therapy, principally ATG alone, 74 (21%) relapsed after a mean of 2.1 years. The actuarial incidence of relapse was 35% at 10 years.[195] Similar results were observed when 227 patients were treated with immunosuppression, primarily ATG alone.[196] The actuarial survival at 15 years was 38% after immunosuppression.[195] However, a combination of immunosuppressive agents provides more effective therapy than ATG alone (see "Combination Immunotherapy" further).

Of 129 patients treated with ALG 28 (22%) saw development of myelodysplasia, leukemia, PNH, or combined disorders.[197] This tendency to relapse and to develop clonal hematologic disorders was reviewed by the European Cooperative Group for Bone Marrow Transplantation in 468 patients, most of whom received ATG.[198] The risk of a hematologic complication increased continuously and reached 57% at 8 years after immunosuppressive therapy. Another survey found 42 (5%) malignancies in 860 patients treated with immunosuppression, whereas only 9 malignancies (1.2% of patients studied) were seen in 748 patients who received marrow transplants.[199]

There are no clinical predictors that augur the risk of clonal evolution in an individual patient, although shorter telomere length at diagnosis and poorer prognosis are associated.[200]

Cyclosporine Administration of cyclosporine, a cyclic polypeptide that inhibits IL-2 production by T lymphocytes and prevents expansion of cytotoxic T cells in response to IL-2, is another approach to immunotherapy. After the initial report in 1984 of its ability to induce remission,[201] several groups have used cyclosporine as either (1) primary treatment,[202-205] (2) in patients refractory to ATG or glucocorticoids,[203-208] (3) in combination with G-CSF,[209,210] or (4) in varying combinations with other modes of therapy.[211] Cyclosporine is administered orally at 10 to 12 mg/kg per day for at least 6 months and with downward dose modification after 6 months for as long as 12 months.

TABLE 4–7. Immunosuppressive Therapy of Aplastic Anemia: Source of Antithymocyte Globulin

Year of Report	Agents Used	No. Pts	Age Range (years)	Percent Response	Percent Survival	Percent Relapse	Comments	Citation
2013	H-ATG + CYA +GM-CSF	46	14-75	48 @ (NR)	84 @ 5 y	23 @ 3 years	H-ATG and R-ATG equivalent	190
	R-ATG +CYA	53	15-66	51 @ (NR)	83 @ 5 y	27 @ 3 years		
2012	R-ATG + CYA + G-CSF + glucocorticoids	24	19-81	64 @ 3 mo	70 @ 5 y	28 @ 5 years		186
2012	R-ATG + CYA	46	2-15	85 @ 1 y	??	??	Pediatric age	188
2012	R-ATG + CYA	35	17-75	60 @ 6 mo	68 @ 27	NR	H-ATG better than R-ATG[a]	189
2011	H-ATG + CYA	60	37 ± 3	68 @ 6 mo	96 @ 3 y	NR	H-ATG better than R-ATG	185
	R-ATG + CYA	60	31 ± 3	37 @ 6 mo	76 @ 3 y	NR		
2011	R-ATG + CYA + glucocorticoids	20	19-80	50 @ 1 y	65 @ 3 y	NR	?R-ATG similar to H-ATG[a]	187
2010	H-ATG	42	1-66	59 @ 6 mo	78 @ 2 y	NR	H-ATG better than R-ATG	183
	R-ATG	29	4-63	34 @ 6 mo	55 @ 2 y	NR		
2009	R-ATG + CYA + G-CSF	13	20-83	92 @ 1y	NR	30 @ 18 mo	?R-ATG better than H-ATG[a]	184
2006	H-ATG +CYA +GM-CSF +EPO	30	2-71	73 @ (NR)	80 @ 5 y	NR	H-ATG better than R-ATG	182
	R-ATG +CYA +GM-CSF +EPO	32	2-71	53 @ (NR)	66 @ 5 y	NR		

Abbreviations: CYA, cyclosporine; EPO, erythropoietin; G-CSF, granulocyte colony-stimulating factor; GM-CSF, granulocyte-monocyte, colony-stimulating factor; H-ATG, horse antithymocyte globulin; No., number; NR, not reported; Pts, patients; R-ATG, rabbit antithymocyte globulin.

[a]Based on prior studies of H-ATG.

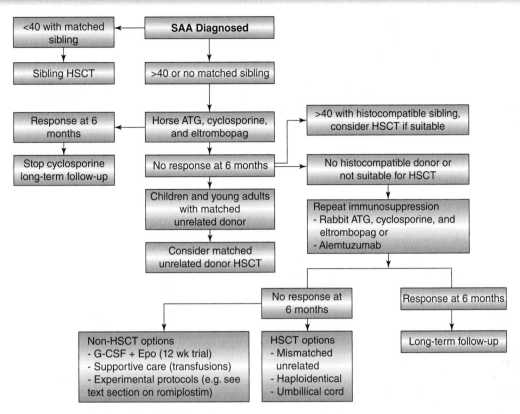

Figure 4–3. Flow chart with general guidelines for treatment. Response to horse ATG plus cyclosporine and eltrombopag is followed for 6 months before deciding the patient has not responded adequately, unless the patient is doing poorly and the neutrophil count remains less than 0.2×10^9/L. In that case, one can proceed to the next suitable option. In general, transplantation options are reassessed at 6 months after immunotherapy and are dependent on donor availability and quality of HLA match, patient age, comorbid conditions that would increase transplantation risk, and the severity of the depression in neutrophil count. In younger patients, a matched, unrelated donor may be appropriate. In older patients, retreating with immunotherapy would be favoured unless the neutrophil count persists in the very-severe-risk category. After two unsuccessful attempts at immunotherapy, therapy is individualized and a high-risk transplantation procedure (slight mismatched-related, haploidentical, umbilical cord blood) may be considered, using the relevant variables (eg, age, comorbidities, performance status, neutrophil count). The age of 40 is an approximate guideline for considering an initial allogeneic hematopoietic cell transplant and may be modified upward somewhat (eg, 41-50 years) based on the clinical status and other features of the patient and donor match. Options other than hematopoietic cell transplant are rarely successful for severe aplastic anemia, refractory to immunotherapy and eltrombopag—and if they are helpful, the effects often are short-lived. *(Modified from permission from Scheinberg P, Young NS. How I treat acquired aplastic anemia,* Blood *2012 Aug 9;120[6]:1185-1196.)*

The drug should be tapered very slowly and, if blood counts remain appropriate, can be given two or three times per week rather than daily during the tapering.[212] Dosage adjustments may be required to maintain trough blood levels of 200 to 400 ng/mL. Renal impairment is common and may require increased hydration or dose adjustments to keep creatinine values below 2 mg/dL. Cyclosporine also may cause moderate hypertension, a variety of neurologic manifestations, and other side effects. Several drug classes interact with cyclosporine to either increase (eg, some antibiotics and antifungals) or decrease (eg, some anticonvulsants) blood levels. Avoidance of other nephrotoxic drugs when using cyclosporine is important, if possible. Responses usually are seen by 3 months and may range from achieving transfusion independence to complete remission. Approximately 25% of patients respond to this agent when it is used alone, but the response rate has ranged from 0% to 80% in various reports.[211]

Although immunosuppression with ALG or ATG has been used the longest and has a better response rate, there are certain advantages to using cyclosporine.[213] The drug does not require patient hospitalization or use of a central venous catheter. Fewer platelet transfusions are required during the first few weeks of therapy compared with treatment with ALG or ATG. A French cooperative trial showed equal effectiveness of cyclosporine compared with ATG plus prednisone.[214] In this crossover study of newly diagnosed patients, survival of approximately 65% was observed 12 months after diagnosis. Cyclosporine has been coupled with ATG as shown in Table 4-8; this combination forms the principal type of immunotherapy for the disease and is the recommended form of immunotherapy at this time.

Eltrombopag Eltrombopag is a TPO receptor agonist used to stimulate platelet production in patients with immune thrombocytopenia. It is a relatively small molecule of the biaryl hydroxone class, is well absorbed from the gastrointestinal tract, and is thus administered orally.[219] It binds to the transmembrane portion of the TPO receptor (cMpl) and induces signal transduction through the mitogen-activated protein kinase and Janus kinase (JAK) pathways. TPO may expand stem cell numbers and promote DNA repair.[220,221] In addition to its use in immune thrombocytopenic purpura, where it can induce megakaryocyte maturation and enhance platelet production, trials of EPAG, given orally, in severe aplastic anemia have found that a multilineage hematopoietic response occurred, leading to restoration of granulopoiesis, erythropoiesis, and megakaryocytopoiesis with a subsequent increase in neutrophil, erythrocyte, and platelet counts, sometimes to normal levels.[222-230] A higher dose of EPAG (150 mg/day) and longer treatment

TABLE 4–8. Response to Immunotherapy in Patients with Severe Aplastic Anemia

Year of Publication	Principal Drugs Used	No. Pts (Age-Range, years)	Significant Response No. (%)	Survival at 5/10 Years (%)	Relapse at 5 Years (Cum%)	Comments	Reference
2011	ATG+CYA	95 (7-80)	63(66)	76[a]/NR	33[a]	Fewer early infections with G-CSF; no difference in response or survival	218
	ATG+CYA+G-CSF	97 (2-81)	71(73)	78[a]/NR	32[a]		
2008	ATG + CYA	77 (<18)	57 (74)	83/80	25	8.5% evolved to clonal myeloid disease	215
2007	ATG + CYA	44 (NR)	31 (70)	NR/88	NR	All cases were associated with hepatitis	216
2007	ATG + CYA	47 (19-75)	31 (66)	80/NR	45	No late clonal diseases at 5 y	217
2007	ATG + CYA + G-CSF	48 (19-74)	37 (77)	90/NR	15	No late clonal diseases at 5 y	217

Abbreviations: ATG, antithymocyte globulin; Cum%, cumulative percent; CYA, cyclosporine; G-CSF, granulocyte colony-stimulating factor; No. Pts, number of patients; NR, not reported; rhuEPO, recombinant human erythropoietin.

[a]At 6 years posttreatment.

(at least 24 weeks) increases the likelihood of response[224,225] MPL receptors are present on hematopoietic stem cells and, presumably, EPAG interacts with marrow stem cells through these receptors, inducing a multilineage progenitor cell proliferative and maturation effect.

Initially, use of EPAG as a single agent in 43 patients with acquired aplastic anemia who did not respond to immunotherapy resulted in improved hematopoiesis and cell counts in 17 (40%), with several having improved bi- or trilineage hematopoiesis and cell counts. Five patients had near normalization of all blood counts and had therapy stopped after 9 to 37 months with maintenance of their blood counts for 1 to 13 months of observation.[223] Many did not normalize their counts, but several became red cell– and platelet transfusion–independent. New cytogenetic abnormalities developed in eight patients (−7 or del[7] developed in 5 of 8 patients), but none progressed to AML. In subsequent studies of patients with aplastic anemia, the response rates improved significantly when EPAG as oral tablets were added to the standard two-drug (ATG and cyclosporine) immunotherapy.[229] The United States Food and Drug Administration approved the use of EPAG for patients with severe aplastic anemia in 2014. Treatment with EPAG, also, improved the cytopenias in 50% of patients with moderate aplastic anemia or unilineage cytopenia.[230]

Combination Immunotherapy (ATG and Cyclosporine) and Eltrombopag Combination immunotherapy of severe aplastic anemia in adults usually includes, for example, ATG (40 mg/kg per day) for 4 days; cyclosporine (6 mg/kg per day in divided doses every 12 hours) for 6 months; and methylprednisolone (1 mg/kg per day) for 2 weeks.[213] The dose of cyclosporine is adjusted to maintain a trough level of 200 to 400 ng/mL. EPAG is given at 150 mg from day 1 for 6 months. Lower doses of EPAG are used for patients of Asian descent and for children.[229] Side effects from treatment include serum sickness from ATG, and hepatotoxicity from ATG, cyclosporine, and EPAG.[224,226,228,229] Prophylaxis for *Pneumocystis carinii* with daily trimethoprim-sulfamethoxazole or with monthly pentamidine inhalations should be considered for these patients as they receive immunosuppressive therapy. In addition, antiviral prophylaxis is recommended for at least 1 month in all patients.[229]

The addition of cyclosporine to the combination of ALG and glucocorticoids improves response rates to approximately 70% of patients,[214,215] and the addition of EPAG further improves it to greater than 90% (Table 4-9). G-CSF added to the combined immunosuppressive therapy does not increase response rate or survival.[216] Response is usually defined as a significant improvement in red cells, white cells, and platelets to eliminate the risk of infection and bleeding and the requirement for red cell transfusions. (See footnote of Table 4-9.)

The 5-year survival after completion of combination immunosuppressive therapy may approximate that after hematopoietic cell transplantation.[237] Forty-eight children treated between 1983 and 1992 had a 10-year survival of approximately 75% for marrow transplantation and approximately 75% for combined immunosuppressive therapy, although there were only half the number of severely affected patients in the immunosuppressive therapy group.[238] In another, report, the 5-year survival and failure-free survivals were 90.5% and 70.4% in 172 children treated with rabbit ATG and cyclosporin.[239] Thus, immunosuppression (now with the addition of EPAG) may be preferable for patients who are older than 30 years and in those who may encounter a delay in finding a suitable donor. Hematopoietic cell transplants are, however, curative for aplastic anemia, whereas more frequent sequelae have been found after immunosuppressive therapy, notably a substantial rate of evolution to a MDS or AML,[240-242] although the effect of adding EPAG to immunotherapy awaits long-term follow-up.

A National Institutes of Health (NIH) protocol was designed to increase immune tolerance by specific deletion of activated T lymphocytes that target primitive hematopoietic progenitor cells.[27] Concurrent administration of cyclosporine with ATG may diminish the ATG effect so that in this program cyclosporine is introduced at a later time. The addition of new immunosuppressive agents, such as mycophenolate mofetil, rapamycin, or monoclonal antibodies, to the IL-2 receptor may be more effective in decreasing cytotoxic T cells, sparing the targeted hematopoietic stem cells.[27]

For the 30% to 40% of patients who relapse after immunotherapy, retreatment with ATG and cyclosporine is effective in 50% to 60% of them.[243,244] Alternatively, alemtuzumab, a monoclonal anti-CD52 antibody that targets the antigen on T lymphocytes, has been an effective immunosuppressive agent in both relapsed and refractory patients, and it may be administered with cyclosporine.[245,246]

In approximately one-quarter to one-third of patients with acquired aplastic anemia, treatment with ATG and cyclosporine fails to restore hematopoiesis and does not result in reasonable blood cell counts. When EPAG was combined with ATG and cyclosporine and administered to previously untreated patients with severe aplastic anemia, the response rate was 94% at 6 months in the group treated from

TABLE 4–9. Studies of Eltrombopag in Patients with Severe Aplastic Anemia

Year	No. Pts.	Oral Dose of EPAG/day	Duration of Treatment	Overall Response[a]	Reference No.
Studies in Which EPAG was Combined with Immunotherapy					
2017	92	150 mg >12 y 75 mg 6-11 y 2.5 mg/kg 2-5 y	24 wk	Cohort 1 Rx Day14-6 mo, 80% Cohort 2 Rx Day 14-3 mo, 87% Cohort 3 Rx Day 1-6 mo, 94%	229
2018	10	150 mg (50-300)	47 wk (14-179)	90%	234
Studies in Which EPAG Was Used in Patients Refractory to or at Relapse After Immunotherapy					
2012	25	150 mg (50-150)	12 wk	44%	223
2018	10	150 mg (50-300)	115 wk (53–253)	50%	234
2018[a]	35	150 mg	2-39 mo	74%	232
2019	40	150 mg (50-150)	24 wk	50%	226

Abbreviations: EPAG, eltrombopag; NIH, U.S. National Institutes of Health.

[a]Overall response is the sum of the complete response and partial response.

Complete response is defined as an absolute neutrophil count ≥1 × 10^9/L, hemoglobin ≥100 g/L, and platelet count ≥100 × 10^9/L. Partial response is defined in some studies as a lesser response in any or all of the platelet, red cell, or neutrophil counts. NIH partial response criteria: platelet response of ≥20 × 10^9/L; hemoglobin response of ≥15 g/L or a reduction of ≥4 units packed red cells transfused during eight consecutive weeks; Neutrophil response of ≥0.5 × 10^9/L.

day 1 with all three agents, compared with a 66% response rate in historical controls treated with ATG and cyclosporine.[229] The overall survival of patients treated with the three agents at 2 years was 97%. This triple-drug approach has not yet been studied widely or for a long follow-up period, but the improvement over ATG and cyclosporine alone is so striking that it is likely to become the treatment of choice in patients not amenable to allogeneic sibling transplantation as a first treatment option (ie, young age and histocompatible sibling donor).[229] Evolution to a clonal myeloid disorder occurred in 8% of patients, similar to historical control patients treated with ATG and cyclosporine without the addition of EPAG. Other studies of EPAG as a treatment for aplastic anemia add weight to its usefulness in its management.[231-237]

Romiplostim This agent is an alternative TPO receptor agonist that is a larger molecule than EPAG and requires parenteral administration. Its mechanism of action differs somewhat from EPAG in that it binds to the TPO receptor site, cMPL, as opposed to the transmembrane region, but stimulates similar metabolic pathways as EPAG does. Patients with immune thrombocytopenia purpura who may not respond to EPAG may respond to romiplastim and vice versa.

A recent phase 2 study of 35 patients with aplastic anemia in Korea indicated benefit of romiplostim as a single agent in some patients who were refractory to standard immunosuppression with ATG and cyclosporine.[247] Only approximately one-half of the patients had "severe" aplastic anemia compared with those in the EPAG studies, which were limited to patients with aplastic anemia classified as severe or very severe (see Table 4-1). Nevertheless, a significant proportion of patients receiving 10 µg/kg body weight of romiplostim, subcutaneously, once weekly, had an increase in hemoglobin, neutrophil, or platelet count or some combination thereof over 52 weeks of therapy. Some patients during the later parts of the study were given 20 µg/week. Some patients were treated for up to 3 years. Patients tolerated the drug with only mild (grade 1 or 2) side effects of fatigue, myalgia, or dizziness. No patients progressed to having clonal cytogenetic evolution or myelodysplasia or AML during the 3 years of study. Marrow cell cytogenetic analysis was done every 6 months.

CD34+, CD38– cells (putative early multipotential hematopoietic or stem cells) and CFU-fibroblasts (putative stromal progenitor cells), CFU-granulocytes or macrophages, CFU-erythroid, BFU-E, and CFU-megakaryocytes were increased in patients with a long-term response, but not in patients without a response. These findings strongly suggest an effect of romiplastim on the reactivation of hematopoietic stem cells. A study is underway to examine the result of combining romiplostim with ATG and cyclosporine at the time of diagnosis.

Other Approaches to Immunotherapy

Alemtuzumab Alemtuzumab is a humanized IgG1 monoclonal antibody directed against the CD52 protein; CD52 is expressed on all lymphocytes and monocytes. Alemtuzumab produces profound and persistent lymphopenia. The antibody has been used to treat severe aplastic anemia that does not respond to or relapses after use of horse antithymocyte globulin.[242,246] It also has been used as a conditioning agent before allogeneic hematopoietic cell transplantation.[170-172]

High-Dose Glucocorticoid Treatment Marrow recovery can occur after very high doses of glucocorticoids.[248,249] Methylprednisolone in the range of 500 to 1000 mg daily for 3 to 14 days has been successful, but the side effects, which include marked hyperglycemia and glycosuria, electrolyte disturbances, gastric irritation, psychosis, increased infections, and aseptic necrosis of the hips, can be severe. Glucocorticoids at lower doses commonly are used only as a component of combination therapy for aplastic anemia to ameliorate the toxic effects of ATG and for providing additional lymphocyte suppression.

High-Dose Cyclophosphamide Therapy High-dose cyclophosphamide has been used as a form of immunosuppression.[250] Although it would seem inappropriate to administer high doses of chemotherapy to patients with severe marrow aplasia, this approach was based on observations of autologous recovery after preparative therapy for allogeneic transplants not followed by transplantation.[6] In an early study, 10 patients who received cyclophosphamide at 45 mg/kg per day intravenously for 4 days with or without cyclosporine for an additional 100 days had gradual neutrophil and platelet recovery over 3 months. Seven patients responded completely and remained in remission 11 years after treatment. High-dose cyclophosphamide treatment may spare hematopoietic stem cells, which have high levels of aldehyde dehydrogenase and are relatively resistant to cyclophosphamide.[26,251,252] Thus, cyclophosphamide in this situation may be more immunosuppressive than myelotoxic. The most extensive trial of high-dose cyclophosphamide resulted in 65% of patients responding completely at 50 months.[253] However, the role of this regimen as initial therapy is not clear because of early toxicity that may exceed that of the ATG and cyclosporine combination.[254] The probability of a durable remission may be superior, but there are insufficient data (comparative clinical trials) to conclude whether high-dose cyclophosphamide provides better long-term results than ATG and cyclosporine. At this writing, the latter approach is favored.

Rituximab A case report of the successful use of the anti-CD20 humanized mouse antibody rituximab has provided preliminary evidence for its potential effectiveness in treating aplastic anemia.[255] Clinical trials have not examined its efficacy compared with standard immunotherapy (ATG and cyclosporine) in patients refractory to standard therapy, or as a third drug in an immunotherapy regimen. Whether B lymphocytes play a role in the pathogenesis of T-cell–mediated aplastic anemia has not been defined, so rituximab does not appear to have a theoretical rationale for use at this time. However, a singular case of antibody-mediated aplastic anemia responded to rituximab, and the autoantibodies became undetectable.[255,256]

Other Nonimmune Therapies

Androgens Randomized trials have not shown efficacy when androgens were used as primary therapy for severe aplastic anemia.[257,258] Androgens stimulate the production of EPO, and their metabolites stimulate erythropoiesis when added to marrow cultures in vitro. High doses of androgens were beneficial in some patients with moderately severe aplasia.[259] A series of studies were reported in which patients' survival seemed improved compared with historical controls, but this could have resulted from improved supportive care.[151] Masculinization and other androgen side effects can be severe, especially in female patients. Long-term survivors after androgen therapy have essentially the same progression to clonal hematologic disorders as patients treated with immunosuppressive agents.[151] These agents have been replaced by immunosuppression or allogeneic hematopoietic cell transplantation as a principal approach to treatment for acquired severe aplastic anemia. Androgens may be useful in the treatment of aplastic anemia syndromes resulting from shortened telomeres.[260]

Cytokines

Granulocyte Colony-Stimulating Factor Despite their effectiveness in accelerating recovery from chemotherapy, these agents have been far less effective in achieving long-term benefits in patients with severe aplastic anemia. Daily treatment with G-CSF[261] has improved marrow cellularity and increased neutrophil counts approximately 1.5- to 10-fold. Unfortunately, in nearly all patients, the blood counts return to baseline within several days of cessation of therapy. Although some patients show evidence of trilineage marrow recovery with long-term therapy, the vast majority do not respond. Therapy with myeloid growth factors is probably best reserved for episodes of severe infection or as a preventive measure before dental work or other procedures that would compromise mucosal barriers in patients who have not responded to hematopoietic cell transplant or immunotherapy. G-CSF in a dose of 5 μg/kg by subcutaneous injection is easiest to administer and seems to be associated with the fewest side effects. The drug can be given daily or fewer times per week depending on the response. Newer pegylated preparations have a longer effect and usually are administered at less frequent, every-other-week intervals. The SAA Working Party of the European Group for Blood and Marrow Transplant reported that G-CSF added to ATG and cyclosporine reduces infection early in treatment,

but does not affect survival or length of remission.[218] Generally, prophylactic use of growth factors is not warranted.

Interleukin-1 or -3 IL-1, a potent stimulator of marrow stromal cell production of other cytokines, and IL-3 have been ineffective in small numbers of patients treated with severe aplastic anemia.[262,263] These disappointing results with cytokines are not unexpected, as previous work has found high serum levels of growth factors in patients with aplastic anemia. Moreover, a majority of patients have suppression of very primitive progenitors, which may be unresponsive to individual factors that act on more mature progenitor cells.

Splenectomy Removal of the spleen does not increase hematopoiesis but may increase neutrophil and platelet counts two- to threefold and improve survival of transfused red cells or platelets in highly sensitized individuals.[264] The surgical morbidity and mortality in patients with few platelets and white cells makes this a questionable therapeutic procedure. Because there are more successful methods of therapy that attack the fundamental problem, this approach is not recommended.

Other Therapy High doses of intravenous γ-globulin have been given to small numbers of patients with severe aplastic anemia[265,266] because of its success in treating certain cases of antibody-mediated pure red cell aplasia. Some improvement was noted in 4 of 6 patients treated. Another treatment that is occasionally successful is lymphocytapheresis to deplete T cells.[267,268]

Course and Prognosis

At diagnosis, the prognosis is largely related to the absolute neutrophil and platelet count. The absolute neutrophil count is the most important prognostic feature, with a count of fewer than 0.5×10^9/L considered to be severe aplastic anemia and a count of fewer than 0.2×10^9/L very severe aplastic anemia, the latter associated with a poor response to immunotherapy and usually a dire prognosis, if early successful allogeneic transplant is not available. In the past, the prognosis appeared worse when the disease followed hepatitis.[77,78] But more comprehensive results with immunosuppression[218] or hematopoietic cell transplantation[269] show an equivalent response to that seen with idiopathic or drug-induced cases.[270,271]

Before hematopoietic cell transplantation and immunosuppressive therapy, more than 25% of patients with severe aplastic anemia died within 4 months of diagnosis; half died within 1 year.[270,272] Hematopoietic cell transplantation is curative for approximately 80% to 90% of patients younger than 20 years, approximately 70% between the ages of 20 and 40 years, and approximately 50% older than 40 years.[169,273] Unfortunately, as many as 40% of transplant survivors experienced the deleterious consequences of chronic graft-versus-host disease,[169] and the risk of subsequent cancer can be as high as 10% in older patients or after immunotherapy before hematopoietic cell transplantation.[274,275] The best outcomes occur in patients who have an allele-based HLA-matched sibling, have not been exposed to immunosuppressive therapy before transplantation, have not been exposed and sensitized to blood cell products, have had a marrow rather than a blood stem cell donor product, and have not been subjected to high-dose radiation in the conditioning regimen for transplantation.[169,274,276,277]

Combination immunosuppressive therapy with ATG and cyclosporine leads to a marked improvement in approximately 70% of patients, and EPAG improves this response to immunotherapy significantly (Table 4-9). Higher initial absolute reticulocyte and lymphocyte counts are predictive of a better response to therapy.[278] The presence of a PNH clone prior to treatment does not diminish resonse to combined immunotherapy.[279] A longer duration of observation for large cohorts of patients who received EPAG as well as immunotherapy are not yet available. Given their higher response rate, one anticipates a better prognosis in patients receiving triple therapy (ATG, cyclosporine, EPAG).

A high proportion of Treg B cells is associated with an increased likelihood of a favorable response to immunotherapy.[42] Treg B lymphocytes can be expanded in vitro with interferon. The addition of low-dose IL-2 to current regimens may improve the results of immunotherapy. This suggestion awaits the results of clinical trials.[42] Although some patients regain normal blood counts, many continue to have moderate anemia or thrombocytopenia. In as many as 40% of patients who initially respond to immunosuppressive therapy, their disease may relapse or progress to PNH, a MDS, or AML over 10 years of observation. Moreover, the beneficial effects of immunotherapy are often lost 10 years after treatment. In 168 transplanted patients, the actual survival rate at 15 years was 69%, and in 227 patients receiving immunosuppressive therapy it was 38%.[195] Long-term survival in pediatric patients younger than 18 years appears better, with approximately one-third having relapse at 10 years.[275]

Treatment with high-dose cyclophosphamide produces early results similar to that seen with the combination of ATG and cyclosporine.[280-282] However, cyclophosphamide has greater early toxicity and slower hematologic recovery but may generate more durable remissions. Its use has been too limited to reach a firm conclusion on its relative merits and it is rarely used as the first choice of immunotherapy. Table 4-10 provides the highlights of management of acquired aplastic anemia.

HEREDITARY APLASTIC ANEMIA

FANCONI ANEMIA

Definition and History

Fanconi anemia (FA) is the most common form of constitutional aplastic anemia and was initially described in three brothers by Fanconi in 1927.[283] It is inherited as an autosomal recessive condition that results from defects in genes that modulate the stability of DNA.

Epidemiology

FA is an uncommon disorder and is estimated to be present in one in 1 million individuals. It is far more frequent in Afrikaners of European descent.[284] This unusually high frequency has been attributed to a founder effect.

Etiology and Pathogenesis

More than 20 complementation groups, defined by somatic cell hybridization, are associated with the development of FA.[285,286] A complementation group is a genetic subgroup. Identifying a complementation group requires adding a gene to the genome of a cell to correct (complement) the genetic defect. This procedure can be done by cell fusion studies. After fusing two cells together, thereby joining their genetic material, one can test the cells for the genetic defect. In the case of FA, this would be with the diepoxybutane test. In this test, diepoxybutane results in chromosome fragmentation in the cells of patients with FA. Hybrids in which the hypersensitivity to diepoxybutane is corrected (complemented) can be assumed to result from the fusion of cells from different genetic subgroups (complementation groups), whereas hybrids that still show the sensitivity are the result of fusion of cells from the same subgroup. Because one can determine the complementation group without knowing the gene involved, this approach is the first step in understanding the genetic basis of a disease. Once the genes are known, one does not need to use cell fusion studies; rather, retroviral vectors can be used to insert corrected genes into the cells.

The complementation groups have been designated *FANCA, B, C, D1, D2, E, F, G, I, J, L, M, N, O, P, Q, R, S, U, V,* and *W.* Table 4-11 lists the gene mutations corresponding to these complementation groups,

---

TABLE 4–10. Summary of Major Therapeutic Considerations in the Management of Severe Aplastic Anemia

- It is important to treat patients in a center with experience in the management of this rare disease.
- Hematopoietic cell transplantation is preferred for children and young adults (<40 y) with an allele-level HLA- matched donor, especially if from a sibling donor.
- ATG and cyclosporine immunotherapy has been used for those patients unable to have a hematopoietic cell transplant (see below addition of eltrombopag).
- Although a remission is common with ATG and cyclosporine (about 75% of treated patients), long-term outlook, as a result of disease relapse or evolution to oligoblastic or polyblastic (acute) myelogenous leukemia, is poor.
- Approximately 15% of patients treated with immunotherapy express an abnormal karyotype or an overt clonal myeloid neoplasm (PNH or oligoblastic or polyblastic [acute] myelogenous leukemia).
- Relapsed patients may respond to a second administration of ATG and cyclosporine. Often, if horse or rabbit ATG is used initially, the alternative is used in retreatment, if available.
- Eltrombopag alone has resulted in a favorable hematologic response in approximately 50% of patients so treated. In adults, 150 mg/d, administered for at least 24 wk is considered appropriate; lower doses are used in adolescents and children and patients of Asian descent
- Discontinuation of eltrombopag has been followed by prolonged improvement in blood counts in some patients; readministration of eltrombopag has restored responses in some patients who lost them after discontinuation.
- The addition of eltrombopag to ATG and cyclosporine at initial treatment has increased the remission rate and the quality of remission substantially, but long-term follow-up has not yet been described.
- Approximately one-fifth of patients treated with eltrombopag develop clonal cytogenetic abnormalities, but progression to a clonal myeloid neoplasm has been uncommon over short-term follow-up.
- Alemtuzumab may be useful in patients who cannot tolerate ATG and cyclosporine, eg, older (>60 y) patients.
- Use of eltrombopag and its role as a single agent or combined with ATG and cyclosporine has advanced management of this disease.
- See the treatment section of this chapter for details of management, Table 4-9, and references 222-236 for details regarding the use of and response to eltrombopag. A meta-analysis of studies treating aplastic anemia with eltrombopag has been published.[235]

Abbreviations: ATG, antithymocyte globulin; HLA, human leukocyte antigen; PNH, paroxysmal nocturnal hemoglobinuria.

TABLE 4–11. Gene Mutations Found in Fanconi Anemia[294,295]

		Comp. Group	Gene	Patient Frequency (%)	Molecular Functions
Genes mutated in FA patients	FA core complex	FANCA		64	Subcomplex with FANCG and FAAP20[a]
		FANCB		2	FA core complex; subcomplex with FAAP100 and FANCL
		FANCC		12	FA core complex; forms a ternary complex with FANCE, FANCF, and FANCD2
		FANCE		1	FA core complex
		FANCF		2	FA Core complex; required for interactions among FANCA, FANCC, and FANCE
		FANCG	XRCC9	8	FA core complex; subcomplex with FANCA and FAAP20; complex with BRCA2, XRCC3, and FANCD2
		FANCL		0.4	RING domain containing E3 ubiquitin ligase within FA core complex
		FANCM		0.1	ATR-mediated checkpoint activation; recruitment of FA core complex and BLM
		FANCT	UBE2T	0.1	FA core complex; E2 ubiquitin-conjugating enzyme
	ID2	FANCP	SLX4	0.5	Master scaffold and regulator of ERCC1-XPF, MUS81-EME1/2, and SLX1 nucleases to excise ICLs
		FANCD2		4	ID2 complex; functions in the ICL excision and bypass step, multiple downstream functions
		FANCI		1	ID2 complex; multiple functions in the ICL repair and replication stress response
	FA/HR	FANCD1	BRCA2	2	HR; stimulates RAD51 recombinase; fork stabilization
		FANCJ	BRIP1	2	Interaction with BRCA1 promotes HR and inhibits TLS; DNA-dependent ATPase and 5′-3′-helicase
		FANCN	PALB2	0.7	HR; stimulates RAD51 recombinase; fork stabilization; links BRCA1 and BRCA2
		FANCO	RAD51C	0.1	HR
		FANCR	RAD51	Rare	HR; fork stabilization
		FANCS	BRCA1	0.1	HR; eviction of CMG (CDC45-MCM-GINS) complex at ICL-induced stalled forks
		FANCU	XRCC2	0.1	HR
	Recent	FANCV	REV7/MAD2L2	One patient	Negatively regulates DNA end resection; promotes end joining; modulates PARPi response
		FANCW	RFWD3	One patient	E3 ubiquitin ligase for regulating turnover of RPA and RAD51 during HR and ICL repair
		FANCQ	ERCC4, XPF	0.1	DNA incision and NER
	FA-associated genes	FAAP10	STRA13/CENPX/MHF2		FA core complex; histone fold–containing protein; constitutive chromatin localization of FANCM
		FAAP16	APITD1/CENPS/MHF1		FA core complex; histone fold–containing protein; constitutive chromatin localization of FANCM
		FAAP20	C1orf86		FANCA stability; binds ubiquitinated TLS polymerase REV1
		FAAP24	C19orf40		FA core complex; interacts with FANCM
		FAAP100	C19orf70		FA core complex
		FAN1			Nuclease; restart of stalled replication forks
		UAF1			ID2 deubiquitination
		UHRF1			Lesion recognition
		USP1			ID2 deubiquitination

Abbreviations: FA, Fanconi anemia; FAAP, FA-associated proteins; HR, homologous recombination; ICL, interstrand cross-link; NER, nucleotide excision repair; PARPi, poly (ADP-ribose) polymerase inhibitor; TLS, translesion synthesis.

[a]FAAPs are important for ICL repair, but to date no FA patient has been found harboring biallelic mutations of them.

Classification of Fanconi anemia genes and their molecular functions.

Genes not named assume the names in the Complementation (Comp.) Group.

Data from Frohnmayer D, Frohnmayer L, Guinan E, et al, eds. Fanconi Anemia Guidelines for Diagnosis and Management, 4th ed. Fanconi Anemia Research Fund; 2014.

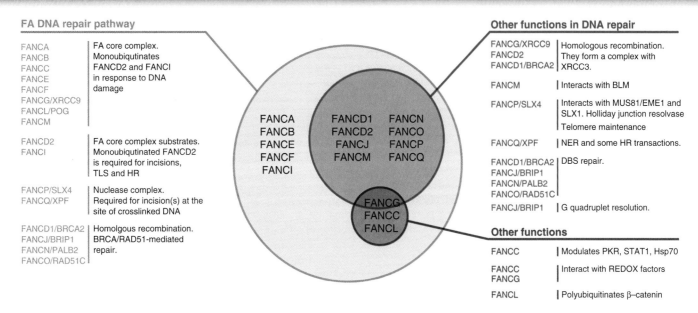

FA DNA repair pathway

Genes	Function
FANCA FANCB FANCC FANCE FANCF FANCG/XRCC9 FANCL/POG FANCM	FA core complex. Monoubiquitinates FANCD2 and FANCI in response to DNA damage
FANCD2 FANCI	FA core complex substrates. Monoubiquitinated FANCD2 is required for incisions, TLS and HR
FANCP/SLX4 FANCQ/XPF	Nuclease complex. Required for incision(s) at the site of crosslinked DNA
FANCD1/BRCA2 FANCJ/BRIP1 FANCN/PALB2 FANCO/RAD51C	Homolgous recombination. BRCA/RAD51-mediated repair.

FANCA	FANCD1 FANCN
FANCB	FANCD2 FANCO
FANCE	FANCJ FANCP
FANCF	FANCM FANCQ
FANCI	
	FANCG
	FANCC
	FANCL

Other functions in DNA repair

Genes	Function
FANCG/XRCC9 FANCD2 FANCD1/BRCA2	Homologous recombination. They form a complex with XRCC3.
FANCM	Interacts with BLM
FANCP/SLX4	Interacts with MUS81/EME1 and SLX1. Holliday junction resolvase Telomere maintenance
FANCQ/XPF	NER and some HR transactions.
FANCD1/BRCA2 FANCJ/BRIP1 FANCN/PALB2 FANCO/RAD51C	DBS repair.
FANCJ/BRIP1	G quadruplet resolution.

Other functions

Genes	Function
FANCC	Modulates PKR, STAT1, Hsp70
FANCC FANCG	Interact with REDOX factors
FANCL	Polyubiquitinates β–catenin

Figure 4–4. Summary of the interactions of the FA proteins. The primary function of this group of proteins is to repair crosslinked DNA and to maintain genomic stability (as shown on the left side of the figure). The FA DNA repair pathway includes a core complex for monoubiquitination of other components (substrates, FANCD2, and FANCI), as well as a nuclease complex and a complex for homologous recombination DNA repair. A number of these FA proteins also participate in other DNA repair functions such as telomere maintenance and interaction with redox proteins as shown in the right side of the figure. *(Reproduced with permission from Garaycoechea JI, Patel KJ: Why does the bone marrow fail in Fanconi Anemia? Blood 2014 Jan 2;123[1]:26-34.)*

and Fig. 4-4 summarizes the functions of the known FA proteins.[286] The great majority of patients have mutations of *FANCA, FANCC,* or *FANCG.*[287] It has been proposed that the A and C gene products, which are cytoplasmic proteins, form an "FA core complex" with the products of genes *B, E, F, G, L,* and *M,* which are adaptors or phosphorylators.[287,288]

The complex translocates to the nucleus, where it is required for the ubiquitination of FANCD2 and protects the cell from DNA cross-linking and participates in DNA repair (Fig. 4-5). DNA damage initiates activation of the FA/BRCA pathway and ubiquitination of FANCD2, which is targeted to the altered DNA and facilitates repair by interacting

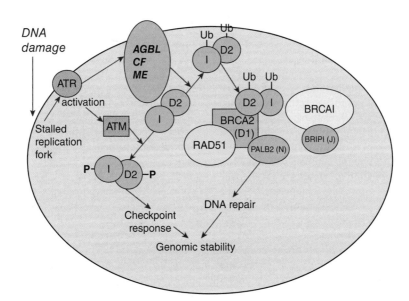

Figure 4–5. Representation of the "FA/BRCA pathway." After DNA damage when a replication fork encounters a DNA cross-link, ATR (ataxia telangiectasia and rad3-related protein) is activated. This leads to the activation of the Fanconi anemia (FA) pathway, as well as cell-cycle checkpoint activation via the ATM (ataxia telangiectasia–mutated) protein. Activation of the FA pathway leads to the formation of the "FA core complex" (consisting of the FA proteins A, B, C, E, F, G, L, and M). This activated FA core complex leads to the monoubiquitination of FANCD2 (FANCD2-Ub) and FANCI (I-Ub). The I-Ub/FANCD2-Ub complex is then targeted to the chromatin containing the cross-link where it interacts with BRCA2 and possibly other DNA repair proteins (eg, RAD51, J, N), leading to the repair of the DNA damage. Proteins mutated in the different FA subtypes are shown in yellow. *(Reproduced with permission from Dokal I, Vulliamy T: Inherited aplastic anaemias/bone marrow failure syndromes, Blood Rev 2008 May;22[3]:141-153.)*

with DNA repair proteins, BRCA1, FANCD1/BRCA2, FANCN/PALB2, and RAD51. In the presence of a mutant gene product, the normal protective and repair functions are disturbed, leading to damaging effects in sensitive tissues, including hematopoietic cells. The genetic damage appears related to the adverse effects of reactive oxygen radicals, such as superoxide and hydrogen peroxide, as well as aldehydes such as formaldehyde produced by normal cellular metabolism.[289-291,292] In addition to the genetic defects leading to DNA instability and an inability to repair DNA, TNF-α and -γ are overexpressed in the marrow of FA patients.[293] The excess TNF-α may play a role in the suppression of erythropoiesis in these patients.

The generation of reactive oxygen radicals and aldehydes, the defective mechanisms of DNA repair, the hypersensitivity to cytokines such as TNF-α, and the age-related shortening of DNA-protective telomeres produce a marked predisposition to clonal evolution and neoplasia in FA patients (see "Therapy and Course" further).

Clinical Features

Growth retardation, resulting in short stature, and skeletal anomalies are common. Absent, misshapen, or supernumerary thumbs and dysplastic radii occur in half the patients. Hip and vertebral abnormalities also may occur. Septal heart defects; eye abnormalities; and absent, misshapen, or fused kidneys may be present. Women may have aplasia of the uterus and vagina, absent ovaries, infertility and late menarche, and early menopause, and men may have hypospermia. Thus, hypogonadism may be evident. Learning disability is frequent, and microcephaly and developmental disability may be features. The skin may be generally hyperpigmented or may have areas of abnormal skin pigmentation referred to as *café-au-lait* spots, which are flat, light brown, and from 1 to 12 centimeters in diameter. Hepatosplenomegaly is not a feature of the disease. Approximately 5% of patients with FA exhibit 3 of 8 features that include vertebral anomalies, anal atresia, congenital heart disease, tracheoesophageal fistula, renal abnormalities, limb abnormalities and hydrocephalus (VACTERL-H phenotype). Some patients have no or minor phenotypic abnormalities and may be diagnosed as a result of the onset of marrow failure or a cancer involving any of many sites in as late as the fifth decade of life.

The onset of marrow failure is gradual and usually is evident during the last half of the first decade of life. The manifestations of anemia, including weakness, fatigue, and dyspnea on exertion, and of thrombocytopenia with epistaxis, purpura, or other unexpected bleeding, are the principal findings. Hematologic and visceral manifestations are combined eventually in more than one-third of patients, but some may have cytopenias and inconspicuous somatic changes, whereas others may have somatic anomalies with no or a nominal disorder of blood cell formation for months or years. Some persons who carry the gene may be virtually unaffected.[296-298] In a review of the more than 1300 patients in the literature, 100 patients (<7%) without anomalies were identified by chromosome breakage studies (see "Laboratory Features" further) because of affected siblings. In the past, children in families with FA history, who had onset of aplastic anemia without congenital somatic abnormalities were thought to have a different disorder termed *Estren-Dameshek syndrome.*[299] However, these children, whose lymphocytes show sensitivity to diepoxybutane, are considered to have FA without skeletal abnormalities. Because patients may present with aplastic anemia later in life and because patients with FA may not have phenotypic features, it has been suggested that all patients with apparent acquired aplastic anemia be screened for chromosome instability (diepoxybutane challenge) as part of their diagnostic evaluation.

Laboratory Features

Blood counts and marrow cellularity in children with FA are often normal until 5 to 10 years of age, when pancytopenia develops over an extended interval. Macrocytosis with anisocytosis and poikilocytosis may be present before any cytopenia occurs. Thrombocytopenia may precede the development of granulocytopenia and anemia. The marrow becomes hypocellular and in vitro colony assays reveal a decrease in CFU-GM and BFU-E.[298]

Random chromatid breaks are present in myeloid cells, lymphocytes, and chorionic villus biopsy samples. This chromosome damage is intensified after exposure to DNA cross-linking agents such as mitomycin C or diepoxybutane. The hypersensitivity of the chromosomes of marrow cells or lymphocytes to the latter agent is used as a diagnostic test for this condition. Cell-cycle progression is prolonged at the G2-to-M transition, and the cells are more susceptible to oxygen toxicity when cultured in vitro. It is important to test the lymphocytes from pediatric patients with aplastic anemia for sensitivity to diepoxybutane, because therapy for FA differs from that used for acquired aplastic anemia.

The FA complex serves as a tumor supressor by stablizing and augmenting DNA repair.[300]

Determining the specific gene mutation responsible in a patient (see Table 4-11) is important because it confirms the diagnosis, identifies the genotype linked to BRCA2 that may predispose to a cancer (eg, breast, ovary), and permits carrier detection.[301]

Differential Diagnosis

The differential diagnosis of FA includes other causes of aplastic anemia; particularly those familial syndromes associated with skeletal anomalies and other dysmorphic features. Other familial types of aplastic anemia have been reported with or without associated anomalies. In those instances, in which no sensitivity to DNA damaging agents is observed, the syndrome does not represent FA. Several uncommon syndromes of this type are described further and are tabulated in Table 4-12.

Therapy and Course

Most patients with FA do not respond to ATG or cyclosporine but do improve with androgen preparations, often for as long as several years. Cytokines may provide some improvement in blood counts, but their effect may wane. Studies in a mouse model also suggest that cytokine effects may not be sustained.[330] The cumulative median survival is approximately 20 years from progressive marrow failure, conversion to MDS, AML (approximately 10% of patients), or the development of a variety of other cancers, such as those involving the genitourinary system, digestive system (especially liver), or head and neck.[331] Multiple cancers in an individual patient also occur. Cancers may occur as late as the fifth decade of life and precede the diagnosis of FA in 25% of patients.[300,331,332] The presence of a clonal cytogenetic abnormality or marrow morphology consistent with myelodysplasia markedly reduces the 5-year survival.[242] Allogeneic hematopoietic cell transplantation is curative for the marrow manifestations of FA.[333-336] Patients transplanted from an identical sibling after 2000 had an 84% survival at 36 months.[337] A marked reduction in the dose of the marrow-conditioning regimen of cyclophosphamide and radiation is necessary, owing to the undue sensitivity of the tissues to DNA-damaging exposures. The risk of cancer is so high that, where practical, surveillance should be used; for example, frequent pelvic examination in women, hepatic ultrasonography to detect adenomas, and careful oropharyngeal examinations. Normal complementary DNA has been transferred into cells from patients with restoration of resistance to DNA-damaging agents.[338,339] Lentiviral vectors and refined gene transfer techniques are being explored for implementation of gene therapy for FA.[340,341] Difficulties in this approach

TABLE 4–12. Other Rare Inherited Syndromes Associated with Aplastic Anemia

Disorder	Findings	Inheritance	Mutated Gene	References
Ataxia-pancytopenia (myelocerebellar disorder)	Cerebellar atrophy and ataxia; aplastic pancytopenia; ± monosomy 7; increased risk of AML	AD	SAMD9/SAMD9L	302-305
Congenital amegakaryocytic thrombocytopenia	Thrombocytopenia; absent or markedly decreased marrow megakaryocytes; hemorrhagic propensity; elevated thrombopoietin; propensity to progress to aplastic pancytopenia; propensity to evolve to clonal myeloid disease	AR (compound heterozygotes or rarely of homozygous mutation of *THPO* gene)	*MPL*	306-309
DNA ligase IV deficiency	Pre- and postnatal growth delay; dysmorphic facies; aplastic pancytopenia	AR (compound heterozygotes)	*LIG4*	314-316
Dubowitz syndrome	Intrauterine and postpartum growth failure; short stature; microcephaly; mental retardation; distinct dysmorphic facies; aplastic pancytopenia; increased risk of AML and ALL	AR	Unknown	317-319
Nijmegen breakage syndrome	Microcephaly; dystrophic facies; short stature; immunodeficiency; radiation sensitivity; aplastic pancytopenia; predisposition to lymphoid malignancy	AR	*NBS1*	320, 321
Reticular dysgenesis (type of severe immunodeficiency syndrome)	Lymphopenia; anemia and neutropenia; corrected by hematopoietic cell transplantation	AR	AK2	322-324
Seckel syndrome	Intrauterine and post partum growth failure; microcephaly; characteristic dysmorphic facies (bird-headed profile); aplastic pancytopenia; possible increased risk of AML	AR	*ATR* (and *RAD3*-related gene); *PCNT*	314, 325-328
WT syndrome	Radial/ulnar abnormalities; aplastic pancytopenia; increased risk of AML	AD	Unknown	329

Abbreviations: AD, autosomal dominant; ALL, acute lymphocytic leukemia; AML, acute myelogenous leukemia; AR, autosomal recessive; XLR, X-linked recessive.

The listed clinical findings in each syndrome are not comprehensive. The designated clinical findings may not be present in all cases of the syndrome. Isolated cases of familial aplastic anemia with or without associated anomalies that are not consistent with FA or other defined syndromes have been reported.

include the paucity of stem cells in these patients, as well as the potential toxicity of the gene transfer method.

DYSKERATOSIS CONGENITA

Definition

This inherited disorder is characterized by cutaneous and mucous membrane abnormalities, progressive marrow insufficiency, and a predisposition to malignant transformation. It is much more common in men than women and occurs in approximately 1 per 1 million persons.[285,342]

Pathogenesis

Dyskeratosis usually is inherited as a recessive X-chromosome–linked disorder, although rare cases can have autosomal dominant or autosomal recessive inheritance (Table 4-13). The disease is a reflection of telomere complex dysfunction[343-346] and results from defective telomerase activity resulting from mutations in the telomerase-related genes (Fig. 4-6).[344,348,349] The telomerase complex maintains the length of telomeres, which are nucleotide tandem repeat structures residing at the termini of eukaryotic chromosomes (eg, 5′-TTAGGG-3′). Telomerase restores the guanine (G)-rich telomere repeats that are lost as a result of end-processing during normal cell division. Combined with protein, located at the ends of chromosomes, they maintain

chromosome integrity by preventing end-to-end chromosome fusion, chromosome degradation, and chromosome instability. In dyskeratosis congenita, the telomeres are markedly shortened, resulting in genomic instability and cell (including marrow cell) apoptosis, and the underlying gene defects may alter Box H/ACA small nucleolar RNAs, such as the TERC, that is central to telomere maintenance.[350,351] Rapidly proliferating cells are at highest risk for dysfunction. Mutations of the *DKC1* gene are responsible for the X-linked recessive form. *DKC1* encodes dyskerin, which is a conserved multifunctional protein component of the telomerase complex. Mutations of the *TERT*, *TERC*, and *TINF2* genes are the principal abnormalities in the autosomal dominant form. TERC is the RNA component of the TERT, the reverse transcriptase, uses to synthesize the 6-bp repeats on the 3′ end of telomeric DNA. Mutations of *TINF2* have been described in patients with dyskeratosis congenita.[352] *TINF2* is a component of the shelterin complex, which prevents end-to-end telomere fusion.[352] It also permits the distinction of telomeres from sites of DNA damage, preventing their inappropriate processing. Recessive mutations in *NHP2* and in *NOP10*, which encode parts of small ribonucleoprotein components associated with the telomerase complex, also have been described in association with dyskeratosis.[353,354] Homozygous recessive mutations in the *TERT* gene produce a severe variant of dyskeratosis, referred to as the *Hoyeraal-Hreidarsson syndrome*.[342]

TABLE 4–13. Gene Mutations in Dyskeratosis Congenita

Gene	Chromosome Location	% of Patients	Inheritance	Protein Function
DKC1	Xq28	30	XLR	Essential part of snoRNPs and telomerase
TERC	3q26	5-10	AD	RNA 3'-end processing and stability
TERT	5p15.33	5-10	AD, AR	Reverse transcriptase component of telomerase
NOP10 (NOLA3)	15q14-q15	<1	AR	RNA binding
TINF2	14q11.2	15	AD	? Binds to TRF1 to regulate telomere length
CTC1	17p13.1	Rare	AR	Telomere maintenance component
NHP2 (NOLA2)	5q35.3	<1	AR	RNA binding protein; associates with NOP10 and DKC1
WRAP53 (TCAB1, WDR79)	17p13.1	Rare	AR	Trafficking of telomerase
331RTEL1 (NHL)	20q13.33	Rare	AD, AR	Regulator of telomere elongation helicase 1
C16orF57 (USB1)	16q21	2	AR	Unknown; Patient telomeres were normal length
hTR	3q	5-10	AD	hTR is the RNA component of telomerase

Abbreviations: AD, autosomal dominant; AR, autosomal recessive; XLR, X-linked recessive.

Table prepared from data in references 285, 288, 343, 346-349, 355 and OMIM (Online Mendelian Inheritance in Man). Percent of patients is approximate because of continuing identification of mutations.

Clinical Findings

The cutaneous findings usually appear after 5 years of age and include reticulated, tan to gray, hyperpigmented and hypopigmented cutaneous macules; alopecia of scalp, eyelashes, and eyebrows; adermatoglyphia (loss of dermal ridges on fingers and toes); hyperkeratosis of palms and soles; mucosal leukoplakia in 75% of patients; and dystrophic nails in more than 85% of patients.[285,342,343] Other mucosal sites, such as conjunctiva, lacrimal duct, esophagus, urethra, vagina, and anus, can be involved, sometimes with stenosis leading to dysphagia or dysuria. Pulmonary vascular involvement occurs in a significant minority of affected children. Aplastic anemia usually develops in late childhood or early adulthood and is evident in the classical blood and marrow findings described under acquired aplastic anemia. Female carriers of X-linked dyskeratosis congenita may have slight abnormalities such as a dystrophic nail, a single area of hypopigmentation, or slight leukoplakia.[342] The clinical manifestations exhibit disease anticipation, occurring earlier in subsequent generations, and this appears related to earlier shortening of the telomeres.[356]

Diagnosis

The diagnosis results from the combination of phenotypic findings and blood cell deficiencies. Genetic analysis for telomerase complex gene

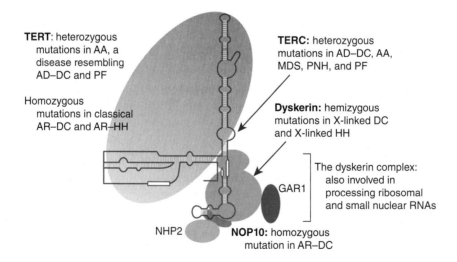

TERT: heterozygous mutations in AA, a disease resembling AD–DC and PF

Homozygous mutations in classical AR–DC and AR–HH

TERC: heterozygous mutations in AD–DC, AA, MDS, PNH, and PF

Dyskerin: hemizygous mutations in X-linked DC and X-linked HH

The dyskerin complex: also involved in processing ribosomal and small nuclear RNAs

GAR1

NHP2

NOP10: homozygous mutation in AR–DC

Figure 4–6. Representation of the interaction between dyskerin and the other molecules (GAR1, NHP2, NOP10, TERC, and TERT) of the telomerase complex (and their association with different disease categories). Telomerase is an RNA-protein complex because TERC is an RNA molecule that is never translated. The other molecules (dyskerin, GAR1, NHP2, NOP10, and TERT) are proteins. The minimal active telomerase enzyme is composed of two molecules each of TERT, TERC, and dyskerin. Dyskerin, GAR1, NHP2, and NOP10 are important for the stability of the telomerase complex. AA, aplastic anemia; AD–DC, autosomal dominant dyskeratosis congenita; AR–DC, autosomal recessive dyskeratosis congenita; AR–HH, autosomal recessive Hoyeraal-Heidarsson syndrome; MDS, myelodysplasia syndrome; PF, pulmonary fibrosis; PNH, paroxysmal nocturnal hemoglobinuria; X-linked DC, X-linked dyskeratosis congenita; X-linked HH, X-linked Hoyeraal-Heidarsson syndrome. *(Reproduced with permission from Dokal I, Vulliamy T: Inherited aplastic anaemias/bone marrow failure syndromes, Blood Rev 2008 May;22[3]:141-153.)*

mutations should be used to confirm the clinical conclusion. Shortened telomere length in leukocytes also can be assessed by flow cytometric fluorescence in situ hybridization studies.[357] The disease may occur without significant or evident phenotypoic features and onset may occur in late childhood or adulthood. Some persons may carry the gene mutation but do not exhibit the disease. For those reasons, patients thought to have acquired aplastic anemia should be tested for telomerase shortening, and if present, for mutaions in the telomerase gene complex.

Management
Hematopoietic cell transplantation has had inconsistent results because of frequent and severe posttransplantation complications, often pulmonary.[358,359] In a series of 109 transplanted patients, the 5- and 10-year survival rates were 57% and 23%, respectively.[360] Nonmyeloablative transplantation may improve results.[361-363] Transplantation might improve the cytopenias, but not the abnormalities of other organs or the frequency of secondary nonhematopoietic cancer.

Course and Prognosis
The incidence of squamous cell carcinoma of mucosal sites has increased, and the squamous cell carcinoma often originates in sites of leukoplakia in the skin, gastrointestinal, or genitourinary tracts.[364] These carcinomas usually develop in patients between the ages of 20 and 30 years. Mortality from neutropenic infection or thrombocytopenic hemorrhage occurs in about two-thirds of patients with aplastic anemia. Median survival is approximately 30 years.

SHWACHMAN-DIAMOND SYNDROME
Definition
This disease is an uncommon inherited disorder that is estimated to occur once in every 75,000 births,[365] manifesting as exocrine pancreatic insufficiency with secondary steatorrhea, blood cell deficiencies, and skeletal abnormalities. It was first described in 1964.[366,367]

Pathogenesis
Shwachman-Diamond syndrome results from mutations in the *SBDS* gene on chromosome 7q11, which induces accelerated cellular apoptosis via the FAS pathway.[368] The resulting hyperproliferation may account for the abnormal telomere shortening that has been documented in the leukocytes in this condition.[369] The pathogenetic mechanism that (1) prevents development of pancreatic acinar cells, (2) results in abnormal bone morphogenesis, and (3) causes marrow impairment of blood cell production is not completely understood. *SBDS* knockdown in experimental animals affects expression of genes involved in brain, bone, and marrow development, and appears to be the result of the gene's role in RNA processing.[370,371] The *SBDS* gene promotes the release of eukaryotic initiation factor 6 (ELF6) from the pre-60s ribosome.[350] This action is necessary for the formation of a mature 80s functional ribosome and production of appropriate ribosome joining. *SBDS* may be mutated by recombination with its pseudogene.[372] The mutations in *SBDS* result in abnormalities in neutrophil motility and chemotaxis, but pus formation in vivo seems adequate. Defects in ELF1 also may result in Schwachman-Diamond syndrome by impairing release of ELF6 from the ribosomes, causing ribosome disruption and impairing protein synthesis.[372] *DNAJ21* and *SRP54* mutations also produce a Schwachman-Diamond phenotype.[373]

Clinical Findings
Pancreatic insufficiency, steatorrhea, and neutropenia are present in most patients at the time of diagnosis.[366,367,374] Pallor may reflect anemia; easy bruising, epistaxis or bleeding from other sites reflect thrombocytopenia. Neutropenia occurs in approximately 95%, anemia in approximately 50%, and thrombocytopenia in approximately 35% of patients.[368] Thus, a substantial plurality of patients has bicytopenia or tricytopenia with hypoplastic marrow. Fetal hemoglobin levels are elevated in approximately 75% of the patients, perhaps secondary to erythroid hypoplasia. Cytogenetic abnormalities involving chromosomes 7 and 20 have been described in marrow cells. Nutritional inadequacies related to intestinal malabsorption result in a failure to thrive. Short stature is characteristic. Skeletal abnormalities are present in most patients, notably osteopenia, but also syndactyly, supernumerary metatarsals, coax vera deformity, and dental enamel defects and caries. Hepatic dysfunction as evidenced by elevated serum aminotransaminase is seen in most young patients and appears to resolve with age.[375] Delayed puberty is common. The neutropenia and chemotactic abnormality may result in recurrent infections, including sinusitis, otitis, pneumonia, osteomyelitis, and others. Pancreatic cell lipase production improves with age, and as many as half the patients may have improvement in lipid absorption in the small bowel over time.

Diagnosis
The diagnosis is based on the clinical findings of failure to thrive, steatorrhea, and neutropenia. Pancreatic insufficiency can be established by low serum trypsinogen in patients younger than 3 years. The marrow may initially be normal but develops evidence of marrow failure and sometimes cytogenetic abnormalities, particularly of chromosome 7, as the child ages. The age of expression of clonal hematopoiesis (eg, MDS or AML) is variable.[376] The *SBDS* gene mutation is present in 90% of patients with Shwachman-Diamond syndrome.[377] The remaining 10% have the clinical features of the syndrome, and some may have *ELF1*, *DNAJ21*, or *SRP54* mutations.[373]

Management
Supportive care, particularly with supplemental pancreatic enzymes, to provide proper nutrition, and appropriate and prompt treatment of bacterial infections with antibiotics is important. Many agents, including G-CSF, glucocorticoids, pancreatic extract, and vitamins have been tried to improve the neutropenia, with unpredictable results. Some agents have potential risks, such as G-CSF fostering clonal evolution and glucocorticoids fostering immunodeficiency. Severe hematopoietic dysfunction and cytopenias can be corrected with allogeneic hematopoietic cell transplantation.[378]

Course and Prognosis
Death from overwhelming sepsis is common. These patients, especially men, have a significant risk of progression to a MDS or AML.[367,379,380] Cytogenetic abnormalities are common, and telomeres are shortened,[381] as in other marrow failure syndromes. Survival is a function of the severity of the cytopenias. If the cytopenias are mild, survival is not uncommon into the fourth or fifth decade of life. It is not clear whether Shwachman-Diamond syndrome is associated with an increased incidence of solid tumors.

● OTHER INHERITED APLASTIC ANEMIAS
Several other rare syndromes are associated with aplastic pancytopenia, and these are described in Table 4-12. Congenital (hereditary) amegakaryocytic thrombocytopenia (CAMT) results from mutations in the TPO receptor gene, *MPL*.[278-281] Affected children can be divided into two groups: CAMT I with mutations leading to complete loss-of-function of the TPO receptor, resulting in more severe thrombocytopenia and a rapid progression to pancytopenia (aplastic anemia); and CAMT II, resulting from a variety of missense mutations, in which affected

children have an increase in platelet count above 50×10^9/L with time and much slower progression to and sometimes less severe pancytopenia.[307] Rarely, homozygous mutations in the *THPO* gene also can cause CAMT, which may respond to romiplostim therapy.[309] A rare homozygous mutation in *MPL* is associated with a familial aplastic anemia syndrome.[310] Reticular dysgenesis results from a pluripotential stem cell defect as both lymphoid and granulocytic progenitors are affected.[322,323] It is a rare autosomal recessive disorder caused by mutations in the adenylate kinase 2 gene *(AK2)* and characterized by bilateral sensorineural deafness, severe combined immunodeficiency, and agranulocytosis, which subjects infants to severe, often, life-threatening infections. *ERCC6L2* homozygous mutations can cause a familial marrow failure syndrome with associated developmental delay microcephaly and cerebellar ataxia in some cases.[311,312] A heterozygous dominant mutation in the SRP72 gene is capable of causing a familial aplastic anemia or MDS.[313] The Seckel syndrome results from mutations in the *ATR* gene, and marrow cells exhibit heightened sister chromatid exchange. The ataxia-telangiectasia–mutated and rad3-related (ATR) kinase mediates cellular responses to DNA damage and replication stress. Most of the eight syndromes delineated in Table 4-12 can be treated by hematopoietic cell transplantation but, if successful, this step does not correct somatic abnormalities, only the hematopoietic and immunologic defect. The restoration of robust lymphohematopoiesis by transplantation may decrease their propensity to undergo clonal evolution to a clonal myeloid or, in some cases, lymphoid disorder.

REFERENCES

1. Incidence of aplastic anemia: the relevance of diagnostic criteria. By the International Agranulocytosis and Aplastic Anemia Study. *Blood.* 1987;70:1718.
2. Ehrlich P. Über einen Fall von Anamie mit Bemerkungen über regenerative Veranderungen des Knochenmarks. *Charite Ann.* 1888;13:300.
3. Chauffard M. Un cas d'anémie pernicieuse aplastique. *Bull Soc Med Hop Paris.* 1904;21:313.
4. Scott JL, Cartwright GE, Wintrobe MM. Acquired aplastic anemia: an analysis of thirty-nine cases and review of the pertinent literature. *Medicine (Baltimore).* 1959;38:119.
5. Thomas ED, Storb R, Fefer A, et al. Aplastic anemia treated by bone marrow transplantation. *Lancet.* 1972;1:284.
6. Thomas ED, Storb R, Giblett B, et al. Recovery from aplastic anemia following attempted marrow transplantation. *Exp Hematol.* 1976;4:97.
7. Champlin RE, Feig SA, Sparkes RS, Gale RP. Bone marrow transplantation from identical twins in the treatment of aplastic anaemia: Implication for the pathogenesis of the disease. *Br J Haematol.* 1984;56:455.
8. Speck B, Gluckman E. Treatment of aplastic anemia by antilymphocyte globulin with and without allogeneic bone marrow infusions. *Lancet.* 1977;2:1145.
9. Mary JY, Baumelou E, Guiguet M. Epidemiology of aplastic anemia in France: a prospective multicentre study. *Blood.* 1990;75:1646.
10. Montané E, Ibáñez L, Vidal X, et al. Epidemiology of aplastic anemia: a prospective multicenter study. *Haematologica.* 2008;93:518.
11. Maluf EM, Pasquini R, Eluf JN, et al. Aplastic anemia in Brazil: incidence and risk factors. *Am J Hematol.* 2002;71:268.
12. McCahon E, Tang K, Rogers PC, et al. The impact of Asian descent on the incidence of acquired severe aplastic anaemia in children. *Br J Haematol.* 2003;121:170.
13. Chongli Y, Ziaobo Z. Incidence survey of aplastic anemia in China. *Chin Med Sci J.* 1991;6:203.
14. Issaragrisil S. Epidemiology of aplastic anemia in Thailand. Thai Aplastic Anemia Study Group. *Int J Hematol.* 1999;70:137.
15. Yong AS, Goh AS, Rahman M, et al. Epidemiology of aplastic anemia in the state of Sabah, Malaysia. *Med J Malaysia.* 1998;53:59.
16. Issaragrisil S, Kaufman DW, Anderson T, et al. The epidemiology of aplastic anemia in Thailand. *Blood.* 2006;107:1299.
17. Young NS, Kaufman DW. The epidemiology of acquired aplastic anemia. *Haematologica.* 2008;93:489.
18. Yin SN, Hayes RB, Linet MS, et al. A cohort study of cancer among benzene-exposed workers in China: overall results. *Am J Ind Med.* 1996;29:227.
19. Locasciulli A, Bacigalupo A, Bruno B, et al. Hepatitis-associated aplastic anaemia: epidemiology and treatment results obtained in Europe. A report of The EBMT aplastic anaemia working party. *Br J Haematol.* 2010;149:890.
20. Mohseny AB, Eikema DA, Neven B, et al. Hematopoietic tem cell ransplantation for hepatitis-associated aplastic anemia following liver transplantation for nonviral hepatitis: A retrospective analysis and a review of the literature by the Severe Aplastic Anemia Working Party of the European Society for Blood and Marrow Transplantation (SAAWP-EBMT). *Pediatr Hematol Oncol.* 2020 Dec 2. doi: 10.1097/MPH.0000000000001991. Online ahead of print.PMID: 33273414
21. Kagan WA, Ascensao J, Pahwa R, et al. Aplastic anemia: presence in human bone marrow of cells that suppress myelopoiesis. *Proc Natl Acad Sci U S A.* 1976;73:2890.
22. Maciejewski JP, Anderson S, Katevas P, Young NS. Phenotypic and functional analysis of bone marrow progenitor cell compartment in bone marrow failure. *Br J Haematol.* 1994;87:227.
23. Scopes J, Bagnara M, Gordon-Smith EC, et al. Haemopoietic progenitor cells are reduced in aplastic anaemia. *Br J Haematol.* 1994;86:427.
24. Maciejewski JP, Selleri C, Sato T, et al. A severe and consistent deficit in marrow and circulating primitive hematopoietic cells (long-term culture-initiating cells) in acquired aplastic anemia. *Blood.* 1996;88:1983.
25. Sugimori C, Yamazaki H, Feng X, et al. Roles of DRB1 ˚1501 and DRB1 ˚1502 in the pathogenesis of aplastic anemia. *Exp Hematol.* 2007;35:13.
26. Young NS, Scheinberg P, Calado RT. Aplastic anemia. *Curr Opin Hematol.* 2008;15:162.
27. Young NS, Calado RT, Scheinberg P. Why does the bone marrow fail in Fanconi anemia? *Blood.* 2006;108:2509.
28. Young NS, Maciejewski J. Mechanisms of disease: the pathophysiology of acquired aplastic anemia. *N Engl J Med.* 1997;336:1365.
29. Laver J, Castro-Malaspina H, Kernan NA, et al. In vitro interferon-gamma production by cultured T-cells in severe aplastic anaemia: correlation with granulomonopoietic inhibition in patients who respond to anti-thymocyte globulin. *Br J Haematol.* 1988;69:545.
30. Gascon P, Zoumbos NC, Scala G, et al. Lymphokine abnormalities in aplastic anemia: implications for the mechanism of action of antithymocyte globulin. *Blood.* 1985;65:407.
31. Hinterberger W, Adolf G, Bettelheim P, et al. Lymphokine overproduction in severe aplastic anemia is not related to blood transfusions. *Blood.* 1989;74:2713.
32. Shinohara K, Ayame H, Tanaka M, et al. Increased production of tumor necrosis factor alpha by peripheral blood mononuclear cells in the patients with aplastic anemia. *Am J Hematol.* 1991;37:75.
33. Nistico A, Young, NS: Gamma-interferon gene expression in the bone marrow of patients with aplastic anemia. *Ann Intern Med.* 1994;120:463.
34. Zoumbos N, Gascon P, Djeu J, Young NS. Interferon is a mediator of hematopoietic suppression in aplastic anemia in vitro and possibly in vivo. *Proc Natl Acad Sci U S A.* 1985;82:188.
35. Sloand E, Kim S, Maciejewski JP, et al. Intracellular interferon-gamma in circulating and marrow T cells detected by flow cytometry and the response to immunosuppressive therapy in patients with aplastic anemia. *Blood.* 2002;100:1185.
36. Solomou EE, Keyvanfar K, Young NS. T-bet, a Th1 transcription factor, is up-regulated in T cells from patients with aplastic anemia. *Blood.* 2006;107:3983.
37. Risitano AM, Maciejewski JP, Green S, et al. In vivo dominant immune responses in aplastic anaemia: molecular tracking of putatively pathogenetic T-cell clones by TCR beta-CDR3 sequencing. *Lancet.* 2004;364:355.
38. Solomou EE, Rezvani K, Mielke S, et al. Deficient CD4+ CD25+ FOXP3+ T regulatory cells in acquired aplastic anemia. *Blood.* 2007;110:1603.
39. Fujisaki J, Wu J, Carlson AL, et al. In vivo imaging of Treg cells providing immune privilege to the haematopoietic stem-cell niche. *Nature.* 2011;474:216.
40. Xiao Y, Zhao S, Li B. Aplastic anemia is related to alterations in T cell receptor signaling. *Stem Cell Investig.* 2017;4:85.
41. Chen J, Ellison FM, Eckhaus MA, et al. Minor antigen h60-mediated aplastic anemia is ameliorated by immunosuppression and the infusion of regulatory T cells. *J Immunol.* 2007;178:4159.
42. Kordasti S, Costantini B, Seidl T, et al. Deep phenotyping of Tregs identifies an immune signature for idiopathic aplastic anemia and predicts response to treatment. *Blood.* 2016;128:1193.
43. Hirano N, Butler MO, Von Bergwelt-Baildon MS, et al. Autoantibodies frequently detected in patients with aplastic anemia. *Blood.* 2003;102:4567.
44. Young NS. Current concepts in the pathophysiology and treatment of aplastic anemia. *Hematology Am Soc Hematol Educ Program.* 2013;2013:76.
45. Townsley DM, Dumitriu B, Young NS. Bone marrow failure and the telomeropathies. *Blood.* 2014;124:2775.
46. Smick K, Condit PK, Proctor RL, Sutcher V. Fatal aplastic anemia: an epidemiological study of its relationship to the drug chloramphenicol. *J Chronic Dis.* 1964;17:899.
47. Modan B, Segal S, Shani M, Sheba C. Aplastic anemia in Israel: evaluation of the etiological role of chloramphenicol on a community-wide basis. *Am J Med Sci.* 1975;270:441.
48. Yunis AA Chloramphenicol toxicity: 25 years of research. *Am J Med.* 1989;87:44N.
49. Custer RP. Aplastic anemia in soldiers treated with Atabrine (quinacrine). *Am J Med Sci.* 1946;212:211.
50. Best WR. Drug-associated blood dyscrasias. *JAMA.* 1963;185:286.
51. Risks of agranulocytosis and aplastic anemia. A first report of their relation to drug use with special reference to analgesics. The International Agranulocytosis and Aplastic Anemia Study. *JAMA.* 1986;256:1749.
52. Retsagi G, Kelly JP, Kaufman DW. Risk of agranulocytosis and aplastic anaemia in relation to use of antithyroid drugs. International Agranulocytosis and Aplastic Anaemia Study. *BMJ.* 1988;297:262.
53. Anti-infective drug use in relation to the risk of agranulocytosis and aplastic anemia. A report from the International Agranulocytosis and Aplastic Anemia Study. *Arch Intern Med.* 1989;149:1036.

54. Kelly JP, Kaufman DW, Shapiro S. Risks of agranulocytosis and aplastic anemia in relation to the use of cardiovascular drugs: the International Agranulocytosis and Aplastic Anemia Study. *Clin Pharmacol Ther.* 1991;49:330.

55. Kaufmann DW, Kelly JP, Jurgelon JM, et al. Drugs in the aetiology of agranulocytosis and aplastic anaemia. *Eur J Haematol.* 1996;57(suppl):23.

56. Baumelou E, Guiguet M, Mary JY, et al. Epidemiology of aplastic anemia in France: a case control study. I. Medical history and medication use. *Blood.* 1993;81:1471.

57. Bithell TC, Wintrobe MM. Drug-induced aplastic anemia. *Semin Hematol.* 1967;4:194.

58. Williams DM, Lynch RE, Cartwright GE. Drug-induced aplastic anemia. *Semin Hematol.* 1973;10:195.

59. Tonkonow B, Hoffman R. Aplastic anemia and cimetidine. *Arch Intern Med.* 1980;140:1123.

60. Volkin RL, Shadduck RK, Winkelstein A, et al. Potentiation of carmustine-cranial-irradiation-induced myelosuppression by cimetidine. *Arch Intern Med.* 1982;142:243.

61. Comito RR, Badu LA, Forcello N. Nivolumab-induced aplastic anemia: a case report and literature review. *J Oncol Pharm Pract.* 2019;25:221-225.

62. Khan HA. Benzene toxicity: a consolidated short review of human and animal studies. *Hum Exp Toxicol.* 2007;26:677.

63. Smith MT. Overview of benzene-induced aplastic anemia. *Eur J Haematol.* 1996;60:107.

64. Snyder R. Benzene and leukemia. *Crit Rev Toxicol.* 2002;32:155.

65. Fleming LE, Timmeny MA. Aplastic anemia and pesticides. An etiologic association? *J Occup Med.* 1993;35:1106.

66. Rugman FP, Cosstick R. Aplastic anaemia associated with organochlorine pesticide: case reports and review of evidence. *J Clin Pathol.* 1990;43:98.

67. Muir KR, Chilvers CE, Harriss C, et al. The role of occupational and environmental exposures in the aetiology of acquired severe aplastic anaemia: a case control investigation. *Br J Haematol.* 2003;123:906.

68. Valdez Salas B, Garcia Duran EI, Wiener MS. Impact of pesticides use on human health in Mexico: a review. *Rev Environ Health.* 2000;15:399.

69. Ahamed M, Anand M, Kumar A, Siddiqui MK. Childhood aplastic anaemia in Lucknow, India: incidence, organochlorines in the blood and review of case reports following exposure to pesticides. *Clin Biochem.* 2006;39:762.

70. Rauch AE, Kowalsky SF, Lesar TS, et al. Lindane (Kwell)-induced aplastic anemia. *Arch Intern Med.* 1990;150:2393.

71. Roberts HJ. Pentachlorophenol-associated aplastic anemia, red cell aplasia, leukemia and other blood disorders. *J Fla Med Assoc.* 1990;77:86.

72. Prager D, Peters C. Development of aplastic anemia and the exposure to Stoddard solvent. *Blood.* 1970;35:286.

73. Powers D. Aplastic anemia secondary to glue sniffing. *N Engl J Med.* 1965;273:700.

74. Kirtadze I, Zurabashvili D. Study of chemical composition of glue "RAZI" used by solvent abusers in Tbilisi. *Georgian Med News.* 2006;133:65.

75. Sabbioni G, Sepai O, Norppa H, et al. Comparison of biomarkers in workers exposed to 2,4,6-trinitrotoluene. *Biomarkers.* 2007;12:21.

76. Crawford MAD. Aplastic anaemia due to trinitrotoluene intoxication. *BMJ.* 1954;2:430.

77. Ajlouni K, Doeblin TD. The syndrome of hepatitis and aplastic anaemia. *Br J Haematol.* 1974;27:345.

78. Hagler L, Pastore RA, Bergin JJ. Aplastic anemia following viral hepatitis: report of 2 fatal cases and literature review. *Medicine (Baltimore).* 1975;54:139.

79. Pol S, Driss F, Devergie A, et al. Is hepatitis C virus involved in hepatitis-associated aplastic anemia? *Ann Intern Med.* 1990;113:435.

80. Hibbs JR, Frickhofen N, Rosenfeld SJ, et al. Aplastic anemia and viral hepatitis: non-A, non-B, non-C? *JAMA.* 1992;267:2051.

81. Honkaniemi E, Gustafsson B, Fischler B, et al. Acquired aplastic anaemia in seven children with severe hepatitis with or without liver failure. *Acta Paediatr.* 2007;96:1660.

82. Tzakis AG, Arditi M, Whitington PF, et al. Aplastic anemia complicating orthotopic liver transplantation for non-A, non-B hepatitis. *N Engl J Med.* 1988;319:393.

83. Brown KE, Tisdale J, Barrett AJ, Dunbar CE, Young NS. Hepatitis-associated aplastic anemia. *N Engl J Med.* 1997;336:1059.

84. Safadi R, Or R, Ilan Y, et al. Lack of known hepatitis virus in hepatitis-associated aplastic anemia and outcome after bone marrow transplantation. *Bone Marrow Transplant.* 2001;27:183.

85. Mishra B, Malhotra P, Ratho RK, et al. Human parvovirus B19 in patients with aplastic anemia. *Am J Hematol.* 2005;79:166.

86. Yetgin S, Cetin M, Ozyürek E, et al. Parvovirus B19 infection associated with severe aplastic anemia in an immunocompetent patient. *Pediatr Hematol Oncol.* 2004;21:223.

87. Wong S, Young NS, Brown KE. Prevalence of parvovirus B19 in liver tissue: no association with fulminant hepatitis or hepatitis-associated aplastic anemia. *J Infect Dis.* 2003;187:1581.

88. Mori T, Onishi Y, Ozawa Y, et al. Outcome of allogeneic hematopoietic stem cell transplantation in adult patients with hepatitis-associated aplastic anemia. *Int J Hematol.* 2019;109:711-717.

89. Locasciulli A, Bacigalupo A, Bruno B, et al. Hepatitis-associated aplastic anaemia: epidemiology and treatment results obtained in Europe. A report of The EBMT aplastic anaemia working party. *Br J Haematol.* 2010;149:890.

90. Rauff B, Idrees M, Shah SAR, et al. Hepatitis associated aplastic anemia: a review. *Virol J.* 2011;8:87.

91. Yang WR, Jing LP, Zhou K, et al. [Hepatitis-associated aplastic anaemia: clinical characteristics and immunosuppressive therapy outcomes]. [Abstract in English] *CMAJ.* 2016;37:399-404.

92. Lazarus KH, Baehner RL. Aplastic anemia complicating infectious mononucleosis: a case report and review of the literature. *Pediatrics.* 1981;67:907.

93. Baranski B, Armstrong G, Truman JT, et al. Epstein-Barr virus in the bone marrow of patients with aplastic anemia. *Ann Intern Med.* 1988;109:695.

94. Vinters HV, Mah V, Mohrmann R, Wiley CA. Evidence for human immunodeficiency virus (HIV) infection of the brain in a patient with aplastic anemia. *Acta Neuropathol.* 1988;76:311.

95. Samuel D, Castaing D, Adam R, et al. Fatal acute HIV infection with aplastic anaemia, transmitted by liver graft. *Lancet.* 1988;1:1221.

96. Morales CE, Sriram I, Baumann MA. Myelodysplastic syndrome occurring as possible first manifestation of human immunodeficiency virus infection with subsequent progression to aplastic anaemia. *Int J STD AIDS.* 1990;1:55.

97. Rosenfeld CS, Rybka WB, Weinbaum D, et al. Late graft failure due to dual bone marrow infection with variants A and B of human Herpesvirus-6. *Exp Hematol.* 1995;23:626.

98. Pavithran K, Raji NL, Thomas M. Aplastic anemia complicating lupus erythematosus—report of a case and review of the literature. *Rheumatol Int.* 2002;22:253.

99. Bailey FA, Lilly M, Bertoli LF, Ball GV. An antibody that inhibits in vitro bone marrow proliferation in a patient with systemic lupus erythematosus and aplastic anemia. *Arthritis Rheum.* 1989;31:901.

100. Chalayer E, Ffrench M, Cathébras P. Aplastic anemia as a feature of systemic lupus erythematosus: a case report and review of the literature. *Rheumatol Int.* 2015;35:1073-82.

101. Sumimoto S, Kawai M, Kasajima Y, Hamamoto T. Aplastic anemia associated with systemic lupus erythematosus. *Am J Hematol.* 1991;38:329.

102. Winkler A, Jackson RW, Kay DS, et al. High-dose intravenous cyclophosphamide treatment of systemic lupus erythematosus-associated aplastic anemia [letter]. *Arthritis Rheum.* 1988;31:693.

103. Kim SW, Rice L, Champlin R, Udden MM. Aplastic anemia in eosinophilic fasciitis: responses to immunosuppression and marrow transplantation. *Haematologica.* 1997;28:131.

104. de Masson A, Bouaziz JD, Peffault de Latour R, et al. Severe aplastic anemia associated with eosinophilic fasciitis: report of four cases and review of the literature. *Medicine (Baltimore).* 2013;92:69-81.

105. Kumar M, Goldman J. Severe aplastic anemia and Grave's disease in a paediatric patient. *Br J Haematol.* 2002;118:327.

106. Tomonari A, Tojo A, Iseki T, et al. Severe aplastic anemia with autoimmune thyroiditis showing no hematological response to intensive immunosuppressive therapy. *Acta Haematol.* 2003;109:90.

107. Aydin Y, Berker D, Ustün I, et al. A very rare cause of aplastic anemia: Graves disease. *South Med J.* 2008;101:666.

108. Lima CS, Zantut Wittmann DE, Castro V, et al. Pancytopenia in untreated patients with Graves' disease. *Thyroid.* 2006;16:403.

109. Das PK, Wherrett D, Dror Y. Remission of aplastic anemia induced by treatment for Graves disease in a pediatric patient. *Pediatr Blood Cancer.* 2007;49:210.

110. Dincol G, Saka B, Aktan M, et al. Very severe aplastic anemia following resection of lymphocytic thymoma: effectiveness of antilymphocyte globulin, cyclosporine A and granulocyte-colony stimulating factor. *Am J Hematol.* 2000;64:78.

111. Ritchie DS, Underhill C, Grigg AP. Aplastic anemia as a late complication of thymoma in remission. *Eur J Haematol.* 2002;68:389.

112. Gaglia A, Bobota A, Pectasides E, et al. Successful treatment with cyclosporine of thymoma-related aplastic anemia. *Anticancer Res.* 2007;27:3025.

113. Trisal V, Nademanee A, Lau SK, Grannis FW Jr. Thymoma-associated severe aplastic anemia treated with surgical resection followed by allogeneic stem-cell transplantation. *J Clin Oncol.* 2007;25:3374.

114. Arcasoy MO, Gockerman JP. Aplastic anaemia as an autoimmune complication of thymoma. *Br J Haematol.* 2007;137:272.

115. Park CY, Kim HJ, Kim YJ, et al. Very severe aplastic anemia appearing after thymectomy. *Korean J Intern Med.* 2003;18:61.

116. Abrams EM, Gibson IW, Blydt-Hansen TD. The concurrent presentation of minimal change nephrotic syndrome and aplastic anemia. *Pediatr Nephrol.* 2009;24:407.

117. Riveros-Perez E, Hermesch AC, Barbour LA. Aplastic anemia during pregnancy: a review of obstetrics and anesthetic considerations. *Int J Womens Health.* 2018;10:117-125.

118. Pajor A, Kelemen E, Szak'acs Z, Lehoczky D. Pregnancy in idiopathic aplastic anemia (report of 10 patients). *Eur J Obstet Gynecol Reprod Biol.* 1992;45:19.

119. Bourantas K, Makrydimas G, Georgiou J, et al. Aplastic anemia: report of a case with recurrent episodes in consecutive pregnancies. *J Reprod Med.* 1997;42:672.

120. Kwon JY, Lee Y, Shin JC, et al. Supportive management of pregnancy-associated aplastic anemia. *Int J Gynaecol Obstet.* 2006;95:115.

121. Thakral B, Saluja K, Sharma RR, et al. Successful management of pregnancy-associated severe aplastic anemia. *Eur J Obstet Gynecol Reprod Biol.* 2007;131:244.

122. Tichelli A, Socie G, Marsh J, et al. Outcome of pregnancy and disease course among women with aplastic anemia treated with immunosuppression. *Ann Intern Med.* 2002;137:164.

123. Court-Brown WM, Doll R. Leukaemia and aplastic anaemia in patients irradiated for ankylosing spondylitis. 1957. *J Radiol Prot.* 2007;27:B15-B154.

124. Darby SC, Doll R, Gill SK, Smith PG. Long term mortality after a single treatment course with x-rays in patients treated with ankylosing spondylitis. *Br J Cancer.* 1987;55:179.

125. Johnson SAN, Bateman CJT, Beard MEJ, et al. Long-term haematological complications of Thorotrast. *Q J Med.* 1977;182:259.

126. Martland HS. The occurrence of malignancy in radioactive persons: a general review of data gathered in the study of the radium dial painters, with special reference to the occurrence of osteogeneic sarcoma and the inter-relationship of certain blood diseases. *Am J Cancer.* 1931;15:2435.

127. Cronkite EP, Haley TJ. Clinical aspects of acute radiation injury. In: *Manual on Radiation Haematology.* International Atomic Energy Agency; 1971:169-173.

128. Mettler FA Jr, Moseley RD Jr. *Medical Effects of Ionizing Irradiation.* Grune and Stratton; 1985:1185.

129. Gale RP. USSR: follow-up after Chernobyl. *Lancet.* 1990;1:401.

130. Green DE, Rubin CT. Consequences of irradiation on bone and marrow phenotypes and its relationship to disruption of hematopoietic precursors. *Bone.* 2014;10:87-94.

131. Nimer SD, Leung DHY, Wolin MJ, Golde DW. Serum stem cell factor levels in patients with aplastic anemia. *Int J Hematol.* 1994;60:185.

132. Kojima S, Matsuyama T, Kodera Y. Plasma levels and production of soluble stem cell factor by marrow stromal cells in patients with aplastic anaemia. *Br J Haematol.* 1997;99:440.

133. Lyman SD, Seaberg M, Hanna R, et al. Plasma/serum levels of flt3 ligand are low in normal individuals and highly elevated in patients with Fanconi anemia and acquired aplastic anemia. *Blood.* 1995;86:4091.

134. Kojima S, Matsuyama T, Kodera Y, et al. Measurement of endogenous plasma granulocyte colony-stimulating factor in patients with acquired aplastic anemia by a sensitive chemiluminescent immunoassay. *Blood.* 1996;87:1303.

135. Kojima S, Matsuyama T, Kodera Y. Circulating erythropoietin in patients with acquired aplastic anaemia. *Acta Haematol.* 1995;94:117.

136. Emmons RVD, Reid DM, Cohen RL, et al. Human thrombopoietin levels are high when thrombocytopenia is due to megakaryocyte deficiency and low when due to increased platelet destruction. *Blood.* 1996;87:4068.

137. Nakao S, Matsushima K, Young N. Deficient interleukin I production by aplastic anaemia monocytes. *Br J Haematol.* 1989;71:431.

138. Holmberg LA, Seidel K, Leisenring W, Torok-Storb B. Aplastic anemia: analysis of stromal cell function in long-term marrow cultures. *Blood.* 1994;84:3685.

139. Medinger M, Drexler B, Lengerke C, Passweg J. Pathogenesis of acquired aplastic anemia. *Front Oncol.* 2018;8:587-597.

140. Stute N, Fehse B, Schroder J, et al. Human mesenchymal stem cells are not of donor origin in patients with severe aplastic anemia who underwent sex-mismatched allogeneic bone marrow transplant. *J Hematother Stem Cell Res.* 2002;11:977.

141. Applebaum FR, Barrall J, Storb R, et al. Clonal cytogenetic abnormalities in patients with otherwise typical aplastic anemia. *Exp Hematol.* 1987;15:1134.

142. Kulasekararaj AG, Jiang J, Smith AE, et al. Somatic mutations identify a subgroup of aplastic anemia patients who progress to myelodysplastic syndrome. *Blood.* 2014;124:2698.

143. Negendank W, Weissman D, Bey TM, et al. Evidence for clonal disease by magnetic resonance imaging in patients with hypoplastic marrow disorders. *Blood.* 1991;78:2872.

144. Schrezenmeier H, Hertenstein B, Wagner B, et al. A pathogenetic link between aplastic anemia and paroxysmal nocturnal hemoglobinuria is suggested by a high frequency of aplastic anemia patients with a deficiency of phosphatidylinositol glycan anchored proteins. *Exp Hematol.* 1995;23:81.

145. Horsley SW, Colman S, McKinley M, et al. Genetic lesions in a preleukemic aplasia phase in a child with acute lymphoblastic leukemia. *Genes Chromosomes Cancer.* 2008;47:333.

146. Suzan F, Terré C, Garcia I, et al. Three cases of typical aplastic anaemia associated with a Philadelphia chromosome. *Br J Haematol.* 2001;112:385.

147. Socie G, Rosenfeld S, Frickhofen N, et al. Late clonal diseases of aplastic anemia. *Semin Hematol.* 2000;37:91101.

148. Gordon-Smith EC, Marsh JC, Gibson FM. Views on the pathophysiology of aplastic anemia. *Int J Hematol.* 2002;76(Suppl 2):163.

149. Maciejewski JP, Risitano A, Sloand EM, et al. Distinct clinical outcomes for cytogenetic abnormalities evolving from aplastic anemia. *Blood.* 2002;99:3129.

150. Socie G, Henryamar M, Bacigalupo A, et al. Malignant tumors occurring after treatment of aplastic anemia. *N Engl J Med.* 1993;329:1152.

151. Najean Y, Haguenauer O. Long-term (5–20 years) evolution of non-grafted aplastic anemias. *Blood.* 1990;76:2222.

152. Ball SE, Gibson FM, Rizzo S. Progressive telomere shortening in aplastic anemia. *Blood.* 1998;91:3582.

153. Rosse WF. New insights into paroxysmal nocturnal hemoglobinuria. *Curr Opin Hematol.* 2001;8:61.

154. Nakakuma H, Kawaguchi T. Pathogenesis of selective expansion of PNH clones. *Int J Hematol.* 2003;77:121.

155. Scheinberg P, Marte M, Nunez O, Young NS. Paroxysmal nocturnal hemoglobinuria clones in severe aplastic anemia patients treated with horse anti-thymocyte globulin plus cyclosporine. *Haematologica.* 2010;95:1075.

156. Stanley N, Olson TS, Babushok DV. Recent advances in understanding clonal haematopoiesis in aplastic anaemia. *Br J Haematol.* 2017;177:509-525.

157. Storb R, Blume KG, O'Donnell MR, et al. Cyclophosphamide and antithymocyte globulin to condition patients with aplastic anemia for allogeneic marrow transplantation: the experience in four centers. *Biol Blood Marrow Transplant.* 2001;7:39.

158. Bayanzay K, Alzoebie L. Reducing the iron burden and improving survival in transfusion-dependent thalassemia patients: current perspectives. *J Blood Med.* 2017;7:159-169.

159. Sagmeister M, Oec L, Gmur J. A restrictive platelet transfusion policy allowing long-term support of outpatients with severe aplastic anemia. *Blood.* 1999;93:3124.

160. Lawrence JB, Yomtovian RA, Hammons T, et al. Lowering the prophylactic platelet transfusion threshold: a prospective analysis. *Leuk Lymphoma.* 2001;41:67.

161. Zeigler ZR. Effects of epsilon aminocaproic acid on primary haemostasis. *Haemostasis.* 1991;21:313.

162. Hod E, Schwartz J. Platelet transfusion refractoriness. *Br J Haematol.* 2008;142:348.

163. Slichter SJ, Davis K, Enright H, et al. Factors affecting posttransfusion platelet increments, platelet refractoriness, and platelet transfusion intervals in thrombocytopenic patients. *Blood.* 2005;105:4106.

164. Drewniak A, Boelens JJ, Vrielink H, et al. Granulocyte concentrates: prolonged functional capacity during storage in the presence of phenotypic changes. *Haematologica.* 2008;93:1058.

165. Armand P, Antin JH. Allogeneic stem cell transplantation for aplastic anemia. *Biol Blood Marrow Transplant.* 2007;13:505.

166. Georges GE, Storb R. Stem cell transplantation for aplastic anemia. *Int J Hematol.* 2002;75:141.

167. Champlin RE, Perez WS, Passweg JR, et al. Bone marrow transplantation for severe aplastic anemia: a randomized controlled study of conditioning regimens. *Blood.* 2007;109:4582.

168. DeZern AE, Zahurak ML, Symons HJ, et al. Haploidentical BMT for severe aplastic anemia with intensive GVHD prophylaxis including posttransplant cyclophosphamide. *Blood Adv* 2020;4:1770-1779.

169. Locasciulli A, Oneto R, Bacigalupo A, et al. Outcome of patients with acquired aplastic anemia given first line bone marrow transplantation or immunosuppressive treatment in the last decade: a report from the European Group for Blood and Marrow Transplantation (EBMT). *Haematologica.* 2007;92:11.

170. Gandhi S, Kulasekararaj AG, Mufti GJ, Marsh JC. Allogeneic stem cell transplantation using alemtuzumab-containing regimens in severe aplastic anemia. *Int J Hematol.* 2013;97:573.

171. Grimaldi F, Potter V, Perez-Abellan P, et al. Mixed T cell chimerism after allogeneic hematopoietic stem cell transplantation for severe aplastic anemia using an alemtuzumab-containing regimen is shaped by persistence of recipient CD8 T cells. *Biol Blood Marrow Transplant.* 2017;23:293.

172. Ngwube A, Hayashi RJ, Murray L, et al. Alemtuzumab based reduced intensity transplantation for pediatric severe aplastic anemia. *Pediatr Blood Cancer.* 2015;62:1270.

173. Viollier R, Socié G, Tichelli A, et al. Recent improvement in outcome of unrelated donor transplantation for aplastic anemia. *Bone Marrow Transplant.* 2008;41:45.

174. Peffault de Latour R, Chevret S, Jubert C, et al; Francophone Society of Bone Marrow Transplantation and Cellular Therapy. Unrelated cord blood transplantation in patients with idiopathic refractory severe aplastic anemia: a nationwide phase 2 study. *Blood.* 2018;132:750-754.

175. Lee SJ, Klein J, Haagenson M, Baxter-Lowe LA, et al. High-resolution donor-recipient HLA matching contributes to the success of unrelated donor marrow transplantation. *Blood.* 2007;110:4576.

176. Pierri F, Dufour C. Management of aplastic anemia after failure of frontline immunosuppression. *Exp Rev Hematol.* 2019;24:1-11.

177. Dubey S, Nityanand S. Involvement of Fas and TNF pathways in the induction of apoptosis of T cells by antithymocyte globulin. *Ann Hematol.* 2003;82:496.

178. Michallet M-C, Saltel F, Preville X, et al. Cathepsin-B-dependent apoptosis triggered by antithymocyte globulins: a novel mechanism of T-cell depletion. *Blood.* 2003; 102:3719.

179. Mangan KF, D'Alessandro L, Mullaney MT. Action of antithymocyte globulin on normal human erythroid progenitor cell proliferation in vitro: erythropoietic growth-enhancing factors are released from marrow accessory cells. *J Lab Clin Med.* 1986;107:353.

180. Kawano Y, Nissen C, Gratwohl A, Speck B. Immunostimulatory effects of different antilymphocyte globulin preparations: a possible clue to their clinical effect. *Br J Haematol.* 1988;68:115.

181. Bielory L, Wright R, Nienhuis AW, et al. Antithymocyte globulin hypersensitivity in bone marrow failure patients. *JAMA.* 1988;260:3164.

182. Zheng Y, Liu Y, Chu Y. Immunosuppressive therapy for acquired severe aplastic anemia (SAA): a prospective comparison of four different regimens. *Exp Hematol.* 2006;34:826.

183. Atta EH, Dias DS, Marra VL, de Azevedo AM. Comparison between horse and rabbit antithymocyte globulin as first-line treatment for patients with severe aplastic anemia: a single-center retrospective study. *Ann Hematol.* 2010;89:851.

184. Garg R, Faderl S, Garcia-Manero G, et al. Phase II study of rabbit anti-thymocyte globulin, cyclosporine and granulocyte colony-stimulating factor in patients with aplastic anemia and myelodysplastic syndrome. *Leukemia.* 2009;23:1297.

185. Scheinberg P, Nunez O, Weinstein B, et al. Horse versus rabbit antithymocyte globulin in acquired aplastic anemia. *N Engl J Med.* 2011;365:430.

186. Kadia TM, Borthakur G, Garcia-Manero G, et al. Final results of the phase II study of rabbit anti-thymocyte globulin, ciclosporin, methylprednisone, and granulocyte colony-stimulating factor in patients with aplastic anaemia and myelodysplastic syndrome. *Br J Haematol.* 2012;157:312.

187. Afable MG 2nd, Shaik M, Sugimoto Y, et al. Efficacy of rabbit anti-thymocyte globulin in severe aplastic anemia. *Haematologica.* 2011;96:2069.

188. Chen, C, Xue HM, Li Y, et al. Rabbit-antithymocyte globulin combined with cyclosporine A as a first-line therapy: improved, effective and safe for children with acquired severe aplastic anemia. *J Cancer Res Clin Oncol.* 2012;138:1105.

189. Marsh JC, Bacigalupo A, Schrezenmeier H, et al. Prospective study of rabbit antithymocyte globulin and cyclosporine for aplastic anemia from the EBMT Severe Aplastic Anaemia Working Party. *Blood.* 2012;119:5391.

190. Shin SH, Yoon JH, Yahng SA, et al. The efficacy of rabbit antithymocyte globulin with cyclosporine in comparison to horse antithymocyte globulin as a first-line treatment in adult patients with severe aplastic anemia: a single-center retrospective study. *Ann Hematol.* 2013;92:817.

191. Scheinberg P, Young NS. How I treat acquired aplastic anemia. *Blood.* 2012;120:1185-1196.

192. Camitta B, O'Reilly RJ, Sensenbrenner L. Antithoracic duct lymphocyte globulin therapy of severe aplastic anemia. *Blood.* 1983;62:883.

193. Champlin R, Ho W, Gale RP. Antithymocyte globulin treatment in patients with aplastic anemia: a prospective randomized trial. *N Engl J Med.* 1983;308:113.

194. Young N, Griffin P, Brittain E, et al. A multicenter trial of antithymocyte globulin in aplastic anemia and related diseases. *Blood.* 1988;72:1861.

195. Schrezenmeier H, Marin P, Raghavachar A, et al. Relapse of aplastic anaemia after immunosuppressive treatment: a report from the European Bone Marrow Transplantation Group SAA Working Party. *Br J Haematol.* 1993;85:371.

196. Doney K, Leisenring W, Storb R, Appelbaum FR. Primary treatment of acquired aplastic anemia: outcomes with bone marrow transplantation and immunosuppressive therapy. *Ann Intern Med.* 1997;126:107.

197. Tichelli A, Gratwohl A, Nissen C, Speck B. Late clonal complications in severe aplastic anemia. *Leuk Lymphoma.* 1994;12:167.

198. De Planque MM, Bacigalupo A, Würsch A, et al. Long-term follow-up of severe aplastic anaemia patients treated with antithymocyte globulin. *Br J Haematol.* 1989;73:121.

199. Socié G, Henry-Amar M, Bacigalupo A, et al. Malignant tumors occurring after treatment of aplastic anemia. *N Engl J Med.* 1993;319:1152.

200. Calado RT, Cooper JN, Padilla-Nash HM, et al. Short telomeres result in chromosomal instability in hematopoietic cells and precede malignant evolution in human aplastic anemia. *Leukemia.* 2012;26:700.

201. Stryckmans PA, Dumont JP, Velu T, Debusscher L. Cyclosporine in refractory severe aplastic anemia [letter]. *N Engl J Med.* 1984;310:655.

202. Lazzarino M, Morra E, Canevari A, et al. Cyclosporine in the treatment of aplastic anaemia and pure red-cell aplasia. *Bone Marrow Transplant.* 1989;4(suppl 4):165.

203. Hinterberger-Fischer M, Höcker P, Lechner K, et al. Oral cyclosporin-A is effective treatment for untreated and also for previously immunosuppressed patients with severe bone marrow failure. *Eur J Haematol.* 1989;43:136.

204. Tötterman TH, Höglund M, Bengtsson M, et al. Treatment of pure red-cell aplasia and aplastic anaemia with cyclosporin: long-term clinical effects. *Eur J Haematol.* 1989;42:126.

205. Leeksma OC, Thomas LLM, van der Lelie J, et al. Effectiveness of low dose cyclosporine in acquired aplastic anaemia with severe neutropenia. *Neth J Med.* 1992;41:143.

206. Leonard EM, Raefsky E, Griffith P, et al. Cyclosporine therapy of aplastic anaemia, congenital and acquired red-cell aplasia. *Br J Haematol.* 1989;72:278.

207. Tong J, Bacigalupo A, Piaggio G, et al. Severe aplastic anemia (SAA): response to cyclosporin A (CyA) in vivo and in vitro. *Eur J Haematol.* 1991;46:212.

208. Nakao S, Yamaguchi M, Shiobara S, et al. Interferon-g gene expression in unstimulated bone marrow mononuclear cells predicts a good response to cyclosporine therapy in aplastic anemia. *Blood.* 1992;79:2531.

209. Kojima S, Fukada M, Miyajima Y, Matsuyama T. Cyclosporine and recombinant granulocyte colony-stimulating factor in severe aplastic anemia [letter]. *N Engl J Med.* 1990;313:920.

210. Bertrand Y, Amri F, Capdeville R, et al. The successful treatment of two cases of severe aplastic anaemia with granulocyte colony-stimulating factor and cyclosporine A [case report]. *Br J Haematol.* 1991;79:648.

211. Schrezenmeier H, Schlander M, Raghavachar A. Cyclosporin A in aplastic anaemia—report of a workshop. *Ann Hematol.* 1992;65:33.

212. Bacigalupo A. How I traet acquired aplastic anemia. *Blood.* 2017;129:1428-1436.

213. Rosenfeld S, Follmann D, Nunez O, et al. Antithymocyte globulin and cyclosporine for severe aplastic anemia: association between hematologic response and long-term outcome. *JAMA.* 2003;289:1130.

214. Gluckman E, Esperou-Bourdeau H, Baruchel A, et al. Multicenter randomized study comparing cyclosporine-A alone and antithymocyte globulin with prednisone for treatment of severe aplastic anemia. *Blood.* 1992;79:2540.

215. Scheinberg P, Wu CO, Nunez O, et al. Long-term outcome of pediatric patients with severe aplastic anemia treated with antithymocyte globulin and cyclosporine. *J Pediatr.* 2008;153:814.

216. Osugi Y, Yagasaki H, Sako M, et al. Antithymocyte globulin and cyclosporine for treatment of 44 children with hepatitis associated aplastic anemia. *Haematologica.* 2007;92:1687.

217. Teramura M, Kimura A, Iwase S, et al. Treatment of severe aplastic anemia with antithymocyte globulin and cyclosporin A with or without G-CSF in adults: a multicenter randomized study in Japan. *Blood.* 2007;110:1756.

218. Tichelli A, Schrezenmeier H, Socié G, et al. A randomized controlled study in patients with newly diagnosed severe aplastic anemia receiving antithymocyte globulin (ATG), cyclosporine, with or without G-CSF: a study of the SAA Working Party of the European Group for Blood and Marrow Transplantation. *Blood.* 2011;117:4434.

219. Lum SH, Grainger GD. Eltrombopag for the treatment of aplastic anemia: current perspectives. *Drug Des Devel Ther.* 2016;10:2833.

220. Hirao A. TPO signal for stem cell genomic integrity. *Blood.* 2014;123:459.

221. de Lavel B, Pawlikowska P, Barbieri D, et al. Thrombopoietin promotes NHEJ DNA repair in hematopoietic stem cells through specific activation of Erk and NF-κB pathways and their target, IEX-1. *Blood.* 2014;123:509.

222. Desmond R, Townsley DM, Dumitriu B, et al. Eltrombopag restores tri-lineage hematopoiesis in refractory severe aplastic anemia which can be sustained on discontinuation of drug. *Blood.* 2014;123:1818.

223. Olnes MJ, Scheinberg P, Calvo KR, et al. Eltrombopag and improved hematopoiesis in refractory aplastic anemia. *N Engl J Med.* 2012;367:11; published correction appears in *N Engl J Med.* 2012;367:284.

224. Scheinberg P. Recent advances and long-term results of medical treatment of acquired aplastic anemia: are patients cured? *Hematol Oncol Clin North Am.* 2018;32:609-618.

225. Keel S. A lot of attention on aplastic anemia. *Hematologist.* 2018;15:1.

226. Winkler T, Fan X, Cooper J, et al. Treatment optimization and genomic outcomes in refractory severe aplastic anemia treated with eltrombopag. *Blood.* 2019;133:2575-2585.

227. Desmond R, Townsley DM, Dunbar C, Young NS. Eltrombopag in aplastic anemia. *Semin Hematol.* 2015;52:31.

228. Boddu PC, Kadia TM. Updates on the pathophysiology and treatment of aplastic anemia: a comprehensive review. *Expert Rev Hematol.* 2017;10:433.

229. Townsley DM, Scheinberg P, Winkler T, et al. Eltrombopag added to standard immunosuppression for aplastic anemia. *N Engl J Med.* 2017;376:1540.

230. Fan X, Desmond R, Winkler T, et al. Eltrombopag for patients with moderate aplastic anemia or uni-lineage cytopenias. *Blood Adv.* 2020;4:1700-1710.

231. Yamazaki H, Ohta K, Lida H, et al. Hematological recovery induced by elotrombopag in Japanese patients with aplastic anemia refractory or intolerant to immunosuppressive therapy. *Int J Hematol.* 2019;110:187-196.

232. Lengline E, Drenou B, Peterlin P, et al. Nationwide survey on the use of eltrombopag in patients with severe aplastic anemia. A report on behalf of the French Reference Center for Aplastic Anemia. *Haematologica.* 2018;103:212-220.

233. Pierri F, Dufour C. Management of aplastic anemia after failure of frontline immunosuppression. *Expert Rev Hematol.* 2019;12(10):809-819.

234. Hwang YY, Gill H, Chan TSY, et al. Eltrombopag in the management of aplastic anaemia: real-world experience in a non-trial setting. *Hematology.* 2018;23:399-404.

235. Hong Y, Li X, Wan B, et al. Efficacy and safety of eltrombopag for aplastic anemia: a systematic review and meta-analysis. *Clin Drug Investig.* 2019;39:141-156.

236. Gill H, Leung GMK, Lopez D, Kwong Y-L. The thrombopoietin mimetics eltrombopag and romiplostim in the treatment of refractory aplastic anemia. *Br J Haematol.* 2017;176:984-999.

237. Bacigalupo A, Brand R, Oneto R, et al. Treatment of acquired severe aplastic anemia: bone marrow transplantation compared with immunosuppressive therapy—The European Group for Blood and Marrow Transplantation experience. *Semin Hematol.* 2000;37:69.

238. Gillio AP, Boulad F, Small TN, et al. Comparison of long-term outcome of children with severe aplastic anemia treated with immunosuppression versus bone marrow transplantation. *Biol Blood Marrow Transplant.* 1997;3:18.

239. Lan Y, Chang L, Yi M, et al. Long-term outcomes of 172 children with severe aplastic anemia treated with rabbit antithymocyte globulin and cyclosporine. *Ann Hematol.* 2021;100:53-61.

240. De Planque MM, Kluin-Nelemans HC, Van Krieken HJM, et al. Evolution of acquired severe aplastic anaemia to myelodysplasia and subsequent leukaemia in adults. *Br J Haematol.* 1988;70:55.

241. Tichelli A, Gratwohl A, Würsch A, et al. Late haematological complications in severe aplastic anaemia. *Br J Haematol.* 1988;69:413.

242. Marsh JC, Kulasekararaj AG. Management of the refractory aplastic anemia patient: what are the options? *Hematology Am Soc Hematol Educ Program.* 2013;2013:87.

243. Tichelli A, Passweg J, Nissen C, et al. Repeated treatment with horse antilymphocyte globulin for severe aplastic anaemia. *Br J Haematol.* 1998;100:393.

244. Scheinberg P, Nunez O, Young NS. Retreatment with rabbit anti-thymocyte globulin and cyclosporin for patients with relapsed or refractory severe aplastic anaemia. *Br J Haematol.* 2006;133:622.

245. Risitano AM, Schrezenmeier H. Alternative immunosuppression in patients failing immunosuppression with ATG who are not transplant candidates: Campath (alemtuzumab). *Bone Marrow Transplant.* 2013;48:186.

246. Scheinberg P, Nunez O, Weinstein B, et al. Activity of alemtuzumab monotherapy in treatment-naive, relapsed, and refractory severe acquired aplastic anemia. *Blood.* 2011;119:345.

247. Lee JW, Lee S-E, Jung CW, et al. Romiplostin in patients with refractory aplastic anemia previously treated with immunosuppressive therapy: a dose-finding and long-term treatment phase 2 trial. *Lancet Haematol.* 2019;6(11):e562.

248. Bacigalupo A, Van Lint MT, Cerri R, et al. Treatment of severe aplastic anemia with bolus 6-methylprednisolone and antilymphocyte globulin. *Blut.* 1980;41:168.

249. Issaragrisil S, Tangnai-Trisorana Y, Siriseriwan T, et al. Methylprednisolone therapy in aplastic anaemia: correlation of in vitro tests and lymphocyte subsets with clinical response. *Eur J Haematol.* 1988;40:343.

250. Brodsky RA, Sensenbrenner LL, Jones RJ. Complete remission in severe aplastic anemia after high-dose cyclophosphamide without bone marrow transplantation. *Blood.* 1996;87:491.

251. Jones RJ, Barber JP, Vala MS, et al. Assessment of aldehyde dehydrogenase in viable cells. *Blood.* 1995;85:2742.

252. Kastan MB, Schlaffer I, Russo JE, et al. Direct demonstration of aldehyde dehydrogenase in human hematopoietic progenitor cells. *Blood.* 1990;75:1947.

253. Brodsky RA, Sensenbrenner LL, Smith BD, et al. Durable treatment-free remission following high-dose cyclophosphamide for previously untreated severe aplastic anemia. *Ann Intern Med.* 2001;135:477.

254. Brodsky RA. High-dose cyclophosphamide for aplastic anemia and autoimmunity. *Curr Opin Oncol.* 2002;14:143.

255. Hansen PB, Lauritzen AM. Aplastic anemia successfully treated with rituximab. *Am J Hematol.* 2005;80:292.

256. Takamatsu H, Yagasaki H, Takahashi Y, et al. Aplastic anemia successfully treated with rituximab: the possible role of aplastic anemia-associated autoantibodies as a marker for response. *Eur J Haematol.* 2011;86:541.

257. Androgen therapy in aplastic anemia: a comparative study of high and low doses of 4 different androgens. French Cooperative Group for the Study of Aplastic and Refractory Anemias. *Scand J Haematol* 1986;36:346.

258. Champlin RE, Ho WG, Feig SA, et al. Do androgens enhance the response to antithymocyte globulin in patients with aplastic anemia? A prospective randomized trial. *Blood.* 1985;66:184.

259. Townsley DM, Dumitriub B, Yping NS. Danazol treatment in telomere disorders. *New Engl J Med.* 2016;375:1095-1996.

260. Bär C, Huber N, Beier F et al. Therapeutic effects of androgen therapy in a mouse model of aplastic anemia produced by short telomere. *Haematologica.* 2015;100:1257-1274.

261. Socie G, Mary JY, Schrezenmeier H, et al. Granulocyte-stimulating factor and severe aplastic anemia: a survey by the European Group for Blood and Marrow Transplantation (EBMT). *Blood.* 2007;109:2794.

262. Ganser A, Lindemann A, Siepelt G, et al. Effects of recombinant human interleukin-3 in aplastic anemia. *Blood.* 1990;76:1287.

263. Walsh CE, Liu JM, Anderson SM, et al. A trial of recombinant human interleukin-1 in patients with severe refractory aplastic anaemia. *Br J Haematol.* 1992;80:106.

264. Speck B, Tichelli A, Widmer E, et al. Splenectomy as an adjuvant measure in the treatment of severe aplastic anaemia. *Br J Haematol.* 1996;92:818.

265. Sadowitz PD, Dubowy RL. Intravenous immunoglobulin in the treatment of aplastic anemia. *Am J Pediatr Hematol Oncol.* 1990;12:198.

266. Bodenstein H. Successful treatment of aplastic anemia with high-dose immunoglobulin [letter]. *N Engl J Med.* 1991;314:1368.

267. Ito T, Haraiwa M, Ishikawa Y, et al. Lymphocytapheresis in a patient with severe aplastic anaemia. *Acta Haematol.* 1988;80:167.

268. Morales-Polanco MR, Sanchez-Valle E, Guerrero-Rivera S, et al. Treatment results of 23 cases of severe aplastic anemia with lymphocytapheresis. *Arch Med Res.* 1997;28:85.

269. Kiem HP, McDonald GB, Myerson D, et al. Marrow transplantation for hepatitis-associated aplastic anemia: a follow-up of long-term survivors. *Biol Blood Marrow Transplant.* 1996;2:93.

270. Lewis SM. Course and prognosis in aplastic anemia. *BMJ.* 1965;1:1027.

271. Alshaibani A, Dufour C, Risitano A, et al. Hepatitis-associated aplastic anemia. *Hematol Oncol Stem Cell Ther.* 2020:S1658-3876(20)30168-0. doi: 10.1016/j.hemonc.2020.10.001.

272. Lynch RE, Williams DM, Reading JC, Cartwright GE. The prognosis in aplastic anemia. *Blood.* 1975;45:517.

273. Horowitz MM. Current status of allogeneic bone marrow transplantation in acquired aplastic anemia. *Semin Hematol.* 2000;37:30.

274. Ades L, Mary J-Y, Robin M, et al. Long-term outcome after bone marrow transplantation for severe aplastic anemia. *Blood.* 2004;103:2490.

275. Sangiolo D, Storb R, Deeg HJ, et al. Outcome of allogeneic hematopoietic cell transplantation from HLA-identical siblings for severe aplastic anemia in patients over 40 years of age. *Biol Blood Marrow Transplant.* 2010;16:1411.

276. Schrezenmeier H, Passweg JR, Marsh JC, et al. Worse outcome and more chronic GVHD with peripheral blood progenitor cells than bone marrow in HLA-matched sibling donor transplants for young patients with severe acquired aplastic anemia. *Blood.* 2007;110:1397.

277. Locasciulli A. Acquired aplastic anemia in children: incidence, prognosis and treatment options. *Paediatr Drugs.* 2002;4:761.

278. Scheinberg P, Wu CO, Nunez O, Young NS. Predicting response to immunosuppressive therapy and survival in severe aplastic anaemia. *Br J Haematol.* 2009;144:206.

279. Wang B, He B, Zhu YD, et al. The predictive value of pre-treatment paroxysmal nocturnal hemoglobinuria clone on response to immunosuppressive therapy in patients with aplastic anemia: a meta-analysis. *Hematology.* 2020;25:464-472.

280. Scheinberg P, Wu CO, Nunez O, Young NS. Long-term outcome of pediatric patients with severe aplastic anemia treated with antithymocyte globulin and cyclosporine. *J Pediatr.* 2008;153:814.

281. Tisdale JF, Dunn DE, Maciejewski J. Cyclophosphamide and other new agents for the treatment of severe aplastic anemia. *Semin Hematol.* 2000;37:102.

282. Brodsky RA, Chen AR, Dorr D, et al. High-dose cyclophosphamide for severe aplastic anemia: long-term follow-up. *Blood.* 2010;115:2136.

283. Fanconi G. Familiäre infantile perniziosaartige anämie (perniziöses blutbild und konstitution). *Jahrbuch Kinderheil.* 1927;117:257.

284. Rosendorff J, Bernstein R, Macdougall L, Jenkins T. Fanconi anemia: another disease of unusually high prevalence in the Afrikaans population of South Africa. *Am J Med Genet.* 1987;27:793.

285. Dokal I, Vulliamy T. Inherited aplastic anaemias/bone marrow failure syndromes. *Blood Rev.* 2008;22:141.

286. Garaycoechea JI, Patel KJ. Why does the bone marrow fail in Fanconi anemia? *Blood.* 2014;123:26.

287. Jacquemont C, Taniguchi T. The Fanconi anemia pathway and ubiquitin. *BMC Biochem.* 2007;22(8 suppl 1):S10.

288. Alter BP, Giri N, Savage SA, et al. Update on inherited bone marrow failure syndromes (IBMFS). *IBMFS Newsletter of the Clinical Genetics Branch.* National Cancer Institute; Summer 2008;1.

289. HGNC: HUGO Gene Nomenclature Committee of the National Human Genome Research Institute: Fanconi Anemia, complementation groups. http://www.genenames.org/genefamilies/fanc. Accessed February 16, 2015.

290. Somyajit K, Subramanya S, Nagaraju G. Distinct roles of FANCO/RAD51C protein in DNA damage signaling and repair. *J Biol Chem.* 2012;287:3366.

291. Kashiyama K, Nakazawa Y, Pliz DT, et al. Malfunction of Nuclease ERCC1-XPF results in diverse clinical manifestations and causes Cockayne syndrome, xeroderma pigmentosa, and Fanconi anemia. *Am J Hum Genet.* 2013;92:807.

292. Xi Shen, Rui Wang, Moon Jong Kim, et al. A surge of DNA damage links transcriptional reprogramming and hematopoietic deficit in Fanconi Anemia. *Mol Cel.* 2020;80:1013-1024.

293. Dufour C, Corcione A, Svahn J, et al. TNF-α and TNF-γ are overexpressed in the bone marrow of Fanconi anemia patients and TNF-α suppresses erythropoiesis in vitro. *Blood.* 2003;102:2053.

294. Frohnmayer D, Frohnmayer L, Guinan E, et al, eds. *Fanconi Anemia Guidelines for Diagnosis and Management,* 4th ed. Fanconi Anemia Research Fund; 2014.

295. Alter BP, Giri N. Thinking of VACTERL-H? Rule out Fanconi anemia according to PHENOS. *Am J Med Genet A.* 2016;170:1520-1524.

296. D'Apolito M, Zelante L, Savoia A. Molecular basis of Fanconi anemia. *Haematologica.* 1998;83:533.

297. Garcia-Higuera I, Kuang Y, D'Andrea AD. The molecular and cellular biology of Fanconi anemia. *Curr Opin Hematol.* 1999;6:83.

298. Young NA, Alter BP. *Aplastic Anemia: Acquired and Inherited.* WB Saunders; 1994.

299. Estren S, Damshek W. Familial hypoplastic anemia of childhood: report of 8 cases in 2 families with beneficial effects of splenectomy in 1 case. *Am J Dis Child.* 1947;73:671.

300. Niraj J, Färkkilä A, D'Andrea AD. The Fanconi anemia pathway in cancer. *Annu Rev Cancer Biol.* 2019;3:457-478.

301. Swhimamura A, D'Andrea AD. Subtyping of Fanconi anemia patients: implications for clinical management. *Blood.* 2003;102:3459.

302. Li FP, Hecht F, Kaiser-McCaw B, et al. Ataxia-pancytopenia: syndrome of cerebellar ataxia, hypoplastic anemia, monosomy 7 and acute myelogenous leukemia. *Cancer Genet Cytogenet.* 1981;4:189.

303. Mahmood F, King MD, Smyth OO, et al. Familial cerebellar hypoplasia and pancytopenia without chromosomal breakages. *Ne antithymocyte globulin uropediatrie.* 1998;29:302.

304. González-del AA, Cervera M, Gomez L, et al. Ataxia-pancytopenia syndrome. *Am J Med Genet.* 2000;90:252.

305. Davidsson J, Puschmann A, Tedgård U, et al. SAMD9 and SAMD9L in inherited predisposition to ataxia, pancytopenia, and myeloid malignancies. *Leukemia.* 2018;32:1106-1115.

306. Geddis AE. Inherited thrombocytopenia: congenital amegakaryocytic thrombocytopenia and thrombocytopenia with absent radii. *Semin Hematol.* 2006;43:196.

307. Germeshausen M, Ballmaier M, Welte K. MPL mutations in 23 patients suffering from congenital amegakaryocytic thrombocytopenia: the type of mutation predicts the course of the disease. *Hum Mutat.* 2006;27:296.

308. King S, Germeshausen M, Strauss G, et al. Congenital amegakaryocytic thrombocytopenia: a retrospective clinical analysis of 20 patients. *Br J Haematol.* 2005;131:636.

309. Pecci A, Ragab I, Bozzi V, et al. Thrombopoietin mutation in congenital amegakaryocytic thrombocytopenia treatable with romiplostim. *EMBO Mol Med.* 2018;10:63-75.

310. Walne AJ, Dokal A, Plagnol V, et al. Exome sequencing identifies MPL as a causative gene in familial aplastic anemia. *Haematologica.* 2012;97:524-528.

311. Tummala H, Kirwan M, Walne AJ et al. ERCC6L2 mutations link a distinct bone–marrow-failure syndrome to DNA repair and mitochondrial function. *Am J Hum Genet.* 2014;94:246-256.

312. Shabanova I, Cohen E, Cda M, et al. ERCC6L2-associated inherited bone marrow failure syndrome. *Mol Genet Genomic Med.* 2018;6:463-468.

313. Kirwan M, Walne AJ, Plagnol V, et al. I. Exome sequencing identifies autosomal-dominant SRP72 mutations associated with familial aplasia and myelodysplasia. *Am J Hum Genet.* 2012:90:888-892.

314. O'Driscoll M, Gennery AR, Seidel J, et al. An overview of three new disorders associated with genetic instability: LIG4 syndrome, RS-SCID and ATR-Seckel syndrome. *DNA Repair (Amst).* 2004;3:1227.

315. Pierce AJ, Jasin M. NHEJ deficiency and disease. *Mol Cell.* 2001;8:1160.

316. O'Driscoll M, Jeggo PA. CSA can induce DNA double-strand breaks: implications for BMT regimens particularly for individuals with defective DNA repair. *Bone Marrow Transplant.* 2008;41:983.

317. Walters TR, Desposito F. Aplastic anemia in Dubowitz syndrome. *J Pediatr.* 1985;106:622.

318. Berthold F, Fuhrmann W, Lampert F. Fatal aplastic anemia in a patient with Dubowitz syndrome. *Eur J Pediatr.* 1987;146:605.

319. Boycott KM, Dyment DA, Innes AM. Unsolved recognizable patterns of human malformation: challenges and opportunities. *Am J Med Genet C Semin Med Genet.* 2018;178:382-386.

320. Gennery AR, Slatter MA, Bhattacharya A, et al. The clinical and biological overlap between Nijmegen breakage syndrome and Fanconi anemia. *Clin Immunol.* 2004;113:214.

321. Gadkowska-Dura M, Dzieranowska-Fangrat K, Dura W, et al. Unique morphological spectrum of lymphomas in Nijmegen breakage syndrome (NBS) patients with high frequency of consecutive lymphoma formation. *J Pathol.* 2008;216:337.

322. Stephan JL, Vlekova V, Le Deist F, et al. Severe combined immunodeficiency: a retrospective single-center study of clinical presentation and outcome in 117 patients. *J Pediatr.* 1993;123:564.

323. Bertrand Y, Muller SM, Casanova JL, et al. Reticular dysgenesis: HLA non-identical bone marrow transplants in a series of 10 patients. *Bone Marrow Transplant.* 2002; 29:759.

324. Hoenig M, Pannicke U, Gaspar HB, Schwarz K. Recent advances in understanding the pathogenesis and management of reticular dysgenesis. *Br J Haematol.* 2018;180:644-653.

325. Esperou-Bourdeau H, Leblanc T, Schaison G, et al. Aplastic anemia associated with "bird-headed" dwarfism (Seckel syndrome). *Nouv Rev Fr Hematol.* 1993;35:99.

326. O'Driscoll M, Ruiz-Perez VL, Woods CG, et al. A splicing mutation affecting expression of ataxia-telangiectasia and RAD3-related protein (ATR) results in Seckel syndrome. *Nat Genet.* 2003;33:497.

327. Griffith E, Walker S, Martin CA, et al. Mutations in pericentrin cause Seckel syndrome with defective ATR-dependent DNA damage signaling. *Nat Genet.* 2008;40:232.

328. Hayani A, Suarez CR, Molnar Z, et al. Acute myeloid leukemia in a patient with Seckel syndrome. *J Med Genet.* 1994;31:148.

329. Gonzalez CH, Durkin-Stamm MV, Geimer NF, et al. The WT syndrome—a "new" autosomal dominant pleiotropic trait of radial/ulnar hypoplasia with high risk of bone marrow failure and/or leukemia. *Birth Defects Orig Artic Ser.* 1977;13:31.

330. Carreau M, Liu L, Gan OI, et al. Short-term granulocyte colony-stimulating factor and erythropoietin treatment enhances hematopoiesis and survival in the mitomycin C-conditioned Fancc(−/−) mouse model, while long-term treatment is ineffective. *Blood.* 2002;100:1499.

331. Nepal M, Che R, Zhang J, et al. Fanconi anemia signaling and cancer. *Trends Cancer.* 2017;3:840-856.

332. Alter BP. Cancer in Fanconi anemia. *Cancer.* 2003;97:425.

333. Alter BP, Caruso JP, Drachtman RA, et al. Fanconi anemia: myelodysplasia as a predictor of outcome. *Cancer Genet Cytogenet.* 2000;117:125.

334. Gluckman E, Wagner JE. Hematopoietic stem cell transplantation in childhood inherited bone marrow failure syndrome. *Bone Marrow Transplant.* 2008;41:127.

335. Huck K, Hanenberg H, Nürnberger W, et al. Favourable long-term outcome after matched sibling transplantation for Fanconi-anemia (FA) and in vivo T-cell depletion. *Klin Padiatr.* 2008;220:147.

336. Ayas M, Al-Jefri A, Al-Seraihi A, et al. Second stem cell transplantation in patients with Fanconi anemia using antithymocyte globulin alone for conditioning. *Biol Blood Marrow Transplant.* 2008;14:445.

337. Bierings M, Bonfim C, Peffault De Latour R, et al. Transplant results in adults with Fanconi anaemia. *Br J Haematol.* 2018;180:100-109.

338. Kelly PF, Radtke S, von Kalle C, et al. Stem cell collection and gene transfer in Fanconi anemia. *Mol Ther.* 2007;15:211.

339. Dufour C, Svahn J. Fanconi anaemia: new strategies. *Bone Marrow Transplant.* 2008;41(suppl 2):S90.

340. Verhoeyen E, Roman-Rodriguez FJ, Cosset FL, et al. Gene therapy in Fanconi anemia: a matter of time, safety and gene transfer tool efficiency. *Curr Gene Ther.* 2017;16:297-308.

341. Hanenberg H, Roellecke K, Wiek C. Stem cell genetic therapy for Fanconi anemia—a new hope. *Curr Gene Ther.* 2017;16(5):309-320.

342. Dokal I. Dyskeratosis congenita in all its forms. *Br J Haematol.* 2000;110:768.

343. Nelson ND, Bertuch AA. Dyskeratosis congenita as a disorder of telomere maintenance. *Mutat Res.* 2012;730:43.

344. Savage SA, Alter BP. The role of telomere biology in bone marrow failure and other disorders. *Mech Ageing Dev.* 2008;129(1-2):35.

345. Keller RB, Gagne KE, Usmani GN, et al. Mutations in a patient with dyskeratosis congenita. *Pediatr Blood Cancer.* 2012;59:311.

346. Ballew B, Yeager M, Jacobs K, et al. Germline mutations of regulator of telomere elongation helicase 1, RTEL1, in dyskeratosis congenita. *Hum Genet.* 2013;132:473.

347. Walne AJ, Vulliamy T, Kirwan M, et al. Constitutional mutations in RTEL1 cause severe dyskeratosis congenita. *Am J Hum Genet.* 2017;92:448-453.

348. Dokal I, Vulliamy T, Mason P, Bessler M. Clinical utility gene card for: dyskeratosis congenital – update 2015. *Eur J Hum Genet.* 2015;23(4).

349. Walne AJ, Bhagat T, Kirwan M, et al. Mutations in the telomere capping complex in bone marrow failure and related syndromes. *Haematologica.* 2013;98:334.

350. Ruggero D, Shimamura A. Marrow failure: a window into ribosome biology. *Blood.* 2014;124:2784.

351. Grill S, Nandakumar J. Molecular mechanisms of telomere biology disorders. *J Biol Chem.* 2020;296:100064. REV120.014017. doi: 10.1074/jbc.REV120.014017.

352. Savage SA, Giri N, Baerlocher GM, et al. TINF2, a component of the shelterin telomere protection complex, is mutated in dyskeratosis congenital. *Am J Hum Genet.* 2008;82:501.

353. Walne AJ, Vulliamy T, Marrone A, et al. Genetic heterogeneity in autosomal recessive dyskeratosis congenita with one subtype due to mutations in the telomerase-associated protein NOP10. *Hum Mol Genet.* 2007;16:1619.

354. Vulliamy T, Beswick R, Kirwan M, et al. Mutations in the telomerase component of NHP2 cause the premature aging syndrome, dyskeratosis congenital. *Proc Natl Acad Sci U S A.* 2008;105:8073.

355. Vulliamy A, Marrone F, Goldman A, et al. The RNA component of telomerase is mutated in autosomal dominant dyskeratosis congenital. *Nature.* 2001;413:432.

356. Vulliamy T, Marrone A, Szydlo R, et al. Disease anticipation is associated with progressive telomere shortening in families with dyskeratosis congenital due to mutations in TERC. *Nat Genet.* 2004;36:447.

357. Alter BP, Baerlocher GM, Savage SA, et al. Very short telomere length by flow fluorescence in situ hybridization identifies patients with dyskeratosis congenital. *Blood.* 2007;110:1439.

358. Ghavamzadeh A, Alimoghadam K, Nasseri P, et al. Correction of bone marrow failure in dyskeratosis congenita by bone marrow transplantation. *Bone Marrow Transplant.* 1999;23:299.

359. Ayas M. Hematopoietic cell transplantation in Fanconi anemia and dyskeratosis congenita: a minireview. *Hematol Oncol Stem Cell Ther.* 2017;10:285-289.

360. Barbaro P, Vedi A. Survival after hematopoietic stem cell transplant in patients with dyskeratosis congenita: systematic review of the literature. *Biol Blood Marrow Transplant.* 2016;22:1152-1158.

361. Cesaro S, Oneto R, Messina C, et al. Haematopoietic stem cell transplantation for Shwachman-Diamond disease: a study from the European Group for Blood and Marrow Transplantation. *Br J Haematol.* 2005;131:231.

362. Güngör T, Corbacioglu S, Storb R, Seger RA. Nonmyeloablative allogeneic hematopoietic stem cell transplantation for treatment of dyskeratosis congenita. *Bone Marrow Transplant.* 2003;31:407.

363. Dror Y, Freedman MH, Leaker M, et al. Low-intensity hematopoietic stem-cell transplantation across human leucocyte antigen barriers in dyskeratosis congenita. *Bone Marrow Transplant.* 2003;31:847.

364. Alter BP, Neelam G, Savage SA, et al. Cancer in dyskeratosis congenital. *Blood.* 2009;113:6549.

365. Goobie S, Popovic M, Morrison J, et al. Shwachman Diamond syndrome with exocrine pancreatic dysfunction and bone marrow failure maps to the centromeric region of chromosome 7. *Am J Hum Genet.* 2001;68:1048.

366. Ginzberg H, Shin J, Ellis L, et al. Shwachman syndrome: phenotypic manifestations of sibling sets and isolated cases in a large patient cohort are similar. *J Pediatr.* 1999;135:81.

367. Shimamura A. Shwachman-Diamond syndrome. *Semin Hematol.* 2006;43:178.

368. Rujkijyanont P, Watanabe K, Ambekar C, et al. SBDS-deficient cells undergo accelerated apoptosis through the FAS pathway. *Haematologica.* 2008;93:363.

369. Thornley I, Dror Y, Sung L, et al. Abnormal telomere shortening in leucocytes of children with Shwachman-Diamond syndrome. *Br J Haematol.* 2002;117:189.

370. Ganapathi KA, Shimamura A. Ribosomal dysfunction and inherited marrow failure. *Br J Haematol.* 2008;141:376.

371. Ganapathi KA, Austin KM, Lee CS, et al. The human Shwachman-Diamond syndrome protein, SBDS, associates with ribosomal RNA. *Blood.* 2007;110:1458.

372. Tan S, Kermasson L, Hoslin A, et al. EFL1 mutations impair eIF6 release to cause Shwachman-Diamond syndrome. *Blood.* 2019;134:277-290.

373. Nelson AS, Myers KC. Diagnosis, treatment, and molecular pathology of Shwachman-Diamond syndrome. *Hematol Oncol Clin North Am.* 2018;32:687-700.

374. Myers KC, Davies SM, Shimamura A. Clinical and molecular pathophysiology of Shwachman-Diamond syndrome: an update. *Hematol Oncol Clin North Am.* 2013;27:117.

375. Toiviainen-Salo S, Durie PR, Numminen K, et al. The natural history of Shwachman Diamond syndrome associated liver disease from childhood to adulthood. *J Pediatr.* 2009;155:807.

376. Dror Y, Durie P, Ginzberg H, et al. Clonal evolution in marrows of patients with Shwachman-Diamond syndrome: a prospective 5-year follow-up study. *Exp Hematol.* 2002;30:659.

377. Woloszynek JR, Rothbaum RJ, Rawis AS, et al. Mutations of the SBDS gene are present in most patients with Shwachman-Diamond syndrome. *Blood.* 2004;104:3588.

378. Bhatla D, Davies SM, Shenoy S, et al. Reduced-intensity conditioning is effective and safe for transplantation of patients with Shwachman-Diamond syndrome. *Bone Marrow Transplant.* 2008;42:159.

379. Dokal I, Rule S, Chen F, et al. Adult onset of acute myeloid leukaemia (M6) in patients with Shwachman-Diamond syndrome. *Br J Haematol.* 1997;99:171.

380. Dror Y, Squire J, Durie P, Freedman MH. Malignant myeloid transformation with isochromosome 7q in Shwachman-Diamond syndrome. *Leukemia.* 1998;12:1591.

381. Thornely I, Dror Y, Sung L, et al. Abnormal telomere shortening in leukocytes of children with Shwachman-Diamond syndrome. *Br J Haematol.* 2002;117:189.

CHAPTER 5
PURE RED CELL APLASIA

Neal S. Young

SUMMARY

Pure red cell aplasia is defined by the combination of anemia, reticulocytopenia, and the absence of erythroid precursors on the marrow examination, but the pathophysiologies are diverse. In children, a genetic defect in ribosome protein genes is responsible for Diamond-Blackfan anemia. In older adults, pure red cell aplasia is usually immune-mediated, sometimes associated with thymoma, and responsive to immunosuppressive therapies. The syndrome can overlap with other diseases, especially large granular lymphocytosis, or complicate them, as with chronic lymphocytic leukemia (CLL) or myelodysplastic syndrome. Parvovirus B19 is an infectious etiology, acutely producing transient aplastic crisis of hemolytic anemia and, when persistent, identical to pure red cell aplasia. The exclusive loss of erythrocyte production is a rare complication of medical drug therapy, but pure red cell aplasia can be iatrogenic, as with anti-erythropoietin antibodies after administration of the hormone and in ABO-incompatible allogeneic transplantation caused by persistence of host isoagglutinins.

INTRODUCTION

Pure red cell aplasia is the diagnosis applied to isolated anemia secondary to failure of erythropoiesis. Cardinal findings are a low hemoglobin level combined with reticulocytopenia and absent or extremely infrequent marrow erythroid precursors. Historical names for pure red cell aplasia include *erythroblast hypoplasia, erythroblastopenia, red cell agenesis, hypoplastic anemia,* and *aregenerative anemia. Aplastic anemia* confers the same meaning, of course, but denotes *pan*cytopenia and an empty marrow (Chap. 4). Pure red cell aplasia as a diagnostic entity was separated from aplastic anemia by Kaznelson in 1922. The association of red cell aplasia and thymoma interested physicians in the 1930s and ultimately led to laboratory studies linking pure red cell aplasia

Acronyms and Abbreviations: B19, primate erythroparvovirus 1; BFU-E, burst-forming unit–erythroid; CD20, a cluster of differentiation molecule expressed on the surface of all mature B cells; CFU-E, colony-forming unit–erythroid; CLL, chronic lymphocytic leukemia; FA, Fanconi anemia; *GATA1* gene, globin transcription factor 1; HLA, human leukocyte antigen; Ig, immunoglobulin; IL, interleukin; LGL, large granular lymphocytosis; NF-KappaB, nuclear factor kappa-light-chain-enhancer of activated B cells; RAS, ra(t) s(arcoma) a group of proteins that are found near cell membranes and regulate cell division and proliferation. *RPS* ribosomal protein genes; *STAT3* gene, signal transducer and activator of transcription 3 gene; T cell, thymus-derived lymphocyte; TP53, tumor protein p53.

to immune mechanisms, including the early identification of antierythroid precursor cell antibodies by Krantz and later characterization of T cells that inhibited erythropoiesis. Red cell aplasia as an acute and life-threatening complication of sickle cell disease and other hemolytic anemias was reported in the 1940s, presaging the role of a specific virus in the etiology of both acute and chronic erythropoietic failure. Despite its infrequency, pure red cell aplasia has been a subject of much laboratory research because of its link to an immune mechanism of erythropoietic failure and as a manifestation of parvovirus B19 infection and viral destruction of red cell progenitors. However, because of its rarity, pure red cell aplasia has not been the subject of large or controlled clinical trials; as a result, therapeutic recommendations are based on single cases or small series. Table 5-1 lists a practical classification of pure red cell aplasia. The clinical pathology of pure red cell aplasia is unique and easily recognized, but there is no typical patient, because the underlying pathophysiology ranges from discrete germline mutations (Diamond-Blackfan anemia); an acquired destructive process (immune pure red cell aplasia and coincident with large granular lymphocytosis); viral infection (acute and persistent B19 parvovirus); drug toxicity (antirecombinant erythropoietin antibodies, checkpoint inhibitors in immunotherapy); and in association with other diseases, especially chronic lymphocytic leukemia (CLL) and thymoma.[1-5]

CONSTITUTIONAL PURE RED CELL APLASIA (DIAMOND-BLACKFAN ANEMIA)

DEFINITION AND HISTORY

Anemia in infancy and early childhood associated with absent reticulocytes in the blood and erythroid precursor cells in the marrow was described by Joseph in 1936[4] as a "failure of erythropoiesis" and by Diamond and Blackfan[5] in 1938 as "congenital hypoplastic anemia." Gasser[6] first reported a response of a patient to glucocorticoids in 1951, and Diamond and associates[7] presented a series of treated patients. Genetic linkage studies have identified etiologic mutations in ribosomal protein genes. Hundreds of cases have been reported, and excellent reviews have been published.[8-10]

EPIDEMIOLOGY

An annual incidence of five cases per 1 million live births has been estimated from registry data.[11] Well-characterized pedigrees are consistent with an autosomal dominant or, less often, recessive inheritance pattern. Sporadic cases are seen most frequently. Retrospective studies may reveal subtle hematologic or biochemical lesions, or an abnormal gene, in an affected parent or another relative without clinical anemia.[12]

ETIOLOGY AND PATHOGENESIS

Genetics

Diamond-Blackfan anemia is a disease of ribosomal biogenesis.[10,13] Linkage analyses of several dozen European families mapped to a site on chromosome 19q13[14] and the finding of a translocation in one individual allowed cloning of the ribosomal protein S19 *(RPS19)* gene, which encodes a protein involved in ribosome assembly. Most mutations are whole-gene deletions, translocations, or truncations; this pattern suggests a mechanism of haploinsufficiency, and *RPS19* behaves as a dominant gene.[15] (Disruption of both copies of the gene in the mouse prevents implantation.[16]) In about 65% of cases, a genetic etiology can be confidently identified: *RPS19* mutations in approximately

TABLE 5–1. Conditions Associated with Red Cell Aplasia

Constitutional

Diamond-Blackfan anemia (ribosome gene mutations [rarely, *GATA1, TSR2*])

Primary

Immune (T-cell autoimmunity)

Large, granular lymphocytosis (T-cell clonal expansion)

Transient erythroblastopenia of childhood

Secondary

Other diseases

Thymoma

Chronic lymphocytic leukemia

Lymphoproliferative malignancies

Collagen vascular diseases

Pregnancy

Infectious

Parvovirus B19

    Transient aplastic crisis of hemolytic anemia (acute infection)

    Chronic PRCA (persistent infection caused by immunodeficiency)

    Hydrops fetalis (infection in utero)

Other viruses (rarely Epstein-Barr virus, hepatitis viruses)

Iatrogenic

Anti-EPO antibodies (erythropoietin treatment)

Monoclonal gammopathy

Post-allogeneic hematopoietic stem cell transplant (donor ABO isoagglutinins)

25% of patients, followed by mutations in other ribosomal biogenesis genes (*RPL5, RPS26, RL11, RPS10, RPL24, RPL35A*, and other genes less frequently).[9,13,17] A globin transcription factor 1 (*GATA1*) gene mutation was identified in a Diamond-Blackfan kindred, implicating a signal transduction pathway of erythroid differentiation as also causative of the syndrome.[18,19] Mutations in *TSR2* affect a gene that represses nuclear factor kappa-light-chain-enhancer of activated B cells (NF-κB) transcription[20] (red cell aplasia is a feature of other genetic syndromes involving the immune system, as for example adenosine deaminase deficiency[21]). There are some correlations of genotype and phenotype: *GATA1* and *TSR2* are X-linked; *RPL11* is associated with thumb abnormalities; *RPL5* with thumb, craniofacial, and heart defects; and *RPS28* and *TSR2* with mandibulofacial dysostosis.

Pathophysiology

Historically, Diamond-Blackfan anemia has been characterized by diminished erythroid progenitor cell numbers.[22,23] In cell culture, early, erythropoietin-independent erythropoiesis is relatively normal; the major defect is in the late stage of erythropoietin-dependent erythroid cell expansion and maturation.[24] A defect in late erythroid differentiation is compatible with the classic findings of macrocytosis and increased hemoglobin F expression in inherited red cell aplasia. Granulopoietic and early hematopoietic progenitors in tissue culture assays are also decreased, but less than are erythroid progenitors.[25] In a zebrafish model, deficiency of *rps19* in early embryogenesis causes a decrease in erythrocytes and also physical anomalies.[26] In tissue culture experiments, silencing of *RPS19* profoundly affects erythropoietic differentiation and, to lesser degrees, myelopoiesis.[27,28] Both in vivo and in

vitro models have implicated accumulation in the cell of free ribosomal proteins, which modulates the inhibitory activity of regulators of tumor protein p53 (TP53), leading to TP53 stabilization and apoptosis.[10] Specificity of this molecular defect for the erythroid pathway may be a result of the extreme requirement of red cell progenitors and precursors for ribosome biogenesis.

Despite the responsiveness of patients to glucocorticoids, there is little evidence of an immune mechanism, cellular or humoral, underlying most constitutional red cell aplasia.

CLINICAL FEATURES

Approximately one-third of patients are diagnosed at birth or within a few weeks of delivery, and almost all are identified within the first year of life.[29] Considerable variations are noted with regard to severity of phenotype, ranging from hydrops fetalis[30] to presentation in adulthood.[31,32] There is no sex predominance. Increased rates of prematurity in patients and of miscarriages in families have been inferred from collected cases.[33] Symptoms of anemia in early childhood include pallor, apathy, poor appetite, and "failure to thrive." Physical anomalies occur in about one-third of cases; most frequent is craniofacial dysmorphism: the classic appearance described by Cathie[34] is "tow-colored hair, snub nose, wide set eyes, thick upper lips, and an intelligent expression." Malformations of the thumbs and short stature are frequent, followed by abnormalities of the urogenital system, web neck, and skeletal and cardiac defects.[11,29,35] Physical anomalies are less prevalent than the abnormalities seen in Fanconi anemia (FA).

LABORATORY FEATURES

The degree of anemia is highly variable at diagnosis. Erythrocytes may be macrocytic or normocytic. Reticulocytopenia is profound. The marrow, which usually is devoid of red blood cell precursors, may show small numbers of megaloblastoid early erythroid cells with apparent "maturation arrest." Platelets are normal or elevated. Leukocytes may be normal or slightly decreased at presentation. Neutrophils often decline with age, and in adult survivors, neutropenia is sometimes severe enough to predispose to fatal infection.[36]

Erythrocyte adenosine deaminase level is elevated in approximately 75% of patients but also may be increased in other aregenerative anemias of childhood. Serum erythropoietin level, serum iron level, and total iron-binding capacity are high. Ferritin increases as patients receive multiple transfusions and develop iron overload unless they are treated with chelation therapy.

DIFFERENTIAL DIAGNOSIS

The characteristic triad consists of the clinical diagnostic features of anemia, reticulocytopenia, and a paucity or absence of erythroid precursors in the marrow. When a constitutional etiology is suspected, germline screening is indicated utilizing genomic panels designed to identify mutations in bone marrow failure genes (testing is available commercially and at academic centers). FA also can be excluded by cytogenetics under clastogenic stress. Transient erythroblastopenia of childhood, which unusually occurs in the first year of life, is established by spontaneous recovery. When presentation occurs at older ages, the clinical distinction between inherited and acquired disease is useful (physical anomalies, family history) but far less reliable than is genomic screening.

THERAPY, COURSE, AND PROGNOSIS

Untreated inherited pure red cell aplasia is fatal; death results from severe anemia and congestive heart failure. Transfusions, glucocorticoids, and allogeneic stem cell transplantation are of proven efficacy.[1,37,38] Supportive care consists of red cell transfusions and iron chelation to avoid transfusional hemosiderosis (Chap. 11). Chelation should be instituted early to prevent injury to visceral organs from iron overload, historically a major cause of death.

Red cell transfusions should be leukocyte-depleted to avoid alloimmunization (Chap. 30). Erythrocytes are administered with the goal of eliminating symptoms and permitting normal growth and sexual development, usually achieved by maintaining hemoglobin levels between 70 and 90 g/dL.

Glucocorticoids are effective. Their mechanism of action in Diamond-Blackfan anemia is not entirely understood: they affect TP53-mediated apoptosis, improve cell-cycle progression, and increase erythroblast proliferation.[39] Predictors of glucocorticoid responsiveness include older age at presentation, a family history, and a normal platelet count, whereas younger age at presentation and premature birth correlate with continued red cell transfusion dependence.[40] In practice, prednisone is administered orally, at 2 mg/kg daily, after definitive diagnosis and in patients older than 1 year.[1,33,38,41-43] A reticulocyte response is seen in most patients 1 to 4 weeks later, followed by a rise in hemoglobin level. Once the hemoglobin reaches 90 to 100 g/L, reduction of the glucocorticoid dose is undertaken with blood count monitoring; although a slow taper is often recommended, lack of tolerance to side effects often necessitates more rapid decreases. Severe anemia and transfusion can be avoided with continued glucocorticoid administration, and 0.5 mg daily or 1 mg on alternative days is considered acceptable.[38] The maintenance dose may be very low (1-2 mg/day). Some patients may remain in remission on complete withdrawal of prednisone, but relapse is frequent and most patients who respond become glucocorticoid-dependent. A variety of patterns of response have been described, ranging from prompt recovery and apparent cure to refractoriness after a long period of responsiveness.[33] Conversely, a second trial of glucocorticoids years after an apparent therapeutic failure may be successful. In a series of 76 patients followed for many years, 59 were treated with prednisone; 31 initially responded, and 2 of the 25 who initially failed to respond later responded to another trial.[41] Glucocorticoid responsiveness is strongly associated with better survival, and patients who require low doses of prednisone, or those few who spontaneously achieve remission, may have normal life expectancies. Glucocorticoid toxicity is substantial, especially with long-term use, and can cause growth retardation, Cushingoid facies, buffalo hump, osteoporosis, aseptic necrosis and fractures, diabetes, hypertension, and cataracts. In some patients, red cell transfusions with iron chelation may be preferable to such outcomes.

Allogeneic stem cell marrow transplantation, when successful, is curative, but the procedure has not been widely applied to children responding to medical measures, whose life expectancy with transfusions and iron chelation is measured in decades.[43] Because of the procedure-related morbidity and mortality, patients often have been transplanted late in their disease course, after large numbers of transfusions, accumulation of heavy iron loads, and alloimmunization. A less favorable outcome has been related to poor compliance and cardiac and hepatic disease from iron overload. In a report from the disease registry in 2006, survival after matched-sibling transplant was 73%.[44] In a Japanese retrospective survey, all of 13 patients had survived long-term.[45] In a report of outcomes in 30 Italian patients, 5-year survival was 75%.[46] In general, children transplanted younger than 10 years fare better, and matched family donors are much preferred over unrelated stem cell donors or use of cord blood stem cells.

Other therapies have had disappointing results in the clinic or have not undergone adequate testing, despite promising preclinical studies[47] and case reports: interleukin (IL)-3, high-dose methylprednisolone, leucine, cyclosporine and other immunosuppressive drugs, and prolactin induction by metoclopramide.

With improved overall survival in Diamond-Blackfan anemia, the risk of late development of leukemia has become apparent.[43,48] Of 76 patients, 4 followed at Children's Hospital in Boston died of acute myelogenous leukemia, with a calculated relative risk of greater than 200 times expected.[41]

Gene transfer in vitro functionally corrects cells defective in *RSP19*,[49] and in animal models corrected cells show improved erythropoiesis and a survival advantage in vivo[27] and the possibility of gene therapy. Zebrafish models offer the opportunity of high throughput screening for drug discovery.[50]

●TRANSIENT APLASTIC CRISIS AND TRANSIENT ERYTHROBLASTOPENIA OF CHILDHOOD

DEFINITIONS AND HISTORY

Temporary failure of erythropoiesis is clinically identical to pure red cell aplasia, except for spontaneous resolution of symptoms and of the laboratory findings of normocytic and normochromic anemia and marrow erythroid hypoplasia, usually over the course of a few weeks. Erythrocyte production is halted: (1) by acute primate erythroparvovirus 1 (B19 parvovirus) infection, typically in the context of underlying hemolytic disease (called *transient aplastic crisis*); (2) in normal children, usually after an infection by another (unknown) childhood virus (transient erythroblastopenia of childhood); or (3) as a drug reaction.

An anemic crisis was described in the 1940s first by Lyngar[51] and then by Owren,[52] Gasser,[6] and Dameshek and Bloom[53] in kindreds with hereditary spherocytosis. Several children within a family suffered anemic crises and exhibited low rather than the usual high reticulocyte numbers. Transient aplastic crisis also was noted as a complication of sickle cell disease.[54,55] Marrow examination showed decrease or absence of erythroid precursor cells, and often giant erythroblasts.[52,53] An infectious etiology was suspected from the history of a preceding febrile illness in families and its simultaneous occurrence in siblings. After the serendipitous discovery of B19 parvovirus in a normal blood donor, Pattison and colleagues screened large numbers of stored sera for evidence of recent infection. Immunoglobulin (Ig) M antibody or viral antigen was found in the blood of Jamaican children in London, all of whom had transient aplastic crisis of sickle cell disease.[56] B19 parvovirus later was established as the agent also responsible for fifth disease.[57] In a large cohort of Jamaican patients with sickle cell, virtually all episodes of transient aplastic crisis could be linked to B19 parvovirus.[58,59] In retrospect, red cell aplasias blamed on kwashiorkor, vitamin deficiency, bacterial infections, and chemical exposures likely represented parvovirus infection.

Gasser[6] described erythroblastopenia in normal children who ultimately recovered[52]; the disease was recognized as an entity in the 1970s.[60] Transient erythroblastopenia of childhood has an unclear etiology but may represent a postviral immune-mediated syndrome. The syndrome is rare and may be declining in incidence.[61]

ETIOLOGY AND PATHOGENESIS

B19 parvovirus, a small DNA virus, commonly infects humans.[57,62] Most of the adult population has IgG antibodies specific to B19. The virus is tropic for erythroid progenitor cells,[63] because of their abundant cell surface P antigen or globoside, the receptor for entry of B19 into the cell (Fig. 5-1).[64,65] Infection lyses the target cell and abrogates erythropoiesis

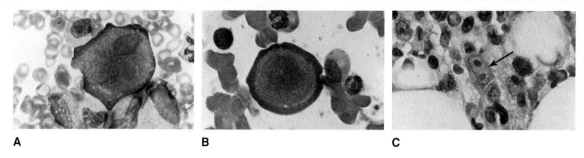

Figure 5-1. A and **B.** Giant early erythroblast precursors in the marrow aspirate of a patient with chronic pure red cell aplasia secondary to persistent B19 parvovirus infection. Note the nuclear inclusions (darker nuclear shading) representing parvovirus infection. **C.** Marrow biopsy section. The arrows point to binucleate erythroid precursor cell with nuclear inclusions representing parvovirus infection. *(Reproduced with permission from Lichtman MA, Shafer MS, Felgar RE, et al: Lichtman's Atlas of Hematology 2016. New York, NY: McGraw Hill; 2017.)*

in vitro and in vivo. Reticulocytopenia probably accompanies B19 parvovirus infection in all infected persons.[66] Significant anemia only manifests if red cell survival is decreased. Infection ordinarily is terminated by production of neutralizing antibodies to the virus (when such antibodies are absent, persistence of the virus produces chronic pure red cell aplasia). B19 parvovirus may appear in epidemics of fifth disease in the normal population and of transient aplastic crisis, for example, in hematology clinics specializing in sickle cell disease.[67,68] In fifth disease, IgM antibody is present in the blood, and virus levels are either low or undetectable. Symptoms and signs of a typical "slapped cheek" cutaneous eruption and arthralgia or arthritis are secondary to antibody–virus immune complex deposition.

In contrast, in transient *aplastic* crisis, high concentrations of virus are present in the circulation, and fifth disease does not develop in patients. In children with sickle cell disease, the incidence of B19 parvovirus infection was estimated to be approximately 11%, and 75% of patients were infected by age 20.[69] In this setting, parvovirus infection was associated with transient aplastic crisis, a higher frequency of fever, pain, acute chest syndrome, and acute splenic sequestration syndrome.[69] As in normal individuals, parvovirus infection can be asymptomatic in sickle cell disease.[70]

The etiology of transient erythroblastopenia of childhood is not understood. An apparent viral prodrome is typical,[71] and temporal and seasonal clustering of cases may occur.[72-74] With rare exception,[75] B19 parvovirus is not the etiology,[76,77] and no other virus has been convincingly implicated.[71] Erythroid colony numbers usually are low.[78] An immune pathophysiology has been inferred from in vitro experiments in which IgG from sera of patients inhibited erythropoiesis[79] in the majority of cases.[80] Cell-mediated mechanisms also may play a causal role. In one report, T-cell depletion led to a dramatic increase in colony-forming unit–erythroid (CFU-E) formation.[81] A possible relationship between transient erythroblastopenia of childhood and inherited red cell aplasia has been suggested by the clustering of polymorphic alleles in familial transient erythroblastopenia.[82]

CLINICAL FEATURES

Transient *aplastic* crisis typically occurs in younger patients who are chronically anemic as a result of hereditary spherocytosis, sickle cell disease, or another hemolytic anemia. The decrease in erythropoiesis results in more evident pallor, fatigue on exertion or at rest, lassitude, and dyspnea on exertion. Gastrointestinal complaints or headache may be associated.[83] Parvovirus infection can unmask previously undiagnosed underlying hemolytic anemia. Physical examination may reveal signs of anemia, such as pallor, tachycardia, and a flow murmur. No rash

or joint swelling is seen. Elevated serum bilirubin or overt icterus may be a clue to underlying hemolysis.

Transient erythroblastopenia of childhood presents as an acute anemia in a previously well child.[84] The syndrome has an estimated incidence rate of 4 to 5 cases per 1 million children.[85-87] Transient erythroblastopenia is a frequent diagnosis in children with severe anemia[86,88] and is the most common cause of acquired red cell aplasia in pediatric patients.[85] Most patients are 1 to 3 years old,[88] but transient erythroblastopenia of childhood can occur in the first year of life and through adolescence. Rare complications include seizures and transient neurologic abnormalities.[89-91]

LABORATORY EVALUATION

In both transient syndromes, acute severe anemia is the hallmark, and hemoglobin levels may be markedly depressed. Reticulocytes usually are absent from the blood, and erythroid precursor cells are not present or markedly decreased in the marrow. Red cell indices are normal. White blood cell and platelet counts are normal or elevated. Occasionally, neutropenia and thrombocytopenia of mild or moderate degree are present (especially if splenic function is intact, as in hereditary spherocytosis and in transient erythroblastopenia of childhood).[88] If the episode is brief and diagnosed during marrow recovery, patients may present with reticulocytosis, and nucleated red blood cells may be seen on the blood film.

DIFFERENTIAL DIAGNOSIS

The reticulocyte count readily distinguishes the cause of increasing anemia in a patient with hemolytic disease as transient aplastic crisis. The most important differential diagnosis for transient erythroblastopenia of childhood is inherited pure red cell aplasia. For the former, the age at presentation is older, the patient usually has no family history (but transient erythroblastopenia of childhood may be familial and can occur simultaneously in siblings),[92] physical anomalies are absent, and the syndrome resolves spontaneously.

In transient erythroblastopenia of childhood (in contrast to inherited red cell aplasia), erythrocyte adenosine deaminase levels are normal, and red cells do not show "stress" patterns of fetal hemoglobin and i antigen (red cell antigen expressed primarily on feral erythrocytes) expression. The patient's medical history, the red cell indices, and appropriate serum assays should allow prompt exclusion of more common causes of anemia in children, such as iron deficiency (Chap. 11) or other nutritional deficiencies (Chap. 12). When transient erythroblastopenia is associated with neutropenia, acute lymphoblastic leukemia and aplastic anemia (Chap. 4) may be suspected; marrow examination clarifies the diagnosis.[93] A record of current medications—more important in adults—may provide the basis for a tentative diagnosis of drug-induced rather than idiopathic disease.

THERAPY, COURSE, AND PROGNOSIS

Transient *aplastic* crisis resolves as neutralizing antibodies to B19 parvovirus are made, usually within 1 to 2 weeks of infection. Ensuing reticulocytosis may be brisk, and the hemoglobin may transiently rise to higher-than-normal values. White cell and platelet numbers may "rebound," and some bone pain from marrow expansion may be present. Severe anemia may require transfusion of red blood cells. In sickle cell disease, parvovirus infection has been associated with other complications, such as acute chest crisis.[94-96] A recombinant vaccine to prevent B19 parvovirus has been tested in healthy volunteers[97,98] and is in early-phase development by the National Institutes of Health.

Transient erythroblastopenia of childhood typically terminates after a few weeks, but anemia may sometimes persist for months. Transfusions may be required during that interval. Overtreatment of a self-limited illness and misdiagnosis of a more serious disease should be avoided.

For drug-associated transient failure of erythropoiesis, use of the suspected offending drug is discontinued and the diagnosis established from subsequent clinical improvement.

●ACQUIRED PURE RED CELL APLASIA

DEFINITION AND HISTORY

Acquired pure red cell aplasia is an uncommon cause of anemia that occurs principally in older adults. The blood counts and marrow appearance are indistinguishable from the picture of Diamond-Blackfan anemia, that is, anemia, severe reticulocytopenia, and absent marrow erythroid precursor cells. The nosologic origins of acquired pure red cell aplasia are obscure. Early descriptions are intermixed with those of aplastic anemia (in retrospect, a poor term for generalized marrow failure). Kaznelson[99] is credited with publishing the first case report in 1922. Early distinction of the two syndromes was stimulated by the relationship of red cell aplasia to thymoma. Although red cell aplasia shares with aplastic anemia an immune pathophysiology and responsiveness to immunosuppressive therapies, the absence of involvement of neutrophils, monocytes, and platelets makes the diagnostic distinction evident. Many of the diverse clinical associations (see Table 5-1) are consistent with an immune-mediated pathophysiology. The mechanism of red cell failure is best understood for T-cell–mediated autoimmune destruction and persistent B19 parvovirus infection.

ETIOLOGY AND PATHOGENESIS

Immune Pure Red Cell Aplasia

Clinical and laboratory evidence supports both antibody and cellular mechanisms of inhibition of erythropoiesis. Red cell aplasia is associated with autoimmune diseases, such as rheumatoid arthritis, systemic lupus erythematosus, myasthenia gravis, autoimmune hemolytic anemia, acquired hypoimmunoglobulinemia, autoimmune polyglandular syndrome, and especially thymoma, and with lymphoproliferative processes, such as CLL and Hodgkin lymphoma, in which immune dysregulation is common. Serum inhibitors can be detected in the laboratory. Krantz and colleagues showed that Ig fractions from the patient's blood inhibited heme synthesis and red cell progenitor assays in vitro.[80] Antibodies that inhibit burst-forming unit–erythroid (BFU-E) and CFU-E colony formation are present in patients with red cell aplasia. A

pathophysiologic role can be inferred, first from the response of patients to specific treatments directed at antibodies, such as plasmapheresis and a monoclonal antibody to a cluster of differentiation molecule expressed on the surface of all mature B cells, CD20, and second from decreased or absent plasma antibody in recovered patients. There, also, have been cases of monoclonal gammopathy associated with erythroid aplasia. Where used the aplasia has resolved after administration of bortezomib or other therapies. The result of therapy strongly supports a role for the monoclonal Ig in the aplasia. However, autoantibodies against erythropoietin were not studied, so assuming this pathogenesis is logical but unproven. Antibodies also may be involved in the red cell aplasia of pregnancy.[100]

Autoantibodies to erythropoietin rarely have caused this disease.[101,102] More frequently, red cell aplasia secondary to antibodies was elicited by administration of certain molecular formulations of recombinant erythropoietin to patients undergoing renal dialysis in Europe[103-105] (current available recombinant erythropoietins do not elicit pathogenic antibodies). Anemia was often profound, and some patients remained transfusion-dependent despite discontinuation of hormone therapy. Glycosylation of recombinant erythropoietin is different from the native molecule, but antibodies are directed against conformational epitopes of the protein and not to the sugar moieties. Erythropoietin immunogenicity is associated with human leukocyte antigen (HLA) specificities.[106]

Pure red cell aplasia after transplant from an erythrocyte antigen-incompatible donor is a second example of specific antibodies etiologic in the destruction of red cell progenitors.[107-112] ABO incompatibility is frequent in allogenic transplant but only occasionally results in hemolytic anemia, delayed erythroid engraftment and late erythropoietic failure, and pure red cell aplasia. Recipient isoagglutinins reactive to donor erythrocyte antigens are usually rapidly cleared without clinical consequences other than a slight increase in transfusions posttransplant. Persistence of isoagglutinins may be related to the persistence of recipient antibody–producing cells, relating to less intensive conditioning, immunosuppressive drug treatment, and the presence of graft-versus-host disease. Transfusion of donor-type red blood cells before transplant may absorb isoagglutinins and lessen transfusion requirements and possibly prevent red cell aplasia.[113] Treatment has been varied and included erythropoiesis-stimulating agents, tapering of immunosuppression or donor lymphocyte infusion to promote a graft-versus-plasma cell effect, glucocorticoids, rituximab, or bortezomib in an effort to decrease isoantibody production or plasmapheresis to remove isoantibodies. These treatments are often ineffective and have side effects. The use of Ig1k anti-CD-38 monoclonal antibody, daratumumab, in two doses 10 days apart was successful in correcting postallogeneic stem cell transplantation in three patients so treated.[114-116]

Suppression of erythropoiesis by T cells may be more common than antibody inhibition as a mechanism of erythropoietic failure.[117] Suggestive clinical observations include the frequent association of red cell aplasia with CLL in approximately 6% of cases[118]; CLL is also associated with autoimmune hemolytic anemia and idiopathic thrombocytopenic purpura,[119] and with large granular lymphocytosis (LGL) in approximately 7% of cases.[120] In a series of 47 patients with red cell aplasia, 4 also had CLL and 9 had LGL.[121] More sensitive flow cytometric and molecular methods may detect clonal T-cell expansion in patients with normal numbers of circulating lymphocytes.[122,123] An attractive molecular mechanism underlying CD8 cell expansion is signal transducer and activator of transcription 3 gene mutations (*STAT3*), leading to constitutive activation of a clone of cytotoxic T cells, which is relatively frequent in patients with LGL[124] and has been described in patients with pure red cell aplasia.[125-127] In one recent study, *STAT3* mutations specifically were identified in 43% of Japanese patients with red cell aplasia and not other marrow failure diseases, restricted to cytotoxic lymphocytes; patients with mutations were younger and less responsive to cyclosporine.[128] Functionally, lymphocytes from patients with idiopathic pure red cell aplasia[129-131] or red cell aplasia associated with CLL,[132] LGL,[133-135] thymoma,[136] other lymphoid malignancies,[137,138] Epstein-Barr virus infection[139] and human T-cell leukemia virus 1 infection[140] suppressed erythropoiesis in colony assays. Several mechanisms of cell killing have been suggested.[120,141] When effector cells show histocompatibility locus A class I–restricted killing, recognition of a specific antigen peptide is implied by a T cell with an αβ T-cell receptor.[142] In a man with red cell aplasia and LGL, erythropoiesis was inhibited by non–major histocompatibility antigen-restricted γδ T cells that lysed CFU-E. T cells downregulated class I histocompatibility antigens and thus were unable to engage the natural killer cell's inhibitory receptors.[135]

Persistent B19 Parvovirus Infection

B19 parvovirus specifically infects and is toxic to erythroid progenitor cells. Parvovirus infection normally is terminated within 1 to 2 weeks of infection by the humoral immune response. Linear neutralizing epitopes are localized to a relatively small region of the capsid protein.[143] In the absence of an effective antibody response, infection persists and causes pure red cell aplasia.[57,143,144] Erythropoietic failure may be the only evidence of parvoviral infection. Persistence of B19 parvovirus infection occurs in the setting of immunodeficiency, most commonly caused by chemotherapeutic and immunosuppressive drugs,[145] human immunodeficiency virus 1 infection,[146] and occasionally Nezelof syndrome's subtle immunologic abnormalities.[147] Parvovirus at one time may have accounted for approximately 15% of severe anemia in patients with AIDS,[148] but highly effective antiretroviral drug regimens have reduced its role.[149,150] There has been one case of red cell aplasia apparently secondary to the antiviral emtricitabine that reversed rapidly on discontinuation.[151] Persistent B19 parvovirus infection can occur in the fetus exposed during the mid-trimester of pregnancy. The infection can cause hydrops fetalis as a result of viral cytotoxicity for erythroid progenitors in the fetal liver and death of the newborn as a result of severe anemia and congestive heart failure.[57] In rare instances, parvovirus-infected or hydropic infants rescued by red cell transfusion show congenital red cell aplasia or dyserythropoietic anemia.[152]

Intrinsic Cellular Defects Leading to Failed Red Blood Cell Production

Red cell aplasia occasionally can be the first or the major manifestation of a myelodysplastic syndrome.[153] Discrete genetic defects can lead to failure of erythropoiesis. Activating point mutations in *N-RAS*, an oncogene in the RAS family, occur in some cases of myelodysplastic syndrome, and mutant *N-RAS* in vitro can induce a proliferative defect in erythroid progenitor cells.[154] Loss of the *RPS14* gene in 5q– deletions leads to red cell aplasia in this myelodysplastic syndrome.[155,156] In vitro colony formation may distinguish such intrinsic cellular defects from immune-mediated marrow failure, with higher BFU-E numbers predicting response to immunosuppressive therapies.[157]

Medications

Idiosyncratic drug reactions are blamed for a far smaller proportion of red cell aplasia than of agranulocytosis. Case reports have implicated diphenylhydantoin, sulfa and sulfonamide drugs, azathioprine, allopurinol, isoniazid, procainamide, ticlopidine, ribavirin, and penicillamine. The same drugs may transiently suppress erythropoiesis as they are associated with chronic pure red cell aplasia.[158] Laboratory investigations of diphenylhydantoin[159] and rifampicin[160] are consistent with a hapten mechanism, in which serum antibody affects erythroid progenitor cells only in the presence of drug. Causality cannot be assigned from case reports; with nonsteroidal anti-inflammatory drugs, gold, and colchicine, the underlying rheumatic syndrome could be the etiologic link.

CLINICAL FEATURES

Symptoms of anemia are pallor, fatigue, lassitude, pulsatile tinnitus, and, in the older patient, sometimes anginal chest pain. Of concomitant diseases, the most important is CLL,[119,161,162] but also associated are lymphomas,[163] autoimmune rheumatologic disorders, myasthenia gravis especially in the setting of thymoma,[164] and cancers. With the introduction of checkpoint inhibitors into clinical practice, autoimmunity is now recognized as a serious toxicity, including pure red cell aplasia, in particular with PD1-PDL1 immunotherapy.[165,166] Pure red cell aplasia and LGL are often observed in the same patient, but this association may represent an extreme of the cytotoxic lymphocyte clonal expansion that is a feature of pure red cell aplasia. Red cell aplasia can also occur with pregnancy.[167]

Persistent B19 parvovirus infection should be suspected in the anemic cancer patient after stem cell transplantation, in patients treated with immunosuppressive drugs, in patients with AIDS, and in patients with a family or personal history suggestive of inherited immune disorder. Pure red cell aplasia is a rare sequela of infectious mononucleosis and seronegative hepatitis.

LABORATORY FEATURES

Anemia is either normocytic or macrocytic, reticulocytopenia is profound, and white cell and platelet counts are generally normal. Marrow examination reveals absent or very few erythroid precursor cells, but normal granulopoiesis and megakaryocytopoiesis. Iron saturation and ferritin level frequently are elevated and rise further after repeated red cell transfusions. Erythroid colony assays may predict responsiveness to immunosuppressive treatment. The presence of marrow or blood BFU-E and CFU-E correlates with hematologic improvement,[129,168,169] but these tests may not be generally available.

Thymomas are frequently associated with autoimmune disease, myasthenia gravis most prominently, and with marrow failure syndromes.[170] In a patient with acquired pure red cell aplasia, a thymoma should be sought by chest imaging, including computed tomographic scan. The association of thymoma and pure red cell aplasia has been emphasized but is uncommon; thymoma in only 2 of 37 patients with red cell aplasia,[171] and only two instances of red cell aplasia in a series of 29 patients with thymoma.[172] The thymomas usually are encapsulated and have a spindle cell histology. In one series, 10 of 56 cases were considered malignant because of their locally infiltrating character[173]; therefore, the tumors should be surgically excised, if feasible.

CLL should be evident based on lymphocyte count and immunophenotyping for monoclonality. LGL, which frequently underlies red cell aplasia, may be more subtle: diagnosis requires careful examination of the blood film for typical lymphocytic forms, flow cytometry for cell surface markers characteristic of natural killer and cytotoxic lymphocytes, and demonstration of monoclonal T-cell proliferation by molecular studies.

Persistent parvovirus infection can be difficult to diagnose. Giant pronormoblasts scattered on the marrow film are the most characteristic of the condition (see Fig. 5-1), but such typical cells may not be observed. Marrow morphologies that are dysplastic or suggestive of leukemia also have been described. Serum antibodies specific to the virus are absent or only IgM is positive. Parvovirus DNA should be present in high concentrations in the blood and readily detected by molecular techniques.

DIFFERENTIAL DIAGNOSIS

The historically difficult diagnostic distinction between constitutional and acquired red cell aplasia has been resolved with comprehensive genomic screening for mutations in the genes responsible for Diamond-Blackfan anemia. Occasionally, pure red cell aplasia is difficult to distinguish from more generalized marrow failure when other blood counts are on borderline. A dysmorphic marrow smear and abnormal chromosomes point to myelodysplasia as responsible for isolated anemia and reticulocytopenia. B19 parvovirus infection should always be suspected and searched for in any immunosuppressed individual who is anemic, because the infection can be treated.

THERAPY, COURSE, AND PROGNOSIS

Transfusion

As with inherited red cell aplasia, transfusions and iron chelation are basic to management.[174] In an adult, 1 unit of packed erythrocytes per week can replace marrow erythropoiesis, which for convenience is usually transfused as 2 units every 2 weeks. The goal of preventing symptoms of anemia is achievable in most patients if the nadir hemoglobin is greater than 70 g/L. A goal greater than 90 g/L may be preferable in patients with cardiac or pulmonary disease and in older patients. Even refractory pure red cell aplasia is consistent with a prolonged and perhaps even normal life expectancy, and iron-chelation therapy can be initiated based on the ferritin level (Chap. 11).

Immunosuppression

Immunosuppressive agents are used to treat disease of suspected immune origin. Response is likely in a majority of patients, but sequential treatment with a variety of agents often is required. Some patients, however, remain refractory to treatment.[114,174-176] Typically, oral prednisone 1 to 2 mg/kg per day is given first, and about half of patients improve. A 1- to 2-month trial can be associated with significant toxicity and evidence of Cushing syndrome. Higher response rates have been cited for cyclosporine, and some experts (and the author) advocate using this drug first.[177-181] Cytotoxic agents, especially azathioprine and cyclophosphamide,[182] can be beneficial but are not first-choice treatments because of their mutagenic and leukemogenic properties. These drugs may be preferred in red cell aplasia associated with LGL, in which cytoreduction may be helpful.[122,183,184] Acquired pure red cell aplasia can respond to antithymocyte globulin.[128,169,185] Monoclonal antibodies have less toxicity than does antilymphocyte globulin, and can be administered without hospitalization. Success has been reported using rituximab (anti-CD20 monoclonal antibody),[186-188] alemtuzumab (anti-CD52),[189-191] and daclizumab (anti–IL-2 receptor,[192] withdrawn from the market). Some patients with refractory disease have responded to fludarabine and cladribine.[193,194] Plasmapheresis has produced long-lasting improvement in few patients, presumably by removing pathogenic antibodies.[195,196] The absence of randomized trials and even case series of adequate sample size makes the extrapolation of case reports to quantitative estimates of response problematic for many of these therapies.[174]

A thymoma should be excised to prevent local spread of a malignant tumor, but thymectomy does not necessarily improve marrow function.[164,173] Red cell aplasia can follow thymectomy. Cyclosporine appears the most effective drug to treat pure red cell aplasia associated with thymoma.[197]

Posttransplant pure red cell aplasia often spontaneously resolves over time, making the interpretation of case reports and small series problematic.[112] Success has been reported with rituximab (anti-CD20 monoclonal antibody), antithymocyte globulins, daratumumab (anti-CD38), and donor lymphocyte infusions[198] (summarized in reference 112).

Hematopoietic Stem Cell Transplantation

Red cell aplasia is rarely an indication for stem cell transplantation because the anemia usually can be managed with less drastic approaches. Although the disease can be cured by infusion of allogeneic stem cells,[199,200] risks are not negligible; in a recent retrospective compilation from European investigators, 5-year survival was disappointing at 51%.[201]

Other Therapies

Despite early favorable case reports, androgens, erythropoietin, and splenectomy are not routinely used to treat pure red cell aplasia.

Persistent parvovirus infection results from the host's inability to mount an effective humoral immune response. It can be effectively treated in almost all cases by administration of commercial immunoglobulin,[202,203] an excellent source of B19 parvovirus neutralizing antibodies present in a large proportion of the normal population. Infusion of immunoglobulin at 0.4 g/kg per day for 5 to 10 days should produce brisk reticulocytosis and restore a hemoglobin level appropriate for the patient. A single course may be adequate to cure long-standing red cell aplasia resulting from an underlying inherited immunodeficiency syndrome, but patients with AIDS may not show complete clearance of parvovirus from the circulation and may relapse, requiring retreatment or maintenance immunoglobulin injections.[146,204] Patients with persistent B19 parvovirus infection do not have typical manifestations of a viral infection, such as fever. In these patients, Ig infusions can induce fifth disease symptoms of variable severity, including cutaneous eruptions and arthritis. Older case reports of red cell aplasia responsive to Ig infusions likely represent treatment of patients with previously unrecognized parvovirus infection.

REFERENCES

1. Narla A, Vlachos A, Nathan DG. Diamond Blackfan anemia treatment: past, present, and future. *Semin Hematol.* 2011;48:117.
2. Means RT Jr. Pure red cell aplasia. *Blood.* 2016;128:2504.
3. Balasubramanian SK, Sadaps M, Thota S, et al. Rational management approach to pure red cell aplasia. *Haematologica.* 2018;103:221.
4. Joseph WH. Anemia of infancy and early childhood. *Medicine.* 1936;15:307.
5. Diamond LK, Blackfan KD. Hypoplastic anemia. *Am J Dis Child.* 1938;56:464.
6. Gasser C. Aplasia of erythropoiesis. *Pediatr Clin North Am.* 1957;4:445.
7. Diamond LK, Wang WC, Alter BB. Congenital hypoplastic anemia. *Adv Pediatr.* 1976;22:349.
8. Vlachos A, Blanc L, Lipton JM. Diamond Blackfan anemia: a model for the translational approach to understanding human disease. *Expert Rev Hematol.* 2014;7:359.
9. Clinton C, Gazda HT. Diamond-Blackfan anemia. In: Adam MP, Ardinger HH, Pagon RA, et al, eds. *GeneReviews®.* University of Washington; 1993 [Updated 2019].
10. Raiser DM, Narla A, Ebert BL. The emerging importance of ribosomal dysfunction in the pathogenesis of hematologic disorders. *Leuk Lymphoma.* 2014;55:491.
11. Ball SE, McGuckin CP, Jenkins G, et al. Diamond-Blackfan anaemia in the U.K.: analysis of 80 cases from a 20-year birth cohort. *Br J Haematol.* 1996;94:645.
12. Orfali KA, Ohene-Abuakwa Y, Ball SE. Diamond Blackfan anemia in the UK: clinical and genetic heterogeneity. *Br J Haematol.* 2004;125:243.
13. Ulirsch JC, Verboon JM, Kazerounian S, et al. The genetic landscape of Diamond-Blackfan anemia. *Am J Hum Genet.* 2018;103:930.
14. Gustavsson P, Willig TN, Van Haederingen A. Diamond-Blackfan anaemia: genetic homogeneity for a gene on chromosome 19q13 restricted to 1.8 Mb. *Nat Genet.* 1997;16:368.
15. Dutt S, Narla A, Lin K, et al. Haploinsufficiency for ribosomal protein genes causes selective activation of p53 in human erythroid progenitor cells. *Blood.* 2011;117:2567.
16. Matsson H, Davey EJ, Draptchinskaia N, et al. Targeted disruption of the ribosomal protein S19 gene is lethal prior to implantation. *Mol Cell Biol.* 2004;24:4032.
17. Boria I, Quarello P, Avondo F, et al. A new database for ribosomal protein genes which are mutated in Diamond-Blackfan anemia. *Hum Mutat.* 2008;29:E263.
18. Sankaran VG, Ghazvinian R, Do R, et al. Exome sequencing identifies *GATA1* mutations resulting in Diamond-Blackfan anemia. *J Clin Investig.* 2012;122:2439.
19. Ling T, Crispino JD. *GATA1* mutations in red cell disorders. *IUBMB Life.* 2020;72:106.
20. Gripp KW, Curry C, Olney AH, et al. Diamond-Blackfan anemia with mandibulofacial dysostosis is heterogeneous, including the novel DBA genes TSR2 and RPS28. *Am J Med Genet A.* 2014;164A:2240.
21. Meyts I, Aksentijevich I: deficiency of adenosine deaminase 2 (DADA2): Updates on the phenotype, genetics, pathogenesis, and treatment. *J Clin Immunol.* 2018;38:569.

22. Perdahl EB, Naprstek BL, Wallace WC, et al. Erythroid failure in Diamond-Blackfan anemia is characterized by apoptosis. *Blood.* 1994;83:645.

23. Casadevall N, Croisille L, Auffray I, et al. Age-related alterations in erythroid and granulopoietic progenitors in Diamond-Blackfan anaemia. *Br J Haematol.* 1994;87:369.

24. Ohene-Abuakwa Y, Orfali KA, Marius C, et al. Two-phase culture in Diamond Blackfan anemia: localization of erythroid defect. *Blood.* 2005;105:838.

25. Giri N, Kang E, Tisdale JF, et al. Clinical and laboratory evidence for a trilineage haematopoietic defect in patients with refractory Diamond-Blackfan anaemia. *Br J Haematol.* 2000;108:167.

26. Uechi T, Nakajima Y, Chakraborty A, et al. Deficiency of ribosomal protein S19 during early embryogenesis leads to reduction of erythrocytes in a zebrafish model of Diamond-Blackfan anemia. *Hum Mol Genet.* 2008;17:3204.

27. Flygare J, Olsson K, Richter J, et al. Gene therapy of Diamond Blackfan anemia CD34+ cells leads to improved erythroid development and engraftment following transplantation. *Exp Hematol.* 2008;36:1428.

28. Miyake K, Flygare J, Kiefer T, et al. Development of cell line models for RPS19 deficient Diamond-Blackfan anemia using drug-inducible expression of siRNA against RPS19. *Mol Ther.* 2005;11:627.

29. Halperin DS, Freedman MH. Diamond-Blackfan anemia: etiology, pathophysiology, and treatment. *Am J Pediatr Hematol Oncol.* 1989;11:380.

30. Scimeca PG, Weinblatt ME, Slepowitz G, et al. Diamond-Blackfan syndrome: an unusual cause of hydrops fetalis. *Am J Pediatr Hematol Oncol.* 1988;10:241.

31. Farrar JE, Dahl N. Untangling the phenotypic heterogeneity of Diamond Blackfan anemia. *Semin. Hematol.* 2011;48:124.

32. Balaban EP, Buchanan GR, Graham M, et al. Diamond-Blackfan syndrome in adult patients. *Am J Med.* 1985;78:533.

33. Alter BP. Diamond-Blackfan anemia. In: Young NS, Alter BP, eds. *Aplastic Anemia, Acquired and Inherited.* W.B. Saunders; 1994:361.

34. Cathie IA. Erythrogenesis imperfecta. *Arch Dis Child.* 1950;25:313.

35. Tisdale J, Dunbar CE. Pure red cell aplasia. In: Young NS. *The Bone Marrow Failure Syndromes.* W.B. Saunders; 2000:135.

36. Schofield KP, Evans DI. Diamond-Blackfan syndrome and neutropenia. *J Clin Pathol.* 1991;44:742.

37. Vlachos A, Muir E. How I treat Diamond-Blackfan anemia. *Blood.* 2010;116:3715.

38. Bartels M, Bierings M. How I manage children with Diamond-Blackfan anaemia. *Br J Haematol.* 2018;184:123.

39. Sjogren SE, Siva K, Soneji S, et al. Glucocorticoids improve erythroid progenitor maintenance and dampen Trp53 response in a mouse model of Diamond-Blackfan anaemia. *Br J Haematol.* 2015;171:517.

40. Willig TN, Niemeyer CM, Leblanc T, et al. Identification of new prognosis factors from the clinical and epidemiologic analysis of a registry of 229 Diamond-Blackfan anemia patients: DBA group of Société d'Hematologie et d'Immunologie Pediatrique (SHIP), Gesellshaft fur Padiatrische Onkologie und Hamatologie (GPOH), and the European Society for Pediatric Hematology and Immunology (ESPHI). *Pediatr Res.* 1999;46:553.

41. Janov AJ, Leong T, Nathan DG, et al. Diamond Blackfan anemia. Natural history and sequelae of treatment. *Medicine (Baltimore).* 1996;75:77.

42. Willig TN, Gazda H, Sieff CA. Diamond-Blackfan anemia. *Curr Opin Hematol.* 2000;7:85.

43. Vlachos A, Ball S, Dahl N, et al. Diagnosing and treating Diamond Blackfan anaemia: results of an international clinical consensus conference. *Br J Haematol.* 2008;142:849.

44. Lipton JM AE, Zyskin I, Vlachos A. Improving clinical care and elucidating the pathophysiology of Diamond Blackfan anemia: an update for the Diamond Blackfan Anemia Registry. *Pediatr Blood Cancer.* 2006;46:558.

45. Mugishima H, Ohga S, Ohara A, et al. Hematopoietic stem cell transplantation for Diamond-Blackfan anemia: a report from the Aplastic Anemia Committee of the Japanese Society of Pediatric Hematology. *Pediatr Transplant.* 2007;11:601.

46. Fagioli F, Quarello P, Zecca M, et al. Haematopoietic stem cell transplantation for Diamond Blackfan anaemia: a report from the Italian Association of Paediatric Haematology and Oncology Registry. *Br J Haematol.* 2014;165:673.

47. Narla A, Payne EM, Abayasekara N, et al. L-Leucine improves the anaemia in models of Diamond Blackfan anaemia and the 5q- syndrome in a TP53-independent way. *Br J Haematol.* 2014;167:524.

48. Lipton J. Diamond Blackfan anemia: new paradigms for a "not so pure" inherited red cell aplasia. *Semin Hematol.* 2006;43:167.

49. Hamaguchi I, Ooka A, Brun A, et al. Gene transfer improves erythroid development in ribosomal protein S19-deficient Diamond-Blackfan anemia. *Blood.* 2002;100:2724.

50. Uechi T, Kenmochi N. Zebrafish models of Diamond-Blackfan anemia: a tool for understanding the disease pathogenesis and drug discovery. *Pharmaceuticals (Basel).* 2019;12(4):151.

51. Lyngar E. Samtidig optreden av anemisk kriser hos 3 barn i en familie med hemolytisk ikterus. *Nordisk Medicin.* 1942;14:1246.

52. Owren PA. Congenital hemolytic jaundice: the pathogenesis of the "hemolytic crisis". *Blood.* 1948;3:231.

53. Dameshek W, Bloom ML. The events in the hemolytic crisis of hereditary spherocytosis, with particular reference to the reticulocytopenia, pancytopenia and an abnormal splenic mechanism. *Blood.* 1948;3:1381.

54. Chernoff AI, Josephson AM. Acute erythroblastopenia in sickle-cell anemia and infectious mononucleosis. *Am J Dis Child.* 1951;82:310.

55. Singer K, Motulsky AG, Wile SA. Aplastic crisis in sickle cell anemia. A study of its mechanism and its relationship to other types of hemolytic crises. *J Lab Clin Med.* 1950;35:721.

56. Pattison JR, Jones SE, Hodgson J, et al. Parvovirus infections and hypoplastic crisis in sickle cell anemia. *Lancet.* 1981;1:664.

57. Young NS, Brown KE. Parvovirus B19. *N Engl J Med.* 2004;350:586.

58. Serjeant GR, Serjeant BE, Thomas PW, et al. Human parvovirus infection in homozygous sickle cell disease. *Lancet.* 1993;341:1237.

59. Serjeant GR, Topley JM, Mason K, et al. Outbreak of aplastic crises in sickle cell anaemia associated with parvovirus-like agent. *Lancet.* 1981;2:595.

60. Wranne L. Transient erythroblastopenia in infancy and childhood. *Scand J Haematol.* 1970;7:76.

61. van den Akker M, Dror Y, Odame I. Transient erythroblastopenia of childhood is an underdiagnosed and self-limiting disease. *Acta Paediatr.* 2014;103:e288.

62. Qiu J, Soderlund-Venermo M, Young NS. Human parvoviruses. *Clin Microbiol Rev.* 2017;30:43.

63. Young NS, Harrison M, Moore JG, et al. Direct demonstration of the human parvovirus in erythroid progenitor cells infected in vitro. *J Clin Investig.* 1984;74:2024.

64. Brown KE, Anderson SM, Young NS. Erythrocyte P antigen: cellular receptor for B19 parvovirus. *Science.* 1993;262:114.

65. Brown KE, Hibbs JR, Gallinella G, et al. Resistance to human parvovirus B19 infection due to lack of virus receptor (erythrocyte P antigen). *N Engl J Med.* 1993;330:1192.

66. Anderson MJ, Higgins PG, Davis LR, et al. Experimental parvoviral infection in humans. *J Infect Dis.* 1985;152:257.

67. Saarinen UM, Chorba TL, Tattersall P, et al. Human parvovirus B19-induced epidemic acute red cell aplasia in patients with hereditary hemolytic anemia. *Blood.* 1986;67:1411.

68. Chorba TL, Coccia P, Holman RC, et al. Role of parvovirus B19 in aplastic crisis and erythema infectiosum (fifth disease). *J Infect Dis.* 1986;154:383.

69. Smith-Whitley K, Zhao H, Hodinka RL, et al. The epidemiology of human parvovirus B19 in children with sickle cell disease. *Blood.* 2003;103:422.

70. Serjeant BE, Hambleton IR, Kerr S, et al. Haematological response to parvovirus B19 infection in homozygous sickle-cell disease. *Lancet.* 2001;358:1779.

71. Skeppner G, Kreuger A, Elinder G. Transient erythroblastopenia of childhood: prospective study of 10 patients with special reference to viral infections. *J Pediatr Hematol Oncol.* 2002;24:294.

72. Beresford CH, MacFarlane SD. Temporal clustering of transient erythroblastopenia (cytopenia) of childhood. *Aust Paediatr J.* 1987;23:351.

73. Bhambhani K, Inoue S, Sarnaik S. Seasonal clustering of transient erythroblastopenia of childhood. *Am J Dis Child.* 1988;142:175.

74. Hays T, Lane PA, Shafer F. Transient erythroblastopenia of childhood. A review of 26 cases and reassessment of indications for bone marrow aspirate. *Am J Dis Child.* 1989;143:605.

75. Prassouli A, Papadakis V, Tsakris A, et al. Classic transient erythroblastopenia of childhood with human parvovirus B19 genome detection in the blood and bone marrow. *J Pediatr Hematol Oncol.* 2005;27:333.

76. Young NS, Mortimer PP, Moore GJ, et al. Characterization of a virus that causes transient aplastic crisis. *J Clin Investig.* 1984;73:224.

77. Rogers BB, Rogers ZR, Timmons CF. Polymerase chain reaction amplification of archival material for parvovirus B19 in children with transient erythroblastopenia of childhood. *Pediatr Pathol Lab Med.* 1996;16:471.

78. Gussetis ES, Peristeri J, Kitra V, et al. Clinical value of bone marrow cultures in childhood pure red cell aplasia. *J Pediatr Hematol Oncol.* 1998;20:120.

79. Koenig HM, Lightsey AL, Nelson DP, et al. Immune suppression of erythropoiesis in transient erythroblastopenia of childhood. *Blood.* 1979;54:742.

80. Dessypris EN, Krantz SB, Roloff JS, et al. Mode of action of the IgG inhibitor of erythropoiesis in transient erythroblastopenia of childhood. *Blood.* 1982;59:114.

81. Tamary H, Kaplinsky C, Shvartzmayer S, et al. Transient erythroblastopenia of childhood: evidence for cell-mediated suppression of erythropoiesis. *Am J Pediatr Hematol.* 1993;15:386.

82. Gustavsson P, Klar J, Matsson H, et al. Familiar transient erythroblastopenia of childhood is associated with the chromosome 19q13.2 region but not caused by mutations in coding sequences of the ribosomal protein S19 (RPS19) gene. *Br J Haematol.* 2002;119:261.

83. Smith JC, Megason GC, Iyer RV, et al. Clinical characteristics of children with hereditary hemolytic anemias and aplastic crisis: a 7-year review. *Southern Med J.* 1994;87:702.

84. Burns RA, Woodward GA. Transient erythroblastopenia of childhood. A review for the pediatric emergency medicine physician. *Pediatr Emerg Care.* 2019;35:237.

85. Kynaston JA, West NC, Reid MM. A regional experience of red cell aplasia. *Eur J Pediatr.* 1993;152:306.

86. Farhi DC, Leubbers E, Rosenthal N. Bone marrow biopsy findings in childhood anemia—prevalence of transient erythroblastopenia of childhood. *Arch Pathol Lab Med.* 1998;122:638.

87. Skeppner G, Wranne L. Transient erythroblastopenia of childhood in Sweden: incident and findings at the time of diagnosis. *Acta Paediatr.* 1993;82:574.

88. Cherrick I, Karayalcin G, Lanzkowsky P. Transient erythroblastopenia of childhood: prospective study of fifty patients. *Am J Pediatr Hematol.* 1994;16:320.

89. Michelson AD, Marshall PC. Transient neurological disorder associated with transient erythroblastopenia of childhood. *Am J Pediatr Hematol.* 1987;9:161.

90. Young RSK, Rannels E, Hilmi A, et al. Severe anemia in childhood presenting as transient ischemic attacks. *Stroke.* 1983;14:622.

91. Chan GCF, Kanwar VS, Wilimas J. Transient erythroblastopenia of childhood associated with transient neurologic deficit: report of a case and review of the literature. *J Paediatr Child Health.* 1998;34:299.

92. Skeppner G, Forestier E, Henter JI, et al. Transient red cell aplasia in siblings: a common environmental or a common hereditary factor? *Acta Paediatr*. 1998;87:43.

93. Leuschner S, Bödewaldt-Radzun S, Rister M. Increase of CALLA-positive stimulated lymphoid cells in transient erythroblastopenia of childhood. *Eur J Pediatr*. 1990;149:551.

94. Hankins JS, Penkert RR, Lavoie P, et al. Parvovirus B19 infection in children with sickle cell disease in the hydroxyurea era. *Exp Biol Med*. 2016;241:749.

95. Bakhshi S, Sarnaik SA, Becker C, et al. Acute encephalopathy with parvovirus B19 infection in sickle cell disease. *Arch Dis Child*. 2004;87:541.

96. Wierenga KJ, Serjeant BE, Serjeant GR. Cerebrovascular complications and parvovirus infection in homozygous sickle cell disease. *J Pediatr*. 2001;139:438.

97. Bernstein DI, El Sahly HM, Keitel WA, et al. Safety and immunogenicity of a candidate parvovirus B19 vaccine. *Vaccine*. 2011;29:7357.

98. Chandramouli S, Medina-Selby A, Coit D, et al. Generation of a parvovirus B19 vaccine candidate. *Vaccine*. 2013;31:3872.

99. Kaznelson P. Zur Enstehung der Blut Plattchen. *Verh Dtsch Ges Inn Med*. 1922;34:557.

100. Baker RI, Manoharan A, De Luca E, et al. Pure red cell aplasia of pregnancy: a distinct clinical entity. *Br J Haematol*. 1993;85:619.

101. Peschle C, Marmont AM, Marone G, et al. Pure red cell aplasia: studies on an IgG serum inhibitor neutralizing erythropoietin. *Br J Haematol*. 1975;30:411.

102. Casadevall N, Dupuy E, Molho-Sabatier P, et al. Autoantibodies against erythropoietin in a patient with pure red cell aplasia. *N Engl J Med*. 1996;334:630.

103. Prabhakar SS, Muhlfelder T. Antibodies to recombinant human erythropoietin causing pure red cell aplasia. *Clin Nephrol*. 1997;47:331.

104. Casadevall N, Nataf J, Viron B, et al. Pure red-cell aplasia and antierythropoietin antibodies in patients treated with recombinant erythropoietin. *N Engl J Med*. 2002;346:469.

105. Barger TE, Wrona D, Goletz TJ, et al. A detailed examination of the antibody prevalence and characteristics of anti-ESA antibodies. *Nephrol Dial Transplant*. 2012;27:3892.

106. Fijal B, Ricci D, Vercammen E, et al. Case-control study of the association between select *HLA* genes and anti-erythropoietin antibody-positive pure red-cell aplasia. *Pharmacogenomics*. 2008;9:157.

107. Bolan CD, Leitman SF, Griffith LM, et al. Delayed donor red cell chimerism and pure red cell aplasia following major ABO-incompatible nonmyeloablative hematopoietic stem cell transplantation. *Blood*. 2001;98:1687.

108. Grigg AP, Juneja SK. Pure red cell aplasia with the onset of graft versus host disease. *Bone Marrow Transplant*. 2003;32:1099.

109. Hayden PJ, Gardiner N, Molloy K, et al. Pure red cell aplasia after a major ABO-mismatched bone marrow transplant for chronic myeloid leukaemia: response to re-introduction of cyclosporin. *Bone Marrow Transplant*. 2003;33:459.

110. Helbig G, Stella-Holowiecka B, Wojnar J, et al. Pure red-cell aplasia following major and bi-directional ABO-incompatible allogeneic stem-cell transplantation: recovery of donor-derived erythropoiesis after long-term treatment using different therapeutic strategies. *Ann Hematol*. 2007;86:677.

111. Staley EM, Schwartz J, Pham HP. An update on ABO incompatible hematopoietic progenitor cell transplantation. *Transfus Apher Sci*. 2016;54:337.

112. Rowley SD, Donato ML, Bhattacharyya P. Red blood cell-incompatible allogeneic hematopoietic progenitor cell transplantation. *Bone Marrow Transplant*. 2011;46:1167.

113. Scholl S, Klink A, Mugge LO, et al. Safety and impact of donor-type red blood cell transfusion before allogeneic peripheral blood progenitor cell transplantation with major ABO mismatch. *Transfusion*. 2005;45:1676.

114. Chapuy CI, Kaufman RM, Alyea EP Connors JM. Daratumumab for delayed red cell engraftment after allogeniec trannspalantation. *N Eng J Med*. 2018;379:1846.

115. Bathini S, Holtzman NG, Koka R, et al. Refractory post-allogeneic stem cell transplant pure red cell aplasia in remission after treatment with daratumumab. *Am J Hematol*. 2019

116. Rautenberg C, Kaivers J, Germing U, et al. Daratumumab for treatment of pure red cell aplasia after allogeneic stem cell transplantation. *Bone Marrow Transplant*. 2020;55:1191.

117. Charles RJ, Sabo KM, Kidd PG, et al. The pathophysiology of pure red cell aplasia: implications for therapy. *Blood*. 1996;87:4831.

118. Chikkappa G, Zarrabi MH, Tsan MF. Pure red-cell aplasia in patients with chronic lymphocytic leukemia. *Medicine (Baltimore)*. 1986;65:339.

119. Visco C, Barcellini W, Maura F, et al. Autoimmune cytopenias in chronic lymphocytic leukemia. *Am J Hematol*. 2014;89:1055.

120. Go RS, Lust JA, Phyliky RL. Aplastic anemia and pure red cell aplasia associated with large granular lymphocyte leukemia. *Semin Hematol*. 2003;40:196.

121. Lacy MQ, Kurtin PJ, Tefferi A. Pure red cell aplasia: association with large granular lymphocyte leukemia and the prognostic value of cytogenetic abnormalities. *Blood*. 1996;87:3000.

122. Yamada O. Clonal T cell proliferation in patients with pure red cell aplasia. *Leuk Lymphoma*. 1999;35:69.

123. Fujishima N, Hirokawa M, Fujishima M, et al. Oligoclonal T cell expansion in blood but not in the thymus from a patient with thymoma-associated pure red cell aplasia. *Haematologica*. 2006;91(suppl 12):ECR47.

124. Koskela HL, Eldfors S, Ellonen P, et al. Somatic STAT3 mutations in large granular lymphocytic leukemia. *N Engl J Med*. 2012;366:1905.

125. Qiu ZY, Fan L, Wang L, et al. STAT3 mutations are frequent in T-cell large granular lymphocytic leukemia with pure red cell aplasia. *J Hematol Oncol*. 2013;6:82.

126. Ghrenassia E, Roulin L, Aline-Fardin A, et al. The spectrum of chronic CD8+ T-cell expansions: clinical features in 14 patients. *PLoS One*. 2014;9:e91505.

127. Ishida F, Matsuda K, Sekiguchi N, et al. STAT3 gene mutations and their association with pure red cell aplasia in large granular lymphocyte leukemia. *Cancer Sci*. 2014;105(3):342.

128. Kawakami T, Sekiguchi N, Kobayashi J, et al. Frequent STAT3 mutations in CD8(+) T cells from patients with pure red cell aplasia. *Blood Adv*. 2018;2:2704.

129. Abkowitz JL, Powell JS, Nakamura JM, et al. Pure red cell aplasia: response to therapy with anti-thymocyte globulin. *Am J Hematol*. 1986;23:363.

130. Abkowitz JL, Kadin ME, Powell JS, et al. Pure red cell aplasia: lymphocyte inhibition of erythropoiesis. *Br J Haematol*. 1986;63:59.

131. Hanada T, Abe T, Nakamura H, et al. Pure red cell aplasia: relationship between inhibitory activity of T cells to CFU-E and erythropoiesis. *Br J Haematol*. 1984;58:107.

132. Mangan KF, D'Alessandro L. Hypoplastic anemia in B cell chronic lymphocytic leukemia: evolution of T cell-mediated suppression of erythropoiesis in early-stage and late-stage disease. *Blood*. 1985;66:533.

133. Hoffman R, Kopel S, Hsu SD, et al. T cell chronic lymphocytic leukemia: presence in bone marrow and peripheral blood of cells that suppress erythropoiesis in vitro. *Blood*. 1978;52:255.

134. Nagasawa T, Abe T, Nakagawa T. Pure red cell aplasia and hypogammaglobulinemia associated with Tr-cell chronic lymphocytic leukemia. *Blood*. 1981;57:1025.

135. Handgretinger R, Geiselhart A, Moris A. Pure red cell aplasia associated with clonal expansion of granular lymphocytes expressing killer-cell inhibitory receptors. *N Engl J Med*. 1999;340:278.

136. Mangan KF, Volkin R, Winkelstein A. Autoreactive erythroid progenitor-T suppressor cells in the pure red cell aplasia associated with thymoma and panhypogammaglobulinemia. *Am J Hematol*. 1986;23:167.

137. Akard LP, Brandt J, Lu L, et al. Chronic T cell lymphoproliferative disorder and pure red cell aplasia. *Am J Hematol*. 1987;83:1069.

138. Reid TJI, Mullancy M, Burrell LM, et al. Pure red cell aplasia after chemotherapy for Hodgkin's lymphoma: in vitro evidence for T cell mediated suppression of erythropoiesis and response to sequential cyclosporin and erythropoietin. *Am J Hematol*. 1994;46:48.

139. Socinski MA, Ershler WB, Frankel J, et al. Pure RBC aplasia and myasthenia gravis. *Arch Intern Med*. 1983;143:543.

140. Levitt LJ, Reyes GR, Moonka DK, et al. Human T cell leukemia virus-I-associated T-suppressor cell inhibition of erythropoiesis in a patient with pure red cell aplasia and chronic T-gamma-lymphoproliferative disease. *J Clin Investig*. 1988;81:538.

141. Fisch P. Pure red cell aplasia. *Br J Haematol*. 2000;111:1010.

142. Lipton JM, Nadler LM, Canellos GP, et al. Evidence for genetic restriction in the suppression of erythropoiesis by a unique subset of T lymphocytes in man. *J Clin Investig*. 1983;72:694.

143. Kurtzman G, Cohen R, Field AM, et al. The immune response to B19 parvovirus infection and an antibody defect in persistent viral infection. *J Clin Investig*. 1989;84:1114.

144. Young NS, Brown KE. Parvovirus B19. *N Engl J Med*. 2004;350:586.

145. Geetha D, Zachary JB, Baldado HM, et al. Pure red cell aplasia caused by Parvovirus B19 infection in solid organ transplant recipients: a case report and review of literature. *Clin Transplant*. 2000;14:586.

146. Frickhofen N, Abkowitz JL, Safford M, et al. Persistent B19 parvovirus infection in patients infected with human immunodeficiency virus type 1 (HIV-1): a treatable cause of anemia in AIDS. *Ann Intern Med*. 1990;113:926.

147. Wiktor JW, Szczylik C, Gornas P, et al. Different marrow cell number requirements for the haemopoietic colony formation and the cure of the W/Wv anemia. *Experientia*. 1979;35:546.

148. Abkowitz JL, Brown KE, Wood RW, et al. Clinical relevance of parvovirus B19 as a cause of anemia in patients with human immunodeficiency virus infection. *J Infect Dis*. 1997;176:269.

149. Mylonakis E, Dickinson BP, Mileno MD, et al. Persistent parvovirus B19 related anemia of seven year's duration in an HIV-infected patient: complete remission associated with highly active antiretroviral therapy. *Am J Hematol*. 1999;60:164.

150. Morelli P, Bestetti G, Longhi E, et al. Persistent parvovirus B19-induced anemia in an HIV-infected patient under HAART. Case report and review of literature. *Eur J Clin Microbiol Infect Dis*. 2007;26:833.

151. Manickchund N, du Plessis C, John MA, et al. Emtricitabine-induced pure red cell aplasia. *South Afr J HIV Med*. 2019;20:983.

152. Brown KE, Green SW, Antunez-de-Mayolo J, et al. Congenital anemia following transplacental B19 parvovirus infection. *Lancet*. 1994;343:895.

153. Garcia-Suárez J, Pascual T, Muñoz MA, et al. Myelodysplastic syndrome with erythroid hypoplasia/aplasia: a case report and review of the literature. *Am J Hematol*. 1998;58:319.

154. Darley RL, Hoy TG, Baines P, et al. Mutant N-RAS induces erythroid lineage dysplasia in human CD34+ cells. *J Exp Med*. 1997;185:1337.

155. Ebert BL, Pretz J, Bosco J, et al. Identification of *RPS1r* as a 5q- syndrome gene by RNA interference screen. *Nature*. 2008;451:335.

156. Vlachos A, Farrar JE, Atsidaftos E, et al. Diminutive somatic deletions in the 5q region lead to a phenotype atypical of classical 5q- syndrome. *Blood*. 2013;122:2487.

157. DeZern AE, Pu J, McDevitt MA, et al. Burst-forming unit-erythroid assays to distinguish cellular bone marrow failure disorders. *Exp Hematol*. 2013;41:808.

158. Thompson DF, Gales MA. Drug-induced pure red cell aplasia. *Pharmacotherapy*. 1996;16:1002.

159. Dessypris EN, Redline S, Harris JW, et al. Diphenylhydantoin-induced pure red cell aplasia. *Blood*. 1985;65:789.

160. Mariette Y, Mitjavila MT, Moulinie PR, et al. Rifampicin-induced pure red cell aplasia. *Am J Med.* 1989;87:459.

161. Tsang M, Parikh SA. A concise review of autoimmune cytopenias in chronic lymphocytic leukemia. *Curr Hematol Malig Rep.* 2017;12:29.

162. De Back TR, Kater AP, Tonino SH. Autoimmune cytopenias in chronic lymphocytic leukemia: a concise review and treatment recommendations. *Expert Rev Hematol.* 2018;11:613.

163. Crickx E, Poullot E, Moulis G, et al. Clinical spectrum, evolution, and management of autoimmune cytopenias associated with angioimmunoblastic T-cell lymphoma. *Eur J Haematol.* 2019;103:35.

164. Wightman SC, Shrager JB. Non-myasthenia gravis immune syndromes and the thymus: is there a role for thymectomy? *Thorac Surg Clin.* 2019;29:215.

165. Michot JM, Lazarovici J, Tieu A, et al. Haematological immune-related adverse events with immune checkpoint inhibitors, how to manage? *Eur J Cancer.* 2019;122:72.

166. Delanoy N, Michot JM, Comont T, et al. Haematological immune-related adverse events induced by anti-PD-1 or anti-PD-L1 immunotherapy: a descriptive observational study. *Lancet Haematol.* 6:e48, 2018.

167. Edahiro Y, Yasuda H, Ando K, et al. Self-limiting pregnancy-associated pure red cell aplasia developing in two consecutive pregnancies: case report and literature review. *Int J Hematol.* 2020;111(4):579.

168. Lacombe C, Casadevall N, Muller O, et al. Erythroid progenitors in adult chronic pure red cell aplasia: relationship of in vitro erythroid colonies to therapeutic response. *Blood.* 1984;64:71.

169. Mangan KF, Shadduck RK. Successful treatment of chronic refractory pure red cell aplasia with antithymocyte globulin: correlation with in vitro erythroid culture studies. *Am J Hematol.* 1984;17:417.

170. Shelly S, Agmon-Levin N, Altman A, et al. Thymoma and autoimmunity. *Cell Mol Immunol.* 2011;8:199.

171. Oski FA. Hematologic consequences of chloramphenicol therapy. *J Pediatr.* 1979;94:515.

172. Holbro A, Jauch A, Lardinois D, et al. High prevalence of infections and autoimmunity in patients with thymoma. *Hum Immunol.* 2012;73:287.

173. Hirst E, Robertson TI. The syndrome of thymoma and erythroblastopenic anemia. *Medicine (Baltimore).* 1967;46:225.

174. Sawada K, Fujishima N, Hirokawa M. Acquired pure red cell aplasia: updated review of treatment. *Br J Haematol.* 2008;142:505.

175. Firkin FC, Maher D. Cytotoxic immunosuppressive drug treatment strategy in pure red cell aplasia. *Eur J Haematol.* 1988;41:212.

176. Kwong YL, Wong KF, Liang RHS, et al. Pure red cell aplasia: Clinical features and treatment results in 16 cases. *Ann Hematol.* 1996;72:137.

177. Mamiya S, Itoh T, Miura AB. Acquired pure red cell aplasia in Japan. *Eur J Haematol.* 1997;59:199.

178. Yamada O, Motoji T, Mizoguchi H. Selective effect of cyclosporine monotherapy for pure red cell aplasia not associated with granular lymphocyte-proliferative disorders. *Br J Haematol.* 1999;106:371.

179. Raghavachar A. Pure red cell aplasia: review of treatment and proposal for a treatment strategy. *Blut.* 1990;61:47.

180. Tötterman TH, Höglund M, Bengtsson M, et al. Treatment of pure red-cell aplasia and aplastic anaemia with ciclosporin: long-term clinical effects. *Eur J Haematol.* 1989;42:126.

181. Sawada K-I, Hirokawa M, Fujishima N, et al. Long-term outcome of patients with acquired primary idiopathic pure red cell aplasia receiving cyclosporine A. A nationwide cohort study in Japan for the PRCA Collaborative Study Group. *Haematologica.* 2007;92(8):1021.

182. Yamada O, Mizoguchi H, Oshimi K. Cyclophosphamide therapy for pure red cell aplasia associated with granular lymphocyte-proliferative disorders. *Br J Haematol.* 1997;97:392.

183. Go RS, Li C-Y, Tefferi A, et al. Acquired pure red cell aplasia associated with lymphoproliferative disease of granular T lymphocytes. *Blood.* 2001;98:483.

184. Fujishima N, Sawada K-I, Hirokawa M, et al. Long-term responses and outcomes following immunosuppressive therapy in large granular lymphocyte leukemia-associated pure red cell aplasia: a nationwide cohort study in Japan for the PRCA Collaborative Study Group. *Haematologica.* 2008;93:1555.

185. Harris SI, Weinberg JB. Treatment of red cell aplasia with antithymocyte globulin: repeated inductions of complete remissions in two patients. *Am J Hematol.* 1985;20:183.

186. Ghazal H. Successful treatment of pure red cell aplasia with rituximab in patients with chronic lymphocytic leukemia. *Blood.* 2002;99:1092.

187. Auner HW, Wolfler A, Beham-Schmid C, et al. Restoration of erythropoiesis by rituximab in an adult patient with primary acquired pure red cell aplasia refractory to conventional treatment. *Br J Haematol.* 2002;116:725.

188. Scaramucci L, Niscola P, Ales M, et al. Pure red cell aplasia associated with hemolytic anemia refractory to standard measures and resolved by rituximab in an elderly patient. *Int J Hematol.* 2008;88:343.

189. Willis F, Marsh JC, Bevan DH, et al. The effect of treatment with Campath-1H in patients with autoimmune cytopenias. *Br J Haematol.* 2001;114:891.

190. Ru X, Liebman HA. Successful treatment of refractory pure red cell aplasia associated with lymphoproliferative disorders with the anti-CD52 monoclonal antibody alemtuzumab (Campath-1H). *Br J Haematol.* 2004;123:278.

191. Chow JKW, Chan TK. Low-dose subcutaneous alemtuzumab is a safe and effective treatment for chronic acquired pure red cell aplasia. *Hong Kong Med J.* 2013;19:549.

192. Sloand EM, Scheinberg P, Maciejewski JP, et al. Brief communication: successful treatment of pure red cell aplasia with an anti-interleukin-2 receptor antibody (Daclizumab). *Ann Intern Med.* 2006;144:181.

193. Ahn JH, Lee KH, Lee JH, et al. A case of refractory idiopathic pure red cell aplasia responsive to fludarabine treatment. *Br J Haematol.* 2001;112:527.

194. Robak T, Kaszn, ki M, et al. Pure red cell aplasia in patients with chronic lymphocytic leukaemia treated with cladribine. *Br J Haematol.* 2001;112:1083.

195. Messner HA, Fauser AA, Curtis JE, et al. Control of antibody-mediated pure red-cell aplasia by plasmapheresis. *N Engl J Med.* 1981;304:1334.

196. Freund LG, Hippe E, Strandgaard S, et al. Complete remission in pure red cell aplasia after plasmapheresis. *Scand J Haematol.* 1985;35:315.

197. Hirokawa M, Sawada J-I, Fujishima N, et al. Long-term response and outcome following immuno-suppressive therapy in thymoma-associated pure red cell aplasia: a nationwide cohort study in Japan by the PRCA collaborative study group. *Haematologica.* 2008;93:27.

198. Verholen F, Stalder M, Helg C, et al. Resistant pure red cell aplasia after allogeneic stem cell transplantation with major ABO mismatch treated by escalating dose donor leukocyte infusion. *Eur J Haematol.* 2004;73:441.

199. Müller BU, Tichelli A, Passweg JR, et al. Successful treatment of refractory acquired pure red cell aplasia (PRCAP) by allogeneic bone marrow transplantation. *Bone Marrow Transplant.* 1999;23:1205.

200. Tseng SB, Lin SF, Chang CS, et al. Successful treatment of acquired pure red cell aplasia (PRCA) by allogeneic peripheral blood stem cell transplantation. *Am J Hematol.* 2003;74:273.

201. Halkes C, de Wreede LC, Knol C, et al. Allogeneic stem cell transplantation for acquired pure red cell aplasia. *Am J Hematol.* 2019;94:E294.

202. Kurtzman GJ, Frickhofen N, Kimble J, et al. Pure red cell aplasia of ten years' duration due to B19 parvovirus infection and its cure with immunoglobulin infusion. *N Engl J Med.* 1989;321:519.

203. Crabol Y, Terrier B, Rozenberg F, et al. Intravenous immunoglobulin therapy for pure red cell aplasia related to human parvovirus b19 infection: a retrospective study of 10 patients and review of the literature. *Clin Infect. Dis.* 2013;56:968.

204. Ramratnam B, Schiffman FJ, Rintels P, et al. Management of persistent B19 parvovirus infection in AIDS. *Br J Haematol.* 1995;91:90.

CHAPTER 6
ANEMIA OF CHRONIC DISEASE

Tomas Ganz

SUMMARY

Most patients who experience chronic infections or chronic inflammation, or some patients with various malignancies, will also have mild to moderate anemia. This anemia, designated *anemia of chronic disease* (ACD) or *anemia of inflammation* (AI), is characterized by a low serum iron level, a low to normal transferrin level, and a high to normal ferritin level. The anemia is caused by the direct and indirect inhibitory effects of inflammatory cytokines on erythrocyte production. Among the cytokines, interleukin-6 has a central role, acting by increasing hepatocyte production of the iron-regulatory hormone hepcidin. Hepcidin then blocks the release of iron from macrophages and hepatocytes, causing the characteristic hypoferremia associated with this anemia and limiting the availability of iron to the developing erythrocytes. Effective treatment of the underlying disease restores normal erythropoiesis. When this is not possible, and treatment is necessary, therapeutic trials have revealed that the anemia is often responsive to pharmacologic doses of erythropoietin (EPO) combined with intravenous iron.

Anemia of chronic kidney disease (CKD) presents similarly to AI but, because the kidneys are the predominant site of EPO production, the pathogenesis of this anemia is frequently dominated by relative EPO deficiency, where EPO concentrations in serum are lower than expected for the severity of anemia. Systemic inflammation from underlying renal disease, or that induced by dialysis treatments and their complications, contributes to pathogenesis in a manner similar to anemia of inflammation. Circulating hepcidin concentrations may also rise because of its decreased renal clearance. Suppressive effects of uremia on erythropoiesis and blood losses from hemodialysis may contribute to anemia in end-stage renal disease. A combination of erythropoiesis-stimulating agents (ESAs) and intravenous iron is usually effective in reversing anemia, but overtreatment may worsen overall outcomes.

Acronyms and Abbreviations: ACD, anemia of chronic disease; AI, anemia of inflammation; CKD, chronic kidney disease; CPG, clinical practice guideline; CRP, C-reactive protein; EPO, erythropoietin; ESA, erythropoiesis-stimulating agent; Hb, hemoglobin; IDA, iron-deficiency anemia; IL, interleukin; KDIGO, The Kidney Disease Improving Global Outcomes; LDH, lactate dehydrogenase; sTfR, soluble transferrin receptor; TfR, transferring receptor; TNF, tumor necrosis factor.

● DEFINITION AND HISTORY

The terms *anemia of chronic disease* (ACD) or *anemia of chronic disorders* refer to mild to moderately severe anemias (hemoglobin [Hb] 7-12) associated with chronic infections and inflammatory disorders and some malignancies.[1,2] The newer name, *anemia of inflammation* (AI), is not only more reflective of the pathophysiology of ACD but also includes *anemia of critical illness*,[3] a condition that presents similarly to ACD but develops within days of the onset of illness. An anemia similar to AI is seen in some older patients in the absence of an identifiable chronic disease; this condition is sometimes referred to as *unexplained anemia of elderlies* or *anemia of aging*.[4]

AI is characterized by inadequate erythrocyte production in the setting of low serum iron and low iron-binding capacity (ie, low transferrin) despite preserved or even increased macrophage iron stores in the marrow. The erythrocytes are usually normocytic and normochromic but can be mildly hypochromic and microcytic. Anemia of critical illness[3] can develop acutely (within days) in intensive care settings where the effects of infection or inflammation are exacerbated by disease-related or iatrogenic blood loss or red cell destruction, which by themselves are not sufficiently severe to cause anemia. Anemia of aging[4] is diagnosed in older adults when a normocytic normochromic anemia with low iron and preserved iron stores develops without an identified underlying disease. Older patients in this defined subset typically have an elevated sedimentation rate and/or elevated C-reactive protein (CRP), a high plasma interleukin-6 (IL-6) concentration, and frailty.

Anemia of chronic kidney disease (anemia of CKD) usually develops as chronic renal disease progresses and generally becomes more severe with decreasing creatinine clearance (Fig. 6-1). The anemia presents similarly to AI but because the kidney is the main site of erythropoietin (EPO) production in adults, the progressive destruction and fibrosis of the kidneys causes relative EPO deficiency, which frequently dominates the pathogenesis of this anemia. Patients with polycystic kidney disease are often at least partially spared, likely because cysts cause local ischemia with resultant increased, local EPO production, whereas patients with bilateral nephrectomy are particularly severely affected by EPO deficiency. Systemic inflammation, true iron deficiency, and decreased clearance of hepcidin are common consequences of the underlying disease and dialysis treatments, and one or more of these factors frequently worsen anemia or diminish the response to EPO therapy.

Physicians have known about the pale appearance of patients with chronic infections for hundreds of years. In 19th-century Europe, tuberculosis was the major killer, and the pallor associated with this disease was romanticized in the art and literature of the time. The first measurements of red cell mass revealed the association between inflammation and anemia. Discussing "the alterations in the condition of the Blood in Inflammation" in Section 372 of the 1859 edition of the *Principles of Human Physiology* by William B. Carpenter[5] described this connection between inflammation and anemia (author's parentheses): "With this increase in the proportion of fibrin and colorless corpuscles (leukocytes), separately or in combination, there is a diminution of in the proportion of the red corpuscles, albumen and the salts of the blood." In 1961, 100 years later, Maxwell Wintrobe, in the fifth edition of *Clinical Hematology*,[6] used the term "simple chronic anemia" for the normocytic anemia associated with the majority of infections and chronic systemic diseases. He described anemia associated with inflammation as a common subtype. Wintrobe proposed "profound alterations in iron and porphyrin metabolism" as the likely cause, and referred to his own experiments that showed a decrease in erythrocyte survival of only 27%, which "could easily be met by increased erythropoiesis if the marrow functional capacity were not impaired." Despite advances in our

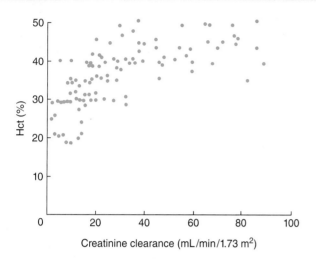

Figure 6–1. Relationship between hematocrit (Hct) and creatinine clearance in patients with chronic kidney disease (CKD). Anemia worsens with decreasing creatinine clearance. *(Reproduced with permission from Radtke HW, Claussner A, Erbes PM, et al. Serum erythropoietin concentration in chronic renal failure: relationship to degree of anemia and excretory renal function. Blood. 1979 Oct;54[4]:877-884.)*

understanding of the pathophysiology of this very common form of anemia, our knowledge is incomplete.

Anemia of CKD became a common problem in the 1960s when hemodialysis became widely available and allowed prolonged survival of patients with end-stage renal failure. Anemia of CKD was usually severe enough to limit activities of daily living and was treated by blood transfusions until the late 1980s, when recombinant EPO became widely available and alleviated the most severe forms of this anemia.

EPIDEMIOLOGY

The high prevalence of infectious diseases worldwide and the high prevalence of inflammatory and malignant disorders in industrialized countries would suggest that AI is the second most common form of anemia after iron-deficiency anemia (IDA).[7] Although the prevalence of iron deficiency in the industrialized countries is now rapidly decreasing,[7,8] AI is expected to increase as the proportion of older adults in the population increases. Table 6-1 lists the most common diseases associated with AI.

TABLE 6-1. Common Conditions Associated with Anemia of Inflammation

Category	Diseases Associated with Anemia of Inflammation
Infection	AIDS/HIV, tuberculosis, malaria (contributory), osteomyelitis, chronic abscesses, sepsis
Inflammation	Rheumatoid arthritis, other rheumatologic disorders, inflammatory bowel diseases, systemic inflammatory response syndrome
Malignancy	Carcinomas, myeloma, lymphomas
Cytokine dysregulation	Anemia of aging

Although anemia can develop early in the progression of CKD, it generally worsens as the kidneys fail.[9-11] Accordingly, the prevalence of patients with anemia of CKD worldwide is influenced by the availability of life-sustaining dialysis therapies. It is estimated that there are currently about 700,000 patients with end-stage renal disease in the United States, and approximately 100,000 new patients each year,[12] the majority of whom are anemic or receive treatment for anemia.[10] Additional patients with milder anemia of CKD are found among the estimated 6.1% of the U.S. population (or approximately 20 million) identified as having likely CKD (estimated glomerular filtration rate <60 mL/min/1.73 m^2) in the National Health and Nutritional Examination Surveys.[10]

ETIOLOGY AND PATHOGENESIS

In the chronic setting, AI predominantly results from the body's inability to increase erythrocyte production to compensate for relatively small decrements in erythrocyte survival.[1] In the steady state, erythrocyte production is sufficiently high so that the resulting anemia is mild to moderate. The anemia associated with acute critical illness has the same pathogenesis as other forms of AI; it develops more rapidly, perhaps because of the more extensive erythrocyte destruction and intensive diagnostic blood draws common in this setting. The key questions about the pathogenesis of AI, still only partially answered, are: (1) What accounts for the inability of the AI marrow to increase erythropoiesis? and (2) How is this deficit connected to the characteristic hypoferremia and sequestration of iron in macrophages and hepatocytes? Anemia of CKD is similar to AI, but the underlying renal pathology also impairs the ability of the kidneys to produce enough EPO, leading to insufficient compensatory erythropoiesis.

RED CELL DESTRUCTION

Human studies indicate that transfused AI erythrocytes have a normal life span in normal recipients, but transfused normal erythrocytes have a decreased life span in AI recipients.[1] This finding suggests that increased erythrocyte destruction is caused by the activation of macrophages that prematurely remove aging erythrocytes from the bloodstream. The explanation is consistent with the predominance of young erythrocytes in AI. Whether extrinsic factors, such as bacterial toxins and medications, or host-derived antibodies or complement, contribute to this process is unknown. The term "consumptive anemia of inflammation" describes rare disorders where hemophagocytosis by activated macrophages is the predominant cause of anemia.[13]

SUPPRESSIVE EFFECTS OF INFLAMMATION ON ERYTHROPOIETIC PRECURSORS

Some cytokines, chiefly tumor necrosis factor-α (TNF-α), IL-1, and the interferons, exert a suppressive effect on erythroid colony formation.[14] Overproduction of interferon-γ suppresses erythropoiesis in a mouse model[15] by reducing erythrocyte life span and decreasing erythropoiesis without any evidence of iron restriction. It is not known to what extent and under what conditions these mechanisms contribute to human AI.

INADEQUATE ERYTHROPOIETIN SECRETION AND RESISTANCE TO ERYTHROPOIETIN

The normal response to increased destruction of erythrocytes is transient anemia followed by an increase in EPO production and subsequent compensatory increase in erythropoiesis. One proposed explanation for the inadequate marrow response in AI is less EPO production than expected based on other types of anemia. Studies of patients with rheumatoid arthritis and AI indicated that EPO levels are increased but less so than in IDA.[16-21] The findings were similar in patients with anemias associated with solid tumors or hematologic malignancies.[22,23] However, these comparisons did not take into account the potentiating effect of iron deficiency on hypoxia sensing (Chap. 2).[24] This effect could increase EPO production in IDA above that in other types of anemia, and make EPO production in AI appear low in comparison. In support of the EPO suppression hypothesis are experiments with EPO-producing cell lines indicating that production of the hormone is inhibited by inflammatory cytokines including TNF-α and IL-1. The inhibition is mediated by the effects of the transcription factor GATA-1 on the EPO promoter, and the suppression of EPO production can be reversed by a GATA inhibitor.[25] Moreover, both baseline and hypoxia-induced EPO gene expression is suppressed in rats treated with bacterial lipopolysaccharide or IL-1β to mimic a septic state.[26] However, suppression of EPO production is not the major mechanism of AI. If it were, administration of relatively small amounts of EPO should be sufficient to reverse the AI.

In contrast, relative EPO deficiency is often a major contributor to anemia of CKD. Most destructive diseases affecting the kidneys also decrease the release of EPO in response to decreased Hb concentration.[27,28] In the kidney, interstitial fibroblasts of neural crest origin[28,29] are the main source of EPO. In response to anemia or hypoxia, the number of renal cells producing EPO increases. In advanced CKD, the kidneys undergo end-stage fibrosis during which these fibroblasts may transdifferentiate into myofibroblasts and lose their ability to produce appropriate amounts of EPO in response to hypoxia.[28,29] However, these or other renal cells can be activated to increase their EPO output by the administration of therapeutic prolyl-hydroxylase inhibitors,[30] as indicated by the lower stimulated EPO production by anephric patients compared with those with end-stage renal disease and retained kidneys. Studies in animal models indicate that the impairment of EPO production in end-stage kidneys may be reversible and could be therapeutically restored.[28,29]

Inflammation is also a strong contributor to the pathogenesis of anemia of CKD. Patients who had renal disease with inflammation, as measured by increased serum CRP greater than 20 mg/L required on average 80% higher doses of EPO than patients with simple primary deficiency from renal disease.[31] In another study, patients with CRP greater than 50 mg/L reached lower concentrations of Hb than patients with CRP lower than 50 mg/L, despite higher doses of erythropoiesis-stimulating agents (ESAs).[32] Inflammation thus induces a state of relative resistance to EPO, contributing to the pathogenesis of anemia of CKD.

ERYTHROPOIESIS RESTRICTION AS A RESULT OF IRON UNAVAILABILITY

Interleukin-6, Hepcidin, and Hypoferremia

Hypoferremia, one of the defining features of AI, develops within hours of the onset of inflammation.[1] The response is dependent on IL-6,[33] which induces the iron-regulatory hormone, hepcidin.[34] Unlike wild-type mice, mice deficient in either hepcidin[35] or IL-6[33] do not become hypoferremic during turpentine-induced inflammation. In human hepatocyte cell cultures, IL-6 is a potent and direct inducer of hepcidin production, and neither IL-1 nor TNF-α share this activity. Infusion of IL-6 into human volunteers induces hepcidin release within hours and causes concomitant hypoferremia.[33] The IL-6–hepcidin axis now appears to be responsible for the induction of hypoferremia during inflammation. However, these studies do not exclude the potential contribution of other cytokines, including activin B and interferon-γ[15,36] to

AI in human diseases or more complex mouse models. In support of multiple pathways of AI in a mouse model of inflammation, either the ablation of hepcidin or the ablation of IL-6 ameliorated the anemia, but neither restored normal Hb.[37,38]

Serum Iron Concentration Is Dependent on Iron Released From Macrophages and Hepatocytes

In the steady state, almost all of the approximately 20 to 25 mg of iron that daily enters the plasma iron/transferrin pool comes from macrophage recycling of senescent erythrocytes and from hepatocyte iron stores; only approximately 1 to 2 mg is derived from dietary iron. Only approximately 2 to 4 mg of iron is bound to transferrin, but the entire daily iron flow transits through this compartment; thus, the iron in this pool turns over every few hours. The concentration of iron in plasma is therefore determined by the balance between iron release from enterocytes, macrophages, and hepatocytes and iron uptake by iron-consuming tissues, predominantly marrow erythroblasts. During inflammation, the release of iron from macrophages and hepatocytes is markedly inhibited.[39-45] Studies in transgenic mice lacking hepcidin and mice overexpressing hepcidin indicate that the peptide is a negative regulator of iron release from macrophages and of intestinal iron uptake.[46,47] During inflammation, IL-6 induces hepcidin production, which inhibits iron release from macrophages and from hepatocytes, leading to hypoferremia (Fig. 6-2). Hepcidin acts by binding to cell membrane–associated ferroportin molecules that are the only conduits for iron export, and inducing ferroportin occlusion, internalization, and degradation.[48,49] As hepcidin concentrations increase, less and less ferroportin is available for iron export and the iron release into plasma from macrophages, hepatocytes, and enterocytes decreases.

Erythropoiesis in Anemia of Inflammation Is Limited by Iron

As an intermediate step during the synthesis of heme, iron becomes incorporated into protoporphyrin IX. Zinc is an alternative protoporphyrin ligand. In iron deficiency, increased amounts of zinc are incorporated into protoporphyrin. In AI, zinc protoporphyrin is also increased.[50] Insufficient iron reaches the sites of heme synthesis in developing erythrocytes, leading to the substitution of zinc. Moreover, the number of sideroblasts, nucleated erythrocyte precursors that stain for iron with Prussian blue, is decreased in AI,[1] a further indication of the limiting role of iron in patients with AI. Clinical evidence that iron deficiency of erythroblasts in AI contributes to anemia is that coadministration of parenteral iron can resolve the resistance of AI to EPO.[51,52] Attempts to treat AI with iron alone generally have been less successful, because iron became rapidly trapped in the macrophage compartment.[1,53,54]

In the context of anemia of CKD, increased zinc protoporphyrin and decreased reticulocyte Hb is also characteristic of functional iron deficiency during intense bursts of erythropoiesis stimulated by pharmacologic doses of EPO derivatives.[55] Here, iron stores are sufficient but iron cannot be delivered rapidly enough to erythroblasts to maintain accelerated erythropoiesis.

Inhibition of Intestinal Absorption of Iron and Other Factors Leading to Systemic Iron Deficiency

In long-standing AI, erythrocytes can become hypochromic and microcytic, partly because progressive depletion of iron stores worsens the iron restriction. As noted before, intestinal absorption of iron is inhibited[56-58] during inflammation, by an IL-6 and hepcidin-mediated mechanism.[35,47,59-61] Only 1 to 2 mg of the daily iron needed for erythropoiesis is supplied from the diet, and most adults have 400 to 1000 mg of iron stores (Chap. 10); therefore, a considerable amount of time is needed to deplete the stored iron. True iron deficiency can eventually

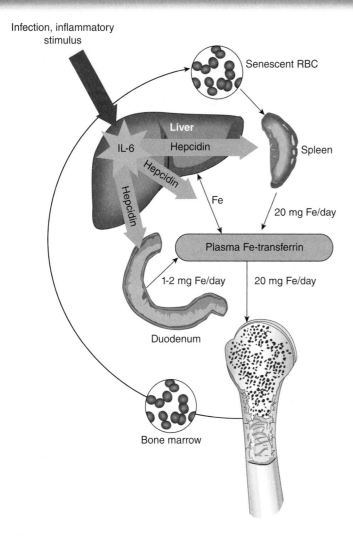

Figure 6–2. Diagram of the effect of inflammation on iron concentrations in plasma. Arrows labeled "Hepcidin" indicate control points where hepcidin inhibits iron flow into the plasma transferrin compartment.

develop in chronic inflammatory diseases, especially in children who have smaller iron stores and additional requirement for iron because of body growth, or in conditions where IL-6 levels are particularly high, such as systemic-onset juvenile chronic arthritis.[62] The anemia in these children was accompanied by an appropriate EPO increase but was unresponsive to oral iron replacement. The anemia was corrected, at least partially, by parenteral iron.

In anemia of CKD, several additional factors may contribute to true iron deficiency, including the blockade of intestinal iron absorption by higher hepcidin concentrations from its decreased renal clearance and the blood losses from hemodialysis, phlebotomy for laboratory studies, and occult gastrointestinal bleeding.

Summary of Pathogenesis

AI is primarily the result of slightly decreased red cell survival and of macrophage iron sequestration, leading to iron-restricted erythropoiesis. Depending on the underlying disease, the condition is compounded by inadequate EPO production, the suppressive effect of inflammation on erythropoietic precursors, and/or the depletion of iron stores. Anemia of CKD is dominated by the effects of relative EPO insufficiency, but inflammation and blood loss contribute importantly to its pathogenesis.

● CLINICAL FEATURES

The clinical manifestations of AI and anemia of CKD are usually obscured by the signs and symptoms of the underlying disease. Moderate anemia (Hb <10 g/dL) can exacerbate the symptoms of preexisting ischemic heart disease or respiratory disease or contribute to fatigue and exertional intolerance. More severe untreated anemia seen mainly with CKD may cause extreme fatigue, exertional dyspnea, and high output congestive heart failure. The diagnosis is based on clinical features found in conjunction with typical laboratory abnormalities.

● LABORATORY FEATURES

The erythrocytes in AI and anemia of CKD are usually normocytic and normochromic but, with increasing severity or duration, can sometimes become hypochromic and eventually microcytic.[1] The absolute reticulocyte count is normal or slightly elevated.

● HYPOFERREMIA AND DECREASED SERUM TRANSFERRIN

Hypoferremia, a decrease in serum iron concentration, is a defining feature of AI and, in the absence of iron therapy, is also commonly seen in anemia of CKD. It develops within hours of the onset of infection or severe inflammation. The concentration of the iron-binding protein, transferrin (measured as total iron-binding capacity or by an immunoassay), is moderately decreased in AI, unlike in IDA, in which transferrin concentration is increased. The decrease in transferrin concentrations develops more slowly than the decrease in serum iron levels because of the longer half-life of transferrin (8-12 days)[63] compared with the turnover of plasma iron (approximately 90 minutes).

INCREASED SERUM FERRITIN

Serum ferritin concentrations, which reflect iron stores and inflammation, are increased in AI but decreased in iron deficiency. Thus, serum ferritin is useful in differential diagnosis in patients with low serum iron concentrations.[64] Depleted iron stores in patients with coexisting inflammation may result in intermediate ferritin levels (Table 6-2 and Fig. 6-3) because ferritin is an acute-phase protein and inflammatory cytokines increase ferritin synthesis. Depending on the severity of inflammation, coexisting iron deficiency should be suspected if ferritin level is less than 100 mcg/L in the presence of significant inflammation. Soluble transferrin receptor (sTfR) levels (Table 6-2) increase with increased demand of the erythroid marrow for iron, but inflammation may have a direct suppressive effect on sTfR. As a result, sTfR is increased in iron deficiency but, unlike ferritin, is unchanged or decreased during infection or inflammation.[65] Although these properties should make sTfR a useful diagnostic parameter alone or in combination with ferritin,[66] the use of sTfr in practice has been hampered by inadequate standardization and inconsistent reports of its clinical utility. Another promising marker that may differentiate AI from systemic iron deficiency is serum hepcidin, because very low serum hepcidin levels in hypoferremia are diagnostic of systemic iron deficiency. However, the assays have not yet been standardized and the clinical utility of hepcidin measurements in differential diagnosis of anemia has not yet been tested in large heterogeneous patient populations.[67]

Low serum ferritin concentrations are indicative of iron deficiency in anemia of CKD, but normal or even high ferritin concentrations do not preclude a clinical response (increased Hb and/or decreased dosage of EPO derivatives) after parenteral iron therapy.[68] In these settings,

TABLE 6–2. Laboratory Studies of Iron Metabolism in Iron-Deficiency Anemia and Anemia of Inflammation

	IDA (n = 48)	AI (n = 58)	COMBI (n = 17)
Hemoglobin, g/L	93 ± 16 (96)	102 ± 12 (103)	88 ± 20 (90)
MCV, fL	75 ± 9 (75)	90 ± 7 (91)	78 ± 9 (79)
Iron, µmol/L (10-40)	8 ± 11 (4)	10 ± 6 (9)	6 ± 3 (6)
Transferrin, g/L (2.1-3.4 m, 2.0-3.1 f)	3.3 ± 0.4 (3.3)	1.9 ± 0.5 (1.8)	2.6 ± 0.6 (2.4)
Transferrin saturation, percent	12 ± 17 (5.7)	23 ± 13 (21)	12 ± 7 (8)
Ferritin, mcg/L (15-306 m, 5-103 f)	21 ± 55 (11)	342 ± 385 (195)	87 ± 167 (23)
TfR, mg/L (0.85-3.05)	6.2 ± 3.5 (5.0)	1.8 ± 0.6 (1.8)	5.1 ± 2.0 (4.7)
TfR/log ferritin	6.8 ± 6.5 (5.4)	0.8 ± 0.3 (0.8)	3.8 ± 1.9 (3.2)

f, Females; m, males; MCV, mean cell volume; TfR, transferrin receptor.

Diagnosis was defined by marrow iron stain and appropriate coexisting disease. Patients with a combination of no stainable marrow iron and either coexisting disease or elevated C-reactive protein (CRP) were classified as "COMBI."

Reference ranges for this laboratory for males and females are indicated. Measurements are presented as mean ± SD (median).

Modified with permission from Punnonen K, Irjala K, Rajamaki A. Serum transferrin receptor and its ratio to serum ferritin in the diagnosis of iron deficiency. *Blood.* 1997 Feb 1;89(3):1052-1057.

high ferritin levels may largely reflect inflammation, and augmented iron supply may be needed to overcome "functional iron deficiency"[55]—that is, to provide sufficient iron supply for pulsatile erythropoiesis stimulated by intermittently administered pharmacologic doses of EPO or its derivatives.[69]

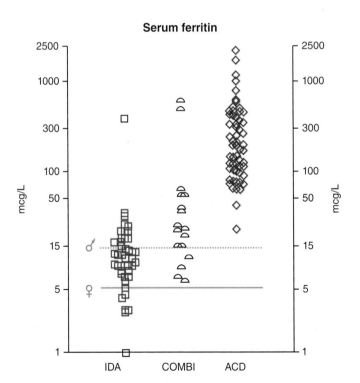

Figure 6–3. Distribution of serum ferritin measurements in patients with iron-deficiency anemia (IDA), anemia of chronic disease (ACD = anemia of inflammation [AI]) and combined IDA and ACD (COMBI). The *horizontal lines* indicate lower normal values for healthy men and women. *(Reproduced with permission from Punnonen K, Irjala K, Rajamaki A: Serum Transferrin Receptor and Its Ratio to Serum Ferritin in the Diagnosis of Iron Deficiency,* Blood *1997 Feb 1;89[3]:1052-1057.)*

MARROW IRON STAIN

Marrow aspiration or biopsy is rarely required for the diagnosis of AI. In general, the marrow is normal, unless the underlying disease alters the picture. The most important information obtained from marrow examination is the content and distribution of iron. Iron in a marrow preparation can be found as storage iron in the cytoplasm of macrophages or as functional iron in nucleated red cells. In normal individuals, a few Prussian blue–staining particles can be found inside or adjacent to many macrophages. Approximately one-third of nucleated red cells contain 1 to 4 blue inclusion bodies by light microscopy, and such cells are called *sideroblasts*. Both sideroblasts and macrophage iron are absent in iron deficiency. In contrast, sideroblasts are decreased or absent, but macrophage iron is increased in AI. The increase in storage iron in association with a decreased level of circulating iron and fewer sideroblasts is characteristic of AI. Although a marrow Prussian blue stain could be considered the gold standard for differential diagnosis of AI and iron deficiency, the discomfort to the patient associated with this procedure, reports of variability in interpretation,[70] and the wide availability of the serum ferritin assay have decreased the use of marrow stain in this setting.

● DIFFERENTIAL DIAGNOSIS

Most patients with chronic infections, inflammatory diseases, or neoplastic disorders are anemic. The diagnosis of AI should only be made if the anemia is mild to moderate, the serum iron and iron-binding capacity are low, and the serum ferritin is elevated. Anemia of CKD is rare in mild renal disease but common and often severe in end-stage renal disease. Underlying diseases, comorbidities, and their treatments can cause many types of anemia, so other potential causes should be considered.

1. *Drug-induced marrow suppression or drug-induced hemolysis* can complicate infections, inflammatory disorders, CKDs, and cancer. When the marrow is suppressed by cytotoxic drugs or an idiopathic toxic reaction, serum iron tends to be high and reticulocyte counts low. In hemolysis, reticulocyte counts, bilirubin, and lactate dehydrogenase (LDH) are increased but haptoglobin is decreased.

2. *Chronic blood loss* depletes iron stores and decreases serum iron and serum ferritin but increases transferrin (Chap. 11). When AI

and chronic blood loss coexist, serum ferritin usually indicates the predominant disorder, although the level can increase as a result of inflammation itself. Chronic blood loss from hemodialysis or occult gastrointestinal bleeding (especially in inflammatory bowel disease) is common in the anemia of CKD, and its lowering effect on ferritin may be masked by coexisting inflammation. Testing stool for occult blood and looking for other sources of overlooked blood loss, including phlebotomy and menorrhagia, often identify the source of bleeding. Once this issue is addressed, a successful trial of iron repletion confirms the diagnosis of iron deficiency complicating AI or anemia of CKD.

3. *Endocrine disorders,* including hypothyroidism and hyperthyroidism, testicular failure, and diabetes mellitus, can be associated with a chronic normocytic, normochromic anemia (Chap. 7). Unless inflammation or associated iron deficiency is present, serum iron should be normal in these disorders.

4. *Anemia resulting from metastatic invasion of the marrow* by tumors can be the presenting symptom of malignancy. The anemia can develop in the setting of a previous diagnosis of carcinoma or lymphoma and by itself is accompanied by normal or increased serum iron (Chap. 13). It often develops in the setting of preexisting malignancy–related AI. The blood film often is abnormal, with poikilocytes, teardrop-shaped red cells, normoblasts, or immature myeloid cells. Direct marrow examination is often necessary to establish the diagnosis.

5. *Thalassemia minor* is a common cause of mild anemia in many parts of the world. It can be confused with AI (Chap. 17). Microcytosis is a lifelong condition and usually is more severe in this group of disorders than in AI.

6. *Dilution anemia* is seen in pregnancy and in patients with severely increased plasma protein levels as a result of myeloma or macroglobulinemia.

●THERAPY, COURSE, AND PROGNOSIS

Anemia that presents in the setting of infection, inflammation, or malignancy requires sufficient diagnostic studies to rule out reversible and potentially more threatening causes, such as occult hemorrhage; iron, B_{12}, and folate deficiency; hemolysis; and drug reaction. If the anemia can be designated as AI after such studies, effective treatment of the underlying disease resolves the anemia. If treatment of the underlying disease is not effective and the patient has symptoms or medical complications attributable to anemia, one or more of the available anemia-specific treatment modalities should be considered (Table 6-3). These recommendations are also applicable to anemia of CKD, where for most patients only renal transplantation can reverse the underlying pathology. However, although anemia generally resolves or improves after renal transplantation, 30% to 40% of patients remain anemic, mainly because of pathologic changes in the transplanted kidney and adverse effects of immunosuppressive drugs.[71-78]

Specific therapies for AI and anemia of CKD are erythrocyte transfusions, ESAs, and intravenous iron (see Table 6-3). Transfusion of erythrocytes is used to correct AI or anemia of CKD when anemia is moderate to severe and the patient is acutely symptomatic. Because treatment with ESAs often effectively treats chronic anemia but increases the risk of thromboembolic events,[79-82] guidelines have been proposed for the appropriate use of these agents. The widespread adjunctive use of intravenous iron with ESAs may increase their effectiveness and reduce the required doses, but evidence as of this writing has not resulted in a consensus on specific indications for intravenous iron or its optimal dosing.[83]

Newer modalities approved in some countries for the treatment of anemia associated with CKD include oral prolyl hydroxylase inhibitors (HIF stabilizers) that act by stimulating hypoxia-sensitive endogenous production of EPO and mobilizing iron from stores and dietary absorption[84,85], and oral iron ferric citrate formulations that control hyperphosphatemia and deliver absorbable iron even in the setting of CKD and inflammation.[86]

THERAPY FOR ANEMIA OF INFLAMMATION

EPO therapy for the treatment of AI has been tested in the setting of various cancers,[87,88] multiple myeloma, and other hematologic malignancies,[23,89,90] rheumatoid arthritis,[93-94] and inflammatory bowel diseases.[95,96] In most reports, more than 50% of the patients experienced Hg increases greater than 2 g/dL. Guidelines for the use of EPO in anemia associated with hematologic and nonhematologic malignancy were published in 2002[97] and then updated in 2007[98] and 2010.[99] Because of shared pathogenesis between anemia of cancer and AI, and the absence

TABLE 6–3. Treatments of Anemia of Inflammation and Anemia of Chronic Kidney Disease

Modality	Indications	Typical Setting	Risks and Side Effects	Specific Benefits
Transfusion	Cardiac ischemia Lack of response to other modalities	Hb <10 g/dL Chest pain and electro-cardiogram changes	Infections Volume overload Transfusion reaction May sensitize for renal transplant rejection	Rapid correction of anemia
Erythropoietin	Fatigue, exertional intolerance	Hb <10 g/dL Anemia symptoms Balance against side effects in Hb 10-12 g/dL	Response takes several weeks Rare red cell aplasia with some forms of erythropoietin[109] May worsen outcome in some cancers[110] Increased thromboembolic events[79-82,99] Expensive	Usually well tolerated, relatively safe
Iron (oral or parenteral)[51]	Coexisting iron deficiency Resistance to erythropoietin (investigational)	Suspected or documented iron deficiency	Gastrointestinal side effects (oral) Systemic and local reactions (parenteral) May decrease resistance to infections[83,106-108]	Inexpensive, relatively safe

Abbreviation: Hb, hemoglobin.

of more specific recommendations, these form a reasonable guide for the EPO treatment of AI. The guidelines (used and quoted or paraphrased here with permission) recommend treating patients with Hb less than 10 g/dL when necessary to avoid red blood cell transfusions, and after discussion of the patient's preferences between transfusion and EPO treatment. Furthermore, the FDA recommends that dosing should be "titrated for each patient to achieve and maintain the lowest Hb level sufficient to avoid the need for blood transfusion." Because of reports of increased risk of thromboembolism in patients receiving these agents, clinicians should carefully weigh the risks of thromboembolism in patients for whom epoetin or darbepoetin are prescribed. An optimal target Hb concentration cannot be definitively determined from the available literature. Modification to reduce the ESA dose is appropriate when Hb reaches a level sufficient to avoid transfusion or the increase exceeds 1 g/dL in any 2-week period to avoid excessive ESA exposure. The FDA-approved starting dose of epoetin is 150 U/kg three times per week or 40,000 U weekly, subcutaneously. The FDA-approved starting dose of darbepoetin is 2.25 mcg/kg weekly or 500 mcg every 3 weeks, subcutaneously. Alternative starting doses or dosing schedules have shown no consistent difference in effectiveness on outcomes including transfusion and Hb response, although they may be considered to improve convenience. Dose escalation should follow FDA-approved labeling; no convincing evidence exists to suggest differences in dose escalation schedules are associated with different effectiveness. Continuing epoetin or darbepoetin treatment beyond 6 to 8 weeks in the absence of response (achieving less than 1-2 g/dL rise in Hb) does not appear to be beneficial and EPO therapy should be discontinued. The most recent specific guidelines for dose reduction are contained in the FDA-approved package insert. Baseline and periodic monitoring of iron, total iron-binding capacity, transferrin saturation, or ferritin levels and instituting iron repletion when indicated may be valuable in limiting the need for ESAs, maximizing symptomatic improvement for patients, and determining the reason for failure to respond adequately to EPO.

THERAPY FOR ANEMIA OF CHRONIC KIDNEY DISEASE

The most up-to-date recommendations are The Kidney Disease Improving Global Outcomes clinical practice guideline for anemia in CKD,[100] based on systematic literature searches last conducted in October 2010, supplemented with additional evidence through March 2012. For adult patients, these guidelines recommend that a newly anemic patient with CKD should have laboratory studies to rule out B_{12} and folate deficiency (Chap. 9), and a therapeutic trial of intravenous iron if their transferrin saturation level is 30% or lower and ferritin is less than 500 ng/mL. After the guidelines were published, the recommendation for a trial of intravenous iron received some support from a randomized trial showing that intravenous iron therapy delays or reduces the need for anemia management including ESAs.[101] However, the entry criteria for this trial were more restrictive than those in the guidelines. The guidelines recommend that individualized therapy with ESAs may be started when Hb concentrations fall below 10 g/dL, and then adjusted to maintain Hb to 11.5 g/dL or lower, unless the patient perceives an increased quality of life at higher Hb levels (not exceeding 13 g/dL) and is willing to accept the increased risks.

ADJUNCTIVE USE OF INTRAVENOUS IRON WITH ERYTHROPOIETIN

This use of intravenous iron is an empiric therapeutic strategy based on the idea that iron becomes limiting when marrow production of erythrocytes is pharmacologically stimulated. In some cases, occult iron deficiency coexists with AI.[65,96] In other situations, limited iron stores may become depleted when EPO is initiated.[93] In hemodialysis patients with high ferritin, low transferrin saturation (<25%), and above-average EPO requirements, iron supplementation of EPO treatment with 1 g loading course of intravenous ferric gluconate was shown to lead to a small increase in Hb and decreased dosage of EPO.[102,103] It is not yet confirmed whether this strategy is applicable to other AI settings. Pending additional studies, the coadministration of iron with EPO in AI in the absence of demonstrated iron deficiency remains to be investigated.[52] Because of its ability to decrease the use of ESAs, the use of intravenous iron is now common practice in CKD patients receiving hemodialysis, with no clear consensus on the indications, dosing, and potential risks of this strategy.[83] Concerns exist that iron supplementation in AI or CKD may increase susceptibility to infections,[104,105] but epidemiologic studies have generally not detected this risk.[83,106,107] However, the use of high-bolus doses of iron in patients with intravenous catheters[108] may be associated with increased infections. Proactive and regular use of intravenous iron appears to reduce cardiovascular events compared with lower-dose reactive administration that exposes the patient to intermittent iron restriction.[68]

REFERENCES

1. Cartwright GE. The anemia of chronic disorders. *Semin Hematol.* 1966;3(4):351-375.
2. Ganz T. Anemia of Inflammation. *N Engl J Med.* 2019;381(12):1148-1157.
3. Corwin HL, Krantz SB. Anemia of the critically ill: "acute" anemia of chronic disease. *Crit Care Med.* 2000;28(8):3098-3099.
4. Ershler WB. Biological interactions of aging and anemia: a focus on cytokines. *J Am Geriatr Soc.* 2003;51(suppl 3):S18-S21.
5. Carpenter WB. *Principles of Human Physiology.* In: Smith FG, ed. New American edition. Blanchard and Lea; 1859.
6. Wintrobe MM. *Clinical Hematology.* 5th ed. Lea & Febiger; 1961.
7. Dallman PR, Yip R, Johnson C. Prevalence and causes of anemia in the United States, 1976 to 1980. *Am J Clin Nutr.* 1984;39(3):437-445.
8. Ramakrishnan U, Yip R. Experiences and challenges in industrialized countries: control of iron deficiency in industrialized countries. *J Nutr.* 2002;132(4):820S-8824.
9. Hsu CY, McCulloch CE, Curhan GC. Epidemiology of anemia associated with chronic renal insufficiency among adults in the United States: results from the Third National Health and Nutrition Examination Survey. *J Am Soc Nephrol.* 2002;13(2):504-510.
10. Stauffer ME, Fan T. Prevalence of anemia in chronic kidney disease in the United States. *PLoS One.* 2014;9(1):e84943.
11. McClellan W, Aronoff SL, Bolton WK, et al. The prevalence of anemia in patients with chronic kidney disease. *Curr Med Res Opin.* 2004;20(9):1501-1510.
12. U.S. Renal Data System, USRDS 2013 Annual Data Report: Atlas of Chronic Kidney Disease and End-Stage Renal Disease in the United States. National Institutes of Health, National Institute of Diabetes and Digestive and Kidney Diseases, Bethesda, MD; 2013.
13. Zoller EE, Lykens JE, Terrell CE, et al. Hemophagocytosis causes a consumptive anemia of inflammation. *J Exp Med.* 2011;208(6):1203-1214.
14. Means RT, Jr., Krantz SB. Inhibition of human erythroid colony-forming units by gamma interferon can be corrected by recombinant human erythropoietin. *Blood.* 1991;78(10):2564-2567.
15. Libregts SF, Gutierrez L, de Bruin AM, et al. Chronic IFN-gamma production in mice induces anemia by reducing erythrocyte life span and inhibiting erythropoiesis through an IRF-1/PU.1 axis. *Blood.* 2011;118(9):2578-2588.
16. Baer AN, Dessypris EN, Goldwasser E, Krantz SB. Blunted erythropoietin response to anemia in rheumatoid arthritis. *Br J Haematol.* 1987;66(4):559-564.
17. Hochberg MC, Arnold CM, Hogans BB, Spivak JL. Serum immunoreactive erythropoietin in rheumatoid arthritis: impaired response to anemia. *Arthritis Rheum.* 1988;31(10):1318-1321.
18. Vreugdenhil G, Wognum AW, van Eijk HG, Swaak AJ. Anemia in rheumatoid arthritis: the role of iron, vitamin B_{12}, and folic acid deficiency, and erythropoietin responsiveness. *Ann Rheum Dis.* 1990;49(2):93-98.
19. Kendall R, Wasti A, Harvey A, et al. The relationship of haemoglobin to serum erythropoietin concentrations in the anemia of rheumatoid arthritis: the effect of oral prednisolone. *Br J Rheumatol.* 1993;32(3):204-208.
20. Noe G, Augustin J, Hausdorf S, Rich IN, Kubanek B. Serum erythropoietin and transferrin receptor levels in patients with rheumatoid arthritis. *Clin ExpRheumatol.* 1995;13(4):445-451.
21. Remacha AF, Rodriguez-de la Serna A, Garcia-Die F, Geli C, Diaz C, Gimferrer E. Erythroid abnormalities in rheumatoid arthritis: the role of erythropoietin. *J Rheumatol.* 1992;19(11):1687-1691.

22. Miller CB, Jones RJ, Piantadosi S, Abeloff MD, Spivak JL. Decreased erythropoietin response in patients with the anemia of cancer. *N Engl J Med.* 1990;322(24):1689-1692.

23. Cazzola M, Messinger D, Battistel V, et al. Recombinant-human-erythropoietin in the anemia associated with multiple-myeloma or non-Hodgkins-lymphoma—dose-finding and identification of predictors of response. *Blood.* 1995;86(12):4446-4453.

24. Safran M, Kaelin WG, Jr. HIF hydroxylation and the mammalian oxygen-sensing pathway. *J Clin Invest.* 2003;111(6):779-783.

25. Imagawa S, Nakano Y, Obara N, et al. A GATA-specific inhibitor (K-7174) rescues anemia induced by IL-1{beta}, TNF-α or L-NMMA. *FASEB J.* 2003;17(12):1742-1744.

26. Frede S, Fandrey J, Pagel H, Hellwig T, Jelkmann W. Erythropoietin gene expression is suppressed after lipopolysaccharide or interleukin-1 beta injections in rats. *Am J Physiol.* 1997;273(3 Pt 2):R1067-R1071.

27. Adamson JW, Eschbach J, Finch CA. The kidney and erythropoiesis. *Am J Med.* 1968;44(5):725-733.

28. Sato Y, Yanagita M. Renal anemia: from incurable to curable. *Am J Physiol Renal Physiol.* 2013;305(9):F1239-F1248.

29. Asada N, Takase M, Nakamura J, et al. Dysfunction of fibroblasts of extrarenal origin underlies renal fibrosis and renal anemia in mice. *J Clin Invest.* 2011;121(10):3981-3990.

30. Bernhardt WM, Wiesener MS, Scigalla P, et al. Inhibition of prolyl hydroxylases increases erythropoietin production in ESRD. *J Am Soc Nephrol.* 2010;21(12):2151-2156.

31. Barany P. Inflammation, serum C-reactive protein, and erythropoietin resistance. *Nephrol Dial Transplant.* 2001;16(2):224-227.

32. Macdougall IC, Cooper AC. Erythropoietin resistance: the role of inflammation and proinflammatory cytokines. *Nephrol Dial Transplant.* 2002;17(90011):39-43.

33. Nemeth E, Rivera S, Gabayan V, et al. IL-6 mediates hypoferremia of inflammation by inducing the synthesis of the iron regulatory hormone hepcidin. *J Clin Invest.* 2004;113(9):1271-1276.

34. Coffey R, Ganz T. Iron homeostasis: an anthropocentric perspective. *J Biol Chem.* 2017;292(31):12727-12734.

35. Nicolas G, Chauvet C, Viatte L, et al. The gene encoding the iron regulatory peptide hepcidin is regulated by anemia, hypoxia, and inflammation. *J Clin Invest.* 2002;110(7):1037-1044.

36. Besson-Fournier C, Latour C, Kautz L, et al. Induction of activin B by inflammatory stimuli upregulates expression of the iron-regulatory peptide hepcidin through Smad1/5/8 signaling. *Blood.* 2012;120(2):431-439.

37. Gardenghi S, Renaud TM, Meloni A, et al. Distinct roles for hepcidin and interleukin-6 in the recovery from anemia in mice injected with heat-killed Brucella abortus. *Blood.* 2014;123(8):1137-1145.

38. Kim A, Fung E, Parikh SG, et al. A mouse model of anemia of inflammation: complex pathogenesis with partial dependence on hepcidin. *Blood.* 2014;123(8):1129-1136.

39. Freireich EM, Miller A, C.P. E, Ross JF. The effect of inflammation on the utilization of erythrocyte and transferrin-bound radio-iron for red cell production. *Blood.* 1957;12:972.

40. Haurani FI, Burke W, Martinez EJ. Defective reutilization of iron in the anemia of inflammation. *J laboratory Clin Med.* 1965;65:560-570.

41. O'Shea MJ, Kershenobich D, Tavill AS. Effects of inflammation on iron and transferrin metabolism. *Br J Haematol.* 1973;25(6):707-714.

42. Hershko C, Cook JD, Finch CA. Storage iron kinetics. VI. The effect of inflammation on iron exchange in the rat. *Br J Haematol.* 1974;28(1):67-75.

43. Zarrabi MH, Lysik R, DiStefano J, Zucker S. The anemia of chronic disorders: studies of iron reutilization in the anemia of experimental malignancy and chronic inflammation. *Br J Haematol.* 1977;35(4):647-658.

44. Feldman BF, Kaneko JJ, Farver TB. Anemia of inflammatory disease in the dog: ferrokinetics of adjuvant-induced anemia. *Am J Vet Res.* 1981;42(4):583-585.

45. Fillet G, Beguin Y, Baldelli L. Model of reticuloendothelial iron metabolism in humans: abnormal behavior in idiopathic hemochromatosis and in inflammation. *Blood.* 1989;74(2):844-851.

46. Nicolas G, Bennoun M, Devaux I, et al. Lack of hepcidin gene expression and severe tissue iron overload in upstream stimulatory factor 2 (USF2) knockout mice. *Proc Natl Acad Sci U S A.* 2001;98(15):8780-8785.

47. Nicolas G, Bennoun M, Porteu A, et al. Severe iron deficiency anemia in transgenic mice expressing liver hepcidin. *Proc Natl Acad Sci U S A.* 2002;99(7):4596-4601.

48. Nemeth E, Tuttle MS, Powelson J, et al. Hepcidin regulates cellular iron efflux by binding to ferroportin and inducing its internalization. *Science.* 2004;306(5704):2090-2093.

49. Aschemeyer S, Qiao B, Stefanova D, et al. Structure-function analysis of ferroportin defines the binding site and an alternative mechanism of action of hepcidin. *Blood.* 2018;131(8):899-910.

50. Hastka J, Lasserre JJ, Schwarzbeck A, Strauch M, Hehlmann R. Zinc protoporphyrin in anemia of chronic disorders. *Blood.* 1993;81(5):1200-1204.

51. Taylor JE, Peat N, Porter C, Morgan AG. Regular low-dose intravenous iron therapy improves response to erythropoietin in haemodialysis patients. *Nephrol Dial Transplant.* 1996;11(6):1079-1083.

52. Goodnough LT, Skikne B, Brugnara C. Erythropoietin, iron, and erythropoiesis. *Blood.* 2000;96(3):823.

53. Hume R, Currie WJ, Tennant M. anemia of rheumatoid arthritis and iron therapy. *Ann Rheum Dis.* 1965;24(5):451-457.

54. Beamish MR, Davies AG, Eakins JD, Jacobs A, Trevett D. The measurement of reticuloendothelial iron release using iron-dextran. *Br J Haematol.* 1971;21(6):617-622.

55. Brugnara C, Chambers LA, Malynn E, Goldberg MA, Kruskall MS. Red blood cell regeneration induced by subcutaneous recombinant erythropoietin: iron-deficient erythropoiesis in iron-replete subjects [see comments]. *Blood.* 1993;81(4):956-964.

56. Gubler CJ, Cartwright GE, Wintrobe MM. The anemis of infection. X. The effect of infection on the absorption and storage of iron by the rat. *J Biol Chem.* 1950;184(2):563-574.

57. Weber J, Werre JM, Julius HW, Marx JJ. Decreased iron absorption in patients with active rheumatoid arthritis, with and without iron deficiency. *Ann Rheum Dis.* 1988;47(5):404-409.

58. Weber J, Julius HW, Verhoef CW, Werre JM. Absorption and retention of iron in rheumatoid arthritis. *Ann Rheum Dis.* 1973;32(1):83.

59. Anderson GJ, Frazer DM, Wilkins SJ, et al. Relationship between intestinal iron-transporter expression, hepatic hepcidin levels and the control of iron absorption. *Biochem Soc Trans.* 2002;30(4):724-726.

60. Roe MA, Collings R, Dainty JR, Swinkels DW, Fairweather-Tait SJ. Plasma hepcidin concentrations significantly predict interindividual variation in iron absorption in healthy men. *Am J Clin Nutr.* 2009;86(4):1088-1091.

61. Young MF, Glahn RP, Riza-Nieto M, et al. Serum hepcidin is significantly associated with iron absorption from food and supplemental sources in healthy young women. *Am J Clin Nutr.* 2009;89(2):533-538.

62. Cazzola M, Ponchio L, de Benedetti F, et al. Defective iron supply for erythropoiesis and adequate endogenous erythropoietin production in the anemia associated with systemic-onset juvenile chronic arthritis. *Blood.* 1996;87(11):4824-4830.

63. Awai M, Brown EB. Studies of the metabolism of I-131-labeled human transferrin. *J laboratory Clin Med.* 1963;61:363-396.

64. Jacobs A, Worwood M. Ferritin in serum. Clinical and biochemical implications. *N Engl J Med.* 1975;292(18):951-956.

65. Punnonen K, Irjala K, Rajamaki A. Serum transferrin receptor and its ratio to serum ferritin in the diagnosis of iron deficiency. *Blood.* 1997;89(3):1052-1057.

66. Skikne BS. Serum transferrin receptor. *Am J Hematol.* 2008;83(11):872-875.

67. Konz T, Montes-Bayon M, Vaulont S. Hepcidin quantification: methods and utility in diagnosis. *Metallomics.* 2014;6(9):1583-1590.

68. Macdougall IC, White C, Anker SD, et al. Intravenous iron in patients undergoing maintenance hemodialysis. *N Engl J Med.* 2019;380(5):447-458.

69. Goodnough LT, Nemeth E, Ganz T. Detection, evaluation, and management of iron-restricted erythropoiesis. *Blood.* 2010;116(23):4754-4761.

70. Barron BA, Hoyer JD, Tefferi A. A bone marrow report of absent stainable iron is not diagnostic of iron deficiency. *Ann Hematol.* 2001;80(3):166-169.

71. Iwamoto H, Nakamura Y, Konno O, et al. Correlation between post kidney transplant anemia and kidney graft function. *Transplant Proc.* 2014;46(2):496-498.

72. Pascual J, Jimenez C, Franco A, et al. Early-onset anemia after kidney transplantation is an independent factor for graft loss: a multicenter, observational cohort study. *Transplantation.* 2013;96(8):717-725.

73. Jones H, Talwar M, Nogueira JM, et al. Anemia after kidney transplantation; its prevalence, risk factors, and independent association with graft and patient survival: a time-varying analysis. *Transplantation.* 2012;93(9):923-928.

74. Kamar N, Rostaing L, Ignace S, Villar E. Impact of post-transplant anemia on patient and graft survival rates after kidney transplantation: a metaanalysis. *Clin Transplant.* 2012;26(3):461-469.

75. Yabu JM, Winkelmayer WC. Posttransplantation anemia: mechanisms and management. *Clin J Am Soc Nephrol.* 2011;6(7):1794-1801.

76. Vanrenterghem Y. Anemia after kidney transplantation. *Transplantation.* 2009;87(9):1265-1267.

77. Ott U, Busch M, Steiner T, Wolf G. Anemia after renal transplantation: an underestimated problem. *Transplant Proc.* 2008;40(10):3481-3484.

78. Ghafari A, Noori-Majelan N. Anemia among long-term renal transplant recipients. *Transplant Proc.* 2008;40(1):186-188.

79. Bennett CL, Silver SM, Djulbegovic B, et al. Venous thromboembolism and mortality associated with recombinant erythropoietin and darbepoetin administration for the treatment of cancer-associated anemia. *JAMA.* 2008;299(8):914-924.

80. Singh AK, Szczech L, Tang KL, et al. Correction of anemia with epoetin alfa in chronic kidney disease. *N Engl J Med.* 2006;355(20):2085-2098.

81. Pfeffer MA, Burdmann EA, Chen CY, et al. A trial of darbepoetin alfa in type 2 diabetes and chronic kidney disease. *N Engl J Med.* 2009;361(21):2019-2032.

82. Solomon SD, Uno H, Lewis EF, et al. Erythropoietic response and outcomes in kidney disease and type 2 diabetes. *N Engl J Med.* 2010;363(12):1146-1155.

83. Gaweda AE, Ginzburg YZ, Chait Y, et al. Iron dosing in kidney disease: inconsistency of evidence and clinical practice. *Nephrol Dial Transplant.* 2014.

84. Sanghani NS, Haase VH. Hypoxia-inducible factor activators in renal anemia: current clinical experience. *Advances in chronic kidney disease.* 2019;26(4):253-266.

85. Yap DYH, McMahon LP, Hao CM, et al. Recommendations by the Asian Pacific society of nephrology (APSN) on the appropriate use of HIF-PH inhibitors. *Nephrology.* 2020;1-14. https://doi.org/10.1111/ nep.13835

86. Ganz T, Bino A, Salusky IB. Mechanism of action and clinical attributes of auryxia((R)) (Ferric Citrate). *Drugs.* 2019;79(9):957-968.

87. Ludwig H, Fritz E, Leitgeb C, Pecherstorfer M, Samonigg H, Schuster J. Prediction of response to erythropoietin treatment in chronic anemia of cancer [see comments]. *Blood.* 1994;84(4):1056-1063.

88. Smith RE, Tchekmedyian NS, Chan D, et al. A dose- and schedule-finding study of darbepoetin alpha for the treatment of chronic anemia of cancer. *Br J Cancer.* 2003;88(12):1851-1858.

89. Dammacco F, Castoldi G, Rodjer S. Efficacy of epoetin alfa in the treatment of anemia of multiple myeloma. *Br J Haematol*. 2001;113(1):172-179.

90. Hedenus M, Adriansson M, San Miguel J, et al. Efficacy and safety of darbepoetin alfa in anaemic patients with lymphoproliferative malignancies: a randomized, double-blind, placebo-controlled study. *Br J Haematol*. 2003;122(3):394-403.

91. Peeters HR, Jongen-Lavrencic M, Bakker CH, Vreugdenhil G, Breedveld FC, Swaak AJ. Recombinant human erythropoietin improves health-related quality of life in patients with rheumatoid arthritis and anemia of chronic disease; utility measures correlate strongly with disease activity measures. *Rheumatol Int*. 1999;18(5-6):201-206.

92. Peeters HR, Jongen-Lavrencic M, Vreugdenhil G, Swaak AJ. Effect of recombinant human erythropoietin on anemia and disease activity in patients with rheumatoid arthritis and anemia of chronic disease: a randomized placebo controlled double blind 52 weeks clinical trial. *Ann Rheum Dis*. 1996;55(10):739-744.

93. Goodnough LT, Marcus RE. The erythropoietic response to erythropoietin in patients with rheumatoid arthritis. *J laboratory Clin Med*. 1997;130(4):381-386.

94. Kaltwasser JP, Kessler U, Gottschalk R, Stucki G, Moller B. Effect of recombinant human erythropoietin and intravenous iron on anemia and disease activity in rheumatoid arthritis. *J Rheumatol*. 2001;28(11):2430-2436.

95. Schreiber S, Howaldt S, Schnoor M, et al. Recombinant erythropoietin for the treatment of anemia in inflammatory bowel disease. *N Engl J Med*. 1996;334(10):619-623.

96. Gasche C, Dejaco C, Reinisch W, et al. Sequential treatment of anemia in ulcerative colitis with intravenous iron and erythropoietin. *Digestion*. 1999;60(3):262-267.

97. Rizzo JD, Lichtin AE, Woolf SH, et al. Use of epoetin in patients with cancer: evidence-based clinical practice guidelines of the American Society of Clinical Oncology and the American Society of Hematology. *J Clin Oncol*. 2002;20(19):4083-4107.

98. Rizzo JD, Somerfield MR, Hagerty KL, et al. Use of epoetin and darbepoetin in patients with cancer: 2007 American Society of Hematology/American Society of Clinical Oncology clinical practice guideline update. *Blood*. 2008;111(1):25-41.

99. Rizzo JD, Brouwers M, Hurley P, et al. American Society of Hematology/American Society of Clinical Oncology clinical practice guideline update on the use of epoetin and darbepoetin in adult patients with cancer. *Blood*. 2010;116(20):4045-4059.

100. Drüeke TB, Parfrey PS. Summary of the KDIGO guideline on anemia and comment: reading between the (guide)line(s). *Kidney Int*. 2012;82(9):952-960.

101. Macdougall IC, Bock AH, Carrera F, et al. FIND-CKD: a randomized trial of intravenous ferric carboxymaltose versus oral iron in patients with chronic kidney disease and iron deficiency anemia. *Nephrol Dial Transplant*. 2014;29(11):2075-2084.

102. Kapoian T, O'Mara NB, Singh AK, et al. Ferric gluconate reduces epoetin requirements in hemodialysis patients with elevated ferritin. *J Am Soc Nephrol*. 2008;19(2):372-379.

103. Coyne DW, Kapoian T, Suki W, et al. Ferric gluconate is highly efficacious in anemic hemodialysis patients with high serum ferritin and low transferrin saturation: results of the Dialysis Patients' Response to IV Iron with Elevated Ferritin (DRIVE) study. *J Am Soc Nephrol*. 2007;18(3):975-984.

104. Jurado RL. Iron, infections, and anemia of inflammation. *Clin Infect Dis*. 1997;25(4):888-895.

105. Oppenheimer SJ. Iron and its relation to immunity and infectious disease. *J Nutr*. 2001;131(2):616S-663S.

106. Susantitaphong P, Alqahtani F, Jaber BL. Efficacy and safety of intravenous iron therapy for functional iron deficiency anemia in hemodialysis patients: a metaanalysis. *Am J Nephrol*. 2014;39(2):130-141.

107. Litton E, Xiao J, Ho KM. Safety and efficacy of intravenous iron therapy in reducing requirement for allogeneic blood transfusion: systematic review and metaanalysis of randomized clinical trials. *BMJ*. 2013;347:f4822.

108. Brookhart MA, Freburger JK, Ellis AR, Wang L, Winkelmayer WC, Kshirsagar AV. Infection risk with bolus versus maintenance iron supplementation in hemodialysis patients. *J Am Soc Nephrol*. 2013;24(7):1151-1158.

109. Jacob S, Nichols J, Macdougall IC, et al. Investigating serious adverse drug reactions in patients receiving erythropoiesis-stimulating agents: A root cause analysis using the "ANTICIPATE" framework. *Am J Ther*. 2018;25:e670-e674.

110. Tiffany MP, Kwanghee K, Erina V, et al. Effects of recombinant erythropoietin on breast cancer-initiating cells. *Neoplasia*. 2007 Dec;9(12):1122-1129. doi: 10.1593/neo.07694.

CHAPTER 7
ERYTHROPOIETIC EFFECTS OF ENDOCRINE DISORDERS

Xylina T. Gregg

SUMMARY

The endocrine system influences homeostasis of virtually every tissue. Thus, it is not unexpected that it also influences hematopoiesis. However, the effect of endocrine disequilibrium is principally on erythropoiesis with limited impact on leukocytes, platelets, and hemostasis. Thus, anemia is the most common hematopoietic abnormality in endocrine disorders and may be the first manifestation of an endocrine disorder. Erythrocytosis is less common but occurs in certain endocrine disorders (eg, congenital adrenal hyperplasia, pheochromocytoma). The pathophysiologic basis of the anemia is often multifactorial, but a direct influence of hormones on erythropoiesis in some instances may contribute to anemia. A decreased plasma volume in some of these disorders may mask the severity of anemia. Some endocrine disorders are associated with an impaired response to the therapeutic use of erythropoietin.

⬤THYROID DYSFUNCTION

THYROID DYSFUNCTION AND INCIDENCE OF ANEMIA

Anemia is a well-recognized complication of thyroidectomy[1] and is associated with hypo- and hyperthyroidism and subclinical thyroid dysfunction. However, the exact frequency of anemia, as well as any causative relationship between thyroid dysfunction and anemia, are not defined.[2-5] In a retrospective review of 412 patients, anemia defined as a hemoglobin less than 130 g/L in men and less than 120 g/L in women was present in 57% of patients with hypothyroidism and 41% of those with hyperthyroidism.[2] Another study found anemia in 43% of an overt group of patients with hypothyroid and 39% in a set of subclinical patients with hypothyroid; however, 26% of the control group also had anemia.[3] A cohort population–based study conducted by the European Prospective Investigation into Cancer-Norfolk (EPIC-Norfolk) of more than 8000 participants, which excluded patients with anemia attributed to chronic kidney disease, inflammation, or iron deficiency, found the highest prevalence of anemia in overt hyperthyroidism (14.6%) compared with 7.7% in overt hypothyroidism and no increase in anemia in those with subclinical hypo- or hyperthyroidism.[4] A subsequent meta-analysis of individual participant data from 16 cohorts (including the EPIC-Norfolk study) found an increased risk of anemia in all categories of abnormal thyroid status compared with euthyroid participants.[5] The odds ratio was 1.84 for overt hypothyroidism, 1.69 for overt hyperthyroidism, 1.21 for subclinical hypothyroidism, and 1.27 for subclinical hyperthyroidism.

HYPOTHYROIDISM

The anemia in hypothyroidism has been described variably as normocytic, macrocytic, or microcytic[1]; coexisting deficiencies of iron, cobalamin (vitamin B_{12}), and folate (Chaps. 9 and 11) may explain some of this heterogeneity. In a study of approximately 60 anemic patients with untreated primary hypothyroidism, 10% had a macrocytic anemia, all of whom had vitamin B_{12} deficiency; 43% had a microcytic anemia and iron deficiency; and the remainder had a normocytic anemia.[6] However, even when these deficiencies are excluded, some patients with hypothyroidism have a macrocytic anemia.[4,7] In one report, the macrocytosis resolved with thyroxine treatment.[7] In addition, although most patients with hypothyroidism have a significant reduction in their red cell mass, anemia is not always evident from hemoglobin and hematocrit values, owing to a concomitant reduction of plasma volume.[8,9]

The relationship between iron and thyroid function is complex. Historically, hypothyroidism has been associated with menorrhagia, which would contribute to the development of iron deficiency but this association is less common than previously thought.[10,11] Because thyroid hormone (TH) may augment iron absorption, iron deficiency in hypothyroidism may also be caused by impaired iron absorption.[12] Patients with chronic autoimmune (Hashimoto disease) thyroiditis have an increased incidence of chronic autoimmune gastritis and celiac disease, with resultant impaired cobalamin and iron absorption.[13] In addition, chronic autoimmune thyroiditis is an inflammatory disease and inflammation is expected to increase hepcidin, which would impair iron availability for erythropoiesis. This was demonstrated in a prospective study of 38 patients with Hashimoto disease whose high hepcidin levels corrected with the establishment of euthyroidism.[14] Conversely, iron deficiency is associated with decreased TH levels. In a retrospective review of pregnant women in China, iron deficiency was an independent risk factor for low serum-free thyroxine levels.[15] Iron deficiency impairs TH synthesis by reducing the activity of heme-dependent thyroid peroxidase[16] and may also alter central nervous system control of thyroid metabolism.[17] In patients with coexisting iron-deficiency anemia and subclinical hypothyroidism, the anemia often does not adequately respond to oral iron therapy. Combined treatment with oral iron and levothyroxine results in superior improvement in hemoglobin and ferritin levels compared with levothyroxine alone in these patients.[18,19] Iron deficiency may reduce the effectiveness of iodized salt programs in areas of endemic goiter. A randomized, placebo-controlled trial of iron supplementation in children with goiter consuming iodized salt showed a statistically significant reduction in thyroid size, although serum thyroxine levels did not differ between the groups.[20]

Even when iron deficiency, cobalamin deficiency, and other confounding causes of anemia have been excluded, anemia can be a direct consequence of TH deficiency.[7] Dogs subjected to thyroidectomy have a normocytic, normochromic anemia that is associated with reticulocytopenia and marrow erythroid hypoplasia.[21] In hypothyroid humans and thyroidectomized animals, the red cell life span is normal, and results of ferrokinetic studies are compatible with hypoproliferative

Acronyms and Abbreviations: BFU-E, burst-forming unit–erythroid; CFU-E, colony forming-unit–erythroid; *EGLN1*, gene encoding proline hydroxylase-2; *EGLN2*, gene encoding proline hydroxylase-1; *EPAS1*, gene encoding HIF2α; EPIC-Norfolk, European Prospective Investigation of Cancer-Norfolk; HepKo, hepcidin knockout; HIF, hypoxia-inducible factor; PCC, pheochromocytoma; PGL, paraganglioma; RTHα, resistance to THα; TH, thyroid hormone; *THRA*, gene encoding thyroid hormone receptor α; *THRB*, gene encoding thyroid hormone receptor β; TRs, thyroid hormone receptors, TRα, thyroid hormone receptor alpha; TSH, thyroid stimulating hormone.

erythropoiesis.[21] Administration of TH increases the rate of red cell production in experimental animals,[22] whereas thyroidectomy decreases red cell production.[23] The terminal erythroid maturation of human erythrocytes in culture requires TH in addition to erythropoietin.[24] Hypothyroidism has been shown to affect the response to erythropoietin therapy for anemia. After adjusting for other variables, the mean monthly erythropoietin dose required to maintain a target hemoglobin level in patients receiving hemodialysis was significantly higher in patients with hypothyroid compared with euthyroid.[25]

The molecular mechanism of the effect of TH on erythropoiesis has been elusive. The action of TH is mediated via binding of the active ligand (T3) to nuclear TH receptors (TRs), TRα and TRβ. TRs are ligand-inducible transcription factors that regulate gene expression by binding to TH response elements in promoters of target genes. The genes encoding these TRs, TH receptor α and β (*THRA* and *THRB*), have several alternatively spliced transcript variants with tissue-specific expression. Both TRα and TRβ proteins are expressed in human CD34+ progenitors, but only TRβ is detectable in late erythroblasts.[26] Knocking out TRα but not TRβ in mice results in reduction in the numbers of early erythroid progenitors in fetal livers and impaired transit of erythroblasts through the final stages of maturation.[27] In in vitro human erythroid cultures, specific depletion of TH blocked terminal erythroid differentiation and enucleation, but this effect appeared to be mediated by TRβ and not TRα.[26] However, *TRα1/TRβ*-knockout female mice, which lack all known TRs, do not have anemia, suggesting that unoccupied TRs may have a negative effect on hematopoiesis.[28]

Anemia is present in patients with rare congenital inactivating mutations of TRα that cause tissue-specific hypothyroidism because of TH resistance. The clinical phenotype of resistance to THα (RTHα) also includes bradycardia, neurodevelopmental delay, constipation, and dysmorphic features.[29] Laboratory studies show a decreased T4/T3 ratio but normal thyroid stimulating hormone (TSH). Erythroid progenitors from patients with resistance to THα have defective maturation capacity; however, there is no apparent relationship between the degree of anemia and the severity of the TRα mutation, nor between red cell number and TH levels.[30]

Treatment of hypothyroidism with TH improves the hemoglobin concentration over a several-month period.[7] White blood cell and platelet counts usually are unaffected in hypothyroidism, but pancytopenia resolving with TH replacement has been reported.[31,32]

HYPERTHYROIDISM

Although TH administration increases red cell production in animals,[33] humans with hyperthyroidism generally do not have erythrocytosis. However, in one report of erythrocytosis associated with hyperthyroidism, elevated levels of erythropoietin and hypoxia-inducible factor (HIF)-1α were described; these levels decreased after treatment of hyperthyroidism.[34] Anemia has been reported in 14% to 47% of patients with hyperthyroidism.[2,4,5,35] This finding may be the result of increased plasma volume[8]; however, decreased red cell survival[36] and ineffective erythropoiesis[37] have also been described. Antithyroid treatment ameliorates the anemia.[35] An association of hyperthyroidism and autoimmune hemolytic anemia that abated with treatment of hyperthyroidism has been described.[38] Pancytopenia rarely occurs but if present may also respond to treatment of hyperthyroidism.[39]

● ADRENAL GLAND DISORDERS

ADRENOCORTICAL INSUFFICIENCY

A normocytic normochromic anemia may be seen in primary adrenal insufficiency (Addison disease),[40,41] but the anemia may also be masked by the concomitant reduction in plasma volume that is common in this disease.[40] In a series of patients with Addison disease, some patients with normal hemoglobin levels developed transient anemia after initiation of hormone replacement therapy, presumably secondary to an increased plasma volume.[40]

In experimental animals, adrenalectomy causes a mild anemia that responds to glucocorticoids.[42] However, the pathophysiologic basis of the anemia and any influence of adrenal cortical hormones on erythropoiesis are not well-defined.

Autoimmune gastric atrophy (pernicious anemia) (Chap. 9) can occur in patients with autoimmune adrenal insufficiency, but is seen primarily in patients with the very rare type I autoimmune polyendocrine syndrome caused by an autosomal recessive mutation of the autoimmune regulator gene. The cardinal manifestations of this syndrome include chronic mucocutaneous candidiasis and hypoparathyroidism.[43] These individuals are susceptible to a variety of autoimmune diseases, including pure red cell aplasia (see Chap. 5).[43] Anemia as a result of primary erythropoietin deficiency was reported in one patient with this syndrome.[44]

CUSHING DISEASE AND ALDOSTERONISM

Glucocorticoids interact with erythropoietin in vitro to enhance erythroid colony proliferation.[45] However, the precise stages of erythroid differentiation at which glucocorticoids exert their effects have been difficult to identify. Dexamethasone treatment of erythroid-differentiated peripheral blood CD34+ progenitors resulted in the expansion of a defined CD34+CD36+CD71hiCD105med immature colony-forming unit–erythroid (CFU-E) population, and proteomics analyses revealed the induction of distinct proteins in dexamethasone-treated erythroid progenitors, specifically, upregulation of p57Kip2, a Cip/Kip cyclin–dependent kinase inhibitor.[46]

Erythrocytosis (Chap. 28) has been reported in Cushing syndrome,[47] primary aldosteronism,[48] and Bartter syndrome.[49] However, a study of 63 women and 17 men with Cushing disease found that although the hemoglobin levels in the women were evenly distributed over the normal range, the hemoglobin levels were in the lowest quartile in 14 of the 17 men, and three of these 14 were anemic.[50] The reduced hemoglobin levels in the male patients correlated with a low testosterone level and slowly improved after treatment of Cushing disease.

CONGENITAL ADRENAL HYPERPLASIA

The most common cause of congenital adrenal hyperplasia is 21-hydroxylase deficiency, which impairs conversion of 17-hydroxyprogesterone to 11-deoxycortisol.[51] Patients with the "classic form" present during the neonatal period with adrenal insufficiency, but others have a late-onset presentation with findings of androgen excess. Erythrocytosis occurs in patients with congenital adrenal hyperplasia resulting from 21-hydroxylase deficiency[52] and may even be the presenting manifestation of this disease.[53] A strong association between testosterone levels and hemoglobin and hematocrit was demonstrated in women with congenital adrenal hyperplasia.[54]

PHEOCHROMOCYTOMA

Pheochromocytomas (PCCs) and paragangliomas (PGLs) are related neuroendocrine tumors that originate from chromaffin cells either in the adrenal medulla (PCCs) or in sympathetic and parasympathetic ganglia (PGLs). PCCs and PGLs are rarely associated with erythrocytosis, which has been attributed to autonomous erythropoietin production by the tumor.[55] Somatic or germline mutations are present in 70% to 80% of PCCs and PGLs, with the majority of the mutations occurring in genes encoding von Hippel–Lindau and other proteins involved in HIF signaling (see Chaps. 2 and 28).[56] Some individuals with PCCs or PGLs have erythrocytosis, which in some cases predated the diagnosis of PCC or PGL.

In several individuals with unexplained congenital polycythemia who subsequently developed recurrent PCCs, PGLs, and sometimes somatostatinomas (Chaps. 3 and 28),[57-60] their tumors were heterozygous for various gain-of-function mutations of the gene encoding HIF-2α (*EPAS1*), and erythropoietin transcript was present not only in tumor tissue but also in the surrounding normal tissue. Consequently, resection of the tumor did not resolve the erythrocytosis. The disease is thought to arise from genomic mosaicism of the gain-of-function *EPAS1* gene, so that adrenal cells with this mutation produce erythropoietin and likely predispose to further PCC-causing mutations, whereas normal adrenal cells do not produce erythropoietin.[59] Since the disease arises from genetic mosaicism, the *EPAS1* mutation is not present in all tissues, and specifically is not found in leukocytes, making the diagnosis of this syndrome difficult.

PGLs and PCCs have been also reported in patients with erythrocytosis and germline mutations in *EPAS1*[61] and the genes encoding proline hydroxylase-1 and -2 (*EGLN1* and *EGLN2*),[62,63] suggesting that germline mutations in the HIF pathway predisposes to development of these tumors.

An erythropoietin-secreting PCC of the adrenal gland associated with erythrocytosis was reported in an African male who had concurrent heterozygous mutations of von Hippel–Lindau and transmembrane-protein-127.[64] In this case, erythrocytosis resolved after surgical resection of the tumor.

● GONADAL HORMONES

ANDROGENS

Sexually mature males have higher hemoglobin levels than prepubertal males, older males, and females.[65] This difference is attributed to the differences in androgen production in those epochs. The male–female difference appears temporally in association with the development of secondary sex characteristics. Testosterone levels directly correlated with hemoglobin levels in a community population of males between the ages 30 and 94 years of age.[66] Orchiectomy results in a median decrease in hemoglobin concentration of 120 g/L.[67] Lowering serum testosterone levels into the castrate range with androgen deprivation therapy also causes anemia, which is reversible on discontinuation of therapy.[68]

The erythropoietic effects of androgens have been widely exploited for the treatment of various anemias, especially before the development of recombinant erythropoietin. Testosterone therapy in hypogonadal men increased the mean hematocrit from 38.0% to 43.1% within 3 months.[69] A meta-analysis of 11 placebo-controlled randomized trials involving 1570 patients showed an increased risk of erythrocytosis with testosterone replacement therapy (relative risk 8.14, 95% CI 1.87, 35.40).[70] Erythrocytosis has rarely been reported as a complication of breast cancer treatment with an aromatase inhibitor, which prevents the conversion of androstenedione and testosterone to estrogen.[71]

The mechanism of androgen action appears to be complex, with evidence for stimulation of erythropoietin secretion[72] and a direct effect on the marrow. Testosterone promotes the differentiation of CD34+ umbilical cord cells into erythroid progenitor cells.[73] Testosterone administration was associated with an increase in erythropoietin levels and a decrease in hepcidin levels.[72] Although erythropoietin levels declined with continued testosterone administration, they

remained inappropriately high despite improved hemoglobin levels, suggesting a new setpoint.[72] Androgen deprivation therapy in non-metastatic prostate cancer was associated with a significant reduction in hemoglobin and hematocrit levels and an increase in hepcidin concentration, but there was no decrease in serum iron levels, suggesting that hepcidin is not the primary driver of the anemia (Chap. 10).[74] There was also no significant change in erythropoietin levels, which might contribute to decreased proliferation of erythroid progenitors. In addition, a study of testosterone administration in a whole-body hepcidin knockout (HepKO) mouse demonstrated that hepcidin suppression is not essential for mediating testosterone's effects on erythropoiesis.[75]

ESTROGENS

Data regarding the role of estrogens in hematopoiesis are conflicting. Administration of large doses of estrogen led to a moderately severe anemia in rats.[76] However, hematopoietic stem cells express estrogen receptor-α and estrogen signaling via this receptor promotes hematopoietic stem cell self-renewal and stimulates erythropoiesis in mice and in human pluripotent stem cells.[77,78]

● PITUITARY GLAND DISORDERS

PITUITARY INSUFFICIENCY

The most common cause of pituitary insufficiency is pituitary tumors or consequences of their therapy.[79] Other etiologies include hypothalamic tumors or dysfunction, sarcoidosis or other infiltrative diseases, pituitary hemorrhage or infarct, genetic causes, and idiopathic pituitary failure. Regardless of the cause, hypopituitarism results in a moderately severe normochromic normocytic anemia, with an average hemoglobin level of 100 g/L.[41] Anemia and erythroid hypoplasia have also been described in hypophysectomized animals.[80]

In rats, removal of the posterior lobe of the pituitary, which secretes vasopressin and oxytocin, does not result in anemia.[81] Thus, the anemia of hypopituitarism presumably results from the absence of the anterior lobe hormones, adrenocorticotropic hormone, TSH, follicle-stimulating hormone, luteinizing hormone, growth hormone, and prolactin, although the exact role of each of these hormones in the pathogenesis of anemia is unknown. The resulting deficiencies of TH, adrenal hormones, and androgens are likely the major contributors to anemia. Combined adrenalectomy and thyroidectomy in animals result in an anemia that is similar but not identical to that seen after hypophysectomy.[82] A correlation between low testosterone levels and anemia has been observed in human males with hypopituitarism resulting from nonfunctioning pituitary adenomas.[83]

Red cell survival is normal in hypopituitarism, but the marrow is hypoplastic. The results of ferrokinetic studies are consistent with decreased erythropoiesis.[41] In addition to anemia, leukopenia and even pancytopenia can occur.[84] Compared with matched healthy controls, 40 women with postpartum ischemic necrosis of the anterior pituitary gland (Sheehan syndrome) had significantly decreased hemoglobin, hematocrit, white cell, and platelet counts.[85] Replacement therapy with a combination of thyroid, adrenal, and gonadal hormones usually effectively corrects anemia and other cytopenias.[84,85] Erythropoietin therapy also was effective in one case of postoperative hypopituitarism refractory to hormone replacement therapy.[86] However, in a mouse pituitary cell line, erythropoietin inhibited adrenocorticotropic hormone secretion.[87]

OTHER PITUITARY HORMONES

Growth Hormone

Growth hormone stimulates erythropoietin-induced erythropoiesis in vitro,[88] and children with isolated growth hormone deficiency become anemic.[89] Growth hormone replacement therapy in both children and adults with growth hormone deficiency increases hemoglobin levels.[90,91]

Prolactin

There is limited information about the influence of prolactin. Prolactin administration in mice increased the number of erythroid and myeloid progenitor cells and partially corrected anemia induced by azidothymidine.[92] Metoclopramide, which stimulates prolactin secretion, improved hemoglobin levels or reduced transfusions in three of nine patients with Diamond-Blackfan anemia (Chap. 4).[93] The prolactin receptor can substitute for the erythropoietin receptor in in vitro studies of erythroid differentiation (Chap. 2).[94]

However, macroprolactinomas have not been associated with erythrocytosis, but with anemia, likely the result of a concomitant decrease in testosterone levels.[95] In a retrospective review of 26 men with prolactinomas, a mild anemia was present in one-third, all of whom had a macroprolactinoma.[96] Hemoglobin levels did not correlate with serum prolactin levels but did correlate with the presence of hypogonadism.[96] Pancytopenia has also been reported in a patient with panhypopituitarism caused by a macroprolactinoma.[97]

Gonadotropins

Pituitary adenomas that secrete gonadotropins are rare but have been associated with erythrocytosis, likely caused by testosterone excess.[98]

●HYPERPARATHYROIDISM

Parathyroid hormone may stimulate hematopoiesis in mice.[99] However, in humans, anemia not attributable to other causes is present in 3% to 5% of patients with primary hyperparathyroidism; these patients usually have severe hyperparathyroidism.[100,101] The anemia is normochromic and normocytic and resolves or improves after parathyroidectomy.[100,101] The cause of the anemia is unknown; marrow fibrosis is present in some but not all patients.[100,102] Although there is no correlation with marrow fibrosis and the duration of hyperparathyroidism, the presence of marrow fibrosis may positively correlate with improvement in anemia after parathyroidectomy.[102]

Although anemia in patients with renal failure is multifactorial, secondary hyperparathyroidism may contribute to refractoriness to erythropoietin therapy. Parathyroidectomy or medical treatment of hyperparathyroidism may improve anemia and decrease requirements for exogenous erythropoietin therapy.[103,104]

REFERENCES

1. Fein HG, Rivlin RS. Anemia in thyroid diseases. *Med Clin North Am*. 1975;59:1133.
2. Omar S, Hadj Taeib S, Kanoun F, et al. Erythrocyte abnormalities in thyroid dysfunction. *Tunis Med*. 2010;88:783.
3. Erdogan M, Kosenli A, Ganidagli S, et al. Characteristics of anemia in subclinical and overt hypothyroid patients. *Endocr J*. 2012;59:213.
4. M'Rabet-Bensalah K, Aubert CE, Coslovsky M, et al. Thyroid dysfunction and anaemia in a large population-based study. *Clin Endocrinol (Oxf)*. 2016;84:627.
5. Wopereis DM, Du Puy RS, van Heemst D, et al. The relation between thyroid function and anemia: a pooled analysis of individual participant data. *J Clin Endocrinol Metab*. 2018;103:3658.
6. Das C, Sahana PK, Sengupta N, et al. Etiology of anemia in primary hypothyroid subjects in a tertiary care center in Eastern India. *Indian J Endocrinol Metab*. 16: S361,2012.
7. Horton L, Coburn RJ, England JM, et al. The haematology of hypothyroidism. *Q J Med*. 1976;45:101.
8. Muldowney FP, Crooks J, Wayne EJ. The total red cell mass in thyrotoxicosis and myxoedema. *Clin Sci*. 1957;16:309.
9. Das KC, Mukherjee M, Sarkar TK, et al. Erythropoiesis and erythropoietin in hypo- and hyperthyroidism. *J Clin Endocrinol Metab*. 1975;40:211.
10. Kakuno Y, Amino N, Kanoh M, et al. Menstrual disturbances in various thyroid diseases. *Endocr J*. 2010;57:1017.
11. Weyand A, Quint EH, Freed GL. Incidence of thyroid disease in adolescent females presenting with heavy menstrual bleeding, *J Pediatr*. 2019;212:232.
12. Donati RM, Fletcher JW, Warnecke MA, et al. Erythropoiesis in hypothyroidism. *Proc Soc Exp Biol Med*. 1973;144:78.
13. Lahner E, Conti L, Cicone F, et al. Thyro-entero-gastric autoimmunity: pathophysiology and implications for patient management. *Best Pract Res Clin Endocrinol Metab*. 2019;101373.
14. Hernik, A, Szczepanek-Parulska, E, Filipowicz, D, et al. The hepcidin concentration decreases in hypothyroid patients with Hashimoto's thyroiditis following restoration of euthyroidism. *Sci Rep*. 2019; 9:16222. https://doi.org/10.1038/s41598-019-52715-3
15. Teng X, Shan Z, Li C, et al. Iron deficiency may predict greater risk for hypothyroxinemia: a retrospective cohort study of pregnant women in China. *Thyroid*. 2018;28:968.
16. Zimmermann MB, Kohrle J. The impact of iron and selenium deficiencies on iodine and thyroid metabolism: biochemistry and relevance to public health. *Thyroid*. 2002;12:867.
17. Beard JL, Brigham DE, Kelley SK, et al. Plasma thyroid hormone kinetics are altered in iron-deficient rats. *J Nutr*. 1998;128:1401.
18. Cinemre H, Bilir C, Gokosmanoglu F, et al. Hematologic effects of levothyroxine in iron-deficient subclinical hypothyroid patients: a randomized, double-blind, controlled study. *J Clin Endocrinol Metab*. 2009;94:151.
19. Ravanbod M, Asadipooya K, Kalantarhormozi M, et al. Treatment of iron-deficiency anemia in patients with subclinical hypothyroidism. *Am J Med*. 2013;126:420.
20. Hess SY, Zimmermann MB, Adou P, et al. Treatment of iron deficiency in goitrous children improves the efficacy of iodized salt in Côte d'Ivoire. *Am J Clin Nutr*. 2002;75:743.
21. Cline MJ, Berlin NI. Erythropoiesis and red cell survival in the hypothyroid dog. *Am J Physiol*. 1963;204:415.
22. Shalet M, Coe D, Reissmann KR. Mechanism of erythropoietic action of thyroid hormone. *Proc Soc Exp Biol Med*. 1966;123:443.
23. Gordon AS, Kadow PC, et al. The thyroid and blood regeneration in the rat. *Am J Med Sci*. 1946;212:385.
24. van den Akker E, Satchwell TJ, Pellegrin S, et al. The majority of the in vitro erythroid expansion potential resides in CD34⁻ cells, outweighing the contribution of CD34(+) cells and significantly increasing the erythroblast yield from peripheral blood samples. *Haematologica*. 2010;95:1594.
25. Ng YY, Lin HD, Wu SC, et al. Impact of thyroid dysfunction on erythropoietin dosage in hemodialysis patients. *Thyroid*. 2013;23:552.
26. Gao X, Lee HY, Li W, et al. Thyroid hormone receptor beta and NCOA4 regulate terminal erythrocyte differentiation. *Proc Natl Acad Sci U S A*. 2017;114:10107.
27. Kendrick TS, Payne CJ, Epis MR, et al. Erythroid defects in TRalpha-/- mice. *Blood*. 2008;111:3245.
28. Sanchez A, Contreras-Jurado C, Rodriguez D, et al. Hematopoiesis in aged female mice devoid of thyroid hormone receptors. *J Endocrinol*. 2020;244:83.
29. Singh BK, Yen PM. A clinician's guide to understanding resistance to thyroid hormone due to receptor mutations in the TRalpha and TRbeta isoforms. *Clin Diabetes Endocrinol*. 2017;3:8.
30. van Gucht ALM, Meima ME, Moran C, et al. Anemia in patients with resistance to thyroid hormone alpha: a role for thyroid hormone receptor alpha in human erythropoiesis. *J Clin Endocrinol Metab*. 2017;102:3517.
31. Tsoukas MA. Pancytopenia in severe hypothyroidism. *Am J Med*. 127:e11,2014.
32. McMahon B, Kamath S. Pancytopenia in a patient with hypothyroidism. *JAMA*. 2016;315:1648.
33. Sullivan PS, McDonald TP. Thyroxine suppresses thrombocytopoiesis and stimulates erythropoiesis in mice. *Proc Soc Exp Biol Med*. 1992;201:271.
34. Liu X, Liu J, Fan L, et al. Erythrocytosis associated with hyperthyroidism: a rare case report and clinical study of possible mechanism. *Endocr Res*. 2015;40:177.
35. Gianoukakis AG, Leigh MJ, Richards P, et al. Characterization of the anaemia associated with Graves' disease. *Clin Endocrinol (Oxf)*. 2009;70:781.
36. Mc CJ, Donegan C, Thorup OA, et al. Survival time of the erythrocyte in myxedema and hyperthyroidism. *J Lab Clin Med*. 1958;51:91.
37. Donati RM, Warnecke MA, Gallagher NI. Ferrokinetics in hyperthyroidism. *Ann Intern Med*. 1965;63:945.
38. Ogihara T, Katoh H, Yoshitake H, et al. Hyperthyroidism associated with autoimmune hemolytic anemia and periodic paralysis: a report of a case in which antihyperthyroid therapy alone was effective against hemolysis. *Jpn J Med*. 1987;26:401.
39. Lima CS, Zantut Wittmann DE, Castro V, et al. Pancytopenia in untreated patients with Graves' disease. *Thyroid*. 2006;16:403.
40. Baez-Villasenor J, Rath CE, Finch CA. The blood picture in Addison's disease. *Blood*. 1948;3:769.
41. Daughaday WH, Williams RH, Daland GA. The effect of endocrinopathies on the blood. *Blood*. 1948;3:1342.
42. Bozzini CE, Barrio Rendo ME, Kofoed JA, et al. Effect of hydrocortisone administration on erythropoiesis in the adrenalectomized dog. *Experientia*. 1968;24:800.
43. Husebye ES, Anderson MS, Kampe O. Autoimmune polyendocrine syndromes. *NEJM*. 2018;378:1132.

44. Toonkel R, Levine M, Gardner L. Erythropoietin-deficient anemia associated with autoimmune polyglandular syndrome type I. *Am J Hematol.* 2004;75:84.

45. von Lindern M, Zauner W, Mellitzer G, et al. The glucocorticoid receptor cooperates with the erythropoietin receptor and c-Kit to enhance and sustain proliferation of erythroid progenitors in vitro. *Blood.* 1999;94:550.

46. Ashley RJ, Yan H, Wang N, et al. Steroid resistance in Diamond Blackfan anemia associates with p57^Kip2 dysregulation in erythroid progenitors. *JCI.* 2020;130:2097.

47. Plotz CM, Knowlton AI, Ragan C. The natural history of Cushing's syndrome. *Am J Med.* 1952;13:597.

48. Mann DL, Gallagher NI, Donati RM. Erythrocytosis and primary aldosteronism. *Ann Intern Med.* 1967;66:335.

49. Erkelens DW, Statius van Eps LW. Bartter's syndrome and erythrocytosis. *Am J Med.* 1973;55:711.

50. Ambrogio AG, De Martin M, Ascoli P, et al. Gender-dependent changes in haematological parameters in patients with Cushing's disease before and after remission. *Eur J Endocrinol.* 2014;170:393.

51. White PC. Update on diagnosis and management of congenital adrenal hyperplasia due to 21-hydroxylase deficiency. *Curr Opin Endocrinol Diabetes Obes.* 2018;25:178.

52. Albareda MM, Rodriguez-Espinosa J, Remacha A, et al. Polycythemia in a patient with 21-hydroxylase deficiency. *Haematologica.* 2008;85:E08.

53. Ramos I, Regadera A, Roman P, et al. [Congenital adrenal hyperplasia owing to 21-hydroxylase deficiency presenting with erythrocytosis]. *Med Clin (Barc).* 2008;131:638.

54. Karunasena N, Han TS, Mallappa A, et al. Androgens correlate with increased erythropoiesis in women with congenital adrenal hyperplasia. *Clin Endocrinol (Oxf).* 2017;86:19.

55. Drenou B, Le Tulzo Y, Caulet-Maugendre S, et al. Pheochromocytoma and secondary erythrocytosis: role of tumour erythropoietin secretion. *Nouv Rev Fr Hematol.* 1995;37:197.

56. Peng S, Zhang J, Tan X, et al. The VHL/HIF axis in the development and treatment of pheochromocytoma/paraganglioma. *Front Endocrinol (Lausanne).* 2020;11:586857.

57. Darr R, Nambuba J, Del Rivero J, et al. Novel insights into the polycythemia-paraganglioma-somatostatinoma syndrome. *Endocr Relat Cancer.* 2016;23:899.

58. Yang C, Sun MG, Matro J, et al. Novel hif2a mutations disrupt oxygen sensing, leading to polycythemia, paragangliomas, and somatostatinomas. *Blood.* 2013;121:2563.

59. Zhuang Z, Yang C, Lorenzo F, et al. Somatic HIF2a gain-of-function mutations in paraganglioma with polycythemia. *N Engl J Med.* 2012;367:922.

60. Liu Q, Wang Y, Tong D, et al. A somatic HIF2alpha mutation-induced multiple and recurrent pheochromocytoma/paraganglioma with polycythemia: clinical study with literature review. *Endocr Pathol.* 2017;28:75.

61. Lorenzo FR, Yang C, Ng Tang Fui M, et al. A novel EPAS1/HIF2a germline mutation in a congenital polycythemia with paraganglioma. *J Mol Med (Berl).* 2013;91:507.

62. Ladroue C, Carcenac R, Leporrier M, et al. PHD2 mutation and congenital erythrocytosis with paraganglioma. *N Engl J Med.* 2008;359:2685.

63. Yang C, Zhuang Z, Fliedner SM, et al. Germ-line PHD1 and PHD2 mutations detected in patients with pheochromocytoma/paraganglioma-polycythemia. *J Mol Med (Berl).* 2015;93:93.

64. Negro A, Graiani G, Nicoli D, et al. Concurrent heterozygous Von-Hippel-Lindau and transmembrane-protein-127 gene mutation causing an erythrocytosis-secreting pheochromocytoma in a normotensive patient with severe erythrocytosis. *J Hypertens.* 2020;38:340.

65. Hawkins WW, Speck E, Leonard VG. Variation of the hemoglobin level with age and sex. *Blood.* 1954;9:999.

66. Yeap BB, Beilin J, Shi Z, et al. Serum testosterone levels correlate with haemoglobin in middle-aged and older men. *Intern Med J.* 2009;39:532.

67. Fonseca R, Rajkumar SV, White WL, et al. Anemia after orchiectomy. *Am J Hematol.* 1998;59:230.

68. Hicks BM, Klil-Drori AJ, Yin H, et al. Androgen deprivation therapy and the risk of anemia in men with prostate cancer. *Epidemiology.* 2017;28:712.

69. Snyder PJ, Peachey H, Berlin JA, et al. Effects of testosterone replacement in hypogonadal men. *J Clin Endocrinol Metab.* 2000;85:2670.

70. Ponce OJ, Spencer-Bonilla G, Alvarez-Villalobos N, et al. The efficacy and adverse events of testosterone replacement therapy in hypogonadal men: a systematic review and meta-analysis of randomized, placebo-controlled trials. *J Clin Endocrinol Metab.* 2018;103(5):1745-1754.

71. Yeruva SL, Nwabudike SM, Ogbonna OH, et al. Aromatase inhibitor-induced erythrocytosis in a patient undergoing hormonal treatment for breast cancer. *Case Rep Hematol.* 2015;2015:784783.

72. Bachman E, Travison TG, Basaria S, et al. Testosterone induces erythrocytosis via increased erythropoietin and suppressed hepcidin: evidence for a new erythropoietin/hemoglobin set point. *J Gerontol A Biol Sci Med Sci.* 2014;69:725.

73. Zhou L, Zhang X, Zhou P, et al. Effect of testosterone and hypoxia on the expansion of umbilical cord blood CD34(+) cells in vitro. *Exp Ther Med.* 2017;14:4467.

74. Gagliano-Juca T, Pencina KM, Ganz T, et al. Mechanisms responsible for reduced erythropoiesis during androgen deprivation therapy in men with prostate cancer. *Am J Physiol Endocrinol Metab.* 2018;315(6):E1185-E1193.

75. Guo W, Schmidt PJ, Fleming MD, Bhasin S. Hepcidin is not essential for mediating testosterone's effects on erythropoiesis. *Andrology.* 2020;8:82.

76. Piliero SJ, Medici PT, Haber C. The interrelationships of the endocrine and erythropoietic systems in the rat with special reference to the mechanism of action of estradiol and testosterone. *Ann N Y Acad Sci.* 1968;149:336.

77. Nakada D, Oguro H, Levi BP, et al. Oestrogen increases haematopoietic stem-cell self-renewal in females and during pregnancy. *Nature.* 2014;505:555.

78. Kim HR, Lee JH, Heo HR, et al. Improved hematopoietic differentiation of human pluripotent stem cells via estrogen receptor signaling pathway. *Cell Biosci.* 2016;6:50.

79. Higham CE, Johannsson G, Shalet SM. Hypopituitarism. *Lancet.* 2016;388:2403.

80. Crafts RC, Meineke HA. The anemia of hypophysectomized animals. *Ann N Y Acad Sci.* 1959;77:501.

81. Van Dyke DC, Garcia JF, Simpson ME, et al. Maintenance of circulating red cell volume in rats after removal of the posterior and intermediate lobes of the pituitary. *Blood.* 1952;7:1005.

82. Crafts RC. The similarity between anemia induced by hypophysectomy and that induced by a combined thyroidectomy and adrenalectomy in adult female rats. *Endocrinology.* 1953;53:465.

83. Ellegala DB, Alden TD, Couture DE, et al. Anemia, testosterone, and pituitary adenoma in men. *J Neurosurg.* 2003;98:974.

84. Lang D, Mead JS, Sykes DB. Hormones and the bone marrow: panhypopituitarism and pancytopenia in a man with a pituitary adenoma. *J Gen Intern Med.* 2015;30:692.

85. Laway BA, Mir SA, Bashir MI, et al. Prevalence of hematological abnormalities in patients with Sheehan's syndrome: response to replacement of glucocorticoids and thyroxine. *Pituitary.* 2011;14:39.

86. Nomiyama J, Shinohara K, Inoue H. Improvement of anemia by recombinant erythropoietin in a patient with postoperative hypopituitarism. *Am J Hematol.* 1994;47:249.

87. Dey S, Scullen T, Noguchi CT. Erythropoietin negatively regulates pituitary ACTH secretion. *Brain Res.* 2015;1608:14.

88. Merchav S, Tatarsky I, Hochberg Z. Enhancement of erythropoiesis in vitro by human growth hormone is mediated by insulin-like growth factor I. *Br J Haematol.* 1988;70:267.

89. Eugster EA, Fisch M, Walvoord EC, et al. Low hemoglobin levels in children with in idiopathic growth hormone deficiency. *Endocrine.* 2002;18:135.

90. Bergamaschi S, Giavoli C, Ferrante E, et al. Growth hormone replacement therapy in growth hormone deficient children and adults: effects on hemochrome. *J Endocrinol Invest.* 2006;29:399.

91. Miniero R, Altomare F, Rubino M, et al. Effect of recombinant human growth hormone (rhGH) on hemoglobin concentration in children with idiopathic growth hormone deficiency-related anemia. *J Pediatr Hematol Oncol.* 2012;34:407.

92. Woody MA, Welniak LA, Sun R, et al. Prolactin exerts hematopoietic growth-promoting effects in vivo and partially counteracts myelosuppression by azidothymidine. *Exp Hematol.* 1999;27:811.

93. Abkowitz JL, Schaison G, Boulad F, et al. Response of Diamond-Blackfan anemia to metoclopramide: evidence for a role for prolactin in erythropoiesis. *Blood.* 2002;100:2687.

94. Socolovsky M, Fallon AE, Lodish HF. The prolactin receptor rescues EpoR-/- erythroid progenitors and replaces epor in a synergistic interaction with c-kit. *Blood.* 1998;92:1491.

95. Shimon I, Benbassat C, Tzvetov G, et al. Anemia in a cohort of men with macroprolactinomas: increase in hemoglobin levels follows prolactin suppression. *Pituitary.* 2011;14:11.

96. Iglesias P, Castro JC, Diez JJ. Clinical significance of anaemia associated with prolactin-secreting pituitary tumours in men. *Int J Clin Pract.* 2011;65:669.

97. Holmes GI, Shepherd P, Walker JD. Panhypopituitarism secondary to a macroprolactinoma manifesting with pancytopenia: case report and literature review. *Endocr Pract.* 17:e32,2011.

98. Ceccato F, Occhi G, Regazzo D, et al. Gonadotropin secreting pituitary adenoma associated with erythrocytosis: case report and literature review. *Hormones (Athens).* 2014;13:131.

99. Lu R, Wang Q, Han Y, et al. Parathyroid hormone administration improves bone marrow microenvironment and partially rescues haematopoietic defects in BMI1-null mice. *PLoS One.* 2014;9(4):e93864.

100. Boxer M, Ellman L, Geller R, et al. Anemia in primary hyperparathyroidism. *Arch Intern Med.* 1977;137:588.

101. Abarca J, Trigonis C, Hamberger B, et al. Anaemia in primary hyperparathyroidism–fantasy or reality. *Ann Chir Gynaecol.* 1985;74:74.

102. Bhadada SK, Bhansali A, Ahluwalia J, et al. Anaemia and marrow fibrosis in patients with primary hyperparathyroidism before and after curative parathyroidectomy. *Clin Endocrinol (Oxf).* 2009;70:527.

103. Trunzo JA, McHenry CR, Schulak JA, et al. Effect of parathyroidectomy on anemia and erythropoietin dosing in end-stage renal disease patients with hyperparathyroidism. *Surgery.* 2008;144:915.

104. Battistella M, Richardson RM, Bargman JM, et al. Improved parathyroid hormone control by cinacalcet is associated with reduction in darbepoetin requirement in patients with end-stage renal disease. *Clin Nephrol.* 2011;76:99.

CHAPTER 8
PAROXYSMAL NOCTURNAL HEMOGLOBINURIA

Charles J. Parker

SUMMARY

In contrast to all other intrinsic abnormalities of the erythrocyte, paroxysmal nocturnal hemoglobinuria (PNH) is an acquired, rather than an inherited, disorder. PNH arises as a consequence of somatic mutation, affecting one or more hematopoietic stem/progenitor cells (HS/PCs), of *PIGA*, a gene located on the X chromosome that is required for synthesis of the glycosyl phosphatidylinositol (GPI) moiety that anchors a functionally diverse group of proteins to the cell surface. Consequently, all GPI-anchored proteins (GPI-APs) that are normally expressed are deficient on the mutant HS/PC stem cell and its progeny. The complement-mediated intravascular hemolytic anemia and the resulting hemoglobinuria that are the clinical hallmarks of PNH are a consequence of deficiency of the GPI-anchored complement regulatory proteins, CD55 and CD59. Although PNH is a clonal disease, it is not a malignant disease in that there is no inexorable proliferation of neoplastic cells (as is the case with acute myeloid leukemia) or invasion of nonmarrow tissue, and the extent to which the mutant clone(s) expand varies greatly among patients. Therefore, the blood cells of patients with PNH is a mosaic of phenotypically normal and abnormal cells. The size of the mutant clone is an important determinant of the clinical manifestations of the disease, which include hemolysis and thrombophilia. An element of immune-mediated marrow failure (of varying degrees and types) is present in all patients, but PNH is a consequence rather than a cause of immune-mediated bone marrow failure. The diagnosis of PNH is determined by using flow cytometry to detect and quantify the percentage of blood erythrocytes and leukocytes (ie, neutrophils and monocytes) that lack GPI-APs as measured by binding of immunoflorescently labeled probes that bind to GPI-anchored cell surface proteins, including CD55 and CD59. The intravascular hemolysis of PNH can be controlled with a humanized monoclonal anticomplement C5 antibody that blocks formation of the cytolytic membrane attack complex of complement (commercially available as eculizumab and ravulizumab). Although treatment with eculizumab/ravulizumab favorably modifies the natural history of PNH, it has no effect on the underlying disease process (ie, on the *PIGA*-mutant HS/PC clone). The *PIGA*-mutant clone can be eradicated and normal hematopoiesis restored by allogeneic hematopoietic stem cell transplantation, but the relatively benign natural history of PNH in patients treated with eculizumab/ravulizumab has tempered enthusiasm for transplantation because of concerns about subjecting patients to the risk of treatment-related morbidity and mortality.

Acronyms and Abbreviations: APC, alternative pathway of complement; CD55, an antigen encoding DAF; CD59, an antigen encoding MAC-inhibitory protein; DAF, decay accelerating factor; EtN, ethanolamine; GPI, glycosyl phosphatidylinositol; GPI-APs, glycosyl phosphatidylinositol-anchored proteins; GLcN, glucosamine; GVHD, graft versus host disease; HS/PC, hematopoietic stem/progenitor cell; HLA, human leukocyte antigen; INR, international normalized ratio of prothrombin assay data; LDH, lactate dehydrogenase; MAC, membrane attack complex of complement; MDS, myelodysplastic syndrome; MIRL, membrane inhibitor of reactive lysis; *PIGA*, phosphatidylinositol glycan class A; PNH, paroxysmal nocturnal hemoglobinuria; PNH-sc, subclinical PNH; RA, refractory anemia; RAEB, refractory anemia with excess of blasts; RAEB-t, refractory anemia with excess of blasts in transformation; RA-PNH+, RA with a population of PNH cells; RA-PNH−, RA without a population of PNH cells; RARS, refractory anemia with ringed sideroblasts; RCMD, refractory cytopenias with multilineage dysplasia; RCMD-RS, RCMD with ringed sideroblasts; US FDA, United States Food and Drug Administration; UTR, untranslated region; WHO, World Health Organization.

● DEFINITION AND HISTORY

Although commonly regarded as a type of hemolytic anemia, paroxysmal nocturnal hemoglobinuria (PNH) is a disorder of hematopoietic stem/progenitor cells (HS/PCs). PNH arises from clonal expansion of one or several hematopoietic HS/PCs that have acquired a somatic mutation of the X-chromosome gene *PIGA* (phosphatidylinositol glycan class A). As a consequence of mutant *PIGA*, any progeny of affected HS/PCs (erythrocytes, granulocytes, monocytes, platelets, and lymphocytes) are deficient in all GPI-APs that are normally expressed on hematopoietic cells. The clinical manifestations of PNH are hemolytic anemia, thrombophilia, and marrow failure, but only the hemolytic anemia is unequivocally a consequence of somatic mutation of *PIGA*. Moreover, the marrow failure component of the disease is likely an antecedent process that creates the conditions that underlie the selection pressure that favors the growth/survival of the GPI-AP–deficient HS/PCs. That the GPI-AP–deficient cells arise as a consequence of Darwinian evolution is supported by the observation that, in some cases, patients have been shown to have multiple, discrete *PIGA*-mutant clones. PNH is a clonal disease, but not a malignant neoplasm in the classical sense of a disease, such as acute leukemia, which is characterized by uncontrolled proliferation of cells with spread to nonmarrow tissues and suppression of normal nonmutated hematopoiesis. The extent to which the mutant clone expands varies widely among patients; however, the basis of the clonal expansion is largely speculative. Thrombosis is the major cause of morbidity and mortality, but the mechanisms that underlie the thrombophilia of PNH are incompletely understood. Rarely, the *PIGA*-mutant clone acquires additional somatic mutations that result in malignant transformation.

Comprehensive, scholarly reviews of the history of PNH are available.[1-4] The first published clinical description of PNH is attributed to William Gull in 1866, but he failed to distinguish definitively PNH from paroxysmal cold hemoglobinuria. In 1882, Paul Strübing clearly recognized PNH as a distinct entity and undertook prescient experiments designed to test his hypothesis that the nocturnal hemoglobinuria was a consequence of acidification of plasma that occurred when carbon dioxide and lactic acid accumulated because of the slowing of respiration during sleep. In 1911, A. A. Hijmans van den Bergh demonstrated that the hemolysis of PNH is caused by a defect in the red cell rather than by the presence of an abnormal plasma factor (as is the case with paroxysmal cold hemoglobinuria; Chap. 26). Thomas Hale Ham is credited with discovering, in the late 1930s, that complement mediates the hemolysis of PNH erythrocytes, although it was not until the alternative pathway of complement was identified and characterized in the mid-1950s by Louis Pillemer that the basis of Ham's original observations became apparent. Ham developed the acidified serum lysis test (Ham test) that, along with the sucrose lysis test (sugar water test) of Robert Hartmann and David Jenkins, was used as the standard diagnostic tests for PNH until it was supplanted in the early 1990s by flow cytometry. Both Hartmann and William Crosby brought attention to the important role that thrombosis (particularly the Budd-Chiari syndrome) plays in the natural history of PNH, and John Dacie and his student and subsequent colleague, S. M. Lewis, first systematically characterized the relationship between PNH and marrow failure.

EPIDEMIOLOGY

The prevalence of PNH is not precisely known. Prevalence estimates are influenced by bias in study design and results differ considerably, largely because of the heterogeneous nature of the disease. The blood of patients with PNH is a mosaic of normal and abnormal cells, and the extent of the mosaicism varies widely among patients (see "Phenotypic Mosaicism is Characteristic of PNH" further). Patients with small PNH clones have few or no symptoms related to hemolysis. Thus, an argument can be made that asymptomatic patients with small clones do not have clinically significant PNH and should be excluded from prevalence estimates. Others, however, argue that any patient with flow cytometric evidence of a population of GPI-AP–deficient cells, regardless of clone size, has PNH and should be included in prevalence estimates. Well-designed, rigorous studies of prevalence that address the issue of disease heterogeneity are needed, but by any definition, PNH is a rare disease. The prevalence of clinically significant PNH (ie, classic PNH) plus patients with relatively large clones that arise in the setting of another marrow failure syndrome (see "Clinical Features" and Table 8-1) are likely in the order of fewer than one case per 200,000 persons, easily fulfilling criteria (ρ1 case per 50,000) for classification as an ultraorphan disease.[5] There is a close association between PNH and aplastic anemia and, to a lesser extent, low-risk myelodysplastic syndrome (MDS). Although PNH has been reported in all age groups, the peak incidence is in the third and fourth decades of life, similar to that of aplastic anemia (Chap. 4). PNH is an acquired disorder, and there is no known inherited risk for development of the disease. Several cases have been reported in which only one of a pair of identical twins was affected.

ETIOLOGY AND PATHOGENESIS

COMPLEMENT AND PNH

The chronic intravascular hemolysis that is the hallmark clinical manifestation of PNH is mediated by the alternative pathway of complement (APC) (Fig. 8-1).[6] The APC is a component of innate immunity.[7] This ancient system evolved to protect the host against invasion by pathogenic microorganisms. Unlike the classical pathway of complement that is part of the system of adaptive immunity and requires antibody for initiation of activation, the APC is in a state of continuous activation, armed at all times to protect the host (see Chap. 26 for a detailed review of the complement system). The APC cascade can be divided into two functional components: the amplification C3 and C5 convertases and the membrane attack complex (MAC). The C3 and C5 convertases (see Fig. 8-1, *top panel*) are enzymatic complexes that initiate and amplify the activity of the APC. Generation of C5b by enzymatic cleavage of C5 by the APC C5 convertase initiates formation of the terminal pathway of complement that results ultimately in assembly of the cytolytic MAC.

Because the APC is always primed for attack, elaborate mechanisms for self-recognition and for protection of the host against APC-mediated injury have evolved. Both fluid-phase and membrane-bound proteins are involved in these processes. Normal human erythrocytes are protected against APC-mediated cytolysis, primarily by decay-accelerating factor (CD55)[8-10] and membrane inhibitor of reactive lysis (CD59).[11] These proteins act at different steps in the complement cascade (see Fig. 8-1, *top panel*). CD55 regulates the formation and stability of the C3 and C5 convertases, whereas CD59 blocks the formation of the MAC. Experimental evidence also supports a role for CD59 in regulation of the C3/C5 convertases.[12] Deficiency of CD55 and CD59

TABLE 8-1. Classification of Paroxysmal Nocturnal Hemoglobinuria[a]

Category	Rate of Intravascular Hemolysis[b]	Marrow	Flow Cytometry	Benefit from Eculizumab
Classic	Florid (macroscopic hemoglobinuria is frequent or persistent)	Cellular marrow with erythroid hyperplasia and normal or near-normal morphology[c]	Large population (>50%) of GPI-AP–deficient PMNs[d]	Yes
PNH in the setting of another marrow failure syndrome[e]	Mild to moderate (macroscopic hemoglobinuria is intermittent or absent)	Evidence of a concomitant marrow failure syndrome[e]	Although variable, the percentage of GPI-AP–deficient PMNs[d] is usually relatively small (<50%)	Dependent on the size of the PNH clone
Subclinical	No clinical or biochemical evidence of intravascular hemolysis	Evidence of a concomitant marrow failure syndrome[e]	Small (<1%) population of GPI-AP–deficient PMNs detected by high-resolution flow cytometry	No

Abbreviations: GPI-AP, glycosyl phosphatidylinositol-anchored protein; PMNs, polymorphonuclear leukocytes; PNH, paroxysmal nocturnal hemoglobinuria.

[a]Based on recommendations of the International PNH Interest Group (Parker C, Omine M, Richards S, et al. Diagnosis and management of paroxysmal nocturnal hemoglobinuria. *Blood.* 2005;106:3699-3709).

[b]Based on macroscopic hemoglobinuria, serum lactate dehydrogenase concentration, and reticulocyte count.

[c]Karyotypic abnormalities are uncommon.

[d]Analysis of PMNs is more informative than analysis of RBCs because of selective destruction of GPI-AP–deficient red blood cells.

[e]Aplastic anemia and refractory anemia/MDS are the most commonly associated marrow failure syndromes.

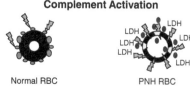

Alternative Pathway of Complement

Complement Activation

Normal RBC   PNH RBC

Figure 8–1. Complement-mediated lysis of paroxysmal nocturnal hemoglobinuria (PNH) erythrocytes. *Upper panel.* The hemolytic anemia of PNH is Coombs'-negative (direct antiglobulin test) because the process is mediated by the antibody-independent alternative pathway of complement (APC). The C3 convertase of the APC consists of activated C3 (C3b), activated factor B (Bb, the enzymatic subunit of the complex that is generated by enzymatic cleavage by factor D), and factor P (a protein that stabilizes the complex, formally called properdin). The C5 convertase has the same components as the C3 convertase, except that two C3b molecules are required to bind and position C5 for cleavage by activated factor B (Bb). C3a and C5a are bioactive peptides that are generated by cleavage of C3 and C5, respectively, by their specific activation convertases. The C3 and C5 convertases greatly amplify complement activation by cleaving multiple substrate molecules. The membrane attack complex (MAC) consists of activated C5 (C5b), C6, C7, C8, and multiple molecules of C9 ($C9_n$). The MAC is the cytolytic unit of the complement system. The glycosyl phosphatidylinositol (GPI)–anchored complement regulatory protein CD55 restricts formation and stability of both the C3 and the C5 amplification convertases by destabilizing the interaction between activated factor B (Bb) and C3b (indicated by the *blue arrow*), whereas GPI-anchored CD59 blocks formation of the MAC by inhibiting the binding of C9 to the C5b-8 complex (indicated by the *brown arrow*). CD59 also regulates the activity of the C3 convertase. Inhibition of MAC formation by the humanized monoclonal anti-C5 antibody eculizumab (indicated by the *red arrow*) ameliorates the intravascular hemolysis of PNH. *Lower panel.* Normal erythrocytes (*left*) are protected against complement-mediated lysis primarily by CD55 (*blue circles*) and CD59 (*green circles*). Deficiency of these GPI-anchored complement regulatory proteins results in APC activation on PNH erythrocytes (*right*). Because of deficiency of CD55 and CD59, the complement cascade activates on the cell surface. Consequently, MACs form pores in the red cell membrane, resulting in colloid osmotic lysis and release of hemoglobin (*red circles*) and other contents of the red cell including lactate dehydrogenase (LDH) into the intravascular space. *(Modified with permission from Parker CJ: The pathophysiology of paroxysmal nocturnal hemoglobinuria. Exp Hematol. 2007 Apr;35[4]:523-533.)*

on the erythrocytes of PNH is the pathophysiologic basis of the direct antiglobulin test–negative, intravascular hemolysis that is the clinical hallmark of the disease (see Fig. 8-1, *bottom panel*). But why are PNH erythrocytes deficient in the two complement regulatory proteins?

THE MOLECULAR PATHOGENESIS AND GENETIC BASIS OF PNH

PNH is a consequence of clonal expansion of one or more hematopoietic HS/PCs with mutant *PIGA* (located on Xp22.1).[13] The protein product of *PIGA* is a glycosyl transferase[13-17] that is an obligate constituent of a complex biochemical pathway required for synthesis of the glycosyl

phosphatidylinositol (GPI) moiety that anchors individual proteins belonging to diverse functional groups to the cell surface (Fig. 8-2). As a result of mutant *PIGA*, progeny of the affected stem cells are deficient in all GPI-APs. Although more than 25 GPI-APs are expressed by hematopoietic cells, it is deficiency on red cells of the two GPI-anchored complement regulatory proteins, CD55 and CD59, that underlies the hemolytic anemia of PNH.[18] Red cells lacking CD55 and CD59 undergo spontaneous intravascular hemolysis as a consequence of unregulated activation of the APC (see Fig. 8-1, *bottom panel*). Thus, the hallmark clinical manifestation of PNH (intravascular hemolysis and the resultant hemoglobinuria) occurs because the two proteins that regulate complement on erythrocytes are GPI-anchored and hence, deficient, because the *PIGA* mutation renders all GPI-APs deficient.

Although the relationship between somatic mutation of *PIGA* and the hemolysis of PNH is understood in detail, the relationship between somatic mutation of *PIGA* (and the consequent deficiency of GPI-APs) and the marrow failure and thrombophilia of PNH remains largely speculative. Especially in the case of marrow failure, the *PIGA* mutation/deficiency of GPI-APs may not be causal. Rather, the prevailing hypothesis posits that the process that causes the marrow failure (proposed as immune attack on HS/PCs) selects for the *PIGA* mutant cell because absence of one or more GPI-APs bestows a survival advantage by allowing the mutant stem cell to either evade or better weather immune attack. Strong support for this hypothesis of immune escape comes from studies of human leukocyte antigen (HLA) patterns in patients with acquired aplastic anemia.[19] Approximately 10% of patients with acquired aplastic anemia has a population of hematopoietic cells that are homozygous for HLA alleles. In most cases, homozygosity is acquired through homologous recombination, resulting in copy number neutral loss of heterozygosity, although somatic mutations that inactivate one allele may cause functional loss of heterogygosity.[20] A patient with PNH may have oligoclonal hematopoiesis due to coexistence of separate clones with mutation of *PIGA* or loss of heterozygosity of HLA.[21]

Whether the thrombophilia of PNH is caused by absence of a GPI-AP that is directly involved in regulation of hemostasis/thrombosis (eg, the receptor for urokinase plasminogen activator) or to indirect consequences of GPI-AP deficiency (eg, complement-mediated activation of the coagulation cascade, generation of procoagulant microparticles as a result of complement-mediated lysis) remains unresolved.[22]

Hypothetically, the PNH phenotype would result from inactivation of any of the more than 25 genes involved in synthesis of the GPI-anchor (see Fig. 8-2) but with one exception,[23,24] somatic mutation of no gene involved in GPI-AP synthesis other than *PIGA* has been reported in patients with PNH. This phenomenon is accounted for by the fact that, of the genes involved in the GPI-anchor synthesis pathway, only *PIGA* is located on the X chromosome. Therefore, somatic mutation of only one allele is required for expression of the phenotype because men have one X chromosome and, as a consequence of X inactivation during embryogenesis, women have only one functional X chromosome in somatic tissues. On the other hand, mutation of two alleles would be required for inactivation of any of the autosomal genes involved in the GPI-anchor synthesis pathway.[23]

Cells with *PIGA* mutations do not appear to have a proliferative advantage in vitro or in hybrid animal models.[25] PIGA mutant cells have been found to be relatively resistant to apoptosis in some studies[26-29] but not others.[30,31] Thus, the basis of clonal selection and clonal expansion of *PIGA*-mutant stem cells in patients with PNH remains largely enigmatic,[32] although a number of hypotheses have been proposed.[17] Studies aimed at identifying somatic mutations in PNH cells of genes involved in myeloid malignancies have been undertaken with a goal of identifying the molecular basis of clonal expansion.[33,34] Although such mutations have been found, they are relatively uncommon, vary in allele

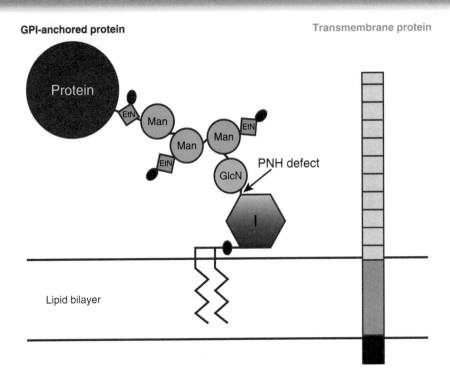

Figure 8–2. The molecular and genetic basis of paroxysmal nocturnal hemoglobinuria (PNH). There are two types of anchoring mechanisms for plasma membrane proteins: transmembrane and GPI. Transmembrane proteins are anchored into the lipid bilayer of the cell by a short series (~25 amino acids) of hydrophobic residues (*blue rectangle*). Transmembrane proteins typically have a short cytoplasmic tail that usually has signaling properties (*red rectangle*). The ectoplasmic portion of the protein is illustrated by the series of *gray-blue squares*. The GPI-APs consist of the following components: phosphatidylinositol (inositol is represented by the *blue hexagon* labeled I and phosphate is represented by the *red oval*); glucosamine (GLcN, *yellow circle*); three mannose (Man, *green circles*); ethanolamine phosphate (EtN, *blue square* with attached phosphate represented by the *red oval*); the protein entity (*blue circle*). The lipid component (indicated by the series of *diagonal lines* within lipid bilayer) is usually 1-alkyl, 2-acylglycerol for mammalian GPI-APs. PNH cells are deficient in all GPI-APs because somatic mutation of the X-chromosome gene *PIGA* disrupts the first step in the biosynthetic pathway (transfer of the nucleotide sugar UDP-GlcNAc to GlcNAc-PI) indicated by the *arrow*.

frequency, and are not specific for PNH.[35] Two patients have been identified whose PNH cells had a concurrent, acquired rearrangement of chromosome 12. In both cases, der(12) had a break within the 3′ untranslated region (UTR) of *HMGA2*, an architectural transcription factor gene that is deregulated in many benign mesenchymal tumors. In both cases, the rearrangement caused ectopic expression of HMGA2 in the marrow. The 3′ UTR contains binding sites for let-7 microRNAs that negatively regulate HMGA2 expression. These observations suggested that ectopic HMGA2 expression, in concert with mutant *PIGA*, accounted for clonal hematopoiesis in these two patients and suggested the concept of PNH as a benign tumor of the bone marrow. Subsequent studies showed that *HMGA2* was aberrantly expressed in the peripheral blood cells of patients with PNH without chromosomal rearrangements,[36] that aberrant expression of *HMGA2* as a consequence of vector integration that disrupts the 3′ UTR during gene therapy for thalassemia results in clonal expansion of hematopoiesis,[37] that truncation of the 3′ UTR of *HMGA2* in murine HSCs results in myeloproliferative-like hematopoiesis,[38] and that *HMGA2* promotes long-term engraftment and myeloerythroid differentiation of human HS/PCs.[39] Together, these observations support the hypothesis that expression of *HMGA2* determines the extent of clonal expansion of *PIGA*-mutant HS/PCs in PNH.

PHENOTYPIC MOSAICISM IS CHARACTERISTIC OF PNH

The blood of patients with PNH is a mosaic of normal and abnormal cells (Fig. 8-3). Although PNH is a clonal disease, the extent to which

the *PIGA*-mutant clone expands varies widely among patients.[18] As an example, in some cases, more than 90% of the blood cells may be derived from the *PIGA*-mutant clone, whereas in others, less than 1% of the blood cells may be GPI-AP–deficient. This unique feature (variability in extent of mosaicism) is clinically relevant because patients with relatively small PNH clones have minimal or no symptoms and require no PNH-specific treatment, whereas those with large clones are often debilitated by the consequences of chronic complement-mediated intravascular hemolysis and respond dramatically to complement inhibitory therapy.

Another remarkable feature of PNH is phenotypic mosaicism (see Fig. 8-3A) based on *PIGA* genotype[40] (see Fig. 8-3B) that determines the degree of GPI-AP deficiency.[18] PNH III cells are completely deficient in GPI-APs, PNH II cells are partially (~90%) deficient, and PNH I cells express GPI-APs at normal density (putatively, these cells are progeny of residual normal stem cells; see Fig. 8-3A). That PNH II cells are approximately 90% deficient in GPI-APs indicates that clonal selection occurs when a deficiency threshold of 90% or higher, based on density of expression of GPI-APs, is reached. Phenotype varies among patients (Fig. 8-4). Some patients have only type I and type III cells (the most common phenotype); some have type I, type II, and type III (the second most common phenotype); and some patients have only type I and type II cells (the least common phenotype). Furthermore, the contribution of each phenotype to the composition of the blood varies. Phenotypic mosaicism is clinically important because PNH II cells are relatively resistant to spontaneous hemolysis, and patients with a high percentage of type II cells have a relatively benign clinical course with respect to hemolysis (see Fig. 8-4).

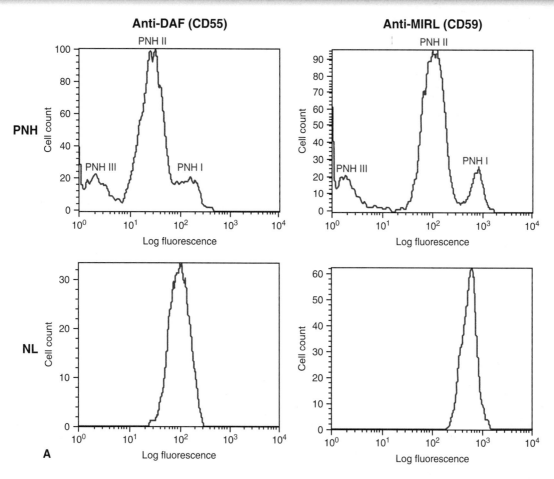

Figure 8–3. Phenotypic mosaicism is a characteristic feature of paroxysmal nocturnal hemoglobinuria (PNH). **A.** The blood of patients with PNH is a mosaic of phenotypically normal and abnormal cells. In some patients, erythrocytes that are partially deficient in GPI-APs (called PNH II) are present in the blood along with cells that are completely deficient (PNH III) and cells that are phenotypically normal (PNH I). In the case illustrated, erythrocytes from a patient with PNH (PNH, *upper panels*) and from a healthy volunteer (NL, *lower panels*) were stained with fluorescently labeled antibodies (anti-CD55, *left panels*; CD59, *right panels*) and analyzed by flow cytometry. **B.** *PIGA* genotype determines PNH phenotype. The PNH II phenotype is a consequence of *PIGA* mutation that partially inactivates enzyme function (*red circles*), whereas any *PIGA* mutation that causes complete loss of enzyme function generates the PNH III phenotype (*green, yellow,* and *blue circles*). PNH I cells have wild-type *PIGA* and are the progeny of normal residual hematopoietic stem cells. In a single individual, multiple discrete *PIGA* mutations can be identified, accounting for the phenotypic mosaicism based on GPI-AP expression.

The anemia of PNH is multifactorial because an element of marrow failure is present in all patients, although the degree of marrow dysfunction is variable.[41] In some patients, PNH arises in the setting of aplastic anemia. In this case, marrow failure is the dominant cause of anemia. In other patients with PNH, evidence of marrow dysfunction may be subtle (eg, an inappropriately low reticulocyte count), with the degree of anemia being determined primarily by the rate of hemolysis that is, in turn, determined by PNH clone size and phenotype.

● CLINICAL FEATURES

The primary clinical manifestations of PNH are hemolysis, thrombosis, and marrow failure.[41] Constitutional symptoms (fatigue, lethargy, malaise, asthenia) dominate the history, with nocturnal hemoglobinuria being a presenting symptom in approximately 25% of patients.[42] Direct questioning frequently elicits a history of episodic dysphagia and odynophagia, abdominal pain, and male impotence. Venous thrombosis, often occurring at unusual sites (Budd-Chiari syndrome, mesenteric, portal vein, dermal or cerebral veins), may complicate PNH. Arterial thrombosis is less common.

● LABORATORY FEATURES

PNH should be suspected in patients with nonspherocytic, direct antiglobulin test–negative intravascular hemolysis (Table 8-2).

Although the clinical manifestations of PNH depend largely on the size of the *PIGA* mutant clone, the extent of the associated marrow failure also contributes to disease manifestations. Thus, PNH is not a binary process and, based on clinical features, marrow characteristics, and the size of the mutant clone as determined by the percentage of GPI-AP–deficient neutrophils, the International PNH Interest Group recognizes three disease subcategories (see Table 8-1).[41]

Reticulocytosis reflects the response to hemolysis, although the reticulocyte count may be lower than expected for the degree of anemia because of underlying marrow failure (see Table 8-2). Serum lactate dehydrogenase (LDH) concentration is always abnormally high in patients with clinically significant hemolysis and serves as an important surrogate marker for estimating and following the rate of intravascular hemolysis. A close association exists between PNH and aplastic anemia and, to a lesser extent, between PNH and low-risk MDS (Chap. 4; and "PNH and Marrow Failure" further). By using high-sensitivity flow cytometry,

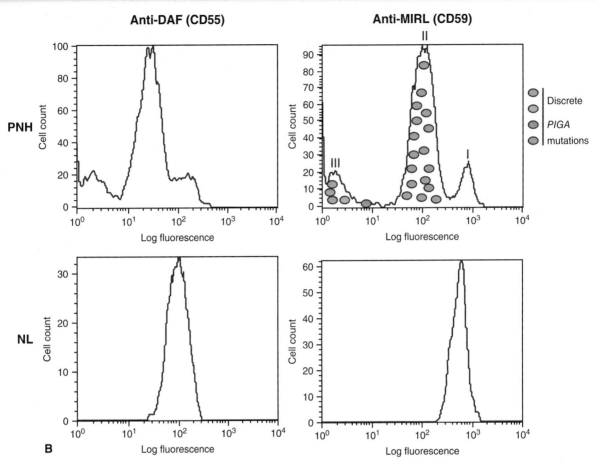

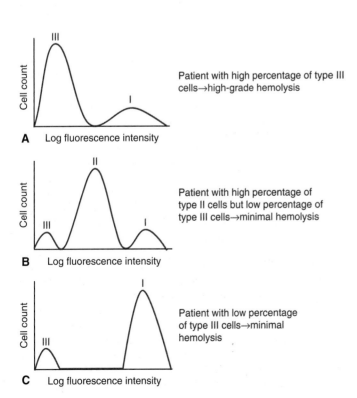

Figure 8–3. (*Continued*)

Figure 8–4. Clinical manifestations of paroxysmal nocturnal hemoglobinuria (PNH) are determined by clone size and erythrocyte phenotype. Mock flow cytometry histograms of erythrocytes from hypothetical patients with PNH stained with anti-CD59 are illustrated. Both the proportion and type of abnormal erythrocytes vary greatly among patients with PNH, and these characteristics are important determinants of clinical manifestations. In general, patients with a high percentage of type III erythrocytes have clinically apparent hemolysis **(A)**. If the erythrocytes are partially deficient in GPI-AP (PNH II cells), hemolysis may be modest even if the percentage of the affected cells is high **(B)**. A patient may have a diagnosis of PNH, but if the proportion of type III cells is low, only biochemical evidence of hemolysis may be observed **(C)**. *(Modified with permission from Parker C, Omine M, Richards S, et al. Diagnosis and management of paroxysmal nocturnal hemoglobinuria. Blood. 2005 Dec 1; 106[12]:3699-3709.)*

TABLE 8-2. Recommendation for Screening Patients for Paroxysmal Nocturnal Hemoglobinuria[a]

History of episodic hemoglobinuria

Evidence of nonspherocytic, Coombs'-negative (direct antiglobulin test) intravascular hemolysis (must have high serum LDH)

Patients with aplastic anemia (screen at diagnosis and once yearly even in the absence of intravascular hemolysis)

Patients with RA or RCMD variants of MDS[b]

Patients with venous thrombosis involving unusual sites (usually have evidence of intravascular hemolysis)
- Budd-Chiari syndrome
- Other intra-abdominal sites
- Cerebral veins
- Dermal veins

Abbreviations: LDH, lactate dehydrogenase; MDS, myelodysplastic syndrome; RA, refractory anemia; RCMD, refractory cytopenias with multilineage dysplasia.

[a]Screening by flow cytometric analysis of glycosyl phosphatidylinositol-anchored proteins (GPI-APs) on red cells and neutrophils.

[b]There is no indication for screening patients with other MDS classifications.

approximately 50% of patients with aplastic anemia and 15% of patients with low-risk MDS have been found to have a detectable population of GPI-AP–deficient erythrocytes and granulocytes.[43-46] In approximately 80% of these cases, the proportion of GPI-AP–deficient cells is smaller than 1% of the total. These patients with very small populations of GPI-AP–deficient erythrocytes have no clinical or biochemical evidence of hemolysis and are designated as subclinical PNH (PNH-sc; see Table 8-1). Varying degrees of leukopenia, thrombocytopenia, and relative reticulocytopenia reflect the extent of marrow insufficiency (see "PNH and Marrow Failure" further).

Once PNH is suspected, diagnosis is straightforward because deficiency of GPI-APs on blood cells is readily demonstrated by flow cytometry (Fig. 8-5).[47,48] Using a combination of fluorochrome-conjugated antibodies against GPI-APs in conjunction with fluorochrome-conjugated antibodies that identify specific peripheral blood elements (erythrocytes, neutrophils, monocytes), populations of GPI-AP–deficient cells as low as 0.005% can be reliably detected using multiparameter flow cytometry.[47,49-51] The pore-forming bacterial protein, aerolysin, secreted from *Aeromonas hydrophila*, binds to the GPI moiety of GPI-APs and, upon oligomerization, forms transmembrane channels that induce osmotic cytolysis. The absence of GPI-APs on PNH cells renders them insusceptible to aerolysin-mediated cytolysis.[52] A genetically modified form of aerolysin has been developed that does not induce cytolysis, and a fluorescently labeled version of this protein (FLAER) can be used in flow cytometric assays to detect GPI-AP–deficient cells.[53] The FLAER assay is useful in identifying GPI-AP–deficient nucleated cells including neutrophils and monocytes, but it cannot be used to identify GPI-AP erythrocytes because red cells lack the proteolytic enzymes necessary to process the protein into its active, binding form. Although they have much biologic and historic importance, the acidified serum lysis test (Ham test) and the sucrose lysis test (sugar water test) have largely been abandoned as diagnostic assays because they are both less sensitive and less quantitative than flow cytometry. Flow cytometric analysis of both red cells and neutrophils is warranted, because clone size will be underestimated if only red cells are examined because GPI-AP–deficient red

cells are selectively destroyed by complement. Recent transfusion will also affect the estimate of clone size, if only red cells are analyzed, but delineation of PNH phenotypes (ie, the percentage of types I, II, and III cells) requires flow cytometric analysis of the erythrocyte population.[47]

In addition to flow cytometric analysis, the basic initial evaluation of a patient with PNH should include complete blood count to assess the effects of the disease on production of leukocytes and platelets, as well as on erythrocytes (Table 8-3). In patients with classic PNH, the leukocyte and platelet counts are usually normal or nearly normal, whereas leukopenia, thrombocytopenia, or both invariably accompany PNH/aplastic anemia and PNH/MDS. The reticulocyte count is needed to assess the ongoing capacity of the marrow to respond to the anemia. Although the reticulocyte count is elevated in patients with classic PNH, as noted earlier, it may be inappropriately low for the degree of anemia, reflecting underlying relative insufficiency of hematopoiesis that is characteristic of the disease. The reticulocyte count is decreased in patients with PNH with concomitant aplastic anemia or low-risk MDS. Serum LDH is always markedly elevated in classic PNH. The degree of serum LDH elevation is variable in patients with PNH/aplastic anemia and PNH/MDS, depending on the size of the PNH clone (see Table 8-1). By definition, patients with PNH-sc have neither clinical nor biochemical evidence of hemolysis (see Table 8-1). Patients with classic PNH are often iron-deficient from chronic iron loss in the form of hemoglobinuria and hemosiderinuria (Chap. 10). Marrow aspirate and biopsy are needed to distinguish classic PNH from PNH in the setting of another marrow abnormality. Nonrandom cytogenetic abnormalities are rare in PNH.[32]

● DIFFERENTIAL DIAGNOSIS

PNH AND MARROW FAILURE

Although the marrow of patients with classic PNH appears to be relatively normal morphologically (see Table 8-1), numerous in vitro studies have shown that the growth characteristics of marrow-derived stem cells are aberrant.[27,54,55] Moreover, when stem cells are sorted into GPI-AP– and GPI-AP+ populations, compared with the GPI-AP+ population, the growth characteristics of the GPI-AP– population more closely approach those of normal control cells.[27,54] One plausible explanation for this observation is that the GPI-AP– cells are relatively protected from the pathophysiologic process that mediates the marrow injury, thereby providing a basis for natural selection of the *PIGA* mutant clone. According to this hypothesis, outgrowth of the *PIGA* mutant clone is an example of Darwinian evolution occurring within the microenvironment of the marrow. Although conceptually appealing, empiric support for this hypothesis is lacking.

A close association exists between PNH and aplastic anemia and to a lesser extent between PNH and low-risk MDS. By using high-resolution flow cytometry,[47] approximately 50% of patients with aplastic anemia and 15% of patients with low-risk MDS have been found to have a detectable population of GPI-AP–deficient erythrocytes and granulocytes.[43,44,47,56,57] In approximately 90% of these cases, the proportion of GPI-AP–deficient blood neutrophils is less than 25% of the total.[58] Patients with very small populations of GPI-AP–deficient erythrocytes (designated subclinical PNH) have no clinical or biochemical evidence of hemolysis and require no specific treatment for PNH (Table 8-1).

Studies have investigated the natural history of PNH clones in the setting of marrow failure.[56,58,59] The threshold that separates subclinical PNH from clinical PNH is reached when the neutrophil clone size is in the range of 25% with a corresponding GPI-AP–deficient erythrocyte population of 3% to 5%.[58] Longitudinal studies indicate that clonal expansion occurs in 15% to 50% of cases.[56,58,59] In 10% to 25% of cases,

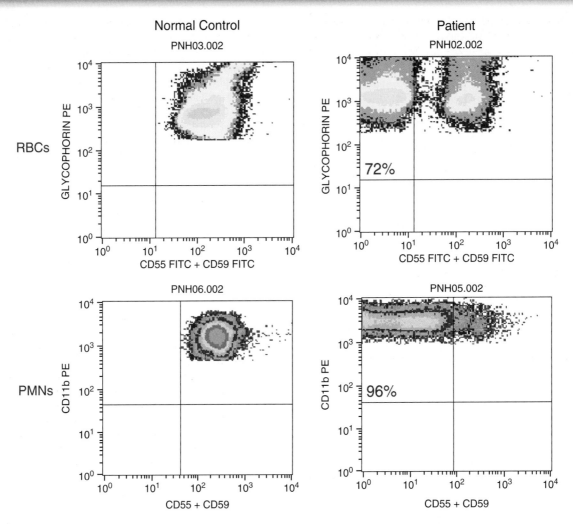

Figure 8–5. Diagnosis of paroxysmal nocturnal hemoglobinuria (PNH) by flow cytometry. Erythrocytes (RBCs) and neutrophils (PMNs) from a healthy volunteer and a patient with PNH were analyzed by flow cytometry using antiglycophorin A (*top row, vertical axis*) to identify RBCs and anti-CD11b (*bottom row, vertical axis*) to identify PMNs. GPI-AP expression was detected using a combination of anti-CD55 and anti-CD59 (*top and bottom rows, horizontal axis*). PNH cells are deficient in both CD55 and CD59 (*upper left quadrant of each histogram*). The percentage of GPI-AP–deficient (PNH) cells is shown for each sample.

TABLE 8–3. Basic Evaluation for PNH

Flow cytometric evidence of a population of erythrocytes and granulocytes partially or completely deficient in multiple GPI-APs[a]

Complete blood count, reticulocyte count, serum concentration of LDH[b], bilirubin (fractionated) and haptoglobin, determination of iron stores

Marrow aspirate, biopsy, and cytogenetics[c]

Abbreviations: GPI-APs, glycosyl phosphatidylinositol-anchored proteins; LDH, lactate dehydrogenase; PNH, paroxysmal nocturnal hemoglobinuria.

[a]PNH clone size is determined by the percentage of GPI-AP–deficient neutrophils.

[b]The most important surrogate marker for intravascular hemolysis.

[c]Marrow aspirate and biopsy are used to distinguish classic PNH from PNH in the setting of another marrow failure syndrome. Nonrandom karyotypic abnormalities are rare in PNH.

the clone disappears, and in 25% to 60% of cases, the clone size remains unchanged.[56,58,59] Available evidence indicates that patients who present with subclinical PNH do not progress to having clinical PNH.[56,58,59] Among patients who present with clinical PNH in the setting of marrow failure, treatment for complications of PNH (eculizumab for hemolysis or anticoagulation for thrombosis) is required in approximately 50% of cases.[59] There is no evidence that treatment with immunosuppressive therapy influences clonal expansion either positively or negatively.

The basis of the relationship between PNH and aplastic anemia is speculative. The vast majority of patients with PNH have some evidence of marrow failure (eg, thrombocytopenia, leukopenia, or both) during the course of their disease.[32,60,61] Therefore, marrow injury may play a central role in the development of PNH by providing the conditions that favor the growth/survival of *PIGA*-mutant, GPI-AP–deficient HS/PCs. Finding a population of GPI-AP–deficient erythrocytes in patients with aplastic anemia is clinically relevant, because these patients, compared with those with aplastic anemia without a PNH clone, have a higher probability of responding to immunosuppress3ive therapy, and the onset of the response is more rapid.[44,46,62]

The presence of PNH cells has also been observed in patients with MDS.[43,46,58,63] Notably, the association between PNH and MDS appears to be confined to low-risk categories of MDS, particularly what had formerly been classified as refractory anemia (RA).[43,46,57] Using high-sensitivity flow cytometry in which more than or at 0.003% of GPI-AP–deficient red cells or neutrophils was classified as abnormal, Wang and colleagues reported that 21 of 119 (18%) patients with RA MDS had a population of PNH cells, whereas GPI-AP–deficient cells were not detected in patients with refractory anemia with ringed sideroblast (RARS), refractory anemia with excess of blasts (RAEB), or refractory anemia with excess of blasts in transformation (RAEB-t).[57] Compared with patients with RA without a population of PNH cells (RA-PNH–), patients with RA with a population of PNH cells (RA-PNH+) had a distinct clinical profile characterized by the following features: (1) less pronounced morphologic abnormalities of blood cells, (2) more severe thrombocytopenia, (3) lower rates of karyotypic abnormalities, (4) higher incidence of human leukocyte antigen (HLA)-DR15, (5) lower rate of progression to acute leukemia, and (6) higher probability of response to cyclosporine therapy.[46]

That a population of PNH cells is associated only with low-risk MDS was confirmed in a North American study of 137 patients classified by World Health Organization (WHO) criteria.[57,64] The study found a population of PNH cells in 1 of 5 (20%) patients with 5q– syndrome, in 6 of 17 (35%) patients with RA, and in 2 of 37 (5%) patients with refractory cytopenias with multilineage dysplasia (RCMD), whereas no patient with RARS (0 of 9), RCMD-ringed sideroblasts (0 of 6), RAEB (0 of 26), MDS unspecified (0 of 10), MDS/myeloproliferative neoplasm (0 of 10), primary myelofibrosis (0 of 5), chronic myelomonocytic leukemia (0 of 5), or acute myeloid leukemia (0 of 6) had a detectable population of GPI-AP–deficient blood cells.[57]

When combined with evidence of polyclonal hematopoiesis (based on the pattern of X-chromosome inactivation in female patients), the presence of a population of PNH cells in patients with MDS predicts a relatively benign clinical course and a higher probability of response to immunosuppressive therapy.[43] A relatively good response to immunosuppressive therapy for patients with MDS and aplastic anemia was also predicted by expression of HLA-DR15 in studies of both North American and Japanese patients.[65,66] Together, these observations provide compelling indirect evidence that aplastic anemia and a subgroup of low-risk MDS are immune-mediated diseases and that the immune pathophysiologic process provides the selection pressure that favors the outgrowth of *PIGA* mutant, GPI-AP–deficient stem cells.

The hypothesis that immune attack is the basis for selection of *PIGA*-mutant HS/PC is supported by observations that loss of heterozygosity of HLA genes is present in some patients with aplastic anemia.[67,68] The altered pattern of HLA expression can occur as a result either of loss of heterozygosity,[68] as a consequence of homologous recombination, or of somatic mutation of the putative causal allele.[67]

●THERAPY

COMPLEMENT INHIBITORY THERAPY

The complement-mediated intravascular hemolysis of PNH can be inhibited by blocking formation of the terminal complement pathway–generated MAC, the cytolytic component of the complement system (see Fig. 8-1). The MAC consists of complement components C5b, C6, C7, C8, and multiple molecules of C9. Eculizumab is a humanized monoclonal antibody that binds to complement C5, preventing its activation to C5b and thereby inhibiting MAC formation (see Fig. 8-1).[69] In 2007, eculizumab was approved by both the US Food and Drug Administration (FDA) and the European Union Commission (now the

European Medicines Agency) for treatment of the hemolysis of PNH. Treatment with eculizumab reduces transfusion requirements, ameliorates the anemia of PNH, and markedly improves quality of life by resolving the debilitating constitutional symptoms (fatigue, lethargy, asthenia) associated with chronic complement-mediated intravascular hemolysis.[70] After treatment, serum LDH concentration returns to normal or near normal, but mild to moderate anemia and reticulocytosis usually persist, likely the result of ongoing extravascular hemolysis mediated by opsonization of PNH erythrocytes by activated complement C3, because eculizumab does not block the activity of the APC C3 convertase (see Fig. 8-1).[71,72] In some cases, extravascular hemolysis is severe enough to require therapy.[73]

Thromboembolic events are the major cause of morbidity and mortality in PNH,[41] and eculizumab appears to ameliorate the thrombophilia of PNH, although the studies supporting that conclusion had a suboptimal design.[74]

Eculizumab is given by intravenous infusion on a biweekly schedule after an initial loading period of five weekly treatments. In general, the drug is well tolerated; however, patients with congenital deficiency of complement C5 have an increased risk of infection with *Neisseria* species. Likewise, patients treated with eculizumab (which blocks the function of C5; see Fig. 8-1) are at risk for meningococcal septicemia. All patients must be inoculated with a meningococcal vaccine 2 weeks before starting therapy, but the vaccine is not 100% effective. Whether prophylactic antibiotic therapy with penicillin aimed at preventing meningococcal infection is justified for patients receiving eculizumab is a matter of debate. Pathologic strains of *Neisseria* that are not recognized by available vaccines have been identified in patients with PNH treated with eculizumab, and penicillin-resist *N meningitides* have appeared in patients receiving prophylactic therapy. Despite the fact that the percentage of GPI-AP–deficient erythrocytes increases during treatment with eculizumab,[75] there have been no reports of catastrophic hemolytic crises in the relatively few PNH patients who have discontinued treatment with eculizumab.[74,76]

Eculizumab is expensive (~$650,000/year in the United States), and it has no effect either on the underlying stem cell abnormality or on the associated marrow failure. Consequently, treatment must continue indefinitely and leukopenia, thrombocytopenia, and reticulocytopenia, if present, persist. Patients treated with eculizumab may become symptomatic (fatigue, lethargy, worsening anemia, hemoglobinuria) near the end of the 14-day treatment cycles. This process, called breakthrough hemolysis, is usually a pharmacokinetic issue, because in some patients, toward the end of the treatment cycle, the concentration of eculizumab falls below that required for complete inhibition of C5. This type of breakthrough hemolysis can be diagnosed by monitoring the CH_{50} or the concentration of free eculizumab.[77] Detectable levels of CH_{50} ($\geq 10\%$ of normal) and concentrations of eculizumab lower than 50 mcg/mL suggest suboptimal dosing of eculizumab. This issue can be addressed by increasing the dose of eculizumab from 900 mg every 2 weeks to 1200 mg every 2 weeks or by shorting the dosing interval from 14 days to 12 days. Breakthrough hemolysis can also occur when a patient has a complication, such as an intercurrent infection, that causes brisk complement activation. These patients may require additional eculizumab to control hemolysis until the inciting event has resolved as the risk of thrombosis increases in this setting.

Patients treated with eculizumab experience varying degrees of extravascular hemolysis as a result of C3 opsonization of PNH erythrocytes. Because affected erythrocytes lack both CD55 and CD59, control of the formation and stability of the APC C3 convertase is lost (see Fig. 8-1). When PNH red cells are protected from complement-mediated hemolysis by treatment with eculizumab, evidence of uncontrolled regulation of the APC C3 convertase in the form of C3 opsonized PNH red cells becomes apparent.[78] Depending upon the extent of C3 opsonization, some eculizumab-treated patients will become direct antiglobulin test–positive for C3, but not immunoglobulin G. The percentage of patients treated with eculizumab who remain transfusion-dependent because of extravascular hemolysis as a result of C3 opsonization is uncertain; however, there is much interest in developing anticomplement therapy aimed at blocking essential components of the APC C3 convertase, including C3 itself, factor B, factor D, and factor P (see Fig. 8-1). Some APC C3 convertase inhibitors are small molecules that are orally available. Conceivable APC C3 convertase inhibition could be used as monotherapy for treatment of PNH because convertase inhibition would also prevent assembly of the C5 convertase and thereby eliminate MAC formation. The APC C3 convertase inhibitors are currently in various stages of clinical development, but they will likely find their place in the treatment of PNH within the next few years.

In December 2018, the FDA approved ravulizumab for treatment of patients with PNH. Like eculizumab, ravulizumab is a humanized, monoclonal antibody that binds to complement C5, thereby preventing enzymatic cleavage by the C5 convertase and subsequent MAC formation. Ravulizumab was engineered to take advantage of immunoglobulin recycling by the neonatal Fc receptor. This modification extended the half-life of ravulizumab, allowing for dosing every 8 weeks (vs every 2 weeks for eculizumab). Clinical trials showed that ravulizumab is noninferior to eculizumab both in the treatment of patients whose disease was well controlled with eculizumab and in patients who were naïve to anticomplement therapy.[79,80] The cost of 1 year of treatment with ravulizumab is approximately 10% less than that of eculizumab.

OTHER TREATMENT FOR PNH

Other than eculizumab/ravulizumab, there is no specific treatment for PNH, and for patients who are not being treated with eculizumab/ravulizumab, treatment is largely supportive.[31] Although hemolysis is ameliorated in some patients by treatment with glucocorticoids or androgens, the use of these steroids in the management of patients with PNH is controversial.[41] The main value of glucocorticoids may be in attenuating acute hemolytic exacerbations. Under these circumstances, brief pulses of prednisone may reduce the severity and duration of the crisis. The value of glucocorticoids in treating chronic hemolysis is limited by toxicity, and the harm that can accrue from long-term use cannot be overemphasized. An every-other-day schedule may attenuate some of the adverse effects of chronic glucocorticoid use,[81] but patients may note worsening of symptoms on the off day.

Androgen therapy, either alone or in combination with glucocorticoids, has been used successfully to treat the anemia of PNH.[81,82] As with glucocorticoids, the mechanism by which androgenic steroids ameliorate the anemia of PNH is not fully understood, although the rapid onset of action is consistent with complement inhibition.[82] Potential complications of androgen therapy include liver toxicity, prostatic hypertrophy, and virilizing effects. The toxicity profile is more favorable for attenuated synthetic androgens such as danazol, making long-term use of this drug a reasonable management option in responding patients. A starting dose of 400 mg twice a day is recommended, but a lower dose (100-400 mg/day) may be adequate to control chronic hemolysis.[41]

Patients with PNH frequently become iron-deficient as a result of both hemoglobinuria and hemosiderinuria.[81,82] Clinically important iron loss from hemosiderinuria can occur (Chap. 11), even in the absence of gross hemoglobinuria. Replacement is often associated with exacerbation of hemolysis, regardless of the route of administration.[81,82] Compared with parenteral replacement, oral administration of iron may be accompanied by less severe hemolytic exacerbations, but urinary iron

loss may be so great that repletion may not be achieved.[81] Concern for inducing a hemolytic exacerbation should not deter iron repletion.[81] If a hemolytic exacerbation occurs in the setting of iron repletion, the episode can be controlled by treatment with glucocorticoids or androgens or by suppression of erythropoiesis by transfusion. There is no concern about iron-replacement therapy inducing a hemolytic exacerbation in patients being treated with eculizumab because hemolysis is inhibited by the drug.

Because the hemolysis is a consequence of a defect intrinsic to a patient's erythrocytes, the anemia of PNH responds to red cell transfusion. Concerns about inducing a hemolytic exacerbation as a consequence of infusion of small amounts of donor plasma that may be included in red cell preparations appear unwarranted.[83] However, hemofiltration is recommended to prevent transfusion reaction arising from the interaction between donor leukocytes and recipient antibodies. Iatrogenic hemochromatosis from chronic transfusion may be delayed in patients with PNH as a result of iron loss from hemoglobinuria/hemosiderinuria,[81] but iron overload remains a concern in patients who require chronic transfusion when the anemia is primarily a consequence of marrow failure rather than intravascular hemolysis.

Supplemental folate (1 mg/day) is recommended to compensate for increased utilization (Chap. 9) associated with heightened erythropoiesis that is a consequence of ongoing hemolysis.[41]

The role of splenectomy in the management of patients with PNH has not been investigated systematically. Reports of amelioration of hemolysis and improvement in cytopenias after splenectomy are anecdotal. Concerns about lack of proven efficacy and the potential for postoperative complications, particularly thrombosis, have led to the argument that splenectomy has no role in the management of PNH.[41]

ALLOGENEIC HEMATOPOIETIC STEM CELL TRANSPLANTATION

Before the availability of eculizumab, the primary indications for transplantation were marrow failure; recurrent, life-threatening thrombosis; and uncontrollable hemolysis (Table 8-4).[41] The latter process can be eliminated by treatment with eculizumab, and the thrombophilia of PNH may also respond to inhibition of intravascular hemolysis by eculizumab.[74,84] Nonetheless, transplant is the only curative therapy for PNH, and the availability of molecularly defined, matched, unrelated donors; less-toxic conditioning regimens; reduction in transplantation-related morbidity and mortality; and improvements in posttransplantation supportive care make this option a viable alternative to anticomplement therapy. Studies (see "Course and Prognosis" further) indicate a normal survival for patients with PNH treated with eculizumab, making the decision of whether to recommend anticomplement therapy or hematopoietic stem cell transplant particularly complex.[84] An understanding of the unique pathobiology of PNH and the input of physicians experienced in transplantation and nontransplant management of PNH are essential to develop an appropriate management plan for transplantation-eligible patients.[85]

For patients who are receiving transplantation for marrow failure, the focus of management is on the etiology of the marrow failure (see Table 8-4). For patients with aplastic anemia and a small PNH clone who undergo matched-sibling donor allotransplantation, the conditioning regimen of antithymocyte globulin and cyclophosphamide coupled with graft-versus-host effects appear sufficient to eradicate the PNH clone.[41] However, in the unusual situation in which the patient has a syngeneic twin, a more intense conditioning regimen is required, as graft-versus-PNH effect does not contribute to clonal eradication in this circumstance.[86] In the event that a patient with low-risk MDS with a PNH clone requires allotransplantation, the MDS conditioning

TABLE 8–4. Hematopoietic Stem Cell Transplantation for PNH

Indications for Transplantation

- Marrow failure—approach to management depends primarily on the underlying marrow abnormality (eg, aplastic anemia) but the treatment regimen must be sufficient to eradicate the PNH clone
- Major complications of PNH
- Refractory, transfusion-dependent hemolytic anemia[a]
- Recurrent, life-threatening thromboembolic complications[b]

Conditioning Regimens and Donors

- Ablative and reduced-intensity conditioning regimens have been successful
- For transplantations involving syngeneic twins, an ablative regimen is recommended[c]
- Matched unrelated donor transplantations have been successful, but experience is limited

Outcomes

- There are no PNH-specific adverse events. Severe, acute graft-versus-host disease occurs in approximately 33% of patients, and the incidence of chronic graft-versus-host disease is roughly 35%
- Overall survival for unselected PNH patients who undergo transplantation using an HLA-matched sibling donor is in the range of 50%-60%

Abbreviations: HLA, human leukocyte antigen; PNH, paroxysmal nocturnal hemoglobinuria.

[a]Treatment with eculizumab controls the intravascular hemolysis of PNH. Mild to moderate extravascular hemolytic anemia persists in most patients with PNH treated with eculizumab, likely as a consequence of opsonization of erythrocytes by activation and degradation products of complement C3.

[b]Eculizumab may ameliorate the thrombophilia of PNH.

[c]Absence of graft-versus-host effect may render nonablative approaches inadequate.

regimen (marrow ablative or reduced intensity) in combination with graft-versus-tumor effects is sufficient to eradicate the PNH clone.

Transplantation for classic PNH is aimed at eradicating the PNH clone, and both marrow-ablative[87-89] and reduced-intensity[90,91] conditioning regimens are effective, although experience with the latter is more limited. Successful outcomes have been reported using matched-unrelated donors and matched-sibling donors.[90,92] There are no PNH-specific adverse events associated with transplantation; severe, acute graft-versus-host disease (GVHD) occurs in more than approximately one-third of the patients, and the incidence of chronic GVHD is about 35%. Overall survival for unselected PNH patients who undergo transplantation using a HLA-matched sibling donor is in the range of 50% to 60%.[41]

MANAGEMENT OF THE THROMBOPHILIA OF PNH

Thromboembolic complications are the leading cause of morbidity and mortality in PNH.[22] Prophylaxis against thromboembolic events in patients with PNH is actively debated.[22] Current estimates of risk are based on retrospective analyses,[74,93-96] but risk may correlate with size of the PNH clone (based on flow cytometric determination of the percentage of GPI-AP–deficient neutrophils), leading to the recommendation that patients with more than 50% to 60% GPI-AP–deficient neutrophils be offered prophylactic anticoagulation.[93,94] Treatment with warfarin with a goal international normalized ratio (INR) of between 2.0 and 3.0 is recommended for patients with PNH who require chronic anticoagulation either for treatment of a thromboembolic event or for prophylaxis. There are no evidence-based data to guide the use of low-molecular-weight heparin or direct oral anticoagulants in these settings, but their use can be considered in patients with adequate renal function in whom warfarin fails or in patients who have difficulty maintaining a consistent therapeutic INR.

Although arterial thrombosis may be observed,[74] thromboembolic events in patients with PNH usually involve the venous system. Acute thrombotic events require anticoagulation with heparin. Systemic thrombolytic therapy,[97,98] or thrombolytic therapy delivered via canalization directly to the affected site,[99] should be strongly considered in patients with acute onset of Budd-Chiari syndrome. In Budd-Chiari syndrome unresponsive to medical therapy, the use of a transjugular intrahepatic shunt should be considered. This technique can lower the portal vein pressure significantly and with periodic nonsurgical revisions as necessary can be effective for over several years in many patients.

Thrombocytopenia often complicates PNH, and this issue must be addressed when formulating an anticoagulation management plan. Thrombocytopenia is a relative contraindication to anticoagulation, and transfusions should be given to maintain the platelet count in a safe range rather than withholding therapy.[100] Patients with PNH who experience a thromboembolic event should be anticoagulated indefinitely. Recurrent, life-threatening thrombosis merits consideration of marrow transplantation, but such patients are at high risk for transplantation-related adverse events (see Table 8-4).[85]

Eculizumab reduces the risk of thromboembolic complications.[74] For patients being treated with eculizumab/ravulizumab who have no prior history of thromboembolic complications, prophylactic anticoagulation may not be necessary.

PREGNANCY AND PNH

Women with PNH can have serious morbidity and increased mortality during pregnancy.[100,101] Because of concerns about fetal/maternal risks from exposure to potentially toxic therapy, anticoagulation and transfusion have been the mainstay of management. Eculizumab has been assigned to pregnancy category C (risk cannot be ruled out) by the FDA; however, recent studies suggest that eculizumab is safe for use during pregnancy.[102,103] A survey involving members of the International PNH Interest Group and physicians participating in an International PNH Registry (75 pregnancies in patients treated with eculizumab) found that 8% (6 cases) of the 75 pregnancies included in the study resulted in a first-trimester miscarriage, stillbirths were reported in 4% (including one case in a set of twins), 54% experienced breakthrough hemolysis and required a higher dose of eculizumab or a decrease in the dosing interval, and 9% required transfusions during pregnancy.[102] The survey reported a 29% rate of premature birth, with no apparent trend for cause of premature delivery. There were no reported thrombotic episodes during pregnancy, but two thrombotic events occurred early in the postpartum period. Low-molecular-weight heparin was used in 88% of pregnancies, with 10 hemorrhagic events reported. Twenty cord-blood samples were assayed for eculizumab; the drug was detected in seven of the samples. A total of 25 infants were breastfed, and in 10 of these cases, breast milk was examined for the presence of eculizumab; the drug was not detected in any of the 10 breast milk samples. Other small series and anecdotal reports suggest that PNH is safe for use during pregnancy.[71,104-106]

Moderate to severe thrombocytopenia may complicate the pregnancy, and clinically significant bleeding in this setting necessitates platelet transfusion. The incidence of clinically apparent venous thromboembolism during pregnancy in women with PNH not treated with eculizumab is approximately 10%,[100] and these events are associated with a high risk of mortality.[100,101] Similar to nonpregnant patients with PNH, cerebral and hepatic veins are commonly involved sites of thrombosis during pregnancy and the postpartum period, and thrombolytic therapy should be considered for those with Budd-Chiari syndrome.

The role of prophylactic anticoagulation for pregnant women with PNH has not been studied prospectively; however, because of the significant morbidity and mortality associated with thromboembolism in this setting, prophylaxis is recommended. Coumadin is contraindicated because of teratogenic potential in the first trimester and hemorrhagic risks later in gestation. Anticoagulation with heparin should begin immediately once pregnancy is confirmed. Low-molecular-weight heparin has a hypothetical advantage over unfractionated heparin because of a lower incidence of drug-induced thrombocytopenia. Careful monitoring of the platelet count is required because thrombocytopenia may worsen during the period of anticoagulation. Anticoagulation can be discontinued briefly around the time of delivery. However, it should be restarted as soon as is feasible and continued for 3 months into the postpartum period, because thrombosis during the puerperium is a major concern.[100-102]

The management team for pregnant patients with PNH should include an obstetrician experienced in the care of patients with high-risk pregnancies, because PNH-associated smooth muscle dystonia may result in uterine/cervical dystocia that may affect labor and delivery.[103] Vaginal delivery is recommended for these patients, and delivery should be planned to accommodate ongoing prophylactic anticoagulation requirements. No PNH-specific treatment is recommended for pregnant patients with subclinical PNH. Treatment with eculizumab is not warranted, and the decision about anticoagulation should not include consideration of the thrombophilic risk associated with PNH. Management involves focusing on the etiology and complications of bone marrow failure, such as thrombocytopenia, anemia, and leukopenia. Approximately 10% of patients with aplastic anemia or low-risk MDS have a PNH clone size smaller than 25%, which is the threshold for biochemical evidence of hemolysis (ie, elevated LDH and bilirubin, decreased haptoglobin). In these patients, treatment with eculizumab and anticoagulation should be initiated or continued during pregnancy. The dose of eculizumab should be modified based on an LDH goal of lower than 1.5 times the upper limit of normal and a CH50 goal of less than 10%. The same treatment paradigm should be used to treat pregnant patients with classic PNH. Despite the many concerns surrounding PNH and pregnancy, successful outcomes appear to be the rule rather than the exception.[95,100,102]

PEDIATRIC PNH

PNH can occur in the young (approximately 10% of patients are younger than 21 years at the time of diagnosis).[41] A retrospective analysis of 26 cases underscored the many similarities between childhood and adult PNH.[107] Signs and symptoms of hemolysis, marrow failure, and thrombosis dominate the clinical picture, although gross hemoglobinuria as a presenting symptom may be less common in young patients. A generally good response to immunosuppressive therapy was observed,[107] but based on poor long-term survival, hematopoietic stem cell transplantation is the recommended treatment for childhood PNH. One study[108] confirmed the common presentation of marrow failure in 11 children with PNH, and reported that 5 patients eventually underwent hematopoietic stem cell transplant (3 matched unrelated donors and 2 matched

family donors), of whom 4 were long-term survivors. In another study of 12 young patients over an 18-year period, 10 presented with evidence of bone marrow failure and only one with hemoglobinuria.[58] There were 6 children with thrombosis and 5 with MDS features, indicating that the clinical presentation may be more similar to adult PNH than previously recognized. Other retrospective studies have reported features similar to those described earlier for pediatric PNH.[109] The safety and effectiveness of eculizumab in pediatric patients younger than 18 years has not been established; however, there are anecdotal reports of its use in pediatric patients with PNH.[110] Although eculizumab is not approved for PNH patients younger than 18 years, approval will likely be sought once pharmacodynamic and pharmacokinetic characteristics of the drug are defined for the pediatric/adolescent population.[111] The availability of eculizumab for pediatric PNH may be particularly advantageous as a bridge before implementation of more definitive therapy (stem cell transplantation). Ravulizumab has not been approved for children with PNH, but has been approved for use in children 1month of age or older with atypical hemolytic uremic syndrome.

COURSE AND PROGNOSIS

As with so many other diseases, initial reports of PNH tended to emphasize the more severely affected patients, so the prognosis was generally deemed to be grave. As physicians developed a higher index of suspicion, and as simplified methods for diagnosis became available, milder cases were diagnosed that had a better long-term outlook. Nonetheless, even today, PNH must be considered a serious disease. The most common lethal event is a thrombotic episode such as the Budd-Chiari syndrome,[19,96,112] but the various complications of pancytopenia may also lead to death,[42,61] and in a few patients, the terminal process is development of acute leukemia.[64] In a study of 220 patients with PNH followed for up to 46 years in the pre-eculizumab era, the Kaplan-Meier survival estimate was 65% at 10 years and 48% at 15 years after diagnosis.[112] In another pre-eculizumab era study of 80 consecutive patients, the outlook was similar: the median survival after diagnosis was 10 years, with 28% of patients surviving for 25 years.[61] Eight-year cumulative incidence rates of the main complications of pancytopenia, thrombosis, and MDS were 15%, 28%, and 5%, respectively. Poor survival was associated with patients older than 55 years at the time of diagnosis; the occurrence of thrombosis as a disease complication; progression to pancytopenia, MDS, or acute leukemia; and thrombocytopenia at diagnosis. The prognosis of patients in whom aplastic anemia antedated PNH was better than in those in whom it did not.[112]

In addition to symptomatic benefit, treatment with eculizumab appears to influence the natural history of PNH. In a retrospective study of the clinical history of 79 patients with classic PNH or PNH/bone marrow failure treated with eculizumab, the median age at diagnosis was 37 years (range, 12-79) and the median age at the time of initiation of treatment with eculizumab was 46 years (range, 14-84).[65] The mean duration of treatment with eculizumab was 39 months (range, 1-98). Based on flow cytometric analysis of blood neutrophils, the average clone size among the treated patients was 96.4% (range, 41.8%-100%). Twenty-four patients (30%) had a history of a marrow failure syndrome at the time of diagnosis (23 with aplastic anemia and 1 with MDS). Thrombotic episodes were reported in 27% of patients before starting eculizumab (including 12 cases of Budd-Chiari syndrome, 4 cases of mesenteric vein thrombosis, and 3 cases of cerebral vein thrombosis). The investigators found that treatment with eculizumab reduced the mean yearly transfusion requirement from 19.3 units to 5.0 units. Of 61 patients who had been treated with eculizumab for more than 1 year, 40 (66%) became transfusion-independent. Thrombosis was observed in two patients while receiving eculizumab. No thrombotic events were reported in 21 patients who discontinued prophylactic anticoagulation after starting treatment with eculizumab.

Survival of the 79 patients treated with eculizumab was the same as that of a group of age- and sex-matched controls from the general population. Meningococcal infection with *N meningitides* serogroup B developed in two patients treated with eculizumab, and thereafter, a program of antibiotic prophylaxis was instituted by the investigators. A multicenter study involving 195 patients followed over 66 months confirmed these findings.[113]

Together, these results demonstrate that treatment with eculizumab alters the natural history of PNH both by reducing or eliminating transfusion requirements through inhibition of intravascular hemolysis and by markedly lessening thromboembolic complications. Eculizumab treatment may also reduce disease-related mortality, although the extent to which the drug enhances survival cannot be accurately determined from these studies, because the experimental design did not include a randomized control group of patients. Eculizumab does not appear to affect either the marrow failure component of the disease or the clonal hematopoiesis that underlies disease pathophysiology. As previously discussed, although PNH is a clonal disease, it is not a malignant disease, and it is this characteristic of PNH that allows for successful long-term symptomatic management in the absence of a treatment strategy aimed at eradicating the *PIGA* mutant hematopoietic stem cells.

REFERENCES

1. Crosby WH. Paroxysmal nocturnal hemoglobinuria; a classic description by Paul Strubling in 1882, and a bibliography of the disease. *Blood.* 1951;6:270-284.
2. Parker CJ. Historical aspects of paroxysmal nocturnal haemoglobinuria: 'defining the disease'. *Br J Haematol.* 2002;117:3-22.
3. Parker CJ. Paroxysmal nocturnal hemoglobinuria: an historical overview. *Hematology Am Soc Hematol Educ Program.* 2008;2008:93-103.
4. Rosse W. *A Brief History of PNH. PNH and the GPI-Linked Proteins.* Academic Press; 2000:1-20.
5. Hughes DA, Tunnage B, Yeo ST. Drugs for exceptionally rare diseases: do they deserve special status for funding? *QJM.* 2005;98:829-836.
6. Parker CJ. Hemolysis in PNH. In: Young NS, Moss J, eds. *Paroxysmal Nocturnal Hemoglobinuria and the GPI-Linked Proteins.* Academic Press; 2000:49-100.
7. Thurman JM, Holers VM. The central role of the alternative complement pathway in human disease. *J Immunol.* 2006;176:1305-1310.
8. Nicholson-Weller A, Burge J, Fearon DT, et al. Isolation of a human erythrocyte membrane glycoprotein with decay-accelerating activity for C3 convertases of the complement system. *J Immunol.* 1982;129:184-189.
9. Nicholson-Weller A, March JP, Rosenfeld SI, Austen KF. Affected erythrocytes of patients with paroxysmal nocturnal hemoglobinuria are deficient in the complement regulatory protein, decay accelerating factor. *Proc Natl Acad Sci U S A.* 1983;80:5066-5070.
10. Pangburn MK, Schreiber RD, Muller-Eberhard HJ. Deficiency of an erythrocyte membrane protein with complement regulatory activity in paroxysmal nocturnal hemoglobinuria. *Proc Natl Acad Sci U S A.* 1983;80:5430-5434.
11. Holguin MH, Fredrick LR, Bernshaw NJ, Wilcox LA, Parker CJ. Isolation and characterization of a membrane protein from normal human erythrocytes that inhibits reactive lysis of the erythrocytes of paroxysmal nocturnal hemoglobinuria. *J Clin Invest.* 1989;84:7-17.
12. Wilcox LA, Ezzell JL, Bernshaw NJ, Parker CJ. Molecular basis of the enhanced susceptibility of the erythrocytes of paroxysmal nocturnal hemoglobinuria to hemolysis in acidified serum. *Blood.* 1991;78:820-829.
13. Kinoshita T, Inoue N, Takeda J. Defective glycosyl phosphatidylinositol anchor synthesis and paroxysmal nocturnal hemoglobinuria. *Adv Immunol.* 1995;60:57-103.
14. Miyata T, Takeda J, Iida Y, et al. The cloning of PIG-A, a component in the early step of GPI-anchor biosynthesis. *Science.* 1993;259:1318-1320.
15. Miyata T, Yamada N, Iida Y, et al. Abnormalities of PIG-A transcripts in granulocytes from patients with paroxysmal nocturnal hemoglobinuria. *N Engl J Med.* 1994;330:249-255.
16. Takahashi M, Takeda J, Hirose S, et al. Deficient biosynthesis of N-acetylglucosaminyl-phosphatidylinositol, the first intermediate of glycosyl phosphatidylinositol anchor biosynthesis, in cell lines established from patients with paroxysmal nocturnal hemoglobinuria. *J Exp Med.* 1993;177:517-521.
17. Takeda J, Miyata T, Kawagoe K, et al. Deficiency of the GPI anchor caused by a somatic mutation of the PIG-A gene in paroxysmal nocturnal hemoglobinuria. *Cell.* 1993;73:703-711.
18. Parker CJ. The pathophysiology of paroxysmal nocturnal hemoglobinuria. *Exp Hematol.* 2007;35:523-533.
19. Takamasa Katagiri, Aiko Sato-Otsubo, Koichi Kashiwase, et al. Frequent loss of HLA alleles associated with copy number-neutral 6pLOH in acquired aplastic anemia. *Blood.* 2011;118:6601-6609.
20. Yasutaka Ueda, Jun-ichi Nishimura, Yoshiko Murakami, et al. Paroxysmal nocturnal hemoglobinuria with copy number-neutral 6pLOH in GPI (+) but not in GPI (−) granulocytes, *Eur J Haematol.* 2013;92:450-453..
21. Daria V. Babushok, Jamie L. Duke, Hongbo M. Xie, et al. Somatic HLA mutations expose the role of class I–mediated autoimmunity in aplastic anemia and its clonal complications. *Blood Adv.* 2017;22:1900-1910.
22. Hill A, Kelly RJ, Hillmen P. Thrombosis in paroxysmal nocturnal hemoglobinuria. *Blood.* 2013;121:4985-4996; quiz 5105.
23. Krawitz PM, Hochsmann B, Murakami Y, et al. A case of paroxysmal nocturnal hemoglobinuria caused by a germline mutation and a somatic mutation in PIGT. *Blood.* 2013;122:1312-1315.
24. Hochsmann B, Murakami Y, Osato M, et al. Complement and inflammasome overactivation mediates paroxysmal nocturnal hemoglobinuria with autoinflammation. *J Clin Invest.* 2019;129:5123-5136.
25. Rosti V, Tremml G, Soares V, Pandolfi PP, Luzzatto L, Bessler M. Murine embryonic stem cells without pig-a gene activity are competent for hematopoiesis with the PNH phenotype but not for clonal expansion. *J Clin Invest.* 1997;100:1028-1036.
26. Brodsky RA, Vala MS, Barber JP, Medof ME, Jones RJ. Resistance to apoptosis caused by PIG-A gene Dear Vivien, mutations in paroxysmal nocturnal hemoglobinuria. *Proc Natl Acad Sci U S A.* 1997;94:8756-8760.
27. Chen R, Nagarajan S, Prince GM, et al. Impaired growth and elevated fas receptor expression in PIGA(+) stem cells in primary paroxysmal nocturnal hemoglobinuria. *J Clin Invest.* 2000;106:689-696.
28. Heeney MM, Ormsbee SM, Moody MA, Howard TA, DeCastro CM, Ware RE. Increased expression of anti-apoptosis genes in peripheral blood cells from patients with paroxysmal nocturnal hemoglobinuria. *Mol Genet Metab.* 2003;78:291-294.
29. Horikawa K, Nakakuma H, Kawaguchi T, et al. Apoptosis resistance of blood cells from patients with paroxysmal nocturnal hemoglobinuria, aplastic anemia, and myelodysplastic syndrome. *Blood.* 1997;90:2716-2722.
30. Ware RE, Nishimura J, Moody MA, Smith C, Rosse WF, Howard TA. The PIG-A mutation and absence of glycosylphosphatidylinositol-linked proteins do not confer resistance to apoptosis in paroxysmal nocturnal hemoglobinuria. *Blood.* 1998;92:2541-2550.
31. Yamamoto T, Shichishima T, Shikama Y, Saitoh Y, Ogawa K, Maruyama Y. Granulocytes from patients with paroxysmal nocturnal hemoglobinuria and normal individuals have the same sensitivity to spontaneous apoptosis. *Exp Hematol.* 2002;30:187-194.
32. Inoue N, Izui-Sarumaru T, Murakami Y, et al. Molecular basis of clonal expansion of hematopoiesis in 2 patients with paroxysmal nocturnal hemoglobinuria (PNH). *Blood.* 2006;108:4232-4236.
33. Shen W, Clemente MJ, Hosono N, et al. Deep sequencing reveals stepwise mutation acquisition in paroxysmal nocturnal hemoglobinuria. *J Clin Invest.* 2014;124:4529-4538.
34. Yoshizato T, Dumitriu B, Hosokawa K, et al. Somatic mutations and clonal hematopoiesis in aplastic anemia. *N Engl J Med.* 2015;373:35-47.
35. Durrani J, Maciejewski JP. Idiopathic aplastic anemia vs hypocellular myelodysplastic syndrome. *Hematology Am Soc Hematol Educ Program.* 2019;2019:97-104.
36. Murakami Y, Inoue N, Shichishima T, et al. Deregulated expression of HMGA2 is implicated in clonal expansion of PIGA deficient cells in paroxysmal nocturnal haemoglobinuria. *Br J Haematol.* 2012;156:383-387.
37. Cavazzana-Calvo M, Payen E, Negre O, et al. Transfusion independence and HMGA2 activation after gene therapy of human beta-thalassaemia. *Nature.* 2010;467:318-322.
38. Ikeda K, Mason PJ, Bessler M. 3'UTR-truncated Hmga2 cDNA causes MPN-like hematopoiesis by conferring a clonal growth advantage at the level of HSC in mice. *Blood.* 2011;117:5860-5869.
39. Kumar P, Beck D, Galeev R, et al. HMGA2 promotes long-term engraftment and myeloerythroid differentiation of human hematopoietic stem and progenitor cells. *Blood Adv.* 2019;3:681-691.
40. Endo M, Ware RE, Vreeke TM, et al. Molecular basis of the heterogeneity of expression of glycosyl phosphatidylinositol anchored proteins in paroxysmal nocturnal hemoglobinuria. *Blood.* 1996;87:2546-2557.
41. Parker C, Omine M, Richards S, et al. Diagnosis and management of paroxysmal nocturnal hemoglobinuria. *Blood.* 2005;106:3699-3709.
42. Dacie JV, Lewis SM. Paroxysmal nocturnal haemoglobinuria: clinical manifestations, haematology, and nature of the disease. *Ser Haematol.* 1972;5:3-23.
43. Ishiyama K, Chuhjo T, Wang H, Yachie A, Omine M, Nakao S. Polyclonal hematopoiesis maintained in patients with bone marrow failure harboring a minor population of paroxysmal nocturnal hemoglobinuria-type cells. *Blood.* 2003;102:1211-1216.
44. Sugimori C, Chuhjo T, Feng X, et al. Minor population of CD55-CD59- blood cells predicts response to immunosuppressive therapy and prognosis in patients with aplastic anemia. *Blood.* 2006;107:1308-1314.
45. Timeus F, Crescenzio N, Longoni D, et al. Paroxysmal nocturnal hemoglobinuria clones in children with acquired aplastic anemia: a multicentre study. *PLoS One.* 2014;9:e101948.
46. Wang H, Chuhjo T, Yasue S, Omine M, Nakao S. Clinical significance of a minor population of paroxysmal nocturnal hemoglobinuria-type cells in bone marrow failure syndrome. *Blood.* 2002;100:3897-3902.
47. Borowitz MJ, Craig FE, Digiuseppe JA, et al. Guidelines for the diagnosis and monitoring of paroxysmal nocturnal hemoglobinuria and related disorders by flow cytometry. *Cytometry B Clin Cytom.* 2010;78:211-230.

48. Richards SJ, Rawstron AC, Hillmen P. Application of flow cytometry to the diagnosis of paroxysmal nocturnal hemoglobinuria. *Cytometry*. 2000;42:223-233.

49. Dezern AE, Borowitz MJ. ICCS/ESCCA consensus guidelines to detect GPI-deficient cells in paroxysmal nocturnal hemoglobinuria (PNH) and related disorders part 1—clinical utility. *Cytometry B Clin Cytom*. 2018;94:16-22.

50. Mevorach D. Paroxysmal nocturnal hemoglobinuria (PNH) and primary p.Cys89Tyr mutation in CD59: Differences and similarities. *Mol Immunol*. 2015;67:51-55.

51. Lee SC, Abdel-Wahab O. The mutational landscape of paroxysmal nocturnal hemoglobinuria revealed: new insights into clonal dominance. *J Clin Invest*. 2014;124:4227-4230.

52. Brodsky RA, Mukhina GL, Nelson KL, Lawrence TS, Jones RJ, Buckley JT. Resistance of paroxysmal nocturnal hemoglobinuria cells to the glycosylphosphatidylinositol-binding toxin aerolysin. *Blood*. 1999;93:1749-1756.

53. Brodsky RA, Mukhina GL, Li S, et al. Improved detection and characterization of paroxysmal nocturnal hemoglobinuria using fluorescent aerolysin. *Am J Clin Pathol*. 2000;114:459-466.

54. Chen D, Kirby M, Zeng W, Young NS, Maciejewski JP. Superior growth of glycophosphatidy linositol-anchored protein-deficient progenitor cells in vitro is due to the higher apoptotic rate of progenitors with normal phenotype in vivo. *Exp Hematol*. 2002;30:774-782.

55. Dunn DE, Liu JM, Young NS. Bone Marrow Failure in PNH. In: Young NS, Moss J, eds. *Paroxysmal Nocturnal Hemoglobinuria and the GPI-Linked Proteins*. Academic Press; 2000:113-138.

56. Sugimori C, Mochizuki K, Qi Z, et al. Origin and fate of blood cells deficient in glycosylphosphatidylinositol-anchored protein among patients with bone marrow failure. *Br J Haematol*. 2009;147:102-112.

57. Wang SA, Pozdnyakova O, Jorgensen JL, et al. Detection of paroxysmal nocturnal hemoglobinuria clones in patients with myelodysplastic syndromes and related bone marrow diseases, with emphasis on diagnostic pitfalls and caveats. *Haematologica*. 2009;94:29-37.

58. Curran KJ, Kernan NA, Prockop SE, et al. Paroxysmal nocturnal hemoglobinuria in pediatric patients. *Pediatr Blood Cancer*. 2012;59:525-529.

59. Scheinberg P, Marte M, Nunez O, Young NS. Paroxysmal nocturnal hemoglobinuria clones in severe aplastic anemia patients treated with horse anti-thymocyte globulin plus cyclosporine. *Haematologica*. 2010;95:1075-1080.

60. de Latour RP, Mary JY, Salanoubat C, et al. Paroxysmal nocturnal hemoglobinuria: natural history of disease subcategories. *Blood*. 2008;112:3099-3106.

61. Hillmen P, Lewis SM, Bessler M, Luzzatto L, Dacie JV. Natural history of paroxysmal nocturnal hemoglobinuria. *N Engl J Med*. 1995;333:1253-1258.

62. Kulagin A, Lisukov I, Ivanova M, et al. Prognostic value of paroxysmal nocturnal haemoglobinuria clone presence in aplastic anaemia patients treated with combined immunosuppression: results of two-centre prospective study. *Br J Haematol*. 2014;164:546-554.

63. Dunn DE, Tanawattanacharoen P, Boccuni P, et al. Paroxysmal nocturnal hemoglobinuria cells in patients with bone marrow failure syndromes. *Ann Intern Med*. 1999;131:401-408.

64. Harris JW, Koscick R, Lazarus HM, Eshleman JR, Medof ME. Leukemia arising out of paroxysmal nocturnal hemoglobinuria. *Leuk Lymphoma*. 1999;32:401-426.

65. Saunthararajah Y, Nakamura R, Nam JM, et al. HLA-DR15 (DR2) is overrepresented in myelodysplastic syndrome and aplastic anemia and predicts a response to immunosuppression in myelodysplastic syndrome. *Blood*. 2002;100:1570-1574.

66. Sugimori C, Yamazaki H, Feng X et al. Roles of DRB1 *1501 and DRB1 *1502 in the pathogenesis of aplastic anemia. *Exp Hematol*. 2007 5:13-20.

67. Imi T, Katagiri T, Hosomichi K, et al. Sustained clonal hematopoiesis by HLA-lacking hematopoietic stem cells without driver mutations in aplastic anemia. *Blood Adv*. 2018;2:1000-1012.

68. Katagiri T, Sato-Otsubo A, Kashiwase K, et al. Frequent loss of HLA alleles associated with copy number-neutral 6pLOH in acquired aplastic anemia. *Blood*. 2011;118:6601-6609.

69. Parker C. Eculizumab for paroxysmal nocturnal haemoglobinuria. *Lancet*. 2009;373:759-767.

70. Hillmen P, Young NS, Schubert J, et al. The complement inhibitor eculizumab in paroxysmal nocturnal hemoglobinuria. *N Engl J Med*. 2006;355:1233-1243.

71. Marasca R, Coluccio V, Santachiara R, et al. Pregnancy in PNH: another eculizumab baby. *Br J Haematol*. 2010;150:707-708.

72. Parker CJ. Thanks for the complement (inhibitor). *Blood*. 2011;118:4503-4504.

73. Risitano AM, Marando L, Seneca E, Rotoli B. Hemoglobin normalization after splenectomy in a paroxysmal nocturnal hemoglobinuria patient treated by eculizumab. *Blood*. 2008;112:449-451.

74. Hillmen P, Muus P, Duhrsen U, et al. Effect of the complement inhibitor eculizumab on thromboembolism in patients with paroxysmal nocturnal hemoglobinuria. *Blood*. 2007;110:4123-4128.

75. Hillmen P, Hall C, Marsh JC, et al. Effect of eculizumab on hemolysis and transfusion requirements in patients with paroxysmal nocturnal hemoglobinuria. *N Engl J Med*. 2004;350:552-559.

76. Ferreira VP, Pangburn MK. Factor H mediated cell surface protection from complement is critical for the survival of PNH erythrocytes. *Blood*. 2007;110:2190-2192.

77. Peffault de Latour R, Fremeaux-Bacchi V, Porcher R, et al. Assessing complement blockade in patients with paroxysmal nocturnal hemoglobinuria receiving eculizumab. *Blood*. 2015;125:775-783.

78. Risitano AM, Notaro R, Marando L, et al. Complement fraction 3 binding on erythrocytes as additional mechanism of disease in paroxysmal nocturnal hemoglobinuria patients treated by eculizumab. *Blood*. 2009;113:4094-4100.

79. Lee JW, Sicre de Fontbrune F, Lee LW, et al. Ravulizumab (ALXN1210) vs eculizumab in adult patients with PNH naive to complement inhibitors: the 301 study. *Blood*. 2019;133:530-539.

80. Kulasekararaj AG, Hill A, Rottinghaus ST, et al. Ravulizumab (ALXN1210) vs eculizumab in C5-inhibitor-experienced adult patients with PNH: the 302 study. *Blood*. 2019;133:540-549.

81. Rosse WF. Treatment of paroxysmal nocturnal hemoglobinuria. *Blood*. 1982;60:20-23.

82. Hartmann RC, Jenkins DE, Jr., McKee LC, Heyssel RM. Paroxysmal nocturnal hemoglobinuria: clinical and laboratory studies relating to iron metabolism and therapy with androgen and iron. *Medicine (Baltimore)*. 1966;45:331-363.

83. Brecher ME, Taswell HF. Paroxysmal nocturnal hemoglobinuria and the transfusio of washed red cells: a myth revisited. *Transfusion*. 1989;29:681-685.

84. Kelly RJ, Hill A, Arnold LM, et al. Long-term treatment with eculizumab in paroxysmal nocturnal hemoglobinuria: sustained efficacy and improved survival. *Blood*. 2011;117:6786-6792.

85. Peffault de Latour R, Schrezenmeier H, Bacigalupo A, et al. Allogeneic stem cell transplantation in paroxysmal nocturnal hemoglobinuria. *Haematologica*. 2012;97:1666-1673.

86. Endo M, Beatty PG, Vreeke TM, Wittwer CT, Singh SP, Parker CJ. Syngeneic bone marrow transplantation without conditioning in a patient with paroxysmal nocturnal hemoglobinuria: in vivo evidence that the mutant stem cells have a survival advantage. *Blood*. 1996;88:742-750.

87. Bemba M, Guardiola P, Garderet L, et al. Bone marrow transplantation for paroxysmal nocturnal haemoglobinuria. *Br J Haematol*. 1999;105:366-368.

88. Hegenbart U, Niederwieser D, Forman S, et al. Hematopoietic cell transplantation from related and unrelated donors after minimal conditioning as a curative treatment modality for severe paroxysmal nocturnal hemoglobinuria. *Biol Blood Marrow Transplant*. 2003;9:689-697.

89. Raiola AM, Van Lint MT, Lamparelli T, et al. Bone marrow transplantation for paroxysmal nocturnal hemoglobinuria. *Haematologica*. 2000;85:59-62.

90. Saso R, Marsh J, Cevreska L, et al. Bone marrow transplants for paroxysmal nocturnal haemoglobinuria. *Br J Haematol*. 1999;104:392-396.

91. Takahashi Y, McCoy JP, Jr., Carvallo C, et al. In vitro and in vivo evidence of PNH cell sensitivity to immune attack after nonmyeloablative allogeneic hematopoietic cell transplantation. *Blood*. 2004;103:1383-1390.

92. Woodard P, Wang W, Pitts N, et al. Successful unrelated donor bone marrow transplantation for paroxysmal nocturnal hemoglobinuria. *Bone Marrow Transplant*. 2001;27:589-592.

93. Hall C, Richards S, Hillmen P. Primary prophylaxis with warfarin prevents thrombosis in paroxysmal nocturnal hemoglobinuria (PNH). *Blood*. 2003;102:3587-3591.

94. Moyo VM, Mukina, G. L., Barrett, E. S., Brodsky, R. A. Natural history of paroxysmal nocturnal haemoglobinuria using modern diagnostic assays. *Br J Haematol*. 2004;126:133-138.

95. Nishimura JI, Kanakura Y, Ware RE, et al. Clinical course and flow cytometric analysis of paroxysmal nocturnal hemoglobinuria in the United States and Japan. *Medicine (Baltimore)*. 2004;83:193-207.

96. Sloand EM, Young NS. Thrombotic complications in PNH. In: Young NS, Moss J, eds. *Paroxysmal Nocturnal Hemoglobinuria and the GPI-Linked Proteins*. Academic Press; 2000:101-112.

97. Griffith JF, Mahmoud AE, Cooper S, Elias E, West RJ, Olliff SP. Radiological intervention in Budd-Chiari syndrome: techniques and outcome in 18 patients. *Clin Radiol*. 1996;51:775-784.

98. McMullin MF, Hillmen P, Jackson J, Ganly P, Luzzatto L. Tissue plasminogen activator for hepatic vein thrombosis in paroxysmal nocturnal haemoglobinuria. *J Intern Med*. 1994;235:85-89.

99. Sholar PW, Bell WR. Thrombolytic therapy for inferior vena cava thrombosis in paroxysmal nocturnal hemoglobinuria. *Ann Intern Med*. 1985;103:539-541.

100. Ray JG, Burows RF, Ginsberg JS, Burrows EA. Paroxysmal nocturnal hemoglobinuria and the risk of venous thrombosis: review and recommendations for management of the pregnant and nonpregnant patient. *Haemostasis*. 2000;30:103-117.

101. Tichelli A, Socie G, Marsh J, et al. Outcome of pregnancy and disease course among women with aplastic anemia treated with immunosuppression. *Ann Intern Med*. 2002;137:164-172.

102. Kelly RJ, Hochsmann B, Szer J, et al. Eculizumab in pregnant patients with paroxysmal nocturnal hemoglobinuria. *N Engl J Med*. 2015;373:1032-1039.

103. Miyasaka N, Miura O. *Pregnancy in Paroxysmal Nocturnal Hemoglobinuria*. Springer; 2017.

104. Miyasaka N, Miura O, Kawaguchi T, et al. Pregnancy outcomes of patients with paroxysmal nocturnal hemoglobinuria treated with eculizumab: a Japanese experience and updated review. *Int J Hematol*. 2016:103:703-712.

105. Danilov AV, Brodsky RA, Craigo S, Smith H, Miller KB. Managing a pregnant patient with paroxysmal nocturnal hemoglobinuria in the era of eculizumab. *Leuk Res*. 2010;34:566-571.

106. Kelly R, Arnold L, Richards S, et al. The management of pregnancy in paroxysmal nocturnal haemoglobinuria on long term eculizumab. *Br J Haematol*. 2010;149:446-450.

107. Ware RE, Hall SE, Rosse WF. Paroxysmal nocturnal hemoglobinuria with onset in childhood and adolescence. *N Engl J Med*. 1991;325:991-996.

108. van den Heuvel-Eibrink MM, Bredius RG, te Winkel ML, et al. Childhood paroxysmal nocturnal haemoglobinuria (PNH), a report of 11 cases in the Netherlands. *Br J Haematol.* 2005;128:571-577.

109. Mercuri A, Farruggia P, Timeus F, et al. A retrospective study of paroxysmal nocturnal hemoglobinuria in pediatric and adolescent patients. *Blood Cells Mol Dis.* 2017;64:45-50.

110. Bauters T, Bordon V, Robays H, Benoit Y, Dhooge C. Successful use of eculizumab in a pediatric patient treated for paroxysmal nocturnal hemoglobinuria. *J Pediatr Hematol Oncol.* 2012;34:e346-e348.

111. Reiss UM, Schwartz J, Sakamoto KM, et al. Efficacy and safety of eculizumab in children and adolescents with paroxysmal nocturnal hemoglobinuria. *Pediatr Blood Cancer.* 2014;61:1544-1550.

112. Socie G, Mary JY, de Gramont A, et al. Paroxysmal nocturnal haemoglobinuria: long-term follow-up and prognostic factors. French Society of Haematology. *Lancet.* 1996;348:573-577.

113. Hillmen P, Muus P, Roth A, et al. Long-term safety and efficacy of sustained eculizumab treatment in patients with paroxysmal nocturnal haemoglobinuria. *Br J Haematol.* 2013;162:62-73.

CHAPTER 9
FOLATE, COBALAMIN, AND MEGALOBLASTIC ANEMIAS

Ralph Green

SUMMARY

Deficiency of either folate or cobalamin (vitamin B_{12}) can lead to macrocytic anemia, with or without other cytopenias, caused by megaloblastic hematopoiesis that results from defective DNA synthesis. Folate in its tetrahydro form is a transporter of 1-carbon fragments, carried at any of three oxidation levels: methanol, formaldehyde, and formic acid. The oxidation levels of the folate-bound 1-carbon fragments can be altered by oxidation and reduction reactions that require nicotinamide adenine dinucleotide phosphate in its oxidized (NADP) or reduced (NADPH) forms, respectively. The original source of the folate-bound 1-carbon fragments is serine which, when it is converted to glycine, passes its terminal carbon to folate. The 1-carbon fragments thus generated are used for biosynthesis of purines, thymidine, and methionine. During biosynthesis of purines and methionine, free folate is released in its tetrahydro form. During biosynthesis of thymidine, tetrahydrofolate is oxidized to the dihydro form and must again be fully reduced by dihydrofolate reductase to continue functioning in 1-carbon metabolism. Methotrexate acts as an anticancer agent because it is an exceedingly powerful inhibitor of dihydrofolate reductase, thereby interdicting the regeneration of reduced folate.

In the cell, folates are serially conjugated to form a chain of 7 or 8 glutamic acid residues by the enzyme folylpolyglutamyl synthase (FPGS). These residues enable the retention of folates as polyglutamates in the cell. When natural food folates are absorbed from the intestine, a process that occurs chiefly in the duodenum and proximal jejunum, all but one of the glutamates are removed by the enzyme glutamate carboxypeptidase II (folate hydrolase). Resulting monoglutamate forms are then taken up by 1 of 2 folate-specific transporters located on the apical brush border, the reduced folate carrier (RFC), or the proton-coupled folate transporter (PCFT). Folates travel in the bloodstream and are taken up by the cells, mainly in the form of methyltetrahydrofolate monoglutamate. The newly absorbed folates are rapidly reglutamylated by FPGS in the cell. If glutamylation is impaired, the folates cannot be retained in the cell, resulting in an intracellular folate deficiency.

Cobalamin is required for two reactions: (1) intramitochondrial conversion of methylmalonyl coenzyme A (CoA), a product of catabolism of odd-carbon fatty acids as well as branched-chain amino acids and ketogenic amino acids, to succinyl CoA, a tricarboxylic acid (Krebs) cycle intermediate; and (2) cytosolic conversion of homocysteine to methionine, a reaction in which the methyl group of methyltetrahydrofolate is transferred to the sulfur atom of homocysteine. In cobalamin deficiency, methyltetrahydrofolate accumulates because, for practical purposes, donation of the methyl group to homocysteine is the only method of regenerating free tetrahydrofolate from methyltetrahydrofolate. Free tetrahydrofolate is an excellent substrate for FPGS; methyltetrahydrofolate is a poor substrate. Consequently, much of the methyltetrahydrofolate taken up by a cobalamin-deficient cell cannot be retained in the cell in the monoglutamated state. The megaloblastic anemia of cobalamin deficiency results from an intracellular folate deficiency that arises because of the cell's limited ability to polyglutamylate methyltetrahydrofolate.

Absorption of cobalamin is a highly complex process. Upon arriving in the stomach, cobalamin is taken up by haptocorrin (HC) binder, a glycoprotein found in virtually all secretions. When the cobalamin HC complex enters the duodenum, the HC is destroyed by tryptic digestion and the released cobalamin is taken up by intrinsic factor, a glycoprotein secreted by the gastric parietal cells. The cobalamin–intrinsic factor complex is absorbed by cells in the ileum through receptor-mediated endocytosis, involving cubilin (CUB) and other proteins. Intracellularly, the cobalamin is released within lysosomes and transported to the bloodstream where it circulates bound to transcobalamin (TC), which delivers its cargo of cobalamin to TC receptors (CD320) located on cell surfaces throughout the body. Folate (vitamin B_9) and cobalamin (vitamin B_{12}) play key roles in the metabolic, synthetic and regulatory machinery of proliferating cells.

Megaloblastic anemia most commonly results from folate or cobalamin (vitamin B_{12}) deficiency. Folate deficiency often had a nutritional basis. Alcoholics and the older poor remain susceptible and it is seen in patients on hyperalimentation, with hemolytic anemia, or hemodialysis. However, in many countries that now practice folic acid fortification of the diet, such as the United States and Canada, the prevalence of folate deficiency has been dramatically reduced and nutritional folate deficiency has been virtually eliminated. Still, in pregnancy, even a mild folate deficiency may be associated with defects in neural tube closure in the fetus, particularly in susceptible groups, so pregnant women should always receive folate supplements. The incidence of neural tube defects has fallen considerably in North America since the introduction of folic acid fortification, but in a substantial proportion of the population, extremely high folate levels are found as a result of the consumption of supplements as well as additionally fortified breakfast cereals. Diagnosis of folate deficiency is based on measurements of folate in serum, which furnishes information about the current level of folate status, and in red cells, which provide data on aggregate folate status over the preceding 120-day period during which those red cells were produced. Nutritional folate deficiency is treated with folic acid by mouth.

Acronyms and Abbreviations: AdoCbl, adenosylcobalamin; AICAR, 5-amino-4-imidazole carboxamide ribotide; AMN, amnionless; ATP, adenosine 5'-triphosphate; ATPase, adenosine triphosphatase; AZT, azidothymidine; CnCbl, cyanocobalamin; CNS, central nervous system; CoA, coenzyme A; CpG, cytosine-phosphate-guanine; CUB, cubilin; CUBAM, the binary ileal cubilin receptor complex consisting of cubilin and amnionless; DEFs, dietary folate equivalents; dTMP, deoxythymidine monophosphate; dU, deoxyuridine; dUMP, deoxyuridine monophosphate; dUTP, deoxyuridine triphosphate; FH_4, tetrahydrofolate; FPGS, folyl polyglutamyl synthase; [^{3}H]Thd, [^{3}H]thymidine; HC, haptocorrin; HCl, hydrochloric acid; HOHCbl, aquocobalamin; IM, intramuscular; LC-MS/MS, liquid chromatography with tandem mass spectrometry; LDH, lactate dehydrogenase; MCV, mean corpuscular volume; MeCbl, methylcobalamin; MRI, magnetic resonance imaging; MRP1, multidrug resistance protein 1; MTHFR, methylenetetrahydrofolate reductase; NADP, nicotinamide adenine dinucleotide phosphate; NADPH, nicotinamide adenine dinucleotide phosphate (reduced form); N_2O, nitrous oxide; OHCbl, hydroxocobalamin; PA, pernicious anemia; PteGlu, pteroylglutamic acid (folic acid); RDA, recommended daily allowance; SAH, S-adenosylhomocysteine; SAM, S-adenosylmethionine; SHMT, serine hydroxymethyltransferase; TC, transcobalamin.

Folate deficiency as a result of malabsorption occurs in tropical and non-tropical sprue. Folate deficiency as a result of tropical sprue is treated with folate supplements and antibiotics. In nontropical sprue the treatment is folate plus a gluten-free diet.

The most common cause of clinically apparent cobalamin deficiency is malabsorption resulting from pernicious anemia (PA), a condition in which the portion of gastric mucosa that contains the parietal cells is destroyed through an autoimmune mechanism. The parietal cells secrete intrinsic factor, which is essential for physiologic cobalamin absorption. Without intrinsic factor, a state of cobalamin deficiency develops over the course of years. Cobalamin deficiency leads not only to megaloblastic anemia but also to a neurological, predominantly demyelinating disease that manifests itself as peripheral neuropathy, spastic paralysis with ataxia (so-called combined system disease of the spinal cord), dementia, psychosis, or some combination of these features. Cobalamin deficiency, which may manifest as neurologic symptoms without anemia, appears to be relatively widespread among older persons. This has been termed atypical, or "subtle" and may result from gastric atrophy with achlorhydria causing malabsorption of natural sources of food B_{12}. The incidence of gastric cancer is increased by a factor of 2 or 3 in patients with PA. Other causes of cobalamin deficiency are gastric resection; stasis of the small intestinal contents as a result of blind loops, strictures, or hypomotility; and disease or resection of the terminal ileum, the site of cobalamin-intrinsic factor complex absorption. Individuals on a vegan diet can become cobalamin-deficient. Cobalamin deficiency is diagnosed by measuring the level of either total or TC-bound vitamin in the blood or by measuring serum methylmalonic acid, which accumulates in the bloodstream in patients with cobalamin deficiency. Cofirmation of cobalamin deficiency in the past was determined by the Schilling test, a measure of cobalamin absorption, but the test is now obsolete and no clinically validated replacement is currently available. In patients with megaloblastic anemia, folate or cobalamin deficiency as the cause of the anemia must be distinguished. If a patient with cobalamin deficiency is treated with folic acid, the anemia may be corrected but the neurologic abnormalities persist, progress, or may be aggravated. Patients with cobalamin deficiency usually are treated with parenteral cobalamin but large doses of oral cobalamin may be used.

Megaloblastic anemia can develop as an acute disorder with rapid development of leukopenia and/or thrombocytopenia. Nitrous oxide anesthesia or abuse is responsible for some cases of acute megaloblastic anemia. The anemia is rarely also seen in patients with a marginal folate status in intensive care units or severe hemolytic anemia through increased folate demand for augmented erythropoiesis. The condition resembles an immune cytopenia but can be ruled out by examining the marrow, which exhibits a floridly megaloblastic picture.

Other causes of megaloblastic anemia include drugs (eg, hydroxyurea, nucleoside analogues) and certain inborn errors of metabolism. Of the inherited conditions, TC deficiency is singled out because it causes a severe megaloblastic anemia in infants who respond completely to high-dose cobalamin. Irreversible neurologic complications supervene if the deficiency is not detected in time. Megaloblastic-like morphologic features of varying degree are seen in the myelodysplastic syndromes, and in acute leukemia of the erythroleukemia type. Megaloblastic anemia seen in association with refractory anemia with excess sideroblasts occasionally responds to very high doses of pyridoxine.

● FOLATE

Folate plays key roles in the metabolism of all cells, particularly proliferating cells, in reactions that involve transfer of 1-carbon units for nucleotide synthesis, amino acid catabolism, conservation of methionine and, in conjunction with cobalamin (vitamin B_{12}), provision of methyl groups for numerous functions including the regulation of gene expression, cell proliferation, mitochondrial respiration, and epigenetic regulation.

CHEMISTRY

The group of compounds referred to as folates consists of folic acid and its various derivatives. *Folic acid* (pteroylglutamic acid) is composed of a pteridine moiety, a *p*-aminobenzoate residue, and an L-glutamic acid residue (Fig. 9-1A). The combination of the pteridine moiety and a *p*-aminobenzoate residue constitutes the *pteroyl* residue or *pteroic acid*.[1] In nature, folates occur largely as conjugates in which multiple glutamic acids are linked by peptide bonds involving their γ-carboxyl groups (Fig. 9-1B). Additionally, the naturally occurring polyglutamated folates are reduced in the 5, 6, 7, and 8 positions of the pteridine ring (see Fig. 9-1B). Conjugates are named according to the length of the glutamate chain (eg, pteroylmonoglutamate, pteroyldiglutamate, pteroylhexaglutamate, etc). Therapeutic folic acid (pteroylglutamic acid) used in supplements and for food fortification, is not naturally occurring, has one glutamic acid and the pteridine ring is not reduced.

To form a functional compound, folates must be in the reduced tetrahydrofolate form (FH_4; see Fig. 9-1B). In this reduction, dihydrofolate (FH_2) is an intermediate. A single enzyme, *dihydrofolate reductase*, catalyzes both $FA \rightarrow FH_2$ and $FH_2 \rightarrow FH_4$.

The folate family consists largely of FH_4 derivatives bearing a 1-carbon substituent (symbolized as FH_4-C). The varieties of FH_4-C differ regarding the identity of the 1-carbon unit and the site of its attachment to FH_4. Figure 9-2 shows 1-carbon substituents of biochemical significance and their major interconversions.

These substituents are attached to FH_4 through N^5, N^{10}, or both (see Fig. 9-2). Specific enzymes interconvert these various FH_4 derivatives through oxidations at any of three levels (methanol, formaldehyde, and formic acid) that require nicotinamide adenine dinucleotide phosphate (NADP) and reductions that use the reduced form NADPH.[2]

Reduced derivatives of folic acid usually are sensitive to oxidation in air and light. An important exception is N^5-formyl FH_4, also called *citrovorum factor, leucovorin,* or *folinic acid,* which, because of its stability, is the form preferred for clinical use.

NUTRITION

Sources

Folate comes from many sources. The richest sources are dark green leafy vegetables including broccoli, spinach, lettuce, asparagus, endive, and lima beans. Each vegetable contains more than 1 mg of folate per 100 g dry weight. The best fruit sources are oranges, lemons, bananas, strawberries, and melons. Folates also are abundant in liver, kidney, yeast, mushrooms, and peanuts. Meat, except for liver, is generally not a good source of folate. Since the advent of folic acid fortification of the food supply, the median daily intake of folate from an average American diet is estimated to be 350 mcg.[3] However, the intake varies considerably with age and with patterns of supplement use and consumption of foods voluntarily fortified beyond the mandatory level of fortification.[4] Foods are readily depleted of folate by excessive cooking[5] especially with large amounts of water discarded before ingestion.

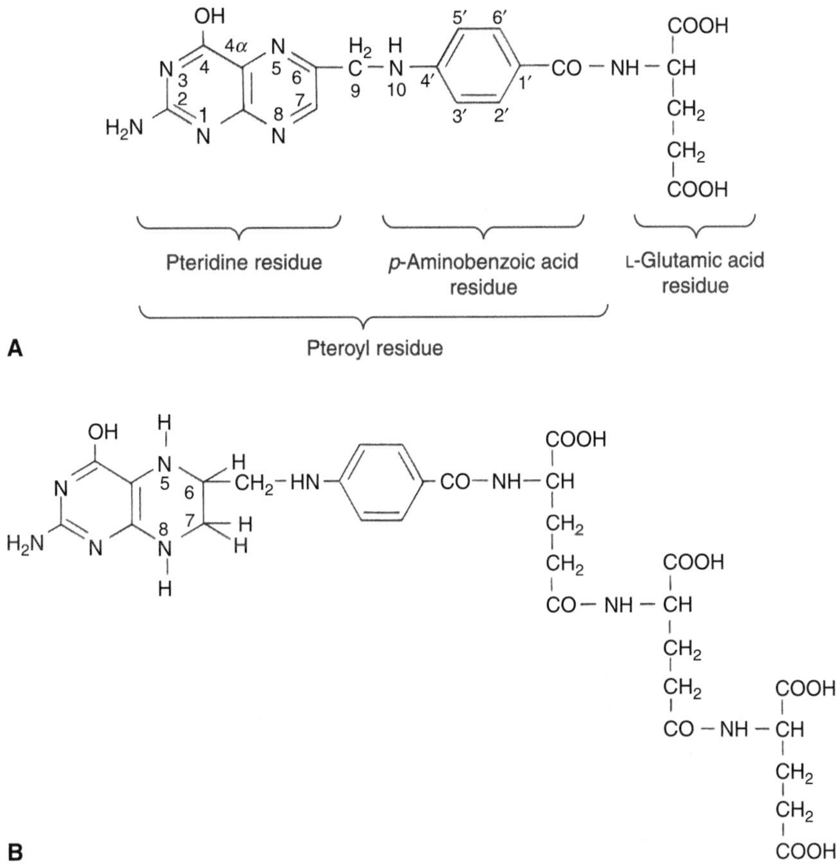

Figure 9–1. Folic acid. **A.** Folic acid (pteroylglutamic acid) and its components. **B.** Tetrahydrofolate triglutamate.

Daily Requirements

In the normal adult, the recommended daily allowance (RDA) for folate is expressed as dietary folate equivalents (DFEs) of folic acid. When expressed as DFEs, all forms of folate are converted to an amount that is equivalent to folic acid.[3,4] One microgram of food folate is the dietary equivalent of 0.6 mcg folic acid added to food. Folic acid is, therefore, on average, 1.7 times more available than food folates. The dietary folate content varies according to region, age, socioeconomic factors, and other demographic factors and some of the folate may have low bioavailability. Accordingly, the officially RDA of *food* folate expressed as DFEs for an adult is 0.4 mg.[3] This figure is derived through considerations of the nutrient requirements to satisfy the needs of 97% to 98% of healthy individuals and the relative differences in absorption and bioavailability between dietary folate and the more bioavailable synthetic folic acid. The body is thought to contain approximately 5 mg of folate.[6] When folate intake is reduced to 5 mcg/day, megaloblastic anemia develops in approximately 4 months.[7]

Folic acid requirements increase with cell turnover as in hemolytic anemia, leukemia, and other malignant diseases, in alcoholism[8] and during growth; in pregnancy and during lactation requirements increase three- to sixfold.[9] Adequate folate supplies are particularly important in pregnant and lactating women, in whom the RDA is increased to 600 and 500 mcg/day, respectively, to meet requirements.[10]

METABOLISM

Folate-Dependent Enzymes

FH_4 is an intermediate in reactions involving the transfer of 1-carbon units from a donor to an acceptor molecule. Table 9-1 summarizes the metabolic systems of animal tissues known to require folic acid coenzymes.

One-carbon units enter the folate pool principally via the serine hydroxymethyltransferase (SHMT) reaction which requires pyridoxal phosphate as a cofactor.[11,12] There are both cytoplasmic (SHMT1) and mitochondrial (SHMT2) isoforms of SHMT, which impart a state of functional redundancy for this important enzyme, the primary source of 1-carbon units for purine and pyrimidine biosynthesis. The cytoplasmic form can undergo sumoylation during S-phase, allowing nuclear localization.[13]

$$\text{Serine} + FH_4 \rightarrow \text{glycine} + N^5,N^{10}\text{-methylene } FH_4 + H_2O$$

Among the several 1-carbon transfers mediated by folic acid, the transfer that is the most important clinically is the methylation of deoxyuridylate to thymidylate, catalyzed by the enzyme thymidylate synthase.[2,13,14] This reaction is an essential step in the synthesis of DNA (Fig. 9-3). In carrying out this reaction, N^5,N^{10}-methylene FH_4 simultaneously transfers and reduces a 1-carbon group, itself serving as the hydrogen donor for the reduction.[15] The reaction generates dihydrofolate, which must be reduced again to FH_4 by dihydrofolate reductase and NADPH before it can again be used as a coenzyme:

$$dUMP + N^5,N^{10}\text{-methylene } FH_4 \rightarrow \text{dihydrofolate}$$
$$+ dTMP \text{ dihydrofolate} + NADPH + H^+ \rightarrow FH_4 + NADP^+$$

where dUMP = deoxyuridine monophosphate; dTMP = deoxythymidine monophosphate; and NADP = nicotinamide adenine dinucleotide phosphate. Limitation of thymidylate synthesis in folic acid deficiency causes incorporation of uracil instead of thymine into DNA (see Fig. 9-3).[16]

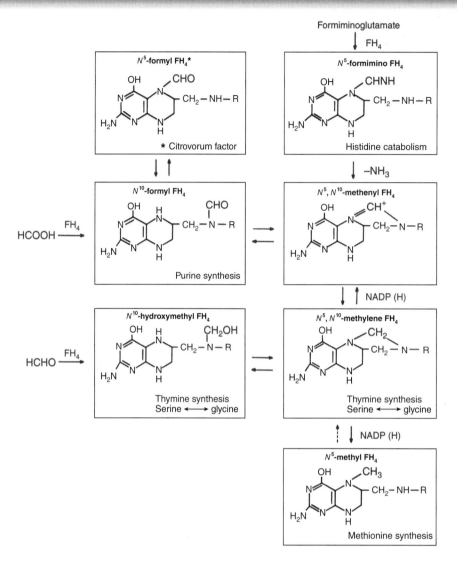

FIGURE 9–2. Derivatives of tetrahydrofolic acid (FH$_4$), their interconversions, and the metabolic pathways in which they participate. One-carbon substituents are shown in *blue*.

TABLE 9–1. Metabolic Systems Requiring Folic Acid Coenzymes in Animal Cells

System	Related Transformations of Folic Acid Coenzymes
Serine → glycine	Serine + FH$_4$ → N^5,N^{10}-methylene FH$_4$ + glycine
Thymidylate synthesis	Deoxyuridylate (dUMP) + N^5,N^{10}-methylene FH$_4$ → FH$_2$ + thymidylate (dTMP)
Histidine catabolism	Formiminoglutamate + FH$_4$ → N^5-formimino FH$_4$ + glutamate
Methionine synthesis	Homocysteine + N^5-methyl FH$_4$ → FH$_4$ + methionine
Purine synthesis	Glycinamide ribotide + N^{10}-formyl FH$_4$ → FH$_4$ + formylglycinamide ribotide
Purine synthesis	5-Amino-4-imidazole carboxamide ribotide + N^{10}-formyl FH$_4$ → FH$_4$ + 5-formamido-4-imidazolecarboxamide ribotide

Abbreviation: FH$_4$, tetrahydrofolate.

The three key enzymes involved in thymidylate synthesis, thymidylate synthase, SHMT, and dihydrofolate reductase undergo sumoylation and nuclear import during cellular S-phase.[13]

A key enzyme, methylenetetrahydrofolate reductase (MTHFR) regulates the distribution of reduced folates by controlling the rate of NADPH-mediated conversion of N^5,N^{10}-methylene FH$_4$ to N5-methyl FH$_4$. Because N^5,N^{10}-methylene FH$_4$ is the obligate 1-carbon donor for thymidylate synthesis, its conversion to N5-methyl FH$_4$ serves as a brake on DNA synthesis and repair, while diverting more folate to the methionine synthase reaction (see Fig. 9-2). Consequently, the activity of MTHFR serves as a checkpoint for intracellular folate trafficking and distribution, and becomes more critical in states of folate depletion.

A polymorphic form of MTHFR, MTHFR 677C → T, is of some clinical importance. The mutation results in a thermolabile form of the enzyme with a higher K$_m$ for its methylene-FH$_4$ substrate. Retardation of the folate methylation cycle makes more methylene-FH$_4$ available for thymidylate synthesis (see Fig. 9-9 below), while affecting the levels of homocysteine, an amino acid that has been linked

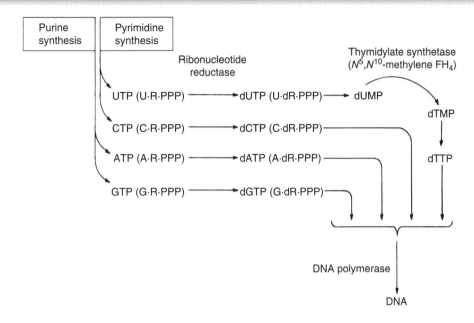

FIGURE 9–3. Pathways of deoxynucleotide and DNA synthesis. ATP, adenosine triphosphate; CTP, cytidine triphosphate; dATP, deoxyadenosine triphosphate; dCTP, deoxycytidine triphosphate; dGTP, deoxyguanosine triphosphate; dTMP, deoxythymidine monophosphate; dTTP, deoxythymidine triphosphate; dUTP, deoxyuridine triphosphate; dUMP, deoxyuridine monophosphate; FH$_4$, tetrahydrofolate; GTP, guanosine triphosphate; UTP, uridine triphosphate.

to disease states and removal of which depends on both methylfolate and cobalamin.

Folate deficiency diminishes purine biosynthesis by slowing (a) the folate-dependent formylation of glycinamide ribotide to *N*-formylglycinamide ribotide, the reaction that places the C-8 in the purine ring, and (b) the folate-dependent conversion of 5-amino-4-imidazole carboxamide ribotide to 5-formamido-4-imidazole carboxy-amide ribotide, the reaction that places the C-2 in the purine ring.[17] Additional reactions dependent on biopterin, a nonfolate pteridine derivative, that are of potential metabolic importance are hydroxylation of phenylalanine to tyrosine, oxidation of long-chain alkyl ethers of glycerol to fatty acid, hydroxylation of tryptophan to 6-hydroxytryptophan (a precursor of serotonin), 17α-hydroxylation of progesterone,[18] and production of nitric oxide.[19] Tetrahydrofolic acid is weakly active in some of these systems in vitro[20]; whether it plays any such role in vivo is unknown.

Significance of Folylpolyglutamates

Intracellular folates exist primarily as polyglutamate conjugates.[21] Approximately 75% of the folate in human erythrocytes and leukocytes is polyglutamylated.[22] Plasma folate consists largely of the monoglutamate N^5-methyl FH$_4$ and is transported into the cells in this form.[23] Inside the cells, the polyglutamate chain is sequentially built up by an adenosine 5′-triphosphate (ATP)-dependent *folylpoly-γ-glutamyl synthase*.[24] The activity of human folylpoly-γ-glutamate synthetase depends greatly on the form of the folate substrate, declining in the order FH$_4$ > N^{10}-formyl FH$_4$ > N^5-methyl FH$_4$, toward which the enzyme is almost inert.[25] In humans, conjugated folates carry, on average, 7 to 8 glutamyl residues.[26] Intracellular folylmonoglutamates leak out of the cells at a fairly rapid rate, whereas polyglutamates do not, presumably because of the highly charged polyglutamate tail.[27] Therefore, attachment of the polyglutamate chain is essential for retaining folates within cells. Additionally, folylpolyglutamates are superior to monoglutamates as substrates for folate-dependent enzyme reactions.[22]

PHYSIOLOGY

Intestinal Absorption

The duodenum and proximal jejunum are the principal sites of folate absorption. Absorption of a dose of either monoglutamate or polyglutamate forms of folate begins within minutes. Peak plasma levels are reached in 1 to 2 hours. Only folylmonoglutamate appears in plasma, suggesting that all folylpolyglutamates must first be hydrolyzed by the enzyme glutamate carboxypeptidase II (folate hydrolase)[28] during absorption across the intestine.[29] This enzyme is located on the brush border membrane and plays an important role in the intestinal absorption of folate.[30] Folylpolyglutamate is hydrolyzed at the brush border of the intestinal cell (Fig. 9-4). Folate hydrolase purified from human

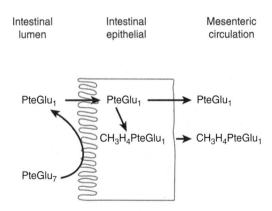

FIGURE 9–4. Digestion and absorption of folate polyglutamate by the intestine. The polyglutamate (in this case, PteGlu$_7$) is hydrolyzed in the intestinal lumen or at the brush border. The resulting pteroylglutamate (PteGlu) is transported into the intestinal cell, where it is reduced and methylated, appearing in the circulation chiefly as N^5-methyl FH$_4$.

jejunum catalyzes the Zn^{2+}-dependent deconjugation of folate polyglutamates ranging from pteroylglutamic acid-2 to at least pteroylglutamic acid-7.[31] It is an exopeptidase that successively removes single glutamate residues from the end of the polyglutamate chain, ultimately yielding the folylmonoglutamate. The monoglutamate forms are then taken up by one of two folate-specific transporters located on the apical brush border, the reduced folate carrier or the proton-coupled folate transporter.[28] While reduced folate carrier has a pH optimum of 7.4, proton-coupled folate transporter is a high-affinity folate transporter that uses a proton-coupled system to facilitate folate absorption and shows maximum transport activity at a low pH.[28,32] This property is consistent with the observation that cancer cells retain a high affinity for the new-generation antifolate pemetrexed (Alimta).[33] Defects in the proton-coupled folate transporter are the underlying cause of hereditary folate malabsorption.[34]

Folate hydrolases also are found outside the intestine. For example, human plasma contains sufficient hydrolase activity to convert polyglutamates containing more than three glutamyl residues to monoglutamates. Other γ-glutamyl hydrolases, appear to be lysosomal carboxypeptidases[35] that are not involved in absorption of folates from the intestine, but which play a role in the release of folate from storage sites in the liver and kidney.[28]

Folate monoglutamates are actively transported across the intestinal epithelium by proton-coupled folate transporter-mediated transport ($K_m = 1–2 \mu M$) that is independent of Na^+, K^+, and transmembrane potential.[36] The mechanism uses the pH gradient between the jejunal lumen (pH ~6) and the interior of the epithelial cell to drive folate into the cell against a concentration gradient.[37] Passive transport also may occur.[38] In the intestinal cell, the absorbed folate monoglutamates are reduced (in the case of folic acid), and then converted to N^5-methyl FH_4 (some N^{10}-formyl FH_4 also is made) and transported into the bloodstream without further change.[39]

Folate undergoes an enterohepatic cycle in which it is first secreted against a concentration gradient into the bile, appearing there chiefly as N^5-methyl FH_4 monoglutamate, and then is reabsorbed from the small intestine.[40] Bile contains approximately 2 to 10 times the folate concentration of normal serum, with biliary excretion accounting for up to 0.1 mg of folate per day. This quantity is sufficiently large that interruption of the enterohepatic cycle by biliary diversion causes serum folate levels to fall by more than 50% in less than 1 day.[40] The enterohepatic cycle has been proposed to redistribute folate between hepatic stores and peripheral tissues according to the availability of exogenous folate supplies.[41]

Physiological Processing

Tritiated folylmonoglutamate (^{3}H-F) administered intravenously is almost completely removed from the bloodstream in a few minutes.[42] Uptake involves two classes of folate-binding proteins[43]: *high-affinity folate receptors*[44] that concentrate folate in intracellular vesicles and a *membrane folate transporter* that transports folate from the vesicles into the cytosol. The high-affinity receptors, which are attached to the outer surface of the cell membrane by glycosylphosphatidylinositol linkages and lack an intracytoplasmic portion,[45] bind very tightly (K_d in the nanomolar range) to most physiologic folate monoglutamates,[46] particularly N^5-methyl FH_4, the major circulating folate.[47] The folate receptors exist in various isoforms (of which α and β are the most important). Folate receptor-α, despite its missing cytoplasmic extension, is effective in mediating endocytosis.[48] Their very high affinity enables the receptors to take up N^5-methyl FH_4 from the plasma, even at its ambient concentration of approximately 10 nM. The membrane folate transporter is a probenecid-inhibitable organic anion carrier that, among other functions, carries reduced folates and methotrexate in and out of the cytoplasm.[43] Its K_m for folate is in the micromolar range.

Once internalized, the folates are retained by the cells partly through polyglutamylation,[49] but also through tight association with a set of intracellular folate-binding proteins.[50] Three of these proteins are enzymes involved in methyl group metabolism: sarcosine dehydrogenase and dimethylglycine dehydrogenase (mitochondrial)[51] and glycine N-methyl transferase (cytosolic).[52] Why these enzymes bind folate so avidly and whether this binding affects overall methyl group metabolism are unknown, although glycine N-methyl transferase is speculated to regulate methyl group metabolism by controlling the tissue concentration of S-adenosylhomocysteine (SAH), one of its reaction products and a potent inhibitor of most methyltransferases.[53] It has been proposed that when glycine N-methyltransferase undergoes nuclear localization, it may also play a role in the regulation of cellular proliferation and serve a tumor suppressor function.[54]

Folates have been found in all body tissues that have been analyzed. The principal form of the vitamin in tissues and in blood appears to be the N^5-methyl form.[55] The total folate pool turns over very slowly.[56,57] Degradation accounts for a portion of this turnover. p-Aminobenzoylglutamate has been identified as a breakdown product. The fate of the pteridine moiety is unknown.

FOLATE-BINDING PROTEINS OF SERUM AND MILK

The soluble folate-binding proteins of serum and milk are high-affinity folate receptors that are released from cell membranes by proteolysis.[58] These proteins can be detected in approximately 15% of normal individuals[59] and are found at increased levels in some pregnant women, women taking oral contraceptives, folate-deficient alcoholics (but, curiously, not patients with cobalamin deficiency),[60] and patients with uremia, hepatic cirrhosis, and chronic myelogenous leukemia.[61] In normal individuals, the proteins are approximately two-thirds saturated and have a total folate-binding capacity of approximately 175 pg/mL of serum.[62] The proteins may not be detectable in some individuals because of complete saturation with endogenous unlabeled folate.[61] Serum folate-binding protein has an Mr of 40,000 and prefers oxidized to reduced folates.[61]

Folate-binding proteins have been found in milk and in normal granulocytes.[63] Folate bound to the milk folate binder in suckling animals is absorbed chiefly in the ileum,[64] rather than the jejunum, the principal site of absorption of free folate. The milk folate binder, a glycoprotein, also promotes folate transport into the liver via the asialoglycoprotein receptor.[65] The milk folate binder is speculated to protect an infant's folate supply by preventing bacteria from sequestering the vitamin away from the intestinal absorptive surface. The folate-binding protein in granulocytes has been localized to the secondary granules, from which it is released when the granulocytes are stimulated and may serve a bacteriostatic effect.[66]

EXCRETION

Folates are both resorbed and secreted by the kidney. Resorption is accomplished by a membrane-bound high-affinity folate receptor (K_m for N^5-methyl FH_4 = 0.4 nM) located in the brush borders of the proximal tubules.[67] Filtered folate may thus be returned to the bloodstream. There is resorption of most, but not all, of the filtered folate. There is evidence that the multiligand receptor megalin plays an additional role in the uptake of folate bound to filtered folate-binding protein.[68]

In humans, intact folates and their cleavage products are excreted by the kidney at a rate of 2 to 5 mcg/day.[69] A small percentage of parenterally administered labeled folate is recoverable in the feces and mainly represents unreabsorbed folate from the enterohepatic cycle.[70]

ASSAY OF SERUM FOLATE

Total folate is measured by chemiluminescent methods using various folate binders. These assays are identical in principle to the radiolig- and binding assays that they have replaced. Measurement of the various folate forms is now possible using liquid chromatography with tandem mass spectrometry (LC-MS/MS).[71]

⬤COBALAMIN

CHEMISTRY

Structure and Nomenclature

The cobalamin molecule has two major portions: a porphyrin-like near-planar macrocycle known as corrin, and a nucleotide that lies almost perpendicular to the corrin ring (Fig. 9-5). The corrin moiety contains four reduced pyrrole rings that bind a central cobalt atom whose two remaining coordination positions are occupied by a 5,6-dimethylbenzimidazolyl group, below the ring and various ligands (in this case, CN) above the ring.[72]

Compounds containing the corrin ring are known as *corrinoids*. The cobalamins are corrinoids whose nucleotide contains 5,6-dimethylbenzimidazolyl. Two connections exist between the corrin and the nucleotide: (1) a bond between the nucleotide phosphate and a side chain in ring D, and (2) a bond between cobalt and a nitrogen atom of benzimidazole. Figure 9-6 summarizes the numbering and ring designations of the corrin system.

The term *vitamin B_{12}* is sometimes used as a generic term for the cobalamins. The term probably is best reserved, however, as an alternative name for cyanocobalamin (CnCbl), the usual therapeutic form of cobalamin.

Four cobalamins are important in animal cell metabolism. Two are CnCbl (vitamin B_{12}) and *hydroxocobalamin* (OHCbl) or *aquocobalamin* (HOHCbl). The other two cobalamins are alkyl derivatives that are synthesized from OHCbl and serve as coenzymes. In one, *adenosylcobalamin* (AdoCbl), a 5′-deoxyadenosyl replaces OH as the cobalt ligand above the ring (Fig. 9-7).[73] In the second, *methylcobalamin* (MeCbl), the upper ligand is a methyl group. MeCbl is the major form of cobalamin in human blood plasma.[74]

NUTRITION

Sources

Cobalamin is synthesized only by certain microorganisms; animals ultimately depend on microbial synthesis for their cobalamin supply.

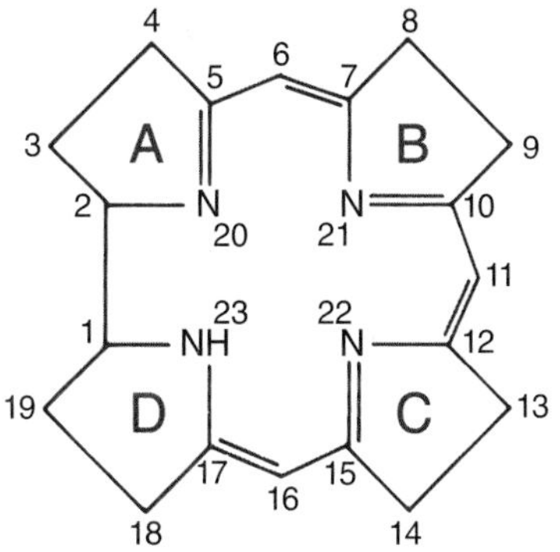

FIGURE 9–6. Corrin ring showing ring designations and standard numbering of the atoms.

Foods that contain cobalamin are of animal origin: meat, liver, seafood, and dairy products. Cobalamin is not known to be synthesized in plants and its presence in foods of plant origin is believed to have come from microbial contamination or through a symbiotic relationship with bacteria.[75,76]

Daily Requirements

The average daily diet in Western countries contains 5 to 30 mcg of cobalamin. Of this, 1 to 5 mcg is absorbed.[77] Less than 250 ng appears in the urine; the unabsorbed remainder appears in the feces. Total body

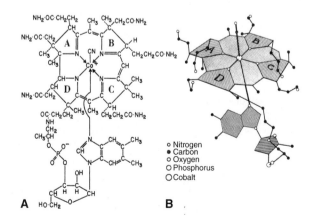

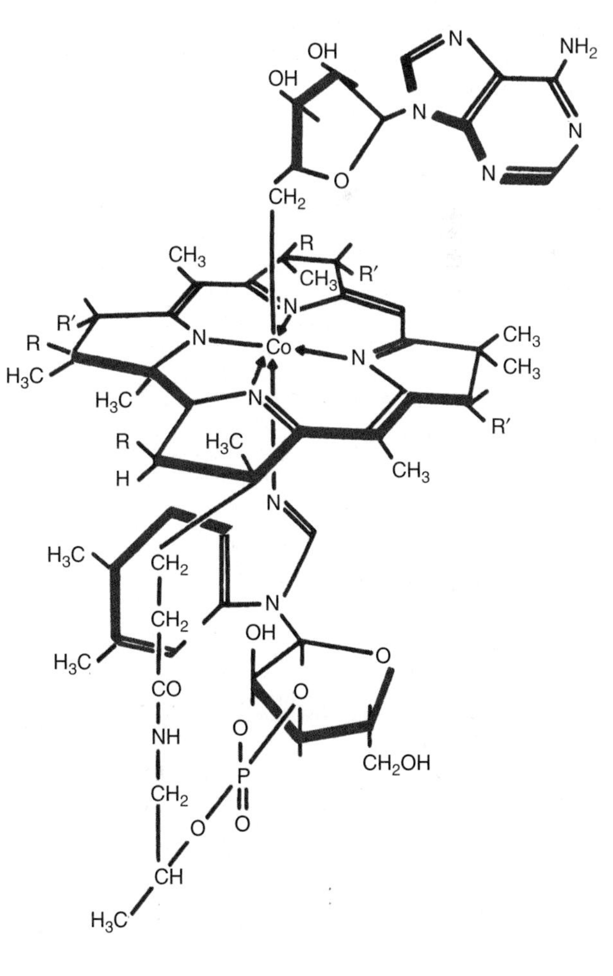

FIGURE 9–5. A. Structure of cyanocobalamin (CnCbl; vitamin B_{12}). **B.** Partial structure of CnCbl showing the relationship between the corrin ring and the nucleotide.

FIGURE 9–7. Adenosylcobalamin (AdoCbl). R, CH_2CONH_2; R′, $CH_2CH_2CONH_2$.

content is 2 to 5 mg in an adult,[78] with approximately 1 mg in the liver. The kidneys also are rich in cobalamin.[79] Relative to the daily requirement, body reserves of cobalamin are much larger than those of folate.

Cobalamin has a daily rate of obligatory loss of approximately 0.1% of the total body pool, irrespective of the pool size. For this reason, a deficiency state does not develop for several years after cessation of cobalamin intake. The official RDA for adults is 2.4 mcg[3]; growth, hypermetabolic states, and pregnancy increase daily requirements. The RDA for children between ages 1 and 13 years is 0.9 to 1.8 mcg. Because of insufficient data, no RDA has been established for infants. Instead, adequate intakes of 0.4 mcg for age 0 to 6 months and 0.5 mcg for age 7 to 12 months have been estimated.

ROLE IN METABOLISM

The only two recognized cobalamin-dependent enzymes in human cells are AdoCbl-dependent *methylmalonyl coenzyme A (CoA) mutase* and MeCbl-dependent *methyltetrahydrofolate-homocysteine methyltransferase*.

Methylmalonyl Coenzyme A Mutase

Methylmalonyl CoA mutase is a mitochondrial enzyme that participates in the disposal of the propionate formed during the breakdown of valine, isoleucine, and odd-carbon fatty acids. The enzyme is a homodimer of a 78-kDa subunit that is encoded by a gene on chromosome 6.[80] In the reaction catalyzed by methylmalonyl CoA mutase, methylmalonyl CoA, which is produced during catabolism of propionate,[81] is converted to succinyl CoA, a Krebs cycle intermediate. During this reaction, hydrogen on the methyl carbon of the substrate exchanges places with the—COSCoA group (Fig. 9-8).

The coenzyme serves as an intermediate hydrogen carrier, accepting the hydrogen from the substrate in the initial phase of the reaction and returning it to the product after migration of COSCoA.

N^5-Methyltetrahydrofolate-Homocysteine Methyltransferase

MeCbl participates in cobalamin-dependent synthesis of methionine from homocysteine by the enzyme N^5-methyl FH_4-homocysteine methyltransferase. *S*-adenosylmethionine (SAM) and a second enzyme, methionine synthase reductase, are required for methyltransferase activity.[82] The reductase converts the oxidized cobalt (Co) to the readily alkalizable Co^{1+}, which then accepts a methyl group from SAM, a powerful biologic methylating agent, thereby restoring activity of the methyltransferase. In humans, this pathway also serves as a mechanism critical for converting N^5-methyltetrahydrofolate to tetrahydrofolate required for synthesis of polyglutamates as well as other important 1-carbon adducts of folate. The demethylation of N^5-methyl FH_4 is a prerequisite for attachment of the polyglutamate chain to newly acquired folate, which is largely taken up by the cell in the form of N^5-methyl FH_4 monoglutamate.[27] Nitrous oxide (N_2O) impairs the methyltransferase by oxidizing cob(I)alamin (a catalytic intermediate in the methyltransferase reaction) to cob(II)alamin. This reaction depletes MeCbl and produces a cobalamin deficiency-like state.[83]

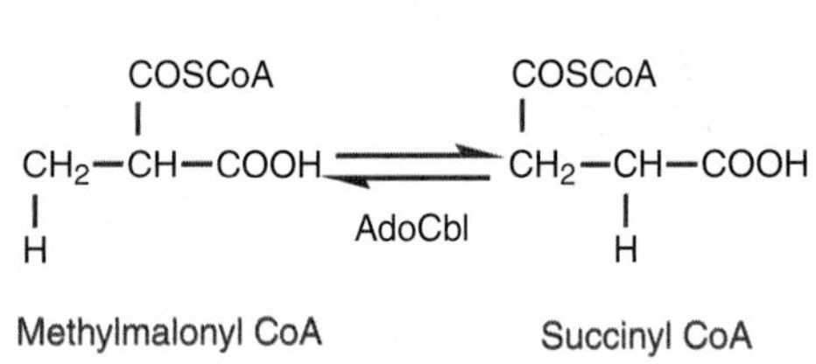

FIGURE 9–8. Methylmalonyl coenzyme A (CoA) mutase reaction. AdoCbl, adenosylcobalamin.

Nonenzymatic Metabolism

Because cobalamin has the capacity to bind cyanide, it may participate in detoxification of cyanide. Tobacco and certain foods (fruits, beans, tubers, and nuts) contain cyanide in the form of thiocyanate. Although the evidence is inconclusive, cobalamin is believed to play a role in neutralizing cyanide taken in via these substances.[72]

FOLATE–COBALAMIN RELATIONSHIP

In either folate deficiency or cobalamin deficiency, the megaloblastic anemia is fully corrected by treatment with the appropriate vitamin. The megaloblastic anemia of cobalamin deficiency also is variably corrected by folic acid supplementation even if no cobalamin is given, although the remission is partial and only temporary. Conversely, the anemia of folate deficiency is generally not helped at all by cobalamin although partial responses to high doses of cobalamin have been reported in some patients with folate deficiency.[84] These clinical observations indicate that the megaloblastic anemia in cobalamin deficiency actually results from a secondary abnormality in folate metabolism.[85] The observation that urinary excretion of formiminoglutamic acid and 5-amino-4-imidazole carboxamide ribotide, normally regarded as a sign of folate deficiency, is seen occasionally in pure cobalamin deficiency,[86] provides further evidence that folate metabolism is deranged by cobalamin deficiency. Figure 9-9 summarizes the metabolic interrelationships between folate and cobalamin. Two explanations have been proposed to account for the folate responsiveness of cobalamin-deficient megaloblastic anemia: (1) the *methylfolate trap* hypothesis, which is accepted by most authorities (Fig. 9-10), and (2) the *formate starvation* hypothesis.

Methylfolate Trap Hypothesis

The methylfolate trap hypothesis[87] is based on the fact that the folate-requiring enzyme N^5-methyl FH_4–homocysteine methyltransferase is also dependent on cobalamin. According to the hypothesis, in cobalamin deficiency tissue folates are gradually diverted into the N^5-methyl FH_4 pool because of slowing of the methyltransferase reaction,[88] the only route out of that pool for folate (see Fig. 9-10). As N^5-methyl FH_4 levels increase, the levels of other forms of folate decline, with a consequent fall in the rates of reactions in which those forms participate. Because the MTHFR reaction is irreversible, methylene tetrahydrofolate (THF) becomes depleted, the synthesis of dTMP is slowed, and megaloblastic anemia ensues.

In its simplest form, the hypothesis predicts that in cobalamin deficiency tissue levels of N^5-methyl FH_4 are abnormally high and those of other forms of folate are abnormally low. Although serum N^5-methyl FH_4 levels are frequently elevated in cobalamin deficiency,[89] tissue folate levels, predominantly polyglutamates, decline.[90] The decreased level is related to the substrate specificity of the folate-conjugating enzyme. This enzyme works very poorly with N^5-methyl FH_4; therefore, it is unable to carry out normal γ-glutamylation of newly internalized N^5-methyl FH_4 monoglutamate in cobalamin-deficient cells because the freshly acquired folate cannot be converted into a suitable substrate (ie, free FH_4 or formyl FH_4). Thus, although sequestration of tissue folates in an expanded N^5-methyl FH_4 pool may account for some of the effects of the blockade in methyltransferase activity, the major problem seems to be a failure to convert newly acquired folate into a form that can be retained by the cell. The upshot is development of tissue folate deficiency as the unconjugated folate leaks out (see Fig. 9-10). The whole process is aggravated by a drop in tissue levels of SAM as the methionine supply is curtailed because of the diminished activity of the methyltransferase.[91] SAM, which is necessary for methyltransferase activity, is also a powerful inhibitor of N^5,N^{10}-methylene FH_4 reductase MTHFR,[92] the enzyme responsible for production of N^5-methyl FH_4. The relief of

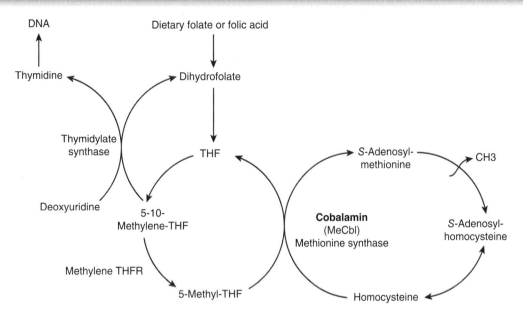

FIGURE 9–9. N^5-methyl FH$_4$–homocysteine methyltransferase reaction. MeCbl, methylcobalamin; THF, tetrahydrofolate; THFR, tetrahydrofolate reductase.

this inhibition as SAM levels fall accelerates the flow of folates toward N^5-methyl FH$_4$, further aggravating the metabolic imbalance resulting from impairment in methyltransferase activity.

This problem could be overcome if N^5-methyl FH$_4$ were converted into a substrate for the conjugating enzyme by another route. In theory, this could be accomplished by reversal of the N^5,N^{10}-methylene FH$_4$ reductase reaction. For practical purposes, however, the N^5,N^{10}-methylene FH$_4$ reductase reaction is irreversible in vivo.[93]

Formate Starvation Hypothesis

This hypothesis holds that formate starvation is the basis for folate-responsive megaloblastic anemia of cobalamin deficiency.[94] This theory is based on the diminished capacity of cobalamin-deficient lymphoblasts to incorporate formaldehyde into purine and methionine[91] and on experiments showing that N^5-formyl FH$_4$ is more effective than FH$_4$ at correcting some of the abnormalities in folate metabolism seen in cobalamin deficiency.[95] The hypothesis states that with the decrease in methionine production under cobalamin-deficient conditions, the generation of formate is depressed (because normally the methyl group of excess methionine is rapidly oxidized to formate),[96] leading to a decline in the production of N^5-formyl FH$_4$.

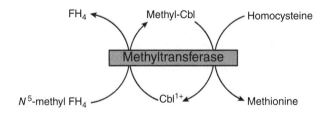

FIGURE 9–10. Cobalamin and folate intersect in the methionine synthase reaction where 5-methyl-THF is able to donate its methyl group to homocysteine to form methionine with cobalamin in the form of MeCbl serving a cofactor in the transfer of the methyl group. In this way, THF is regenerated. Cbl, cobalamin; MeCbl, methylcobalamin; THF, tetrahydrofolate.

INTESTINAL ABSORPTION

Intrinsic Factor

Intrinsic factor is one of several binding proteins in which cobalamin is ensconced as it makes its way through the body (Table 9-2). Intrinsic factor is needed for the absorption of cobalamins taken orally at physiologic dosage levels. Human intrinsic factor is a glycoprotein (Mr approximately 44,000) encoded by a gene on chromosome 11.[97] It has binding sites for cobalamin and a specific ileal receptor, the former situated near the carboxyterminus and the latter near the aminoterminus of the intrinsic factor molecule.[98] Binding to cobalamin is very tight, and involves the 5,6-dimethylbenzimidazolyl lower axial ligand of the molecule. This specificity for cobalamin allows for the exclusion of other noncobalamin corrinoids during the tightly regulated absorptive process.[72,85] The entrapment of the vitamin alters the conformation of intrinsic factor, to produce a more compact form that is resistant to proteolytic digestion.

In humans, intrinsic factor is synthesized and secreted by the parietal cells of the cardiac and fundic mucosa.[99] Secretion of intrinsic factor usually parallels that of hydrochloric acid (HCl). It is enhanced by the presence of food in the stomach, vagal stimulation, histamine, and gastrin. Gastric juice also contains other cobalamin-binding glycoproteins.[100] These proteins were known as the *R proteins* because of their rapid electrophoretic mobility compared with intrinsic factor.

TABLE 9–2. Cobalamin-Binding Proteins

Protein	Source	Function
Intrinsic factor	Gastric parietal cells	Promotes absorption uptake of cobalamin by ileum
Transcobalamin	Probably all cells	Promotes uptake of cobalamin by cells
Haptocorrin	Exocrine glands, phagocytes	Helps dispose of cobalamin analogues; possible antimicrobial function(?)

Elucidation of the primary protein structure of the R proteins reveals that they belong to the same family of isoproteins as the plasma haptocorrin (HC) binder (previously known as transcobalamin [TC] I and TC III).[101] These HC-like proteins are also produced by the salivary glands.

Absorption of Cobalamin: Cubilin

Cobalamins in foods are liberated in the stomach by peptic digestion.[102] They are first bound to the HC-like protein because cobalamin binds much more tightly to HC than to intrinsic factor at the acid pH of the stomach.[103] Upon entering the duodenum, cobalamin is released from the cobalamin–HC protein complex through digestion by pancreatic proteases, which, in normal individuals, act by selectively degrading HC and the cobalamin–HC complex while sparing intrinsic factor.[103] Only at this point can cobalamin bind to intrinsic factor to form the intrinsic factor–cobalamin complex.

The intrinsic factor–cobalamin complex, which is very resistant to digestion,[105] traverses the intestine until it reaches the intrinsic factor receptor, *cubilin* (CUB),[105] a 460-kDa peripheral membrane glycoprotein located in the microvillus pits of the ileal mucosa brush border. CUB forms part of a multifunctional epithelial receptor complex also found in the yolk sac and renal proximal tubule cells.[106] In the kidney, it serves a role in the overall body economy of cobalamin through tubular reabsorption,[107] but the function of the CUB receptor complex in the kidney and other polarized epithelial surfaces extends beyond cobalamin. The ileal CUB receptor complex consists of two proteins, CUB and amnionless (AMN), the product of two distinct genes, *CUB* and *AMN*. Both proteins, which together have been designated the "CUBAM complex," colocalize in the endocytic compartment and are required for the process of assimilation of cobalamin,[108] AMN serving as a chaperone for endosomal targeting. Mutations affecting either of the two proteins disrupt the normal process of the intestinal phase of cobalamin absorption. In addition to the tightly embracing components of the CUBAM complex, a distinct, large, multifunctional protein, megalin, which belongs to the low-density lipoprotein family,[109] also participates in the conformational changes that accompany internalization. The concentration of the CUBAM intrinsic factor receptor complex rises progressively to a maximum near the terminal ileum.[110] A specific site on the intrinsic factor molecule avidly attaches to the receptor in a binding reaction that requires a pH of 5.4 or greater and Ca^{2+} (or other divalent cations) but no energy.[111]

The intrinsic factor–cobalamin receptor complex is taken into the ileal mucosal cells over 30 to 60 minutes by endocytosis,[112] where the vitamin is processed and released into the portal blood over several hours. The receptors recycle to the microvillus surface to shuttle another load of intrinsic factor–cobalamin complex.[112] That this process has a limited capacity is evident from estimates of the maximum amount of cobalamin that can be absorbed from a single dose via this physiologic pathway.[72,113] Defects in the genes that regulate the complex mechanism of ileal absorption are implicated in autosomal recessive megaloblastic anemia, caused by intestinal malabsorption of cobalamin[85] (see "Selective Malabsorption of Cobalamin, Autosomal Recessive Megaloblastic Anemia, Imerslund-Gräsbeck Disease" further).

During its sojourn in the ileal enterocyte, the vitamin first appears in the lysosomes, but by 4 hours most of the vitamin is located in the cytosol.[114] During absorption, the entire intrinsic factor–cobalamin complex appears to be taken into the cell, where the cobalamin is released while the intrinsic factor is degraded.[115]

Cobalamin from a small oral dose (10-20 mcg) starts to appear in the blood after 3 to 4 hours, and the vitamin reaches a peak level in 6 to 12 hours. In the portal blood, the cobalamin is complexed with a cobalamin-transporting protein known as TC previously known as TC II.[116] There is evidence that cobalamin leaves the enterocyte through a portal that is part of the adenosine triphosphate binding cassette (ABC) drug transport system, ABCC1 (also known as the multidrug resistance protein 1 [MRP1]) located on the basolateral surface of the intestinal epithelium, as well as other polar cells, and nonpolar cells (macrophages).[117] The cobalamin–TC complex forms as it exits the ileal enterocyte, one of a variety of cells that synthesize TC, including the neighboring vascular endothelial cells in the submucosa.[118] Large oral doses (1 mg) of cobalamin are absorbed inefficiently (1%-2% of an oral dose) through any mucosal surface by simple diffusion, not mediated by intrinsic factor.[113] In these instances, the vitamin appears in blood within minutes following ingestion.

Like the folates, the cobalamins undergo appreciable enterohepatic recycling.[119,120] In humans, between 0.5 and 9 mcg/day of cobalamin is secreted into the bile, where it is bound to HC.[121] After entering the intestine, the cobalamin–HC complexes of biliary origin are treated exactly like those delivered from the stomach following ingestion. The cobalamin is released by digestion of the HC by pancreatic proteases, and then is taken up by intrinsic factor and reabsorbed. From 65% to 75% of biliary cobalamin is estimated to be reabsorbed by this mechanism.[122] Because of the size of the cobalamin storage pool and the existence of this enterohepatic circulation, a very long time—as long as 10 to 20 years, depending on the amount of stored cobalamin—is required for a clinically significant cobalamin deficiency to develop from a diet providing insufficient cobalamin (eg, a strictly vegetarian diet).[123] Patients who are unable to absorb the vitamin, however, become clinically deficient in only 3 to 6 years because the absorption of both biliary and dietary cobalamin are interdicted.[124]

COBALAMIN IN THE CELL: TRANSCOBALAMIN

Uptake of Cobalamin by Cells

TC is the plasma protein that mediates the transport of cobalamin into the tissues.[125] A β-globulin protein with a calculated molecular weight of 45,538 from the deduced amino acid sequence,[126,127] TC binds cobalamin with exceedingly high affinity ($K_a = 10^{-11}\ M$).[128] Unlike intrinsic factor, whose binding is highly specific for cobalamins, TC shows some promiscuity and also can bind certain corrins that are chemically related to the cobalamins but have no function in mammalian systems and are known as cobalamin "analogues."[129] TC is synthesized by many types of cells, including enterocytes, hepatocytes, endothelial cells, mononuclear phagocytes, fibroblasts, glial cells, and hematopoietic precursors in the marrow.[72] Although circulating TC carries only a minor fraction of the cobalamin in the plasma, it is the protein on which cobalamin absorbed through the intestine is transported into the portal blood as the preformed cobalamin–TC complex. It also is the protein with which cobalamin given parenterally associates almost immediately.[130] These cobalamin–TC complexes are transported into the tissues within minutes of appearing in the bloodstream.[131] The transport process begins with binding of the cobalamin–TC complex to a specific membrane receptor that is present on a wide variety of cells.[132] The protein and gene encoding the TC receptor has been purified from placental membranes and characterized.[133] Designated as CD320, the receptor belongs to the low-density lipoprotein receptor family and its internalization involves megalin. The receptor-bound complex is internalized by receptor-mediated endocytosis and delivered to lysosomes, where the TC is digested and the cobalamin is freed.[134,135] There is some evidence that TC may play a role in cobalamin absorption at the apical surface of the intestinal mucosa.[136-138]

Formation of Adenosylcobalamin and Methylcobalamin

To become metabolically active, CnCbl and OHCbl must first be converted to AdoCbl and MeCbl, the coenzymatically active cobalamins.

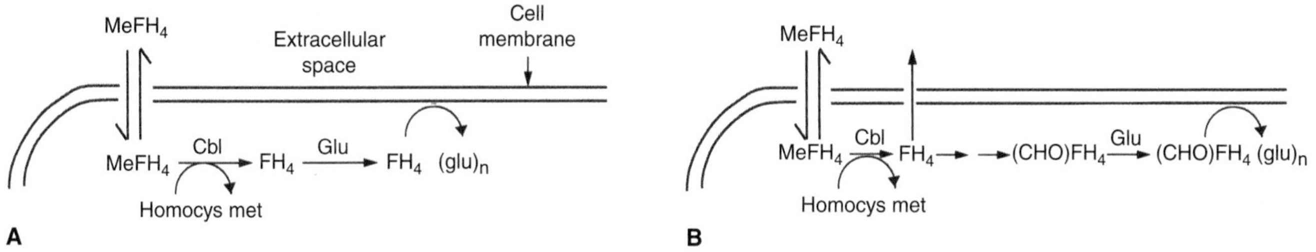

FIGURE 9–11. Methods by which cobalamin deficiency decreases intracellular folate levels. Methyltetrahydrofolate ($MeFH_4$), the principal form of folate in the bloodstream, circulates in the unconjugated form (ie, it has no polyglutamate side chain). This and other forms of unconjugated FH_4 can be taken into cells but leak out again unless they are conjugated. Methyl FH_4 is not a substrate for the conjugating enzyme, so conjugation cannot occur until the methyl FH_4 is converted to another form of folate. Cobalamin is necessary for this process because it is the cofactor for the reaction that converts methyl FH_4 to FH_4. In cobalamin deficiency, the conversion of methyl FH_4 to FH_4 is defective. Newly transported folate remains in the form of methyl FH_4, which cannot be conjugated and leaks back out the cell. **A.** According to the *methylfolate trap hypothesis*, all forms of FH_4 other than methyl FH_4 can be conjugated, so methyl FH_4 is the only folate species that leaks out the cell. **B.** The *formate starvation hypothesis* differs from the methylfolate trap hypothesis solely in assuming that only the formylated folates (N^{10}-formyl FH_4 and/or N^5,N^{10}-methenyl FH_4) can be conjugated, so newly transported methyl FH_4, N^5,N^{10}-methylene FH_4 and free FH_4 leak out of the cell. $(CH_2) FH_4 = N^5,N^{10}$-methylene FH_4; $(CHO) FH_4 = N^{10}$-formyl FH_4 or N^5,N^{10}-methenyl FH_4. Cbl, cobalamin; FH_4, tetrahydrofolate; Glu, glutamate; Homocys met, homocysteine methyltransferase.

The conversion is accomplished by reduction and alkylation. CnCbl and OHCbl are first reduced to the Co^{2+} form [cob(II)alamin] by NADPH-dependent and NADH-dependent reductases that are present in mitochondria and microsomes.[139] CN^- and OH^- are displaced from the metal during reduction. Some of the cob(II)alamin is reduced further in the mitochondria to the intensely nucleophilic Co^+ form [cob(I)alamin]. This molecule is then alkylated by ATP to form AdoCbl in a reaction in which the 5′-deoxyadenosyl moiety of ATP is transferred to the cobalamin and the three phosphates of ATP are released as inorganic triphosphate (Figs. 9-11 and 9-12). The rest of the reduced cobalamin binds to cytosolic N^5-methyltetrahydrofolate-homocysteine methyltransferase, where it is converted to MeCbl. The several steps involved in the conversion of cobalamin to its coenzymatically active forms are regulated by genes that play a critical role in the processing of the vitamin. There are several inherited metabolic errors that correspond to one or more of these specific steps and that result in characteristic syndromes affecting aspects of cobalamin metabolism that are discussed later in this chapter.

PLASMA HAPTOCORRIN (TRANSCOBALAMINS I AND III; "R" PROTEINS)

The HCs (previously known as R proteins or TC I and TC III) are a group of immunologically related proteins of apparent Mr approximately 60,000 consisting of a single polypeptide species variably substituted with oligosaccharides that terminate with different quantities of sialic acid.[140] They are found in milk, plasma, saliva, gastric juice, and numerous other body fluids. They appear to be synthesized by mucosal cells of the organs that secrete them[141] and by phagocytes.[142] Although the HCs bind cobalamin, unlike intrinsic factor, they are unable to promote the intestinal absorption of the vitamin.

Plasma HC carries most (70%-90%) of the circulating cobalamin. It contains nine potential glycosylation sites[143] and is encoded by a gene on chromosome 11, the same chromosome that carries the intrinsic factor gene.[144] In contrast to TC, HC clearance from the plasma is very slow (terminal half-life: 9-10 days).[145] The asialoglycoprotein receptor carries the cobalamin–HC complexes into the hepatocytes, where the complexes are degraded, and their load of cobalamins is excreted in the bile.[119,146] HC binds its ligands more tightly than does either intrinsic factor or TC. Furthermore, HC is less restrictive than either intrinsic factor or TC with respect to ligand specificity; it avidly takes up corrinoids of widely varying structure.[147] The ligand-binding properties of HC and its mode of clearance by the liver suggest that HC helps clear the system of nonphysiologic cobalamin analogues that may have been acquired or may have arisen through degradation of cobalamin.[148] As the liver metabolizes analogue–HC complexes, it secretes the analogues into the bile. Because these analogues are bound poorly by intrinsic factor,[147] they are poorly reabsorbed from the intestine and are eliminated in the feces. The precise role of HC is unknown, although it may play

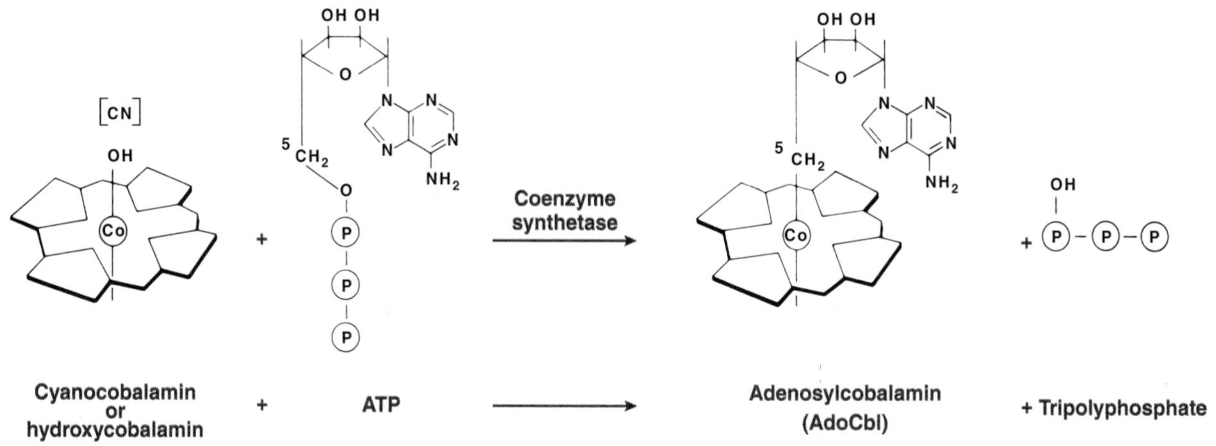

FIGURE 9–12. Biosynthesis of adenosylcobalamin (AdoCbl).

a role in the body economy of cobalamin by facilitating excretion of cobalamin analogues while conserving cobalamin through enterohepatic recycling. Additionally, it has been proposed that HC may serve an antimicrobial role.[72]

ASSAY OF SERUM COBALAMIN AND THE TRANSCOBALAMINS

As with folate, cobalamin is usually measured with automated competitive displacement assays using intrinsic factor as a cobalamin-binding protein. The misleading results previously provided by competitive ligand displacement assays were explained by the discovery in serum and tissue of a class of cobalamin analogues that are detected by the radioisotope assay when HC-type proteins and not intrinsic factor were used as the binding protein.[149] Current assays use intrinsic factor as the binder and give more reliable values for serum cobalamin. The chemical nature and biologic significance of the analogues are unknown,[150] but evidence suggests that they may arise in the gastrointestinal tract.[148]

TC and HC are present in plasma in trace quantities (approximately 7 and 20 mcg/L, respectively). In fasting plasma, at least 70% of the circulating cobalamin is bound to HC.[151] TC binds only 10% to 25% of the total plasma cobalamin,[152] but provides the majority (approximately 75%) of the total unsaturated cobalamin-binding capacity of plasma.[151] Table 9-3 lists alterations in unsaturated cobalamin-binding capacity, and in HC and TC levels in various disease states. The assays have been developed that measure the fraction of the plasma cobalamin that is bound to TC. This component, known as holotranscobalamin, shows some evidence of improved specificity compared with the standard cobalamin assay for identifying true cobalamin deficiency, although the assays appear to be generally comparable with respect to sensitivity.[153-159]

● MEGALOBLASTIC ANEMIAS

DEFINITION

Megaloblastic anemias are disorders caused by impaired DNA synthesis. The presence of megaloblastic cells is the morphologic hallmark of this group of anemias. Megaloblastic red cell precursors are larger than normal and have more cytoplasm relative to the size of the nucleus. Promegaloblasts show a blue granule-free cytoplasm and a fine "salt and pepper" granular chromatin that contrasts with the ground-glass

TABLE 9–3. Levels and Binding Capacity of Cobalamin-Binding Proteins in Disease

Binder	Disease
Increased haptocorrin (transcobalamin I, R protein)	Myeloproliferative disorders
	Polycythemia vera
	Myelofibrosis
	Benign neutrophilia
	Chronic myelocytic leukemia
	Hepatoma (occasionally)
	Metastatic cancer
Increased transcobalamin	Liver disease
	Inflammatory disorders
	Gaucher disease

Data from Lawler S, Roberts P, Hoffbrand A. Chromosome studies in megaloblastic anaemia before and after treatment. *Scand J Haematol.* 1971;8(4):309-320.

texture of its normal counterpart. As the cell matures, the chromatin condenses more slowly than normal into darker aggregates that coalesce, but do not fuse homogeneously, giving the nucleus a characteristic fenestrated appearance. Continuing maturation of the cytoplasm as it acquires hemoglobin contrasts with the immature-looking nucleus—a feature termed *nuclear-cytoplasmic asynchrony.*[160]

Megaloblastic granulocyte precursors are also larger than normal and show nuclear-cytoplasmic asynchrony. A characteristic cell is the *giant metamyelocyte*, which has a large horseshoe-shaped nucleus, sometimes irregularly shaped, containing ragged open chromatin.

Megaloblastic megakaryocytes may be abnormally large and polylobated, with deficient granulation of the cytoplasm. In severe megaloblastosis, the nucleus may show detached lobes. Further details are provided in "Laboratory Features" and in Figs. 9-13 and 9-14.

ETIOLOGY AND PATHOGENESIS

Table 9-4 lists the causes of megaloblastic anemia. By far the most common causes worldwide are folate deficiency and cobalamin deficiency. There has been, however, a marked reduction in the prevalence of folate deficiency in countries that have implemented folic acid fortification of the food supply.

Megaloblastic cells have much more cytoplasm and RNA than do their normal counterparts, but they have a relatively normal amount of DNA,[161] suggesting that synthesis of cytoplasmic constituents (RNA and protein) proceed faster than DNA. Evidence that maturation is retarded in megaloblastic precursors supports this conclusion.[162] DNA synthesis is impaired,[163] migration of the DNA replication fork and the joining of DNA fragments synthesized from the lagging strand (Okazaki fragments) are delayed,[164] and S phase is prolonged.[163]

Slowing of DNA replication in the megaloblastic anemias of folate and cobalamin deficiency appears to arise from failure of the folate-dependent conversion of dUMP to dTMP. This reaction is nuclear, in contradistinction to folate-dependent purine synthesis which is cytoplasmic and in cobalamin-deficient cell model systems; de novo dTMP biosynthesis capacity is substantially reduced, concomitant with a marked increase in nuclear N^5-methyl FH4.[165] Because of this failure, deoxyuridine triphosphate levels become abundant and because DNA polymerase is promiscuous with respect to its substrate specificity, this allows deoxyuridine triphosphate to become incorporated into the DNA of folate-deprived cells in place of deoxythymidine triphosphate.[166] DNA excision-repair mechanisms to mend the DNA by replacing uridine with thymidine fail for the same reason that uridine triphosphate was incorporated into the DNA in the first place. The result is a repetitive iteration of flawed DNA repair that ultimately leads to DNA strand breaks, fragmentation, and apoptotic cell death.[167]

Addition of deoxyuridine to marrow cells in culture normally decreases the incorporation of tritiated thymidine into DNA, because the deoxyuridine is converted via dUMP → dTMP to unlabeled deoxythymidine triphosphate, which competes with the tritiated thymidine. In megaloblastic cells, this effect of added deoxyuridine is greatly diminished. This finding is consistent with impairment in the dUMP → dTMP reaction in the megaloblastic cells and was the basis for the now defunct *deoxyuridine suppression test.*[168] The failed excision-repair model following deoxyuridine triphosphate misincorporation into DNA also explains the chromosome breaks and other abnormalities that occur in megaloblastic cells.[169]

CLINICAL FEATURES

All megaloblastic anemias share certain general clinical features.[160] Because the anemia develops slowly, with opportunity for cardiopulmonary and intraerythrocytic compensatory changes,[170] it produces few symptoms

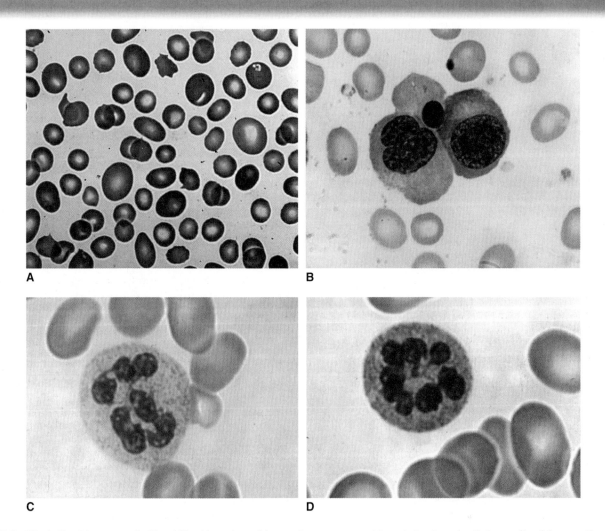

FIGURE 9–13. A. Pernicious anemia. Blood film. Note the striking oval macrocytes, wide variation in red cell size, and poikilocytes. Despite the anisocytosis and microcytes, the mean red cell volume is usually elevated, as in this case (mean corpuscular volume [MCV] = 121 fL). **B.** Marrow precursors in pernicious anemia. Note very large size of erythroblasts (megaloblasts) and asynchronous maturation. Cell on *right* is a polychromatophilic megaloblast with an immature nucleus for that stage of maturation. Cell on *left* is an orthochromatic megaloblast with a lobulated immature nucleus. An orthochromatic megaloblast with a condensed nucleus is between and above those two cells. **C** and **D.** Two examples of hypersegmented neutrophils characteristic of megaloblastic anemia. The morphology of blood and marrow cells in folate-deficient and vitamin B_{12}-deficient patients is identical. The extent of the morphologic changes in each case is related to the severity of the vitamin deficiency. *(Reproduced with permission from Lichtman MA, Shafer MS, Felgar RE, et al: Lichtman's Atlas of Hematology 2016. New York, NY: McGraw Hill; 2017.)*

until the blood hemoglobin concentration is severely depressed. Symptoms, when they appear, are those of anemia: weakness, palpitation, fatigue, light-headedness, and shortness of breath. The blending of severe pallor and slight jaundice caused by a combination of intramedullary and extravascular hemolysis produce a characteristic lemon-yellow skin tint. Leukocyte and platelet counts may be low, but rarely cause clinical problems. Details of the clinical manifestations are given in the sections on the specific forms of megaloblastic anemia later in this chapter.

LABORATORY FEATURES

Blood Cells

All cell lines are affected. Erythrocytes vary markedly in size and shape, often are large and oval, and in severe cases can show basophilic stippling and nuclear remnants (Cabot rings, and Howell-Jolly bodies). Erythroid activity in the marrow is increased, although ineffective because the megaloblastic cells usually undergo apoptosis before they

are released, accounting for the reduced reticulocyte count. The more severe the anemia, the more pronounced the morphologic changes in the red cells. When the hematocrit is less than 20%, erythroblasts with megaloblastic nuclei, including an occasional promegaloblast, may appear in the blood. The anemia is usually macrocytic (mean corpuscular volume [MCV] is 100-150 fL or more), although coexisting iron deficiency, thalassemia trait,[171] or inflammation can prevent macrocytosis.[172] Because of the progressive nature of gradual replacement of normocytic red cells with the macrocytic progeny of a megaloblastic marrow, the earliest observable change in red cell indices is an increase in the red cell distribution width, reflecting an increase in anisocytosis.

Neutrophil nuclei often have more than the usual three to five lobes (see Fig. 9-13).[173] Typically, more than 5% of the neutrophils have five lobes. Cells may contain six or more lobes, a morphology rarely seen in normal neutrophils but not pathognomonic of megaloblastic hematopoiesis. In nutritional megaloblastic anemias caused by folate deficiency, hypersegmented neutrophils are an early sign

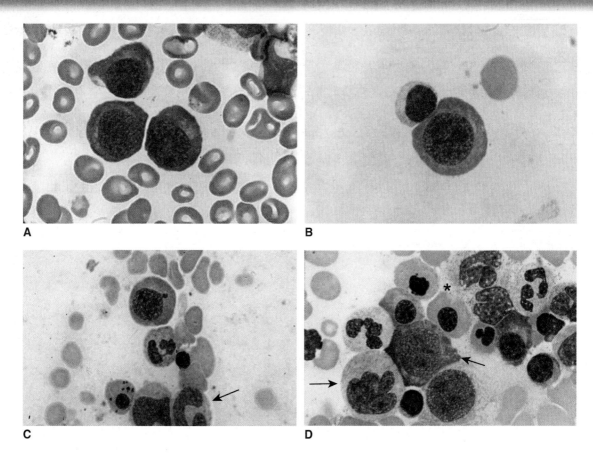

FIGURE 9–14. Marrow films. Megaloblastic anemia. Patient with pernicious anemia (vitamin B$_{12}$ deficiency). **A.** Basophilic megaloblasts. Large cell size, very characteristic nuclear chromatin pattern with exaggerated proportion of euchromatin. **B.** Polychromatophilic megaloblast. Very large cell size for maturational stage. Large nuclear size and abnormally large proportion of euchromatin without appropriate nuclear condensation at this stage of maturation. Adjacent lymphocyte. **C.** Polychromatophilic megaloblast with small nuclear fragment. *Arrow* indicates giant band neutrophil. At lower left is orthochromatic megaloblast with multiple nuclear fragments. **D.** *Oblique arrow* indicates promegaloblast. *Horizontal arrow* indicates giant band neutrophil. To the left of and below the *asterisk* are 4 orthochromatic megaloblasts—large cell size for maturational stage—2 with delayed nuclear condensation and 2 with condensed nuclei with abnormal nuclear margins showing small or large budding nuclei. To the right of the asterisk are 2 giant band neutrophils. On the right at midfield is a plasma cell below which is a lymphocyte. *(Reproduced with permission from Lichtman MA, Shafer MS, Felgar RE, et al: Lichtman's Atlas of Hematology 2016. New York, NY: McGraw Hill; 2017.)*

of megaloblastosis[6] and persist in the blood for many days after treatment.[173] Neutrophil hypersegmentation was not found to be a sensitive test for mild cobalamin deficiency.[174] Cytogenetic studies are nonspecific and show chromosomes that are elongated and broken. Specific therapy corrects these abnormalities, usually within 2 days, although some abnormalities do not disappear for months.[160,169,175] Platelets are often reduced in number and slightly smaller than normal with a wider variation in size (increased platelet distribution width).[176] The morphologic features of megaloblastic anemia may be grossly exaggerated in patients who have been splenectomized or lack a functional spleen as occurs in celiac disease or sickle cell anemia. Numerous circulating megaloblasts and bizarre red cell morphology may be present.[177]

Marrow

Aspirated marrow is cellular and shows striking megaloblastic changes, especially in the erythroid series with well-hemoglobinized erythroblasts containing nuclei that possess less mature, more open nuclear chromatin than their normal counterparts. There is a preponderance of earlier basophilic erythroblasts over more mature forms, which gives the overall impression of a maturation arrest (see Fig. 9-14).[160]

Sideroblasts are increased in number and contain increased numbers of iron granules. The ratio of myeloid to erythroid precursors falls to 1:1 or lower, and granulocyte reserves may be decreased. In severe cases, promegaloblasts containing an unusually large number of mitotic figures are plentiful. Macrophage iron content often is increased, caused by ineffective erythropoiesis with consequent reduced iron utilization. Megaloblastic features in the granulocytic series are also usually present with giant forms and large horseshoe-shaped nuclei. Occasionally megakaryocytes with hyperlobated nuclei are present.

Coexisting Microcytic Anemia

Many features of megaloblastic anemia may be masked when megaloblastic anemia is combined with a microcytic anemia.[172] The anemia can be normocytic or even microcytic, whereas the blood film may show both microcytes and macroovalocytes (a "dimorphic anemia"). The marrow may contain "intermediate" megaloblasts[178] that are smaller and look less "megaloblastic" than usual. In this kind of mixed anemia, the microcytic component usually is iron-deficiency anemia,[172] but it may be thalassemia minor[171] or the anemia of chronic inflammation. Even megaloblastic anemia masked by a severe microcytic anemia usually shows hypersegmented neutrophils in the blood and giant

TABLE 9–4. Causes of Megaloblastic Anemias

I. Folate Deficiency
  A. Decreased intake
    1. Poor nutrition
    2. Old age, poverty, alcoholism
    3. Hyperalimentation
    4. Hemodialysis
    5. Premature infants
    6. Spinal cord injury
    7. Children on synthetic diets
    8. Goat's milk anemia
  B. Impaired absorption
    1. Nontropical sprue
    2. Tropical sprue
    3. Other disease of the small intestine
  C. Increased requirements
    1. Pregnancy
    2. Increased cell turnover
    3. Chronic hemolytic anemia
    4. Exfoliative dermatitis
II. Cobalamin Deficiency
  A. Impaired absorption
    1. Gastric causes
      a. Pernicious anemia
      b. Gastrectomy
      c. Gastric reduction surgery
      d. Zollinger-Ellison syndrome
    2. Intestinal causes
      a. Ileal resection or disease
      b. Blind loop syndrome
      c. Fish tapeworm
    3. Pancreatic insufficiency
  B. Decreased intake
    1. Vegans

III. Acute Megaloblastic Anemia
  A. Nitrous oxide exposure
  B. Severe illness with
    1. Extensive transfusion
    2. Dialysis
    3. Total parenteral nutrition
IV. Drugs
  A. Dihydrofolate reductase inhibitors
  B. Antimetabolites
  C. Inhibitors of deoxynucleotide synthesis
  D. Anticonvulsants
  E. Oral contraceptives
  F. Others, such as long-term exposure to weak folate antagonists (eg, trimethoprim or low-dose methotrexate)
V. Inborn Errors
  A. Cobalamin deficiency
    1. Imerslund-Gräsbeck disease
    2. Congenital deficiency of intrinsic factor
    3. Transcobalamin deficiency
  B. Errors of cobalamin metabolism
    1. "Cobalamin mutant" syndromes with homocystinuria and/or methylmalonic acidemia
  C. Errors of folate metabolism
    1. Congenital folate malabsorption
    2. Dihydrofolate reductase deficiency
    3. N^5-methyl FH_4 homocysteine-methyltransferase deficiency
  D. Other errors
    1. Hereditary orotic aciduria
    2. Lesch-Nyhan syndrome
    3. Thiamine-responsive megaloblastic anemia
VI. Unexplained
  A. Congenital dyserythropoietic anemia
  B. Refractory megaloblastic anemia
  C. Erythroleukemia

metamyelocytes and bands in the marrow. Neutrophil myeloperoxidase levels are high.[179]

Less commonly, the megaloblastic component of a mixed iron-deficiency anemia can be overlooked, and the patient may be treated only with iron. In this situation, the anemia may respond only partly to therapy, and megaloblastic features become more conspicuous as hypoferremic erythropoiesis is corrected and iron stores fill. The masking of macrocytosis in these situations may be responsible for delay or difficulty in diagnosis of pernicious anemia (PA), particularly in certain geographic areas and ethnic groups where there is a high incidence of thalassemia and microcytic hemoglobinopathies.[171,180,181] There are several situations that favor the coexistence of a megaloblastic state with iron deficiency. Both folate and iron deficiency occur in celiac disease,[181] and cobalamin and iron deficiency both complicate gastric reduction surgery for morbid obesity.[182,184] Furthermore, *Helicobacter pylori* infection is associated with gastric atrophy that can result first in iron deficiency and later lead to cobalamin malabsorption and perhaps even predispose to PA.[185,186]

Incomplete Megaloblastic Anemia

If a patient with a full-blown megaloblastic anemia receives cobalamin or folate before marrow aspiration, the anemia persists but the megaloblastic changes may be obscured. Attenuated megaloblastic changes also are seen in patients with early megaloblastic anemia, in patients with coexisting infection,[172] or in patients after transfusion. Rarely, cases with megaloblastic anemia caused either by cobalamin or folate deficiency have been reported with erythroid hypoplasia and inappropriately low levels of serum lactate dehydrogenase (LDH).[187]

Megaloblastic Anemia Misdiagnosed as Acute Leukemia

Occasionally, very severe megaloblastic anemia produces marrow morphology so bizarre as to be mistaken for acute leukemia. In some cases, the erythroid series does not mature, and the megaloblastic pronormoblast dominates the marrow with prominent mitotic figures and dysmorphic forms, raising the possibility of erythroid leukemia.[160]

Megaloblastic Changes in Other Cells

In most forms of megaloblastic anemia, cytologic abnormalities resembling megaloblastosis may appear in other proliferating cells. Epithelial cells from the mouth, stomach, small intestine, and cervix uteri may look megaloblastic, appearing larger than their normal counterparts and containing atypical immature-looking nuclei. Distinguishing these cytological "megaloblastic" changes from the changes of malignancy may be difficult.[188]

Chemical Changes in Body Fluids

Plasma bilirubin, iron, and ferritin levels are increased.[189] Serum LDH-1 and LDH-2, both found in red cells, are markedly elevated as a result of rapid intramedullary erythroblast turnover and increase with the severity of the anemia.[190] In megaloblastic anemia isoenzyme LDH-1 is greater than LDH-2, whereas in other anemias LDH-2 is greater than LDH-1.[191] Serum muramidase (lysozyme) levels are high,[192] whereas serum glutamic oxaloacetic transaminase (aspartate transaminase) is normal.[193] Erythropoietin levels rise, but less than in other anemias of similar severity.[194] Surprisingly, the elevated erythropoietin levels fall sharply within 1 day of beginning treatment, an interval too short to have been mediated by the hemoglobin concentration.

Cytokinetics

Megaloblastic anemia is associated with two pathophysiologic abnormalities: *ineffective erythropoiesis* (exaggerated apoptosis of precursor cells) and *hemolysis*. Ineffective erythropoiesis increases the red cell precursor to reticulocyte ratio, plasma iron turnover,[195] LDH-1 and LDH-2 levels,[191] and "early labeled" bilirubin.[196] Both intramedullary and extramedullary hemolysis occur in megaloblastic anemia, with red cell life span decreased by 30% to 50%.[197]

Increased serum muramidase in megaloblastic anemia can be caused by increased granulocyte turnover,[192] possibly resulting from exaggerated apoptosis of granulocyte precursors in the marrow (ineffective granulopoiesis). In cobalamin deficiency, platelet production is only 10% of that expected from the megakaryocyte mass,[198] perhaps reflecting ineffective thrombopoiesis. Platelets in severe cobalamin deficiency are functionally abnormal.[199]

FOLIC ACID DEFICIENCY

Etiology and Pathogenesis

Folate deficiency is caused by (1) dietary deficiency, (2) impaired absorption, and (3) increased requirements or losses (see Table 9-4).

Decreased Intake Caused by Poor Nutrition Prior to the mid-1990s, inadequate dietary intake was the major cause of folate deficiency. However, in the era of folic acid fortification, the prevalence of folate deficiency has fallen dramatically. In the United States, the prevalence of low plasma folate has dropped from 22% to 1.7% of the population.[200] However, a caveat to the impression that clinical folate deficiency is rare throughout the world is based on the notion that in resource-limited countries, where dietary folate deficiency can coexist with vitamin B_{12} deficiency or malaria or both, the serum folate concentration can be spuriously elevated and range from normal to high, leading to serious underestimation of tissue folate status.[201] Because folate reserves are limited, deficiency develops rapidly in malnourished persons, typically the old, the poor, and the alcoholic. Folate deficiency can also occur during hyperalimentation[202] and subclinical folate deficiency has been reported in subtotal gastrectomy.[203] Folate deficiency can occur in premature infants, especially with infection, diarrhea, or hemolytic anemia[204]; in children on a synthetic diet because of inherited metabolic disorders[205]; and in infants raised on goat's milk, which is poor in available folate.[205-207] Destruction of folate through excessive cooking can aggravate folate deficiency.[5]

In alcoholic cirrhosis, megaloblastic anemia usually is caused by folate deficiency.[208] Alcohol may acutely depress serum folate, even if folate stores are replete,[209] and accelerates the development of megaloblastic anemia in persons with early folate deficiency.[210] Alcohol causes acute marrow suppression, decreases in reticulocyte, platelet, and granulocyte levels[211]; reversible vacuolation of erythroid and myeloid precursors; and dysfunction of granulocytes.[212] These changes occur even if large doses of folate are given with the alcohol.[213]

Celiac Disease

Nontropical sprue It is related to ingestion of wheat gluten.[214] Pathologically, nontropical sprue shows atrophy and chronic inflammation of the small intestinal mucosa that is severest proximally. Findings include weight loss; glossitis; other signs of a generalized vitamin deficiency; diarrhea; and passage of light-colored, bulky stools with a particularly foul odor caused by steatorrhea. Iron deficiency, hypocalcemia, osteoporosis, and osteomalacia may occur.

Folate malabsorption occurs in most patients with this disorder.[215] Serum folate levels are low,[216] and megaloblastic anemia occurs frequently. Malabsorption with resulting deficiency of other hematologically important micronutrients, including cobalamin and iron are often also present and patients with celiac disease are at increased risk of developing mucosa-associated lymphoid tumors.[217]

Tropical Sprue Tropical sprue was previously endemic in the West Indies, southern India, parts of Southern Africa, and Southeast Asia. It was acquired by travelers to those regions and persisted for many years after the traveler's return.[218] Typically there is malabsorption of other nutrients as well, notably cobalamin and fat.[219] Tropical sprue is rapidly corrected by folate therapy, even though folate deficiency is not the primary cause of the disease. The precise etiology of tropical sprue is unknown, although the response of the disease to antibiotics suggests that an underlying infection or disturbance of the microbiome may be involved.[220] Although now less commonly encountered than in the past, tropical sprue is still widely prevalent in some parts of the world and is a common cause of malabsorption syndrome.[221]

Clinically and pathologically, tropical sprue is like nontropical sprue, except that tropical sprue is more severe in the distal small intestine.[222] Tropical sprue eventually also leads to cobalamin deficiency[223] and should be considered a possible cause of cobalamin deficiency in former residents of the tropics, even though they have been away from the tropics for 20 years or more. Folate malabsorption may occur,[224] possibly because the diseased intestine fails to deconjugate folate polyglutamates.[224] Consequently, megaloblastic anemia is very common in patients with this disease,[225] and may result from both folate and cobalamin deficiency.

Other Intestinal Disorders Malabsorption of folic acid commonly occurs in regional enteritis,[225] after extensive resections of the small intestine,[226] and in conditions such as lymphomatous or leukemic infiltration of the small intestine,[227] Whipple disease,[221] scleroderma and amyloidosis,[228] and diabetes mellitus.[229] Systemic bacterial infections may impair folate absorption.[230]

Increased Folate Requirements in Pregnancy During pregnancy,[231] folate requirements increase 5- to 10-fold because of transfer of folate to the growing fetus,[232] which depletes maternal folate stores. This transfer occurs even in the face of severe maternal folate deficiency.[233] Further increases in requirements may result from the presence of multiple fetuses, a poor diet, infection, coexisting hemolytic anemia, or anticonvulsant medication.[234] Lactation aggravates folate deficiency.[235] Consequently, folate deficiency is very common in pregnancy and is the major cause of the megaloblastic anemia of pregnancy,[236] particularly in developing countries.[237]

Folate deficiency is difficult to diagnose in pregnancy because the signs of deficiency are obscured by the normal hematologic changes of pregnancy. During pregnancy, a physiologic "anemia" develops because of increased plasma volume that is only partly offset by an accompanying increase in red cell mass. Hemoglobin levels may fall to 100 g/L. The anemia is also associated with a physiologic macrocytosis; MCV may increase to 120 fL, although the average at term is 104 fL.[238] Serum and red cell folate levels fall steadily during pregnancy, even in well-nourished women who are not taking a folic acid supplement.[239,240] Conversely, hypersegmented neutrophils, usually a reliable clue to early megaloblastic anemia, are inconspicuous in early megaloblastic anemia of pregnancy.[241]

Increased Cell Turnover Because of increased marrow cell turnover, the folate requirement rises sharply in chronic *hemolytic anemia*.[242] During bouts of acute hemolysis that can occur in these anemias, the marrow may become megaloblastic within days.

Folic acid deficiency may arise in chronic *exfoliative dermatitis*, in which folate losses of 5 to 20 mcg/day may occur.[243] Patients with psoriasis who are treated with methotrexate have an added reason for developing signs of folate deficiency. Pretreating such patients with folate may prevent these signs without impairing the therapeutic effect of methotrexate.[243] During hemodialysis, folate is lost in the dialysis fluid.[244]

Clinical Features

The clinical picture of folate deficiency includes all the general manifestations of megaloblastic anemia *plus* the following specific features: (1) a history and laboratory studies indicating folate deficiency, (2) absence of the neurologic signs of cobalamin deficiency (see "Cobalamin Deficiency" further), and (3) a full response to *physiologic* doses of folate.

Laboratory Features

The earliest specific indicator of folate deficiency is a low serum or plasma folate. Raised plasma levels of homocysteine may precede any lowering of plasma folate below the reference range. However, elevated homocysteine has poor specificity as there are several causes of a raised plasma homocysteine.[245] Plasma folate follows folate intake closely, so an isolated low serum folate (less than approximately 3 ng/mL) may simply indicate a drop in folate intake over the preceding few days.[7] Similarly, a low plasma folate caused by inadequate intake rather than malabsorption, rises quickly on refeeding.

A more stable indicator of the tissue folate status is the red cell folate,[246] which remains relatively unchanged during the red cell life span and thus reflects aggregate folate status over the preceding 2 to 3 months. Red cell folate usually is low in folate-deficient megaloblastic anemia. However, red cell folate also is low in more than 50% of patients with cobalamin-deficient megaloblastic anemia[113] owing to impaired synthesis of polyglutamates and the poor retention of methyl THF monoglutamate within the cells; consequently, red cell folate cannot be reliably used to distinguish between folate and cobalamin deficiencies. Conversely, red cell folate may be normal in the megaloblastic state that occurs, often with little accompanying anemia, in rapidly developing folate deficiency (see "Acute Megaloblastic Anemia" further).[247]

The deoxyuridine suppression test has been used in research on pathogenetic mechanisms in megaloblastic states. It adds little to the clinical evaluation of a megaloblastic anemia. The test is further discussed in "Deoxyuridine Suppression" further.

Differential Diagnosis

Macrocytosis without megaloblastic anemia occurs in alcoholism, liver disease, hypothyroidism, aplastic anemia, certain forms of myelodysplasia, pregnancy, and any condition associated with reticulocytosis (eg, autoimmune hemolytic anemia).[248] Macrocytosis also has been reported among smokers.[249] However, MCV rarely exceeds 110 fL in these conditions, whereas in folate deficiency, uncomplicated by causes of microcytosis, the MCV is usually higher than 110 fL.

A full hematologic response to physiologic doses of folate (ie, 200 mcg daily) distinguishes folate deficiency from cobalamin deficiency, in which a response occurs only at pharmacologic doses of folate (typically 5 mg daily or more). This is not recommended as a diagnostic test because neurologic problems may develop in cobalamin-deficient patients treated with folate alone. High doses of cobalamin may produce a partial response in folate deficiency.[84]

The diagnosis of nontropical sprue rests on (1) the demonstration of malabsorption, (2) a jejunal biopsy showing villus atrophy, and (3) the response to a gluten-free diet. In 80% of patients, a gluten-free diet gradually reverses the functional disorder by correcting folate malabsorption.[250]

Combined Megaloblastic and Sideroblastic Anemia Consumption of goat's milk can not only cause folate deficiency with resulting megaloblastic anemia but also can cause vitamin B_6 deficiency and present as a combined clinicopathologic picture of megaloblastic and sideroblastic anemia.[207] In the marrow megaloblastic changes with increased mitotic figures are seen along with ring (pathologic) sideroblasts in the marrow aspirate iron stain.

Nonhematologic Effects of Folate Deficiency

The hematologic problems associated with folate deficiency have been recognized for decades. However, folate deficiency has been associated with several serious disorders not involving the hematopoietic system. Moreover, these disorders occur at folate levels usually regarded as low normal. They include developmental, neurologic, cardiovascular, and neoplasmic disorders.[251]

Abnormalities of Neural Tube Closure

A close association exists between mild folate deficiency and congenital anomalies of the fetus, most notably defects in neural tube closure, but also abnormalities involving the heart, urinary tract, limbs, and other sites.[252] A portion of the neural tube closure defects are associated with antibodies against folate receptors that may be overcome by higher folate intake.[253] Mutations and polymorphisms affecting enzymes of folate metabolism, especially the common 677C → T polymorphism of the *MTHFR* gene (also designated as *MTHFR* 677C → T),[254] also predispose to congenital anomalies. As noted earlier, this polymorphism results in diminished conversion of its substrate methylene THF to methyl THF, supporting the view that it is the role of folate in methylation through methionine synthesis (see Table 9-1) that is critical in embryonic neurodevelopment. Folic acid fortification programs, which were mandated in the United States and Canada in the mid-1990s, have been highly successful as a public health measure in reducing the incidence of neural tube defect births by between 20% and 50%.[255,256]

Cobalamin also plays a significant role as a risk factor for neural tube defects. Levels of TC in normal pregnant women correlate with their likelihood of bearing an infant with a defect in neural tube closure. Patients in the lowest quintile of TC concentration are 5 times more likely to give birth to a defective infant as patients in the highest quintile.[257] In populations exposed to folic acid fortification, there is an approximately threefold increase in the risk of neural tube defects in offspring of mothers in the lowest quartile of TC.[258]

Several poorly defined neuropsychiatric abnormalities that respond to folate therapy occur in patients with folate deficiency. The most convincing associations are with depressive illness.[251,259]

Vascular Disease

A mildly elevated homocysteine level is a major independent risk factor for atherosclerosis and venous thrombosis, possibly because of an effect on the vascular endothelium.[260] The effect of lowering homocysteine levels by the use of folate, cobalamin, and pyridoxine supplements, on the risk of recurrent vascular disease is unclear. While there is some evidence that such supplements reduce risk,[261] contradictory evidence suggests that supplement use may actually increase the risk of in-stent coronary restenosis[262] or other adverse cardiovascular outcome.[263] An accelerated rate of decrease in stroke mortality has been observed in the United States and Canada that coincided with the introduction of folic acid fortification in these countries.[264] The disparate designs of these studies makes it difficult to draw firm conclusions regarding the question of whether lowering of plasma homocysteine in individuals at risk for cardiovascular disease has any ameliorative or deleterious effect on outcome. In a meta-analysis of 8 randomized trials involving more than 37,000 individuals, the authors concluded that supplementation with folic acid in various combinations with cobalamin and vitamin B_6 for periods of up to 7.3 years, despite an overall reduction of plasma homocysteine of 22% in folic acid-fortified populations and 25% in folic acid-nonfortified populations, there were no significant effects on cardiovascular events, overall cancer, or mortality.[265] Critical factors might relate to several considerations, including the preexisting degree of vascular damage in relation to the time of the intervention and the form and dosage of administered vitamins. A more compelling association of elevated homocysteine is with cognitive decline. Several studies indicate that moderately elevated plasma homocysteine is a strong modifiable risk factor for vascular dementia and Alzheimer disease.[266]

The *MTHFR* polymorphism *MTHFR* 677C → T leads to increased homocysteine levels in individuals with low folate or cobalamin levels,[267] although controversy exists as to whether *MTHFR* 677C → T contributes to an increased incidence of vascular disease. Like folate, cobalamin seems to be important in decreasing the risk of vascular disease.[268] A 1561C → T polymorphism in the gene for glutamate carboxypeptidase-II increases serum folate and decreases serum homocysteine in the homozygote, possibly protecting against vascular disease.[269]

HELLP Syndrome

Severe folate deficiency reportedly mimics the hemolysis, elevated liver enzymes, low platelets (HELLP) syndrome (preeclampsia with liver swelling and abnormal liver function studies in pregnant women;.[270] In these patients, the diagnosis of severe folate deficiency can be made based on the presence of anemia and a megaloblastic blood film and marrow. Serum and red cell folate, serum cobalamin, homocysteine, and methylmalonic acid levels all should be assayed before treatment is started.[271] The patient should immediately be given high doses of folate plus cobalamin; cobalamin should be given in case the megaloblastic anemia actually results from cobalamin deficiency, a possibility rendered more likely in folic acid-fortified populations. A major goal of treatment is preventing preterm delivery of the fetus.

Colon Cancer

A large study of nurses in the United States indicated that supplementation with more than 400 mcg of folic acid per day reduces the incidence of colon cancer by 31%.[272] Furthermore, individuals who are homozygous for the 677C → T *MTHFR* mutation also have a decreased incidence for colon cancer compared with 677C → T heterozygotes and normal controls.[273] On the other hand, other evidence points to possible deleterious effect of folic acid on colon cancer incidence. Although only circumstantial, an epidemiologic study reported that after several successive years of a declining incidence of colorectal cancer in the United States and Canada, there was a significant increase in the rate in both countries that coincided with and followed the introduction of folic acid fortification.[274] These apparently contradictory observations may be reconcilable because of the several roles of folate on cellular proliferation and repair as well as on the stage of tumorigenesis.[275] Because folate is critical for de novo thymidine synthesis, it plays an important part

in DNA repair, thus correcting mutations and DNA strand breaks that could initiate cancer. On the other hand, the growth of established neoplastic clones might be accelerated by additional folate, allowing more rapid tumor progression. The situation is rendered even more complex if the potential role of folate in epigenetic regulation of gene expression is considered. Folate is necessary for synthesis of the universal methyl donor, SAM, which is required for both cytosine and histone methylation. In this pathway, too, the role of folate theoretically may be cancer promoting or cancer protective, depending on whether oncogenes or tumor suppressor genes are silenced by methylation of cytosine-phosphate-guanine (CpG) islands in DNA or by conformational changes in chromatin resulting from histone methylation. Another possible link between increased intake of folic acid and cancer has been raised by observations linking increased plasma levels of unmetabolized folic acid with reduced natural killer cell cytotoxicity.[276,277] The question of a possible effect of increased folate intake through the use of folic acid supplements on overall and site-specific cancer incidence was examined in a metaanalysis of 50,000 individuals. The authors concluded that there was no substantial increase or decrease in incidence over a 5-year period of folic acid supplement use.[278]

Therapy, Course, and Prognosis

Folate, usually in the form of folic acid, 1 to 5 mg/day, is given orally, although 1 mg usually is sufficient. At this dose, anemia usually is corrected even in patients with malabsorption. A parenteral preparation containing 5 mg/mL of folate also is available.

Treatment for tropical sprue consists of the usual doses of folate, plus cobalamin if indicated. To prevent relapse, treatment should be maintained for at least 2 years. Broad-spectrum antibiotics are helpful adjuncts, although antibiotics alone fail to correct the condition.

Pregnant women must be given at least 400 mcg of folate per day.[279] As to the possibility of overlooking cobalamin deficiency resulting from folate administration, although PA in women of childbearing age is rare in whites, this is not the case among Black people and Hispanics.[280,281] In pregnant women at risk for cobalamin deficiency (eg, vegans or patients with malabsorption), the risk of an associated cobalamin deficiency is easily prevented with vitamin B_{12}, 1 mg given parenterally every 3 months during the pregnancy.

Therapeutic doses of folate partially and temporarily correct the hematologic abnormalities in cobalamin deficiency, but the neurologic manifestations can progress, with disastrous results.[282] Therefore, both folate status and cobalamin status must be evaluated early in the workup of a megaloblastic anemia. If treatment is urgent and the nature of the deficiency is unclear, both folate and cobalamin should be given after suitable specimens have been obtained for measurement.

Patients who receive low-dose methotrexate therapy as an immunosuppressant may develop side effects, the worst of which is hepatotoxicity. The incidence of side effects, including hepatotoxicity, has been correlated with reduced folate levels.[283] Administration of folic or folinic acid can prevent or greatly diminish the major side effects without reducing the therapeutic effect of low-dose methotrexate. Coadministration of folic acid together with vitamin B_{12} also reduces side effects without adversely affecting the therapeutic efficacy of the newer multi-targeted antifolate drug, pemetrexed.[284]

COBALAMIN DEFICIENCY

Etiology and Pathogenesis

There are several causes and varying degrees of severity of cobalamin depletion and deficiency. From the hematologic standpoint, it is convenient to divide the causes of B_{12} deficiency into those that frequently lead to megaloblastic anemia and those that usually do not.[85,285,286] Table 9-4 lists disorders that lead to cobalamin deficiency.

Decreased Uptake Caused by Impaired Absorption Cobalamin deficiency most often results from defective absorption, most commonly PA, a condition characterized by failure of gastric intrinsic factor production. Many other causes of defective cobalamin absorption involve mainly the stomach, or small intestine and to lesser extent, the pancreas.

Gastric Disorders Pernicious Anemia PA is a disease of insidious onset that usually begins after age 40.[287] In this condition, intrinsic factor secretion fails because of gastric mucosal atrophy. PA is an autoimmune disease. The gastric atrophy of PA probably results from immune destruction of the acid-secreting and pepsin-secreting portion of the gastric mucosa. The term PA sometimes is used as a synonym for cobalamin deficiency, but it should be reserved for the condition resulting from defective secretion of intrinsic factor by an atrophic gastric mucosa caused by an autoimmune process primarily directed against the parietal cells and their products.

In patients with PA, antibodies occur that recognize the H^+/K^+-ATPase, which resides in the secretory membrane of the parietal cell and is responsible for acidifying the stomach contents. These antiparietal cell antibodies occur in approximately 60% of patients with simple atrophic gastritis and in 90% of patients with PA, but in only 5% of a random 30- to 60-year-old population.[288] Antiparietal cell antibodies also occur in a significant percentage of patients with thyroid disease.[289] Conversely, patients with PA have a higher than expected incidence of antibodies against thyroid epithelium, lymphocytes, and renal collecting duct cells.[290,291]

Antiparietal cell antibodies are not thought to be responsible for the pathogenesis of PA. Rather, studies in mice suggest the gastric atrophy in PA is caused by CD4+ T cells whose receptors recognize the H^+/K^+-ATPase. Thus, thymectomized BALB/c mice develop an autoimmune atrophic gastritis similar to that seen in PA patients. CD4+ T cells from these mice produce atrophic gastritis when injected into nude mice.[292]

Antibodies to intrinsic factor ("type I," or "blocking," antibodies) or the intrinsic factor–cobalamin (Cbl) complex ("type II," or "binding," antibodies) are highly specific to PA patients.[291,293] Blocking antibodies, which prevent formation of the intrinsic factor–Cbl complex, are found in up to 70% of PA sera.[293] Binding antibodies, which prevent the intrinsic factor–Cbl complex from binding to its ileal receptors, are found in approximately half the sera that contain blocking antibody. Some findings in humans support the idea that T cells are responsible for the gastric atrophy in PA. First, lymphocytes from patients with PA are hyperresponsive to gastric antigens.[294] Second, the incidence of PA is higher than expected in patients with agammaglobulinemia, even though their sera contain none of the antibodies typical of PA.[295]

Other Autoimmune Diseases The coexistence of several other autoimmune diseases and PA is further evidence that PA is an autoimmune disease. Antiparietal cell antibodies and PA are unexpectedly frequent in patients with other autoimmune diseases,[291,295] including autoimmune thyroid disorders (thyrotoxicosis, hypothyroidism, and Hashimoto thyroiditis),[296] type I diabetes mellitus, hypoparathyroidism,[297] Addison disease, postpartum hypophysitis,[298] vitiligo,[299] pure red cell aplasia,[300] acquired agammaglobulinemia,[295] infertile female patients younger than 40 years,[301] and hypospermia and infertility in men.[302,303] Infertility may, however, relate to impairment of DNA synthesis in gonadal cells rather than to an autoimmune mechanism.

Inherited Predisposition to Pernicious Anemia Predisposition to PA can be inherited. The disease is associated with human leukocyte antigen types A2, A3, B7, and B12[304] and with blood group A.[305] PA and antiparietal cell antibodies occur more frequently than expected in the families of PA patients.[306] In one study, gastric atrophy was found in more than 30% of the relatives of patients with PA; of these relatives, 65% had antiparietal cell antibodies and 22% had anti-intrinsic factor antibodies.[307] PA occurs relatively frequently in northern Europeans

(especially Scandinavians)[308] as well as Africans,[181,309] but is uncommon in Asians. In Americans of African descent, the disease tends to begin early, occurs with high frequency in women, and often is severe.[181,281]

Stomach and Intestine in Pernicious Anemia Gastric manifestations of PA include achlorhydria, acquired intrinsic factor deficiency previously demonstrable through showing malabsorption of cobalamin by the Schilling test, and an increased incidence of certain malignancies. There is an approximately twofold increase in the incidence of gastric cancer, similar increases in the incidence of certain hematologic malignancies, and an increase in the incidence of gastric carcinoid.[308] Achlorhydria may precede by many years the loss of intrinsic factor secretion and the development of PA.[310] The absence of achlorhydria excludes the diagnosis of PA. *H. pylori*, a microorganism that infects the gastric mucosa, is a major cause of gastritis and peptic ulcers. Evidence is conflicting regarding the role of *H. pylori* in PA. In two studies, cultures of gastric biopsies showed a very low incidence of *H. pylori* infection in patients with PA.[311] One study reported that anti–*H. pylori* antibodies were found in only a small fraction of the sera from these patients. The other study reported that these antibodies were present in most of the PA sera, indicating that most of the patients described in the study had been infected previously. Whether *H. pylori* participates in the pathogenesis of PA is an open question. An intriguing hypothesis has been advanced that chronic infection with *H. pylori* may be responsible for triggering an autoimmune reaction directed against the host H+/K+-ATPase protein as a result of molecular mimicry.[185,186,312] The nexus among *H. pylori*, PA, and gastric cancer provides possible insights into the connections between this gastric pathogen and a major cause of cobalamin deficiency.[185,313]

Fasting plasma gastrin levels are high in most patients with PA, whereas somatostatin levels are low.[314] In biopsies from PA patients' stomachs, however, fundal gastrin and somatostatin levels were high, correlating with increases in argyrophilic cells in the basal crypts; antral gastrin and somatostatin were normal. Gastrin levels are high in simple achlorhydria without PA.[315]

The stomach shows characteristic histologic abnormalities in PA (Fig. 9-15). The mucosa of the cardia and fundus is atrophic, containing few chief (ie, pepsin-secreting) or parietal cells. The withered mucosa is infiltrated with lymphocytes[316] and plasma cells. In contrast, the antral and pyloric mucosa are normal. Gastric atrophy is partly reversible by glucocorticoid treatment, with some regeneration and return of intrinsic factor secretion, further evidence for the autoimmune nature of PA.[317] Clinical response to administration of glucocorticoids or adrenocorticotropic hormone in patients with neurologic disease may reflect temporary amelioration of underlying and undiagnosed PA.[318]

Megaloblastic changes reversible by cobalamin are seen in the gastrointestinal epithelium. Cells recovered by lavage are large[188] and show atypical nuclei resembling early malignant change.[319] Small intestinal biopsy shows decreased mitoses in crypts, shortening of villi, megaloblastic changes in epithelial cells, and infiltration in the lamina propria.[320] These changes may account for the malabsorption of D-xylose and carotene observed in PA.[321]

Recognizing PA may be difficult. PA combines the general features of megaloblastic anemia and features specific for cobalamin deficiency with unique clinical features related to its (probable) autoimmune etiology and gastric pathology. The disease is easily missed because of its (1) insidious onset, (2) tendency to be masked by the use of multivitamin preparations containing folic acid,[322] and (3) many atypical presentations,[323,324] including its presentation as a neurologic disease without hematologic findings,[89,325] absence of macrocytosis because of coexistent iron deficiency or thalassemia minor,[171,172] and its tendency to be overlooked in patients with another autoimmune disease.

Antiparietal cell and anti-intrinsic factor antibodies are rarely measured, even though anti-intrinsic factor antibodies in particular approximately 25% to 50% have low serum cobalamin levels, and many have varying degrees of decreased cobalamin absorption.[327] Achlorhydria not present before surgery often develops some years after gastrectomy. Postgastrectomy patients with low serum cobalamin levels usually have low serum iron levels,[328] in contrast to the high iron levels otherwise typical of cobalamin deficiency.

Cobalamin deficiency after partial gastrectomy can be caused by mucosal atrophy in the unresected remnant of the stomach[329] or, if a gastrojejunostomy was performed, by bacterial overgrowth in the afferent loop (see "Competing Intestinal Flora and Fauna: 'Blind Loop Syndrome'" further). A surgical procedure that has gained popularity for the treatment of morbid obesity is gastric reduction surgery. This procedure results in multiple deficiencies of micronutrients, including cobalamin.[184,330]

Of the various causes of cobalamin malabsorption described, those that most often lead to megaloblastic anemia include PA, total or partial gastrectomy, intestinal blind loop syndrome, fish tapeworm (see further), ileal resection, Crohn disease, and tropical sprue.[72] In addition, several of the inherited disorders affecting cobalamin absorption and metabolism, such as congenital intrinsic factor deficiency, selective cobalamin malabsorption, and congenital TC deficiency, can also result in megaloblastic anemia.

Zollinger-Ellison Syndrome In Zollinger-Ellison syndrome, a gastrin-producing tumor, usually in the pancreas, stimulates the gastric mucosa to secrete immense amounts of HCl. The major clinical problem is a severe ulcer diathesis. Malabsorption of cobalamin occurs when the vast quantities of HCl secreted by the overactive gastric mucosa cannot be completely neutralized by the pancreatic secretions. The resulting acidification of the duodenal contents prevents transfer of Cbl from HC binder to intrinsic factor and inactivates pancreatic proteases.[331]

Intestinal Diseases Because the terminal ileum is the site for physiologic cobalamin absorption, a number of intestinal disorders can lead to cobalamin deficiency, including: (1) extensive resection of the ileum[332]; (2) inflammatory bowel disease or regional ileitis or other disease affecting the ileum (eg, lymphoma, radiation damage[333]); (3) cobalamin malabsorption associated with hypothyroidism,[334] or certain drugs[335]; (4) the effects of cobalamin deficiency itself[336]; and (5) sprue, either tropical or, less often, nontropical.[223] In each of these disorders, administration of exogenous intrinsic factor, as was carried out in the Schilling test, would fail to correct a subnormal cobalamin absorption test result.

Competing Intestinal Flora and Fauna: "Blind Loop Syndrome" The *blind loop syndrome* is a state of cobalamin malabsorption with megaloblastic anemia caused by intestinal stasis from anatomic lesions (strictures, diverticula, anastomoses, surgical blind loops) or impaired motility (scleroderma, amyloid).[337] Serum cobalamin is low, but intrinsic factor secretion is normal. Cobalamin malabsorption was not corrected by exogenous intrinsic factor in a Schilling test but could be corrected by antibiotic treatment. The defect in cobalamin absorption is caused by colonization of the diseased small intestine by bacteria that take up ingested cobalamin before it can be absorbed from the intestine.[338] Cobalamin analogues found in the feces point to the possibility that intestinal microbiota disassemble cobalamin, retaining portions of the molecule for their own use.[147,148] Steatorrhea is also seen in the blind loop syndrome.

Another cause of cobalamin deficiency is infestation with the fish tapeworm *Diphyllobothrium latum*. Prevalence is highest near the Baltic Sea, Canada, and Alaska where raw or undercooked fish is consumed. Cobalamin deficiency results from competition between the worm and the host for ingested cobalamin.[339] The clinical picture of *D. latum* infestation ranges from no symptoms to a full-blown megaloblastic anemia with neurologic changes. The infestation is diagnosed by finding tapeworm ova in the feces.

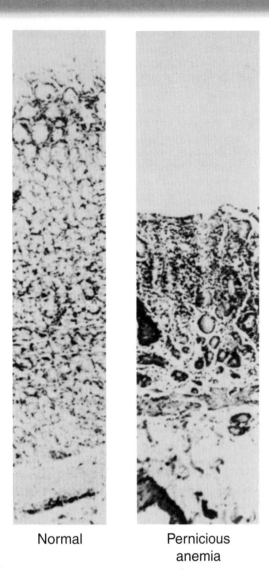

Normal   Pernicious anemia

FIGURE 9–15. Gastric histology in pernicious anemia. (*Left*) Normal fundus. The thick mucosa is packed with gastric glands composed mostly of chief cells and parietal cells. The mucus-secreting cells are concentrated in the necks of the glands. (*Right*) Fundus in pernicious anemia. Gastric glands in the atrophic mucosa are sparse and consist mainly of mucus-secreting cells. The mucosa is densely infiltrated by lymphocytes.

could be of considerable diagnostic value.[247] In the absence of a reliable method to assess vitamin B_{12} absorption, following the demise of the Schilling test, measurement of antiintrinsic factor antibodies in serum represents the only available method to positively confirm a diagnosis of PA. Anti-intrinsic factor antibody is highly specific for PA (although its sensitivity is only a modest 60%-70%), and its presence in a megaloblastic anemia makes the diagnosis of PA almost certain.

Gastrectomy Syndromes Gastric surgery often leads to anemia. Iron-deficiency anemia is most common, but cobalamin deficiency with megaloblastic anemia can occur. After *total gastrectomy*, cobalamin deficiency develops within 5 or 6 years because the operation removes the source of intrinsic factor.[326] The delay between surgery and the onset of cobalamin deficiency reflects the time needed to exhaust cobalamin stores after cobalamin absorption ceases. This may occur more rapidly because of abrogation of the enterohepatic reabsorption of biliary cobalamin.[122]

After *partial gastrectomy*, few patients show frank cobalamin deficiency, but approximately 5% show some degree of megaloblastosis,

Acquired Immunodeficiency Syndrome A substantial number of patients with AIDS have low serum cobalamin levels with associated evidence of cobalamin malabsorption.[340] In addition, individuals testing seropositive for HIV infection may also have low serum cobalamin and evidence of cobalamin malabsorption.[340] The cause of the malabsorption may be intestinal or gastric or a combination of both.[341,342]

Pancreatic Disease Some degree of cobalamin malabsorption has been demonstrated in 50% to 70% of patients with exocrine pancreatic insufficiency.[343] Cobalamin malabsorption in pancreatic insufficiency is caused by a deficiency in pancreatic proteases, resulting in a partial failure to destroy HC–Cbl complexes whose destruction is a prerequisite for the transfer of cobalamin to intrinsic factor.[344] Pancreatic insufficiency rarely causes clinically significant cobalamin deficiency.[345]

Dietary Cobalamin Deficiency Dietary cobalamin deficiency was previously considered very unusual and restricted largely to complete vegetarians who also do not consume dairy products and eggs (vegans).[346] Low serum cobalamin levels occur in 50% to 60% of individuals in this group. The onset of cobalamin deficiency in vegans is slower than in conditions associated with cobalamin malabsorption. Thus it may take 10 to 20 years for an individual consuming a vegan diet to manifest features of cobalamin deficiency.[347] This is because the enterohepatic pathway for biliary cobalamin absorption remains intact, which conserves body cobalamin stores.[72] Breastfed infants of vegan mothers also may develop cobalamin deficiency.[348] Cobalamin deficiency in vegans presents with mild megaloblastic anemia, glossitis, and neurologic disturbances. In addition to vegans, however, there is mounting evidence of cobalamin inadequacy in children and young adults in developing countries that cannot be explained on the basis of cobalamin malabsorption, and has therefore been attributed to inadequate dietary intake.[349]

Cobalamin deficiency may occur in severe general malnutrition. A megaloblastic anemia not related to cobalamin deficiency may accompany kwashiorkor or marasmus.[350] This may be related to other associated micronutrient deficiencies (Chap. 12).

Neurologic Effects of Cobalamin Deficiency

Previously, the neurologic abnormalities of cobalamin deficiency were attributed to disordered metabolism of myelin lipids caused by an impaired methylmalonyl CoA mutase reaction.[351] Similar neurologic abnormalities do not, however, occur in patients with inherited methylmalonyl CoA mutase deficiency.[288,352] Authentic combined system disease has occurred in a patient with nutritional folate deficiency[353] and in a patient with MTHFR deficiency.[354] The latter reports suggest the neurologic lesions of cobalamin deficiency result from deranged methyl group metabolism. Animal studies support this hypothesis. Neurologic disorders closely resembling combined system disease develop in cobalamin-deficient fruit bats,[355] pigs, and monkeys.[356] The development of these disorders is prevented by methionine, which is produced in a cobalamin-dependent reaction and is the precursor of the biologic methylating reagent SAM.[357] A finding that further supports a methylation defect is that brains from cobalamin-deficient pigs contain increased levels of SAH,[358] a powerful methylation inhibitor produced in SAM-dependent methylation reactions:

$$SAM + RH \rightarrow SAH + RCH_3$$

Against the methylation defect hypothesis is the finding that cobalamin deficiency had no effect on SAM, SAH, or methylation of phospholipids or myelin basic protein[359] in the brains of fruit bats.

Clinical Features

The clinical manifestations of cobalamin deficiency have been reviewed.[85,286,360] The more typical clinical picture of cobalamin deficiency includes the nonspecific manifestations of megaloblastosis, such as anemia, thrombocytopenia, neutropenia, smooth tongue, cardiomyopathy, pale yellow skin and/or weight loss, plus specific features caused by the lack of cobalamin, chiefly neurologic abnormalities. Disturbances in either or both cellular and hormonal immune functions have been reported in cobalamin deficiency.[361,362] Cobalamin deficiency may also contribute to the risk of vascular disease through elevation of homocysteine levels. Other disease associations with cobalamin deficiency have been described. These include a possible increase in breast cancer risk in premenopausal women[363] and of osteoporosis.[363,365] Because cobalamin reserves are large, years may pass between the cessation of cobalamin absorption and the appearance of deficiency symptoms.

Neurologic Abnormalities Cobalamin deficiency causes a neurologic syndrome that is particularly dangerous because the syndrome can develop insidiously and in isolation,[366] with no megaloblastic anemia to suggest a lack of cobalamin,[325,367] and because the syndrome cannot be reversed by treatment when it is sufficiently far advanced. The syndrome usually begins with paresthesias in feet and fingers as a result of early peripheral neuropathy and disturbances of vibratory sense and proprioception. The earliest signs, which precede other neurologic findings by months, are loss of position sense in the second toe and loss of vibration sense for a 256-Hz but not a 128-Hz tuning fork.[368] Left untreated, the neurologic disorder progresses to spastic ataxia resulting from demyelination of the dorsal and lateral columns of the spinal cord, so-called combined system disease (Fig. 9-16).[369]

The peripheral nerves, the spinal cord, and the brain are affected by cobalamin deficiency. Somnolence and perversion of taste, smell, and vision with occasional optic atrophy are accompanied by slow waves on the electroencephalogram. A dementia mimicking Alzheimer disease can develop.[370] There is evidence linking low cobalamin status with brain volume loss and cerebral white matter lesions.[371,372] Psychological derangements, including psychotic depression and paranoid schizophrenia, can occur.[373] Frank psychosis in cobalamin deficiency has been given the sobriquet *megaloblastic madness*.[374] In a description of PA in the classical text *The Red Cell*, Harris and Kellermeyer described the metamorphosis as "The patient, formerly a pleasant individual, is now a cantankerous curmudgeon."[375]

The neurologic lesions of cobalamin deficiency can be detected by magnetic resonance imaging (MRI). Demyelination appears as T2-weighted hyperintensity of the white matter.[376,377] MRI is particularly useful for confirming the diagnosis of a neurologic disorder resulting from cobalamin deficiency. MRI also has been used to follow the progress of neurologic abnormalities during treatment of cobalamin-deficient patients.[376]

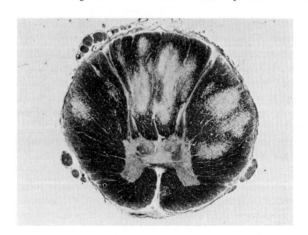

FIGURE 9–16. Degeneration of spinal cord in combined system disease. (*Reproduced with permission from Harris JW, Kellermeyer RW. The Red Cell: Production, Metabolism, Destruction: Normal and Abnormal, rev ed. Cambridge: Harvard University Press; 1970.*)

Subtle Cobalamin Deficiency Some observations suggest the existence of a large group of patients who are hematologically normal, with a normal hematocrit and MCV, but who have cobalamin-responsive neuropsychiatric disease.[325] Neuropsychiatric findings include peripheral neuropathy, gait disturbance, memory loss, and psychiatric symptoms, often with abnormal evoked potentials. Serum cobalamin may be normal, borderline, or low, but tissue cobalamin deficiency is suggested by consistently high levels of serum methylmalonic acid and/or homocysteine. Most of the neuropsychiatric abnormalities appear to respond to cobalamin therapy.

Thrombotic Microangiopathy Cases of thrombotic microangiopathy with severe vitamin B_{12} deficiency resulting from the inborn errors of metabolism have been described and referred to as cblC or cblG disease.[378] cblG is characterized by mutation in the *MTR* gene leading to a dysfunctional methionine synthase enzyme and cblC disease involves a defect in the enzyme responsible for conversion of cobalamin into its metabolically active reduced forms causing accumulation of homocysteine. However, other causes of hyperhomocysteinemia do not lead to thrombotic microangiopathy per se. Patients with cblG disease and associated methionine synthase (MTR) deficiency may represent the development of vasculopathies with thrombotic consequences in cblG disease. In patients with thrombotic microangiopathy associated with cblC, treatment with hydroxycobalamin resulted in improved kidney function and overall survival.[379]

Laboratory Features

Plasma or Serum Cobalamin Levels Plasma or serum cobalamin is low in most but not all patients with cobalamin deficiency.[245] Cobalamin levels are usually normal in cobalamin deficiency resulting from exposure to nitrous oxide,[82] TC deficiency, and inborn errors of cobalamin metabolism.[380] Levels also may be normal in cobalamin-deficient patients with high HC levels resulting from myeloproliferative diseases.[324] Conversely, plasma cobalamin levels may be low in the presence of normal tissue cobalamins in vegetarians, in individuals taking megadoses of ascorbic acid,[381] in pregnancy (25%), in the presence of HC deficiency,[382,383] and in 30% of patients with megaloblastic anemia resulting from folate deficiency (30%).[245] On the other hand, plasma folate may be high in cobalamin deficiency because of the methyl folate "trap" resulting in retardation in conversion of methyl-THF, which is the predominant form in plasma.[6] Patients deficient in both cobalamin and folate may therefore show normal serum folate levels.[201]

Serum Holotranscobalamin The fraction of the cobalamin in plasma that is bound to TC constitutes only 10% to 30% of the total plasma cobalamin. Even so, it is this fraction that is functionally important and also better reflects the integrity of the cobalamin absorptive status of an individual.[158,384,385] The major fraction of plasma cobalamin bound to HC is considered functionally inert and is therefore less relevant for the consideration of cobalamin status. Consequently, and with the development of assays to measure the TC-bound fraction of the plasma cobalamin, an increasing body of evidence has accumulated to support the usefulness of TC-associated cobalamin (holotranscobalamin).[72,153,156,384]

Methylmalonic Acid Except when caused by an inborn error, methylmalonic aciduria is a reliable indicator of cobalamin deficiency.[386] Normal individuals excrete only traces of methylmalonate (0-3.4 mg/day). In cobalamin deficiency, urine methylmalonate usually is elevated.[387] Cobalamin therapy restores excretion to normal in a few days. Another possible advantage of measurement of urine rather than plasma methylmalonic acid is that in conditions of impaired renal function, when plasma methylmalonic acid may give misleadingly elevated levels, measurement of the metabolite in urine when correlated with creatinine obviates this problem.[388]

Serum or Plasma Methylmalonic Acid and Homocysteine Elevated plasma or serum methylmalonic acid and homocysteine levels are indicators of *tissue* cobalamin deficiency. Their levels are high in more than 90% of cobalamin-deficient patients and rise before plasma cobalamin falls to subnormal levels.[245,389] Elevated plasma methylmalonic acid and/or elevated homocysteine are both indicators of cobalamin deficiency in patients without a congenital metabolic disorder. Of the two, methylmalonic acid measurement is both more sensitive and more specific, and elevated methylmalonic acid will persist for several days, even after cobalamin treatment is instituted. Unlike homocysteine levels that rise in folate and pyridoxine deficiencies, as well as in hypothyroidism, methylmalonic acid elevation occurs only in cobalamin deficiency.[245] In renal diseases, however, both homocysteine and methylmalonate, acid levels are frequently elevated. Additionally, intestinal bacteria synthesize propionate, a precursor of methylmalonate, and in conditions of bacterial overgrowth, microbially derived methylmalonic acid may contribute to elevations in plasma methylmalonic acid.[389,390] Although measurement of these metabolites may be used for population screening for evidence of cobalamin deficiency, the finding of an isolated elevation of plasma methylmalonate cannot be taken as a priori evidence of clinically attributable cobalamin deficiency, absent any demonstration of a therapeutic response to the administration of cobalamin.[390,391] A combined indicator using several tests provide improved clinical predictive value for the confirmation of presumed cobalamin deficiency.[392,393]

A common polymorphism in the gene for 3-hydroxyisobutyryl-CoA hydrolase (*HIBCH*) has been identified. The polymorphism results in higher methylmalonic acid concentrations unrelated to B_{12} status.[394] It is not clear whether this could be clinically important with regard to defining cutpoints for cobalamin deficiency in individuals with this single-nucleotide polymorphism.

Spinal fluid methylmalonic acid levels are markedly elevated in cobalamin deficiency.[395]

Assays of Cobalamin Absorption and Intrinsic Factor Despite its numerous shortcomings the previous "gold standard" for assessment of cobalamin absorption was the Schilling test. The Schilling test assessed cobalamin absorption by measuring urinary radioactivity after an oral dose of radioactive cobalamin. The test could be performed even after cobalamin deficiency had been corrected. The test consisted of administering a physiologic dose of radiolabeled Co-CnCbl by mouth followed 2 hours later by injection of a large "flushing" dose of unlabeled CnCbl and determination of radioactivity in a 24-hour collection of urine. Subjects with normal absorption excreted 7% or more of the radioactivity in the urine. Subjects with subnormal urinary excretion of the label would have the test repeated with addition of an animal-derived intrinsic factor to determine whether the malabsorption could be corrected.[396] The use of the Schilling test has become obsolete as a consequence of reduced availability of the test components, cost, radioactive waste disposal, and concern about the use of animal-derived tissues for human use, which were required for the intrinsic factor administered in the second part of the test.[72] Replacements for the Schilling test are needed and some attempts have been made. One approach uses measurement of the change in holotranscobalamin following oral administration of nonradiolabeled cobalamin.[384,385,397] A different approach involves the use of accelerator mass spectrometry and microbially produced CnCbl labeled with C-14 in the 5,6-dimethylbenzimidazolyl lower axial ligand at attomolar concentrations.[398] In this approach, C-14 is measured in blood at the time of peak appearance 6 to 8 hours following the dose. Both methods show promise but have not been approved or validated for routine clinical use. In a modification of the C-14 label approach, a method using C13 has been described.[399,400]

Deoxyuridine Suppression Test The deoxyuridine suppression test is based on the finding that unlabeled deoxyuridine can suppress the uptake of [^{3}H]thymidine into the DNA of cultured lymphocytes or marrow cells through dilution of the label in the thymidine pool.[401]

This occurs when the thymidylate synthase reaction is functionally intact, which requires adequate quantities of both folate and cobalamin. In deficiencies of either vitamin, suppression of [³H]thymidine by deoxyuridine fails.

The deoxyuridine suppression test is chiefly a research tool. It can help diagnose certain special clinical problems,[401] but these problems also can be diagnosed using other laboratory tests, therapeutic trials with vitamins or iron, or watchful waiting. Furthermore, the test has not moved from the research laboratory into the clinic and seems unlikely to enjoy more widespread clinical use in the future.

Therapy, Course, and Prognosis

Treatment of cobalamin deficiency consists of parenteral CnCbl (vitamin B_{12}) or OHCbl to replace daily losses and restore cobalamin reserves, which normally contain 2 to 5 mg of cobalamin.[402] Toxicity is highly unusual, and there is no defined upper limit.[2] A nested case-control study found an association of high levels of serum cobalamin with lung cancer risk.[403] Another Dutch study suggested that higher levels of plasma concentrations of vitamin B_{12} were associated with increased risk of all-cause mortality.[404] This association, though without any any cause and effect validity, was widely publicized, with resulting deleterious effect on the compliance of patients who require regular supplemental cobalamin. A subsequent study reporting on 24,262 subjects in the NHANES cohort has somewhat mitigated the alarm caused by the Dutch study. This study concluded that there was a small but significant increase in cardiovascular mortality in the groups with either low or high serum B_{12}. However, high intake of vitamin B_{12} in the form of supplements was not associated with any adverse effect on mortality and therefore can be regarded as safe.[405] Doses exceeding 100 mcg saturate the cobalamin-binding proteins (TC and HC), and the excess is lost in the urine. A typical treatment schedule consists of 1000 mcg cobalamin intramuscularly daily for 2 weeks, then weekly until the hematocrit is normal or symptoms improve, and then monthly for life. For neurologic manifestations, 1000 mcg every 2 weeks for 6 months is recommended. Higher doses are given for certain inherited disorders (eg, TC deficiency). *Transfusion* occasionally is required when the hematocrit is less than 15% or the patient is debilitated, infected, or in heart failure. In such instances, packed cells should be given slowly to avoid circulatory overload and pulmonary edema. Infections can impair the response to cobalamin and must be treated vigorously.

Response to Treatment and Therapeutic Trial Following parenteral administration of cobalamin to deficient patients, elevated plasma bilirubin, iron, and LDH levels fall rapidly (Fig. 9-17).[406] Decreasing plasma iron turnover and fecal urobilinogen reflect cessation of ineffective erythropoiesis. Within 12 hours, the marrow begins to change from megaloblastic to normoblastic, a process that is complete in 2 to 3 days. Consequently, morphologic diagnosis may be difficult after treatment is initiated.[160] Reticulocytosis begins on days 3 to 5 and peaks on days 4 to 10.[407] The new red cells come from new normoblasts, not from the old megaloblasts, most of which die before leaving the marrow.[167] Blood hemoglobin concentration becomes normal within 1 to 2 months. If normal values are not achieved by 2 months, another cause of anemia should be sought.

Other changes include: (1) prompt and dramatic improvement in the sense of well-being; (2) normalization of leukocyte and platelet counts, although neutrophil hypersegmentation may persist for 10 to 14 days; and (3) rise in serum cobalamin and folate; return to normal of plasma homocysteine and methylmalonate levels. Cobalamin deficiency does not respond to a physiologic dose of folate (100-400 mcg/day), although this dose produces a complete response in folate deficiency. Larger doses of folate (5-15 mg/day) can produce a reticulocytosis and partially or temporarily correct the anemia in cobalamin deficiency. To avoid the risk of masking an underlying cobalamin deficiency by inducing a hematologic remission in response to folate, doses

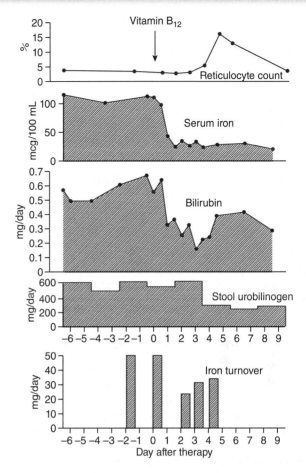

FIGURE 9–17. Effect of cyanocobalamin on reticulocyte count, serum iron, serum bilirubin, stool urobilinogen, and plasma iron turnover. *(Adapted with permission from Coleman D, Donohue D, Finch C, et al. Erythrokinetics in pernicious anemia. Blood. 1956 Sep;11[9]:807-820.)*

in excess of 1 mg folic acid daily should be shunned until an underlying cobalamin deficiency has been ruled out.[3]

Special Circumstances

After Gastrectomy Cobalamin should always be given after total gastrectomy. Cobalamin administration is not necessary after partial gastrectomy, but patients need to be watched for megaloblastic anemia, bearing in mind that this anemia can be masked by postgastrectomy iron deficiency.[390,408]

Blind Loop Syndrome The anemia of the blind loop syndrome can be treated by parenteral cobalamin therapy. It also responds after approximately 1 week to oral broad-spectrum antibiotics (cephalexin monohydrate [Keflex] 250 mg QID plus metronidazole 250 mg TID for 10 days),[409] and cobalamin absorption is restored. Successful surgical correction of an anatomic lesion also ameliorates the condition.

Fish Tapeworm Treatment consists of a single oral dose of vermicide in the form of 50 mg/kg of niclosamide or a dose of 5 to 10 mg/kg of praziquantel.

Rekindled Use of Oral Cobalamin Interest was rekindled[410] regarding the possibility of treating cobalamin deficiency with oral cobalamin as had been proposed previously.[411] Oral cobalamin can be used not only for treatment of dietary cobalamin deficiency that occurs in vegans and in patients with very severe general malnutrition, but also for patients with food cobalamin malabsorption[412] and for patients with PA, provided the patients are followed carefully.[413] In patients lacking intrinsic factor, approximately 1% to 2% of an oral dose of the vitamin crosses the intestinal epithelium by mass action. Therefore, 1000 to 2000 mcg/day of oral cobalamin supplies most PA patients with their daily cobalamin requirement without the need for injections and their accompanying pain and expense. Cobalamin should be given by mouth to patients with dietary cobalamin deficiency and patients (eg, hemophiliacs, the frail elderly) who cannot take intramuscular injections.

Reported Refractoriness to Treatment Though anecdotal, it is worthy of mention that numbers of patients diagnosed with cobalamin deficiency complain of persistent, mainly neurological, symptoms unless the frequency of replacement of injected B_{12} is more frequent than the standard protocol. This apparent refractoriness has no known scientific basis but requires further investigation.

ACUTE MEGALOBLASTIC ANEMIA

Megaloblastic anemia usually is a chronic condition that requires weeks or months to develop, but a potentially fatal megaloblastic state resulting from acute tissue folate or cobalamin deficiency can arise over the course of only a few days. Patients with acute megaloblastic anemia present with rapidly developing thrombocytopenia and/or leukopenia and counts that sometimes fall to very low levels, but little change in red cell levels unless another cause of anemia is present. The discrepancy between platelet and leukocyte counts on the one hand and red cells on the other hand reflects the much longer red cell life span. The clinical picture can suggest an immune cytopenia. The diagnosis is made from the marrow aspirate, which is floridly megaloblastic, and confirmed by the rapid response to appropriate replacement therapy.

The most common cause of acute megaloblastic anemia is N_2O anesthesia.[414] N_2O rapidly destroys MeCbl,[415] leading to a megaloblastic state. AdoCbl eventually is lost, SAM and total folate levels decline, and the proportion of folate in the form of N^5-methyl FH_4 increases.[416] Clinical findings develop quickly. Grossly megaloblastic changes are seen in the marrow after 12 to 24 hours.[417] Hypersegmented neutrophils do not appear until 5 days after exposure but then persist for several days.[418] The effects of N_2O disappear spontaneously after a few days; disappearance can be hastened by administration of folinic acid or cobalamin.[419] Fatalities resulting from N_2O-induced megaloblastosis have occurred in patients with tetanus given N_2O for weeks.[420] Long-term recreational use of N_2O has led to a neurologic disorder similar to combined system disease.[421]

Acute megaloblastic anemia occurs in other clinical settings. A rapidly developing megaloblastic state with acute thrombocytopenia has occurred in seriously ill patients, often in intensive care units.[422] Especially at risk are patients who are transfused extensively at surgery,[423] those on dialysis or total parenteral nutrition, and those receiving weak folate antagonists such as trimethoprim. Morphologic clues to the diagnosis (eg, hypersegmented neutrophils) often are absent from the blood film. Both red cell folate and serum cobalamin levels may be normal, but the marrow is always megaloblastic. A rapid response to therapeutic doses of parenteral folate (5 mg/day) and cobalamin (1 mg) is the rule.

MEGALOBLASTIC ANEMIA CAUSED BY DRUGS

Table 9-5 lists the drugs that cause megaloblastic anemia. *Aminopterin* and *methotrexate* are structurally almost identical to folic acid. After they enter cells via the folate carrier[424] and acquire a polyglutamate chain,[425] they act as very powerful inhibitors of dihydrofolate reductase.[426] By blocking the $FH_2 \rightarrow FH_4$ reaction and perhaps inhibiting other enzymes of folate metabolism, they effect the rapid withdrawal of folates from the 1-carbon fragment carrier pool, causing a fall in nucleotide (especially thymidine) biosynthesis that leads to a major derangement in DNA replication.[427] The methyl group donated by 5,10-methylene tetrahydrofolate is an essential step of purine/pyrimidine synthesis. Formation of tetrahydrofolate from dihydrofolate with acquisition of a carbon unit from serine leading to 5,10-methylene tetrahydrofolate

leads to the generation of thymidylate via thymidylate synthase. If there is interference with this crucial step in the synthesis of thymidylate as a result of either folate or cobalamin deficiency, the cells are deprived of thymidylate and DNA synthesis is slowed down. This pathway is generally targeted by anticancer agents (purine/pyrimidine antagonists), and certain antiviral agents. Occasionally, drugs such as 5-fluorouracil and 5-fluorodeoxyuridine can cause irreversible inhibition of thymidylate synthase, ultimately causing cellular "suicide" through apoptosis. Certain antimetabolites may mimic purine/pyrimidines (eg azathioprine, mycophenolate mofetil, methotrexate, and allopurinol) and either inhibit DNA polymerase or become falsely incorporated into the DNA during its synthesis preventing further elongation of the DNA strand. Similarly, drugs that inhibit pyrimidine synthesis, such as leflunomide for inflammatory arthritis and teriflunomide for multiple sclerosis, inhibit dihydroorotate dehydrogenase.[428] Megaloblastosis as a result of the anesthetic gas N_2O causing oxidation damage of cobalamin is discussed in "Acute Megaloblastic Anemia" earlier.

Generalized toxic effects of drugs that disrupt nucleotide synthesis include necrotic mouth lesions; ulcerations of the esophagus, small intestine, and colon, with abdominal pain, vomiting, and diarrhea; megaloblastic anemia; alopecia; and hyperpigmentation. The drug is excreted by the kidney, so effects and toxicity are prolonged and aggravated if renal function is impaired. Toxicity caused by dihydrofolate antagonists is treated with folinic acid (N^5-formyl FH_4). Folic acid itself is useless in this setting because the blocked reductase cannot convert folic acid and dihydrofolate to the active tetrahydro form. Folinic acid is already in the tetrahydro form, so is effective despite reductase blockade. The usual dose of folinic acid is 3 to 6 mg/day intramuscularly. Larger doses are given in chemotherapy protocols that use folinic acid to rescue patients deliberately treated with otherwise highly toxic and even fatal doses of methotrexate. Folinic acid has been used successfully intrathecally in a patient in whom a large overdose of methotrexate was accidentally delivered into the subarachnoid space.[429]

Zidovudine (azidothymidine [AZT]) is used for HIV infections (AIDS).[430] Its principal toxic effect is severe megaloblastic anemia. Anemia or neutropenia produced by zidovudine limits use of this drug.[431]

HIV infection itself suppresses hematopoiesis, leading to pancytopenia with myelodysplastic features. The blood film shows vacuolated monocytes. Megaloblastosis in HIV infection may result from folate or cobalamin deficiency[432] or AZT or trimethoprim toxicity.

Hydroxyurea is used at high doses to treat chronic myelogenous leukemia, polycythemia vera, and essential thrombocythemia, and at lower doses to treat psoriasis, rheumatoid arthritis, and sickle cell disease. It inhibits conversion of ribonucleotides to deoxyribonucleotides.[433] Marked megaloblastic changes are routinely found in the marrow 1 to 2 days after initiating hydroxyurea therapy. These changes are rapidly reversed after the drug is withdrawn. Long-term use of omeprazole and other H^+/K^+-ATPase inhibitors is associated with reduced serum cobalamin levels, presumably because of the ability of these drugs to inhibit parietal cell function with consequent malabsorption of food cobalamin.[434] Reduced serum cobalamin levels are not a problem when these drugs are used for short intervals.[435]

Pemetrexed is an antifolate approved for use in mesothelioma and for treatment of non–small cell lung cancer. Like other antifolate agents, pemetrexed can result in a megaloblastic anemia that is treated with cobalamin and folate. Coadministration of the drug with cobalamin and folate also reduces toxicity. Trimethoprim is a dihydrofolate reductase inhibitor that is designed to act on the microbial rather than the mammalian enzyme. Still, in patients with borderline folate status, trimethoprim can precipitate a state of folate deficiency.[436] A much-disputed topic is the use of contraceptives leading to inhibition of folate absorption. Contraceptives, to some extent, restrict the intestinal

TABLE 9–5. Drugs That Cause Megaloblastic Anemia

Agents	Comments	Reference
Antifolates		
Methotrexate	Very potent inhibitor of dihydrofolate reductase	484
Aminopterin	Treat overdose with folinic acid	438
Pyrimethamine	Much weaker than methotrexate and aminopterin	
Trimethoprim	Treat with folinic acid or by withdrawing the drug	437, 485
Sulfasalazine	Can cause acute megaloblastic anemia in susceptible patients, especially those with low folate stores	486
Chlorguanide (Proguanil)		484
Triamterene	Use of folate and cobalamin during pemetrexed treatment reduces toxicity	
Pemetrexed (Alimta)		485
Purine analogues		
6-Mercaptopurine	Megaloblastosis precedes hypoplasia, usually mild	486
6-Thioguanine	Responds to folinic acid but not folic acid	489
Azathioprine		488
Acyclovir	Megaloblastosis at high doses	489
Pyrimidine analogues		
5-Fluorouracil	Mild megaloblastosis	493
Floxuridine (5-fluorodeoxyuridine)		493
6-Azauridine	Blocks uridine monophosphate production by inhibiting orotidyl decarboxylase; occasional megaloblastosis with orotic acid and orotidine in urine	492
Zidovudine (AZT)	Severe megaloblastic anemia is the major side effect	432
Ribonucleotide reductase inhibitors		
Hydroxyurea	Marked megaloblastosis within 1-2 days of starting therapy; quickly reversed by withdrawing drug	492
Cytarabine (cytosine arabinoside)	Early megaloblastosis is routine	493
Anticonvulsants		
Phenytoin (diphenylhydantoin)	Occasional megaloblastosis, associated with low folate levels; responds to high-dose folate (1-5 mg/day); how anticonvulsants cause low folate is not understood, but may be related to a drug-induced rise in cytochrome P450	497
Phenobarbital		497
Primidone		497
Carbamazepine		497
Other drugs that depress folates		
Oral contraceptives	Occasional megaloblastosis; sometimes dysplasia of uterine cervix, corrected with folate	498
Glutethimide		
Cycloserine		
H+/K+-ATPase inhibitors		
Omeprazole	Long-term use causes decreased serum cobalamin levels	435
Lansoprazole		
Miscellaneous		
Nitrous oxide (N$_2$O)	See "Acute Megaloblastic Anemia"	421
p-Aminosalicylic acid	Causes cobalamin malabsorption with occasional mild megaloblastic anemia	499
Metformin		500
Phenformin	Causes cobalamin malabsorption but not anemia	
Colchicine		501
Neomycin		502
Arsenic	Causes myelodysplastic hematopoiesis, sometimes with megaloblastic changes	503

deconjugation of polyglutamyl forms of folic acid,[437,438] so in normal healthy women receiving contraceptives, this might not be a problem. However, women who have some additional factors inhibiting folate absorption or have dietary deficiency may be at risk of contraceptives contributing to inhibition of folate absorption.

MEGALOBLASTIC ANEMIA IN CHILDHOOD

Although cobalamin deficiency and megaloblastic anemia in childhood may occur as a result of the various causes that affect adults, it is often the result of genetic disorders affecting either the cobalamin binding proteins or the enzymes concerned with intracellular trafficking of cobalamin or its conversion to coenzymatically active forms. Several reviews have dealt comprehensively with this topic.[352,380,439]

Defects Involving Cobalamin-Binding Proteins

Several genetic mutations and polymorphisms exist that affect the key binding proteins for cobalamin. Their effects range from being clinically benign to causing severe cobalamin deficiency with megaloblastic anemia and neurologic complications usually manifesting in infancy or early childhood, occasionally in adolescence or early adulthood. In general, the mutations and deletions affecting the encoded proteins cause serious health consequences whereas the polymorphic variants may be totally inconspicuous or result only in a modified likelihood of disease risk.

Cobalamin malabsorption occurs in four childhood conditions associated with a genetic component: (1) cobalamin malabsorption in the presence of normal intrinsic factor secretion, (2) congenital abnormality of intrinsic factor, (3) TC deficiency, and (4) true PA of childhood. The management of cobalamin deficiency in childhood has been comprehensively reviewed.[380]

Selective Malabsorption of Cobalamin, Autosomal Recessive Megaloblastic Anemia, Imerslund-Gräsbeck Disease Imerslund-Gräsbeck disease[440] is an inherited failure of transport of the intrinsic factor–Cbl complex by the ileum, usually accompanied by proteinuria, mostly of albumin.[380] It may be the most common cause of cobalamin deficiency in infancy in some populations.[441] Cobalamin deficiency usually is seen in patients younger than 2 years, but may appear earlier or later. Cobalamin malabsorption is not corrected by addition of intrinsic factor. Endogenous intrinsic factor and HCl secretion, TC and HC levels, and gastric and intestinal histology are all normal. Intrinsic factor antibodies are absent. The molecular defect responsible for this disease has been elucidated. For the ileal phase of cobalamin absorption, two genes code distinct proteins that form part of the cobalamin–intrinsic factor receptor complex. The first, *CUBN*, is affected by several mutations that were described in Finnish patients with recessive megaloblastic anemia.[108,442] The second, affecting the protein AMN results in a milder recessive megaloblastic anemia phenotype and is found in Norwegian patients.[108,443] Again, several mutations in this gene have been described.[108] Patients are treated with intramuscular cobalamin. The anemia is corrected, but proteinuria persists.

Congenital Intrinsic Factor Deficiency Congenital intrinsic factor deficiency is an autosomal recessive disease in which parietal cells fail to produce functionally normal intrinsic factor.[444] Patients present with irritability and megaloblastic anemia when cobalamin stores (<25 mcg at birth) are exhausted. The disease usually presents at age 6 to 24 months. HCl secretion and gastric histology are normal, proteinuria is not present, and anti-intrinsic factor antibodies are absent.[445] In the Schilling test, abnormal cobalamin absorption was corrected by oral intrinsic factor.[446] Treatment consists of standard doses of intramuscular cobalamin.

Transcobalamin Deficiency TC deficiency is an autosomal recessive disorder causing a flagrant megaloblastic anemia that generally presents in early infancy.[445] The disease is dangerously deceptive because it results from a very severe deficiency of tissue cobalamin, usually with serum cobalamin levels in the reference range because most of the plasma cobalamin is bound to HC, resulting in a misleading test result if reliance is placed simply on serum cobalamin measurement. Undiagnosed TC deficiency causes irreversible central nervous system (CNS) damage.[447] Patients are healthy at birth but over the next few weeks develop signs and symptoms of cobalamin deficiency, such as rapidly progressive pancytopenia, mouth ulcers, vomiting, and diarrhea. Recurrent bacterial infections may occur.[445] Neurologic findings are not prominent in the early stages of the disease.[447]

Serum folate and cobalamin are normal (the latter because most cobalamin is carried by HC). Homocysteine and/or methylmalonic acid levels are elevated in the plasma.[448] The marrow is megaloblastic and the cobalamin absorption is usually but not always abnormal and is not corrected by intrinsic factor, although correction of malabsorption using exogenous orally administered rabbit TC has been reported.[138] The diagnosis is made by measuring plasma TC.[380] Prenatal diagnosis is possible.[449] Serum should be obtained prior to treatment because TC levels in normal individuals drop sharply after cobalamin is given which could result in a false-positive result. TC deficiency is treated with cobalamin doses sufficiently large to force enough vitamin into the cells to allow normal function. Initial therapy can consist of oral CnCbl or OHCbl 500 to 1000 mcg twice a week, or intramuscular OHCbl 1000 mcg/week. The parenteral route is preferable to ensure adequate replenishment of cobalamin. Blood counts and symptoms should be monitored and doses adjusted upward if necessary.

Several single nucleotide polymorphisms in the TC gene have been described and the allele frequency of the most common form (776 C>G) is high in certain populations.[450,451] Holotranscobalamin levels are lower in individuals homozygous for the G allele[450] and methylmalonate levels are higher,[451] indicating that this genotype is associated with potentially less-favorable cobalamin status.[72]

Haptocorrin Deficiency Congenital deficiency is not associated with clinically manifested cobalamin deficiency, although the plasma or serum cobalamin levels are well-below normal,[383] and this is how the condition is recognized. The absence of morbidity in these patients indicates that HCs do not appear to be essential for maintenance health.

True Juvenile Pernicious Anemia True PA, with gastric atrophy and a defect in intrinsic factor secretion, is exceedingly rare in childhood.[452] Patients usually present in their teens with cobalamin deficiency. Serum anti-intrinsic factor antibodies usually are present.[294] The diagnosis and treatment are the same as for PA in adults.

INBORN ERRORS OF COBALAMIN METABOLISM

Cobalamin is converted to AdoCbl and MeCbl by a complex series of transformations involving several steps.[439,448,453] Eight disorders affecting this cobalamin transformation pathway have been described, one for each of the steps. Because the molecular causes of these disorders have not yet been fully characterized, the disorders themselves are not named for a defective protein but instead are designated by sequential capital letters preceded by a *cbl* prefix. The identification of specific gene mutations within these more broadly categorized entities is now possible using genome-wide and whole-exome sequencing.[454] The disorders can be grouped into three broad clinical syndromes based on the abnormal metabolites in the patient's urine (Table 9-6). These disorders are usually discovered during investigation of infants with unexplained developmental delay, acidosis, anemia, or unexplained neurologic difficulties. Typically, they have normal plasma cobalamin levels.

TABLE 9–6. Cobalamin Mutant Class Syndromes

Syndrome	Methylmalonic Aciduria	Homocystinuria	Megaloblastic Anemia
cblA, cblB, cblH	+	–	–
cblC, cblE	–	+	+
cblC, cblD, cblF	+	+	±

Abbreviation: cbl, Cobalamin.

Methylmalonic Aciduria Only (cblA, cblB, and cblH)

In cblA and cblB, AdoCbl production is impaired but MeCbl production is normal. This may result either from an abnormal methylmalonyl CoA mutase (designated mut° or mut⁻) or from a defect in activation or production of its cofactor, AdoCbl. The cblH variant appears to represent an interallelic variant of cblA.[455] Patients present in infancy with acidosis because they cannot catabolize methylmalonic acid. Symptoms include lethargy and failure to thrive, vomiting, and neurologic problems. Mental retardation is not prominent, and megaloblastic anemia is absent. Most patients respond to 1000 mcg/day of OHCbl or CnCbl, although mut° and mut⁻ patients are unresponsive.

Homocystinuria Only (cblE and cblG)

In these disorders, N^5-methyltetrahydrofolate-homocysteine methyltransferase (methionine synthase) is defective and lacks the capacity to produce MeCbl.[456] In patients with cblG, methionine synthase is missing or defective.[457] cblE results from failure to reactivate methionine synthase that was inactivated by oxidation of its bound cobalamin.[458] Patients present in infancy with vomiting, mental retardation, and megaloblastic anemia. They have marked homocystinuria and hyperhomocysteinemia without methylmalonic aciduria or methylmalonic acidemia. They respond well to 1000 mcg/week intramuscularly. Infants diagnosed prenatally and treated from birth usually show normal development. On rare occasions, this disorder may first become apparent in adult life.

Methylmalonic Aciduria and Homocystinuria (cblC, cblD, and cblF)

In these disorders, the defect in Cbl transformation affects both AdoCbl and MeCbl, probably because reduction of cobalt from Co^{2+} to Co^{1+} is defective. These patients have both hyperhomocysteinemia and methylmalonic acidemia. The age at initial presentation ranges from early infancy to adolescence. In addition to lethargy and failure to thrive, affected infants present with serious neurologic difficulties. Older patients present with psychological problems, progressive dementia, and motor signs and symptoms. cblC disease is the most common of the cobalamin inborn errors. In cblF the defect lies in an inability to release cobalamin from lysosomes.[459] Megaloblastic anemia occurs in about half the cases. Patients respond partially to 1000 mcg/day, administered intramuscularly, of OHCbl or CnCbl.

A tentative diagnosis of a cobalamin mutation can be made by demonstrating methylmalonic aciduria and/or homocystinuria in a patient with the clinical findings described earlier in "Methylmalonic Aciduria Only" or "Homocystinuria Only," respectively. Previously, establishing a diagnosis required a specialized laboratory equipped to do cultured fibroblast complementation studies.[439] However, diagnosis is now possible through the use of whole-exome sequencing and novel mutations can now be identified.[454] In a patient suspected of having a cobalamin mutation, treatment should be started pending the test results because early high-dose cobalamin treatment is risk-free and may reduce the chance of damage to the CNS. Fetuses with these diseases have been successfully treated in utero with very large doses (22.5 mg/day in three doses) of CnCbl given parenterally to the mother.[460]

INBORN ERRORS OF FOLATE METABOLISM

Megaloblastic anemia in infancy has been described in three inherited disorders of folate metabolism.[34,380,461]

Hereditary Folate Malabsorption

Hereditary folate malabsorption is a rare inherited disorder in which patients cannot absorb folate from the gastrointestinal tract or transport it across the choroid plexus and into the cerebrospinal fluid.[32,34] The molecular basis for this disorder is caused by abnormalities in the proton-coupled folate transporter.[32] Patients present with severe megaloblastic anemia, seizures, mental retardation, and other CNS findings.[462] Folate levels are low in the serum and nil in the cerebrospinal fluid. Folate given parenterally has corrected the anemia and seizures in some patients but has had no effect on other CNS symptoms or on the cerebrospinal fluid folate level. Treatment with daily folinic acid by injection maintains the spinal fluid level and can lead to normal development.[380]

Dihydrofolate Reductase Deficiency

Dihydrofolate reductase deficiency may present isolated megaloblastic anemia within days or weeks after birth. The anemia responds to folinic acid but not to folic acid.[463] Identification of novel mutations of this gene associated with megaloblastic anemia and severe cerebral folate deficiency have been carried out using genome-wide sequencing techniques.[464]

N^5-Methyl FH₄–Homocysteine Methyltransferase Deficiency

Decreased methyltransferase activity was described in a liver biopsy from a child with megaloblastic anemia and mental retardation. The anemia failed to respond to folate, cobalamin, or pyridoxal phosphate.[465] The phenotype of this disorder resembles the inborn errors of cobalamin metabolism affecting the methionine synthesis reaction.

Methylene Tetrahydrofolate Reductase Deficiency

In this rare autosomal recessive disorder, there is a severe hyperhomocysteinemia and homocystinuria with low plasma methionine. Patients have neurologic and vascular complications, but no megaloblastic anemia or methylmalonic aciduria.[380] The less serious polymorphic variations in MTHFR were discussed earlier (see "Vascular Disease" earlier), as well as their influence on disease susceptibility and the influence of the enzyme on the distribution of major folate species toward either methylation or DNA synthetic pathways.

Formiminoglutamic Aciduria

Formiminoglutamic aciduria is another important inborn error of folate metabolism. It has a reported incidence of approximately 1:46,000,[466] and is the second most common inherited folate disorder.

There is a mutation in the gene encoding glutamate formiminotransferase (*FTCD*), required for the conversion of formiminoglutamate to 5-formiminotetrahydrofolate followed by cyclodeamination of the formimino group forming 5,10-methenyltetrahydrofolate and ammonia.[467] The patients present with increased urinary formiminoglutamate excretion. Patients generally present with a wide clinical spectrum of mild to severe developmental delays with megaloblastic anemia.[465,468] Nowadays, newborn screening panels can identify mutations in *FTCD* by whole-exome sequencing.[469] Identification of a mutation makes it possible to monitor such patients with appropriate long-term biochemical and clinical follow-up to prevent development delays.

OTHER INBORN ERRORS

Hereditary Orotic Aciduria
Hereditary orotic aciduria is an autosomal recessive disorder of pyrimidine metabolism[470] characterized by megaloblastic anemia, growth impairment, and excretion of orotic acid in the urine. Cobalamin and folate levels are normal.

Lesch-Nyhan Syndrome
The Lesch-Nyhan syndrome is an X-linked disorder of purine metabolism characterized by hyperuricemia, hyperuricosuria, and a neurologic disease with self-mutilation. It is caused by a hypoxanthine-guanine phosphoribosyltransferase deficiency. One patient described had megaloblastic anemia.[471]

Thiamine-Responsive Megaloblastic Anemia
Several children with severe megaloblastic anemia, sensorineural deafness, and non-autoimmune diabetes mellitus, all presenting symptoms in the early childhood or adolescence, have been reported (also known as Rogers syndrome).[472] The anemia and diabetes responds to thiamine

(25-100 mg/day).[473] The marrow was reported as myelodysplastic in two patients with the disorder.[474] The gene for this puzzling disorder has been mapped to the long arm of chromosome 1, and the underlying biochemical defect is caused by reduced nucleic acid production through impairment of the thiamine-dependent pentose cycle enzyme transketolase that results in cell-cycle arrest and the megaloblastic phenotype.[475] (Chap. 12)

OTHER CAUSES OF MEGALOBLASTIC ANEMIA

Congenital Dyserythropoietic Anemia
The congenital dyserythropoietic anemias are lifelong anemias. They often are mild, showing dysplastic changes affecting the red cell line only, most typically multinuclearity of the normoblasts. They appear to result from defects in glycosylation of polylactosaminoglycans linked to membrane proteins and ceramides.[476] Of the three types, two (type I usually[477] and type III occasionally[478]) show megaloblastic red cell precursors (Chap. 14).

Refractory Megaloblastic Anemia
Refractory megaloblastic anemia is regarded as a manifestation of some sideroblastic anemias (Chap. 20) and myelodysplastic disorders.[479] The megaloblastic changes are atypical. Dysplastic features are confined to the erythroid series. Giant metamyelocytes and bands are absent from the marrow. A few patients with refractory megaloblastic anemia respond to pharmacologic doses of pyridoxine (200 mg/day),[480] perhaps because of an effect on serine transformylase, which requires both pyridoxine and folate.

Acute Erythroid Leukemia
In acute erythroid leukemia, a variety of acute myelogenous leukemia[481] nucleated red cells appear on the blood film, there is usually marked

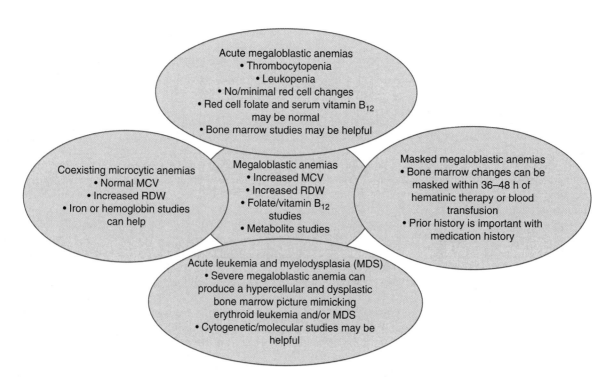

FIGURE 9–18. Diagnostic challenges in megaloblastic anemia. The major causes of conditions that may obscure the typical changes of megaloblastic anemia or cause potential difficulties in the differential diagnosis when megaloblastic changes are identified. MCV, mean corpuscular volume; RDW, red cell distribution width.

anisocytosis and anisochromia, and macrocytes are usually present. The marrow shows pronounced erythroid hyperplasia involving very bizarre looking megaloblast-like red cell precursors, often containing multiple nuclei or nuclear fragments together with increased numbers of blasts. The megaloblastoid erythroid precursors frequently appear vacuolated.

Consideration of the rarer causes of megaloblastic anemia is important when the common and correctable causes due to folate or cobalamin deficiencies have been excluded. This is particularly important in the pediatric age group, but also in patients who are refractory to treatment with either folate or cobalamin.

DIAGNOSTIC CHALLENGES IN MEGALOBLASTIC ANEMIA

There are several diagnostic challenges already discussed earlier. In this section a few important considerations in the differential diagnosis (Fig. 9-18) that should be borne in mind when dealing with patients presenting with atypical megaloblastic anemias are highlighted. These fall into the broad categories of benign variations versus malignant mimickers of megaloblastic anemias. Among the benign conditions we include concurrent microcytic anemias where, the megaloblastic picture in the marrow or blood can be missed in the presence of concurrent microcytic anemia that was caused by iron deficiency, chronic disease, or thalassemia.[171,172] There will be aniso-poikilocytosis, normal MCV, and markedly increased red cell distribution width with hypersegmented neutrophils. The marrow will typically not have large megaloblastic erythroid precursors but will be comprised of intermediate cells, giant metamyelocytes, and bands.[178] Likewise, patients receiving hematinic or transfusion therapies for severe megaloblastic anemias can have fading signs of megaloblastic changes in the marrow within 36 to 48 hours of institution of therapy.[160]

Also, as noted earlier, an acute deficiency of folate and vitamin B_{12} can cause a decrease in platelet and white blood cell counts without immediately affecting the red blood cell counts. Hypersegmented neutrophils in the blood film with marrow megaloblastic changes are typically noted. These patients generally respond to parenteral doses of folate and vitamin B_{12}.[160,418,419,423]

Megaloblastic anemias may, when morphology is extreme or bizarre mimic leukemias and myelodysplastic syndromes. The marrow morphology may be hypercellular with severe dysplastic features mimicking leukemia or myelodysplasia.[482,483] There is rare to absent maturation in the erythroid precursors with a preponderance of megaloblastic pronormoblasts. Dysmorphic erythroid precursors with frequent mitotic figures are also noted, resembling erythroid leukemia. Distinguishing erythroid leukemia from severe megaloblastic anemia caused by nutritional deficiency is not always obvious and can at times befuddle the unwary. Because of the vast differences in the treatment and prognosis for both these entities, a high level of caution should be exercised to avoid misdiagnosing these conditions by performing appropriate tests before starting chemotherapy.

REFERENCES

1. Butterworth CJ, Santini RJ, Frommeyer WJ. The pteroylglutamate components of American diets as determined by chromatographic fractionation. *J Clin Invest.* 1963;42:1929-1939.
2. Stover PJ, Field MS. Trafficking of intracellular folates. *Adv Nutr.* 2011;2(4):325-331.
3. Institute of Medicine (US) Standing Committee on the Scientific Evaluation of Dietary Reference Intakes and its Panel on Folate, Other B Vitamins, and Choline. *Dietary Reference Intakes for Thiamin, Riboflavin, Niacin, Vitamin B₆, Folate, Vitamin B₁₂, Pantothenic Acid, Biotin, and Choline.* National Academies Press; 1998:446.
4. Bailey LB, da Silva V, West AA, Caudill MA. Folate. In: Zempleni J, Stover PJ, Gregory JF III, Suttie K, eds. *Handbook of Vitamins.* 5th ed. CRC Press; 2014:421-446.
5. Colman N, Green R, Metz J. Prevention of folate deficiency by food fortification. II. Absorption of folic acid from fortified staple foods. *Am J Clin Nutr.* 1975;28:459-464.
6. von der Porten AE, Gregory JF 3rd, Toth JP, et al. In vivo folate kinetics during chronic supplementation of human subjects with deuterium-labeled folic acid. *J Nutr.* 1992;122(6):1293-1299.
7. Herbert V. Experimental nutritional folate deficiency in man. *Trans Assoc Am Physicians.* 1962;75:307-320.
8. Halsted C. Folate deficiency in alcoholism. *Am J Clin Nutr.* 1980;33(12):2736-2740.
9. Alperin J, Hutchinson H, Levin W. Studies of folic acid requirements in megaloblastic anemia of pregnancy. *Arch Intern Med.* 1966;117(5):681-688.
10. Schwarz R, Johnston RJ. Folic acid supplementation—when and how. *Obstet Gynecol.* 1996;88(5):886-887.
11. Ulevitch R, Kallen R. Purification and characterization of pyridoxal 5???-phosphate dependent serine hydroxymethylase from lamb liver and its action upon beta-phenylserines. *Biochemistry.* 1977;16(24):5342-5350.
12. Zheng Y, Cantley LC. Toward a better understanding of folate metabolism in health and disease. *J Exp Med.* 2019;216:253-266.
13. Anderson DD, Stover PJ. SHMT1 and SHMT2 are functionally redundant in nuclear de novo thymidylate biosynthesis. *PLoS One.* 2009;4(6):e5839.
14. Deacon R, Chanarin I, Perry J, Lumb M. Marrow cells from patients with untreated pernicious anaemia cannot use tetrahydrofolate normally. *Br J Haematol.* 1980;46(4):523-528.
15. Wahba A, Friedkin M. The enzymatic synthesis of thymidylate. I. Early steps in the purification of thymidylate synthetase of *Escherichia coli. J Biol Chem.* 1962;237:3794-3801.
16. Fenech M. The role of folic acid and vitamin B_{12} in genomic stability of human cells. *Mutat Res.* 2001;475(1-2):57-67.
17. Huennekens F. Folic acid coenzymes in the biosynthesis of purines and pyrimidines. *Vitam Horm.* 1968;26:375-394.
18. Kaufman S. The phenylalanine hydroxylating system from mammalian liver. *Adv Enzymol Relat Areas Mol Biol.* 1971;35:245-319.
19. Kwon N, Nathan C, Stuehr D. Reduced biopterin as a cofactor in the generation of nitrogen oxides by murine macrophages. *J Biol Chem.* 1989;264(34):20496-20501.
20. Banerjee S, Snyder S. Methyltetrahydrofolic acid mediates N- and O-methylation of biogenic amines. *Science.* 1973;182(107):74-75.
21. Bird O, McGlohon V, Vaitkus J. Naturally occurring folates in the blood and liver of the rat. *Anal Biochem.* 1965;12(1):18-35.
22. Shane B. Folylpolyglutamate synthesis and role in the regulation of one-carbon metabolism. *Vitam Horm.* 1989;45:263-335.
23. Pratt R, Cooper B. Folates in plasma and bile of man after feeding folic acid—3H and 5-formyltetrahydrofolate (folinic acid). *J Clin Invest.* 1971;50(2):455-462.
24. Kisliuk R. Pteroylpolyglutamates. *Mol Cell Biochem.* 1981;39:331-345.
25. Atkinson I, Garrow T, Brenner A, Shane B. Human cytosolic folylpoly-gamma-glutamate synthase. *Methods Enzymol.* 1997;281:134-140.
26. Sussman D, Milman G, Shane B. Characterization of human folylpolyglutamate synthetase expressed in Chinese hamster ovary cells. *Somat Cell Mol Genet.* 1986;12(12):531-540.
27. Shane B, Stokstad E. Vitamin B_{12}-folate interrelationships. *Annu Rev Nutr.* 1985;5:115-141.
28. Visentin M, Diop-Bove N, Zhao R, Goldman ID. The intestinal absorption of folates. *Annu Rev Physiol.* 2014;76:251-274.
29. Butterworth CJ, Baugh C, Krumdieck C. A study of folate absorption and metabolism in man utilizing carbon-14–labeled polyglutamates synthesized by the solid phase method. *J Clin Invest.* 1969;48(48):1131-1142.
30. Rosenberg I, Godwin H. The digestion and absorption of dietary folate. *Gastroenterology.* 1971;60(3):445-463.
31. Chandler C, Wang T, Halsted C. Pteroylpolyglutamate hydrolase from human jejunal brush borders. Purification and characterization. *J Biol Chem.* 1986;261(2):928-933.
32. Qiu A, Jansen M, Sakaris A, et al. Identification of an intestinal folate transporter and the molecular basis for hereditary folate malabsorption. *Cell.* 2006;127(5):917-928.
33. Wilson MR, Hou Z, Yang S, et al. Targeting nonsquamous nonsmall cell lung cancer via the proton-coupled folate transporter with 6-substituted pyrrolo[2,3-d]pyrimidine thienoyl antifolates. *Mol Pharmacol.* 2016;89(1):425-434.
34. Zhao R, Matherly L, Goldman I. Membrane transporters and folate homeostasis: intestinal absorption and transport into systemic compartments and tissues. *Expert Rev Mol Med.* 2009;11:e4.
35. Elsenhans B, Ahmad O, Rosenberg I. Isolation and characterization of pteroylpolyglutamate hydrolase from rat intestinal mucosa. *J Biol Chem.* 1984;259(10):6364-6368.
36. Schron C. pH modulation of the kinetics of rabbit jejunal, brush-border folate transport. *J Membr Biol.* 1991;120(2):192-200.
37. Schron C, Washington CJ, Blitzer B. The transmembrane pH gradient drives uphill folate transport in rabbit jejunum. Direct evidence for folate/hydroxyl exchange in brush border membrane vesicles. *J Clin Invest.* 1985;76(5):2030-2033.
38. Zimmerman J, Selhub J, Rosenberg I. Role of sodium ion in transport of folic acid in the small intestine. *Am J Physiol.* 1986;251(2, pt 1):G218-G222.
39. Perry J, Chanarin I. Intestinal absorption of reduced folate compounds in man. *Br J Haematol.* 1970;18(3):329-339.
40. Steinberg S, Campbell C, Hillman R. Kinetics of the normal folate enterohepatic cycle. *J Clin Invest.* 1979;64(1):83-88.
41. Steinberg S. Mechanisms of folate homeostasis. *Am J Physiol.* 1984;246(4, pt 1):G319-G324.
42. Johns D, Sperti S, Burgen A. The metabolism of tritiated folic acid in man. *J Clin Invest.* 1961;40:1684-1695.

43. Antony A. The biological chemistry of folate receptors. *Blood.* 1992;79(11):2807-2820.

44. Weitman S, Weinberg A, Coney L, et al. Cellular localization of the folate receptor: potential role in drug toxicity and folate homeostasis. *Cancer Res.* 1992;52(23):6708-6711.

45. Luhrs C, Slomiany B. A human membrane-associated folate binding protein is anchored by a glycosyl-phosphatidylinositol tail. *J Biol Chem.* 1989;264(36):21446-21449.

46. Green T, Ford HC. Human placental microvilli contain high-affinity binding sites for folate. *Biochem J.* 1984;218(1):75-80.

47. Rothberg K, Ying Y, Kolhouse J, et al. The glycophospholipid-linked folate receptor internalizes folate without entering the clathrin-coated pit endocytic pathway. *J Cell Biol.* 1990;110(3):637-649.

48. Moestrup SK. New insights into carrier binding and epithelial uptake of the erythropoietic nutrients cobalamin and folate. *Curr Opin Hematol.* 2006;13(3):119-123.

49. Hilton J, Cooper B, Rosenblatt D. Folate polyglutamate synthesis and turnover in cultured human fibroblasts. *J Biol Chem.* 1979;254(17):8398-8403.

50. Zamierowski M, Wagner C. High molecular weight complexes of folic acid in mammalian tissues. *Biochem Biophys Res Commun.* 1974;60(1):81-87.

51. Duch D, Bowers S, Nichol C. Analysis of folate cofactor levels in tissues using high-performance liquid chromatography. *Anal Biochem.* 1983;130(2):385-392.

52. Cook R, Wagner C. Glycine N-methyltransferase is a folate binding protein of rat liver cytosol. *Proc Natl Acad Sci U S A.* 1984;81(12):3631-3634.

53. Wang YC, Tang FY, Chen SY, et al. Glycine-N methyltransferase expression in HepG2 cells is involved in methyl group homeostasis by regulating transmethylation kinetics and DNA methylation. *J Nutr.* 2011;141(5):777-782.

54. DebRoy S, Kramarenko II, Ghose S, et al. A novel tumor suppressor function of glycine N-methyltransferase is independent of its catalytic activity but requires nuclear localization. *PLoS One.* 2013;8:e70062.

55. Rosenblatt D, Cooper B, Lue-Shing S, et al. Folate distribution in cultured human cells. Studies on 5,10-CH2-H4PteGlu reductase deficiency. *J Clin Invest.* 1979;63(5):1019-1025.

56. Stites T, Bailey L, Scott K, et al. Kinetic modeling of folate metabolism through use of chronic administration of deuterium-labeled folic acid in men. *Am J Clin Nutr.* 1997;65(1):53-60.

57. Lin Y, Dueker SR, Follett JR, et al. Quantitation of in vivo human folate metabolism. *Am J Clin Nutr.* 2004;80(3):680-691.

58. Elwood P, Deutsch J, Kolhouse J. The conversion of the human membrane-associated folate binding protein (folate receptor) to the soluble folate binding protein by a membrane-associated metalloprotease. *J Biol Chem.* 1991;266(4):2346-2353.

59. Colman N, Herbert V. Total plasma binding capacity of normal human plasma, and variations in uremia, cirrhosis, and pregnancy. *Blood.* 1976;48(6):911-921.

60. Waxman S. Folate binding proteins. *Br J Haematol.* 1975;29(1):23-29.

61. Waxman S, Schreiber C. Measurement of serum folate levels and serum folic acid-binding protein by 3H-PGA radioassay. *Blood.* 1973;42(2):281-290.

62. Colman N, Herbert V. Folate-binding proteins. *Annu Rev Med.* 1980;31:433-439.

63. Rothenberg S. A macromolecular factor in some leukemic cells which binds folic acid. *Proc Soc Exp Biol Med.* 1970;133(2):428-432.

64. Mason J, Selhub J. Folate-binding protein and the absorption of folic acid in the small intestine of the suckling rat. *Am J Clin Nutr.* 1988;48(3):620-625.

65. Rubinoff M, Abramson R, Schreiber C, Waxman S. Effect of a folate-binding protein on the plasma transport and tissue distribution of folic acid. *Acta Haematol.* 1981;65(3):145-152.

66. Hoier-Madsen M, Holm J, Hansen SI. Alpha Isoforms of soluble and membrane-linked folate-binding protein in human blood. *Biosci Rep.* 2008;28(3):153-160.

67. Selhub J, Nakamura S, Carone F. Renal folate absorption and the kidney folate binding protein. II. Microinfusion studies. *Am J Physiol.* 1987;252(4 Pt 2):F757-F760.

68. Birn H. The kidney in vitamin B12 and folate homeostasis: characterization of receptors for tubular uptake of vitamins and carrier proteins. *Am J Physiol Renal Physiol.* 2006;291:F22-F36.

69. O'Brien J. Urinary excretion of folic and folinic acids in normal adults. *Proc Soc Exp Biol Med.* 1960;104:354-355.

70. Clifford A, Arjomand A, Dueker S, et al. The dynamics of folic acid metabolism in an adult given a small tracer dose of 14C-folic acid. *Adv Exp Med Biol.* 1998;445:239-251.

71. Fazili Z, Whitehead RD Jr, Paladugula N, Pfeiffer CM. A high-throughput LC-MS/MS method suitable for population biomonitoring measures five serum folate vitamers and one oxidation product. *Anal Bioanal Chem.* 2013;405:4549-4560.

72. Green R, Miller JW. Vitamin B12. In: Zempleni J, Stover PJ, Gregory JF III, Suttie K, eds. *Handbook of Vitamins.* 5th ed. CRC Press; 2014:447-490.

73. Lenhert P, Hodgkin D. Structure of the 5,6-dimethyl-benzimidazolylcobamide coenzyme. *Nature.* 1961;192:937-938.

74. Lindstrom K. Isolation of methylcobalamin from natural source material. *Nature.* 1964;204:188-189.

75. Croft MT, Lawrence AD, Raux-Deery E, et al. Algae acquire vitamin B12 through a symbiotic relationship with bacteria. *Nature.* 2005;438(7064):90-93.

76. Sela I, Yaskolka Meir A, Brandis A, et al. Wolffia globosa-Mankai plant-based protein contains bioactive vitamin B12 and is well absorbed in humans. *Nutrients.* 2020;12(10):3067.

77. Heyssel R, Bozian R, Darby W, Bell M. Vitamin B12 turnover in man. The assimilation of vitamin B12 from natural foodstuff by man and estimates of minimal daily dietary requirements. *Am J Clin Nutr.* 1966;18(3):176-184.

78. Grasbeck R. Calculations on vitamin B12 turnover in man. With a note on the maintenance treatment in pernicious anemia and the radiation dose received by patients ingesting radiovitamin B12. *Scand J Clin Lab Invest.* 1959;11:250-258.

79. Hsu JM, Kawin B, Minor P, Mitchell JA. Vitamin B12 concentrations in human tissues. *Nature.* 1966;210(5042):1264-1265.

80. Nham S, Wilkemeyer M, Ledley F. Structure of the human methylmalonyl-CoA mutase (MUT) locus. *Genomics.* 1990;8(4):710-716.

81. Beck W, Flavin M, Ochoa S. Metabolism of propionic acid in animal tissues. III. Formation of succinate. *J Biol Chem.* 1957;229(2):997-1010.

82. Taylor R, Weissbach H. Enzymic synthesis of methionine: formation of a radioactive cobamide enzyme with N5-methyl-14C-tetrahydrofolate. *Arch Biochem Biophys.* 1967;119(1):572-579.

83. Oussalah A, Julien M, Levy J, et al. Global Burden related to nitrous oxide exposure in medical and recreational settings: a systematic review and individual patient data meta-analysis. *J Clin Med.* 2019;8:551.

84. Zalusky R, Herbert V, Castle W. Cyanocobalamin therapy effect in folic acid deficiency. *Arch Intern Med.* 1962;109:545-554.

85. Green R, Allen LH, Bjorke-Monsen AL, et al. Correction: Vitamin B12 deficiency. *Nat Rev Dis Primers.* 2017;3:17054.

86. Knowles J, Prankerd T. Abnormal folic acid metabolism in vitamin B12 deficiency. *Clin Sci.* 1962;22:233-238.

87. Herbert V, Zalusky R. Interrelations of vitamin B12 and folic acid metabolism: folic acid clearance studies. *J Clin Invest.* 1962;41:1263-1276.

88. Kano Y, Sakamoto S, Hida K, et al. 5-Methyltetrahydrofolate related enzymes and DNA polymerase alpha activities in bone marrow cells from patients with vitamin B12 deficient megaloblastic anemia. *Blood.* 1982;59(4):832-837.

89. Waters A, Mollin D. Observations on the metabolism of folic acid in pernicious anaemia. *Br J Haematol.* 1963;9:319-327.

90. Jeejeebhoy K, Pathare S, Noronha J. Observations on conjugated and unconjugated blood folate levels in megaloblastic anemia and the effects of vitamin B12. *Blood.* 1965;26:354-359.

91. Boss G. Cobalamin inactivation decreases purine and methionine synthesis in cultured lymphoblasts. *J Clin Invest.* 1985;76(1):213-218.

92. Finkelstein JD, Martin JJ. Methionine metabolism in mammals. Adaptation to methionine excess. *J Biol Chem.* 1986;261(4):1582-1587.

93. Katzen H, Buchanan J. Enzymatic synthesis of the methyl group of methionine. 8. Repression-derepression, purification, and properties of 5,10-methylenetetrahydrofolate reductase from *Escherichia coli. J Biol Chem.* 1965;240:825-835.

94. Chanarin I, Deacon R, Lumb M, Perry J. Vitamin B12 regulates folate metabolism by the supply of formate. *Lancet.* 1980;2(8193):505-507.

95. Taheri M, Wickremasinghe R, Jackson B, Hoffbrand A. The effect of folate analogues and vitamin B12 on provision of thymine nucleotides for DNA synthesis in megaloblastic anemia. *Blood.* 1982;59(3):634-640.

96. Chanarin I, Deacon R, Lumb M, Perry J. Cobalamin and folate: recent developments. *J Clin Pathol.* 1992;45(4):277-283.

97. Hewitt J, Gordon M, Taggart R, et al. Human gastric intrinsic factor: characterization of cDNA and genomic clones and localization to human chromosome 11. *Genomics.* 1991;10(2):432-440.

98. Tang L, Chokshi H, Hu C, et al. The intrinsic factor (IF)-cobalamin receptor binding site is located in the amino-terminal portion of IF. *J Biol Chem.* 1992;267(32):22982-22986.

99. Levine JS, Nakane PK, Allen RH. Immunocytochemical localization of human intrinsic factor: the nonstimulated stomach. *Gastroenterology.* 1980;79(3):493-502.

100. Stenman U. Vitamin B12-binding proteins of r-type, cobalophilin. *Scand J Haematol.* 1975;14(2):91-107.

101. Morkbak AL, Poulsen SS, Nexo E. Haptocorrin in humans. *Clin Chem Lab Med.* 2007;45(12):1751-1759.

102. Cooper B, Castle W. Sequential mechanisms in the enhanced absorption of vitamin B12 by intrinsic factor in the rat. *J Clin Invest.* 1960;39:199-214.

103. Allen R, Seetharam B, Podell E, Alpers D. Effect of proteolytic enzymes on the binding of cobalamin to R protein and intrinsic factor. In vitro evidence that a failure to partially degrade R protein is responsible for cobalamin malabsorption in pancreatic insufficiency. *J Clin Invest.* 1978;61(1):47-54.

104. Abels J, Schilling R. Protection of intrinsic factor by vitamin B12. *J Lab Clin Med.* 1964;64:375-384.

105. Moestrup S, Kozyraki R, Kristiansen M, et al. The intrinsic factor-vitamin B12 receptor and target of teratogenic antibodies is a megalin-binding peripheral membrane protein with homology to developmental proteins. *J Biol Chem.* 1998;273(9):5235-5242.

106. Barth JL, Argraves WS. Cubilin and megalin: partners in lipoprotein and vitamin metabolism. *Trends Cardiovasc Med.* 2001;11(1):26-31.

107. Birn H, Willnow T, Nielsen R, et al. Megalin is essential for renal proximal tubule reabsorption and accumulation of transcobalamin-B(12). *Am J Physiol Renal Physiol.* 2002;282(3):F408-F416.

108. Fyfe J, Madsen M, Højrup P, et al. The functional cobalamin (vitamin B12)-intrinsic factor receptor is a novel complex of cubilin and amnionless. *Blood.* 2004;103(5):1573-1579.

109. Christensen E, Birn H. Megalin and cubilin: multifunctional endocytic receptors. *Nat Rev Mol Cell Biol.* 2002;3(4):256-266.

110. Hagedorn C, Alpers D. Distribution of intrinsic factor-vitamin B12 receptors in human intestine. *Gastroenterology.* 1977;73(5):1019-1022.

111. Kapadia C, Serfilippi D, Voloshin K, Donaldson RJ. Intrinsic factor-mediated absorption of cobalamin by guinea pig ileal cells. *J Clin Invest.* 1983;71(3):440-448.

112. Robertson J, Gallagher N. In vivo evidence that cobalamin is absorbed by receptor-mediated endocytosis in the mouse. *Gastroenterology.* 1985;88(4):908-912.

113. Chanarin I. *The Megaloblastic Anaemias.* Blackwell Scientific; 1969.

114. Horadagoda N, Batt R. Lysosomal localisation of cobalamin during absorption by the ileum of the dog. *Biochim Biophys Acta.* 1985;838(2):206-210.

115. Rothenberg S, Weisberg H, Ficarra A. Evidence for the absorption of immunoreactive intrinsic factor into the intestinal epithelial cell during vitamin B_{12} absorption. *J Lab Clin Med.* 1972;79(4):587-597.

116. Hall C. Transcobalamins I and II as natural transport proteins of vitamin B_{12}. *J Clin Invest.* 1975;56(5):1125-1131.

117. Beedholm-Ebsen R, van de Wetering K, Hardlei T, et al. Identification of multidrug resistance protein 1 (MRP1/ABCC1) as a molecular gate for cellular export of cobalamin. *Blood.* 2010;115(8):1632-1639.

118. Quadros E, Regec A, Khan K, et al. Transcobalamin II synthesized in the intestinal villi facilitates transfer of cobalamin to the portal blood. *Am J Physiol.* 1999;277(1, pt 1):G161-G166.

119. Green R, Jacobsen D, van Tonder S, et al. Enterohepatic circulation of cobalamin in the nonhuman primate. *Gastroenterology.* 1981;81(4):773-776.

120. Kanazawa S, Herbert V. Mechanism of enterohepatic circulation of vitamin B_{12}: movement of vitamin B_{12} from bile R-binder to intrinsic factor due to the action of pancreatic trypsin. *Trans Assoc Am Physicians.* 1983;96:336-344

121. Grasbeck R, Nyberg W, Reizenstein P. Biliary and fecal vit. B_{12} excretion in man: an isotope study. *Proc Soc Exp Biol Med.* 1958;97(4):780-784.

122. Green R, Jacobsen D, Van Tonder S, et al. Absorption of biliary cobalamin in baboons following total gastrectomy. *J Lab Clin Med.* 1982;100(5):771-777.

123. Antony A. Vegetarianism and vitamin B-12 (cobalamin) deficiency. *Am J Clin Nutr.* 2003;78(1):3-6.

124. Doscherholmen A, Hagen P. A dual mechanism of vitamin B_{12} plasma absorption. *J Clin Invest.* 1957;36(11):1551-1557.

125. Seetharam B, Alpers D. Cellular uptake of cobalamin. *Nutr Rev.* 1985;43(4):97-102.

126. Quadros EV, Rothenberg SP, Pan YC, Stein S. Purification and molecular characterization of human transcobalamin II. *J Biol Chem.* 1986;261(33):15455-15460.

127. Platica O, Janeczko R, Quadros E, et al. The cDNA sequence and the deduced amino acid sequence of human transcobalamin II show homology with rat intrinsic factor and human transcobalamin I. *J Biol Chem.* 1991;266(12):7860-7863.

128. Hippe E, Olesen H. Nature of vitamin B 12 binding. 3. Thermodynamics of binding to human intrinsic factor and transcobalamins. *Biochim Biophys Acta.* 1971;243(1):83-88.

129. Kolhouse J, Allen R. Absorption, plasma transport, and cellular retention of cobalamin analogues in the rabbit. Evidence for the existence of multiple mechanisms that prevent the absorption and tissue dissemination of naturally occurring cobalamin analogues. *J Clin Invest.* 1977;60(6):1381-1392.

130. Donaldson RJ, Brand M, Serfilippi D. Changes in circulating transcobalamin II after injection of cyanocobalamin. *N Engl J Med.* 1977;296(25):1427-1430.

131. Schneider R, Burger R, Mehlman C, Allen R. The role and fate of rabbit and human transcobalamin II in the plasma transport of vitamin B_{12} in the rabbit. *J Clin Invest.* 1976;57(1):27-38.

132. Youngdahl-Turner P, Rosenberg L, Allen R. Binding and uptake of transcobalamin II by human fibroblasts. *J Clin Invest.* 1978;61(1):133-141.

133. Quadros E, Nakayama Y, Sequeira J. The protein and the gene encoding the receptor for the cellular uptake of transcobalamin-bound cobalamin. *Blood.* 2009;113(1):186-192.

134. Peters TJ, Quinlan A, Hoffbrand AV. Subcellular localization of radioactive vitamin B_{12} during absorption by guinea-pig ileum. *Clin Sci.* 1969;37(2):568-569.

135. Pletsch Q, Coffey J. Properties of the proteins that bind vitamin B 12 in subcellular fractions of rat liver. *Arch Biochem Biophys.* 1972;151(1):157-167.

136. Hine B, Boggs I, Green R, et al. Transcobalamin derived from bovine milk stimulates apical uptake of vitamin B_{12} into human intestinal epithelial cells. *J Cell Biochem.* 2014;115(11):1948-1954.

137. Juul CB, Fedosov SN, Nexo E, Heegaard CW. Kinetic analysis of transcellular passage of the cobalamin-transcobalamin complex in Caco-2 monolayers. *Mol Biol Cell.* 2019;30(4):467-477.

138. Barshop B, Wolff J, Nyhan W, et al. Transcobalamin II deficiency presenting with methylmalonic aciduria and homocystinuria and abnormal absorption of cobalamin. *Am J Med Genet A.* 1990;35(2):222-228.

139. Watanabe F, Nakano Y. Comparative biochemistry of vitamin B_{12} (cobalamin) metabolism: biochemical diversity in the systems for intracellular cobalamin transfer and synthesis of the coenzymes. *Int J Biochem.* 1991;23(12):1353-1359.

140. Burger R, Allen R. Characterization of vitamin B_{12}-binding proteins isolated from human milk and saliva by affinity chromatography. *J Biol Chem.* 1974;249(22):7220-7227.

141. Hurlimann J, Zuber C. Vitamin B12-binders in human body fluids. II. Synthesis in vitro. *Clin Exp Immunol.* 1969;4(1):141-148.

142. Simons K, Weber T. The vitamin B_{12}-binding protein in human leukocytes. *Biochim Biophys Acta.* 1966;117(1):201-208.

143. Johnston J, Bollekens J, Allen R, Berliner N. Structure of the cDNA encoding transcobalamin I, a neutrophil granule protein. *J Biol Chem.* 1989;264(27):15754-15757.

144. Johnston J, Yang-Feng T, Berliner N. Genomic structure and mapping of the chromosomal gene for transcobalamin I (TCN1): comparison to human intrinsic factor. *Genomics.* 1992;12(3):459-464.

145. Burger R, Schneider R, Mehlman C, Allen R. Human plasma R-type vitamin B_{12}-binding proteins. II. The role of transcobalamin I, transcobalamin III, and the normal granulocyte vitamin B_{12}-binding protein in the plasma transport of vitamin B_{12}. *J Biol Chem.* 1975;250(19):7707-7713.

146. Guéant J, Monin B, Boissel P, et al. Biliary excretion of cobalamin and cobalamin analogues in man. *Digestion.* 1984;30(3):151-157.

147. Gottlieb C, Retief F, Herbert V. Blockade of vitamin B_{12}-binding sites in gastric juice, serum and saliva by analogues and derivatives of vitamin B_{12} and by antibody to intrinsic factor. *Biochim Biophys Acta.* 1967;141(3):560-572.

148. Allen R, Stabler S. Identification and quantitation of cobalamin and cobalamin analogues in human feces. *Am J Clin Nutr.* 2008;87(5):1324-1335.

149. Kolhouse J, Kondo H, Allen N, et al. Cobalamin analogues are present in human plasma and can mask cobalamin deficiency because current radioisotope dilution assays are not specific for true cobalamin. *N Engl J Med.* 1978;299(15):785-792.

150. Kondo H, Kolhouse J, Allen R. Presence of cobalamin analogues in animal tissues. *Proc Natl Acad Sci U S A.* 1980;77(2):817-821.

151. Hom B. Plasma turnover of 57cobalt-vitamin B_{12} bound to transcobalamin I and II. *Scand J Haematol.* 1967;4(5):321-332.

152. Carmel R. The distribution of endogenous cobalamin among cobalamin-binding proteins in the blood in normal and abnormal states. *Am J Clin Nutr.* 1985;41(4):713-719.

153. Nexo E, Hvas A, Bleie Ø, et al. Holo-transcobalamin is an early marker of changes in cobalamin homeostasis. A randomized placebo-controlled study. *Clin Chem.* 2002;48(10):1768-1771.

154. Hvas A, Nexo E. Holotranscobalamin as a predictor of vitamin B_{12} status. *Clin Chem Lab Med.* 2003;41(11):1489-1492.

155. Lloyd-Wright Z, Hvas A, Møller J, et al. Holotranscobalamin as an indicator of dietary vitamin B_{12} deficiency. *Clin Chem.* 2003;49(12):2076-2078.

156. Obeid R, Herrmann W. Holotranscobalamin in laboratory diagnosis of cobalamin deficiency compared to total cobalamin and methylmalonic acid. *Clin Chem Lab Med.* 2007;45(12):1746-1750.

157. Herzlich B, Herbert V. Depletion of serum holotranscobalamin II. An early sign of negative vitamin B_{12} balance. *Lab Invest.* 1988;58(3):332-337.

158. Lindgren A, Kilander A, Bagge E, Nexø E. Holotranscobalamin—a sensitive marker of cobalamin malabsorption. *Eur J Clin Invest.* 1999;29(4):321-329.

159. Miller JW, Garrod MG, Rockwood AL, et al. Measurement of total vitamin B_{12} and holotranscobalamin, singly and in combination, in screening for metabolic vitamin B_{12} deficiency. *Clin Chem.* 2006;52(2):278-285.

160. Green R, Datta Mitra A. Megaloblastic anemias: nutritional and other causes. *Med Clin North Am.* 2017;101(2):297-317.

161. Bertaux O, Mederic C, Valencia R. Amplification of ribosomal DNA in the nucleolus of vitamin B_{12}-deficient Euglena cells. *Exp Cell Res.* 1991;195(1):119-128.

162. Rondanelli E, Gorini P, Magliulo E, Fiori G. Differences in proliferative activity between normoblasts and pernicious anemia megaloblasts. *Blood.* 1964;24:542-552.

163. Steinberg S, Fonda S, Campbell C, Hillman R. Cellular abnormalities of folate deficiency. *Br J Haematol.* 1983;54(4):605-612.

164. Wickremasinghe R, Hoffbrand A. Reduced rate of DNA replication fork movement in megaloblastic anemia. *J Clin Invest.* 1980;65(1):26-36.

165. Palmer AM, Kamynina E, Field MS, Stover PJ. Folate rescues vitamin B_{12} depletion-induced inhibition of nuclear thymidylate biosynthesis and genome instability. *Proc Natl Acad Sci U S A.* 2017;114(20):E4095-E4102.

166. Duthie S, McMillan P. Uracil misincorporation in human DNA detected using single cell gel electrophoresis. *Carcinogenesis.* 1997;18(9):1709-1714.

167. Koury M, Horne D, Brown Z, et al. Apoptosis of late-stage erythroblasts in megaloblastic anemia: association with DNA damage and macrocyte production. *Blood.* 1997;89(12):4617-4623.

168. Metz J, Kelly A, Swett V, et al. Deranged DNA synthesis by bone marrow from vitamin B-12-deficient humans. *Br J Haematol.* 1968;14(6):575-592.

169. Das K, Mohanty D, Garewal G. Cytogenetics in nutritional megaloblastic anaemia: prolonged persistence of chromosomal abnormalities in lymphocytes after remission. *Acta Haematol.* 1986;76(2-3):146-154.

170. Fernandes-Costa F, Green R, Torrance J. Increased erythrocytic diphosphoglycerate in megaloblastic anaemia. A compensatory mechanism? *S Afr Med J.* 1978;53(18):709-712.

171. Green R, Kuhl W, Jacobson R, et al. Masking of macrocytosis by alpha-thalassemia in blacks with pernicious anemia. *N Engl J Med.* 1982;307(21):1322-1325.

172. Spivak JL. Masked megaloblastic anemia. *Arch Intern Med.* 1982;142(12):2111-2114.

173. Lindenbaum J, Nath BJ. Megaloblastic anaemia and neutrophil hypersegmentation. *Br J Haematol.* 1980;44(3):511-513.

174. Carmel R, Green R, Jacobsen DW, Qian GD. Neutrophil nuclear segmentation in mild cobalamin deficiency: relation to metabolic tests of cobalamin status and observations on ethnic differences in neutrophil segmentation. *Am J Clin Pathol.* 1996;106(1):57-63.

175. Lawler S, Roberts P, Hoffbrand A. Chromosome studies in megaloblastic anaemia before and after treatment. *Scand J Haematol.* 1971;8(4):309-320.

176. Bessman J, Williams L, Gilmer PJ. Platelet size in health and hematologic disease. *Am J Clin Pathol.* 1982;78(2):150-153.

177. Marsh GW, Stewart JS. Splenic function in adult coeliac disease. *Br J Haematol.* 1970;19(4):445-457.

178. Fudenberg H, Estren S. Non-Addisonian megaloblastic anemia; the intermediate megaloblast in the differential diagnosis of pernicious and related anemias. *Am J Med.* 1958;25(2):198-209.

179. Gulley M, Bentley S, Ross D. Neutrophil myeloperoxidase measurement uncovers masked megaloblastic anemia. *Blood.* 1990;76(5):1004-1007.

180. Solanki DL, Jacobson RJ, McKibbon J, Green R. Racial patterns in pernicious anemia. *N Engl J Med.* 1978;298(24):1365.

181. Solanki D, Jacobson R, Green R, et al. Pernicious anemia in blacks. A study of 64 patients from Washington, D. C., and Johannesburg, South Africa. *Am J Clin Pathol.* 1981;75(1):96-99.

182. Harper JW, Holleran SF, Ramakrishnan R, et al. Anemia in celiac disease is multifactorial in etiology. *Am J Hematol.* 2007;82(11):996-1000.

183. Green R. Anemias beyond B12 and iron deficiency: the buzz about other B's, elementary, and nonelementary problems. *Hematology Am Soc Hematol Educ Program.* 2012;2012:492-498.

184. Chen M, Krishnamurthy A, Mohamed AR, Green R. Hematological disorders following gastric bypass surgery: emerging concepts of the interplay between nutritional deficiency and inflammation. *Biomed Res Int.* 2013;2013:205467.

185. Bunn HF. Vitamin B12 and pernicious anemia—the dawn of molecular medicine. *N Engl J Med.* 2014;370(8):773-776.

186. Hershko C, Ronson A, Souroujon M, et al. Variable hematologic presentation of autoimmune gastritis: age-related progression from iron deficiency to cobalamin depletion. *Blood.* 2006;107(4):1673-1679.

187. Pezzimenti JF, Lindenbaum J. Megaloblastic anemia associated with erythroid hypoplasia. *Am J Med.* 1972;53(6):748-754.

188. Boddington M, Spriggs A. The epithelial cells in megaloblastic anaemias. *J Clin Pathol.* 1959;12(3):228-234.

189. Hussein S, Laulicht M, Hoffbrand A. Serum ferritin in megaloblastic anaemia. *Scand J Haematol.* 1978;20(3):241-245.

190. Emerson P, Wilkinson J. Lactate dehydrogenase in the diagnosis and assessment of response to treatment of megaloblastic anaemia. *Br J Haematol.* 1966;12(6):678-688.

191. Winston R, Warburton F, Stott A. Enzymatic diagnosis of megaloblastic anaemia. *Br J Haematol.* 1970;19(5):587-592.

192. Hansen N, Karle H. Blood and bone-marrow lysozyme in neutropenia: an attempt towards pathogenetic classification. *Br J Haematol.* 1971;21(3):261-270.

193. Heller P, Weinstein H, West M, Zimmerman H. Enzymes in anemia: a study of abnormalities of several enzymes of carbohvdrate metabolism in the plasma and erythrocytes in patients with anemia, with preliminary observations of boen marrow enzymes. *Ann Intern Med.* 1960;53:898-913.

194. de Klerk G, Rosengarten P, Vet R, Goudsmit R. Serum erythropoietin (ESF) titers in polycythemia. *Blood.* 1981;58(6):1171-1174.

195. Myhre E. Studies on the erythrokinetics in pernicious anemia. *Scand J Clin Lab Invest.* 1964;16:391-402.

196. Lindahl J. Quantification of ineffective erythropoiesis in megaloblastic anaemia by determination of endogenous production of 14CO after administration of glycine-2-14C. *Scand J Haematol.* 1980;24(4):281-291.

197. Hamililton H, Sheets R, Degowin E. Studies with inagglutinable erythrocyte counts. VII. Further investigation of the hemolytic mechanism in untreated pernicious anemia and the demonstration of a hemolytic property in the plasma. *J Lab Clin Med.* 1958;51(6):942-955.

198. Harker L, Finch C. Thrombokinetics in man. *J Clin Invest.* 1969;48(6):963-974.

199. Obeid R, Geisel J, Schorr H, et al. The impact of vegetarianism on some haematological parameters. *Eur J Haematol.* 2002;69(5-6):275-279.

200. Jacques P, Selhub J, Bostom A, et al. The effect of folic acid fortification on plasma folate and total homocysteine concentrations. *N Engl J Med.* 1999;340(19):1449-1454.

201. Antony AC. Evidence for potential underestimation of clinical folate deficiency in resource-limited countries using blood tests. *Nutr Rev.* 2017;75:600-615.

202. Ballard H, Lindenbaum J. Megaloblastic anemia complicating hyperalimentation therapy. *Am J Med.* 1974;56(5):740-742.

203. Mollin D, Hines J. Late post-gastrectomy syndromes. Observations on the nature and pathogenesis of anaemia following partial gastrectomy. *Proc R Soc Med.* 1964;57:575-580.

204. Hoffbrand A. Folate deficiency in premature infants. *Arch Dis Child.* 1970;45(242):441-444.

205. Royston NJ, Parry TE. Megaloblastic anaemia complicating dietary treatment of phenylketonuria in infancy. *Arch Dis Child.* 1962;37(194):430-435.

206. Ford JD, Scott KJ. The folic acid activity of some milk foods for babies. *J Dairy Res.* 1968;35(1):85-90.

207. Datta-Mitra A, Vali-Betts E, Green R, et al. Combined megaloblastic and sideroblastic anemia in an infant fed with goat's milk. *J Pediatr Hematol Oncol.* 2017;39(4):319-320.

208. Savage D, Lindenbaum J. Anemia in alcoholics. *Medicine (Baltimore).* 1986;65(5):322-338.

209. Eichner E, Hillman R. Effect of alcohol on serum folate level. *J Clin Invest.* 1973;52(3):584-591.

210. Lieber C. Metabolism and metabolic effects of alcohol. *Semin Hematol.* 1980;17(2):85-99.

211. Post R, Desforges J. Thrombocytopenia and alcoholism. *Ann Intern Med.* 1968;68(6):1230-1236.

212. Liu Y. Effects of alcohol on granulocytes and lymphocytes. *Semin Hematol.* 1980;17(2):130-136.

213. Lindenbaum J, Lieber C. Hematologic effects of alcohol in man in the absence of nutritional deficiency. *N Engl J Med.* 1969;281(7):333-338.

214. Trier J. Celiac sprue. *N Engl J Med.* 1991;325(24):1709-1719.

215. Halsted C, Reisenauer A, Romero J, et al. Jejunal perfusion of simple and conjugated folates in celiac sprue. *J Clin Invest.* 1977;59(5):933-940.

216. Hjelt K, Krasilnikoff P. The impact of gluten on haematological status, dietary intakes of haemopoietic nutrients and vitamin B12 and folic acid absorption in children with coeliac disease. *Acta Paediatr Scand.* 1990;79(10):911-919.

217. Halfdanarson TR, Litzow MR, Murray JA. Hematologic manifestations of celiac disease. *Blood.* 2007;109(2):412-421.

218. Klipstein F. Tropical sprue in New York City. *Gastroenterology.* 1964;47:457-470.

219. Klipstein F. Folate in tropical sprue. *Br J Haematol.* 1972;23(suppl):119-133.

220. Klipstein F, Schenk E, Samloff I. Folate repletion associated with oral tetracycline therapy in tropical sprue. *Gastroenterology.* 1966;51(3):317-332.

221. Ghoshal UC, Srivastava D, Verma A, Ghoshal U. Tropical sprue in 2014: the new face of an old disease. *Curr Gastroenterol Rep.* 2014;16(6):391.

222. Klipstein F. Progress in Gastroenterology: tropical sprue. *Gastroenterology.* 1968;54:275-293.

223. Sheehy T, Perez-Santiago E, Rubini M. Tropical sprue and vitamin B12. *N Engl J Med.* 1961;265:1232-1236.

224. Corcino J, Coll G, Klipstein F. Pteroylglutamic acid malabsorption in tropical sprue. *Blood.* 1975;45(4):577-580.

225. Chanarin I, Bennett M. Absorption of folic acid and D-xylose as tests of small-intestinal function. *Br Med J.* 1962;1(5283):985-989.

226. Booth C. The metabolic effects of intestinal resection in man. *Postgrad Med J.* 1961;37:725-739.

227. Pitney W, Joske R, Mackinnon N. Folic acid and other absorption tests in lymphosarcoma, chronic lymphocytic leukaemia, and some related conditions. *J Clin Pathol.* 1960;13:440-447.

228. Hoskins L, Norris H, Gottlieb L, Zamcheck N. Functional and morphologic alterations of the gastrointestinal tract in progressive systemic sclerosis (scleroderma). *Am J Med.* 1962;33:459-470.

229. Vinnik I, Kern FJ, Struthers JJ. Malabsorption and the diarrhea of diabetes mellitus. *Gastroenterology.* 1962;43:507-520.

230. Cook G, Morgan J, Hoffbrand A. Impairment of folate absorption by systemic bacterial infections. *Lancet.* 1974;2(7894):1416-1417.

231. Shojania AM. Folic acid and vitamin B12 deficiency in pregnancy and in the neonatal period. *Clin Perinatol.* 1984;11(2):433-459.

232. Landon M, Eyre D, Hytten F. Transfer of folate to the fetus. *Br J Obstet Gynaecol.* 1975;82(1):12-19.

233. Pritchard J, Scott D, Whalley P, Haling RJ. Infants of mothers with megaloblastic anemia due to folate deficiency. *JAMA.* 1970;211(12):1982-1984.

234. Reynolds EH, Green R. Valproate and folate: congenital and developmental risks. *Epilepsy Behav.* 2020;108:107068.

235. Shapiro J, Alberts H, Welch P, Metz J. Folate and vitamin B-12 deficiency associated with lactation. *Br J Haematol.* 1965;11:498-504.

236. Streiff R, Little A. Folic acid deficiency in pregnancy. *N Engl J Med.* 1967;276(14):776-779.

237. de Benoist B. Conclusions of a WHO Technical Consultation on folate and vitamin B12 deficiencies. *Food Nutr Bull.* 2008;29(2 suppl): S238-S244.

238. Chanarin I, McFadyen I, Kyle R. The physiological macrocytosis of pregnancy. *Br J Obstet Gynaecol.* 1977;84(7):504-508.

239. Avery B, Ledger W. Folic acid metabolism in well-nourished pregnant women. *Obstet Gynecol.* 1970;35(4):616-624.

240. Colman N, Barker M, Green R, Metz J. Prevention of folate deficiency in pregnancy by food fortification. *Am J Clin Nutr.* 1974;27(4):339-344.

241. Giles C. An account of 335 cases of megaloblastic anaemia of pregnancy and the puerperium. *J Clin Pathol.* 1966;19(1):1-11.

242. Lindenbaum J, Klipstein F. Folic acid deficiency in sickle-cell anemia. *N Engl J Med.* 1963;269:875-882.

243. Hild D. Folate losses from the skin in exfoliative dermatitis. *Arch Intern Med.* 1969;123(1):51-57.

244. Whitehead V, Comty C, Posen G, Kaye M. Homeostasis of folic acid in patients undergoing maintenance hemodialysis. *N Engl J Med.* 1968;279(18):970-974.

245. Green R. Metabolite assays in cobalamin and folate deficiency. *Baillieres Clin Haematol.* 1995;8(3):533-566.

246. Hoffbrand A, Newcombe F, Mollin D. Method of assay of red cell folate activity and the value of the assay as a test for folate deficiency. *J Clin Pathol.* 1966;19(1):17-28.

247. Lindenbaum J. Status of laboratory testing in the diagnosis of megaloblastic anemia. *Blood.* 1983;61(4):624-627.

248. Green R, Dwyre DM. Evaluation of macrocytic anemias. *Semin Hematol.* 2015;52:279-286.

249. McNamee T, Hyland T, Harrington J, et al. Haematinic deficiency and macrocytosis in middle-aged and older adults. *PLoS One.* 2013;8(11):e77743.

250. Kinnear D, Macintosh P, Cameron D, et al. Intestinal absorption of tritum-labelled folic acid in idiopathic steatorrhea: effect of a glutenfree diet. *Can Med Assoc J.* 1963;89:975-979.

251. Green R, Miller JW. Folate deficiency beyond megaloblastic anemia: hyperhomocysteinemia and other manifestations of dysfunctional folate status. *Semin Hematol.* 1999;36(1):47-64.

252. Prevention of neural tube defects: results of the Medical Research Council Vitamin Study. MRC Vitamin Study Research Group. *Lancet.* 1991;338(8760):131-137.

253. Rothenberg S, da Costa M, Sequeira J, et al. Autoantibodies against folate receptors in women with a pregnancy complicated by a neural-tube defect. *N Engl J Med.* 2004;350(2):134-142.

254. van der Put N, Gabreës F, Stevens E, et al. A second common mutation in the methylenetetrahydrofolate reductase gene: an additional risk factor for neural-tube defects? *Am J Hum Genet.* 1998;62(5):1044-1051.

255. Honein M, Paulozzi L, Mathews T, et al. Impact of folic acid fortification of the US food supply on the occurrence of neural tube defects. *JAMA.* 2001;285(23):2981-2986.

256. De Wals P, Tairou F, Van Allen M, et al. Reduction in neural-tube defects after folic acid fortification in Canada. *N Engl J Med.* 2007;357(2):135-142.

257. Afman L, Van Der Put N, Thomas C, et al. Reduced vitamin B_{12} binding by transcobalamin II increases the risk of neural tube defects. *QJM.* 2001;94(3):159-166.

258. Thompson M, Cole D, Ray J. Vitamin B-12 and neural tube defects: the Canadian experience. *Am J Clin Nutr.* 2009;89(2):697S-701S.

259. Ramos MI, Allen LH, Haan MN, et al. Plasma folate concentrations are associated with depressive symptoms in elderly Latina women despite folic acid fortification. *Am J Clin Nutr.* 2004;80(4):1024-1028.

260. D'Angelo A, Selhub J. Homocysteine and thrombotic disease. *Blood.* 1997;90(1):1-11.

261. Schnyder G, Roffi M, Pin R, et al. Decreased rate of coronary restenosis after lowering of plasma homocysteine levels. *N Engl J Med.* 2001;345(22):1593-1600.

262. Lange H, Suryapranata H, De Luca G, et al. Folate therapy and in-stent restenosis after coronary stenting. *N Engl J Med.* 2004;350(26):2673-2681.

263. Bonaa KH, Njolstad I, Ueland PM, et al. Homocysteine lowering and cardiovascular events after acute myocardial infarction. *N Engl J Med.* 2006;354(15):1578-1588.

264. Yang Q, Botto LD, Erickson JD, et al. Improvement in stroke mortality in Canada and the United States, 1990 to 2002. *Circulation.* 2006;113(10):1335-1343.

265. Clarke R, Halsey J, Lewington S, et al. Effects of lowering homocysteine levels with B vitamins on cardiovascular disease, cancer, and cause-specific mortality: meta-analysis of 8 randomized trials involving 37 485 individuals. *Arch Intern Med.* 2010;170(18):1622-1631.

266. Smith AD, Refsum H. Homocysteine, B vitamins, and cognitive impairment. *Annu Rev Nutr.* 2016;36:211-239.

267. Kluijtmans L, Young I, Boreham C, et al. Genetic and nutritional factors contributing to hyperhomocysteinemia in young adults. *Blood.* 2003;101(7):2483-2488.

268. Quinlivan E, McPartlin J, McNulty H, et al. Importance of both folic acid and vitamin B_{12} in reduction of risk of vascular disease. *Lancet.* 2002;359(9302):227-228.

269. Lievers K, Kluijtmans L, Boers G, et al. Influence of a glutamate carboxypeptidase II (GCPII) polymorphism (1561C—>T) on plasma homocysteine, folate and vitamin B(12) levels and its relationship to cardiovascular disease risk. *Atherosclerosis.* 2002;164(2):269-273.

270. Walker S, Wein P, Ihle B. Severe folate deficiency masquerading as the syndrome of hemolysis, elevated liver enzymes, and low platelets. *Obstet Gynecol.* 1997;90(4, pt 2):655-657.

271. Hartong SC, Steegers EA, Visser W. Hemolysis, elevated liver enzymes and low platelets during pregnancy due to vitamin B_{12} and folate deficiencies. *Eur J Obstet Gynecol Reprod Biol.* 2007;131(2):241-242.

272. Giovannucci E, Stampfer M, Colditz G, et al. Multivitamin use, folate, and colon cancer in women in the Nurses' Health Study. *Ann Intern Med.* 1998;129(7):517-524.

273. Ma J, Stampfer M, Giovannucci E, et al. Methylenetetrahydrofolate reductase polymorphism, dietary interactions, and risk of colorectal cancer. *Cancer Res.* 1997;57(6):1098-1102.

274. Mason JB, Dickstein A, Jacques PF, et al. A temporal association between folic acid fortification and an increase in colorectal cancer rates may be illuminating important biological principles: a hypothesis. *Cancer Epidemiol Biomarkers Prev.* 2007;16(7):1325-1329.

275. Kim Y. Will mandatory folic acid fortification prevent or promote cancer? *Am J Clin Nutr.* 2004;80(5):1123-1128.

276. Troen AM, Mitchell B, Sorensen B, et al. Unmetabolized folic acid in plasma is associated with reduced natural killer cell cytotoxicity among postmenopausal women. *J Nutr.* 2006;136(1):189-194.

277. Paniz C, Bertinato JF, Lucena MR, et al. A daily dose of 5 mg folic acid for 90 days is associated with increased serum unmetabolized folic acid and reduced natural killer cell cytotoxicity in healthy brazilian adults. *J Nutr.* 2017;147:1677-1685.

278. Vollset SE, Clarke R, Lewington S, et al. Effects of folic acid supplementation on overall and site-specific cancer incidence during the randomised trials: meta-analyses of data on 50,000 individuals. *Lancet.* 2013;381(9871):1029-1036.

279. Rosenberg I. Folic acid and neural-tube defects—time for action? *N Engl J Med.* 1992;327(26):1875-1877.

280. Hibbard E, Spencer W. Low serum B_{12} levels and latent Addisonian anaemia in pregnancy. *J Obstet Gynaecol Br Commonw.* 1970;77(1):52-57.

281. Carmel R, Johnson C. Racial patterns in pernicious anemia. Early age at onset and increased frequency of intrinsic-factor antibody in black women. *N Engl J Med.* 1978;298(12):647-650.

282. Vilter CF, Vilter RW, Spies TD. The treatment of pernicious and related anemias with synthetic folic acid; observations on the maintenance of a normal hematologic status and on the occurrence of combined system disease at the end of one year. *J Lab Clin Med.* 1947;32(3):262-273.

283. Andersen L, Hansen E, Knudsen J, et al. Prospectively measured red cell folate levels in methotrexate treated patients with rheumatoid arthritis: relation to withdrawal and side effects. *J Rheumatol.* 1997;24(5):830-837.

284. Kim YS, Sun JM, Ahn JS, et al. The optimal duration of vitamin supplementation prior to the first dose of pemetrexed in patients with non-small-cell lung cancer. *Lung Cancer.* 2013;81(2):231-235.

285. Stabler SP. Clinical practice. Vitamin B_{12} deficiency. *N Engl J Med.* 2013;368(2):149-160.

286. Green R. Vitamin B_{12} deficiency from the perspective of a practicing hematologist. *Blood.* 2017;129(19):2603-2611.

287. Toh B, van Driel I, Gleeson P. Pernicious anemia. *N Engl J Med.* 1997;337(20):1441-1448.

288. Kano Y, Sakamoto S, Miura Y, Takaku F. Disorders of cobalamin metabolism. *Crit Rev Oncol Hematol.* 1985;3(1):1-34.

289. Irvine W, Davies S, Teitelbaum S, et al. The clinical and pathological significance of gastric parietal cell antibody. *Ann N Y Acad Sci.* 1965;124(2):657-691.

290. Gaarder P, Heier H. A human autoantibody to renal collecting duct cells associated with thyroid and gastric autoimmunity and possibly renal tubular acidosis. *Clin Exp Immunol.* 1983;51(1):29-37.

291. Toh BH. Pathophysiology and laboratory diagnosis of pernicious anemia. *Immunol Res.* 2017;65(1):326-330.

292. Suri-Payer E, Kehn P, Cheever A, Shevach E. Pathogenesis of post-thymectomy autoimmune gastritis. Identification of anti-H/K adenosine triphosphatase-reactive T cells. *J Immunol.* 1996;157(4):1799-1805.

293. Kapadia C, Donaldson RJ. Disorders of cobalamin (vitamin B_{12}) absorption and transport. *Annu Rev Med.* 1985;36:93-110.

294. Chanarin I, James D. Humoral and cell-mediated intrinsic-factor antibody in pernicious anaemia. *Lancet.* 1974;1(7866):1078-1080.

295. Conn H, Binder H, Burns B. Pernicious anemia and immunologic deficiency. *Ann Intern Med.* 1968;68(3):603-612.

296. Ardeman S, Chanarin I, Krafchik B, Singer W. Addisonian pernicious anaemia and intrinsic factor antibodies in thyroid disorders. *Q J Med.* 1966;35(139):421-431.

297. Comin D, Hines J, Wieland R. Coexistent pernicious anemia and idiopathic hypoparathyroidism in a women. *JAMA.* 1969;207(6):1147-1149.

298. Mazzone T, Kelly W, Ensinck J. Lymphocytic hypophysitis. Associated with antiparietal cell antibodies and vitamin B_{12} deficiency. *Arch Intern Med.* 1983;143(9):1794-1795.

299. Howitz J, Schwartz M. Vitiligo, achlorhydria, and pernicious anaemia. *Lancet.* 1971;1(7713):1331-1334.

300. Robins-Browne RM, Green R, Katz J, Becker D. Thymoma, pure red cell aplasia, pernicious anaemia and candidiasis: a defect in immunohomeostasis. *Br J Haematol.* 1977;36:5-13.

301. Jackson I, Doig W, McDonald G. Pernicious anaemia as a cause of infertility. *Lancet.* 1967;2(7527):1159-1160.

302. Watson A. Seminal vitamin B_{12} and sterility. *Lancet.* 1962;2(7257):644.

303. Pront R, Margalioth EJ, Green R, et al. Prevalence of low serum cobalamin in infertile couples. *Andrologia.* 2009;41(1):46-50.

304. Ungar B, Mathews J, Tait B, Cowling D. HLA-DR patterns in pernicious anaemia. *Br Med J (Clin Res Ed).* 1981;282(6266):768-770.

305. Hoskins L, Loux H, Britten A, Zamcheck N. Distribution of ABO blood groups in patients with pernicious anemia, gastric carcinoma and gastric carcinoma associated with pernicious anemia. *N Engl J Med.* 1965;273(12):633-637.

306. Wangel A, Callender S, Spray G, Wright R. A family study of pernicious anaemia. I. Autoantibodies, achlorhydria, serum pepsinogen and vitamin B_{12}. *Br J Haematol.* 1968;14(2):161-181.

307. Varis K, Ihamäki T, Härkönen M, et al. Gastric morphology, function, and immunology in first-degree relatives of probands with pernicious anemia and controls. *Scand J Gastroenterol.* 1979;14(2):129-139.

308. Eriksson S, Clase L, Moquist-Olsson I. Pernicious anemia as a risk factor in gastric cancer. The extent of the problem. *Acta Med Scand.* 1981;210(6):481-484.

309. Savage D, Gangaidzo I, Lindenbaum J, et al. Vitamin B_{12} deficiency is the primary cause of megaloblastic anaemia in Zimbabwe. *Br J Haematol.* 1994;86(4):844-850.

310. Wilkinson JF. The gastric secretions in pernicious anemia. *Q J Med.* 1932;1:361-386.

311. Karnes WJ, Samloff I, Siurala M, et al. Positive serum antibody and negative tissue staining for *Helicobacter pylori* in subjects with atrophic body gastritis. *Gastroenterology.* 1991;101(1):167-174.

312. Green R. Protean *H pylori:* perhaps "pernicious" too? *Blood.* 2006;107(4):1247.

313. Lichtman MA. A bacterial cause of cancer: an historical essay. *Oncologist.* 2017;22(5):542-548.

314. Slingerland D, Cardarelli J, Burrows B, Miller A. The utility of serum gastrin levels in assessing the significance of low serum B_{12} levels. *Arch Intern Med.* 1984;144(6):1167-1168.

315. Ganguli P, Cullen D, Irvine W. Radioimmunoassay of plasmagastrin in pernicious anaemia, achlorhydria without pernicious anaemia, hypochlorhydria, and in controls. *Lancet.* 1971;1(7691):155-158.

316. Kaye M, Whorwell P, Wright R. Gastric mucosal lymphocyte subpopulations in pernicious anemia and in normal stomach. *Clin Immunol Immunopathol.* 1983;28(3):431-440.

317. Rodbro P, Dige-Petersen H, Schwartz M, Dalgaard O. Effect of steroids on gastric mucosal structure and function in pernicious anemia. *Acta Med Scand.* 1967;181(4):445-452.

318. Ransohoff R, Jacobsen D, Green R. Vitamin B_{12} deficiency and multiple sclerosis. *Lancet.* 1990;335(8700):1285-1286.

319. Nieburgs H, Glass G. Gastric-cell maturation disorders in atrophic gastritis, pernicious anemia, and carcinoma. Histologic site of origin and diagnostic significance of abnormal cells. *Am J Dig Dis.* 1963;8:135-159.

320. Foroozan P, Trier J. Mucosa of the small intestine in pernicious anemia. *N Engl J Med.* 1967;277(11):553-559.

321. Bezman A, Kinnear D, Zamcheck N. D-xylose and potassium iodide absorption and serum carotene in pernicious anemia. *J Lab Clin Med.* 1959;53(2):226-232.

322. Ellison A. Pernicious anemia masked by multivitamins containing folic acid. *JAMA.* 1960;173:240-243.

323. Carmel R. Subtle and atypical cobalamin deficiency states. *Am J Hematol.* 1990;34(2):108-114.

324. Green R. Typical and atypical manifestations of pernicious anemia. In: M. Besser, R. Bhatt, V.H.T. James, H. Keen, eds. *Thomas Addison and His Diseases: 200 Years On.* J Endocrinol. 1994;1:377-390.

325. Lindenbaum J, Healton E, Savage D, et al. Neuropsychiatric disorders caused by cobalamin deficiency in the absence of anemia or macrocytosis. *N Engl J Med.* 1988;318(26):1720-1728.

326. Maclean L, Sundberg R. Incidence of megaloblastic anemia after total gastrectomy. *N Engl J Med.* 1956;254(19):885-893.

327. Gozzard D, Dawson D, Lewis M. Experiences with dual protein bound aqueous vitamin B₁₂ absorption test in subjects with low serum vitamin B₁₂ concentrations. *J Clin Pathol.* 1987;40(6):633-637.

328. Van der Weyden M, Rother M, Firkin B. Megaloblastic maturation masked by iron deficiency: a biochemical basis. *Br J Haematol.* 1972;22(3):299-307.

329. Lees F, Grandjean L. The gastric and jejunal mucosae in healthy patients with partial gastrectomy. *AMA Arch Intern Med.* 1958;101(5):943-951.

330. Engebretsen KV, Blom-Hogestol IK, Hewitt S, et al. Anemia following Roux-en-Y gastric bypass for morbid obesity; a 5-year follow-up study. *Scand J Gastroenterol.* 2018;53(8):917-922.

331. Shimoda S, Rubin C. The Zollinger-Ellison syndrome with steatorrhea. I. Anticholinergic treatment followed by total gastrectomy and colonic interposition. *Gastroenterology.* 1968;55(6):695-704.

332. Kennedy H, Callender S, Truelove S, Warner G. Haematological aspects of life with an ileostomy. *Br J Haematol.* 1982;52(3):445-454.

333. Anderson C, Walton K, Chanarin I. Megaloblastic anaemia after pelvic radiotherapy for carcinoma of the cervix. *J Clin Pathol.* 1981;34(2):151-152.

334. Tudhope G, Wilson G. Deficiency of vitamin B₁₂ in hypothyroidism. *Lancet.* 1962;1(7232):703-706.

335. Waxman S, Corcino J, Herbert V. Drugs, toxins and dietary amino acids affecting vitamin B₁₂ or folic acid absorption or utilization. *Am J Med.* 1970;48(5):599-608.

336. Lindenbaum J, Pezzimenti JF, Shea N. Small-intestinal function in vitamin B 12 deficiency. *Ann Intern Med.* 1974;80(3):326-331.

337. Cameron D, Watson G, Witts L. The clinical association of macrocytic anemia with intestinal stricture and anastomosis. *Blood.* 1949;4(7):793-802.

338. Murphy M, Sourial N, Burman J, et al. Megaloblastic anaemia due to vitamin B₁₂ deficiency caused by small intestinal bacterial overgrowth: possible role of vitamin B₁₂ analogues. *Br J Haematol.* 1986;62(1):7-12.

339. Nyberg W. The influence of *Diphyllobothrium latum* on the vitamin B₁₂-intrinsic factor complex. I. In vivo studies with Schilling test technique. *Acta Med Scand.* 1960;167:185-187.

340. Harriman G, Smith P, Horne M, et al. Vitamin B₁₂ malabsorption in patients with acquired immunodeficiency syndrome. *Arch Intern Med.* 1989;149(9):2039-2041.

341. Herzlich B, Schiano T, Moussa Z, et al. Decreased intrinsic factor secretion in AIDS: relation to parietal cell acid secretory capacity and vitamin B₁₂ malabsorption. *Am J Gastroenterol.* 1992;87(12):1781-1788.

342. Remacha A, Cadafalch J. Cobalamin deficiency in patients infected with the human immunodeficiency virus. *Semin Hematol.* 1999;36(1):75-87.

343. Guéant J, Champigneulle B, Gaucher P, Nicolas J. Malabsorption of vitamin B₁₂ in pancreatic insufficiency of the adult and of the child. *Pancreas.* 1990;5(5):559-567.

344. Toskes P, Deren J, Conrad M. Trypsin-like nature of the pancreatic factor that corrects vitamin B₁₂ malabsorption associated with pancreatic dysfunction. *J Clin Invest.* 1973;52(7):1660-1664.

345. Henderson J, Simpson J, Warwick R, Shearman D. Does malabsorption of vitamin B 12 occur in chronic pancreatitis? *Lancet.* 1972;2(7771):241-243.

346. Gilois C, Wierzbicki A, Hirani N, et al. The hematological and electrophysiological effects of cobalamin. Deficiency secondary to vegetarian diets. *Ann N Y Acad Sci.* 1992;669:345-348.

347. Ford M. Megaloblastic anaemia in a vegetarian. *Br J Clin Pract.* 1980;34(7):222.

348. Michaud J, Lemieux B, Ogier H, Lambert M. Nutritional vitamin B₁₂ deficiency: two cases detected by routine newborn urinary screening. *Eur J Pediatr.* 1992;151(3):218-220.

349. Allen LH. How common is vitamin B-12 deficiency? *Am J Clin Nutr.* 2009;89(2):693S-696S.

350. Wickramasinghe S, Akinyanju O, Grange A, Litwinczuk R. Folate levels and deoxyuridine suppression tests in protein-energy malnutrition. *Br J Haematol.* 1983;54(1):135-143.

351. Frenkel E. Abnormal fatty acid metabolism in peripheral nerves of patients with pernicious anemia. *J Clin Invest.* 1973;52(5):1237-1245.

352. Watkins D, Rosenblatt DS. Inborn errors of cobalamin absorption and metabolism. *Am J Med Genet C Semin Med Genet.* 2011;157C(1):33-44.

353. Lever E, Elwes R, Williams A, Reynolds E. Subacute combined degeneration of the cord due to folate deficiency: response to methyl folate treatment. *J Neurol Neurosurg Psychiatry.* 1986;49(10):1203-1207.

354. Clayton P, Smith I, Harding B, et al. Subacute combined degeneration of the cord, dementia and parkinsonism due to an inborn error of folate metabolism. *J Neurol Neurosurg Psychiatry.* 1986;49(8):920-927.

355. Green R, Van Tonder S, Oettle G, et al. Neurological changes in fruit bats deficient in vitamin B₁₂. *Nature.* 1975;254(5496):148-150.

356. Weir D, Keating S, Molloy A, et al. Methylation deficiency causes vitamin B₁₂-associated neuropathy in the pig. *J Neurochem.* 1988;51(6):1949-1952.

357. van der Westhuyzen J, Fernandes-Costa F, Metz J. Cobalamin inactivation by nitrous oxide produces severe neurological impairment in fruit bats: protection by methionine and aggravation by folates. *Life Sci.* 1982;31(18):2001-2010.

358. Molloy A, Orsi B, Kennedy D, et al. The relationship between the activity of methionine synthase and the ratio of S-adenosylmethionine to S-adenosylhomocysteine in the brain and other tissues of the pig. *Biochem Pharmacol.* 1992;44(7):1349-1355.

359. Deacon R, Purkiss P, Green R, et al. Vitamin B₁₂ neuropathy is not due to failure to methylate myelin basic protein. *J Neurol Sci.* 1986;72(1):113-117.

360. Stabler SP. Vitamin B₁₂ deficiency. *N Engl J Med.* 2013;368(21):2041-2042.

361. Kätkä K. Immune functions in pernicious anaemia before and during treatment with vitamin B₁₂. *Scand J Haematol.* 1984;32(1):76-82.

362. Kätkä K, Eskola J, Granfors K, et al. Serum IgA deficiency and anti-IgA antibodies in pernicious anemia. *Clin Immunol Immunopathol.* 1988;46(1):55-60.

363. Zhang S, Willett W, Selhub J, et al. Plasma folate, vitamin B6, vitamin B₁₂, homocysteine, and risk of breast cancer. *J Natl Cancer Inst.* 2003;95(5):373-380.

364. Dhonukshe-Rutten R, Lips M, de Jong N, et al. Vitamin B-12 status is associated with bone mineral content and bone mineral density in frail elderly women but not in men. *J Nutr.* 2003;133(3):801-807.

365. Stone K, Bauer D, Sellmeyer D, Cummings S. Low serum vitamin B-12 levels are associated with increased hip bone loss in older women: a prospective study. *J Clin Endocrinol Metab.* 2004;89(3):1217-1221.

366. Beck W. Neuropsychiatric consequences of cobalamin deficiency. *Adv Intern Med.* 1991;36:33-56.

367. Victor M, Lear A. Subacute combined degeneration of the spinal cord; current concepts of the disease process; value of serum vitamin B₁₂; determinations in clarifying some of the common clinical problems. *Am J Med.* 1956;20(6):896-911.

368. Herbert V. Megaloblastic anemias. *Lab Invest.* 1985;52(1):3-19.

369. Di Lazzaro V, Restuccia D, Fogli D, et al. Central sensory and motor conduction in vitamin B₁₂ deficiency. *Electroencephalogr Clin Neurophysiol.* 1992;84(5):433-439.

370. Fraser T. Cerebral manifestations of Addisonian pernicious anaemia. *Lancet.* 1960;2(7148):458-459.

371. Vogiatzoglou A, Refsum H, Johnston C, et al. Vitamin B₁₂ status and rate of brain volume loss in community-dwelling elderly. *Neurology.* 2008;71(11):826-832.

372. de Lau L, Smith A, Refsum H, et al. Plasma vitamin B₁₂ status and cerebral white-matter lesions. *J Neurol Neurosurg Psychiatry.* 2009;80(2):149-157.

373. Shulman R. Psychiatric aspects of pernicious anaemia: a prospective controlled investigation. *Br Med J.* 1967;3(5560):266-270.

374. Smith ADM. Megaloblastic madness. *Br Med J.* 1960; 2(5216):1840-1845.

375. Harris JW, Kellermeyer RW. *The Red Cell.* Harvard University Press. 1970.

376. Stojsavljević N, Lević Z, Drulović J, Dragutinović G. A 44-month clinical-brain MRI follow-up in a patient with B₁₂ deficiency. *Neurology.* 1997;49(3):878-881.

377. Scherer K. Images in clinical medicine. Neurologic manifestations of vitamin B₁₂ deficiency. *N Engl J Med.* 2003;348(22):2208.

378. Mullikin D, Pillai N, Sanchez R, et al. Megaloblastic anemia progressing to severe thrombotic microangiopathy in patients with disordered vitamin B₁₂ metabolism: case reports and literature review. *J Pediatr.* 2018;202:315-319.e2.

379. Beck BB, van Spronsen F, Diepstra A, et al. Renal thrombotic microangiopathy in patients with cblC defect: review of an under-recognized entity. *Pediatr Nephrol.* 2017;32(5):733-741.

380. Whitehead V. Acquired and inherited disorders of cobalamin and folate in children. *Br J Haematol.* 2006;134(2):125-136.

381. Herbert V, Jacob E, Wong KT, et al. Low serum vitamin B₁₂ levels in patients receiving ascorbic acid in megadoses: studies concerning the effect of ascorbate on radioisotope vitamin B₁₂ assay. *Am J Clin Nutr.* 1978;31(2):253-258.

382. Carmel R. R-binder deficiency. A clinically benign cause of cobalamin pseudodeficiency. *JAMA.* 1983;250(14):1886-1890.

383. Carmel R. Mild transcobalamin I (haptocorrin) deficiency and low serum cobalamin concentrations. *Clin Chem.* 2003;49(8):1367-1374.

384. Bor MV, Nexø E, Hvas A-M. Holo-transcobalamin concentration and transcobalamin saturation reflect recent vitamin B₁₂ absorption better than does serum vitamin B₁₂. *Clin Chem.* 2004;50(6):1043-1049.

385. von Castel-Roberts K, Morkbak A, Nexo E, et al. Holo-transcobalamin is an indicator of vitamin B-12 absorption in healthy adults with adequate vitamin B-12 status. *Am J Clin Nutr.* 2007;85(4):1057-1061.

386. Kahn SB, Williams WJ, Barness LA, et al. Methylmalonic acid excretion: a sensitive indicator of vitamin B₁₂ deficiency. *Transl Res.* 1965;66(1):75-83.

387. Norman E, Morrison J. Screening elderly populations for cobalamin (vitamin B₁₂) deficiency using the urinary methylmalonic acid assay by gas chromatography mass spectrometry. *Am J Med.* 1993;94(6):589-594.

388. Norman E, Martelo O, Denton M. Cobalamin (vitamin B₁₂) deficiency detection by urinary methylmalonic acid quantitation. *Blood.* 1982;59(6):1128-1131.

389. Lindenbaum J, Savage D, Stabler S, Allen R. Diagnosis of cobalamin deficiency: II. Relative sensitivities of serum cobalamin, methylmalonic acid, and total homocysteine concentrations. *Am J Hematol.* 1990;34(2):99-107.

390. Green R. Screening for vitamin B₁₂ deficiency: caveat emptor. *Ann Intern Med.* 1996;124(5):509-511.

391. Solomon LR. Cobalamin-responsive disorders in the ambulatory care setting: unreliability of cobalamin, methylmalonic acid, and homocysteine testing. *Blood.* 2005;105(3):978-985; author reply 1137.

392. Fedosov SN. Biochemical markers of vitamin B₁₂ deficiency combined in one diagnostic parameter: the age-dependence and association with cognitive function and blood hemoglobin. *Clin Chim Acta.* 2013;422:47-53.

393. Fedosov SN, Brito A, Miller JW, et al. Combined indicator of vitamin B₁₂ status: modification for missing biomarkers and folate status and recommendations for revised cut-points. *Clin Chem Lab Med.* 2015;53(8):1215-1225.

394. Molloy AM, Pangilinan F, Mills JL, et al. A common polymorphism in HIBCH influences methylmalonic acid concentrations in blood independently of cobalamin. *Am J Hum Genet.* 2016;98(5):869-882.

395. Stabler S, Allen R, Barrett R, et al. Cerebrospinal fluid methylmalonic acid levels in normal subjects and patients with cobalamin deficiency. *Neurology.* 1991;41(10):1627-1632.

396. Fairbanks V, Wahner H, Phyliky R. Tests for pernicious anemia: the "Schilling test." *Mayo Clin Proc.* 1983;58(8):541-544.

397. Bor M, Cetin M, Aytaç S, et al. Nonradioactive vitamin B_{12} absorption test evaluated in controls and in patients with inherited malabsorption of vitamin B_{12}. *Clin Chem.* 2005;51(11):2151-2155.

398. Carkeet C, Dueker S, Lango J, et al. Human vitamin B_{12} absorption measurement by accelerator mass spectrometry using specifically labeled (14)C-cobalamin. *Proc Natl Acad Sci U S A.* 2006;103(15):5694-5699.

399. Devi S, Pasanna RM, Shamshuddin Z, et al. Measuring vitamin B-12 bioavailability with [13C]-cyanocobalamin in humans. *Am J Clin Nutr.* 2020;112:1504-1515.

400. Miller JW, Green R. Assessing vitamin B-12 absorption and bioavailability: read the label. *Am J Clin Nutr.* 2020;112:1420-1421.

401. Metz J. The deoxyuridine suppression test. *Crit Rev Clin Lab Sci.* 1984;20(3):205-241.

402. Boddy K, King P, Mervyn L, et al. Retention of cyanocobalamin, hydroxocobalamin, and coenzyme B_{12} after parenteral administration. *Lancet.* 1968;2(7570):710-712.

403. Fanidi A, Carreras-Torres R, Larose TL, et al. Is high vitamin B_{12} status a cause of lung cancer? *Int J Cancer.* 2019;145(6):1499-1503.

404. Flores-Guerrero JL, Minovic I, Groothof D, et al. Association of plasma concentration of vitamin B_{12} with all-cause mortality in the general population in the Netherlands. *JAMA Netw Open.* 2020;3(1):e1919274.

405. Wolffenbuttel BHR, Heiner-Fokkema MR, Green R, Gans ROB. Relationship between serum B_{12} concentrations and mortality: experience in NHANES. *BMC Med.* 2020;18(1):307.

406. Coleman D, Donohue D, Finch C, et al. Erythrokinetics in pernicious anemia. *Blood.* 1956;11(9):807-820.

407. Hillman R, Adamson J, Burka E. Characteristics of vitamin B_{12} correction of the abnormal erythropoiesis of pernicious anemia. *Blood.* 1968;31(4):419-432.

408. Sumner A, Chin M, Abrahm J, et al. Elevated methylmalonic acid and total homocysteine levels show high prevalence of vitamin B_{12} deficiency after gastric surgery. *Ann Intern Med.* 1996;124(5):469-476.

409. Paulk EJ, Farrar WJ. Diverticulosis of the small intestine and megaloblastic anemia: intestinal microflora and absorption before and after tetracycline administration. *Am J Med.* 1964;37:473-480.

410. Kuzminski A, Del Giacco E, Allen R, et al. Effective treatment of cobalamin deficiency with oral cobalamin. *Blood.* 1998;92(4):1191-1198.

411. Crosby W. Improvisation revisited. Oral cyanocobalamin without intrinsic factor for pernicious anemia. *Arch Intern Med.* 1980;140(12):1582.

412. Andrès E, Kurtz J, Perrin A, et al. Oral cobalamin therapy for the treatment of patients with food-cobalamin malabsorption. *Am J Med.* 2001;111(2):126-129.

413. Lederle F. Oral cobalamin for pernicious anemia: back from the verge of extinction. *J Am Geriatr Soc.* 1998;46(9):1125-1127.

414. Oussalah A, Julien M, Levy J, et al. Global burden related to nitrous oxide exposure in medical and recreational settings: a systematic review and individual patient data meta-analysis. *J Clin Med.* 2019;8(4):551.

415. Kondo H, Osborne M, Kolhouse J, et al. Nitrous oxide has multiple deleterious effects on cobalamin metabolism and causes decreases in activities of both mammalian cobalamin-dependent enzymes in rats. *J Clin Invest.* 1981;67(5):1270-1283.

416. Lumb M, Sharer N, Deacon R, et al. Effects of nitrous oxide-induced inactivation of cobalamin on methionine and S-adenosylmethionine metabolism in the rat. *Biochim Biophys Acta.* 1983;756(3):354-359.

417. O'Sullivan H, Jennings F, Ward K, et al. Human bone marrow biochemical function and megaloblastic hematopoiesis after nitrous oxide anesthesia. *Anesthesiology.* 1981;55(6):645-649.

418. Skacel P, Hewlett A, Lewis J, et al. Studies on the haemopoietic toxicity of nitrous oxide in man. *Br J Haematol.* 1983;53(2):189-200.

419. Kano Y, Sakamoto S, Sakuraya K, et al. Effects of leucovorin and methylcobalamin with N_2O anesthesia. *J Lab Clin Med.* 1984;104(5):711-717.

420. Amess J, Burman J, Rees G, et al. Megaloblastic haemopoiesis in patients receiving nitrous oxide. *Lancet.* 1978;2(8085):339-342.

421. Layzer R, Fishman R, Schafer J. Neuropathy following abuse of nitrous oxide. *Neurology.* 1978;28(5):504-506.

422. Easton D. Severe thrombocytopenia associated with acute folic acid deficiency and severe hemorrhage in two patients. *Can Med Assoc J.* 1984;130(4):418-420, 422.

423. Beard M, Hatipov C, Hamer J. Acute onset of folate deficiency in patients under intensive care. *Crit Care Med.* 1980;8(9):500-503.

424. Henderson G, Suresh M, Vitols K, Huennekens F. Transport of folate compounds in L1210 cells: kinetic evidence that folate influx proceeds via the high-affinity transport system for 5-methyltetrahydrofolate and methotrexate. *Cancer Res.* 1986;46(4, pt 1):1639-1643.

425. Schoo M, Pristupa Z, Vickers P, Scrimgeour K. Folate analogues as substrates of mammalian folylpolyglutamate synthetase. *Cancer Res.* 1985;45(7):3034-3041.

426. Huennekens FM Duffy TH, Pope LE, et al. Biochemistry of methotrexate: teaching an old drug new tricks. In: Cory JG, Szentivanyi A, eds. *Cancer Biology and Therapeutics.* Springer; 1987:43-61.

427. Kesavan V, Sur P, Doig M, et al. Effects of methotrexate on folates in Krebs ascites and L1210 murine leukemia cells. *Cancer Lett.* 1986;30(1):55-59.

428. He D, Zhang C, Zhao X, et al. Teriflunomide for multiple sclerosis. *Cochrane Database Syst Rev.* 2016;3:CD009882.

429. Spiegel R, Cooper P, Blum R, et al. Treatment of massive intrathecal methotrexate overdose by ventriculolumbar perfusion. *N Engl J Med.* 1984;311(6):386-388.

430. Yarchoan R, Broder S. Development of antiretroviral therapy for the acquired immunodeficiency syndrome and related disorders. A progress report. *N Engl J Med.* 1987;316(9):557-564.

431. Richman D, Fischl M, Grieco M, et al. The toxicity of azidothymidine (AZT) in the treatment of patients with AIDS and AIDS-related complex. A double-blind, placebo-controlled trial. *N Engl J Med.* 1987;317(4):192-197.

432. Boudes P, Zittoun J, Sobel A. Folate, vitamin B_{12}, and HIV infection. *Lancet.* 1990;335(8702):1401-1402.

433. Krakoff I, Brown N, Reichard P. Inhibition of ribonucleoside diphosphate reductase by hydroxyurea. *Cancer Res.* 1968;28(8):1559-1565.

434. Termanini B, Gibril F, Sutliff VE, et al. Effect of long-term gastric acid suppressive therapy on serum vitamin B_{12} levels in patients with Zollinger-Ellison syndrome. *Am J Med.* 1998;104(5):422-430.

435. Koop H, Bachem M. Serum iron, ferritin, and vitamin B_{12} during prolonged omeprazole therapy. *J Clin Gastroenterol.* 1992;14(4):288-292.

436. Spector I, Green R, Bowes D, et al. Trimethoprim-sulphamethoxazole therapy and folate nutrition. *S Afr Med J.* 1973;47(28):1230-1232.

437. Prasad AS, Lei KY, Moghissi KS, et al. Effect of oral contraceptives on nutrients. III. Vitamins B_6, B_{12}, and folic acid. *Am J Obstet Gynecol.* 1976;125(8):1063-1069.

438. Holzgreve W, Pietrzik K, Koletzko B, Eckmann-Scholz C. Adding folate to the contraceptive pill: a new concept for the prevention of neural tube defects. *J Matern Fetal Neonatal Med.* 2012;25(9):1529-1536.

439. Rosenblatt DS, Fenton WA. Inherited disorders of folate and cobalamin transport and metabolism. In: Scriver CR, Beaudet AL Sly WS, et al, eds. *The Metabolic and Molecular Bases of Inherited Metabolic Disease.* 8th ed. McGraw-Hill; 2001:3897-3933.

440. Grasbeck R, Gordin R, Kantero I, Kuhlback B. Selective vitamin B_{12} malabsorption and proteinuria in young people. A syndrome. *Acta Med Scand.* 1960;167:289-296.

441. Zimran A, Hershko C. The changing pattern of megaloblastic anemia: megaloblastic anemia in Israel. *Am J Clin Nutr.* 1983;37(5):855-861.

442. Aminoff M, Carter J, Chadwick R, et al. Mutations in CUBN, encoding the intrinsic factor-vitamin B_{12} receptor, cubilin, cause hereditary megaloblastic anaemia 1. *Nat Genet.* 1999;21(3):309-313.

443. He Q, Madsen M, Kilkenney A, et al. Amnionless function is required for cubilin brush-border expression and intrinsic factor-cobalamin (vitamin B_{12}) absorption in vivo. *Blood.* 2005;106(4):1447-1453.

444. Carmel R. Gastric juice in congenital pernicious anemia contains no immunoreactive intrinsic factor molecule: study of three kindreds with variable ages at presentation, including a patient first diagnosed in adulthood. *Am J Hum Genet.* 1983;35(1):67-77.

445. Cooper B, Rosenblatt D. Inherited defects of vitamin B_{12} metabolism. *Annu Rev Nutr.* 1987;7:291-320.

446. Miller D, Bloom G, Streiff R, et al. Juvenile "congenital" pernicious anemia. Clinical and immunologic studies. *N Engl J Med.* 1966;275(18):978-983.

447. Thomas P, Hoffbrand A, Smith I. Neurological involvement in hereditary transcobalamin II deficiency. *J Neurol Neurosurg Psychiatry.* 1982;45(1):74-77.

448. Carmel R, Green R, Rosenblatt D, Watkins D. Update on cobalamin, folate, and homocysteine. *Hematology Am Soc Hematol Educ Program.* 2003:62-81.

449. Rosenblatt D, Hosack A, Matiaszuk N. Expression of transcobalamin II by amniocytes. *Prenat Diagn.* 1987;7(1):35-39.

450. Namour F, Olivier J, Abdelmoutaleb I, et al. Transcobalamin codon 259 polymorphism in HT-29 and Caco-2 cells and in Caucasians: relation to transcobalamin and homocysteine concentration in blood. *Blood.* 2001;97(4):1092-1098.

451. Miller JW, Ramos MI, Garrod MG, et al. Transcobalamin II 775G>C polymorphism and indices of vitamin B_{12} status in healthy older adults. *Blood.* 2002;100(2):718-720.

452. Mcintyre O, Sullivan L, Jeffries G, Silver R. Pernicious anemia in childhood. *N Engl J Med.* 1965;272:981-986.

453. Fowler B. Genetic defects of folate and cobalamin metabolism. *Eur J Pediatr.* 1998;157 Suppl 2: S60-6.

454. Pupavac M, Watkins D, Petrella F, et al. Inborn error of cobalamin metabolism associated with the intracellular accumulation of transcobalamin-bound cobalamin and mutations in ZNF143, which codes for a transcriptional activator. *Hum Mutat.* 2016;37(9):976-982.

455. Watkins D, Matiaszuk N, Rosenblatt D. Complementation studies in the cblA class of inborn error of cobalamin metabolism: evidence for interallelic complementation and for a new complementation class (cblH). *J Med Genet.* 2000;37(7):510-513.

456. Rosenblatt D, Cooper B, Pottier A, et al. Altered vitamin B_{12} metabolism in fibroblasts from a patient with megaloblastic anemia and homocystinuria due to a new defect in methionine biosynthesis. *J Clin Invest.* 1984;74(6):2149-2156.

457. Leclerc D, Campeau E, Goyette P, et al. Human methionine synthase: cDNA cloning and identification of mutations in patients of the cblG complementation group of folate/cobalamin disorders. *Hum Mol Genet.* 1996;5(12):1867-1874.

458. Gulati S, Chen Z, Brody L, et al. Defects in auxiliary redox proteins lead to functional methionine synthase deficiency. *J Biol Chem.* 1997;272(31):19171-19175.

459. Watkins D, Rosenblatt DS. Failure of lysosomal release of vitamin B_{12}: a new complementation group causing methylmalonic aciduria (cblF). *Am J Hum Genet.* 1986;39(3):404-408.

460. van der Meer S, Spaapen L, Fowler B, et al. Prenatal treatment of a patient with vitamin B$_{12}$-responsive methylmalonic acidemia. *J Pediatr.* 1990;117(6):923-926.

461. Erbe R. Inborn errors of folate metabolism (second of two parts). *N Engl J Med.* 1975;293(16):807-812.

462. Min S, Oh S, Karp G, et al. The clinical course and genetic defect in the PCFT gene in a 27-year-old woman with hereditary folate malabsorption. *J Pediatr.* 2008;153(3):435-437.

463. Zittoun J. Congenital errors of folate metabolism. *Baillieres Clin Haematol.* 1995;8(3):603-616.

464. Banka S, Blom HJ, Walter J, et al. Identification and characterization of an inborn error of metabolism caused by dihydrofolate reductase deficiency. *Am J Hum Genet.* 2011;88(2):216-225.

465. Arakawa T, Narisawa K, Tanno K, et al. Megaloblastic anemia and mental retardation associated with hyperfolic-acidemia: probably due to N5 methyltetrahydrofolate transferase deficiency. *Tohoku J Exp Med.* 1967;93(1):1-22.

466. Majumdar R, Yori A, Rush PW, et al. Allelic spectrum of formiminotransferase-cyclodeaminase gene variants in individuals with formiminoglutamic aciduria. *Mol Genet Genomic Med.* 2017;5(6):795-799.

467. Hilton JF, Christensen KE, Watkins D, et al. The molecular basis of glutamate formiminotransferase deficiency. *Hum Mutat.* 2003;22(1):67-73.

468. Perry TL, Applegarth DA, Evans ME, et al. Metabolic studies of a family with massive formiminoglutamic aciduria. *Pediatr Res.* 1975;9(3):117-122.

469. Yang Y, Muzny DM, Xia F, et al. Molecular findings among patients referred for clinical whole-exome sequencing. *JAMA.* 2014;312(18):1870-1879.

470. Fox R, Wood M, Royse-Smith D, O'Sullivan W. Hereditary orotic aciduria: types I and II. *Am J Med.* 1973;55(6):791-798.

471. van der Zee S, Schretlen E, Monnens L. Megaloblastic anaemia in the Lesch-Nyhan syndrome. *Lancet.* 1968;1(7557):1427.

472. Porter FS, Rogers LE, Sidbury JB Jr. Thiamine-responsive megaloblastic anemia. *J Pediatr.* 1969;74(4):494-504.

473. Habeb AM, Flanagan SE, Zulali MA, et al. Pharmacogenomics in diabetes: outcomes of thiamine therapy in TRMA syndrome. *Diabetologia.* 2018;61(5):1027-1036.

474. Bazarbachi A, Muakkit S, Ayas M, et al. Thiamine-responsive myelodysplasia. *Br J Haematol.* 1998;102(4):1098-1100.

475. Boros L, Steinkamp M, Fleming J, et al. Defective RNA ribose synthesis in fibroblasts from patients with thiamine-responsive megaloblastic anemia (TRMA). *Blood.* 2003;102(10):3556-3561.

476. Zdebska E, Mendek-Czajkowska E, Ploski R, et al. Heterozygosity of CDAN II (HEMPAS) gene may be detected by the analysis of erythrocyte membrane glycoconjugates from healthy carriers. *Haematologica.* 2002;87(2):126-130.

477. Maeda K, Saeed S, Rebuck J, Monto R. Type I dyserythropoietic anemia. A 30-year follow-up. *Am J Clin Pathol.* 1980;73(3):433-438.

478. Wickramasinghe S, Parry T, Williams C, et al. A new case of congenital dyserythropoietic anaemia, type III: studies of the cell cycle distribution and ultrastructure of erythroblasts and of nucleic acid synthesis in marrow cells. *J Clin Pathol.* 1982;35(10):1103-1109.

479. Najfeld V, McArthur J, Shashaty G. Monosomy 7 in a patient with pancytopenia and abnormal erythropoiesis. *Acta Haematol.* 1981;66(1):12-18.

480. Camaschella C. Recent advances in the understanding of inherited sideroblastic anaemia. *Br J Haematol.* 2008;143(1):27-38.

481. Roggli V, Saleem A. Erythroleukemia: a study of 15 cases and literature review. *Cancer.* 1982;49(1):101-108.

482. Dalsania CJ, Khemka V, Shum M, et al. A sheep in wolf's clothing. *Am J Med.* 2008;121(2):107-109.

483. Parmentier S, Meinel J, Oelschlaegel U, et al. Severe pernicious anemia with distinct cytogenetic and flow cytometric aberrations mimicking myelodysplastic syndrome. *Ann Hematol.* 2012;91(12):1979-1981.

484. Boots M, Phillips M, Curtis JR. Megaloblastic anemia and pancytopenia due to proguanil in patients with chronic renal failure. *Clin Nephrol.* 1982;18(2):106-108.

485. Fossella FV. Pemetrexed for treatment of advanced non-small cell lung cancer. *Semin Oncol.* 2004;31(1)(suppl 1):100-105.

486. Bethell FH, Thompson DS. Treatment of leukemia and related disorders with 6-mercaptopurine. *Ann N Y Acad Sci.* 1954;60(2):436-438.

487. Christoph R, Pirnay D, Hartl W. Megaloblastic anemia following treatment of rheumatoid arthritis with azathioprine. Article in German. *Med Welt.* 1971;46:1824-1827.

488. Klippel JH, Decker JL. Relative macrocytosis in cyclophosphamide and azathioprine therapy. *JAMA.* 1974;229(2):180-181.

489. Amos RJ, Amess JAL. Megaloblastic hematopoiesis due to acyclovir. *Lancet.* 1983;1(8318):242-243.

490. Reyes P, Heidelberger C. Fluorinated pyrimidines. XXV. The inhibition of thymidylate synthetase from Ehrlich ascites carcinoma cells by pyrimidine analogs. *Biochim Biophys Acta.* 1965;103:177-179.

491. Cornell RC, Milstein HG, Fox RM, Stoughton RB. Anemia of azaribine in the treatment of psoriasis. *Arch Dermatol.* 1976;112(12):1717-1723.

492. Frenkel EP, Arthur C. Induced ribotide reductive conversion defect by hydroxyurea and its relationship to megaloblastosis. *Cancer Res.* 1967;27(6):1016-1019.

493. Papac RJ. Clinical and hematologic studies with 1-beta-D-arabinosylcytosine. *J Natl Cancer Inst.* 1968;40(5):997-1002.

494. Druskin MS, Bohagura L, Wallen MH. Anticonvulsant-associated megaloblastic anemia-response to 25 microgm. of folic acid administered by mouth daily. *N Engl J Med.* 1962;267(10):483-485.

495. Gerson CD, Brown N, Herbert V, et al. Inhibition by diphenylhydantoin of folic-acid absorption in man. *Gastroenterology.* 1972;63(2):246-251.

496. Carl GF, Smith ML, Furman GM, et al. Phenytoin-treatment and folate supplementation affect folate concentrations and methylation capacity in rats. *J Nutr.* 1991;121(8):1214-1221.

497. Isojarvi JIT, Pakarinen AJ, Myllyla VV. Basic haematological parameters, serum gammaglutamyl-transferase activity, and erythrocyte folate and serum vitamin B-12 levels during carbamazepine and oxcarbazepine therapy. *Seizure.* 1997;6(3):207-211.

498. Lindenbaum J, Whitehead N, Reyner F. Oral-contraceptive hormones, folate metabolism, and cervical epithelium. *Am J Clin Nutr.* 1975;28(4):346-353.

499. Heinivaa O, Palva IP. Malabsorption and deficiency of vitamin B$_{12}$ caused by treatment with para-aminosalicylic acid. *Acta Med Scand.* 1965;177(3):337-341.

500. Callaghan TS, Hadden DR. Megaloblastic-anemia due to vitamin-B$_{12}$ malabsorption associated with long-term metformin treatment. *BMJ.* 1980;280(6225):1214-1215.

501. Webb DI, Chodos RB, Mahar CQ, Faloon WW. Mechanism of vitamin B$_{12}$ malabsorption in patients receiving colchicine. *N Engl J Med.* 1968;279(16):845-850.

502. Dobbins WO, Herrero BA, Mansbach CM. Morphologic alterations associated with neomycin induced malabsorption. *Am J Med Sci.* 1968;255:63-77.

503. Lerman BB, Ali N, Green D. Megaloblastic, dyserythropoietic anemia following arsenic ingestion. *Ann Clin Lab Sci.* 1980;10(6):515-517.

CHAPTER 10
IRON METABOLISM

Tomas Ganz

SUMMARY

Iron is a component of nearly all living organisms. It plays an important metabolic role, particularly in electron transfer reactions. Most of the iron in the human body is in the hemoglobin of circulating red cells, which contain approximately 1 mg of iron per 1 mL of packed cells. Smaller amounts of iron are present in myoglobin and in many enzymes. Iron is stored within cells inside ferritin and circulates in plasma bound to transferrin. Most of the iron flow into the plasma is generated by the release of iron recycled from senescent erythrocytes by splenic and hepatic macrophages. Plasma iron is largely destined for hemoglobin synthesis in marrow erythroblasts, with much smaller amounts serving the needs of other tissues. Because little iron is lost from the body under normal circumstances, the iron content of the body is controlled by modulating dietary iron absorption. Iron absorption increases in the presence of iron deficiency and it decreases when there is iron overload. The absorption of inorganic iron involves a ferrireductase and a divalent iron transporter, DMT-1, on the gastrointestinal luminal apical membranes of enterocytes, and ferroportin and hephaestin, located on the basolateral enterocyte membranes, in contact with blood. In contrast to elemental iron, heme iron is absorbed by a distinct pathway, which is still not well understood.

Systemic iron homeostasis is orchestrated by the hepatic peptide hormone hepcidin, which regulates plasma iron concentrations, the absorption of dietary iron, and the release of iron from macrophages involved in iron recycling and storage and from hepatocytes that store iron. The cellular iron exporter ferroportin serves as the receptor for hepcidin and is occluded and then destroyed when the complex is formed. This impairs transport from intestinal mucosal cells, from macrophages and from hepatocytes into the plasma, and lowers iron absorption and release from stores. Hepcidin therefore decreases plasma iron levels by causing iron to be sequestered within cells, predominantly in macrophages or enterocytes, the latter of which are then shed along with their absorbed iron.

Acronyms and Abbreviations: ABCB10, ATP-binding cassette (ABC) transporter in the inner membrane of mitochondria; ALA synthase, aminolevulinic acid synthase; BMP, bone morphogenetic protein; dcytb, duodenal cytochrome b; DMT, divalent metal transporter; Fpn, ferroportin; Fe-Tf, transferrin bound iron; GDF15, growth differentiation factor 15; HCP1, heme carrier protein 1; HFE, human hemochromatosis protein; HRG1, heme transporter; IL, interleukin; IRE, iron-responsive element; IRP, iron-regulatory protein; NADPH, nicotinamide adenine dinucleotide phosphate; Nramp1, natural resistance-associated macrophage protein one; O_2, oxygen; PCBP1,poly(rC)-binding protein 1; SMAD 1the abbreviation refers to the homologies to the *Caenorhabditis elegans* SMA ("small" worm phenotype) and Drosophila MAD ("Mothers Against Decapentaplegic"); STEAP3, six-transmembrane epithelial antigen of prostate 3; TfR, transferrin receptor; Tmprss6, transmembrane serine protease 6.

Once ferric iron enters the plasma, it is bound by transferrin, which after forming a complex with the transferrin receptor, transports the metal into cells. The transferrin receptor is internalized together with bound transferrin and iron, and the iron is released inside the cell into an acidified vacuole. The transferrin receptor then recycles to the cell surface.

Cellular iron homeostasis is largely achieved through posttranscriptional regulation of key proteins involved in iron transport, storage, and utilization. The synthesis of these proteins is regulated by binding of one of the iron-regulatory proteins (IRPs) to iron-responsive elements (IREs) located within stem loop structures of the corresponding messenger ribonucleic acids (mRNAs). IRP-1 is cytoplasmic aconitase that binds to the IRE when it is not complexed with iron and does not bind when iron is present; IRP-2, a closely related protein, is destabilized by the presence of iron. When IRPs bind to IREs at the 5′ end of the mRNA, they prevent translation; when they bind at the 3′ end, they stabilize the mRNA.

INTRODUCTION

Iron is a key element in the metabolism of nearly all living organisms. Iron is a component of heme, which is the active site of electron transport in cytochromes and cytochrome oxidase involved in mitochondrial energy generation. The heme moiety of hemoglobin and myoglobin binds oxygen (O_2), providing the means to transfer O_2 from the lungs to tissues and to store it. Heme is also the active site of peroxidases that protect cells from oxidative injury by reducing peroxides to water or generate microbicidal hypochlorite in granulocytes. DNA synthesis requires the enzyme ribonucleotide reductase to convert ribonucleotides to deoxyribonucleotides. Neither bacteria nor nucleated cells proliferate when the supply of iron is insufficient.

DISTRIBUTION OF IRON IN THE AVERAGE PERSON

Table 10-1 summarizes the most important iron compartments.

HEMOGLOBIN

Hemoglobin, which is 0.34% iron by weight, contains approximately 2 g of body iron in men and 1.5 g in women. One milliliter of packed erythrocytes contains approximately 1 mg of iron. Because the life span of human erythrocytes is approximately 120 days, every day 1/120 of the iron in hemoglobin is recycled by macrophages in the spleen and the liver, and returned to the plasma, from where it is largely delivered to marrow erythroblasts for incorporation into newly synthesized hemoglobin (Fig. 10-1).

STORAGE COMPARTMENT

Iron is stored either as ferritin or as hemosiderin. The former is water-soluble; the latter is water-insoluble. The protein ferritin is composed of 24 similar or identical subunits arranged as 12 dimers forming a dodecahedron that approximates a hollow sphere with a cavity capable of storing up to 4500 Fe atoms as hydrous ferric oxide polymers.[1,2] The ferritin subunits are of H (heavy) or L (light) type. H subunits have ferroxidase activity, thereby enabling ferritin to take up or release iron quite rapidly. Ferritin that is rich in H subunits takes up iron more readily but retains it less avidly than does ferritin composed predominantly

TABLE·10–1. Iron Compartments in the Average Person[a]

Compartment	Iron Content (mg)	Total Body Iron (%)
Hemoglobin iron	2000	67
Storage iron (ferritin, hemosiderin)	1000	27
Myoglobin iron	130	3.5
Labile pool	80	2.2
Other tissue iron	8	0.2
Transport iron	3	0.08

[a]These values represent estimates for an "average" person, ie, 70 kg (154 lb) in weight and 177 cm (70 inches) in height. The values are derived from data in several sources.

of L subunits. Much of the storage iron in the liver and spleen is in ferritin containing mostly L subunits.

Ferritin is found in virtually all cells of the body and in tissue fluids. In plasma, ferritin is present in minute concentrations. It is glycosylated and largely composed of L subunits. Except under conditions of inflammation, the plasma (serum) ferritin concentration usually correlates with total-body iron stores, making measurement of serum ferritin levels important in the diagnosis of disorders of iron metabolism.

The size of the iron storage compartment is quite variable. Normally, in adult men, it amounts to 800 to 2000 mg; in adult women it is a few hundred milligrams. The mobilization of storage iron from ferritin

involves its autophagy followed by lysosomal degradation.[3] The cargo protein NCOA4, a ferritin receptor, is increased during iron deficiency and delivers ferritin to lysosomes.[4] To a lesser extent, iron can exit ferritin through the reduction of Fe^{3+} to Fe^{2+}, its release from the core crystal, and its diffusion out of the apoferritin shell.

Hemosiderin is found predominantly in macrophages. Microscopically, in unstained tissue sections or marrow films, it appears as clumps or granules of golden refractile pigment. Under pathologic conditions, it may accumulate in large quantities in almost every tissue of the body. Hemosiderin is chemically similar to the iron core of ferritin and may be derived from ferritins whose protein shells have been digested in lysosomes.

MYOGLOBIN

Myoglobin is structurally similar to hemoglobin, but it is monomeric rather than tetrameric: each myoglobin molecule consists of a heme group nearly surrounded by polypeptide loops of the 154 amino acid proteins. It is present in small amounts in all skeletal and cardiac muscle cells, where it may serve as an oxygen reservoir to protect against cellular injury during periods of oxygen deprivation, and may scavenge nitric oxide and reactive oxygen species.[5]

LABILE IRON POOL

The existence of a cellular labile iron pool was postulated from studies of the rate of clearance of injected ^{59}Fe from plasma.[6] Iron leaves the plasma and enters the interstitial and intracellular fluid compartments for a brief time before it is incorporated into heme or storage

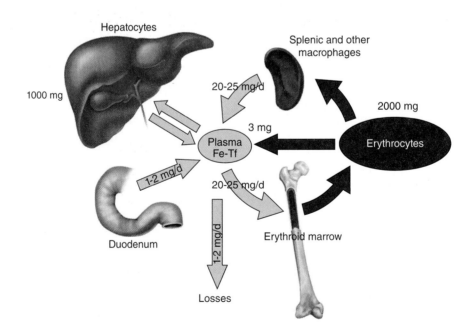

FIGURE 10–1. The iron cycle in humans. Iron is tightly conserved in a nearly closed system in which each iron atom cycles repeatedly from plasma and extracellular fluid ("plasma") to the marrow, where it is incorporated into hemoglobin. Then it moves into the blood within erythrocytes and circulates for 120 days. It then travels to phagocytes of the mononuclear phagocyte system ("splenic and other macrophages"), where senescent erythrocytes are engulfed and destroyed, hemoglobin is digested, and iron is released to plasma, where the cycle continues. With each cycle, a small proportion of iron is transferred to storage sites, where it is incorporated into ferritin or hemosiderin, a small proportion of storage iron is released to plasma; a small proportion is lost in urine, sweat, feces, or blood; and an equivalent small amount of iron is absorbed from the intestinal tract. In addition, a small proportion (~10%) of newly formed erythrocytes normally is destroyed within the marrow and its iron released, bypassing the circulating blood part of the cycle (ineffective erythropoiesis). During the life span of erythroblasts and erythrocytes, surplus iron is released into plasma. The numbers indicate the approximate amount of iron (in mg) in various compartments and fluxes of iron (mg/d) that enter and leave each of these iron compartments in healthy adults who do not have bleeding or other blood disorders.

compounds. Some of the iron reenters plasma, causing a biphasic curve of ^{59}Fe clearance 1 to 2 days after injection. The change in slope defines the size of the labile pool, normally 80 to 90 mg of iron. It is now sometimes considered to be equivalent to the chelatable iron pool.[7]

TISSUE IRON COMPARTMENT

Tissue iron (exclusive of hemoglobin, ferritin, hemosiderin, myoglobin, and the labile compartment) normally amounts to 6 to 8 mg. This includes cytochromes and other iron-containing enzymes. Although a small compartment, it is vital and sensitive to iron deficiency.[8,9]

TRANSPORT COMPARTMENT

From the standpoint of its total iron content, normally about 3 mg, the transport compartment of plasma is the smallest but the most active of the iron compartments. Its iron, almost entirely carried by transferrin, normally turns over at least 10 times each day. This is the common pathway for interchange of iron between compartments. The predominant iron flow is from hepatic and splenic macrophages that recycle iron from senescent erythrocytes to the erythroblasts in the marrow that use iron to produce hemoglobin.

Transferrin

Transferrin is a dumbbell-shaped glycoprotein with a molecular weight of approximately 80 kDa where each of the two globular domains contains a binding cleft for Fe^{3+}.[10-12] Normally, approximately one-third of the transferrin iron-binding sites are occupied by iron. Human plasma normally contains approximately 25 to 45 µM (200-360 mg/dL) transferrin, capable of binding 50 to 90 µM iron but carrying only 10 to 30 µM (50-180 mcg/dL) iron. Apotransferrin (transferrin devoid of iron) is synthesized by hepatocytes and by cells of the monocyte macrophage system.[13,14]

● DIETARY IRON

CONTENT

Average American adult men and women ingest 9 to 10 mg and 12 to 14 mg of iron daily, respectively.[15] The amount of iron absorbed by a normal adult male need only balance the small amount that is excreted, mostly in the stool (~1 mg/day).[16] More iron is needed during growth periods or after blood loss. In women, absorbed iron must be sufficient to replace that lost through menstruation or utilized to support the fetus and expanded maternal erythrocyte mass during pregnancy and milk production afterward. Table 10-2 shows the age- and gender-specific recommended dietary allowances for iron.[17]

BIOAVAILABILITY

In meat-eaters in Western countries, heme from hemoglobin and myoglobin normally comprises approximately 15% of dietary iron, but is much more efficiently absorbed than nonheme iron, and promotes the absorption of nonheme iron.[18] The absorption of nonheme dietary iron is strongly affected by iron-binding components of food. Oxalates, phytates, and phosphates complex with iron and retard its absorption, whereas simple reducing substances, such as hydroquinone, ascorbate, lactate, pyruvate, succinate, fructose, cysteine, and sorbitol, increase iron absorption.[19] Iron-fortified cereals are major sources of iron in countries where fortification is practiced, but cooking in iron pots may also provide important exogenous iron.[18] Gastric acid secretion, the transit time, and mucus secretion all play roles in iron absorption. Red wine, contrary to popular belief, inhibits iron absorption, probably

Age	Male	Female	Pregnancy	Lactation
TABLE 10–2. Recommended Dietary Allowances (RDAs) for Iron				
Birth to 6 mo	0.27 mg[a]	0.27 mg[a]		
7-12 mo	11 mg	11 mg		
1-3 y	7 mg	7 mg		
4-8 y	10 mg	10 mg		
9-13 y	8 mg	8 mg		
14-18 y	11 mg	15 mg	27 mg	10 mg
19-50 y	8 mg	18 mg	27 mg	9 mg
51+ y	8 mg	8 mg		

[a]Adequate intake (AI).

Reproduced with permission from Dubach R, Moore CV, Callender S: Studies in iron transportation and metabolism. IX. The excretion of iron as measured by the isotope technique, *J Lab Clin Med.* 1955 Apr;45(4):599-615.

because of the presence of polyphenols.[20] In mice, alcohol suppresses the response of hepcidin to iron,[21] and this may contribute to iron loading that is seen in some alcoholic subjects.

● IRON ABSORPTION

Iron normally enters the body through the gastrointestinal tract, through the enterocytes mostly in the duodenum. The amount of iron absorbed is normally tightly regulated according to body needs. Active erythropoiesis and/or iron deficiency increase absorption; iron overload and systemic inflammation decrease absorption. Nevertheless, the amount of iron absorbed increases with the administered dose even though the percentage absorbed decreases (Fig. 10-2).[22] Accidental or

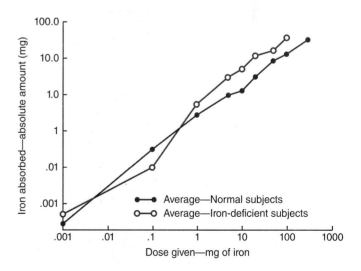

FIGURE 10–2. The relationship between oral iron dosage and amount of iron absorbed in humans. When the logarithm of the dose is plotted against the logarithm of the amount of iron absorbed, a rectilinear relationship is observed. Thus, at all levels, the greater the dose of iron, the more is absorbed, although the percent of the dose that is absorbed progressively declines. (*Data from Smith MD, Pannacciulli IM. Absorption of inorganic iron from graded doses: its significance in relation to iron absorption tests and mucosal block theory. Br J Haematol. 1958 Oct;4[4]:428-434.*)

deliberate ingestion of large doses of medicinal iron can therefore cause iron intoxication.

MECHANISM OF TRANSPORT ACROSS THE INTESTINAL MUCOSA

Heme Iron

Understanding the mechanism of iron absorption has been made more difficult by the fact that the pathways for the uptake of inorganic iron and of heme by enterocytes are different but seem to merge within the intestinal cell, where heme is converted to inorganic iron. How much heme (if any) is exported intact by enterocytes and bound by plasma heme-binding protein hemopexin is not clear, but hemopexin knockout mice show minor retention of iron in duodenal enterocytes without any effect on systemic iron homeostasis,[23] arguing against a major contribution from this mechanism, at least in mice. Efforts to identify the apical heme import mechanism in enterocytes have not yet been definitive,[24] in part because laboratory rodents are herbivores and may not use this mechanism.

Ferric Iron

After the reduction of ferric iron to ferrous iron, in part by duodenal cytochrome b (Dcytb) reductase,[25] ferrous iron is transported into the intestinal villus cell by the divalent metal transporter (DMT)-1.[26,27] Iron transport by DMT-1 requires an acid milieu on the luminal side to provide sufficient protons to drive the transport. Although acid gastric secretions have an important role in increasing the solubility of luminal iron, the protons in the mucosal brush border are supplied by a sodium-proton exchanger, NHE3, that transfers protons from the cytoplasm of duodenal enterocytes into the mucosa.[28] How iron transits within the enterocytes is not yet known, but recent studies implicate PCBP1 and 2 (poly(rC)-binding proteins 1 and 2, as cytoplasmic iron chaperones for iron delivery to proteins involved in iron utilization,

storage, and transport.[29,30] Basolateral export of ferrous iron is mediated by ferroportin[31-33] in association with hephaestin[34] and plasma ceruloplasmin[35] to oxidize iron to the ferric state. Ferric iron is taken up by plasma apotransferrin. Figure 10-3 illustrates some of the steps that are thought to regulate iron transport across the mucosal cell.[36,37]

IRON RECYCLING

Role of the Monocyte–Macrophage System

In humans, the destruction and production of erythrocytes generates most of the iron flux in and out of plasma (20-25 mg/day recycled in adults vs 1-2 mg/day absorbed). A smaller amount of iron, some of which may originate from damaged hemoglobin, can be exported by erythroblast and erythrocyte ferroportin[38] directly to plasma (see Fig. 10-1). Iron from other cell types is likely also recycled, but this source contributes little to iron flux and has not been studied. Destruction of aged erythrocytes and hemoglobin degradation was thought to occur within macrophages but this view was recently challenged by evidence of shear-induced extracellular release of hemoglobin from senescent erythrocytes as they squeeze through the walls of sinusoids in the spleen.[39] Recycling proceeds at a rate sufficient to release approximately 20% of the hemoglobin iron from the cell to the plasma compartment within a few hours. Approximately 80% of this iron is rapidly reincorporated into hemoglobin. Thus, 20% to 70% of the hemoglobin iron of nonviable erythrocytes reappears in circulating red cells in 12 days. The remainder of the iron enters the storage pool as ferritin or hemosiderin and then turns over very slowly. In normal subjects, approximately 40% of this iron remains in storage after 140 days. When there is an increased iron demand for hemoglobin synthesis, however, storage iron may be mobilized more rapidly.[40] Conversely, in the presence of infection or another inflammatory process (eg, rheumatoid arthritis or malignancy), iron is much more slowly reused in hemoglobin synthesis, a condition associated with anemia (Chaps. 3 and 17).[41,42]

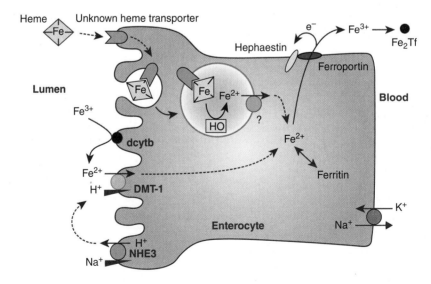

FIGURE 10–3. Schematic of iron uptake from the intestine and transfer to the plasma by an intestinal villus cell. Nonheme dietary iron includes Fe(II) and Fe(III) salts and organic complexes. Fe^{3+} is reduced to Fe^{2+} by ascorbic acid and apical membrane ferrireductases that include duodenal cytochrome b (dcytb). The acid microclimate at the brush-border provides an H^+ electrochemical potential gradient to drive transport of Fe^{2+} via the divalent metal-ion transporter (DMT-1) into the enterocyte. DMT-1 can also transport other nutritionally important metal ions (eg, Mn^{2+}) but is not required for this function.[36] Heme can be taken up by endocytosis, and Fe^{2+} is liberated within the endosome/lysosome, but the molecular identity of proteins involved, including heme carrier protein 1 (HCP1), is yet to be elucidated. Basolateral export of Fe^{2+} may be mediated by ferroportin in association with hephaestin. HO, heme oxygenase; Fe_2Tf, diferric transferrin. *(Reproduced with permission from Mackenzie B, Garrick MD. Iron Imports. II. Iron uptake at the apical membrane in the intestine. Am J Physiol Gastrointest Liver Physiol. 2005 Dec;289[6]:G981-G986.)*

Erythrophagocytosis

As human erythrocytes age during their average 120-day life span, they shrink, stiffen, and their membranes accumulate markers of senescence (Chap. 2).[43] These changes make them more susceptible to shear-induced damage and leakage of hemoglobin as they transit into the sinusoids[1] and may eventually trigger phagocytosis by splenic or hepatic sinusoidal macrophages. Macrophages also take up the products of intravascular hemolysis, including hemoglobin (bound by haptoglobin) and heme (bound by hemopexin), using specific endocytic receptors for these complexes.[44] The vesicles involved in phagocytosis and endocytosis must fuse with lysosomes to digest cellular materials or protein complexes and to free heme from hemoglobin. The membrane complex of nicotinamide adenine dinucleotide phosphate cytochrome c reductase, heme oxygenase 1, and biliverdin reductase releases ferrous iron from heme and simultaneously protects erythrocyte-recycling macrophages from heme-induced toxicity.[45] The subcellular location of the conversion of heme to iron is not known with certainty. Heme oxygenase 1 is mostly located in the endoplasmic reticulum in erythrophagocytic macrophages[46] with the catalytic face in the cytosol, and little, if any, heme oxygenase in the phagosomal membrane. Moreover, the phagosomal membrane is enriched in the heme transporter HRG1,[47] and macrophage heme has a signaling role in inducing various proteins involved in macrophage iron metabolism, indicating that it may leave the phagosome, and the heme oxygenase-1–mediated release of iron may occur in the cytoplasm. However, the ferrous iron transporter Nramp1, and perhaps DMT-1, may also participate in subcellular iron transport.[48] Ultimately, depending on systemic iron requirements, the released ferrous iron is either exported to plasma via ferroportin[49] or trapped in macrophage cytoplasmic ferritin. By a mechanism potentially important at the low oxygen tensions found in some tissues, plasma ceruloplasmin[50-56] catalyzes the conversion of ferrous to ferric iron, the form of iron loaded to plasma transferrin for systemic distribution.

SYSTEMIC IRON HOMEOSTASIS

The mechanism by which body iron content is regulated by the modulation of iron absorption has been a subject of intense interest for the past 65 years. It has now become clear that intestinal iron absorption, plasma iron concentrations, and tissue distribution of iron are subject to endocrine regulation similar to that of other simple nutrients, for example, glucose or calcium.

Hepcidin and Ferroportin

Hepcidin, a 25-amino-acid peptide hormone with four disulfide bonds,[53-56] is produced predominantly by hepatocytes and plays a central role in systemic iron homeostasis. Hepcidin regulates plasma iron concentrations by controlling the absorption of iron by the intestinal epithelial enterocytes and its release from iron-recycling macrophages and hepatocytes involved in iron storage. The structural similarity of hepcidin and a class of antimicrobial peptides termed *defensins* suggests that the hormone may have evolved from a defensin-like peptide to modulate iron homeostasis as a mechanism of body defense against microorganisms. Overexpression of hepcidin causes hypoferremia and marked iron-deficiency anemia in mice[57] and hypoferremia and refractory anemia resembling the anemia of chronic inflammation in humans,[58] and injection of synthetic hepcidin rapidly lowers plasma iron concentrations.[59] Because many microorganisms are dependent on plasma iron for survival in the circulation, the hypoferremic effects of hepcidin can contribute to host defense. In fact, patients with iron overload and high plasma iron levels are susceptible to gram-negative infections, such as with *Vibrio vulnificus* and *Yersinia enterocolitica,* and this susceptibility is reproduced in mouse models of hepcidin deficiency.[60]

Hepcidin exerts its iron-regulatory effect by binding to ferroportin, a transmembrane iron-export protein expressed on enterocytes, macrophages, and hepatocytes. Hepcidin binding to ferroportin occludes[61,62] ferroportin, which is then internalized, and undergoes proteolysis.[49,63] With membrane ferroportin occluded and depleted, iron cannot be exported from the enterocyte, the macrophage, or the hepatocyte into the plasma (Fig. 10-4). This results in decreased iron absorption from the gastrointestinal tract and a fall in the plasma iron concentration. Hepcidin production is stimulated by inflammatory cytokines such as interleukin (IL)-6,[64,65] and the overproduction of hepcidin is an important factor in the pathogenesis of the anemia of chronic inflammation (Chaps. 1 and 6).

The regulation of hepcidin production seems to be entirely transcriptional. In humans and laboratory rodents, hepcidin mRNA and

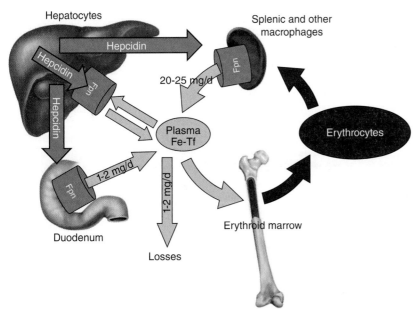

FIGURE 10–4. Regulation of iron flows into plasma by hepcidin. Ferroportin is the only known transporter that exports iron from cells to plasma (and extracellular fluid). Hepcidin induces ferroportin endocytosis and proteolysis and thereby controls the transfer of iron to plasma from all its major sources: iron-absorbing duodenal enterocytes, iron-storing hepatocytes, and iron-recycling macrophages. Fpn, ferroportin; Fe-Tf, transferrin bound iron.

plasma hepcidin levels increase in parallel with iron-loading and inflammatory stimuli,[53,66,67] and are decreased by erythropoietic activity[68] and iron deficiency.[69]

Regulation of Hepcidin by Iron

Both elevated plasma iron concentrations and increased liver stores are sensed in the intact organism and regulate hepcidin transcription,[70,71] but the relevant mechanisms are only partially understood. Isolated hepatocytes do not show consistently increased hepcidin synthesis after iron treatment, although small effects were observed when the cells were freshly harvested from mice.[72] One reason for this unexpected behavior is that sinusoidal endothelial cells that are largely removed during hepatocyte isolation provide essential regulatory signals to hepatocytes for hepcidin regulation. Important clues are provided by hereditary disorders in which hepcidin transcription is dysregulated. As indicated in Table 10-3, impairment of the function of several genes is associated with iron overload in humans and in experimental animals. In addition to genes that encode the hormone hepcidin itself and its receptor, ferroportin, or encode proteins primarily involved in iron transport, there are several genes whose products are likely to function in iron sensing, signal transduction, and transcriptional regulation. These include human hemochromatosis protein (HFE), transferrin receptor-2, bone morphogenetic proteins (BMPs), BMP receptor and its signaling pathway, and hemojuvelin, all of which encode proteins that normally stimulate hepcidin transcription to prevent iron overload. In the best-supported model (Fig. 10-5), hepcidin transcription is regulated in an iron-dependent manner by the BMP pathway. Complexes of HFE, transferrin receptor-1, and transferrin receptor-2 may be involved in sensing the concentration of iron-transferrin and interact in an as yet unknown manner with the BMP receptor to stimulate the transcription of hepcidin.[73-76] In addition, the receptor ligands BMP2 and BMP6 (and possibly others) are secreted by sinusoidal endothelial cells in response to hepatic iron loading, transit the space of Disse, and bind to the hepatocyte BMP receptor complex. Hemojuvelin, whose autosomal recessive mutations cause a very severe form of hereditary hemochromatosis, serves as a coreceptor for the BMPs.[77,78] A soluble fragment of hemojuvelin acts as an inhibitor of the interaction of BMP with the receptor, but it is not clear whether it has a physiologic regulatory role.[79,80] Regulation of hepcidin transcription itself is complex, involving the formation of a complex of liver- and response-specific transcription factors.[81] The epigenetic mechanisms of histone acetylation and deacetylation also play a role in the regulation of hepcidin transcription by iron.[82] An inhibitory effect of hepcidin transcription is exerted by Tmprss6 (also called matriptase 2), a membrane serine protease that likely acts by proteolysis of hemojuvelin[83,84] and perhaps also other proteins in the BMP receptor complex.[85] This function was discovered when random mutagenesis in mice produced an iron-deficient animal with mutagenized Tmprss6.[86] Subsequently, humans with mutations of the Tmprss6 ortholog were shown to manifest iron-refractory iron-deficiency anemia,[58] which does not improve with oral iron therapy and responds only partially to parenteral iron therapy.

Regulation of Hepcidin by Erythropoiesis

Intestinal iron absorption is increased several-fold after hemorrhage or erythropoietin administration, and is chronically increased in patients with ineffective erythropoiesis but not in aplastic anemia.[87] These observations led to the hypothesis that the marrow generates an "erythroid regulator"[87] that modulates intestinal iron absorption. Later studies in mouse models[68] provided evidence that the erythroid regulator is a marrow-derived suppressor of hepcidin. Erythroferrone is an erythropoietin-induced erythroblast-secreted glycoprotein that acts on hepatocytes to suppress their hepcidin production and is required for

rapid suppression of hepcidin after hemorrhage or erythropoietin administration.[88] It also contributes to hepcidin suppression and iron overload in murine models of β-thalassemia intermedia. Growth differentiation factor 15, a member of the BMP family, may also contribute to pathologic hepcidin suppression in anemias with ineffective erythropoiesis.[89] Erythroferrone binds BMP2/6 secreted by sinusoidal endothelial cells in the space of Disse and thereby inhibits BMP signaling and hepcidin transcription in hepatocytes (Fig. 10-6).[90,91]

Regulation of Hepcidin by Inflammation

Within hours after the onset of systemic infection, plasma iron concentration decreases. This response is thought to contribute to host defense, particularly against microbes with high dependence on environmental iron,[92] some of which are common pathogens.[93] This response, hypoferremia of inflammation, is also triggered by noninfectious causes of acute and chronic inflammation. Hypoferremia of inflammation is mediated by cytokine-induced increase in plasma hepcidin concentrations,[66] causing hepcidin-induced sequestration of iron in macrophages. The main human cytokine responsible for hepcidin induction is IL-6,[64,65] acting via the JAK2-STAT3 pathway,[94-96] but other cytokines may also contribute. Chronic inflammation impairs iron supply to erythropoiesis and combines with other effects of inflammation to cause anemia of inflammation (anemia of chronic disease, Chap. 6).

TRANSPORT OF IRON

Once an atom of iron enters the blood plasma from dietary iron absorption, it is virtually trapped in the body and cycles almost endlessly from the plasma to the developing erythroblast (where it is used in hemoglobin synthesis), and then into the circulating blood for approximately four months, and then to macrophages. Here it is removed from heme by heme oxygenase and released back into the plasma to repeat the cycle. The major function of the transport protein transferrin is to move iron from wherever it enters the plasma (intestinal villi, splenic, and hepatic sinusoids) to the erythroblasts of the marrow and to other sites of utilization.

ENDOCYTOSIS OF TRANSFERRIN

Diferric (holo)transferrin binds to the transferrin receptor (TfR)-1 on the cell surface, and the holotransferrin-TfR1 complex forms clusters in pits on the cell membrane.[136] The complex is then internalized by endocytosis (Fig. 10-7). Within the cytosol, the holotransferrin-TfR1 complex is in a clathrin-coated vesicle. The vesicles fuse with endosomes and become acidified to pH 5, which releases iron from transferrin. Iron-depleted (apo)transferrin and TfR1 remain complexed as they return to the cell membrane, where at neutral pH, apotransferrin separates from its receptor and is released to the interstitial fluid to reenter plasma and take up more iron.

TfR1 is a protein consisting of two subunits that are linked by disulfide bonds.[10] Its aminoterminus is on the cytoplasmic side of the membrane, and its carboxyl-terminus is on the outer surface. Because of the role of TfR1 in the binding and endocytosis of diferric transferrin, control of TfR1 biosynthesis is a major mechanism for regulation of iron metabolism. Synthesis of TfR1 is induced by iron deficiency. Iron inhibits TfR1 synthesis by destabilizing TfR1 mRNA by a mechanism that involves the iron-responsive element/iron-regulatory protein (IRE/IRP) regulatory system (Fig. 10-8).[85,86] TfR1 binds to HFE[73] using a binding site that overlaps that of holotransferrin. According to a current model of iron sensing, high concentrations of holotransferrin would therefore displace HFE from its complex with TfR1, leaving HFE to signal to the BMP receptor complex to increase hepcidin transcription. This model

TABLE 10–3. Proteins That Play a Role in Iron Homeostasis in Humans or in Animal Models

Proteins That Affect Iron Homeostasis	Effect of Deficiency or Mutation (Human Disease)	References to Human Data	References to Murine Data	Comments
HFE	Parenchymal Fe increased (hereditary hemochromatosis)	97	98, 99	Most patients with hereditary hemochromatosis are homozygous for the 845 A→G (C282Y) mutation of this gene In signaling pathway to hepcidin
Ferroportin (SLC40A1, SLC11A3)	Macrophage Fe increased (loss of function), ("ferroportin disease")	100	101	Autosomal dominant, hepcidin receptor, cellular iron exporter
	Parenchymal Fe increased, resistance to hepcidin, (dominant form of hereditary hemochromatosis)	102, 103	104	Autosomal dominant
β_2-Microglobulin	Parenchymal Fe increased	Unknown	105, 106	Facilitates transport of *HFE* to membrane
Transferrin	Parenchymal Fe increased	107-109	110, 111	Plasma iron transporter, holotransferrin concentrations regulate hepcidin
Transferrin receptor-1	Lethal; increased CNS Fe (severe combined immunodeficiency)	112	113	Mediates cellular iron uptake, essential for erythropoiesis, may be involved in signaling for hepcidin regulation, essential for clonal expansion of lymphocytes
Transferrin receptor-2	Parenchymal Fe increased (hereditary hemochromatosis)	114, 115	116	Signaling for hepcidin regulation
Hephaestin	Fe deficiency	Unknown	34	Sex-linked gene; deletion of exons is cause of *sla* mouse
Ceruloplasmin	Fe increased (CNS disease)	117	51	Brain iron accumulation and neurologic disease
Ferritin H chain	Fe increased (systemic iron overload)	118	Unknown	Dominant IRE mutation
Duodenal cytochrome b (dcytb)	Unknown	Unknown	25	Mild iron restriction under erythropoietic stress
Nramp1 (SLC11A1)	Alters iron distribution in macrophages	Unknown	48	Deficiency increases susceptibility to infection in mice
Nramp2 (DMT-1, SLC11A2)	Hypochromic microcytic anemia and hepatic siderosis in people; Fe deficiency in rodents	119-121	122, 123	Anemia is ameliorated by erythropoietin therapy in humans; same naturally occurring mutations found in the *mk* mouse and the Belgrade rat
Hepcidin	Parenchymal Fe increased (juvenile hereditary hemochromatosis)	124	55, 125	The hormone regulating iron absorption, plasma iron concentration and systemic distribution
Hemojuvelin	Parenchymal Fe increased (juvenile hereditary hemochromatosis)	77	126, 127	Signaling for hepcidin regulation
Tmprss6	Fe deficiency (iron-refractory iron-deficiency anemia)	58	83, 86	Signaling for hepcidin regulation, membrane protease, cleaves hemojuvelin
BMP6	Parenchymal Fe increased	Unknown	128, 129	Necessary for iron regulation in mice
BMP2	Parenchymal Fe increased	Unknown	130	
BMP receptor subunit	Parenchymal Fe increased	Unknown	131	Necessary for iron regulation in mice
SMAD4 in the liver	Parenchymal Fe increased	Unknown	132	In signaling pathway for hepcidin regulation
Neogenin	Parenchymal Fe increased	Unknown	133, 134	Necessary for hepcidin regulation
Erythroferrone	Transient anemia during rapid growth, slow recovery from hemorrhage	Unknown	88, 135	Necessary for rapid suppression of hepcidin after hemorrhage, excess contributes to iron overload in β-thalassemia intermedia and other iron-loading anemias

Abbreviations: BMP, bone morphogenetic protein; CNS, central nervous system; HFE, human hemochromatosis protein.

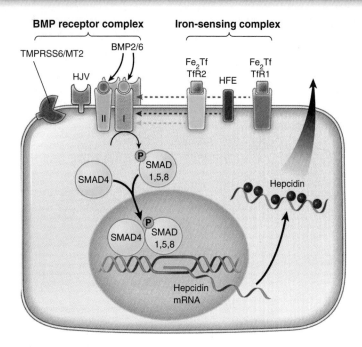

FIGURE 10–5. Regulation of hepatocyte hepcidin synthesis by hepatic iron stores and plasma holotransferrin concentration. The bone morphogenetic protein (BMP) receptor (BMPR) complex, consisting of a heterotetramer of two BMP type I (I) and two BMP type II (II) receptors, is activated by ligands BMP2 and BMP6, produced by nearby hepatic sinusoidal endothelial cells in proportion to hepatic iron stores. Hemojuvelin (HJV), a BMP coreceptor, strongly potentiates BMP signaling while the transmembrane serine protease TMPRSS66/MT2 inhibits it. Two types of transferrin receptors, TfR1 and TfR2, sense the concentration of diferric transferrin (Fe_2Tf) in plasma and, aided by the hemochromatosis protein HFE, stimulate BMPR signaling proportionately to plasma holotransferrin concentration. Activated BMPRI phosphorylates SMAD 1, 5, and 8, which then complex with SMAD4 to regulate hepcidin gene transcription and ultimately the synthesis and secretion of hepcidin.

is supported by studies in which the expression of HFE or its binding site on TfR1 are manipulated.[73]

A second TfR, TfR2, also endocytic for holotransferrin, is not thought to be involved in delivering iron to cells but its hepatic expression is necessary for normal hepcidin expression and regulation.[115] TfR2 influences the BMP complex and its signaling pathway to regulate hepcidin transcription, but the molecular mechanism of this effect is not yet understood. TfR2 is also expressed in erythroid precursors where it interacts with the erythropoietin receptor via the receptor control molecule Scribble to limit erythroblast proliferation and differentiation during iron deficiency.[137,138]

INTRACELLULAR IRON HOMEOSTASIS

Each cell must regulate its iron uptake and subcellular distribution, both to assure adequate iron for a multitude of cellular enzymes and to prevent excessive iron accumulation that could be injurious or deny adequate iron to other cells. Accordingly, the synthesis of key cellular proteins involved in iron transport, storage, and utilization is regulated posttranscriptionally by cellular iron concentrations.[85,86] The mRNA for each of these proteins contains one or several IREs. If the IRE is located at the 5' end of the mRNA, it serves to regulate translation; 3' IREs regulate the stability of the mRNA. Each IRE consists of a stem-and-loop structure. IRE/IRP-regulated mRNAs include those encoding ferritin, TfR1, aminolevulinic acid (ALA) synthase, transferrin, aconitase, DMT-1, and ferroportin. The ferritin mRNA has as its IRE a single stem-loop structure in the 5' (upstream) region. In contrast to the ferritin IRE, there are as many as five stem-loops in the 3' untranslated portion of TfR mRNA. The IREs are targeted by specific RNA-binding proteins, IRPs. IRP-1 is cytoplasmic aconitase with four iron-sulfur clusters and the ability to bind iron, which is required for its aconitase activity; IRP-2 is highly homologous to IRP-1 but differs by the presence of a 73-amino-acid insertion in the N-terminus and a lack of aconitase activity. In the absence of iron, IRP-1 binds to IREs, but in its presence becomes a cytoplasmic aconitase and does not bind IREs. IRP-2 (also to some extent IRP-1) undergoes ubiquitination and proteasomal

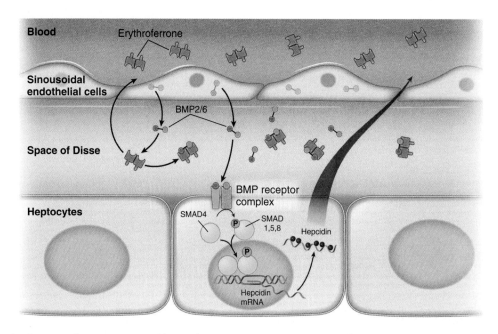

FIGURE 10-6. Erythroferrone, a hormone secreted by erythropoietin-stimulated erythroblasts, suppresses hepcidin production by hepatocytes. Erythroferrone acts by binding BMP2/6 in the space of Disse and preventing the bone morphogenetic proteins (BMPs) from stimulating hepcidin transcription.

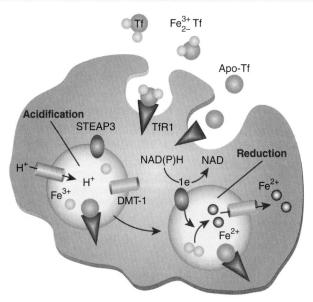

FIGURE 10–7. The transferrin cycle. Holotransferrin (Fe^{3+}_2-Tf) binds to transferrin receptors (TfR1) on the cell surface. The complexes localize to clathrin-coated pits, which invaginate to initiate endocytosis. Specialized endosomes form and become acidified through the action of a proton pump. Acidification leads to protein conformational changes that release iron from transferrin. STEAP3 (six-transmembrane epithelial antigen of prostate 3) reduces ferric iron to ferrous iron, enabling iron transport out of the endosomes through the activity of the divalent metal transporter-1 protein (DMT-1). Subsequently, apotransferrin (Apo-Tf) and the transferrin receptor both return to the cell surface, where they dissociate at neutral pH. Both proteins participate in further rounds of iron delivery. In nonerythroid cells, iron is stored as ferritin and hemosiderin. *(Reproduced with permission from McKie AT. A ferrireductase fills the gap in the transferrin cycle. Nat Genet. 2005 Nov;37[11]:1159-60.)*

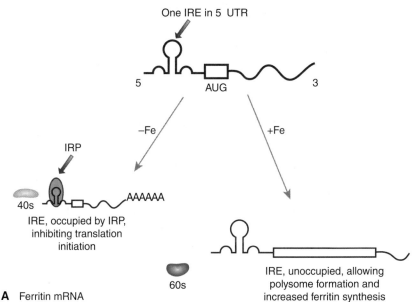

A Ferritin mRNA

FIGURE 10–8. The regulation of iron metabolism at the cytoplasmic mRNA level by interaction of iron-regulatory protein (IRP)-1 and the iron-responsive elements (IREs) to apoferritin mRNA **(A)** and transferrin receptor (TfR) mRNA **(B).** When the cytoplasmic iron concentration is low (*left side of illustration*), IRP-1 binds to the IREs of both mRNAs. This represses the translation of apoferritin mRNA, where the IRE is at the 5′ end of the mRNA, thereby reducing the amount of apoferritin formed. It stabilizes and increases the translation of TfR mRNA where the IRE is at the 3′ end of the mRNA, thereby increasing the amount of TfR formed. Conversely, when there is an abundance of iron in the cytoplasm (*right side of illustration*), IRP-1 is displaced from both species of mRNA. This results in derepression of apoferritin synthesis and destabilization and degradation of TfR mRNA. *(Reproduced with permission from Rouault T, Klausner R. Regulation of iron metabolism in eukaryotes. Curr Top Cell Regul. 1997;35:1-19.)*

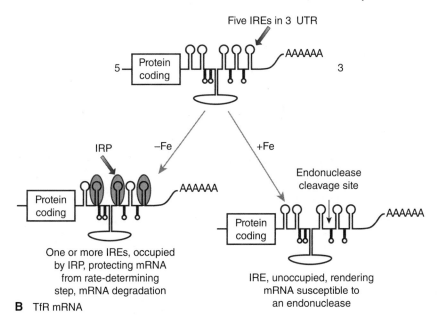

B TfR mRNA

degradation in the presence of iron.[139,140] The effect of binding of IRPs to 5′ IREs is to inhibit protein translation; the effect of binding of IRPs to 3′ IREs is to increase the stability of the mRNA and thus to enhance the synthesis of the gene product. The cytoplasmic endonuclease regnase-1 degrades mRNAs with unbound 3′IRE.[141] Figure 10-8 illustrates these relationships for the regulation of synthesis of ferritin and TfR. The net effect of the IRE/IRP system is to balance cellular iron uptake with storage, utilization, and, in some cell types, export of iron.

IRON IN THE ERYTHROBLAST

Once within the developing erythroblast, iron must be transported to mitochondria to be incorporated into heme, or taken up by ferritin within siderosomes. Within the vesicle, STEAP3 (six-transmembrane epithelial antigen of prostate 3) effects the reduction of ferric (Fe3+) to ferrous (Fe++) iron, and another protein DMT-1 (the same transporter as in intestinal iron absorption) transports Fe++ into the cytosol, where it is taken up by mitochondria by a complex of mitoferrin-1, Abcb10, and ferrochelatase for heme synthesis.[142] Physical interaction between mitochondria and endosomes ("kiss and run") may also be required.[143]

Mitochondrial Iron

Mitochondria, working together with cellular cytoplasm, supply each cell with heme. Although heme synthesis is important for all cells, erythroblasts synthesize much more heme than any other cell type. The final steps of heme synthesis take place in mitochondria, where iron is inserted into protoporphyrin by the enzyme ferrochelatase. When heme synthesis is impaired, as in lead poisoning or in the sideroblastic anemias (Chap. 20), the mitochondria accumulate excessive amounts of amorphous iron aggregates. The mitochondria can then be stained by the Prussian blue reaction and are seen by light microscopy as a ring of large blue siderotic granules encircling the erythroblast nucleus (ringed sideroblast). In normal, iron-replete marrow, much smaller siderotic granules are also demonstrable, scattered in the cytoplasm of about one-third of erythroblasts (Chap. 1). These normal siderotic granules are ferritin aggregates located in lysosomal organelles designated *siderosomes*.[144] Erythroblasts containing these siderotic granules, sideroblasts, normally represent 20% to 50% of the erythrocyte precursors of the marrow and as visualized by light microscopy. In iron deficiency and in the anemia that accompanies chronic disorders, sideroblasts almost disappear from the marrow. Conversely, in some states of iron overload, they may become more numerous and contain excessive numbers of granules, some of which may be considerably larger than normal.

IRON EXCRETION

The body conserves iron with remarkable efficiency. Most iron loss occurs by way of desquamated intestinal cells in the feces and it normally amounts to about 1 mg per day,[16,145] less than one-thousandth of the body's total iron. Exfoliation of skin and dermal appendages and perspiration result in much smaller losses. Even in tropical climates, the loss of iron in sweat is minimal. Very small amounts of iron are lost in the urine. Lactation may cause excretion of approximately 1 mg of iron daily, thus doubling the overall rate of iron loss. Blood loss by normal menstruation contributes to negative iron balance.

Although total daily iron loss is normally approximately 1 mg for men,[16] it averages approximately 2 mg for menstruating women. Persons with marked iron overload, as in hemochromatosis, may lose as much as 4 mg of iron daily, probably because of the shedding of iron-laden cells.

REFERENCES

1. Arosio P, Levi S. Cytosolic and mitochondrial ferritins in the regulation of cellular iron homeostasis and oxidative damage. *Biochim Biophys Acta.* 2010;1800(8):783-792.
2. Koorts AM, Viljoen M. Ferritin and ferritin isoforms I: structure-function relationships, synthesis, degradation and secretion. *Arch Physiol Biochem.* 2007;113(1):30-54.
3. Mancias JD, Wang X, Gygi SP, et al. Quantitative proteomics identifies NCOA4 as the cargo receptor mediating ferritinophagy. *Nature.* 2014;509(7498):105-109.
4. Mancias JD, Pontano Vaites L, Nissim S, et al. Ferritinophagy via NCOA4 is required for erythropoiesis and is regulated by iron dependent HERC2-mediated proteolysis. *Elife.* 2015;4.
5. Ordway GA, Garry DJ. Myoglobin: an essential hemoprotein in striated muscle. *J Exp Biol.* 2004;207(20):3441-3446.
6. Hosain F, Marsaglia G, Finch CA. Blood ferrokinetics in normal man. *J Clin Invest.* 1967;46(1):1-9.
7. Breuer W, Shvartsman M, Cabantchik ZI. Intracellular labile iron. *Int J Biochem Cell Biol.* 2008;40(3):350-354.
8. Dallman PR, Beutler E, Finch CA. Effects of iron deficiency exclusive of anaemia. *Br J Haematol.* 1978;40(2):179-184.
9. Radlowski EC, Johnson RW. Perinatal iron deficiency and neurocognitive development. *Front Hum Neurosci.* 2013;7:1-11.
10. Cheng Y, Zak O, Aisen P, et al. Structure of the human transferrin receptor-transferrin complex. *Cell.* 2004;116(4):565-576.
11. Bailey S, Evans RW, Garratt RC, et al. Molecular structure of serum transferrin at 3.3-A resolution. *Biochemistry.* 1988;27(15):5804-5812.
12. Aisen P, Brown EB. Structure and function of transferrin. *Prog Hematol.* 1975;9:25-56.
13. Thorbecke GJ, Liem HH, Knight S, et al. Sites of formation of the serum proteins transferrin and hemopexin. *J Clin Invest.* 1973;52(3):725-731.
14. Haurani FI, Meyer A, O'Brien R. Production of transferrin by the macrophage. *J Reticuloendothel Soc.* 1973;14(3):309-316.
15. Egan SK, Tao SS, Pennington JA, et al. US Food and Drug Administration's Total Diet Study: intake of nutritional and toxic elements, 1991-96. *Food Addit Contam.* 2002;19(2):103-125.
16. Dubach R, Moore CV, Callender S. Studies in iron transportation and metabolism. IX. The excretion of iron as measured by the isotope technique. *J Lab Clin Med.* 1955;45(4):599-615.
17. Trumbo P, Yates AA, Schlicker S, et al. Dietary reference intakes: vitamin A, vitamin K, arsenic, boron, chromium, copper, iodine, iron, manganese, molybdenum, nickel, silicon, vanadium, and zinc. *J Am Diet Assoc.* 2001;101(3):294-301.
18. Heath AL, Fairweather T. Clinical implications of changes in the modern diet: iron intake, absorption and status. *Best Pract Res Clin Haematol.* 2002;15(2):225-241.
19. Hurrell R, Egli I. Iron bioavailability and dietary reference values. *Am J Clin Nutr.* 2010;91(5):1461S-1467S.
20. Cook JD, Reddy MB, Hurrell RF. The effect of red and white wines on nonheme-iron absorption in humans. *Am J Clin Nutr.* 1995;61(4):800-804.
21. Anderson ER, Taylor M, Xue X, et al. The hypoxia-inducible factor-C/EBPalpha axis controls ethanol-mediated hepcidin repression. *Mol Cell Biol.* 2012;32(19):4068-4077.
22. Smith MD, Pannacciulli IM. Absorption of inorganic iron from graded doses: its significance in relation to iron absorption tests and mucosal block theory. *Br J Haematol.* 1958;4(4):428-434.
23. Fiorito V, Geninatti CS, Silengo L, et al. Lack of plasma protein hemopexin results in increased duodenal iron uptake. *PLoS One.* 2013;8(6):e68146.
24. Korolnek T, Hamza I. Like iron in the blood of the people: the requirement for heme trafficking in iron metabolism. *Front Pharmacol.* 2014;5:126.
25. Choi J, Masaratana P, Latunde-Dada GO, et al. Duodenal reductase activity and spleen iron stores are reduced and erythropoiesis is abnormal in Dcytb knockout mice exposed to hypoxic conditions. *J Nutr.* 2012;142(11):1929-1934.
26. Gunshin H, Mackenzie B, Berger UV, et al. Cloning and characterization of a mammalian proton-coupled metal-ion transporter. *Nature.* 1997;388(6641):482-488.
27. Shawki A, Knight PB, Maliken BD, et al. H(+)-coupled divalent metal-ion transporter-1: functional properties, physiological roles and therapeutics. *Curr Top Membr.* 2012;70:169-214.
28. Shawki A, Engevik MA, Kim RS, et al. Intestinal brush-border Na+/H+ exchanger-3 drives H+-coupled iron absorption in the mouse. *Am J Physiol Gastrointest Liver Physiol.* 2016;311(3):G423-430.
29. Yanatori I, Richardson DR, Imada K, et al. Iron export through the transporter ferroportin 1 is modulated by the iron chaperone PCBP2. *J Biol Chem.* 2016;291(33):17303-17318.
30. Leidgens S, Bullough KZ, Shi H, et al. Each member of the poly-r(C)-binding protein (PCBP) family exhibits iron chaperone activity toward ferritin. *J Biol Chem.* 2013;288(24):17791-17802.
31. Donovan A, Brownlie A, Zhou Y, et al. Positional cloning of zebrafish ferroportin1 identifies a conserved vertebrate iron exporter. *Nature.* 2000;403(6771):776-781.
32. McKie AT, Marciani P, Rolfs A, et al. A novel duodenal iron-regulated transporter, IREG1, implicated in the basolateral transfer of iron to the circulation. *Mol Cell.* 2000;5(2):299-309.
33. Abboud S, Haile DJ. A novel mammalian iron-regulated protein involved in intracellular iron metabolism. *J Biol Chem.* 2000;275(26):19906-19912.

34. Vulpe CD, Kuo YM, Murphy TL, et al. Hephaestin, a ceruloplasmin homologue implicated in intestinal iron transport, is defective in the sla mouse. *Nat Genet.* 1999;21(2):195-199.

35. Cherukuri S, Potla R, Sarkar J, et al. Unexpected role of ceruloplasmin in intestinal iron absorption. *Cell Metab.* 2005;2(5):309-319.

36. Shawki A, Anthony SR, Nose Y, et al. Intestinal DMT1 is critical for iron absorption in the mouse but is not required for the absorption of copper or manganese. *Am J Physiol Gastrointest Liver Physiol.* 2015;309(8):G635-647.

37. Mackenzie B, Garrick MD. Iron imports. II. Iron uptake at the apical membrane in the intestine. *Am J Physiol Gastrointest Liver Physiol.* 2005;289(6):G981-G986.

38. Zhang D-L, Wu J, Shah BN, et al. Erythrocytic ferroportin reduces intracellular iron accumulation, hemolysis, and malaria risk. *Science.* 2018;359(6383):1520-1523.

39. Klei TRL, Dalimot J, Nota B, et al. Hemolysis in the spleen drives erythrocyte turnover. *Blood.* 2020;136(14):1579-1589.

40. Noyes WD, Bothwell TH, Finch CA. The role of the reticulo-endothelial cell in iron metabolism. *Br J Haematol.* 1960;6:43-55.

41. Haurani FI, Burke W, Martinez EJ. Defective reutilization of iron in the anemia of inflammation. *J Lab Clin Med.* 1965;65:560-570.

42. O'Shea MJ, Kershenobich D, Tavill AS. Effects of inflammation on iron and transferrin metabolism. *Br J Haematol.* 1973;25(6):707-714.

43. Bosman GJCG, Werre JM, Willekens FLA, et al. Erythrocyte ageing in vivo and in vitro: structural aspects and implications for transfusion. *Transfus Med.* 2008;18(6):335-347.

44. Beaumont C, Delaby C. Recycling iron in normal and pathological states. *Semin Hematol.* 2009;46(4):328-338.

45. Kovtunovych G, Eckhaus MA, Ghosh MC, et al. Dysfunction of the heme recycling system in heme oxygenase-1 deficient mice: effects on macrophage viability and tissue iron distribution. *Blood.* 2010;116(26):6054-6062.

46. Delaby C, Rondeau C, Pouzet C, et al. Subcellular localization of iron and heme metabolism related proteins at early stages of erythrophagocytosis. *PLoS One.* 2012;7(7):e42199.

47. White C, Yuan X, Schmidt PJ, et al. HRG1 is essential for heme transport from the phagolysosome of macrophages during erythrophagocytosis. *Cell Metab.* 2013;17(2):261-270.

48. Soe-Lin S, Apte SS, Andriopoulos B, Jr., et al. Nramp1 promotes efficient macrophage recycling of iron following erythrophagocytosis in vivo. *Proc Natl Acad Sci U S A.* 2009;106(14):5960-5965.

49. Knutson MD, Oukka M, Koss LM, et al. Iron release from macrophages after erythrophagocytosis is up-regulated by ferroportin 1 overexpression and down-regulated by hepcidin. *Proc Natl Acad Sci U S A.* 2005;102(5):1324-1328.

50. Cherukuri S, Tripoulas NA, Nurko S, et al. Anemia and impaired stress-induced erythropoiesis in aceruloplasminemic mice. *Blood Cells Mol Dis.* 2004;33(3):346-355.

51. Harris ZL, Durley AP, Man TK, et al. Targeted gene disruption reveals an essential role for ceruloplasmin in cellular iron efflux. *Proc Natl Acad Sci U S A.* 1999;96(19):10812-10817.

52. Sarkar J, Seshadri V, Tripoulas NA, et al. Role of ceruloplasmin in macrophage iron efflux during hypoxia. *J Biol Chem.* 2003;278(45):44018-44024.

53. Pigeon C, Ilyin G, Courselaud B, et al. A new mouse liver-specific gene, encoding a protein homologous to human antimicrobial peptide hepcidin, is overexpressed during iron overload. *J Biol Chem.* 2001;276(11):7811-7819.

54. Park CH, Valore EV, Waring AJ, et al. Hepcidin, a urinary antimicrobial peptide synthesized in the liver. *J Biol Chem.* 2001;276(11):7806-7810.

55. Nicolas G, Bennoun M, Devaux I, et al. Lack of hepcidin gene expression and severe tissue iron overload in upstream stimulatory factor 2 (USF2) knockout mice. *Proc Natl Acad Sci U S A.* 2001;98(15):8780-8785.

56. Ganz T. Hepcidin and iron regulation, 10 years later. *Blood.* 2011;117(17):4425-4433.

57. Nicolas G, Bennoun M, Porteu A, et al. Severe iron deficiency anemia in transgenic mice expressing liver hepcidin. *Proc Natl Acad Sci U S A.* 2002;99(7):4596-4601.

58. Finberg KE, Heeney MM, Campagna DR, et al. Mutations in TMPRSS6 cause iron-refractory iron deficiency anemia (IRIDA). *Nat Genet.* 2008;40(5):569-571.

59. Rivera S, Nemeth E, Gabayan V, et al. Synthetic hepcidin causes rapid dose-dependent hypoferremia and is concentrated in ferroportin-containing organs. *Blood.* 2005; 106(6):2196-2199.

60. Stefanova D, Raychev A, Arezes J, et al. Endogenous hepcidin and its agonist mediate resistance to selected infections by clearing non-transferrin-bound iron. *Blood.* 2017;130(3):245-257.

61. Aschemeyer S, Qiao B, Stefanova D, et al. Structure-function analysis of ferroportin defines the binding site and an alternative mechanism of action of hepcidin. *Blood.* 2018;131(8):899-910.

62. Billesbolle CB, Azumaya CM, Kretsch RC, et al. Structure of hepcidin-bound ferroportin reveals iron homeostatic mechanisms. *Nature.* 2020;586(7831):807-811.

63. Nemeth E, Tuttle MS, Powelson J, et al. Hepcidin regulates cellular iron efflux by binding to ferroportin and inducing its internalization. *Science.* 2004;306(5704):2090-2093.

64. Nemeth E, Rivera S, Gabayan V, et al. IL-6 mediates hypoferremia of inflammation by inducing the synthesis of the iron regulatory hormone hepcidin. *J Clin Invest.* 2004;113(9):1271-1276.

65. Rodriguez R, Jung CL, Gabayan V, et al. Hepcidin induction by pathogens and pathogen-derived molecules is strongly dependent on interleukin-6. *Infect Immun.* 2014;82(2):745-752.

66. Nicolas G, Chauvet C, Viatte L, et al. The gene encoding the iron regulatory peptide hepcidin is regulated by anemia, hypoxia, and inflammation. *J Clin Invest.* 2002;110(7):1037-1044.

67. Nemeth E, Valore EV, Territo M, et al. Hepcidin, a putative mediator of anemia of inflammation, is a type II acute-phase protein. *Blood.* 2003;101(7):2461-2463.

68. Pak M, Lopez MA, Gabayan V, et al. Suppression of hepcidin during anemia requires erythropoietic activity. *Blood.* 2006;108(12):3730-3735.

69. Ganz T, Olbina G, Girelli D, et al. Immunoassay for human serum hepcidin. *Blood.* 2008;112(10):4292-4297.

70. Ramos E, Kautz L, Rodriguez R, et al. Evidence for distinct pathways of hepcidin regulation by acute and chronic iron loading in mice. *Hepatology.* 2011;53(4):1333-1341.

71. Corradini E, Meynard D, Wu Q, et al. Serum and liver iron differently regulate the bone morphogenetic protein 6 (BMP6)-SMAD signaling pathway in mice. *Hepatology.* 2011;54(1):273-284.

72. Lin L, Valore EV, Nemeth E, et al. Iron transferrin regulates hepcidin synthesis in primary hepatocyte culture through hemojuvelin and BMP2/4. *Blood.* 2007;110(6):2182-2189.

73. Schmidt PJ, Toran PT, Giannetti AM, et al. The transferrin receptor modulates Hfe-dependent regulation of hepcidin expression. *Cell Metab.* 2008;7(3):205-214.

74. Schmidt PJ, Huang FW, Wrighting DM, et al. Hepcidin expression is regulated by a complex of hemochromatosis-associated proteins. *ASH Annu Meet Abstr.* 2006;108(11):267.

75. D'Alessio F, Hentze MW, Muckenthaler MU. The hemochromatosis proteins HFE, TfR2, and HJV form a membrane-associated protein complex for hepcidin regulation. *J Hepatol.* 2012;57(5):1052-1060.

76. Rishi G, Crampton EM, Wallace DF, et al. In situ proximity ligation assays indicate that hemochromatosis proteins Hfe and transferrin receptor 2 (Tfr2) do not interact. *PLoS One.* 2013;8(10):e77267.

77. Papanikolaou G, Samuels ME, Ludwig EH, et al. Mutations in HFE2 cause iron overload in chromosome 1q-linked juvenile hemochromatosis. *Nat Genet.* 2004;36(1):77-82.

78. Babitt JL, Huang FW, Wrighting DM, et al. Bone morphogenetic protein signaling by hemojuvelin regulates hepcidin expression. *Nat Genet.* 2006;38(5):531-539.

79. Lin L, Nemeth E, Goodnough JB, et al. Soluble hemojuvelin is released by proprotein convertase-mediated cleavage at a conserved polybasic RNRR site. *Blood Cells Mol Dis.* 2008;40(1):122-131.

80. Lin L, Goldberg YP, Ganz T. Competitive regulation of hepcidin mRNA by soluble and cell-associated hemojuvelin. *Blood.* 2005;106(8):2884-2889.

81. Truksa J, Lee P, Beutler E. Two BMP responsive elements, STAT, and bZIP/HNF4/COUP motifs of the hepcidin promoter are critical for BMP, SMAD1, and HJV responsiveness. *Blood.* 2009;113(3):688-695.

82. Pasricha SR, Lim PJ, Duarte TL, et al. Hepcidin is regulated by promoter-associated histone acetylation and HDAC3. *Nat Commun.* 2017;8(1):403.

83. Silvestri L, Pagani A, Nai A, et al. The serine protease matriptase-2 (TMPRSS6) inhibits hepcidin activation by cleaving membrane hemojuvelin. *Cell Metab.* 2008;8(6):502-511.

84. Truksa J, Gelbart T, Peng H, et al. Suppression of the hepcidin-encoding gene Hamp permits iron overload in mice lacking both hemojuvelin and matriptase-2/TMPRSS6. *Br J Haematol.* 2009;147(4):571-581.

85. Wahedi M, Wortham AM, Kleven MD, et al. Matriptase-2 suppresses hepcidin expression by cleaving multiple components of the hepcidin induction pathway. *J Biol Chem.* 2017;292(44):18354-18371.

86. Du X, She E, Gelbart T, et al. The serine protease TMPRSS6 is required to sense iron deficiency. *Science.* 2008;320(5879):1088-1092.

87. Finch C. Regulators of iron balance in humans. *Blood.* 1994;84(6):1697-1702.

88. Kautz L, Jung G, Valore EV, et al. Identification of erythroferrone as an erythroid regulator of iron metabolism. *Nat Genet.* 2014;46(7):678-684.

89. Tanno T, Bhanu NV, Oneal PA, et al. High levels of GDF15 in thalassemia suppress expression of the iron regulatory protein hepcidin. *Nat Med.* 2007;13(9):1096-1101.

90. Arezes J, Foy N, McHugh K, et al. Erythroferrone inhibits the induction of hepcidin by BMP6. *Blood.* 2018;132(14):1473-1477.

91. Wang CY, Xu Y, Traeger L, et al. Erythroferrone lowers hepcidin by sequestering BMP2/6 heterodimer from binding to the BMP type I receptor ALK3. *Blood.* 2020;135(6):453-456.

92. Drakesmith H, Prentice AM. Hepcidin and the iron-infection axis. *Science.* 2012;338(6108):768-772.

93. Stefanova D, Raychev A, Deville J, et al. Hepcidin protects against lethal *Escherichia coli* sepsis in mice inoculated with isolates from septic patients. *Infect Immun.* 2018;86(7).

94. Wrighting DM, Andrews NC. Interleukin-6 induces hepcidin expression through STAT3. *Blood.* 2006;108(9):3204-3209.

95. Pietrangelo A, Dierssen U, Valli L, et al. STAT 3 is required for IL-6-gp130-dependent activation of hepcidin in vivo. *Gastroenterology.* 2007;132(1):294-300.

96. Verga Falzacappa MV, Vujic SM, Kessler R, et al. STAT3 mediates hepatic hepcidin expression and its inflammatory stimulation. *Blood.* 2007;109(1):353-358.

97. Feder JN, Gnirke A, Thomas W, et al. A novel MHC class I-like gene is mutated in patients with hereditary haemochromatosis. *Nat Genet.* 1996;13(4):399-408.

98. Zhou XY, Tomatsu S, Fleming RE, et al. HFE gene knockout produces mouse model of hereditary hemochromatosis. *Proc Natl Acad Sci U S A.* 1998;95(5):2492-2497.

99. Ahmad KA, Ahmann JR, Migas MC, et al. Decreased liver hepcidin expression in the Hfe knockout mouse. *Blood Cells Mol Dis.* 2002;29(3):361-366.

100. Montosi G, Donovan A, Totaro A, et al. Autosomal-dominant hemochromatosis is associated with a mutation in the ferroportin (SLC11A3) gene. *J Clin Invest.* 2001;108(4):619-623.

101. Zohn IE, De Domenico I, Pollock A, et al. The flatiron mutation in mouse ferroportin acts as a dominant negative to cause ferroportin disease. *Blood.* 2007;109(10):4174-4180.

102. Njajou OT, Vaessen N, Joosse M, et al. A mutation in SLC11A3 is associated with autosomal dominant hemochromatosis. *Nat Genet.* 2001;28(3):213-214.

103. Sham RL, Phatak PD, Nemeth E, et al. Hereditary hemochromatosis due to resistance to hepcidin: high hepcidin concentrations in a family with C326S ferroportin mutation. *Blood.* 2009;114(2):493-494.

104. Altamura S, Groene HJ, Kessler R, et al. In vivo disruption of the hepcidin-ferroportin regulatory circuitry causes fatal systemic and exocrine pancreatic iron overload. *ASH Annu Meet Abstr.* 2013:175.

105. De Sousa M, Reimao R, Lacerda R, et al. Iron overload in beta 2-microglobulin-deficient mice. *Immunol Lett.* 1994;39(2):105-111.

106. Rothenberg BE, Voland JR. Beta2 knockout mice develop parenchymal iron overload: a putative role for class I genes of the major histocompatibility complex in iron metabolism. *Proc Natl Acad Sci U S A.* 1996;93(4):1529-1534.

107. Goya N, Miyazaki S, Kodate S, et al. A family of congenital atransferrinemia. *Blood.* 1972;40(2):239-245.

108. Bernstein SE. Hereditary hypotransferrinemia with hemosiderosis, a murine disorder resembling human atransferrinemia. *J Lab Clin Med.* 1987;110(6):690-705.

109. Hamill RL, Woods JC, Cook BA. Congenital atransferrinemia. A case report and review of the literature. *Am J Clin Pathol.* 1991;96(2):215-218.

110. Trenor CC, III, Campagna DR, Sellers VM, et al. The molecular defect in hypotransferrinemic mice. *Blood.* 2000;96(3):1113-1118.

111. Bartnikas TB, Andrews NC, Fleming MD. Transferrin is a major determinant of hepcidin expression in hypotransferrinemic mice. *Blood.* 2011;117(2):630-637.

112. Lo B. The requirement of iron transport for lymphocyte function. *Nat Genet.* 2016; 48(1):10-11.

113. Levy JE, Jin O, Fujiwara Y, et al. Transferrin receptor is necessary for development of erythrocytes and the nervous system. *Nat Genet.* 1999;21(4):396-399.

114. Camaschella C, Roetto A, Cali A, et al. The gene TFR2 is mutated in a new type of haemochromatosis mapping to 7q22. *Nat Genet.* 2000;25(1):14-15.

115. Nemeth E, Roetto A, Garozzo G, et al. Hepcidin is decreased in TFR2 hemochromatosis. *Blood.* 2005;105(4):1803-1806.

116. Fleming RE, Ahmann JR, Migas MC, et al. Targeted mutagenesis of the murine transferrin receptor-2 gene produces hemochromatosis. *Proc Natl Acad Sci U S A.* 2002;99(16):10653-10658.

117. Harris ZL, Takahashi Y, Miyajima H, et al. Aceruloplasminemia: molecular characterization of this disorder of iron metabolism. *Proc Natl Acad Sci U S A.* 1995;92(7):2539-2543.

118. Kato J, Fujikawa K, Kanda M, et al. A mutation, in the iron-responsive element of H ferritin mRNA, causing autosomal dominant iron overload. *Am J Hum Genet.* 2001;69(1):191-197.

119. Mims MP, Guan Y, Pospisilova D, et al. Identification of a human mutation of DMT1 in a patient with microcytic anemia and iron overload. *Blood.* 2005;105(3):1337-1342.

120. Iolascon A, De FL. Mutations in the gene encoding DMT1: clinical presentation and treatment. *Semin Hematol.* 2009;46(4):358-370.

121. Blanco E, Kannengiesser C, Grandchamp B, et al. Not all DMT1 mutations lead to iron overload. *Blood Cells Mol Dis.* 2009;43(2):199-201.

122. Fleming MD, Trenor CC, III, Su MA, et al. Microcytic anaemia mice have a mutation in Nramp2, a candidate iron transporter gene. *Nat Genet.* 1997;16(4):383-386.

123. Fleming MD, Romano MA, Su MA, et al. Nramp2 is mutated in the anemic Belgrade (b) rat: evidence of a role for Nramp2 in endosomal iron transport. *Proc Natl Acad Sci U S A.* 1998;95(3):1148-1153.

124. Roetto A, Papanikolaou G, Politou M, et al. Mutant antimicrobial peptide hepcidin is associated with severe juvenile hemochromatosis. *Nat Genet.* 2003;33(1):21-22.

125. Lesbordes-Brion JC, Viatte L, Bennoun M, et al. Targeted disruption of the hepcidin 1 gene results in severe hemochromatosis. *Blood.* 2006;108(4):1402-1405.

126. Niederkofler V, Salie R, Arber S. Hemojuvelin is essential for dietary iron sensing, and its mutation leads to severe iron overload. *J Clin Invest.* 2005;115(8):2180-2186.

127. Huang FW, Pinkus JL, Pinkus GS, et al. A mouse model of juvenile hemochromatosis. *J Clinv Invest.* 2005;115(8):2187-2191.

128. Meynard D, Kautz L, Darnaud V, et al. Lack of the bone morphogenetic protein BMP6 induces massive iron overload. *Nat Genet.* 2009;41(4):478-481.

129. Andriopoulos B, Jr., Corradini E, Xia Y, et al. BMP6 is a key endogenous regulator of hepcidin expression and iron metabolism. *Nat Genet.* 2009;41(4):482-487.

130. Koch PS, Olsavszky V, Ulbrich F, et al. Angiocrine Bmp2 signaling in murine liver controls normal iron homeostasis. *Blood.* 2017;129(4):415-419.

131. Steinbicker AU, Bartnikas TB, Lohmeyer LK, et al. Perturbation of hepcidin expression by BMP type I receptor deletion induces iron overload in mice. *Blood.* 2011;118(15):4224-4230.

132. Wang RH, Li C, Xu X, et al. A role of SMAD4 in iron metabolism through the positive regulation of hepcidin expression. *Cell Metab.* 2005;2(6):399-409.

133. Lee DH, Zhou LJ, Zhou Z, et al. Neogenin inhibits HJV secretion and regulates BMP-induced hepcidin expression and iron homeostasis. *Blood.* 2010;115(15):3136-3145.

134. Enns CA, Ahmed R, Zhang AS. Neogenin interacts with matriptase-2 to facilitate hemojuvelin cleavage. *J Biol Chem.* 2012;287(42):35104-35117.

135. Kautz L, Jung G, Nemeth E, et al. Erythroferrone contributes to recovery from anemia of inflammation. *Blood.* 2014;124(16):2569-2574.

136. Aisen P. Transferrin receptor 1. *Int J Biochem Cell Biol.* 2004;36(11):2137-2143.

137. Silvestri L, Nai A, Pagani A, et al. The extrahepatic role of TFR2 in iron homeostasis. *Front Pharmacol.* 2014;5:93.

138. Khalil S, Delehanty L, Grado S, et al. Iron modulation of erythropoiesis is associated with Scribble-mediated control of the erythropoietin receptor. *J Exp Med.* 2018;215(2):661-679.

139. Vashisht AA, Zumbrennen KB, Huang X, et al. Control of iron homeostasis by an iron-regulated ubiquitin ligase. *Science.* 2009;326(5953):718-721.

140. Salahudeen AA, Thompson JW, Ruiz JC, et al. An E3 ligase possessing an iron-responsive hemerythrin domain is a regulator of iron homeostasis. *Science.* 2009;326(5953):722-726.

141. Yoshinaga M, Nakatsuka Y, Vandenbon A, et al. Regnase-1 maintains iron homeostasis via the degradation of transferrin receptor 1 and prolyl-hydroxylase-domain-containing protein 3 mRNAs. *Cell Rep.* 2017;19(8):1614-1630.

142. Chen W, Dailey HA, Paw BH. Ferrochelatase forms an oligomeric complex with mitoferrin-1 and Abcb10 for erythroid heme biosynthesis. *Blood.* 2010;116(4):628-630.

143. Sheftel AD, Zhang AS, Brown C, et al. Direct interorganellar transfer of iron from endosome to mitochondrion. *Blood.* 2007;110(1):125-132.

144. Cartwright GE, Deiss A. Sideroblasts, siderocytes, and sideroblastic anemia. *N Engl J Med.* 1975;292(4):185-193.

145. Green R, Charlton R, Seftel H, et al. Body iron excretion in man: a collaborative study. *Am J Med.* 1968;45(3):336-353.

CHAPTER 11
IRON DEFICIENCY AND OVERLOAD

Tomas Ganz

SUMMARY

Iron deficiency and iron-deficiency anemia are common nutritional and hematologic disorders. In infants and young children, iron deficiency is most commonly caused by insufficient dietary iron. Rarely, it can result from mutations in *TMPRSS6*, a gene encoding a membrane protease that serves normally as a transcriptional suppressor of the primary negative regulator of iron absorption, hepcidin. In young women, iron deficiency is most often the result of blood loss in menstruation or from blood loss during pregnancy, childbirth, and lactation. In older adults, bleeding is often the cause of iron deficiency and may originate from the gastrointestinal tract, as from hemorrhoids, peptic ulcer, hiatus hernia, colon cancer, or angiodysplasia; from the genitourinary tract; from uterine leiomyomas or carcinoma, or a renal tumor; or from the pulmonary tree, through chronic hemoptysis caused by infection or malignancy, or as a result of idiopathic pulmonary hemosiderosis. Iron deficiency in infants can result in impairment of growth and intellectual development. The hematologic features of iron deficiency are nonspecific and too often confused with other causes of microcytic anemia such as thalassemias and chronic inflammation. A low serum ferritin concentration is a good indicator of iron deficiency, but ferritin levels are increased by inflammation and can be particularly high in cancer, macrophage activation syndromes, hepatitis, or chronic kidney disease, which may mask iron deficiency coexisting with the anemia of chronic inflammation. The plasma iron is decreased and the iron-binding capacity increased in severe iron deficiency, but these alterations are not uniformly present in mild iron deficiency, and low plasma iron levels are also characteristic of the anemia of inflammation. Other laboratory tests that are useful include assays for serum transferrin receptor, reticulocyte hemoglobin (Hb) content, percent hypochromic erythrocytes and erythrocyte zinc protoporphyrin. Diagnosis of iron deficiency, particularly in an adult, obliges the clinician to determine the

Acronyms and Abbreviations: BMP, bone morphogenetic protein; cDNA, complementary DNA; DMT, divalent metal transporter; ESPGHAN, European Society for Pediatric Gastroenterology, Hepatology, and Nutrition; Hgb, hemoglobin; FGF23, fibroblast growth factor 23; HJV, hemojuvelin; HFE, high iron (*high Fe*)—a mutated protein associated with common hereditary hemochromatosis; HLA, human leukocyte antigen; IL, interleukin; IRE, iron-responsive element; IRP, iron-regulatory protein; IV, intravenous; MCV, mean corpuscular volume; MRI, magnetic resonance imaging; O_2, oxygen; RDA, recommended daily allowance; RDW, red cell distribution width; sTfR, serum transferrin receptor; TfR, transferrin receptor; TIBC, total iron-binding capacity; Tmprss6, the membrane serine protease; UIBC, unsaturated iron-binding capacity; VO_2max, peak oxygen consumption.

site and cause of blood loss, and to rectify it whenever possible. Ferrous salts, in doses of 100 to 200 mg of elemental iron daily, are the initial treatment in most patients with iron deficiency. Enteric-coated and prolonged-release preparations should be avoided. If the patients take the iron preparation as instructed, complete correction of anemia is expected in 8 to 12 weeks, depending on the patient's age. If this response is not achieved, the patient, their compliance with the oral iron regimen, and the diagnosis require reevaluation. Administration of iron should be continued for 12 months after correction of anemia, or for as long as bleeding continues. Parenteral iron is used in patients who need more iron than can be delivered by the oral route, patients who do not tolerate oral iron salts, patients with gastrointestinal disease or after certain forms of bariatric surgery, noncompliant patients, and patients undergoing renal dialysis. All current parenteral iron preparations are much less likely to cause serious adverse events than was the case for the high-molecular-weight iron dextran formulations used in the past.

At the opposite end of the iron disorder spectrum, iron storage disease (hemochromatosis) can be the result of mutations of genes that are involved in regulation of iron homeostasis or transport, including the genes encoding high iron (*high Fe*; HFE), transferrin receptor 2, ferroportin, hemojuvelin (HJV), and hepcidin. Because iron is not substantially excreted, iron overload commonly results from chronic erythrocyte transfusions for those anemias that are not caused by blood loss or iron deficiency.

Alternatively, iron overload resembling hereditary hemochromatosis can be the result of hyperabsorption of iron induced by ineffective erythropoiesis, including in β-thalassemias, dyserythropoietic anemias, pyruvate kinase deficiency, congenital dyserythropoietic anemias, and some sideroblastic anemias. Here iron overload can develop even in the absence of erythrocyte transfusions or the (ill-advised) administration of medicinal iron, but it is further aggravated by these events.

The diagnosis of systemic iron overload depends, in large part, on increased serum ferritin levels accompanied by increased transferrin saturation, which tend to reflect increased iron stores. However, ferritin levels are also increased in patients with chronic inflammation or neoplasia or with the hyperferritinemia cataract syndrome, a disorder caused by mutations in the iron-responsive element (IRE) of the ferritin light chain. The transferrin saturation is usually increased in patients with hereditary hemochromatosis even when the ferritin level is normal.

Many subjects with genetic hemochromatosis never progress to having organ dysfunction, but in those who do, clinically significant cirrhosis of the liver, darkening of the skin, diabetes, cardiomyopathies, and arthropathies predominate and contribute to significant morbidity and mortality if left untreated. Iron deposition is primarily in hepatocytes, with macrophages and intestinal mucosal cells being relatively iron poor. The most common causes of genetic hemochromatosis are mutations of the *HFE* gene. Two common mutations are involved: the c.854G→A (C282Y) and c.187C→G (H63D) substitutions. Increased transferrin saturation values, serum ferritin levels, and iron stores were found in a majority of homozygotes for the C282Y mutation and in many compound heterozygotes for C282Y/H63D or, rarely, in homozygotes for H63D. However, clinical manifestations even among homozygotes for the C282Y mutation are rare, in contrast to biochemical and/or histologic manifestations of the increased iron levels, which are common. Only a few percent of C282Y homozygous patients develop clinically significant disease, and cofactors including male gender and alcohol intake potentiate disease development. Juvenile hemochromatosis, an earlier-onset and more severe type of hemochromatosis with high penetrance, is the result of mutations of the HJV or the hepcidin gene. Ferroportin mutations produced two types of autosomal dominant iron overload. In one of these, the iron is chiefly retained in macrophages; the other is similar to classical hereditary hemochromatosis with iron deposition in hepatocytes and other parenchymal cells.

Iron can be removed from patients with hereditary hemochromatosis by serial phlebotomy, but in patients with iron-loading anemias, iron chelation therapy with either parenteral desferrioxamine infusions or the oral chelators deferiprone or deferasirox is required.

●IRON DEFICIENCY

DEFINITION AND HISTORY

Iron deficiency is the state in which the content of iron in the body is less than normal. Iron depletion is the earliest stage of iron deficiency, in which storage iron is decreased or absent but serum iron concentration, transferrin saturation, and blood Hb levels are normal. Iron deficiency without anemia is a somewhat more advanced stage of iron deficiency, characterized by absent storage iron, usually low serum iron concentration and transferrin saturation, but without frank anemia. Iron-deficiency anemia, the most advanced stage of iron deficiency, is characterized by absent iron stores, low serum iron concentration, low transferrin saturation, and low blood Hb concentration.

Chlorosis, or "green sickness," was well known to European physicians after the middle of the 16th century. In France, by the middle of the 17th century, iron salts and other remedies (including, oddly enough, phlebotomy) were used in its treatment. Not long thereafter, iron was recommended by Sydenham as a specific remedy for chlorosis. For the 100 years preceding 1930, iron was used in the treatment of chlorosis, often in ineffective doses, although the mechanism of action of iron and the appropriateness of its use were highly controversial. By the beginning of the 20th century, it had been established that chlorosis was characterized by a decrease in the iron content of the blood and by the presence of hypochromic erythrocytes, but it was not until the classic 1932 studies by Heath, Strauss, and Castle[1] that it was shown that the response of anemia to iron was stoichiometrically related to the amount of iron given and that chlorosis was, indeed, iron deficiency. The history of iron deficiency has been reviewed in greater detail elsewhere.[2,3]

EPIDEMIOLOGY

Iron-deficiency anemia is the most common anemia worldwide and is especially prevalent in women and children in regions where meat intake is low, food is not fortified with iron, and malaria, intestinal infections, and parasitic worms are common.[4-6] Women with frequent pregnancies may be particularly susceptible. In the United States, iron deficiency is most common in children between ages 1 and 4 years and in adolescent, reproductive-age, or pregnant women.[7-9]

ETIOLOGY AND PATHOGENESIS

Etiology

Iron deficiency may occur as a result of chronic blood loss, diversion of iron to fetal and infant erythropoiesis during pregnancy and lactation, inadequate dietary iron intake, malabsorption of iron, intravascular hemolysis with hemoglobinuria, diversion of iron to nonhematopoietic tissues such as the lung, genetic factors, or a combination of these

factors. Of these, gastrointestinal or menstrual blood loss is most common. As discussed in Chapter 10, the average adult male has approximately 1000 mg of iron in stores but, on average, women have less than half of this amount. The average daily dietary intake of iron is 10 to 12 mg, but much of this is not absorbed, even when absorption is maximal. Blood loss of each milliliter of packed erythrocytes represents 1 mg of iron. Thus, chronic daily blood loss greater than 5 mL of erythrocytes will deplete iron reserves over weeks to months, and even if bleeding stops completely, the repletion of lost iron, including the restoration of iron stores (around 1000 mg in the average adult man) will take many months.

Blood Loss

Gastrointestinal Blood Loss In men and in postmenopausal women, iron deficiency is most commonly caused by chronic bleeding from the gastrointestinal tract. Table 11-1 lists the causes of such blood loss. After history and physical examination rule out an obvious bleeding source in the genitourinary or respiratory tracts, evaluation of the gastrointestinal tract[10] is necessary because of the potential that the pathologic process causing the blood loss is life-threatening. In the adult, the most common causes are peptic ulcer, erosion in a hiatal hernia, gastritis (including that caused by alcohol or aspirin ingestion), hemorrhoids, vascular anomalies (such as angiodysplasia), and neoplasms.

Gastritis, Varices, Ulcers, and Inflammation Gastritis caused by drug ingestion is a common cause of bleeding. Aspirin, indomethacin, ibuprofen, or other nonsteroidal anti-inflammatory drugs cause gastritis but may also cause bleeding by inducing gastric or duodenal ulcers, or lesions in the small intestine[11] and even the colon. Gastritis caused by alcohol ingestion[12] can also cause significant blood loss. Chronic blood loss is often the cause of anemia in rheumatoid arthritis (perhaps because of the use of nonsteroidal anti-inflammatory medications), in inflammatory bowel disease, and in chronic kidney disease even in patients who are not on hemodialysis.

Chronic blood loss from esophageal or gastric varices can lead to iron-deficiency anemia. Hemorrhoidal bleeding may lead to severe iron-deficiency anemia. Chronic blood loss may result from diffuse gastric mucosal hypertrophy (Ménétrier disease).[13] Peptic ulcers of the stomach or duodenum are common causes of iron deficiency, and an association between infection with *Helicobacter pylori* and iron-deficiency anemia has been documented in numerous studies.[14] Some of these iron-deficient patients who are infected with *H. pylori* do not respond to oral iron therapy alone but do respond to eradication of *H. pylori*.[15]

Gastric ulceration and bleeding can also occur in disorders of hypergastrinemia, as in Zollinger-Ellison syndrome and pseudo–Zollinger-Ellison syndrome. Although concerns were raised that long-term medical therapy of these disorders with proton pump inhibitors would also cause iron deficiency by raising gastric pH and making iron less soluble, this does not seem to be the case.[16] Anemia that follows subtotal gastrectomy is usually attributed to reduced absorption of dietary iron (see "Malabsorption of Iron," further), but occult intermittent gastrointestinal bleeding from gastrointestinal lesions may also be a contributory factor and requires endoscopic evaluation.[17]

Diaphragmatic Hernia Diaphragmatic (hiatal) hernia is often associated with gastrointestinal bleeding.[18-20] The frequency of anemia ranges from 8% to 38%. Bleeding is much more likely to occur in patients with paraesophageal or large hernias than in those with sliding hernias or small ones. Mucosal changes cannot always be demonstrated by esophagoscopy or gastroscopy in patients who have had blood loss from hiatus hernia. However, a linear gastric erosion, also called a "Cameron ulcer," commonly occurs on the crests of mucosal folds at the level of the diaphragm and appears to be the site of bleeding.[21]

TABLE 11–1. Sources of Blood Loss

Alimentary Tract

Esophagus

Varices

Stomach and duodenum

   Ulcer

   Hiatus hernia

   Gastritis

   Carcinoma

   Varices

   Angiodysplasia

   Hemangioma

   Leiomyoma (Ménétrier disease)

   Mucosal hypertrophy

   Hypergastrinemia

   Antral vascular ectasia

   "Watermelon stomach"

Small intestine

   Vascular ectasia

   Tumors

   Ulceration

   Meckel's diverticulum

Colon and anorectal

   Hemorrhoids

   Carcinoma

   Polyp

   Diverticulum

   Ulcerative colitis

   Angiodysplasia

   Hemangioma

   Telangiectasia

   Amebiasis

Biliary Tract

Intrahepatic bleeding

Carcinoma

Cholelithiasis

Trauma

Ruptured aneurysm

Aberrant pancreas

Genitourinary Tract

Menorrhagia

Uterine fibroids

Endometriosis

Carcinoma

Vascular abnormalities

Respiratory Tract

Epistaxis

Carcinoma

Infections

Telangiectases

Idiopathic pulmonary hemosiderosis

Intestinal Parasitism Hookworms are a major cause of gastrointestinal blood loss in many parts of the world.[22]

Vascular Anomalies The lesions of angiodysplasia may occur in any part of the gastrointestinal tract.[23] These tiny vascular anomalies may be the cause of significant blood loss. Endoscopy is usually required for diagnosis, and often needs to be repeated because bleeding can be intermittent. Gastric antral vascular ectasia[24] exhibits a characteristic endoscopic appearance ("watermelon stomach") and is another cause of blood loss. Hemorrhage into the biliary tract is a rare cause of chronic iron-deficiency anemia.[25]

Tortuous, dilated sublingual venous structures, the cherry hemangiomas commonly seen in the elderly, and the spider telangiectases of chronic liver disease are usually easily distinguished from the lesions of hereditary hemorrhagic telangiectasia. Bleeding from intestinal telangiectases has also been observed in scleroderma[26] and Turner syndrome[27] as a manifestation of bleeding from abnormal blood vessels. Cutaneous hemangiomas (blue rubber bleb nevus) may be associated with hemorrhage from intestinal hemangiomas.[28]

In hereditary hemorrhagic telangiectasia, characteristic lesions commonly occur on fingertips, nasal septum, tongue, lips, margins (helices) of ears, oral and pharyngeal mucosa, palms and soles, and other epithelial and cutaneous surfaces throughout the body. Those lesions that occur in the gastrointestinal tract are particularly likely to bleed and to cause intractable iron deficiency.

Meckel Diverticulum Meckel diverticulum is a very common abnormality representing a vestigial remnant of the omphalomesenteric duct. In children, bleeding from this structure accounts for a small proportion of cases of iron-deficiency anemia.[29]

Genitourinary Tract Heavy menstrual bleeding[30] is a common cause of iron deficiency. The amount of blood lost with menstruation[31] varies markedly from one woman to another and is often difficult to evaluate by questioning the patient. The average menstrual blood loss is approximately 40 mL per cycle. Blood loss exceeds 80 mL (equivalent to ~30 mg of iron) per cycle in only 10% of women. The volume of blood lost during one menstrual cycle may be as high as 495 mL in apparently healthy, nonanemic women who do not regard their menstrual flow to be excessive. The amount of menstrual blood lost does not seem to vary markedly from one cycle to another for any given individual. Oral contraceptives reduce menstrual blood loss, but the use of an intrauterine coil for contraception increases menstrual blood loss, especially during the first year of use. Because the daily dietary intake of iron is usually between 10 and 12 mg and only a few milligrams of this can be absorbed, iron balance in many menstruating women is precarious.

Excessive bleeding may be caused by uterine fibroids and malignant neoplasms. Neoplasms, stones, or inflammatory disease of the kidney, ureter, or bladder may cause enough chronic blood loss to produce iron deficiency.

In the absence of hematuria, urinary iron losses as high as 1 mg/day have been reported in rare patients with nephrotic syndrome, some of whom had hypoferremia and hypochromic anemia.[32] We found only one report of a patient in whom abnormally high urinary iron loss may have caused anemia without proteinuria or hematuria.[33]

Bleeding Disorders Hemostatic defects, particularly those related to abnormal platelet function or number may lead to gastrointestinal bleeding, although unless the thrombocytopenia or platelet dysfunction is severe, gastrointestinal bleeding usually signifies an abnormality in the gastrointestinal tract. Gastrointestinal bleeding is common in von Willebrand disease but often because of coexistent peptic ulcer disease. Polycythemia vera is typically associated with iron deficiency as a result of the shift of iron into the increased erythrocyte mass, spontaneous gastrointestinal hemorrhage that commonly occurs in this disorder, or phlebotomy therapy, or a combination of these mechanisms.

When a patient with a disorder of hemostasis suffers from gastrointestinal bleeding, one must consider the possibility that the bleeding may not be caused by a hemostatic defect alone, but that an anatomic lesion of the gastrointestinal tract may also be present.

Nosocomial (Iatrogenic) Anemia Iatrogenic anemia is particularly prevalent in intensive care units,[34] where repetitive blood sampling may result in removal of 40 to 70 mL of blood daily, and this iatrogenic phlebotomy can result in iron-deficiency anemia.

The use of extracorporeal dialysis for treatment of chronic renal disease may cause iron deficiency,[35,36] often superimposed upon the anemia of chronic renal disease (Chaps. 3 and 6). Patients treated with chronic hemodialysis who experience multiple sources of blood loss with the dialysis equipment is a major cause, along with gastrointestinal bleeding, blood sampling, and bleeding related to vascular access.

Anemia from Blood Donation Each whole-blood donation removes approximately 200 mg of iron from the body. Lesser amounts of iron are removed in the course of donating platelets or leukocytes. Potential donors are screened in blood banks, so that those with frank anemia are not phlebotomized. Yet, by the time they are excluded from donation, some blood donors are iron-depleted[37-39] and may readily develop iron-deficiency anemia with relatively small additional blood loss. High school-age donors (16-18 years old) may be particularly susceptible to the development of iron deficiency after blood donation.[40]

Factitious Anemia Factitious anemia caused by self-inflicted bleeding may present a formidable diagnostic and therapeutic problem. This rare condition has also been called, in literary allusion to a fictitious character, "Lasthénie de Ferjol syndrome" (in Barbey d'Aurevilly's gloomy novel, *Une Histoire Sans Nom*), or part of Munchausen syndrome (based on the Rudolf Raspe book, *The Surprising Adventures of Baron Münchausen*).[41,42] Most patients are women, and patients are often employed in a medical setting. There is often a history of numerous blood transfusions. The anemia is chronic and may be severe. The site of induced blood loss is obscure. Hence, patients are subjected to numerous radiographic and endoscopic examinations, usually to no avail. The patients are usually refractory to medical advice and therapy. The patients may be depressed and suicidal; some also suffer anorexia nervosa. Psychiatric care is needed, but often is unsuccessful. Rarely, the outcome of self-bleeding may be fatal.[43]

Cow's-Milk Anemia Ingestion of whole cow's milk may induce protein-losing enteropathy and gastrointestinal bleeding in infants,[44,45] probably on the basis of hypersensitivity or allergy. In four such cases observed endoscopically, erosive gastritis or gastroduodenitis was demonstrated as the probable source of bleeding. At least during the first year of life, children should not be given whole bovine milk, either raw or pasteurized. More protracted heating, as in preparation of infant formulas, eliminates this problem. Intrinsic lesions of the gastrointestinal tract, such as those listed earlier, may cause bleeding in infants and older children.

Respiratory Tract Persistent recurrent hemoptysis may lead to iron-deficiency anemia. It may be a result of congenital anomalies of the respiratory tract, endobronchial vascular anomalies, chronic infections, neoplasms, or valvular heart disease. Severe iron-deficiency anemia is a manifestation of idiopathic pulmonary hemosiderosis[46] and of Goodpasture syndrome (progressive glomerulonephritis with intrapulmonary hemorrhage). In some of these disorders, hemoptysis may not be observed, but sufficient amounts of blood-laden sputum may be swallowed to result in positive tests for occult blood in the stools. Iron deficiency occurs in a large proportion of patients with cystic fibrosis[47,48] and occurs even in the absence of hemoptysis, suggesting that inflammatory inhibition of dietary iron absorption and iron loss in purulent sputum could contribute to the deficiency.

Pregnancy and Parturition

Although physiologic decrease in Hb concentration is an expected consequence of hemodilution associated with pregnancy, true iron deficiency frequently results in more severe anemia. In pregnancy, the average iron loss resulting from diversion of iron to the fetus, blood loss at delivery (equivalent to an average of 150-200 mg of iron), and lactation is altogether approximately 900 mg; in terms of iron content, this is equivalent to the loss of more than 2 L of blood. Approximately 30 mg of iron may be expended monthly in lactation. Because most women begin pregnancy with low iron reserves, these additional demands frequently result in iron-deficiency anemia. Iron depletion has been reported in some 85% to 100% of pregnant women. Iron-deficient mothers are likely to have smaller babies. The incidence of anemia and iron deficiency is lower in women who take oral iron supplementation, daily or intermittently.[49-52] In regions with endemic malaria, iron supplementation may increase the risk of malaria and some experts recommend that it be combined with malarial prophylaxis.[53] Most agree that oral iron supplementation during pregnancy is desirable despite its side effects. Increasing safety and convenience of parenteral iron therapy may lead to reevaluation of its role in the prevention and treatment of iron-deficiency anemia of pregnancy.[54]

Dietary Iron Deficiency

In infants, iron deficiency is most often a result of the use of unsupplemented milk diets, which contain an inadequate amount of iron. During the first year of life, a full-term infant requires approximately 160 mg and the premature infant approximately 240 mg of iron to meet the needs of an expanding red cell mass. Approximately 50 mg of this need is fulfilled by the destruction of erythrocytes that occurs physiologically during the first week of life (Chap. 2). The rest must come from the diet. Milk products are very poor sources of iron, and prolonged breast- or bottle-feeding of infants frequently leads to iron-deficiency anemia unless iron supplementation is implemented. This is especially true of premature infants. The European Society for Pediatric Gastroenterology, Hepatology, and Nutrition (ESPGHAN) Committee on Nutrition has urged that all infant formulas be iron-fortified[55]; in North America, the use of iron-fortified formula is now generally accepted, but there is controversy about the appropriate level of fortification.[56] In older children, an iron-poor diet may also contribute to the development of iron-deficiency anemia, particularly during rapid growth periods.

Infants and young women are usually in precarious iron balance, their iron intake being less than 80% of the recommended daily allowance (RDA).[57] Fortification of bread and cereals with ferrous sulfate or metallic iron is commonplace. This practice was suspended in Sweden because of concern for the possibility of increasing iron storage in patients with the hemochromatosis genotype, resulting in increased incidence of iron-deficiency anemia.[58]

The scant iron supply of the American diet places young women and children at particular risk of negative iron balance. Because the adult male needs to absorb only approximately 1 mg iron daily from his diet to maintain normal iron balance, iron deficiency in older men is very rarely caused by insufficient dietary intake alone.

Malabsorption of Iron

Gastric secretion of hydrochloric acid is often reduced in iron deficiency.[59] Histamine-fast achlorhydria has been found in as much as 43% of patients with iron deficiency. In persons older than 30 years, the achlorhydria is usually irreversible. Furthermore, when atrophic gastritis coexists with iron deficiency, no improvement in gastric secretory function has followed iron therapy. Autoimmune gastritis often associated with *H. pylori* infection[14,15] may play an important role in both iron-deficiency anemia and, in later life, in the development of pernicious anemia.

Intestinal malabsorption of iron is quite an uncommon cause of iron deficiency except after gastrointestinal surgery and in malabsorption syndromes. Iron-deficiency anemia develops years later in 10% to 34% of patients who have undergone subtotal gastric resection. Many such patients have impaired absorption of food iron, caused in part by more rapid gastrojejunal transit and in part by partially digested food bypassing some of the duodenum as a result of the location of the anastomosis. Fortunately, medicinal iron is well absorbed in post–partial gastrectomy patients. Moreover, gastrointestinal blood loss may also play an important role in anemia after gastric resection (see "Gastrointestinal Blood Loss," earlier). In malabsorption syndromes, absorption of iron may be so limited that iron-deficiency anemia develops over a period of years. Celiac disease, whether overt or occult, may be associated with iron-deficiency anemia.[14,15,60,61]

Intravascular Hemolysis and Hemoglobinuria

Iron-deficiency anemia may occur in paroxysmal nocturnal hemoglobinuria (Chap. 8) and in hemolysis resulting from mechanical erythrocyte trauma from intracardiac myxomas, valvular prostheses, or patches (Chaps. 3 and 22). In these disorders, up to 10 mg/day of iron is lost in the urine as hemosiderin and ferritin in desquamated tubular cells, and as Hb dimers, an amount sufficient to cause systemic iron deficiency.[62,63]

Iron deficiency occurs frequently in athletes engaged in a variety of sports (Chaps. 3 and 22), affecting female athletes especially.[64] There may be mild anemia. Increased intravascular hemolysis, presumably with some renal loss of iron, may play a role, but gastrointestinal blood loss has also been demonstrated in persons engaged in strenuous athletic pursuits. Hemoglobinuria and hemosiderinuria is also seen in competitive and recreational runners, that is, *march hemoglobinuria* (Chaps. 3 and 22). Strenuous exercise also elicits a rise in serum IL-6 and hepcidin, and this could decrease dietary iron absorption.[64]

Women soldiers undergoing basic training experience iron depletion as determined by serum ferritin measurements, and this can be partially reversed by iron supplementation.[65] The etiology may be comparable to the iron deficiency seen in athletes.

Genetic Factors

Based on twin studies,[66] genetic factors play a role in iron deficiency. Mutations in multiple genes including *HFE* (*high Fe*) and transferrin show weak associations with iron measures but only mutations of the membrane serine protease Tmprss6[67] have been identified in genome-wide association studies as genetic factors that cause or predispose to iron deficiency. The genetic syndrome of iron-refractory iron-deficiency anemia is mediated by inappropriately increased hepcidin as a result of homozygous or compound heterozygous mutations in Tmprss6.[68-70] Increased hepcidin diminishes iron absorption and causes inappropriate retention of available iron in splenic macrophages and Kupffer cells.

PATHOGENESIS

As iron deficiency develops, different compartments are depleted in iron in an overlapping sequence, as illustrated schematically in Fig. 11-1.

Iron-Containing Proteins

As the body becomes depleted of iron, changes occur in many tissues. Hemosiderin and ferritin virtually disappear from marrow and other storage sites. Hb synthesis in the marrow decreases, first as a result of fewer erythroblasts[71] but eventually also per erythroblast if iron deficiency becomes more severe, resulting in Hb-deficient erythrocytes. The concentration of many other iron-containing proteins is affected;

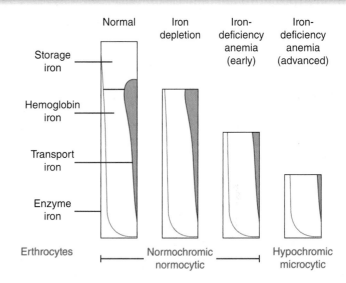

FIGURE 11–1. Stages in the development of iron deficiency. Early iron deficiency (iron depletion) is usually not accompanied by any abnormalities in blood; at this stage, serum iron concentration is occasionally below normal values and storage iron is markedly depleted. As iron deficiency progresses, development of anemia precedes appearance of morphologic changes in blood, although some cells may be smaller and paler than normal; serum iron concentration is usually low at this time, but it may be normal. With advanced iron depletion, classic changes of hypochromic, microcytic, hypoferremic anemia become manifest.

often in an organ-specific manner.[72] Studies in laboratory animals on defined iron-deficient diets are most informative about this process, because human iron deficiency is often confounded by other forms of malnutrition. In such models of severe (pure) iron deficiency, skeletal muscle myoglobin is mildly depleted but cardiac myoglobin is not. Cytochromes and other mitochondrial ferroproteins are depleted but selectively so. Because these classical studies were performed, it has become apparent that the synthesis of many ferroproteins is regulated in an iron-dependent manner, mainly via the iron-responsive element/iron-regulatory protein (IRE/IRP) system (Chap. 10). The selective changes in iron-containing proteins may thus be adaptive[73] to allow the survival of the organism until more iron becomes available.

Muscular Function and Exercise Tolerance

Decrements in high-intensity exercise performance can be detected even during nonanemic iron deficiency,[64] and then worsen with increasing anemia.[74] The limitation of high-level exercise by oxygen (O_2) delivery and therefore Hb content of blood is well known, and has given rise to surreptitious blood doping and erythropoietin abuse by athletes. The impairment of performance during nonanemic iron deficiency consists of decreased spontaneous activity (seen in humans and in animal models) and decreased ventilatory threshold, that is, the point at which ventilation starts increasing more rapidly than O_2 consumption.[75] Other deficits that have been reported include decreased endurance and increased muscle fatigue. The biochemical basis of the deficits associated with nonanemic iron deficiency is not well understood but has been attributed to the depletion of iron-containing mitochondrial proteins that are involved in energy metabolism.[64] The condition is reversible with iron supplementation.

Neurologic Changes

Iron deficiency is associated with both developmental abnormalities in children and with restless leg syndrome in adults but in neither case has iron deficiency been established as the primary cause.[76,77] The substantia nigra is a particularly iron-rich region of the brain and contains dopaminergic neurons that are suspected of involvement in restless leg syndrome. In mouse models of iron deficiency, iron depletion of the substantia nigra is highly strain-dependent,[78] suggesting that iron deficiency, and as yet incompletely characterized genetic variations, may cooperate in the pathogenesis of restless leg syndrome by allowing the depletion of iron from susceptible brain regions involved in dopaminergic signaling.[79]

Host Defense and Inflammation

In multiple publications, iron deficiency was reported to impair various immune functions, but the effects appeared to be minor and inconsistent.[80] Certain transferrin receptor-1 mutations were found to cause mild anemia with severe combined immunodeficiency,[81] which was shown to be caused by iron deficiency that disproportionately affected lymphocytes. Systematic studies of responses to vaccination documented the deleterious effects of iron deficiency on the efficacy of common vaccines,[82] effects which could be reversed by iron administration. The likely common mechanism[83] by which iron deficiency impairs adaptive immunity is the high requirement of lymphocytes for iron during clonal expansion induced by antigen recognition. Perhaps surprisingly, the evidence for a narrowly protective and proinflammatory effect of iron deficiency appears strong also. Iron deficiency decreases the risk and severity of malaria (Chap. 24),[84,85] and iron supplementation may have the opposite effect, especially when not targeted to patients with iron deficiency.[53,86] The mechanism of this effect is of great interest but is not yet well understood.[87] There are some indications that iron deficiency may have a proinflammatory effect. In a mouse model, iron deficiency potentiated the systemic effect of lipopolysaccharide in a hepcidin-dependent manner,[88] and in a mouse model of asthma, iron deficiency promoted allergic inflammation.[89]

Growth and Metabolism

Iron-deficient children have been reported to suffer from growth retardation, but it is difficult to isolate the effect of iron deficiency from other nutritional and environmental causes of stunting. Two comprehensive analyses of randomized controlled trials did not detect an effect on growth of iron supplementation alone.[90,91] Decreased thermoregulation in response to cold exposure is seen in both humans and laboratory models.[92] It has been attributed to the conflicting effects on blood flow of decreased O_2 content of blood and the need to minimize heat loss, as well as the effect of iron deficiency on thyroid function.

Histologic Findings

Severe iron deficiency may lead to histologic changes in various organs. The rapidly proliferating cells of the upper part of the alimentary tract seem particularly susceptible to the effect of iron deficiency. There may be atrophy of the mucosa of the tongue and esophagus,[93] stomach,[94] and small intestine.[95] The epithelium of the lateral margins of the tongue is reduced in thickness despite an increase in the progenitor compartment. This thinning presumably reflects accelerated exfoliation of epithelial cells.[96] Buccal mucosa has shown thinning and keratinization of epithelium and increased mitotic activity.[97,98] However, light microscopic and electron microscopic examination of exfoliated oral mucosal cells showed no aberrations in morphology of nuclei or cytoplasm of the cells of patients with iron-deficiency anemia.[99] In iron-deficiency anemia resulting from idiopathic pulmonary hemosiderosis, characteristic pathologic changes are found in the lungs, including intense deposition of iron in the littoral cells of the alveoli and interstitial fibrosis.[46]

Widening of diploic spaces of bones, particularly those of the skull and hands,[100-102] may be a consequence of chronic iron deficiency

beginning in infancy. In the skull, this is of the same character as in thalassemia, except that in β-thalassemia major there is maxillary hypertrophy, whereas in severe iron-deficiency anemia, maxillary growth and pneumatization are normal.

CLINICAL FEATURES

Clinical Manifestations of Anemia

The anemia in iron-deficient patients can be severe, with blood Hb levels lower than 4 g/dL reported in some patients. Severe iron-deficiency anemia is associated with all of the various symptoms of anemia, resulting from hypoxia and the body's response to hypoxia, as described in Chap. 3. Thus, tachycardia with palpitations and pounding in the ears, headache, light-headedness, and even angina pectoris may all occur in patients who are severely anemic.

Clinical Manifestations That May Be Unrelated to Anemia

In addition to symptoms caused by the anemia, there are clinical features attributed to iron deficiency itself. Several controlled studies showed that various manifestations of iron deficiency can occur in individuals whose Hb is within the accepted normal range.

Decreased Work Performance Objective measurements of work performance and studies using O_2 consumption as an index of work performance have given contradictory results, but a comprehensive review led to the conclusion that severe iron-deficiency anemia (Hb <80 g/L) and mild iron-deficiency anemia (Hb between 80 and 120 g/L) led to decreased work performance, primarily as estimated by peak O_2 consumption (VO_2max) measurements, but the evidence that nonanemic iron deficiency had such an effect was less convincing.[103] However, in athletes with low ferritin levels but normal Hb levels, iron-supplemented subjects showed an increased VO_2max without a change in their red cell mass, and in other studies nonanemic subjects treated with iron showed improved performance and/or VO_2max.[64]

Infant and Childhood Development It has been reported that in infants and children, iron deficiency is associated with poor attention span, poor response to sensory stimuli, and retarded behavioral and developmental achievement even in the absence of anemia. The causality of these associations is confounded by other coexisting nutritional deficits and socioeconomic deprivation, so reversibility by iron supplementation would be important in establishing causality. However, in systematic meta-analyses, iron supplementation had weak or no effects on these deficits.[90,104-106]

Hyperactivity Syndromes It has been speculated that there is a relationship between restless legs syndrome, Tourette syndrome, and attention-deficit/hyperactivity disorder and that iron deficiency contributes to their pathophysiology. Restless legs syndrome, a common nocturnal problem, especially in older adults, has been associated with iron deficiency and has reportedly improved with iron therapy, but the beneficial effects have been inconsistent and not well predicted by blood ferritin or transferrin saturation.[76,107,108] It is possible that iron deficiency is an important contributor to the pathogenesis of the disorder in a specific subgroup of patients with restless leg syndrome and, if so, identifying such patients is important because treatment with iron causes fewer side effects than other therapeutic modalities.[109] In children there may be a relationship between iron deficiency and attention-deficit/hyperactivity disorder but the association is inconsistent.[110]

Other Neurologic Symptoms Breath holding in children, headaches, and paresthesia have been attributed to iron deficiency, but there are no controlled studies to support this impression. Anecdotal reports of intracranial hypertension with papilledema are supported by apparent response to iron therapy.[111-114] Stroke in children and in adults, possibly triggered by thrombocytosis, has been associated with iron-deficiency anemia.[115-119]

Oral and Nasopharyngeal Symptoms Burning of the tongue has also been described anecdotally in many accounts of iron deficiency, and although this symptom has been observed to diminish with treatment, no controlled studies have been performed. The tongue symptoms could be a result of concurrent pyridoxine deficiency. Although iron deficiency has been proposed as a cause of atrophic rhinitis, the evidence for this is weak.

Dysphagia In the laryngopharynx, mucosal atrophy may lead to web formation in the postcricoid region, thereby giving rise to dysphagia (Paterson-Kelly or Plummer-Vinson syndrome).[120] If these alterations are of long duration, they may lead to pharyngeal carcinoma. Although it has been generally thought that these changes are secondary to long-standing iron deficiency, this mechanism is not universally accepted. The frequency of the condition is considered to have decreased considerably, and it is remarkably rare in many parts of the world where iron deficiency is common.

Pica The craving to eat unusual substances, for example, dirt, clay, ice, laundry starch, salt, cardboard, and hair, is a well-documented manifestation of iron deficiency and is usually cured promptly by iron therapy.[121-124]

Hair Loss Although the association of hair loss with iron deficiency is controversial,[125] low ferritin levels were a risk factor for hair loss in a large multivariate analysis.[126] Remarkably, hair loss sparing the face ("mask mouse") is a sign of iron deficiency in mice.[127]

Physical Findings

The physical findings in iron-deficiency anemia include pallor, glossitis (smooth, red tongue), stomatitis, and angular cheilitis. Koilonychia (spoon nails), once a common finding, is now encountered rarely. Retinal hemorrhages and exudates may be seen in severely anemic patients (eg, Hb concentration <50 g/L). Splenomegaly has occasionally been attributed to iron-deficiency anemia, but when it occurs, it is probably from other causes.

LABORATORY FEATURES

In severe, uncomplicated iron-deficiency anemia, the erythrocytes are hypochromic and microcytic, the plasma iron concentration is diminished, the iron-binding capacity is increased, the serum ferritin concentration is low, the serum transferrin receptor (sTfR) and erythrocyte zinc protoporphyrin concentrations are increased, and the marrow is depleted of stainable iron. However, the classic combination of laboratory findings occurs consistently only when iron-deficiency anemia is far advanced, when there are no complicating factors such as infection or malignant neoplasms, and when there has not been previous therapy with transfusions or parenteral iron.

Blood Cells

Erythrocytes Anisocytosis is the earliest recognizable morphologic change of erythrocytes in iron-deficiency anemia (Fig. 11-2).[128] The anisocytosis is typically accompanied by mild ovalocytosis. As the iron deficiency worsens, a mild normochromic, normocytic anemia often develops. With further progression, Hb concentration, erythrocyte count, mean corpuscular volume (MCV), and mean erythrocyte Hb content all decline together.[129,130] As the indices change, the erythrocytes appear microcytic and hypochromic on stained blood films. Target cells may sometimes be present. Elongated hypochromic elliptocytes may be seen, in which the long sides are nearly parallel. Such cells have been called "pencil cells," although they more nearly resemble cigars in shape.

The red cell indices are consistently abnormal in adults only when iron-deficiency anemia is moderate or severe (eg, in men with Hb concentrations <120 g/L or in women with Hb concentrations <100 g/L) (Fig. 11-3). The distribution of erythrocyte volume (eg, red cell distribution width [RDW]) is usually increased in established iron-deficiency anemia. The RDW is reported often as the coefficient of variation (in percent) of erythrocyte volume (see "Differential Diagnosis," further).

Leukocytes Leukopenia has been found in some patients with iron-deficiency anemia, but the overall distribution of leukocyte counts in iron-deficient patients seems to be approximately normal.

Platelets Both thrombocytopenia[131] and thrombocytosis[132] have been associated with iron deficiency. Platelet abnormalities correct with iron therapy. Thrombotic complications of iron deficiency have been reported but are rare.[133] The etiology of either abnormality is not known. A low-iron diet induced iron-deficiency anemia in a rat model within 2 weeks and this was accompanied by a sustained 50% increase in platelet count with increased platelet size, but without significant changes in known megakaryocyte growth factors (thrombopoietin, interleukin [IL] 6, or IL 11). It has been suggested that high erythropoietin levels may stimulate thrombopoietin receptors because the two hematopoietic

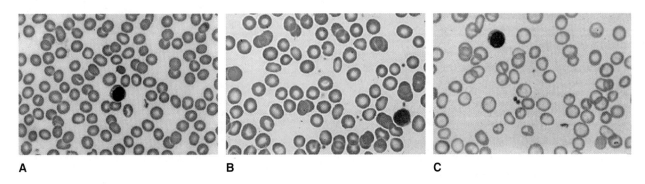

A   **B**   **C**

FIGURE 11–2. Variability in morphologic diagnosis of iron-deficiency anemia from blood film. As in all deficiency states leading to anemia, the blood film morphology and blood cell changes are a function of the severity of the deficiency. **A.** Normal blood film. Normocytic-normochromic red cells with normal shape. **B.** Mild iron deficiency. Serum iron, ferritin, and transferring saturation were consistent with mild iron deficiency. Cannot discern if mean red cell size has decreased. There may be a few red cells that have larger central pallor, but that is arguable. A few cells have oval or elliptical shape. **C.** Severe iron deficiency. Serum iron, ferritin, and transferring saturation were consistent with severe iron deficiency. Note obvious increase in overtly hypochromic cells and higher frequency of microcytes. *(Reproduced with permission from Lichtman MA, Shafer MS, Felgar RE, et al: Lichtman's Atlas of Hematology 2016. New York, NY: McGraw Hill; 2017.)*

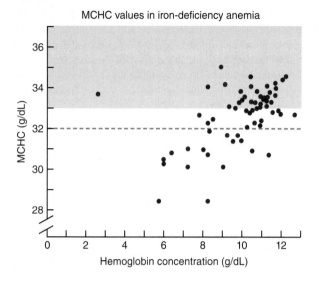

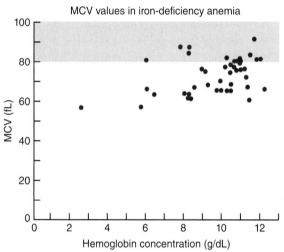

FIGURE 11–3. Erythrocyte indices in iron-deficiency anemia of adults; data obtained with Coulter Counter, Model S. Normal ranges of indices observed in approximately 500 healthy adults using the same instrument are indicated by shading. The *dashed line* in the *top panel* indicates the more widely accepted lower normal limit of mean corpuscular hemoglobin concentrations (MCHCs) stated in this text. *(Top)* Correlation between venous blood hemoglobin concentration and MCHC. More than half of 62 patients with iron-deficiency anemia had MCHC values clearly in the normal range. *(Bottom)* Correlation between venous blood hemoglobin concentrations and mean corpuscular volume (MCV). Nearly 70% of cases exhibited distinct microcytosis. Thus, when indices are determined by automated cell-counting methods, the MCV is much more sensitive than is the MCHC in detecting changes of iron deficiency. However, at least 30% of cases of iron-deficiency anemia will be misdiagnosed if physicians rely on the erythrocyte indices. *(Data from Klee GG. Decision Rules for Accelerated Hematology Laboratory Investigation. Thesis, University of Minnesota.)*

factors are structurally related, but this does not seem to be the case.[134] Most recent studies suggest that low iron biases the commitment of megakaryocytic-erythroid progenitors toward the megakaryocytic lineage in both human and mouse.[135]

Reticulocytes Reticulocyte count is often mildly increased,[136] a finding consistent with the increased erythroid activity of the marrow (see "Marrow," next).

Marrow

Because most of the iron in the body is normally in erythrocytes, and iron is not excreted, decrease in erythrocyte mass generally results in increased storage iron. Iron-deficiency anemia is the exception, because iron stores are depleted before the red cell mass is compromised. Thus, evaluation of iron stores should be a sensitive and usually reliable means for the differentiation between iron-deficiency anemia and all other anemias. Decreased or absent hemosiderin in the marrow is characteristic of iron deficiency and is readily evaluated after staining by the Prussian blue method. Stored iron in the macrophages of the marrow can be seen in marrow spicules in marrow sections, or in marrow aspirate films. Iron granules, normally found in the cytoplasm of approximately 30% of erythroblasts, become rare but may not be entirely absent.

Evaluation of the amount of iron in marrow macrophages has long been considered the "gold standard" for the diagnosis of iron deficiency. There are, however, technical barriers to the accurate histochemical determination of marrow iron. First, an invasive procedure, marrow aspiration, is required. Second, identifying the differentiation of iron within macrophages from artifacts takes experience and skill. In one study, only 74 of 108 cases had been accurately reported.[137] Moreover, misleading results may be obtained in patients who have been transfused or who have been treated with parenteral iron.[138] The marrow of such patients may contain normal, or even increased, quantities of stainable iron in the face of typical iron-responsive iron-deficiency anemia. In such patients, iron that is seen on marrow examination is not readily available for erythropoiesis. As serum markers of iron deficiency became widely available, the reasons for the primacy of marrow iron estimation have been questioned.[139]

Serum Iron Concentration

The serum iron concentration is usually low in untreated iron-deficiency anemia but may rarely be normal.[130,140,141] Iron in blood plasma turns over every few hours and constitutes less than 0.1% of total body iron in adults, so iron concentrations are readily perturbed by transient changes in iron supply or demand. Physiologically, the serum iron concentration has a diurnal rhythm; it decreases in late afternoon and evening, reaching a nadir near 9 pm and increases to its maximum between 7 am and 10 am. This effect is rarely of sufficient magnitude to influence diagnosis.[142] Serum iron levels decrease at about the time of menstrual bleeding[143,144] regardless of whether the bleeding is physiologic or induced by withdrawal of contraceptive hormonal preparations.

Importantly, the serum iron concentration is reduced in the presence of either acute or chronic inflammatory processes[145] or malignancy[146] and after acute myocardial infarction.[147,148] The serum iron concentration under these circumstances may be decreased sufficiently to suggest iron deficiency. Conversely, during chemotherapy of malignancy, the serum iron concentration may be quite elevated, because cytotoxic effects of the drugs on erythroblasts inhibit erythropoiesis and related iron consumption. This effect is observed from the third to the seventh day after inception of chemotherapy of a variety of tumors.[149]

Normal or high concentrations of serum iron are commonly observed even in patients with iron-deficiency anemia if such patients receive iron medication before blood is drawn for these measurements. Even multivitamin preparations, which commonly contain approximately 18 mg of elemental iron per tablet, can cause this effect. Oral iron medication should be withheld for 24 hours before blood samples are obtained. Parenteral injection of iron dextran may result in a very high serum iron concentration (eg, 500-1000 mcg/dL), at least with some methods,[150] for several weeks. The elevation of serum iron levels after infusion of sodium ferric gluconate or iron sucrose is of much shorter duration.[151]

Iron-Binding Capacity and Transferrin Saturation

The iron-binding capacity is a measure of the amount of transferrin in circulating blood. Normally, there is enough transferrin present in 1 L of serum to bind 44 to 80 μmol (2.5-4.5 mg) of iron; because the normal serum iron concentration is approximately 18 μmol/L (1 mg/L), transferrin may be found to be approximately one-third saturated with iron. The unsaturated or latent iron-binding capacity (UIBC) is easily measured with radioactive iron or by spectrophotometric techniques. The sum of the UIBC and the plasma iron represents total iron-binding capacity (TIBC). TIBC may also be measured directly. In iron-deficiency anemia, UIBC and TIBC are often increased and serum iron concentrations are decreased so that transferrin saturation of 15% or less is usually found. Because transferrin concentration and TIBC are decreased during inflammation, a normal value for transferrin saturation often accompanies a low serum iron concentration in the anemia of chronic inflammation.

Serum Ferritin

Serum ferritin, secreted mainly by macrophages[152] and hepatocytes, contains relatively little iron, yet serum ferritin concentration empirically correlates with total body iron stores,[153] for reasons that are still obscure. Serum ferritin concentrations of 10 mcg/L or less are characteristic of iron-deficiency anemia. In iron deficiency without anemia, serum ferritin concentration is typically in the range of 10 to 20 mcg/L. An increase in serum ferritin concentration occurs in inflammatory disorders, such as rheumatoid arthritis, in chronic renal disease, and in malignancies.[154] When one of these conditions coexists with iron deficiency, as they often do, the serum ferritin concentration is commonly in the normal range; interpretation of results of this assay then becomes difficult. In patients with rheumatoid arthritis who are anemic, some suggest that concomitant iron deficiency may be suspected when the serum ferritin concentration is less than 60 mcg/L,[155] but such empiric guidelines cannot possibly apply to the full spectrum of severity of inflammation. Increased serum ferritin concentrations are also characteristic of some malignancies, acute and chronic liver disease, and chronic renal failure.[156-159] In Gaucher disease, juvenile rheumatoid arthritis and various macrophage activation syndromes, and in ferroportin disease characterized by massive iron loading of macrophages, the serum ferritin concentration is commonly in the range of thousands of micrograms per liter and may mask iron deficiency.[160-164]

Erythrocyte Zinc Protoporphyrin

Erythrocyte protoporphyrin, principally zinc protoporphyrin, is increased in disorders of heme synthesis, including iron deficiency, lead poisoning, and sideroblastic anemias, as well as other conditions.[165-167] This assay analyzes the fluorescence of erythrocytes and utilizes small blood samples. It is quite sensitive in the diagnosis of iron deficiency and practical for large-scale screening programs designed to identify children with either iron deficiency or lead poisoning.[59,165] It does not differentiate between iron deficiency and anemia that accompanies inflammatory or malignant processes.[168] However, the specificity for iron deficiency of fluorescence-based determination of erythrocyte protoporphyrin is low, presumably because of interference by other fluorescent substances in blood.[169]

Serum Transferrin Receptor

The transferrin receptor (TfR) transports transferrin iron into cells (see "*SLC40A1* [Ferroportin] Mutations"). The circulating soluble receptor is a truncated form of the cellular receptor, lacking the transmembrane and cytoplasmic domains of the cellular receptor. It circulates bound to transferrin. Sensitive immunologic methods can detect approximately 5 mg/L of receptor in serum. The levels of circulating TfR mirror the amount of cellular receptor, and therefore are proportional to the number of erythroblasts expressing the receptor and the number of receptors per erythroblast. Because receptor synthesis is greatly increased when cells lack iron, the amount of the circulating receptor increases in iron deficiency.[170,171] In anemia of inflammation, the synthesis of the TfR is suppressed by cytokines, and this negates the opposing stimulatory effect of iron restriction, resulting in a lower sTfR concentration than in pure iron deficiency.[172] This test for iron deficiency has gradually come into clinical use, but the methodology is incompletely standardized, making laboratory-to-laboratory comparisons difficult. A method for performing reproducible assays for the soluble TfR has been standardized.[173] Like the serum ferritin and serum iron, sTfR assay results may be confounded by poorly understood variations in patients with malignancies; in patients in whom the sTfR concentration is reduced; and in patients with asymptomatic malaria or thalassemia trait,[174,175] in whom it is increased in the absence of iron deficiency. The ratio of sTfR to serum ferritin seems to be a useful but not infallible reflection of body iron stores.[176] Moreover, several studies show that the soluble transferrin index calculated as a ratio of the sTfR/log ferritin (TfR-F Index) may be superior to other means for detection of iron deficiency.[177-179]

Reticulocyte Hemoglobin Content and Other Novel Erythrocyte Indices

Many automated hematology instruments offer a method for diagnosis of iron deficiency: an assay of Hb content within reticulocytes. This parameter is an indicator of iron restriction of Hb synthesis during 3 to 4 days before the test.[180,181] The percentage of hypochromic erythrocytes offers a longer-term assessment of iron restriction during the preceding few months.[180,182]

Serum Hepcidin

The iron-regulatory hormone hepcidin is feedback-regulated by plasma iron and hepatic iron stores, causing a rapid decrease of serum hepcidin concentrations during uncomplicated iron deficiency.[183-185] However, like ferritin, hepcidin is potently induced by inflammation and infection, diminishing its utility for the diagnosis of iron deficiency in complex settings. One potential advantage of serum hepcidin measurement over serum ferritin assay is that, as the iron regulatory hormone, hepcidin controls duodenal iron absorption and therefore predicts the effectiveness of oral iron therapeutics.[186] Multiple sensitive and specific methods for assaying serum or plasma hepcidin have been developed, and are undergoing worldwide harmonization[187] but as of early 2021, their use is limited to research settings and the diagnosis of rare iron disorders. Future technical advances and additional clinical validation should increase the usefulness of this assay.

DIFFERENTIAL DIAGNOSIS

Iron-deficiency anemia is characterized by many abnormal laboratory features. Because none of these are unique, a small deviation from normal will detect most cases of iron deficiency (high sensitivity), but also falsely identify non–iron-deficient subjects as being iron-deficient (low specificity). On the other hand, a large deviation from normal will exclude most nondeficient patients (high specificity) but miss many iron-deficient subjects (low sensitivity). This trade-off is shown graphically in so-called *receiver operator characteristic curves*. These curves are constructed by plotting the sensitivity against the false-positive rate (1-specificity) at various values of the analyte. Figure 11-4 shows a receiver operator characteristic curve for some tests for iron deficiency. The situation is complicated in the case of iron deficiency by the fact that the diagnostic problem faced by the physician is not one of differentiating a patient with iron-deficiency anemia from a normal person,

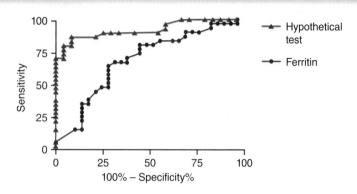

FIGURE 11–4. Two receiver operator curves. As the specificity increases, the sensitivity decreases. The receiver-operator properties of serum ferritin are far from ideal. When the specificity is high (to the *left on the abscissa*) the sensitivity is low; only when the specificity is low is the sensitivity adequate. The curve that would be obtained with a nearly ideal test for iron deficiency gives high specificity and high sensitivity. In the curve shown, a cutoff value could be found that allows one to identify 75% of patients with iron deficiency with a specificity of greater than 90%. Unfortunately, no such test exists.

TABLE 11–2. Microcytic Disorders Other Than Iron Deficiency	
Mechanisms	**Diseases**
Impaired globin chain synthesis or highly unstable hemoglobin	β-thalassemia or trait, α-thalassemia minima or minor, hemoglobin H, hemoglobin E or trait, combinations of above
Drugs or toxins that inhibit heme synthesis	Lead, isoniazid, pyrazinamide, sirolimus
Disorders that impair heme synthesis directly or by decreased iron delivery to erythroblasts, or decreased uptake or utilization of iron by erythroblasts	sideroblastic anemias, erythropoietic porphyrias, atransferrinemia,[212] aceruloplasminemia,[293] DMT-1 mutations,[216] STEAP3 deficiency[294]

Abbreviations: DMT, divalent metal transporter; STEAP3, six-transmembrane epithelial antigen of prostate 3.

but rather from a patient who has an anemia with a different etiology. It is partly for this reason that a simple algorithm for the diagnosis of iron deficiency does not exist. In a severely anemic patient, microcytosis would have very high specificity and high sensitivity compared with a normal patient, but compared with a patient with thalassemia, the specificity would be very low. Similarly, a low serum ferritin level is an excellent test in the general population, but it is of relatively little value in patients with chronic renal disease. Another problem that is inherent in evaluating diagnostic tests for iron deficiency is the standard that is applied to decide who is iron-deficient and who is not. Marrow iron has served as one "gold standard" but has limitations, as discussed earlier (see "Marrow"). Alternatively, the response to iron therapy serves as a powerful indicator of which anemia is actually the result of an iron deficiency. Here, there are also limitations in that some iron-deficient patients may fail to respond adequately because of factors such as infection, and high doses of intravenous (IV) iron may be effective in some patients with anemia of inflammation. Lacking an absolute test for iron deficiency, the ability of the physician to use judgment relevant to a particular patient's circumstances is of paramount importance.

The forms of anemia that must be distinguished from iron-deficiency anemia most frequently include those of thalassemia minor, chronic inflammatory disease, malignancy, chronic liver disease, and chronic renal disease. It is the microcytic anemias that are most likely to be confused with iron deficiency. These include other conditions in which Hb synthesis is impaired,[188] including inflammation (Chap. 6) and thalassemias (Chap. 17), drug- or toxin-induced impairments of heme synthesis, sideroblastic anemias (Chap. 20), and rare defects in the delivery of iron to erythrocytes or erythrocyte iron uptake and utilization (Table 11-2).

Thalassemia Minor

In many parts of the world and in many communities of North America, the frequency of β-thalassemia minor is second only to that of iron deficiency as a cause of hypochromic microcytic anemia (Chap. 17). In African Americans, homozygosity for α-thalassemia-2, that is, the state in which only a single α-globin gene is present on each chromosome, is a common cause of microcytosis. Approximately 3% of African Americans are homozygous for α-thalassemia-2 (Chap. 17). The condition is associated with only a very modest lowering of the blood Hb

level.[189] Heterozygotes may also have microcytosis, although usually they are hematologically normal. Among persons of Mediterranean ancestry both α- and β-thalassemia are very prevalent, particularly the latter. Among Asians, particularly in those from Southeast Asia, β-thalassemia minor, α-thalassemia minor, and Hb E trait, all occur frequently. All are characterized by microcytosis, and none can be distinguished reliably from the others on the basis of erythrocyte morphology or erythrocyte indices alone. In each of these conditions, there may be only mild to moderate microcytosis without any other distinctive changes. However, in the majority of patients with α- or β-thalassemia minor, Hb Lepore trait, and Hb E trait, the erythrocyte count is greater than 5×10^{12} per L (5,000,000/μL), despite low Hb concentration.[190,191] Homozygous Hb E is also characterized by marked hypochromia, microcytosis, abundant target cells, and elevated erythrocyte count, but usually not by more than minimal anemia (Chap. 18).[190]

In contrast to the findings in these hemoglobinopathies, erythrocyte counts of 5×10^{12}/L (5,000,000/μL) or higher are relatively uncommon among adults with iron-deficiency anemia.[192] However, erythrocytosis may be seen in children with iron-deficiency anemia or in polycythemia vera patients who have become iron-deficient after hemorrhage or therapeutic phlebotomy. Consequently, although the mean MCV is almost always reduced in α- or β-thalassemia minor and in homozygous Hb E, with values of 60 to 70 fL being the rule, values this low are seen only in severe iron-deficiency anemia. In Hb Lepore trait and Hb E trait, only minimal microcytosis is observed.[190,191,193] Algorithmic rules based on red cell counts, MCV, or RDW are not sufficiently reliable for distinguishing iron deficiency from thalassemia in populations with a high prevalence of iron deficiency compared with thalassemias.

Mild reticulocytosis, polychromatophilia, and basophilic stippling are more likely to be encountered in β-thalassemia minor, δβ-thalassemia minor, and Hb Lepore trait than in iron-deficiency anemia, but they also may be absent in these disorders. The serum iron concentration is usually normal or increased in thalassemic syndromes and is usually low in iron-deficiency anemia. Similarly, examination of marrow iron stores helps differentiate these disorders. The presence of β-thalassemia trait is substantiated by the demonstration of increased proportions of Hb A_2 and F, or by the presence on electrophoresis of Hb H or Lepore (Chaps. 17 and 18). The diagnosis of α-thalassemia minor should be made on the basis of exclusion of other causes of microcytosis and confirmed by direct demonstration of mutations in α-globin genes by DNA-based techniques.

Iron deficiency may mask concurrent thalassemia. The amounts of both Hb A_2 and Hb H are diminished disproportionately to the reduction in Hb A in the presence of iron deficiency (Chap. 17)[194]; however, usually the Hb A_2 level remains above the normal range.

Anemia of Inflammation (Anemia of Chronic Disease)

The anemia of inflammation (Chap. 6) is usually normochromic and normocytic, but hypochromic microcytic anemia occurs in 20% to 30% of patients with chronic infections or malignancies.[145] Thus these disorders cannot be distinguished from iron-deficiency anemia by examination of the blood film. Furthermore, the serum iron concentration is usually decreased in these disorders,[145] sometimes severely. In uncomplicated iron deficiency, the TIBC is usually increased, whereas in inflammatory and neoplastic diseases it is commonly decreased, but there is considerable overlap among TIBC values of normal subjects, those with iron-deficiency anemia, and those with chronic inflammatory diseases.

Transferrin saturation may be normal in iron-deficiency anemia and, conversely, low saturation is sometimes observed in chronic inflammation. However, circulating soluble TfR increases in iron deficiency but not in the anemia of inflammation.[178] The serum ferritin level is usually diminished in iron deficiency, but it is generally increased in chronic inflammatory and neoplastic disorders.[153] Measurement of the ratio of soluble TfR to ferritin has been found to be useful in distinguishing the anemia of chronic inflammation from that of iron deficiency,[178] but meta-analysis of the relevant clinical studies suggested that the ratio may not be better than soluble TfR alone at discriminating between iron-deficiency anemia and anemia of inflammation.[195] Examination of the marrow for stainable iron is invasive and requires skilled reading but may be helpful in an occasional patient. Iron staining of marrow macrophages is greatly decreased in amount or absent in iron-deficiency anemia and normal or increased in the other disorders. Low serum hepcidin concentrations are characteristic of iron deficiency, and high serum hepcidin indicates anemia of inflammation, but this assay is not yet widely available and its clinical value is unknown. As would be expected from the inhibitory effect of hepcidin on the absorption of iron, high hepcidin levels predict a poor response to oral iron therapy[186] and low incorporation of dietary iron into erythrocytes.[196]

Anemia of Chronic Liver Disease

The erythrocytes in the blood film from patients with chronic liver disease may be normochromic and normocytic, macrocytic, or hypochromic. Target cells are frequently present in large numbers. Because the blood film in iron-deficiency anemia may also display these features, differential diagnosis must be based on other observations. Low serum ferritin levels are useful in detecting iron deficiency in the setting of cirrhosis,[197] but normal or even increased serum ferritin does not exclude iron deficiency, especially in the presence of active liver injury.[197,198]

Anemia of Chronic Renal Disease

Iron-deficiency anemia is frequent in patients with chronic renal disease (Chaps. 3 and 6) but is often difficult to diagnose in this setting, because iron delivery to the marrow is inadequate because of coexisting inflammation and because of increased demands from pulsatile erythropoiesis caused by erythropoiesis-stimulating agents. Because the problem is fairly common, and perhaps because of interest in identifying those patients who can benefit from iron therapy and decrease their usage of erythropoiesis-stimulating agents, a large number of studies have been done to determine the best way to diagnose iron deficiency in patients undergoing extracorporeal dialysis. The diagnostic problem is further complicated by the common occurrence of "functional iron deficiency,"[199] that is, a state in which iron stores are adequate but

iron delivery to the marrow is insufficient to meet the increased kinetic requirements of erythropoiesis stimulated by intermittent use of erythropoietin and related agents. If Hb response to IV iron therapy is used to diagnose iron deficiency, even many patients with abnormally high ferritin levels will be iron-deficient.[158,200] High serum ferritins do not preclude a response to IV iron, not even patients with chronic kidney disease who are not on hemodialysis.[201] Although measurements of reticulocyte Hb and percent of hypochromic erythrocytes show promise as markers of response to iron therapy, there is insufficient evidence currently that any individual biomarker or combination of biomarkers can reliably predict the response to iron treatment in chronic kidney disease.[202]

Anemia of Hemolytic Disease

Hemolytic disease can usually be distinguished from iron-deficiency anemia on the basis of the blood film. The marked poikilocytosis, polychromatophilia, spherocytosis, Heinz bodies, basophilic stippling, and other morphologic features characteristic of various types of hemolysis usually are not seen in iron-deficiency anemia. Furthermore, reticulocytosis is usually marked in hemolytic disorders but is minimal or absent in iron-deficiency anemia. However, there are some outstanding exceptions to these generally valid principles.

In unstable Hb disorders, such as Hb H disease or Hb Köln disease (Chap. 18), erythrocytic hypochromia may be pronounced. In these disorders, there is moderate reticulocytosis, which helps differentiate them from iron-deficiency anemia. The serum iron concentration is normal or increased.

When there is chronic intravascular hemolysis, erythrocytes in the blood film may display marked morphologic abnormalities, such as burr cells and schistocytes. Yet, because of loss of iron in the urine, iron deficiency may be the dominant cause of the resulting anemia. Evaluation of iron content in marrow aspirates or measurement of serum iron concentration and TIBC may clarify the diagnosis in this form of anemia.

Hypoplastic and Aplastic Anemia

In their early phases, these disorders cannot reliably be differentiated from mild iron-deficiency anemia on the basis of erythrocyte morphology alone (Chaps. 1 and 4). The reticulocyte count is generally less than 0.5% in hypoplastic or aplastic anemia. The presence of neutropenia and thrombocytopenia suggests a diagnosis of aplastic anemia, but mild neutropenia may also occur in iron-deficiency anemia. The serum iron concentration is usually increased in aplastic anemia; and the percentage transferrin saturation is then elevated. Marrow aspiration may produce scant material for cytologic study, and marrow biopsy is necessary. An iron stain usually reveals increased amounts of hemosiderin in aplastic or hypoplastic anemia. However, if chronic bleeding has occurred, for example, as a consequence of thrombocytopenia, iron stores may be depleted.

Sideroblastic Anemia

In this heterogeneous group of disorders (Chap. 20), the blood findings often simulate those of iron-deficiency anemia. Reticulocytosis is usually absent, and the serum iron concentration and serum ferritin are generally normal or increased. Marrow examination shows increased amounts of stainable iron.

Congenital Dyserythropoietic Anemia

In the rare congenital dyserythropoietic anemias (Chap. 14), erythrocyte morphologic abnormalities may resemble those of iron deficiency or thalassemia (Chap. 17). In general, in congenital dyserythropoietic anemias, poikilocytosis is very striking and occurs with less reduction in MCV than in iron deficiency or thalassemias. However, such cases are often believed to be thalassemic until the marrow is examined.

Megaloblastic Anemia

In pernicious anemia and other types of megaloblastic anemia (Chap. 9), the blood film usually shows sufficiently distinctive changes so there is little difficulty in making a differential diagnosis. One potential source of error is the change in serum iron concentration that occurs after therapy. In the patient with pernicious anemia or folic acid deficiency, early after starting treatment, the serum iron concentration decreases markedly as iron is utilized rapidly for Hb synthesis.[203] Thus, the finding of a low serum iron concentration in such circumstances should not be taken as evidence of iron deficiency. Iron-deficiency anemia and anemia as a consequence of folic acid or vitamin B_{12} deficiency may coexist. During the course of treatment, with the rapid increase in the number of red cells, the typical manifestations of severe iron deficiency may develop. The mixture of microcytic-hypochromic and normocytic-normochromic cells has been called *dimorphic anemia* (see "Coexisting Microcytic Anemia" in Chap. 20).

Anemia of Hypothyroidism

The anemia of severe hypothyroidism (myxedema; Chap. 7) is usually normochromic and normocytic and may be accompanied by mild to moderate depression of serum iron concentration. Marrow examination may be required to determine whether iron deficiency is present, especially because iron deficiency often complicates myxedema because of menorrhagia, which is common in this disorder.

Therapeutic Trial

In the final analysis, the response to iron therapy is the proof of correctness of diagnosis of iron-deficiency anemia. Furthermore, some physicians or patients may not have access to all the techniques described for diagnosis of iron-deficiency anemia. In this event, the patient's response to therapy may become a primary diagnostic measure. Iron administration in such a therapeutic trial is usually via the oral route, but IV iron can be used if there is evidence or strong suspicion of coexisting inflammation, iron malabsorption, or intolerance of oral iron preparations. The only caveat is that large doses of IV iron may increase Hb not only in iron-deficiency anemia but, by overwhelming the sequestration of iron in reticuloendothelial macrophages, also in conditions where total body iron is maldistributed, as in anemia of inflammation or anemia associated with chronic renal disease. A therapeutic trial under any circumstances should be followed carefully. If the cause of anemia is iron deficiency, adequate iron therapy should result in reticulocytosis, with a peak occurring after 1 to 2 weeks of therapy, although if anemia is mild, the reticulocyte response may be minimal. A significant increase in the Hb concentration of the blood should be evident 3 to 4 weeks later, and the Hb concentration should attain a normal value within 2 to 4 months. Unless there is evidence of continued substantial blood loss, the absence of response to oral or, when appropriate, parenteral iron must be taken as evidence that iron deficiency is not the cause of anemia. Iron therapy should be discontinued and another cause for the anemia sought.

Special Studies to Delineate the Cause of Iron Deficiency

The physician who establishes a diagnosis of iron deficiency resulting from blood loss has the obligation to determine the site and cause of hemorrhage. Examination of the stool for the presence of blood is particularly helpful in determining what additional studies should be carried out. Specimens should be examined on different days, because bleeding may be intermittent. Occasionally, it is helpful to label the patient's erythrocytes with chromium-51 (^{51}Cr) sodium chromate and

to determine quantitatively the amount of blood lost daily. When there is reason to believe that bleeding is from the gastrointestinal tract, roentgenographic and other imaging studies and endoscopic investigation are indicated. The latter often include gastroscopy, esophagoscopy, and colonoscopy, capsule endoscopy, and, rarely, angiography or scintigraphic studies. Numerous clinical studies indicate that intensive investigation of patients, particularly men and postmenopausal women, reveals unexpected bleeding lesions, many of which are curable or treatable.[10,204] *H. pylori* infection should be sought, particularly in patients who are iron-deficient but who do not seem to respond to therapy.[14,15] An iron stain of sputum may reveal hemosiderin-laden macrophages when there is intrapulmonary bleeding.

THERAPY

Once it has been established that a patient is deficient in iron, replacement therapy should be instituted. Iron may be administered orally, as simple iron salts; parenterally, as an iron-carbohydrate complex; or, very rarely, as a blood transfusion. Historically, the oral route has been preferred but the IV route is increasingly used because of the improved safety and convenience of new parenteral iron preparations. In most patients, iron-deficiency anemia is a disorder of long duration and slow progression, and restoration of normal Hb is not urgent unless the patient suffers from acute cardiac problems, in which case blood transfusion is appropriate. There is usually time to wait for normal mechanisms of erythropoiesis to respond to the body's needs, and for gradual adjustment of the cardiovascular system, to re-expansion of the total circulating erythrocyte volume.

Oral Iron Therapy

Dietary Therapy The patient should be encouraged to eat a diversified diet supplying all nutritional requirements. Nonetheless, it must be emphasized that neither meat nor any other dietary article contains enough iron to be useful therapeutically. Meat contains small amounts of myoglobin and Hb and insignificant amounts of iron in other proteins. Although heme iron is better absorbed than inorganic iron, the quantity of heme iron in meat is actually quite small. In fact, an average (3-oz) serving of steak provides only about 3 mg of iron, that is, the equivalent of only 3 mL of packed erythrocytes. Provision of sufficient dietary iron to permit a maximal rate or recovery from iron-deficiency anemia might require a daily intake of at least 10 pounds of steak. For these and other reasons, medicinal iron is superior to dietary iron in the therapy of iron deficiency.

Iron Preparations The pharmaceutical market is glutted with iron preparations in nearly every conceivable form; each promoted to appeal to physician or patient for one reason or another. The following simple principles may help the physician find a way through this chaos.

1. Each dose of an inorganic iron preparation for an adult should contain between 30 and 100 mg of ferrous iron. Doses of this magnitude cause unpleasant side effects relatively infrequently.[205] Smaller doses have been popular in the past, but these may result in a slower recovery of the patient or no recovery at all. Contrary to older literature, ferric iron as citrate is also well tolerated and sufficiently absorbed,[206] and in the chronic renal disease setting has the potential benefit of acting as a phosphate binder.
2. The iron should be readily released in acidic or neutral gastric juice or duodenal juice (usually pH 5-6), because maximal absorption occurs when iron is presented to the duodenal mucosa. Enteric-coated and prolonged-release preparations dissolve slowly in any of these fluids. Thus, with such preparations the iron that eventually is released may be presented to a portion of the intestinal mucosa in which absorption is least efficient. Some patients who have been

treated unsuccessfully with enteric-coated or prolonged-release iron preparations respond promptly to the administration of non–enteric-coated ferrous salts.

3. Side effects should be infrequent. This seems not to be a problem for any of the common commercially available iron compounds. Despite the claims of pharmaceutical companies, there is no convincing evidence that any one effective preparation is superior in this respect to any other.

4. Inexpensive iron preparations can be as effective as the more costly ones. The use of preparations containing several therapeutic agents is unnecessary and may increase side effects. Physicians should be aware that if ferrous sulfate is prescribed generically, the choice of preparation is left to the pharmacist who may dispense enteric-coated tablets. It is advisable to specify "nonenteric" or to prescribe by brand name a product that is not enteric-coated. Although substances such as ascorbic acid, succinate, and fructose enhance iron absorption, the gain is offset to a large extent by the increase in frequency of side effects, cost of therapy, or both. There is no convincing evidence to support the use of chelated forms of iron or of iron in combination with wetting agents.

Dosage

For therapy of iron deficiency in adults, the dosage should be sufficient to provide between 150 and 200 mg of elemental iron daily. Traditionally, the iron is taken orally in three or four doses 1 hour before meals. Infants may be given 6 mg/kg[207] daily in divided doses for therapy, or a daily dose of 12.5 mg daily for prophylaxis of iron deficiency. However, data support an alternative approach to iron administration. In women with iron deficiency from menstrual blood loss with or without anemia,[208,209] a single 100- or 200-mg iron dose alternate-day treatment was effective, well-tolerated, and more efficiently absorbed than daily treatment. This dosing scheme avoids the transient inhibitory effect of hepcidin induction by each iron dose on iron absorption of the next dose. It is likely that alternate-day dosing will be effective in other moderately iron-deficient patients, but its applicability to dosing in more severe iron deficiency remains to be established.

Side Effects Mild gastrointestinal side effects may occur in the form of nausea, heartburn, constipation, or changes in stool consistency and color. A metallic taste may be experienced. Most patients tolerate the usual therapeutic doses of iron without the least side effect. However, there is no doubt that some patients, perhaps 10% to 20%, have symptoms that may be ascribed to the iron preparation and may be dose-dependent. In such cases, reduction of the frequency of administration to one tablet per day for a few days may alleviate the symptoms; later, the patient may be able to tolerate a full-dose treatment. Alternate-day dosing can also be tried in this setting. It might also be useful to change to another iron preparation, especially one with a different external appearance.

Carbonyl iron has been proposed as an alternative to iron salts, on the assertion that it can be given in large doses with minimal side effects. This substance is actually metallic iron powder, with a particle size less than 5 μm. Because it is insoluble, it is not absorbed until it is converted to the ionic form. The bioavailability of carbonyl iron has been estimated to be approximately 70% of that of an equivalent amount of ferrous sulfate,[210] but oral doses of 1 to 3 g/day may be required for optimal therapy. Oral doses as high as 600 mg three times daily did not produce toxic effects.[210]

Oral ferric citrate formulated to enhance solubility and containing 210 mg of ferric iron in each tablet[211] has been approved for the treatment of iron deficiency in the setting of chronic kidney disease, and it appears to be effective and well tolerated at doses of 3 to 12 tablets per day.

Widespread iron supplementation in regions where malaria and gastrointestinal infections are highly endemic has been associated with increased malaria transmission and childhood mortality, presumably from increased infections.[212] Although there is not yet a consensus on optimal strategy in such settings, it seems reasonable to target iron supplementation to children who are iron-deficient.

Acute Iron Poisoning Acute iron poisoning is usually a consequence of the accidental ingestion by infants or small children of iron-containing medications intended for adults. Any potent oral preparation may cause acute iron poisoning, and this serious disorder remains a problem, despite public awareness campaigns and safer packaging of medications.[213] In the United States, there were more than 6000 reported incidents in 2017. The earliest manifestation of iron poisoning is vomiting, usually within 1 hour of the ingestion. There may be hematemesis or melena. Restlessness, hypotension, tachypnea, and cyanosis may develop soon thereafter, and may be followed within a few hours by coma and death, but fatal outcomes are now extremely rare. Usually, medical aid is sought early, and with proper treatment, most iron-poisoned children survive. The initial treatment is prompt evacuation of the stomach. In the home, this may be induced by digital stimulation of the pharyngeal gag reflex. If the patient arrives in the emergency department within minutes of ingestion, gastric intubation and lavage should be performed promptly. Whole-bowel irrigation[213] is currently recommended for all heavy metal intoxications. Supportive measures should be used as needed for shock or for metabolic acidosis should these develop. IV desferrioxamine is the agent of choice for specific therapy of hyperferremia, at a maximum rate of 15 mg/kg per hour for 1 hour, then lowered to 125 mg/h. Improvement often appears several hours to a few days after the onset of iron poisoning. Children who survive for 3 or 4 days usually recover without sequelae. However, gastric strictures and fibrosis or intestinal stenosis may occur as later complications.

Parenteral Iron Therapy

Indications As parenteral iron preparations have become safer and easier to administer, the use of parenteral iron is increasing. Established indications for the use of parenteral rather than oral iron include malabsorption, either because of systemic inflammation or gastrointestinal pathology, intolerance to iron taken orally, iron need in excess of an amount that can be absorbed in the intestine, and noncompliance. Parenteral iron administration has an erythropoietin-sparing effect in anemic patients on long-term hemodialysis for chronic renal disease.[35,214,215] Because of systemic inflammation and possibly other factors, these patients do not respond adequately to oral iron therapy.

Calculating Dosage The amount of iron that should be given is readily estimated by noting that 1 mL of red cells contains approximately 1 mg of iron. However, various formulas have been used for estimating total dose required for treatment. Because total blood volume is approximately 65 mL/kg and the iron content of Hb is 0.34% by weight, the simplest formula for estimating the total dose required for correction of anemia only is as follows:

$$\text{The dose of iron (mg)} = \text{whole-blood hemoglobin deficit (g/dL)} \times \text{body weight (lbs)}$$

Assuming a normal mean Hb concentration of 16 g/dL, a male weighing 170 pounds, whose Hb concentration is 7 g/dL, would require $170 \times (16 - 9) = 1530$ mg iron to correct this anemia. To this should be added enough iron to replete iron stores, approximately 1000 mg for men and approximately 600 mg for women. Thus, a 170-pound male with a Hb concentration of 7 g/dL should receive 2530 mg iron.

Parenteral Iron Preparations Because iron salts are highly toxic when given parenterally, all iron preparations consist of a colloidal (nanoparticulate) complex of iron with carbohydrates. To make the iron bioavailable for erythropoiesis and other biological processes, the iron complexes must be ingested by macrophages and digested so that the administered iron can be gradually delivered to plasma transferrin. Currently available preparations include iron sucrose, low-molecular-weight iron dextran, ferric gluconate, ferumoxytol, ferric carboxymaltose, and ferric derisomaltose (iron isomaltoside). High-molecular-weight dextran was associated with anaphylactoid adverse events compared with the other preparations, is no longer available in most countries and should be avoided.[216] Other reports indicate that ferric carboxymaltose may cause clinically important phosphate wasting and hypophosphatemia,[217] which can result in osteomalacia after chronic repeated use. The mechanism involves increased plasma concentrations of the active form of the phosphaturic hormone fibroblast growth factor 23. The less-used iron polymaltose and the older saccharated ferric oxide preparations are also reported to cause phosphate wasting. Patients with inflammatory bowel disease appear to be more susceptible, whereas those with chronic renal disease may be protected. Thus, it is important to check serum phosphate levels before repeat administration of ferric carboxymaltose, iron polymaltose, or saccharated ferric oxide. The remaining preparations are safe, and serious adverse events are extremely rare.[218] Although the recommended methods of administration, including the use of test dosing, the amount of iron per infusion, and infusion rates, differ among the preparations, these are not based on comparative studies. Premedication to prevent allergic responses was commonly used with the older preparations, but it is neither needed nor known to be effective with the newer formulations and may introduce side effects of its own.

Unlike IV iron preparations that require processing by reticuloendothelial macrophages, ferric pyrophosphate citrate transfers iron directly to transferrin and has been approved for iron supplementation during hemodialysis.[219] Here the iron salt is added to the dialysate fluid at 2 μM concentration that avoids saturation of transferrin with iron and delivers about 6.5 mg of iron in each dialysis session, an amount that may be sufficient to replace ongoing iron losses in the hemodialysis population. Another version of this iron compound can be administered intravenously at the same low dose 6.75 mg to replace losses during hemodialysis. As the ferric iron from this compound is delivered directly to transferrin, greater doses than those approved should not be given as they may cause the appearance of large amounts of unbound drug in the circulation, with as yet unknown consequences.

COURSE AND PROGNOSIS

Course

If therapy is adequate, the correction of iron-deficiency anemia is usually gratifying. Symptoms such as headache, fatigue, pica, paresthesias, and burning sensation of the oropharyngeal mucosa may abate within a few days. In the blood, the reticulocyte count begins to increase after a few days, usually reaches a maximum at about 7 to 12 days, and thereafter decreases. When anemia is mild, little or no reticulocytosis may be observed. Little change in Hb concentration or hematocrit value is to be expected for the first 2 weeks, but then the anemia is corrected rapidly. The Hb concentration in the blood may be halfway back to normal after 4 to 5 weeks of therapy. The relatively slow response to iron therapy compared with a more rapid response to the treatment of megaloblastic anemias (Chap. 9) with folate or vitamin B_{12} is related to the state of the marrow at the time of treatment. Iron deficiency suppresses hematopoiesis, so when iron therapy commences, several days are required for hematopoietic stem/progenitor cells to differentiate into erythroid progenitors in which the iron can be used to produce Hb. In contrast, the marrow of a patient with megaloblastic anemia is hypercellular and,

once replete with the appropriate vitamin, can rapidly convert the megaloblastic erythroid progenitors into reticulocytes that are released into the blood. By the end of 2 months of therapy, and often much sooner, the Hb concentration should have reached a normal level.

When iron-deficiency anemia does not resolve with oral iron treatment, careful inquiry into the nature, duration, and regularity of iron therapy may reveal a reason for the failure of therapy and permit a gratifying response to be elicited with adequate therapy. Other questions that should be asked in evaluation of such a case are as following:

1. Has bleeding been controlled?
2. Has the patient been on iron therapy long enough to show a response?
3. Has the dose of iron been adequate?
4. Are there other factors—inflammatory disease, neoplastic disease, hepatic or renal disease, prior gastrointestinal surgery, concomitant deficiencies (vitamin B_{12}, folic acid, thyroid)—that might retard response? Prominent among these are *H. pylori* infection, autoimmune gastritis and celiac disease.[15]
5. Is the diagnosis of iron deficiency correct?
6. Is the patient taking the iron preparation as prescribed?

IV iron should be effective in patients with established iron deficiency who do not respond to oral iron after several weeks. Continued loss of blood or, rarely, the genetic disorder iron-refractory iron-deficiency anemia,[15] may account for incomplete response to IV iron.

Prognosis

When the cause of the iron deficiency is a benign disorder, the prognosis is excellent, provided bleeding is controlled or can be compensated for by continual iron therapy. If there is a benign cause of recurrent bleeding that cannot be alleviated, such as hiatal hernia, menorrhagia, or hereditary hemorrhagic telangiectasia, oral iron therapy may be continued indefinitely; if the bleeding is especially brisk, supplementation with parenterally administered iron or, rarely, with transfusion may be needed. Continuous iron administration may also be required in patients with iron deficiency secondary to intravascular hemolysis with hemoglobinuria.

● IRON STORAGE DISEASE

DEFINITION AND HISTORY

The terms *iron storage disease* and *hemochromatosis* are used to designate an increase of tissue iron resulting in a disease state; *hemosiderosis* denotes an increase of tissue iron stores with or without tissue damage. Classically, hemochromatosis has been characterized by bronzing of the skin, cirrhosis, and diabetes, and was once called *bronzed diabetes*. Since the 1970s, usage of the term *hemochromatosis* has expanded well beyond its original meaning. This diagnosis is now commonly applied to persons who have increased body iron as suggested by increased serum ferritin levels, and even to those who merely have the hemochromatosis *HFE* genotype, regardless of the level of their iron stores.

Hemochromatosis may be divided into genetic forms and acquired forms. The former has sometimes been designated as *primary* and the latter as *secondary* forms. The disorder once designated *idiopathic hemochromatosis* and now as *hereditary hemochromatosis* usually is applied to the common genetic form of the disorder, found principally in those of northern European ancestry, and as a result of mutations in the *HFE* gene (type I hemochromatosis). In the United States, this is by far the most common form of the disease. *Juvenile hemochromatosis* from HJV and hepcidin mutations (type 2), hemochromatosis as a result of transferrin receptor-2 mutations (type 3), hemochromatosis caused by ferroportin mutations (type 4), and *African iron overload* are

TABLE 11-3. Classification of Hemochromatosis

I. Hereditary hemochromatosis
  A. Classical hemochromatosis (HFE hemochromatosis) (type 1)
  B. Juvenile hemochromatosis (type 2)
    1. Abnormality in hemojuvelin
    2. Abnormality of hepcidin
  C. Transferrin receptor-2 deficiency (type 3)
  D. Ferroportin abnormalities (type 4)
    1. Gain of function (systemic iron overload)
    2. Loss of function (macrophage iron overload)
  E. Ferritin H-chain iron-responsive element mutation
  F. African iron overload
II. Secondary hemochromatosis

among these types. Table 11-3 classifies hereditary hemochromatosis. *Secondary hemochromatosis* occurs in patients who receive multiple blood transfusions, particularly when they have ineffective erythropoiesis and hence hyperabsorb dietary iron.

Systemic iron overload and hepatic iron accumulation similar to hemochromatosis is also characteristic of atransferrinemia[220-223] and of human divalent metal transporter (DMT)-1 mutations.[224,225] A fetal and neonatal disorder termed *neonatal hemochromatosis* is characterized by hepatic and extrahepatic iron deposition and fulminant hepatitis caused by the maternal immune response to fetal antigens.[226]

Iron accumulation in localized sites, particularly the brain, occurs in disorders other than hemochromatosis. Increased quantities of brain iron are characteristic of aceruloplasminemia, and are found in Alzheimer disease, parkinsonism, Friedreich ataxia, Hallervorden-Spatz disease, and multiple-system atrophy. Because none of these are primarily hematologic disorders, and because the role of iron deposition in the pathology of the disorders is uncertain, they are not discussed further here.

Hemochromatosis was first described by Trousseau in 1865. The massive accumulation of iron that occurred in this disease was recognized as its hallmark. The ingenious development of serial phlebotomy as treatment for the disease suggested by Finch in 1949 and implemented on a larger scale in 1952,[227] made it clear that iron accumulation was the most important pathogenetic factor. Alcohol consumption and other environmental factors were also commonly found in patients with hemochromatosis.[228] The existence of a long suspected hereditary factor was firmly established when the disease was tightly linked to the human leukocyte antigen (HLA locus). Then, the gene proved to be *HFE* (initially named *HLA-H*), one of the many HLA-like genes, also located on chromosome 6.[229]

The identification of the *HFE* gene made it possible, for the first time, to accurately assess the gene frequency and penetrance of the *HFE* mutations. This brought about a fusion of the apparently contrasting views of genetic and environmental causes. The penetrance of the homozygous state is so low that it could be considered an essential risk factor that requires other genetic or environmental factors for disease development.[230]

EPIDEMIOLOGY

The prevalence of mutations of the *HFE* gene is very high. The most important of these is the c.845 A→G (C282Y) mutation, and with a gene frequency of approximately 0.07 in the northern European population, approximately 5 in 1000 northern Europeans are homozygous for the mutation. The C282Y and S65C mutations are almost entirely confined to individuals with European ancestry. The H63D mutation is more widespread geographically but is also most common in Europeans. Within Europe, the highest gene frequencies of the C282Y mutation are encountered in the southern British Isles and in northern France, but other northern Europeans, including Scandinavians, also have high gene frequencies, consistent with a mutation of Celtic or possibly Viking origin.[231]

Although earlier studies attributed nonspecific symptoms in patients to hemochromatosis, large controlled series have shown that most such symptoms are not present in homozygotes for the C282Y mutation at a higher frequency than in controls,[232-234] or a borderline increase, at most, invariably in groups of patients who were aware of their diagnosis when answering questions about symptoms. These findings are consistent with the very low prevalence of hemochromatosis reported in autopsy series and in hospital surveys. The prevalence of symptomatic clinical hemochromatosis in northern European populations is probably only approximately 5 in 100,000 individuals. If patients with abnormal liver function tests and/or fibrosis on liver biopsy are included, the number of affected persons may be several-fold higher.[235-238] The factors that determine whether disease develops in a patient with the C282Y homozygous genotype are not well understood. The patient's gender is clearly a modifying factor, with more severe manifestations observed in men, because pregnancy and menstrual iron losses tend to ameliorate the disease in women. Other genetic factors that might interact with the C282Y homozygous genotype in producing clinically significant iron storage disease have been sought but not found, except rare instances in which coinheritance of mutations of the hepcidin gene may be responsible. An increased proportion of severely affected patients have a large alcohol intake.[239,240]

The widespread perception that classical hereditary hemochromatosis frequently led to clinical disease resulted in enthusiasm for population-based screening. However, the cost–benefit analysis used was based on the assumptions that life-threatening disease manifestations will occur in 43% of men and 28% of women, estimates that were based on the prevalence of disease in patients, most of whom had been diagnosed clinically with hemochromatosis. With the realization that the clinical penetrance is much lower, interest in screening the general population for hemochromatosis has largely disappeared.

The prevalence of other forms of hemochromatosis, including juvenile hemochromatosis, hemochromatosis caused by ferroportin deficiency, and atransferrinemia, is much lower than that of the prevalence of classical hereditary hemochromatosis. These forms of hemochromatosis are rare.

ETIOLOGY AND PATHOGENESIS

Toxicity of Iron

In living organisms, iron associates with proteins to function in O_2 storage and transport and in various metabolic reactions as an electron donor or electron acceptor. The capacity to catalyze oxidation-reduction reactions appears to cause iron-mediated cellular and tissue injury. One of the pathways considered to be of greatest importance is the Haber-Weiss reaction:

$$Fe^{++} + H_2O_2 \rightarrow Fe^{+++} + OH^- + HO^{\cdot}$$
$$O_2^- + Fe^{+++} \rightarrow O_2 + Fe^{++}$$

The sum of these two reactions is the Fenton reaction:

$$O_2^- + H_2O_2 \rightarrow O_2 + OH^- + HO^{\cdot}$$

The hydroxyl radical (HO$^{\cdot}$) has been implicated in producing damage to polysaccharides, DNA, and enzymes, and in causing lipid peroxidation.[241] Although there is no direct evidence that HO˙ generation is the main pathway of tissue damage in hemochromatosis, this common conjecture seems reasonable. Demonstrating a damaging effect of iron alone on experimental animals has been difficult. Although subtle biochemical defects have been documented in mouse models of genetic, parenteral, or dietary iron overload, frank cirrhotic changes have not been found. In gerbils, parenteral iron overload causes hepatic necrosis, fibrosis, and nodular regeneration, as well as cardiac damage.[242] In rats, iron alone does not cause fibrosis, and alcohol alone causes only minor liver abnormalities. However, administration of both excess iron and alcohol results in fibrosis.[243] These findings in rats are quite consistent with the strong association that has been demonstrated to exist between alcohol ingestion and cirrhosis in patients with the hemochromatosis genotype. In a number of species, including birds, rhinoceros, tapirs, fruit bats, and others, iron overload has been observed in zoos or other restricted settings, where a diet other than the animal's native diet is fed.

Iron is stored in ferritin in the cytoplasm of all cells. The multiple isoferritins found in human tissues comprise variable proportions of two subunits: L-ferritin (light) and H-ferritin (heavy).[244] Because free iron is potentially harmful to the cell, it is sequestered and detoxified to the less-soluble ferric form by ferroxidase activity; H-ferritin exerts most of its ferroxidase activity in the cytosol. The mitochondrial ferritin, expressed in the mitochondrial matrix, also has potent ferroxidase activity and is markedly upregulated in sideroblastic anemias (Chap. 20).

Causes of Iron Overload

Because body iron content is maintained by regulating absorption, excess body iron can accumulate only when absorption is increased above iron requirements, or when iron is injected into the body, either in the form of medicinal iron or as transfused erythrocytes.

Excessive Iron Absorption A variety of mutations are known to cause increased iron absorption in experimental animals and in man, as summarized in Table 11-3. Mutations in the genes encoding HFE, transferrin receptor-2, ferroportin, HJV, and hepcidin are all associated with iron overload (Chap. 10). The common pathway that causes hyperabsorption of iron is deficiency of hepcidin, which allows excessive activity of the iron exporter ferroportin in the duodenum and in macrophages of the reticuloendothelial system. Normally, hepcidin is upregulated when body iron increases. However, this response is blunted or absent in either *Hfe-, Tfr2-,* or *Hjv*-deficient mice[245] or in the human disease,[246-248] all of which exhibit disproportionately low hepcidin levels for the degree of iron overload. Although the biochemistry of their interactions is not known, there is increasing evidence that HFE, TfR2, and HJV are part of the signaling pathway that regulates hepcidin expression. In autosomal dominant hereditary hemochromatosis (class 4), ferroportin mutations interfere with binding of hepcidin to ferroportin[249,250] or with the resulting ferroportin endocytosis, so that hepcidin cannot exert its bioactivity.

Ineffective Erythropoiesis Anemias with ineffective erythropoiesis commonly cause systemic iron overload with damage to the liver, heart, and endocrine system. Iron storage disease is particularly common in disorders such as β-thalassemia, hereditary dyserythropoietic anemia, and pyruvate kinase deficiency. The amount of body iron may greatly exceed the quantity that can be accounted for through blood transfusion, and iron overload is common even in patients who are rarely or never transfused.

The iron overload commonly observed in β-thalassemia intermedia and major patients likely results, at least in part, from suppression of the iron regulatory hormone hepcidin by erythroid factors secreted by massively proliferating erythropoietin-stimulated erythroblasts. The erythroid suppressors of hepcidin include GDF-15[251] and erythroferrone.[252] GDF-15[253,254] and erythroferrone[255] overexpression was also observed in congenital dyserythropoietic anemia (Chap. 14).

Transfusion or Iron Therapy Iron overload can be iatrogenic in origin. Because erythrocytes contain 1 mg of iron per milliliter, transfusion of 450 mL of whole blood or 200 mL of red cells adds 200 mg of total iron to the body—iron that will not be excreted. Thus, a patient who receives two units of blood monthly for an anemia that is not a result of blood loss will accumulate 4.8 g of iron per year. If the need for transfusion is caused by a disorder in which ineffective erythropoiesis plays a prominent role, the accumulation of iron is even greater. Thalassemia is the most common anemia with ineffective erythropoiesis, and iron overload has been the most important cause of death in patients with this disorder (Chap. 17).

The homeostatic mechanisms of the body are such that the inappropriate administration of iron by the oral route is very unlikely to produce clinically significant iron overload. Of the few cases that have been described, all but one were documented before the cloning of the *HFE* gene, raising the possibility that the patients had genetic hemochromatosis that was accelerated by excess iron intake. Documented iron overload after iron injection is even less common and has not been accompanied by demonstrable tissue damage.

Pathology

Affected tissues and organs exhibit a deep brown color. Histologic examination reveals prominent hemosiderin deposition in many tissues and organs.

Liver The liver is often enlarged. After cirrhosis has developed, the organ becomes granular or coarsely nodular. In the liver of patients with classical hemochromatosis, TfR2 mutations and in juvenile hemochromatosis, hemosiderin is found primarily in hepatocytes. Kupffer cells are relatively spared. Before the development of cirrhosis, the hemosiderin accumulates primarily in periportal hepatocytes and is less toward the central veins. The iron of cirrhotic livers is mostly in the periphery of regenerative nodules. Fibrosis begins periportally, then fibrous septa traverse the lobules. Usually, the distortion of the architecture is not as severe or as uniform as in alcoholic cirrhosis. The cirrhosis of hemochromatosis usually has a micronodular appearance. Iron in bile duct epithelium has sometimes been considered a specific marker for hemochromatosis but is not reliable. The amount of iron in the liver is always greatly increased. This is apparent on inspection of sections stained for iron with the Prussian blue reaction and can be quantitated on liver biopsy specimens. An iron concentration of more than 300 μmol/g dry weight (or about 50 μmol/g wet weight) is considered strong evidence for hemochromatosis when factors such as transfusions are eliminated as the cause.

In the original description of African iron overload, the liver pathology was deemed to be indistinguishable from that of classical hemochromatosis, but in newer studies[256] it seems that only some of the affected patients manifest iron storage, primarily in the hepatocytes; some have storage primarily in Kupffer cells. In the case of patients with ferroportin mutations that prevent transport of iron, storage of iron takes place mostly in the Kupffer cells, and fibrosis seems to be absent; ferroportin mutations that prevent interaction with hepcidin, on the other hand, are associated with hepatocyte iron overload, as is seen in classical hemochromatosis.[250,257]

Heart Iron accumulates more slowly in the myocardium than in the liver but the heart is more sensitive to its toxic effects. Myocardial damage is seen when iron loading is rapid, for example, in β-thalassemic patients dying of transfusional iron overload in their 20s and 30s[259] before effective chelation therapy, and in juvenile hemochromatosis patients who usually present with iron-induced cardiomyopathy and endocrinopathy rather than liver failure.[260] The myocardium is thickened and the heart is often enlarged; arrhythmias and myocardial failure follow. Accumulation of cardiac iron is the leading cause of death in transfused patients with β-thalassemia major. Patients with transfusion-dependent anemias, such as congenital dyserythropoietic anemia and Diamond-Blackfan syndrome, also develop iron overload–induced cardiomyopathy. In transfused patients with myelodysplastic syndrome, transfusion threshold guidelines of 75 units of blood was suggested as a risk factor of cardiac iron overload but this is not based on firm data. Direct cardiac iron measurement using magnetic resonance imaging (MRI) predicts cardiac complications and can stratify the risk of subsequent cardiac dysfunction.[261] This technique measures the half-life, T2`, of cardiac muscle darkening (with respect to echo time) produced by magnetically active stored cardiac iron.

Marrow The quantity of iron in the marrow of patients with classical hereditary hemochromatosis is only modestly increased, if at all. The iron is characteristically distributed into small, equal-size granules located in endothelial lining cells rather than in macrophages. In classical hereditary hemochromatosis, both macrophages[262] and intestinal mucosal cells are iron-poor relative to the overall iron burden.

Genetics

Genetic factors play an important role in the etiology of iron storage disease. This is true not only in the primary forms of the disorder, but also in secondary hemochromatosis, where genetic disorders of erythropoiesis are the most common causes. The genetics of these disorders, including the thalassemias, dyserythropoietic anemias, and red cell enzymopathies and membrane disorders are described in Chaps. 14, 15, 16, and 17. Mutations of several genes that play an important role in iron homeostasis have been found to lead to iron storage disease.[263]

HFE **Mutations** The most common cause of hereditary hemochromatosis is a mutation of the *HFE* gene. This HLA-like gene resides on chromosome 6. Three polymorphic mutations have been identified. These are located at nucleotides 187, 193, and 845 of the complementary DNA and at the protein level encode the H63D, S65C, and C282Y mutations, respectively. The phenotypic severity of these mutations on iron homeostasis is manifested in the following order: C282Y > H63D > S65C. Hereditary hemochromatosis is essentially an autosomal recessive disorder. Approximately two-thirds of homozygotes for the C282Y, and a slightly lower percentage of compound heterozygotes for the C282Y and H63D mutations, manifest increased serum transferrin saturations and serum ferritin levels. Individuals heterozygous for either the C282Y or the H63D mutation have, on average, significantly higher transferrin saturations and serum ferritin levels than do wild-type homozygotes. However, the magnitude of this increase is very low.[264] For example, the average transferrin saturation of man with the wild-type genotype is 26.69% and heterozygotes for the C282Y mutation have a transferrin saturation averaging 30.63%. The effect of the H63D mutation is even less, and that of the S65C mutation is barely perceptible.

Despite the minimal effect of the heterozygous state for *HFE* mutations on iron homeostasis, a number of investigators have proposed that heterozygotes are at increased risk for a variety of disorders. What has not been taken into account in the studies is that the *HFE* gene is in close proximity to (and therefore likely to be coinherited with) many immune-response genes on chromosome 6; consequently, it is not possible to distinguish the minor effects that *HFE* mutations may have on iron homeostasis from variation in the immune response.

Hamp **(Hepcidin) Mutations** Mutations of hepcidin are rare and associated with severe juvenile hemochromatosis.[265]

SLC40A1 **(Ferroportin) Mutations** Mutations of the gene encoding ferroportin cause an autosomal dominant iron storage disease of two types. Gain of function mutations, for example, the C326S mutation, interfere with hepcidin binding to ferroportin or with the resulting ferroportin endocytosis, so that mutant ferroportin molecules continue exporting iron from enterocytes and macrophages to plasma, even in the face of high hepcidin levels[249] that normally cause ferroportin endocytosis and proteolysis. A mouse model of this condition shows that a heterozygous mutation is sufficient to cause severe iron overload but that homozygosity for this mutation is even more severe.[266] Loss-of-function mutations are more common and include ferroportin mutations that do not localize to the cell surface, or prevent transport of iron. Here storage of iron takes place mostly in the Kupffer cells and splenic macrophages, and cirrhosis does not occur. It is not clear why these act in a dominant manner and why all of the reported mutations encode amino acid substitutions and none are completely destructive (frameshift or stop codons).[164,267] An attractive explanation is that these mutations act in a dominant negative manner but this mechanism has not yet been supported by convincing biochemical data. A common polymorphism, c.744G→T (Gln284His), shows an association with African iron overload[256,268,269] but is clearly not present in all patients who manifest this syndrome.

TfR2 **Mutations** Mutations of *TfR2* cause an autosomal recessive disorder that is indistinguishable clinically from the common HFE-related form of hereditary hemochromatosis.[247,270-272]

Hemojuvelin Mutations Several different mutations of a gene designated as *HFE2* and as *HJV* cause juvenile hemochromatosis.[248,273-277] HJV belongs to the class of glycosylphosphatidylinositol-anchored repulsive-guidance molecules and may act as a coreceptor for bone morphogenetic proteins. Bone morphogenetic protein receptor is now known to be a key regulator of hepcidin transcription.[278]

DMT-1 Human Mutations DMT-1 human mutations are all associated with hepatic hemosiderosis[224,225,279] and most with abnormal liver function tests in addition to microcytic hypochromic anemia. This is in contrast to mice and rats with DMT-1 mutations, because these DMT-1–deficient rodents are iron-deficient. This is likely because humans, unlike rodents, can also absorb heme-containing iron, at least to a small degree in a DMT-1–independent manner.

Animal Models

Naturally Occurring Models When kept in zoos or other nonnative habitats, a number of animal species, such as mynah birds, the toco toucan, Salers cattle, lemurs, and the browsing rhinoceros, are iron-loaded. Rhinoceroses may represent an interesting paradigm for iron storage in captive species. Although the browsing rhinoceros species are iron-loaded, grazing species are not, even when kept under similar conditions. It seems likely that because iron is not readily available in the leaves and twigs eaten by the browsing species, these species have evolved to more efficiently take up iron from its diet—more efficiently than needed when fed a zoo diet. Molecular comparisons of iron-regulatory genes in browser versus grazer rhinoceroses identified some promising candidates, but the ultimate cause of the differences in iron handling has not yet been established.[280]

Models Produced by Iron Loading Numerous efforts have been made to create models of hemochromatosis by loading laboratory animals with iron, either by the oral or parenteral route. A few of these appear to simulate the human disease in one respect or another. For example, the iron-loaded gerbil[281-284] develops heart disease, features of which resemble the human disease. Such models have been used for the study of potential chelating agents.

Targeted Disruption Models Targeted disruption of most of the genes associated with human iron disorders has been achieved. Included are *HFE*,[285] TfR 2,[271] ferroportin,[286] HJV,[274,275] and hepcidin.[287] The targeted disruption of several genes, including those encoding bone morphogenetic protein-6,[288,289] or the components of the bone morphogenetic protein receptor,[278] caused iron overload in mice, but the equivalent human diseases have not yet been found.

CLINICAL FEATURES

HFE-Related (Type 1) Hereditary Hemochromatosis

Onset The clinical features of the most common form of hereditary hemochromatosis are cirrhosis of the liver, darkening of the skin, cardiomyopathies, and diabetes. These features are only seen in the fully penetrant form of the disease and may depend on additional cofactors such as alcohol consumption. In contrast to the juvenile form of the disease, in which onset is usually in the second or third decade of life, classical hereditary hemochromatosis associated with mutations of the *HFE* gene generally is diagnosed in the fifth or sixth decade of life.

General Symptomatology Many symptoms are attributed to hereditary hemochromatosis, including abdominal pain, weakness, lethargy, fatigue, loss of libido, impotence, and arthropathies. However, all of these symptoms are common in an aging population, and epidemiologic studies show that none of them are more common in patients with the HFE hemochromatosis, even those with the biochemical phenotype, than they are in the general population.

Arthropathies The arthropathy of patients with hemochromatosis has characteristic features.[235,290,291] It tends to begin at the small joints of the hands, especially the second and third metacarpal joints, and in some cases, episodes of acute synovitis may occur as in calcium pyrophosphosphate dehydrate deposition arthropathy (pseudogout; chondrocalcinosis). Radiologically, the arthropathy resembles that of osteoarthritis with joint space loss, subchondral cysts, sclerosis, and osteophytosis. The features that have been considered distinctive include the joint distribution, the presence of shape osteophytes emerging from the radial sides of the metacarpal distal epiphysis, and the presence of radiolucent zones in the subchondral area of the femoral head. It is generally recognized that arthritis does not respond to phlebotomy therapy. The possibility that this type of arthritis depends on linkage of HFE to other HLA genes is made less likely by the occurrence of similar arthritis in juvenile hemochromatosis,[292] which is genetically independent of the HLA locus. Hip arthritis at an early age was also noted in a family with hepcidin-resistant ferroportin mutation and iron overload.[257]

Liver Patients with hepatic iron overload are at a greatly increased risk of development of hepatocellular carcinoma[258], especially when cirrhosis is present.[293] Some patients with hereditary hemochromatosis have been reported to develop hepatocellular carcinoma even in the absence of cirrhosis, suggesting that iron overload could be directly carcinogenic.

Porphyria Cutanea Tarda Porphyria cutanea tarda is a disease well known to be associated with mild iron overload and that responds to phlebotomy treatment (Chap. 21). Numerous studies document that the prevalence of patients with this disorder who also have mutations of the HFE gene has considerably increased.[294]

Juvenile Hemochromatosis

The penetrance of the rare juvenile form of the disease seems to be high, and cardiomyopathies and endocrine deficiencies are the major clinical features.[295] Joint manifestations were found to be relatively common in patients with juvenile hemochromatosis.[292]

African Iron Overload

It is not clear to what extent African iron overload is symptomatic. Among the Bantu, where the disorder was originally described, there are many complicating factors, including malnutrition and high alcohol intake. Among African Americans, various associated disorders have been noted, but a cause-and-effect relationship is not clear.

Secondary Hemochromatosis

The clinical findings in patients with hemochromatosis secondary to blood transfusion and/or disorders of erythropoiesis are, in general, indistinguishable from those found in patients with the primary hemochromatosis.[296]

LABORATORY FEATURES

The main laboratory features of hereditary hemochromatosis are abnormally high transferrin saturation and increased serum ferritin level. In secondary hemochromatosis, anemia and the other manifestations of the underlying disorder are found. Macrocytosis of the erythrocytes and slightly increased blood Hb[297] is a common feature; this finding is also seen in mouse models of hemochromatosis and could be caused by increased transferrin saturation relieving the slight baseline iron restriction in healthy populations.

Differential Diagnosis

A large number of methods have been introduced that allow the amount of storage iron to be estimated.[298] The suspicion that a patient may have primary hemochromatosis is generally raised by an increased serum transferrin saturation, particularly when it is found together with an elevated serum ferritin level. An increased transferrin saturation commonly occurs in patients with chronic liver disease who have no mutations in the *HFE* gene.[299] Ferritin is an acute-phase protein and levels are elevated in a variety of disorders. Particularly high levels are encountered in patients with macrophage activation syndromes, loss-of-function ferroportin mutations, acute hepatitis, Gaucher disease, some malignancies, and in patients with the hyperferritinemia-cataract syndrome.[300] The latter disorder is an uncommon autosomal dominant defect in which a mutation in the 5′ IRP of the ferritin light chain prevents binding of the IRPs, resulting in unrestrained constitutive production of the ferritin chains.

Many clinicians have considered a liver biopsy the "gold standard" for the diagnosis of iron overload. The material obtained at biopsy not only provides the opportunity to assess the histopathology of the liver of the patient, but also to quantitate the amount of nonheme iron in the specimen. Dividing the iron content by the patient's age provides an iron index; a value greater than 2 implies the presence of hemochromatosis. Although in some situations, liver biopsy may provide useful information, it is an invasive procedure that, although low risk, is no longer required for the diagnosis of hemochromatosis. Enthusiasm for subjecting every patient with potential hemochromatosis to liver biopsy has diminished with the ready availability of genetic analysis. Moreover, a simple way to determine whether a patient is iron-overloaded is to institute a program of phlebotomies. This is an essentially harmless way to determine how much storage iron the body contains. MRI can detect and reliably quantify increased amounts of iron in the liver.[301] For detection of cardiac iron overload, T2* MRI[261] is a superior diagnostic approach.

THERAPY

The treatment of hemochromatosis consists of removing the accumulated iron. In the case of patients who are able to mount an erythropoietin response to phlebotomy, removal of blood is generally the treatment of choice. When the patient has marked impairment of erythropoiesis, as in thalassemia and dyserythropoietic anemia, it is necessary to employ chelating agents to remove iron, although occasionally serial phlebotomy will stimulate sufficient erythropoiesis to make it a viable therapy.

Phlebotomy

Each milliliter of packed red cells contains approximately 1 mg of iron. Thus, the removal of 500 mL of blood with a hematocrit of 40% removes approximately 200 mg of iron, and after phlebotomies iron is mobilized from the stores. When the stores have been exhausted, the signs of iron deficiency develop, and this is the end point of the initial part of the phlebotomy program. The patient is then followed and a schedule of maintenance phlebotomies is established, with the frequency of phlebotomies tailored to maintain the serum ferritin level, the best indicator of body stores, below 100 ng/mL.

The actual volume of blood removed at each phlebotomy depends on the patient's size. Most average-size patients tolerate removal of 500 mL, but patients who weigh 50 kg or less are better treated by the removal of correspondingly smaller volumes of blood. Many patients may complain of symptoms after the first few phlebotomies. Better compliance is achieved if such symptoms are minimized by performing phlebotomies only every 14 days initially, increasing the frequency to weekly phlebotomies once the patient has become accustomed to the procedure and the activity of the marrow has been stimulated so as to replace the lost erythrocytes rapidly. The hematocrit or Hb and the MCV of the red cells should be measured before each phlebotomy is undertaken. If there has been a substantial decrease in the hematocrit or Hb, the phlebotomy should be deferred. The MCV may rise early in the treatment program, but as iron deficiency develops, it will fall, signaling that the end point has been reached or is near. The transferrin saturation and serum ferritin level should be measured every 2 or 3 months. When the transferrin saturation is less than 10% and the serum ferritin less than 10 ng/mL, phlebotomy should be discontinued and the patient be monitored every 3 to 6 months so that the rate of ferritin rise can be estimated. When the serum ferritin is in the 50 to 100 ng/mL range, the maintenance phase should be initiated. Some patients may require phlebotomies monthly to maintain a normal ferritin value, whereas others may only require one to three phlebotomies per year.

Chelation Therapy

Chelation therapy instituted in a timely manner can decrease the potential morbidity caused by iron overload and prolong the life of patients with hereditary chronic iron-loading disorders such as β-thalassemia major or intermedia. It also has a place in the management of some patients with acquired marrow dysplasias provided the prognosis of the underlying disorder warrants the potential risks and burdens.[302] Although the availability of oral chelating agents has made this option much more practical, the prospect of long-term benefit is often uncertain.

Desferrioxamine

Desferrioxamine is a naturally occurring iron-chelating compound synthesized by the microorganism *Streptomyces pilosus,* having evolved to enable the microbe to obtain iron from its environment. One molecule of this chelator binds one atom of iron. Its molecular weight is 560 Da. The iron complex is excreted into the urine and feces. Urine iron is derived primarily from red cells broken down by macrophages, whereas fecal iron is believed to be from iron chelated in the liver.[303]

Desferrioxamine is poorly absorbed from the gastrointestinal tract and must therefore be given parenterally, either by the subcutaneous or IV route. The effectiveness of chelation is proportional to the duration of exposure of iron-loaded tissue to the drug. Rapid IV or intramuscular injection results in relatively little iron mobilization; instead, it is necessary to administer desferrioxamine by slow IV or subcutaneous infusion over a period of 8 to 10 hours. Increasing doses of desferrioxamine result in increased iron excretion, and the usual recommended dose is 30 to 50 mL/kg.[303,304] Vitamin C (up to 200 mg daily) may be given to enhance iron excretion. The amount of iron excreted will vary per patient and depends largely on the iron burden. Because the treatment is cumbersome and costly, one should be reasonably certain that sufficient good is being accomplished to justify the effort. This can be achieved by measuring urine output of iron after a test desferrioxamine infusion, bearing in mind that urinary excretion may account for only one-third of the iron excreted, fecal excretion accounting for the rest.

Desferrioxamine is usually well tolerated. Minor local reactions such as local pruritus, induration, or pain at the site of infusion are not uncommon. Large doses are associated with hearing loss, night blindness and other visual abnormalities, growth retardation, and skeletal changes. At very high doses, occasional cases of kidney and lung abnormalities have been reported.[303] About 20% of patients on desferrioxamine alone will continue to have cardiac iron overload.

Oral Chelating Agents

The inconvenience and high cost of administration with desferrioxamine has stimulated an intensive search for safe, orally active chelating agents. Deferiprone is an orally effective bidentate chelating agent; three molecules of deferiprone bind one iron atom. Its molecular weight is only 139 Da and it is excreted almost entirely in the urine. The usual dose is 75 mg/kg per day divided into three doses. Deferiprone administration is associated with several toxic effects, including gastrointestinal disturbances, arthropathy, transient increases in the serum levels of liver enzymes, and zinc deficiency. The main concern has centered on the propensity of the drug to produce neutropenia and agranulocytosis. The latter complication occurs in approximately 1% of patients. It appears to be idiosyncratic, is more common in women, and appears to be reversible. Neutropenia with a granulocyte level between 0.5 and 1.5×10^9/L (500 and 1500/μL) recurs in an additional 5% of patients. Treatment should be stopped at the first sign of a fall in the leukocyte count.[303] It has been suggested that deferiprone may be more effective in removing iron from the heart and desferrioxamine more effective with respect to liver iron accumulations.[304] Preliminary investigations suggest that a combination of desferrioxamine and deferiprone may be more effective than either alone. It has been proposed that deferiprone enters cells and removes their iron and then passes the iron to desferrioxamine.[305] The combination may be particularly useful in patients with heart failure from iron overload, where it may decrease mortality, and in patients with endocrinopathies.[305]

Deferasirox (Exjade and Jadenu, formulated as an oral suspension and a film-coated tablet, respectively), a tridented triazole component, is a newer oral iron-chelating agent with a long plasma half-life.[305] At a dose of 30 mg/kg per day, it was found to be as efficient as desferrioxamine and is generally well tolerated. It has been recommended for patients who are noncompliant with desferrioxamine and, like deferiprone, may be effective at removing cardiac iron. The main toxicities are renal and hepatic, but it may also cause gastrointestinal hemorrhage.[305] Combination therapy with the two oral chelators is still experimental.

COURSE AND PROGNOSIS

The outlook in this disease has changed in the current century to one in which the life span of patients with hemochromatosis is normal or nearly so. This is largely a result of the change in the definition of the disorder. In the early 20th century, the diagnosis was reserved for the rare patient with full-blown bronzed diabetes. Today, the diagnosis is applied to any person found to be homozygous for the C282Y mutation or anyone with an increased transferrin saturation and elevated serum ferritin level. Realistically, patients with a diagnosis of hemochromatosis based on genetic and/or biochemical criteria have a normal life span. This is not to suggest that patients do not die of hereditary hemochromatosis; it is simply that the penetrance of the disorder as detected on genetic or biochemical bases is so low that the few deaths that do occur cannot be detected even in very sizable series.

For those patients with classical hereditary hemochromatosis who are clinically affected, it is likely that removal of iron by phlebotomy prevents further complications and prolongs life span. Although controlled studies of the effect of phlebotomy are not ethically feasible, serial observations in patients undergoing phlebotomy suggest that cirrhosis is either stabilized or may, at least in some patients, improve. The course of untreated juvenile hemochromatosis seems much less benign. Cardiac deaths seem to be particularly common,[296] and in a few cases, cardiac transplantation has been performed successfully. If patients can be supported in intensive care units, the cardiac dysfunction appears to be reversible with intensive chelation therapy.[306]

Institution of iron chelation has greatly improved outcomes in β-thalassemia major and similar disorders, but the prognosis is grim when iron chelation is not performed (Chap. 17). Death is most frequently a result of cardiac failure.

REFERENCES

1. Heath CW, Strauss MB, Castle WB. Quantitative aspects of iron deficiency in hypochromic anemia: (the parenteral administration of iron). *J Clin Invest.* 1932;11(6):1293-1312.
2. Beutler E. History of iron in medicine. *Blood Cells Mol Dis.* 2002;29(3):297-308.
3. Poskitt EM. Early history of iron deficiency. *Br J Haematol.* 2003;122(4):554-562.
4. Stoltzfus RJ. Iron interventions for women and children in low-income countries. *J Nutr.* 2011;141(4):756S-762S.
5. McLean E, Cogswell M, Egli I, et al. Worldwide prevalence of anaemia, WHO Vitamin and Mineral Nutrition Information System, 1993-2005. *Public Health Nutr.* 2009;12(4):444-454.
6. Pasricha SR, Drakesmith H, Black J, et al. Control of iron deficiency anemia in low- and middle-income countries. *Blood.* 2013;121(14):2607-2617.
7. Cogswell ME, Looker AC, Pfeiffer CM, et al. Assessment of iron deficiency in US preschool children and nonpregnant females of childbearing age: National Health and Nutrition Examination Survey 2003-2006. *Am J Clin Nutr.* 2009;89(5):1334-1342.
8. Looker AC, Dallman PR, Carroll MD, et al. Prevalence of iron deficiency in the United States. *JAMA.* 1997;277(12):973-976.
9. Mei Z, Cogswell ME, Looker AC, et al. Assessment of iron status in US pregnant women from the National Health and Nutrition Examination Survey (NHANES), 1999-2006. *Am J Clin Nutr.* 2011;93(6):1312-1320.
10. Rockey DC. Occult and obscure gastrointestinal bleeding: causes and clinical management. *Nat Rev Gastroenterol Hepatol.* 2010;7(5):265-279.
11. Blackler RW, Gemici B, Manko A, et al. NSAID-gastroenteropathy: new aspects of pathogenesis and prevention. *Curr Opin Pharmacol.* 2014;19C:11-16.
12. Bode C, Christian Bode J. Effect of alcohol consumption on the gut. *Best Pract Res Clin Gastroenterol.* 2003;17(4):575-592.
13. Coffey RJ, Washington MK, Corless CL, et al. Menetrier disease and gastrointestinal stromal tumors: hyperproliferative disorders of the stomach. *J Clin Invest.* 2007;117(1):70-80.
14. Hershko C, Skikne B. Pathogenesis and management of iron deficiency anemia: emerging role of celiac disease, *Helicobacter pylori*, and autoimmune gastritis. *Semin Hematol.* 2009;46(4):339-350.
15. Hershko CC. How I treat unexplained refractory iron deficiency anemia. *Blood.* 2013;123(3):326-333.
16. Stewart, Termanini, Sutliff, et al. Iron absorption in patients with Zollinger-Ellison syndrome treated with long-term gastric acid antisecretory therapy. *Aliment Pharmacol Ther.* 1998;12(1):83-98.
17. Bini EJ, Unger JS, Weinshel EH. Outcomes of endoscopy in patients with iron deficiency anemia after Billroth II partial gastrectomy. *J Clin Gastroenterol.* 2002;34(4):421-426.
18. Ruhl CE, Everhart JE. Relationship of iron-deficiency anemia with esophagitis and hiatal hernia: hospital findings from a prospective, population-based study. *Am J Gastroenterol.* 2001;96(2):322-326.
19. Panzuto F, Di Giulio E, Capurso G, et al. Large hiatal hernia in patients with iron deficiency anaemia: a prospective study on prevalence and treatment. *Aliment Pharmacol Ther.* 2004;19(6):663-670.
20. Haurani C, Carlin A, Hammoud Z, et al. Prevalence and resolution of anemia with paraesophageal hernia repair. *J Gastrointest Surg.* 2012;16(10):1817-1820.
21. Camus M, Jensen DM, Ohning GV, et al. Severe upper gastrointestinal hemorrhage from linear gastric ulcers in large hiatal hernias: a large prospective case series of Cameron ulcers. *Endoscopy.* 2013;45(05):397-400.
22. Crompton DWT, Nesheim MC. nutritional impact of intestinal helminthiasis during the human life cycle. *Annu Rev Nutr.* 2002;22(1):35-59.
23. Hemingway AP. Angiodysplasia as a cause of iron deficiency anaemia. *Blood Rev.* 1989;3(3):147-151.
24. Kar P, Mitra S, Resnick JM, et al. Gastric antral vascular ectasia: case report and review of the literature. *Clin Med Res.* 2013;11(2):80-85.
25. Chin MW, Enns R. Hemobilia. *Curr Gastroenterol Rep* 2010;12(2):121-129.
26. Duchini A, Sessoms S. Gastrointestinal hemorrhage in patients with systemic sclerosis and CREST syndrome. *Am J Gastroenterol.* 1998;93(9):1453-1456.
27. Bang JY, Peter S. Obscure gastrointestinal bleeding and Turner syndrome. *Dig Endosc.* 2013;25(4):462-464.
28. Wong CH, Tan YM, Chow WC, et al. Blue rubber bleb nevus syndrome: a clinical spectrum with correlation between cutaneous and gastrointestinal manifestations. *J Gastroenterol Hepatol.* 2003;18(8):1000-1002.
29. Sparberg M. Chronic iron deficiency anemia due to Meckel's diverticulum. *Am J Dis Child.* 1967;113(2):286-287.
30. Pai M, Chan A, Barr R. How I manage heavy menstrual bleeding. *Br J Haematol.* 2013;162(6):721-729.
31. Hallberg L, Rossander-Hulten L. Iron requirements in menstruating women. *Am J Clin Nutr.* 1991;54(6):1047-1058.
32. Brown EA, Sampson B, Muller BR, et al. Urinary iron loss in the nephrotic syndrome-an unusual cause of iron deficiency with a note on urinary copper losses. *Postgrad Med J.* 1984;60(700):125-128.
33. Kildahl-Andersen O, Dahl IM, Thorstensen K, et al. Iron deficiency anemia in a patient with excessive urinary iron loss. *Eur J Haematol.* 2000;64(3):204-205.
34. Hayden SJ, Albert TJ, Watkins TR, et al. Anemia in critical illness: insights into etiology, consequences, and management. *Am J Respir Crit Care Med.* 2012;185(10):1049-1057.
35. Fishbane S, Frei GL, Maesaka J. Reduction in recombinant human erythropoietin doses by the use of chronic intravenous iron supplementation. *Am J Kidney Dis.* 1995;26(1):41-46.
36. Eschbach JW, Cook JD, Scribner BH, et al. Iron balance in hemodialysis patients. *Ann Intern Med.* 1977;87(6):710-713.
37. Salvin HE, Pasricha SR, Marks DC, et al. Iron deficiency in blood donors: a national cross-sectional study. *Transfusion.* 2014;54(10):2434-2444.
38. Baart AM, van Noord PAH, Vergouwe Y, et al. High prevalence of subclinical iron deficiency in whole blood donors not deferred for low hemoglobin. *Transfusion.* 2013;53(8):1670-1677.
39. Brittenham GM. Iron deficiency in whole blood donors. *Transfusion.* 2011;51(3):458-461.
40. Spencer BR, Bialkowski W, Creel DV, et al. Elevated risk for iron depletion in high-school age blood donors. *Transfusion.* 2019;59(5):1706-1716.
41. Bernard J. [Lasthenie de Ferjol, Marie de Saint-Vallier, Emilie de Tourville or the novelist and anemia]. *Nouv Rev Fr Hematol.* 1982;24(1):43-44.
42. Karamanou M, Androutsos G. Lasthenie de Ferjol syndrome: a rare disease with fascinating history. *Intern Med J.* 2010;40(5):381-382.
43. Hirayama Y, Sakamaki S, Tsuji Y, et al. Fatality caused by self-bloodletting in a patient with factitious anemia. *Int J Hematol.* 2003;78(2):146-148.
44. Coello-Ramirez P, Larrosa-Haro A. Gastrointestinal occult hemorrhage and gastroduodenitis in cow's milk protein intolerance. *J Pediatr Gastroenterol Nutr.* 1984;3(2):215-218.
45. Kokkonen J, Simila S. Cow's milk intolerance with melena. *Eur J Pediatr.* 1980;135(2):189-194.
46. Milman N, Pedersen FM. Idiopathic pulmonary haemosiderosis. Epidemiology, pathogenic aspects and diagnosis. *Respir Med.* 1998;92(7):902-907.
47. Reid DW, Withers NJ, Francis L, et al. Iron deficiency in cystic fibrosis: Relationship to lung disease severity and chronic pseudomonas aeruginosa infection. *Chest.* 2002;121(1):48-54.
48. von Drygalski A, Biller J. Anemia in cystic fibrosis: incidence, mechanisms, and association with pulmonary function and vitamin deficiency. *Nutr Clin Pract.* 2008;23(5):557-563.
49. Pena-Rosas JP, De-Regil LM, Dowswell T, et al. Daily oral iron supplementation during pregnancy. *Cochrane Database Syst Rev.* 2012;12:CD004736.
50. Pena-Rosas JP, De-Regil LM, Dowswell T, et al. Intermittent oral iron supplementation during pregnancy. *Cochrane Database Syst Rev.* 2012;7:CD009997.
51. Reveiz L, Gyte GM, Cuervo LG, et al. Treatments for iron-deficiency anaemia in pregnancy. *Cochrane Database Syst Rev.* 2011;(10):CD003094.
52. Pena-Rosas JP, Viteri FE. Effects and safety of preventive oral iron or iron+folic acid supplementation for women during pregnancy. *Cochrane Database Syst Rev.* 2009;(4):CD004736.
53. Sangare L, van Eijk AM, Ter Kuile FO, et al. The association between malaria and iron status or supplementation in pregnancy: a systematic review and meta-analysis. *PLoS One.* 2014;9(2):e87743.
54. Auerbach M. IV Iron in pregnancy: an unmet clinical need. *Am J Hematol.* 2014;89(7):789-789.
55. Domellof M, Braegger C, Campoy C, et al. Iron requirements of infants and toddlers. *J Pediatr Gastroenterol Nutr.* 2014;58(1):119-129.
56. Baker RD, Greer FR, Nutrition TCo. Diagnosis and prevention of iron deficiency and iron-deficiency anemia in infants and young children (0-3 years of age). *Pediatrics.* 2010;126(5):1040-1050.

57. Egan SK, Tao SS, Pennington JA, et al. US Food and Drug Administration's Total Diet Study: intake of nutritional and toxic elements, 1991-96. *Food Addit Contam.* 2002;19(2):103-125.

58. Hallberg L, Hulthqn L. Perspectives on iron absorption. *Blood Cells Mol Dis.* 2002;29(3):562-573.

59. Jacobs A, Lawrie JH, Entwistle CC, et al. Gastric acid secretion in chronic iron-deficiency anaemia. *Lancet.* 1966;2(7456):190-192.

60. Schmitz U, Ko Y, Seewald S, et al. Iron-deficiency anemia as the sole manifestation of celiac disease. *Clin Investig.* 1994;72(7):519-521.

61. Kilpatrick ZM, Katz J. Occult celiac disease as a cause of iron deficiency anemia. *JAMA.* 1969;208(6):999-1001.

62. Sears DA, Anderson PR, Foy AL, et al. Urinary iron excretion and renal metabolism of hemoglobin in hemolytic diseases. *Blood.* 1966;28(5):708-725.

63. Roeser HP, Powell LW. Urinary iron excretion in valvular heart disease and after heart valve replacement. *Blood.* 1970;36(6):785-792.

64. McClung JP. Iron status and the female athlete. *J Trace Elem Med Biol.* 2012;26(2-3):124-126.

65. Karl JP, Lieberman HR, Cable SJ, et al. Randomized, double-blind, placebo-controlled trial of an iron-fortified food product in female soldiers during military training: relations between iron status, serum hepcidin, and inflammation. *Am J Clin Nutr.* 2010;92(1):93-100.

66. Whitfield JB, Treloar S, Zhu G, et al. Relative importance of female-specific and non-female-specific effects on variation in iron stores between women. *Br J Haematol.* 2003;120(5):860-866.

67. An P, Wu Q, Wang H, et al. TMPRSS6, but not TF, TFR2 or BMP2 variants are associated with increased risk of iron-deficiency anemia. *Hum Mol Genet.* 2012;21(9):2124-2131.

68. Finberg KE, Heeney MM, Campagna DR, et al. Mutations in TMPRSS6 cause iron-refractory iron deficiency anemia (IRIDA). *Nat Genet.* 2008;40(5):569-571.

69. Guillem F, Lawson S, Kannengiesser C, et al. Two nonsense mutations in the TMPRSS6 gene in a patient with microcytic anemia and iron deficiency. *Blood.* 2008;112(5):2089-2091.

70. Du X, She E, Gelbart T, et al. The serine protease TMPRSS6 is required to sense iron deficiency. *Science.* 2008;320(5879):1088-1092.

71. Kimura H, Finch CA, Adamson JW. Hematopoiesis in the rat: quantitation of hematopoietic progenitors and the response to iron deficiency anemia. *J Cell Physiol.* 1986;126(2):298-306.

72. Dallman PR. Biochemical basis for the manifestations of iron deficiency. *Annu Rev Nutr.* 1986;6:13-40.

73. Eisenstein RS, Ross KL. Novel roles for iron regulatory proteins in the adaptive response to iron deficiency. *J Nutr.* 2003;133(5):1510S-1516S.

74. Woodson RD, Wills RE, Lenfant C. Effect of acute and established anemia on O2 transport at rest, submaximal and maximal work. *J Appl Physiol Respir Environ Exerc Physiol.* 1978;44(1):36-43.

75. Crouter SE, DellaValle DM, Haas JD. Relationship between physical activity, physical performance, and iron status in adult women. *Appl Physiol Nutr Metab.* 2012;37(4):697-705.

76. Allen RP, Auerbach S, Bahrain H, et al. The prevalence and impact of restless legs syndrome on patients with iron deficiency anemia. *Am J Hematol.* 2013;88(4):261-264.

77. McCann JC, Ames BN. An overview of evidence for a causal relation between iron deficiency during development and deficits in cognitive or behavioral function. *Am J Clin Nutr.* 2007;85(4):931-945.

78. Jellen LC, Lu L, Wang X, et al. Iron deficiency alters expression of dopamine-related genes in the ventral midbrain in mice. *Neuroscience.* 2013;252(0):13-23.

79. Earley CJ, Allen RP, Beard JL, et al. Insight into the pathophysiology of restless legs syndrome. *J Neurosci Res.* 2000;62(5):623-628.

80. Oppenheimer SJ. Iron and its relation to immunity and infectious disease. *J Nutr.* 2001;131(2):616S-663S.

81. Jabara HH, Boyden SE, Chou J, et al. A missense mutation in TFRC, encoding transferrin receptor 1, causes combined immunodeficiency. *Nat Genet.* 2016;48(1):74-78.

82. Stoffel NU, Uyoga MA, Mutuku FM, et al. Iron deficiency anemia at time of vaccination predicts decreased vaccine response and iron supplementation at time of vaccination increases humoral vaccine response: a birth cohort study and a randomized trial follow-up study in Kenyan infants. *Front Immunol.* 2020:11:1313.

83. Lo B. The requirement of iron transport for lymphocyte function. *Nat Genet.* 2016;48(1):10-11.

84. Gwamaka M, Kurtis JD, Sorensen BE, et al. Iron deficiency protects against severe Plasmodium falciparum malaria and death in young children. *Clin Infect Dis.* 2012;54(8):1137-1144.

85. Kabyemela ER, Fried M, Kurtis JD, et al. Decreased susceptibility to *Plasmodium falciparum* infection in pregnant women with iron deficiency. *J Infect Dis.* 2008;198(2):163-166.

86. Stoltzfus RJ, Heidkamp R, Kenkel D, et al. Iron supplementation of young children: learning from the new evidence. *Food Nutr Bull.* 2007;28(suppl 4):S572-S584.

87. Spottiswoode N, Duffy P, Drakesmith H. Iron, anemia and hepcidin in malaria. *Front Pharmacol.* 2014;30;5:125.

88. Pagani A, Nai A, Corna G, et al. Low hepcidin accounts for the proinflammatory status associated with iron deficiency. *Blood.* 2011;118(3):736-746.

89. Hale LP, Kant EP, Greer PK, et al. Iron supplementation decreases severity of allergic inflammation in murine lung. *PLoS One.* 2012;7(9):e45667.

90. Thompson J, Biggs BA, Pasricha SR. Effects of daily iron supplementation in 2- to 5-year-old children: systematic review and meta-analysis. *Pediatrics.* 2013;131(4):739-753.

91. Sachdev H, Gera T, Nestel P. Effect of iron supplementation on physical growth in children: systematic review of randomised controlled trials. *Public Health Nutr.* 2006;9(7):904-920.

92. Beard JL, Borel MJ, Derr J. Impaired thermoregulation and thyroid function in iron-deficiency anemia. *Am J Clin Nutr.* 1990;52(5):813-819.

93. Baird IM, Dodge OG, Palmer FJ, et al. The tongue and oesophagus in iron-deficiency anaemia and the effect of iron therapy. *J Clin Pathol.* 1961;14:603-609.

94. Lees F, Rosenthal FD. Gastric mucosal lesions before and after treatment in iron deficiency anaemia. *Q J Med.* 1958;27(105):19-26.

95. Naiman JL, Oski FA, Diamond LK, et al. The gastrointestinal effects of iron-deficiency anaemia. *Pediatrics.* 1964;33:83-99.

96. Scott J, Valentine JA, St Hill CA, et al. A quantitative histological analysis of the effects of age and sex on human lingual epithelium. *J Biol Buccale.* 1983;11(4):303-315.

97. Jacobs A. The buccal mucosa in anaemia. *J Clin Pathol.* 1960;13:463-468.

98. Boddington MM. Changes in buccal cells in the anaemias. *J Clin Pathol.* 1959;12(3):222-227.

99. Macleod RI, Hamilton PJ, Soames JV. Quantitative exfoliative oral cytology in iron-deficiency and megaloblastic anemia. *Anal Quant Cytol Histol.* 1988;10(3):176-180.

100. Burko H, Mellins HZ, Watson J. Skull changes in iron deficiency anemia simulating congenital hemolytic anemia. *Am J Roentgenol Radium Ther Nucl Med.* 1961;86:447-452.

101. Moseley JE. Skull changes in chronic iron deficiency anemia. *Am J Roentgenol Radium Ther Nucl Med.* 1961;85:649-652.

102. Shahidi NT, Diamond LK. Skull changes in infants with chronic iron-deficiency anemia. *N Engl J Med.* 1960;262:137-139.

103. Haas JD, Brownlie T. Iron deficiency and reduced work capacity: a critical review of the research to determine a causal relationship. *J Nutr.* 2001;131(2):676S-690S.

104. Wang B, Zhan S, Gong T, et al. Iron therapy for improving psychomotor development and cognitive function in children under the age of three with iron deficiency anaemia. *Cochrane Database Syst Rev.* 2013;6:CD001444.

105. Abdullah K, Kendzerska T, Shah P, et al. Efficacy of oral iron therapy in improving the developmental outcome of pre-school children with non-anaemic iron deficiency: a systematic review. *Public Health Nutr.* 2013;16(8):1497-1506.

106. Hermoso M, Vucic V, Vollhardt C, et al. The effect of iron on cognitive development and function in infants, children and adolescents: a systematic review. *Ann Nutr Metab.* 2011;59(2-4):154-165.

107. Hornyak M, Scholz H, Kohnen R, et al. What treatment works best for restless legs syndrome? Meta-analyses of dopaminergic and non-dopaminergic medications. *Sleep Med Rev.* 2014;18(2):153-164.

108. Trotti LM, Bhadriraju S, Becker LA. Iron for restless legs syndrome. *Cochrane Database Syst Rev.* 2012;5:CD007834.

109. Trenkwalder C, Allen R, Högl B, et al. Comorbidities, treatment, and pathophysiology in restless legs syndrome. *Lancet Neurol.* 2018;17(11):994-1005.

110. Cortese S, Angriman M, Lecendreux M, et al. Iron and attention deficit/hyperactivity disorder: what is the empirical evidence so far? A systematic review of the literature. *Expert Rev Neurother.* 2012;12(10):1227-1240.

111. Trujillo MH, Desenne JJ, Pinto HB. Reversible papilledema in iron deficiency anemia. Two cases with normal spinal fluid pressure. *Ann Ophthalmol.* 1972;4(5):378-380.

112. Knizley H Jr, Noyes WD. Iron deficiency anemia, papilledema, thrombocytosis, and transient hemiparesis. *Arch Intern Med.* 1972;129(3):483-486.

113. Stoebner R, Kiser R, Alperin JB. Iron deficiency anemia and papilledema. Rapid resolution with oral iron therapy. *Am J Dig Dis.* 1970;15(10):919-922.

114. Lubeck MJ. Papilledema caused by iron-deficiency anemia. *Trans Am Acad Ophthalmol Otolaryngol.* 1959;63(3):306-310.

115. Kim LJ, Coelho FM, Tufik S, et al. New perspectives of iron deficiency as a risk factor for ischemic stroke. *Ann Hematol.* 2014;93(7):1243-1244.

116. Chang YL, Hung SH, Ling W, et al. Association between ischemic stroke and iron-deficiency anemia: a population-based study. *PLoS One.* 2013;8(12):e82952.

117. Munot P, De VC, Hemingway C, et al. Severe iron deficiency anaemia and ischaemic stroke in children. *Arch Dis Child.* 2011;96(3):276-279.

118. Maguire JL, deVeber G, Parkin PC. Association between iron-deficiency anemia and stroke in young children. *Pediatrics.* 2007;120(5):1053-1057.

119. Yager JY, Hartfield DS. Neurologic manifestations of iron deficiency in childhood. *Pediatr Neurol.* 2002;27(2):85-92.

120. Novacek G. Plummer-Vinson syndrome. *Orphanet J Rare Dis.* 2006;1:36.

121. Lumish RA, Young SL, Lee S, et al. Gestational iron deficiency is associated with pica behaviors in adolescents. *J Nutr.* 2014;144(10):1533-1539.

122. Uchida T, Kawati Y. Pagophagia in iron deficiency anemia. *Rinsho Ketsueki.* 2014;55(4):436-439.

123. Spencer BR, Kleinman S, Wright DJ, et al. Restless legs syndrome, pica, and iron status in blood donors. *Transfusion.* 2013;53(8):1645-1652.

124. Barton J, Barton JC, Bertoli L. Pica associated with iron deficiency or depletion: clinical and laboratory correlates in 262 non-pregnant adult outpatients. *BMC Blood Disord.* 2010;10(1):9.

125. Olsen EA, Reed KB, Cacchio PB, et al. Iron deficiency in female pattern hair loss, chronic telogen effluvium, and control groups. *J Am Acad Dermatol.* 2010;63(6):991-999.

126. Deloche C, Bastien P, Chadoutaud S, et al. Low iron stores: a risk factor for excessive hair loss in non-menopausal women. *Eur J Dermatol.* 2007;17(6):507-512.

127. Beutler E, Lee P, Gelbart T, et al. The mask mutation identifies TMPRSS6 as an essential suppressor of hepcidin gene expression, required for normal uptake of dietary iron. *ASH Annu Meet Abstr.* 2007;110(11):3.

128. Bessman JD, Feinstein DI. Quantitative anisocytosis as a discriminant between iron deficiency and thalassemia minor. *Blood.* 1979;53(2):288-293.

129. England JM, Ward SM, Down MC. Microcytosis, anisocytosis and the red cell indices in iron deficiency. *Br J Haematol.* 1976;34(4):589-597.

130. Beutler E. The red cell indices in the diagnosis of iron-deficiency anemia. *Ann Intern Med.* 1959;50(2):313-322.

131. Verma V, Ayalew G, Sidhu G, et al. An analysis of the relationship between severe iron deficiency anemia and thrombocytopenia. *Ann Hematol.* 2014;1-3.

132. Dan K. Thrombocytosis in iron deficiency anemia. *Intern Med.* 2005;44(10):1025-1026.

133. Keung YK, Owen J. Iron deficiency and thrombosis: literature review. *Clin Appl Thromb Hemost.* 2004;10(4):387-391.

134. Geddis AE, Kaushansky K. Cross-reactivity between erythropoietin and thrombopoietin at the level of Mpl does not account for the thrombocytosis seen in iron deficiency. *J Pediatr Hematol Oncol.* 2003;25(11):919-920.

135. Xavier-Ferrucio J, Scanlon V, Li X, et al. Low iron promotes megakaryocytic commitment of megakaryocytic-erythroid progenitors in humans and mice. *Blood.* 2019;134(18):1547-1557.

136. Kasper CK, Whissell DY, Wallerstein RO. Clinical aspects of iron deficiency. *JAMA.* 1965;191:359-363.

137. Barron BA, Hoyer JD, Tefferi A. A bone marrow report of absent stainable iron is not diagnostic of iron deficiency. *Ann Hematol.* 2001;80(3):166-169.

138. Thomason RW, Lavelle J, Nelson D, et al. Parenteral iron therapy is associated with a characteristic pattern of iron staining on bone marrow aspirate smears. *Am J Clin Pathol.* 2007;128(4):590-593.

139. Cavill IA. Iron status indicators: hello new, goodbye old? *Blood.* 2013;101(1):372-373.

140. Ellis LD, Jensen WN, Westerman MP. Marrow iron. An evaluation of depleted stores in a series of 1,332 needle biopsies. *Ann Intern Med.* 1964;61:44-49.

141. Garby L, Irnell L, Werner I. Iron deficiency in women of fertile age in a Swedish community. II. Efficiency of several laboratory tests to predict the response to iron supplementation. *Acta Med Scand.* 1969;185(1-2):107-111.

142. Dale JC, Burritt MF, Zinsmeister AR. Diurnal variation of serum iron, iron-binding capacity, transferrin saturation, and ferritin levels. *Am J Clin Pathol.* 2002;117(5):802-808.

143. Mardell M, Zilva JF. Effect of oral contraceptives on the variations in serum-iron during the menstrual cycle. *Lancet.* 1967;2(7530):1323-1325.

144. Zilva JF, Patston VJ. Variations in serum-iron in healthy women. *Lancet.* 1966;1(7435):459-462.

145. Cartwright GE. The anemia of chronic disorders. *Semin Hematol.* 1966;3(4):351-375.

146. Adamson JW. The anemia of inflammation/malignancy: mechanisms and management. *Hematology Am Soc Hematol Educ Program.* 2008;159-165.

147. Huang CH, Chang CC, Kuo CL, et al. Serum iron concentration, but not hemoglobin, correlates with TIMI risk score and 6-month left ventricular performance after primary angioplasty for acute myocardial infarction. *PLoS One.* 2014;9(8):e104495.

148. Syrkis I, Machtey I. Hypoferremia in acute myocardial infarction. *J Am Geriatr Soc.* 1973;21(1):28-30.

149. Follezou JY, Bizon M. Cancer chemotherapy induces a transient increase of serum-iron level. *Neoplasma.* 1986;33(2):225-231.

150. Seligman PA, Schleicher RB. Comparison of methods used to measure serum iron in the presence of iron gluconate or iron dextran. *Clin Chem.* 1999;45(6 Pt 1):898-901.

151. Geisser P, Burckhardt S. The pharmacokinetics and pharmacodynamics of iron preparations. *Pharmaceutics.* 2011;3(1):12-33.

152. Cohen LA, Gutierrez L, Weiss A, et al. Serum ferritin is derived primarily from macrophages through a nonclassical secretory pathway. *Blood.* 2010;116(9):1574-1584.

153. Lipschitz DA, Cook JD, Finch CA. A clinical evaluation of serum ferritin as an index of iron stores. *N Engl J Med.* 1974;290(22):1213-1216.

154. Sears DA. Anemia of chronic disease. *Med Clin North Am.* 1992;76(3):567-579.

155. Hansen TM, Hansen NE. Serum ferritin as indicator of iron responsive anaemia in patients with rheumatoid arthritis. *Ann Rheum Dis.* 1986;45(7):596-602.

156. Fishbane S, Kalantar-Zadeh K, Nissenson AR. Serum ferritin in chronic kidney disease: reconsidering the upper limit for iron treatment. *Semin Dial.* 2004;17(5):336-341.

157. Milman N, Graudal N, Hegnhøj J, et al. Relationships among serum iron status markers, chemical and histochemical liver iron content in 117 patients with alcoholic and non-alcoholic hepatic disease. *Hepatogastroenterology.* 1994;41(1):20-24.

158. Milman N, Graudal N. Serum ferritin in acute viral hepatitis. *Scand J Gastroenterol.* 1984;19(1):38-40.

159. Matzner Y, Konijn AM, Hershko C. Serum ferritin in hematologic malignancies. *Am J Hematol.* 1980;9(1):13-22.

160. Medrano-Engay B, Irun P, Gervas-Arruga J, et al. Iron homeostasis and inflammatory biomarker analysis in patients with type 1 Gaucher disease. *Blood Cells Mol Dis.* 2014;53(4):171-175.

161. Mekinian A, Stirnemann J, Belmatoug N, et al. Ferritinemia during type 1 Gaucher disease: mechanisms and progression under treatment. *Blood Cells Mol Dis.* 2012;49(1):53-57.

162. Moore C Jr, Ormseth M, Fuchs H. Causes and significance of markedly elevated serum ferritin levels in an academic medical center. *J Clin Rheumatol.* 2013;19(6):324-328.

163. Lehmberg K, McClain KL, Janka GE, et al. Determination of an appropriate cut-off value for ferritin in the diagnosis of hemophagocytic lymphohistiocytosis. *Pediatr Blood Cancer.* 2014;61(11):2101-2103.

164. Mayr R, Janecke AR, Schranz M, et al. Ferroportin disease: a systematic meta-analysis of clinical and molecular findings. *J Hepatol.* 2010;53(5):941-949.

165. Magge H, Sprinz P, Adams WG, et al. Zinc protoporphyrin and iron deficiency screening: trends and therapeutic response in an urban pediatric center. *JAMA Pediatr.* 2013;167(4):361-367.

166. Mei Z, Parvanta I, Cogswell ME, et al. Erythrocyte protoporphyrin or hemoglobin: which is a better screening test for iron deficiency in children and women? *Am J Clin Nutr.* 2003;77(5):1229-1233.

167. Braun J. Erythrocyte zinc protoporphyrin. *Kidney Int Suppl.* 1999;69:S57-S60.

168. Hastka J, Lasserre JJ, Schwarzbeck A, et al. Zinc protoporphyrin in anemia of chronic disorders. *Blood.* 1993;81(5):1200-1204.

169. Mwangi MN, Maskey S, Andang'o PEA, et al. Diagnostic utility of zinc protoporphyrin to detect iron deficiency in Kenyan pregnant women. *BMC Medicine.* 2014;12(1):229.

170. Skikne BS, Flowers CH, Cook JD. Serum transferrin receptor: a quantitative measure of tissue iron deficiency. *Blood.* 1990;75(9):1870-1876.

171. Skikne BS. Serum transferrin receptor. *Am J Hematol.* 2008;83(11):872-875.

172. Pettersson T, Kivivuori SM, Siimes MA. Is serum transferrin receptor useful for detecting iron-deficiency in anaemic patients with chronic inflammatory diseases? *Br J Rheumatol.* 1994;33(8):740-744.

173. Thorpe SJ, Heath A, Sharp G, et al. A WHO reference reagent for the serum transferrin receptor (sTfR): international collaborative study to evaluate a recombinant soluble transferrin receptor preparation. *Clin Chem Lab Med.* 2010;48(6):815-820.

174. Uaprasert N, Rojnuckarin P, Bhokaisawan N, et al. Elevated serum transferrin receptor levels in common types of thalassemia heterozygotes in Southeast Asia: a correlation with genotypes and red cell indices. *Clin Chim Acta.* 2009;403(1-2):110-113.

175. Mockenhaupt FP, May J, Stark K, et al. Serum transferrin receptor levels are increased in asymptomatic and mild *Plasmodium falciparum*-infection. *Haematologica.* 1999;84(10):869-873.

176. Cook JD, Flowers CH, Skikne BS. The quantitative assessment of body iron. *Blood.* 2003;101(9):3359-3363.

177. Skikne BS, Punnonen K, Caldron PH, et al. Improved differential diagnosis of anemia of chronic disease and iron deficiency anemia: a prospective multicenter evaluation of soluble transferrin receptor and the sTfR/log ferritin index. *Am J Hematol.* 2011;86(11):923-927.

178. Suominen P, Punnonen K, Rajamaki A, et al. Serum transferrin receptor and transferrin receptor-ferritin index identify healthy subjects with subclinical iron deficits. *Blood.* 1998;92(8):2934-2939.

179. Punnonen K, Irjala K, Rajamaki A. Serum transferrin receptor and its ratio to serum ferritin in the diagnosis of iron deficiency. *Blood.* 1997;89(3):1052-1057.

180. Brugnara C, Mohandas N. Red cell indices in classification and treatment of anemias: from M.M. Wintrobe's original 1934 classification to the third millennium. *Curr Opin Hematol.* 2013;20(3):222-230.

181. Brugnara C, Schiller B, Moran J. Reticulocyte hemoglobin equivalent (Ret He) and assessment of iron-deficient states. *Clin Lab Haematol.* 2006;28(5):303-308.

182. Bovy C, Gothot A, Krzesinski JM, et al. Mature erythrocyte indices: new markers of iron availability. *Haematologica.* 2005;90(4):549-551.

183. Wang CY, Babitt JL. Liver iron sensing and body iron homeostasis. *Blood.* 2019;133(1):18-29.

184. Ganz T. Systemic iron homeostasis. *Physiol Rev.* 2013;93(4):1721-1741.

185. Ganz T, Olbina G, Girelli D, et al. Immunoassay for human serum hepcidin. *Blood.* 2008;112(10):4292-4297.

186. Bregman DB, Morris D, Koch TA, et al. Hepcidin levels predict nonresponsiveness to oral iron therapy in patients with iron deficiency anemia. *Am J Hematol.* 2013;88(2):97-101.

187. van der Vorm LN, Hendriks JC, Laarakkers CM, et al. Toward worldwide hepcidin assay harmonization: identification of a commutable secondary reference material. *Clin Chem.* 2016;62(7):993-1001.

188. Iolascon A, De FL, Beaumont C. Molecular basis of inherited microcytic anemia due to defects in iron acquisition or heme synthesis. *Haematologica.* 2009;94(3):395-408.

189. Beutler E, West C. Hematologic differences between African-Americans and whites: the roles of iron deficiency and alpha-thalassemia on hemoglobin levels and mean corpuscular volume. *Blood.* 2005;106(2):740-745.

190. Fairbanks VF, Oliveros R, Brandabur JH, et al. Homozygous hemoglobin E mimics beta-thalassemia minor without anemia or hemolysis: hematologic, functional, and biosynthetic studies of first North American cases. *Am J Hematol.* 1980;8(1):109-121.

191. Fairbanks VF, Gilchrist GS, Brimhall B, et al. Hemoglobin E trait reexamined: a cause of microcytosis and erythrocytosis. *Blood.* 1979;53(1):109-115.

192. Johnson CS, Tegos C, Beutler E. Thalassemia minor: routine erythrocyte measurements and differentiation from iron deficiency. *Am J Clin Pathol.* 1983;80(1):31-36.

193. Duma H, Efremov G, Sadikario A, et al. Study of nine families with haemoglobin-Lepore. *Br J Haematol.* 1968;15(2):161-172.

194. Cartei G, Chisesi T, Cazzavillan M, et al. Relationship between Hb and HbA2 concentrations in beta-thalassemia trait and effect of iron deficiency anaemia. *Biomedicine.* 1976;25(8):282-284.

195. Infusino I, Braga F, Dolci A, et al. Soluble transferrin receptor (sTfR) and sTfR/log ferritin index for the diagnosis of iron-deficiency anemia: a meta-analysis. *Am J Clin Pathol.* 2012;138(5):642-649.

196. Prentice AM, Doherty CP, Abrams SA, et al. Hepcidin is the major predictor of erythrocyte iron incorporation in anemic African children. *Blood.* 2012;119(8):1922-1928.

197. Intragumtornchai T, Rojnukkarin P, Swasdikul D, et al. The role of serum ferritin in the diagnosis of iron deficiency anaemia in patients with liver cirrhosis. *J Intern Med.* 1998;243(3):233-241.

198. Prieto J, Barry M, Sherlock S. Serum ferritin in patients with iron overload and with acute and chronic liver diseases. *Gastroenterology.* 1975;68(3):525-533.

199. Macdougall IC, Hutton RD, Cavill I, et al. Poor response to treatment of renal anaemia with erythropoietin corrected by iron given intravenously. *BMJ.* 1989;299(6692):157-158.

200. Dukkipati R, Kalantar-Zadeh K. Should we limit the ferritin upper threshold to 500 ng/mL in CKD patients? *Nephrol News Issues.* 2007;21(1):34-38.

201. Macdougall IC, Bock AH, Carrera F, et al. FIND-CKD: a randomized trial of intravenous ferric carboxymaltose versus oral iron in patients with chronic kidney disease and iron deficiency anaemia. *Nephrol Dial Transplant.* 2014;29(11):2075-2084.

202. Chung M, Chan JA, Moorthy D, et al. Biomarkers for assessing and managing iron deficiency anemia in late-stage chronic kidney disease. *Comparative Effectiveness Reviews, No. 83. AHRQ Publication* 2013;12(13).

203. Hilal H, McCurdy PR. A pitfall in the interpretation of serum iron values. *Ann Intern Med.* 1967;66(5):983-988.

204. Rockey DC. Occult Gastrointestinal Bleeding. *Gastroenterol Clin North Am.* 2005;34(4):699-718.

205. Hallberg L, Ryttinger L, Solvell L. Side-effects of oral iron therapy. A double-blind study of different iron compounds in tablet form. *Acta Med Scand Suppl.* 1966;459:3-10.

206. Fishbane S, Block GA, Loram L, et al. Effects of ferric citrate in patients with nondialysis-dependent CKD and iron deficiency anemia. *J Am Soc Nephrol.* 2017;28(6):1851-1858.

207. Leung AK, Chan KW. Iron deficiency anemia. *Adv Pediatr.* 2001;48:385-408.

208. Stoffel NU, Cercamondi CI, Brittenham G, et al. Iron absorption from oral iron supplements given on consecutive versus alternate days and as single morning doses versus twice-daily split dosing in iron-depleted women: two open-label, randomised controlled trials. *Lancet Haematol.* 2017;4(11):e524-e533.

209. Stoffel NU, Zeder C, Brittenham GM, et al. Iron absorption from supplements is greater with alternate day than with consecutive day dosing in iron-deficient anemic women. *Haematologica.* 2020;105(5):1232-1239.

210. Gordeuk VR, Brittenham GM, Hughes M, et al. High-dose carbonyl iron for iron deficiency anemia: a randomized double-blind trial. *Am J Clin Nutr.* 1987;46(6):1029-1034.

211. Ganz T, Bino A, Salusky IB. Mechanism of action and clinical attributes of Auryxia((R)) (ferric citrate). *Drugs.* 2019;79(9):957-968.

212. Harding KB, Neufeld LM. Iron deficiency and anemia control for infants and young children in malaria-endemic areas: a call to action and consensus among the research community. *Adv Nutr.* 2012;3(4):551-554.

213. Chang TP, Rangan C. Iron poisoning: a literature-based review of epidemiology, diagnosis, and management. *Pediatr Emerg Care.* 2011;27(10):978-985.

214. Susantitaphong P, Alqahtani F, Jaber BL. Efficacy and safety of intravenous iron therapy for functional iron deficiency anemia in hemodialysis patients: a meta-analysis. *Am J Nephrol.* 2014;39(2):130-141.

215. Taylor JE, Peat N, Porter C, et al. Regular low-dose intravenous iron therapy improves response to erythropoietin in haemodialysis patients. *Nephrol Dial Transplant.* 1996;11(6):1079-1083.

216. Rodgers GM, Auerbach M, Cella D, et al. High-molecular weight iron dextran: a wolf in sheep's clothing? *J Am Soc Nephrol.* 2008;19(5):833-834.

217. Wolf M, Chertow GM, Macdougall IC, et al. Randomized trial of intravenous iron-induced hypophosphatemia. *JCI Insight.* 2018;3(23).

218. Bircher AJ, Auerbach M. Hypersensitivity from intravenous iron products. *Immunol Allergy Clin North Am.* 2014;34(3):707-723.

219. Fishbane SN, Singh AK, Cournoyer SH, et al. Ferric pyrophosphate citrate (Triferic) administration via the dialysate maintains hemoglobin and iron balance in chronic hemodialysis patients. *Nephrol Dial Transplant.* 2015;30(12):2019-2026.

220. Aslan D, Crain K, Beutler E. A new case of human atransferrinemia with a previously undescribed mutation in the transferrin gene. *Acta Haematol.* 2007;118(4):244-247.

221. Chen C, Wen S, Tan X. Molecular analysis of a novel case of congenital atransferrinemia. *Acta Haematol.* 2009;122(1):27-28.

222. Knisely AS, Gelbart T, Beutler E. Molecular characterization of a third case of human atransferrinemia. *Blood.* 2004;104(8):2607.

223. Shamsian BS, Rezaei N, Arzanian MT, et al. Severe hypochromic microcytic anemia in a patient with congenital atransferrinemia. *Pediatr Hematol Oncol.* 2009;26(5):356-362.

224. Iolascon A, De FL. Mutations in the gene encoding DMT1: clinical presentation and treatment. *Semin Hematol.* 2009;46(4):358-370.

225. Mims MP, Guan Y, Pospisilova D, et al. Identification of a human mutation of DMT1 in a patient with microcytic anemia and iron overload. *Blood.* 2005;105(3):1337-1342.

226. Whitington PF. Gestational alloimmune liver disease and neonatal hemochromatosis. *Semin Liver Dis.* 2012;32(4):325-332.

227. Davis WD Jr, Arrowsmith WR. The treatment of hemochromatosis by massive venesection. *Ann Intern Med.* 1953;39(4):723-734.

228. MacDonald RA. Hemochromatosis: a perlustration. *Am J Clin Nutr.* 1970;23(5):592-603.

229. Feder JN, Gnirke A, Thomas W, et al. A novel MHC class I-like gene is mutated in patients with hereditary haemochromatosis. *Nat Genet.* 1996;13(4):399-408.

230. Beutler E. Iron storage disease: facts, fiction and progress. *Blood Cells Mol Dis.* 2007;39(2):140-147.

231. Lucotte G, Dieterlen F. A European allele map of the C282Y mutation of hemochromatosis: Celtic versus Viking origin of the mutation? *Blood Cells Mol Dis.* 2003;31(2):262-267.

232. Adams PC, Deugnier Y, Moirand R, et al. The relationship between iron overload, clinical symptoms, and age in 410 patients with genetic hemochromatosis. *Hepatology.* 1997;25(1):162-166.

233. McDonnell SM, Preston BL, Jewell SA, et al. A survey of 2,851 patients with hemochromatosis: symptoms and response to treatment. *Am J Med.* 1999;106(6):619-624.

234. Waalen J, Felitti V, Gelbart T, et al. Prevalence of hemochromatosis-related symptoms among individuals with mutations in the HFE gene. *Mayo Clin Proc.* 2002;77(6):522-530.

235. Allen KJ, Gurrin LC, Constantine CC, et al. Iron-overload-related disease in HFE hereditary hemochromatosis. *N Engl J Med.* 2008;358(3):221-230.

236. Beutler E. The HFE Cys282Tyr mutation as a necessary but not sufficient cause of clinical hereditary hemochromatosis. *Blood.* 2003;101(9):3347-3350.

237. Rossi E, Olynyk JK, Jeffrey GP. Clinical penetrance of C282Y homozygous HFE hemochromatosis. *Expert Rev Hematol.* 2008;1(2):205-216.

238. Bacon BR, Britton RS. Clinical penetrance of hereditary hemochromatosis. *N Engl J Med.* 2008;358(3):291-292.

239. Fletcher LM, Powell LW. Hemochromatosis and alcoholic liver disease. *Alcohol.* 2003;30(2):131-136.

240. Fletcher LM, Dixon JL, Purdie DM, et al. Excess alcohol greatly increases the prevalence of cirrhosis in hereditary hemochromatosis. *Gastroenterology.* 2002;122(2):281-289.

241. McCord JM. Iron, free radicals, and oxidative injury. *Semin Hematol.* 1998;35(1):5-12.

242. Carthew P, Dorman BM, Edwards RE, et al. A unique rodent model for both the cardiotoxic and hepatotoxic effects of prolonged iron overload. *Lab Invest.* 1993;69(2):217-222.

243. Tsukamoto H, Horne W, Kamimura S, et al. Experimental liver cirrhosis induced by alcohol and iron. *J Clin Invest.* 1995;96(1):620-630.

244. Arosio P, Ingrassia R, Cavadini P. Ferritins: a family of molecules for iron storage, anti-oxidation and more. *Biochim Biophys Acta.* 2009;1790(7):589-599.

245. Ramos E, Kautz L, Rodriguez R, et al. Evidence for distinct pathways of hepcidin regulation by acute and chronic iron loading in mice. *Hepatology.* 2011;53(4):1333-1341.

246. Bridle KR, Frazer DM, Wilkins SJ, et al. Disrupted hepcidin regulation in *HFE*-associated haemochromatosis and the liver as a regulator of body iron homoeostasis. *Lancet.* 2003;361:669-673.

247. Nemeth E, Roetto A, Garozzo G, et al. Hepcidin is decreased in TFR2 hemochromatosis. *Blood.* 2005;105(4):1803-1806.

248. Papanikolaou G, Samuels ME, Ludwig EH, et al. Mutations in HFE2 cause iron overload in chromosome 1q-linked juvenile hemochromatosis. *Nat Genet.* 2004;36(1):77-82.

249. Sham RL, Phatak PD, Nemeth E, et al. Hereditary hemochromatosis due to resistance to hepcidin: high hepcidin concentrations in a family with C326S ferroportin mutation. *Blood.* 2009;114(2):493-494.

250. Fernandes A, Preza GC, Phung Y, et al. The molecular basis of hepcidin-resistant hereditary hemochromatosis. *Blood.* 2009;114(2):437-443.

251. Tanno T, Bhanu NV, Oneal PA, et al. High levels of GDF15 in thalassemia suppress expression of the iron regulatory protein hepcidin. *Nat Med.* 2007;13(9):1096-1101.

252. Kautz L, Jung G, Valore EV, et al. Identification of erythroferrone as an erythroid regulator of iron metabolism. *Nat Genet.* 2014;46(7):678-684.

253. Tamary H, Shalev H, Perez-Avraham G, et al. Elevated growth differentiation factor 15 expression in patients with congenital dyserythropoietic anemia type I. *Blood.* 2008;112(13):5241-5244.

254. Casanovas G, Swinkels DW, Altamura S, et al. Growth differentiation factor 15 in patients with congenital dyserythropoietic anaemia (CDA) type II. *J Mol Med(Berl).* 2011;89(8):811-816.

255. Andolfo I, Rosato BE, Marra R, et al. The BMP-SMAD pathway mediates the impaired hepatic iron metabolism associated with the ERFE-A260S variant. *Am J Hematol.* 2019;94(11):1227-1235.

256. Barton JC, Acton RT, Rivers CA, et al. Genotypic and phenotypic heterogeneity of African Americans with primary iron overload. *Blood Cells Mol Dis.* 2003;31(3):310-319.

257. Sham RL, Phatak PD, West C, et al. Autosomal dominant hereditary hemochromatosis associated with a novel ferroportin mutation and unique clinical features. *Blood Cells Mol Dis.* 2005;34(2):157-161.

258. Atkins JL, Pilling LC, Masoli JAH, et al. Association of hemochromatosis HFE p.C282Y homozygosity with hepatic malignancy. *JAMA.* 2020;324(20):2048-2057.

259. Porter JB, Garbowski M. The pathophysiology of transfusional iron overload. *Hematol Oncol Clin North Am.* 2014;28(4):683-701, vi.

260. Pietrangelo A. Juvenile hemochromatosis. *J Hepatol.* 2006;45(6):892-894.

261. Anderson LJ. Assessment of iron overload with T2* magnetic resonance imaging. *Prog Cardiovasc Dis.* 2011;54(3):287-294.

262. Herring WB, Gay RM. Absence of stainable bone marrow iron in hemochromatosis. *South Med J.* 1981;74(9):1088-1089, 1094.

263. Camaschella C, Poggiali E. Inherited disorders of iron metabolism. *Curr Opin Pediatr.* 2011;23(1):14-20.

264. Beutler E, Felitti VJ, Ho NJ, et al. Commentary on HFE S65C Variant Is Not Associated with Increased Transferrin Saturation in Voluntary Blood Donors by Naveen Arya, Subrata Chakrabrati, Robert A. Hegele, Paul C. Adams. *Blood Cells Mol Dis.* 1999;25(6):358-360.

265. Roetto A, Papanikolaou G, Politou M, et al. Mutant antimicrobial peptide hepcidin is associated with severe juvenile hemochromatosis. *Nat Genet.* 2003;33(1):21-22.

266. Altamura S, Kessler R, Gröne HJ, et al. Resistance of ferroportin to hepcidin binding causes exocrine pancreatic failure and fatal iron overload. *Cell Metab.* 2014;20(2):359-367.

267. Wallace DF, Harris JM, Subramaniam VN. Functional analysis and theoretical modeling of ferroportin reveals clustering of mutations according to phenotype. *Am J Physiol Cell Physiol.* 2010;298(1):C75-C84.

268. Barton JC, Acton RT, Lee PL, et al. SLC40A1 Q248H allele frequencies and Q248H-associated risk of non-HFE iron overload in persons of sub-Saharan African descent. *Blood Cells Mol Dis.* 2007;39(2):206-211.

269. Rivers CA, Barton JC, Gordeuk VR, et al. Association of ferroportin Q248H polymorphism with elevated levels of serum ferritin in African Americans in the Hemochromatosis and Iron Overload Screening (HEIRS) Study. *Blood Cells Mol Dis.* 2007;38(3):247-252.

270. Girelli D, Trombini P, Busti F, et al. A time course of hepcidin response to iron challenge in patients with HFE and TFR2 hemochromatosis. *Haematologica.* 2011;96(4):500-506.

271. Kawabata H, Fleming RE, Gui D, et al. Expression of hepcidin is down-regulated in TfR2 mutant mice manifesting a phenotype of hereditary hemochromatosis. *Blood.* 2005;105(1):376-381.

272. Camaschella C, Roetto A, Cali A, et al. The gene TFR2 is mutated in a new type of haemochromatosis mapping to 7q22. *Nat Genet.* 2000;25(1):14-15.

273. Huang FW, Babitt JL, Wrighting DM, et al. Hemojuvelin acts as a bone morphogenetic protein co-receptor to regulate hepcidin expression. *ASH Annu Meet Abstr.* 2005;106(11):511.

274. Niederkofler V, Salie R, Arber S. Hemojuvelin is essential for dietary iron sensing, and its mutation leads to severe iron overload. *J Clin Invest.* 2005;115(8):2180-2186.

275. Huang FW, Pinkus JL, Pinkus GS, et al. A mouse model of juvenile hemochromatosis. *J Clin Invest.* 2005;115(8):2187-2191.

276. Lee PL, Beutler E, Rao SV, et al. Genetic abnormalities and juvenile hemochromatosis: mutations of the HJV gene encoding hemojuvelin. *Blood.* 2004;103(12):4669-4671.

277. Lanzara C, Roetto A, Daraio F, et al. Spectrum of hemojuvelin gene mutations in 1q-linked juvenile hemochromatosis. *Blood.* 2004;103(11):4317-4321.

278. Steinbicker AU, Bartnikas TB, Lohmeyer LK, et al. Perturbation of hepcidin expression by BMP type I receptor deletion induces iron overload in mice. *Blood.* 2011;118(15):4224-4230.

279. Blanco E, Kannengiesser C, Grandchamp B, et al. Not all DMT1 mutations lead to iron overload. *Blood Cells Mol Dis.* 2009;43(2):199-201.

280. Ganz T, Goff J, Klasing K, et al. IOD in rhinos--immunity group report: report from the Immunity, Genetics and Toxicology Working Group of the International Workshop on Iron Overload Disorder in Browsing Rhinoceros (February 2011). *J Zoo Wildl Med.* 2012;43(suppl 3):S117-S119.

281. Yang T, Brittenham GM, Dong WQ, et al. Deferoxamine prevents cardiac hypertrophy and failure in the gerbil model of iron-induced cardiomyopathy. *J Lab Clin Med.* 2003;142(5):332-340.

282. Brittenham GM, Kuryshev YA, Obejero-Paz CA, et al. Yang et al response. *J Lab Clin Med.* 2003;141(6):420-422.

283. Wood JC, Otto-Duessel M, Gonzalez I, et al. Deferasirox and deferiprone remove cardiac iron in the iron-overloaded gerbil. *Transl Res.* 2006;148(5):272-280.

284. Hershko C, Link G, Konijn AM, et al. The iron-loaded gerbil model revisited: effects of deferoxamine and deferiprone treatment. *J Lab Clin Med.* 2002;139(1):50-58.

285. Zhou XY, Tomatsu S, Fleming RE, et al. HFE gene knockout produces mouse model of hereditary hemochromatosis. *Proc Natl Acad Sci U S A.* 1998;95(5):2492-2497.

286. Donovan A, Lima CA, Pinkus JL, et al. The iron exporter ferroportin/Slc40a1 is essential for iron homeostasis. *Cell Metab.* 2005;1(3):191-200.

287. Lesbordes-Brion JC, Viatte L, Bennoun M, et al. Targeted disruption of the hepcidin 1 gene results in severe hemochromatosis. *Blood.* 2006;108(4):1402-1405.

288. Meynard D, Kautz L, Darnaud V, et al. Lack of the bone morphogenetic protein BMP6 induces massive iron overload. *Nat Genet.* 2009;41(4):478-481.

289. Andriopoulos B Jr, Corradini E, Xia Y, et al. BMP6 is a key endogenous regulator of hepcidin expression and iron metabolism. *Nat Genet.* 2009;41(4):482-487.

290. Carroll GJ, Breidahl WH, Bulsara MK, et al. Hereditary hemochromatosis is characterized by a clinically definable arthropathy that correlates with iron load. *Arthritis Rheum.* 2011;63(1):286-294.

291. Elmberg M, Hultcrantz R, Simard JF, et al. Increased risk of arthropathies and joint replacement surgery in patients with genetic hemochromatosis: a study of 3,531 patients and their 11,794 first-degree relatives. *Arthritis Care Res (Hoboken).* 2013;65(5):678-685.

292. Vaiopoulos G, Papanikolaou G, Politou M, et al. Arthropathy in juvenile hemochromatosis. *Arthritis Rheum.* 2003;48(1):227-230.

293. Ko C, Siddaiah N, Berger J, et al. Prevalence of hepatic iron overload and association with hepatocellular cancer in end-stage liver disease: results from the National Hemochromatosis Transplant Registry. *Liver Int.* 2007;27(10):1394-1401.

294. Ryan CF, Sendi H, Bonkovsky HL. Hepatitis C, porphyria cutanea tarda and liver iron: an update. *Liver Int.* 2012;32(6):880-893.

295. Camaschella C, Roetto A, De GM. Juvenile hemochromatosis. *Semin Hematol.* 2002;39(4):242-248.

296. Bottomley SS. Secondary iron overload disorders. *Semin Hematol.* 1998;35(1):77-86.

297. Ernest B, Vincent F, Terri G, et al. Haematological effects of the C282Y HFE mutation in homozygous and heterozygous states among subjects of northern and southern European ancestry. *Br J Haematol.* 2003;120(5):887-893.

298. Jensen PD. Evaluation of iron overload. *Br J Haematol.* 2004;124(6):697-711.

299. Poullis A, Moodie SJ, Ang L, et al. Routine transferrin saturation measurement in liver clinic patients increases detection of hereditary haemochromatosis. *Ann Clin Biochem.* 2003;40(Pt 5):521-527.

300. Yin D, Kulhalli V, Walker AP. Raised serum ferritin concentration in hereditary hyperferritinemia cataract syndrome is not a marker for iron overload. *Hepatology.* 2014;59(3):1204-1206.

301. Brissot P, Bardou-Jacquet E, Jouanolle AM, et al. Iron disorders of genetic origin: a changing world. *Trends Mol Med.* 2011;17(12):707-713.

302. Angelucci E, Li J, Greenberg P, et al. Iron chelation in transfusion-dependent patients with low- to intermediate-1-risk myelodysplastic syndromes: a randomized trial. *Ann Intern Med.* 2020;172(8):513-522.

303. Porter JB. Practical management of iron overload. *Br J Haematol.* 2001;115(2):239-252.

304. Hoffbrand AV, Taher A, Cappellini MD. How I treat transfusional iron overload. *Blood.* 2012;120(18):3657-3669.

305. Cooray SD, Heerasing NM, Selkrig LA, et al. Reversal of end-stage heart failure in juvenile hemochromatosis with iron chelation therapy: a case report. *J Med Case Rep.* 2018;12(1):18.

CHAPTER 12
ANEMIA RESULTING FROM OTHER NUTRITIONAL DEFICIENCIES

Ralph Green and Ananya Datta Mitra

SUMMARY

The anemia that results from deficiencies of vitamin B_{12}, folic acid (Chap. 9), or iron (Chap. 11) is, in general, clearly defined and is relatively common. In contrast, the characteristics of anemia that may occur with deficiencies of other micronutrients, including other vitamins and minerals, are poorly defined and relatively rare in humans. When present, they usually exist not as isolated deficiencies of one vitamin or one mineral but rather as a combination of deficiencies resulting from malnutrition or malabsorption. In this context, it is difficult to deduce which abnormalities are results of a particular deficiency. Studies in experimental animals may not accurately reflect the role of micronutrients in humans. Accordingly, our knowledge of the effect of many micronutrients on hematopoiesis is fragmentary and based on clinical observations and interpretations that may be flawed. Inborn metabolic errors that affect single micronutrient pathways may shed light on the specific effects of those micronutrients on hematopoiesis. The levels of relevant micronutrients normally found in the serum, red cell, and leukocytes are provided in this chapter.

INTRODUCTION

Apart from iron, folate (vitamin B_9), and cobalamin (vitamin B_{12}), other trace mineral and vitamin micronutrients play an essential role in the prevention of anemia. Red cell numbers are adequately maintained by regulated continuous red cell production to counterbalance red cell loss due to the physiologic process of elimination of aged or damaged red cells from circulation or due to acute or chronic hemorrhage. Erythroid precursors in the marrow require adequate nutritional support to produce red cells to match the replacement of approximately 1% of the total red cell mass daily under steady-state conditions.

Deficiencies of other nutrients are not as common as folate, vitamin B_{12}, and iron, but reports in the literature indicate that lack of other micronutrients can also lead to or exacerbate anemia. Leading examples of such nutrient deficiencies include protein-energy malnutrition, deficiencies of other B-group vitamins, riboflavin, pyridoxine

Acronyms and Abbreviations: EGRa, erythrocyte glutathione reductase activity; IBD, inflammatory bowel disease; IRIDA, iron-refractory iron-deficiency anemia; MCV, mean cell volume; MCHC, mean cell hemoglobin concentration; RDW, red cell distribution width; T_3, triiodothyronine; T_4, thyroxine.

and thiamine, ascorbic acid, the fat-soluble vitamins, A and E, and other trace elements such as copper, zinc, and selenium. Anemia caused by deficiencies of these micronutrients constitutes only a small fraction of the total burden of anemia accounted for by folate, vitamin B_{12}, and iron deficiencies. Moreover, anemia resulting from vitamin B_{12}, folic acid, or iron deficiencies is generally well defined and is relatively common; however, the characteristics of anemia arising from other micronutrient deficiencies are poorly defined and are infrequent in humans.

Miscellaneous micronutrient deficiencies can coexist, and it is often difficult to pinpoint which abnormalities are results of which nutrient deficiency. An overview of these less common micronutrient deficiencies associated with anemia is provided in this chapter. Table 12-1 contains the normal values for the micronutrient deficiencies discussed in this chapter.

VITAMIN-DEFICIENCY ANEMIAS

VITAMIN A DEFICIENCY

Chronic deprivation of vitamin A results in anemia resembling that observed in iron deficiency.[1-4]

Mean cell volume (MCV) and mean cell hemoglobin concentration (MCHC) are reduced. Anisocytosis and poikilocytosis may be present, and serum iron levels are low. Unlike iron-deficiency anemia, but like the anemia of chronic disease, the iron stores in the liver and marrow are increased, the serum transferrin concentration usually is normal or decreased, and administration of medicinal iron does not correct the anemia. However, vitamin A deficiency may result in impaired iron absorption or utilization[5] and this may be mediated through effects on expression of genes involved in the regulation of intestinal iron absorption.[6] The suggestion that vitamin A may facilitate iron absorption[7] has not been confirmed.[8] Supplementation with vitamin A alone may ameliorate the anemia, although coadministration of vitamin A and iron resulted in a better response than with either nutrient alone.[9] Regarding mechanism, it has also been suggested that vitamin A plays an important role in regulation of the growth and differentiation of erythroid progenitor cells.[13]

Surveys conducted in developing countries find that vitamin A deficiency represents a public health problem among infants, schoolchildren, and women of childbearing age.[10,11] The prevalence of vitamin A deficiency closely coincides with the prevalence of iron deficiency in this demographic setting.[12] However, there is no known causal relationship between the two nutrients beyond both occurring in a setting of generalized malnutrition. Although vitamin A deficiency is recognized to occur in the United States, the relationship between it and anemia is not known.

DEFICIENCIES OF MEMBERS OF THE VITAMIN B GROUP

Isolated nutritional deficiencies of members of the vitamin B group resulting in morbidity, apart from folate and cobalamin, are very uncommon in humans. Evidence linking isolated nutritional deficiencies of pyridoxine, riboflavin, pantothenic acid, and niacin to anemia in patients is inconclusive. In animals, experimentally induced deficiency states are more consistently associated with hematologic abnormalities.

Vitamin B_6 Deficiency

Vitamin B_6 includes the vitamers pyridoxal, pyridoxine, and pyridoxamine. These components are converted to pyridoxal 5-phosphate, which acts as a cofactor in the decarboxylation and transamination of amino acids and in the synthesis of aminolevulinic acid, a primary precursor in the porphyrin synthetic pathway (Chap. 21). Vitamin B_6 deficiency in infants is associated with a hypochromic microcytic anemia.[14]

TABLE 12-1. Blood Vitamin and Mineral Levels (Adult Values)

Vitamin or Mineral	Serum Level	Plasma Level	Red Cell Level	White Cell Level
Copper	11-24 µmol/L		14-24 µmol/L	
Folate	7-45 nmol/L		>320 nmol/L	
Riboflavin (B$_2$)	110-640 nmol/L		265-1350 nmol/L	
Vitamin A	1-3 µmol/L			
Vitamin B$_6$		20-122 nmol/L		
Vitamin C		25-85 µmol/L		11-30 attomol/cell
Vitamin E	12-40 µmol/L			
Selenium	1200-2000 nmol/L			
Zinc	11-18 µmol/L			

Data from Burtis CA and Ashwood EF. *Tietz Textbook of Clinical Chemistry,* 3rd ed. Philadelphia, PA: WB Saunders; 1999.

A malnourished patient with a hypochromic anemia who failed to respond to iron therapy but subsequently responded to administration of vitamin B$_6$ has been described.[15] In some anemic pregnant women who did not respond to iron supplementation alone, vitamin B$_6$ administration resulted in subsequent improvement in hemoglobin level.[16] Occasionally, patients receiving therapy with the antituberculosis agent, isoniazid, which interferes with vitamin B$_6$ metabolism, develop a microcytic anemia that can be corrected with large doses of pyridoxine.[17] Pyridoxine is, therefore, usually prescribed with isoniazid to prevent such an effect. Some patients with sideroblastic anemias (Chap. 20) respond to the administration of large doses of pyridoxine, but these patients are not deficient in this vitamin.[18] A review of more than 200 patients with acquired sideroblastic anemia reported that fewer than 7% showed greater than 15 g/L improvement in hemoglobin concentration.[19] Pyridoxine is involved in many metabolic processes. Derangements in these pathways, sometimes involving anemia, are usually the result of inborn errors affecting the pathways of vitamin B$_6$ metabolism and specific pyridoxal phosphate-dependent enzymes or the result of inborn errors that lead to accumulation of small molecules that react with pyridoxal phosphate and inactivate it.[20] Pyridoxine-responsive anemia has been reported in two patients after pancreaticoduodenectomy.[21] Pyridoxine deficiency has also been reported in conjunction with folate deficiency in an infant fed with goat's milk.[22] Other acquired conditions that may influence pyridoxine metabolism include drugs that react with pyridoxal phosphate or that affect its metabolism, malabsorptive states such as celiac disease, nephrosis with proteinuria, and renal dialysis, which leads to increased losses of vitamin B$_6$ vitamers from the circulation because these vitamers are bound to plasma albumin.[23]

Riboflavin Deficiency

Riboflavin deficiency results in a decrease in red cell glutathione reductase activity because this enzyme requires flavin adenine dinucleotide for activation. The glutathione reductase deficiency induced by riboflavin deficiency is not associated with a hemolytic anemia or increased susceptibility to oxidant-induced injury (Chap. 16).[24] Human volunteers maintained on a semisynthetic riboflavin-deficient diet and fed the riboflavin antagonist galactoflavin develop pure red cell aplasia.[25] Vacuolated erythroid precursors are evident before the development of aplasia. This anemia is reversed specifically by administration of riboflavin. It has been suggested that riboflavin deficiency causes anemia, possibly by interfering with iron release from ferritin.[25,26] Although the relationship between dietary riboflavin deficiency and anemia is not clear, inadequate riboflavin intake increased the risk of anemia in Chinese adults and was associated with a high probability of anemia when iron intake was low.[19] Thus, poor riboflavin status may interfere with iron handling and contribute to the development of anemia when iron intakes are low. A study in healthy nonpregnant, nonbreastfeeding women in Canada and Malaysia reported an association between erythrocyte glutathione reductase activity (EGRac) and hemoglobin concentration after adjusting for other known risk factors for anemia in this demographic group and concluded that the women with riboflavin deficiency were twice as likely to present with anemia than those with normal riboflavin status assessed by EGRac.[27] There is also evidence to indicate that riboflavin may exert its effects secondarily on other nutrients of primary hematologic interest, such as folate and cobalamin, since riboflavin is also required for the methionine synthase reaction.[28]

Pantothenic Acid Deficiency

Pantothenic acid deficiency, when artificially induced in humans, is not associated with anemia.[29]

Niacin Deficiency

Pellagra (niacin deficiency) is associated with anemia, which responds to treatment with niacin.[30] However, it is not clear whether the anemia is a direct or an indirect effect of niacin deficiency.

Thiamine Deficiency

Megaloblastic anemia, responsive to thiamine, occurs in a childhood syndrome in association with diabetes and sensorineural deafness (Rogers syndrome). There is usually profound anemia and megaloblastic changes with or without ringed sideroblasts in the marrow and occasionally thrombocytopenia.[31] Most cases have been reported in patients of Middle and Far Eastern origin. The underlying defect in this condition has been identified as being the result of a defect in the high-affinity thiamine transporter, which primarily affects the synthesis of the ribose-5-phosphate portion of nucleic acids as a consequence of the thiamine-dependent pentose-cycle enzyme transketolase.[32] A decrease in ribose synthesis resulting in reduced nucleic acid production appears to be the underlying biochemical disturbance that likely induces cell-cycle arrest or apoptosis in marrow cells and leads to the thiamine-responsive megaloblastic anemia syndrome in these patients. Anemia in these patients responds to the lifelong administration of oral thiamine (25-100 mg/day). The *SLC19A2* gene on chromosome 1q23.3 is implicated in all cases of thiamine-responsive megaloblastic anemia.[33] It is of interest that the reduced folate carrier and the thiamine transporters appear to have evolved from the same family of solute carriers.[34]

VITAMIN C (ASCORBIC ACID) DEFICIENCY

Although approximately 80% of patients with scurvy[35] are anemic, attempts to induce anemia in human volunteers by severely restricting dietary ascorbic acid have been unsuccessful.[36] Anemia observed in subjects with scurvy is not simply the result of a deficiency of ascorbic acid but rather a result of blood loss resulting from the scorbutic capillary defect or an associated deficiency of folate.[35] Human subjects with scurvy and megaloblastic anemia fail to correct their anemia with vitamin C administration if they are maintained on a folic acid-deficient diet. When folic acid is given to these subjects in a dose of 50 mcg/day, a prompt hematologic response has been observed.[37]

Ascorbic acid, in common with other compounds that contribute to cellular reducing potential, participates in the maintenance of dihydrofolate reductase in its reduced, or active, form. Impaired dihydrofolate reductase activity results in an inability to form tetrahydrofolate, the metabolically active, reduced form of folic acid (Chap. 9). Patients with scurvy and megaloblastic anemia excrete 10-formylfolate as the major urinary folate metabolite. After ascorbic acid therapy, 5-methyltetrahydrofolate becomes the major urinary folate metabolite. This observation has led to the suggestion that ascorbic acid prevents the irreversible oxidation of methyltetrahydrofolate to formylfolate.[38] Failure to synthesize tetrahydrofolate or protect it from oxidation ultimately results in megaloblastic anemia. Under these circumstances, ascorbic acid therapy produces a hematologic response, but only if enough folate is present to interact with the ascorbic acid.[39]

Dietary iron deficiency in children often occurs in association with dietary ascorbate deficiency. Iron balance may be compromised by ascorbic acid deficiency because the vitamin serves to facilitate intestinal iron absorption by maintaining iron in the more soluble reduced or ferrous (Fe^{2+}) state. Patients with scurvy, particularly children, may require both iron and vitamin C to correct a hypochromic microcytic anemia.[40] Ascorbate affects oxido-reduction involved in compartmental iron release and may stimulate iron mobilization from endosomes as well as transferrin-dependent iron uptake. There is a role for ascorbate as a novel modulator of the classical transferrin-iron uptake pathway, which provides almost all iron for cellular demands and erythropoiesis. Ascorbate acts to stimulate transferrin-dependent iron uptake through an intracellular reductive mechanism by stimulating iron mobilization from endosomes. This role of ascorbate might explain how ascorbate deficiency contributes to anemia in iron deficiency.[41] Scurvy itself may contribute to iron deficiency because of external bleeding. Another potential intersection of ascorbate with iron deficiency has been noted in patients with the iron-refractory iron-deficiency anemia (IRIDA) phenotype caused by genetic defects in the *TMPRSS6* gene (Chap. 11). Improvement in hematologic response to oral iron and vitamin C combination in children with IRIDA has been described.[42]

In patients with iron overload from repeated blood transfusions, the level of vitamin C in leukocytes is often decreased because of rapid conversion of ascorbate to oxalate.[43] Deferoxamine (desferrioxamine)-induced iron excretion is diminished when stores of vitamin C are reduced, but excretion returns to expected values with vitamin C supplementation.[44,45] Large doses of ascorbic acid may be harmful in patients with iron overload and should be given only after an infusion of deferoxamine mesylate has been initiated (Chap. 11). The presence of scurvy in patients with iron overload may protect them from tissue damage.[46] In scorbutic guinea pigs and in Southern African subjects with nutritional vitamin C deficiency and dietary hemosiderosis, iron accumulates in the monocyte–macrophage system rather than in the parenchymal cells of the liver.[47,48]

VITAMIN E DEFICIENCY

Vitamin E, α-tocopherol, is a fat-soluble vitamin that functions as an antioxidant in humans. It is not a recognized cofactor in any essential reactions. Nutritional deficiency of vitamin E in humans is extremely uncommon because of the widespread occurrence of α-tocopherol in food. The daily requirement of *d*-α-tocopherol for adults' ranges from 5 to 7 mg, but the requirement varies with the polyunsaturated fatty acid content of the diet and the content of peroxidizable lipids in tissues. Hematologic manifestations of vitamin E deficiency in humans are limited to the neonatal period and to pathologic states associated with chronic fat malabsorption.

Low-birth-weight infants are born with low serum and tissue concentrations of vitamin E. When these infants are fed a diet unusually rich in polyunsaturated fatty acids and inadequate in vitamin E, a hemolytic anemia frequently develops by 4 to 6 weeks of age, particularly if iron supplements are being administered.[49] The anemia often is associated with fragmentation and other morphologic alterations of the erythrocytes,[50] thrombocytosis, and edema of the dorsum of the feet and pretibial area.[51] Treatment with vitamin E produces a prompt increase in hemoglobin level, a decrease in the elevated reticulocyte count, normalization of the red cell life span, and disappearance of thrombocytosis and edema. Although it has been reported that modifications of infant formulas have all but eliminated vitamin E deficiency in preterm infants,[52] a recent study of preterm infants in an intensive care unit noted hemolytic anemia that responded to vitamin E supplementation.[53]

Vitamin E deficiency is common in patients with cystic fibrosis if the patients are not receiving daily supplements of the water-soluble form of the vitamin.[54] The life span of red cell in such patients is shortened to an average ^{51}Cr half-life of 19 days (normal, ~30 days). After vitamin E therapy, the red cell half-life increases to 27.5 days.[55] Severe anemia may be present.[54] A Cochrane review emphasizes that vitamin E supplementation is widely recommended in cystic fibrosis because of the serious complications that can arise from vitamin E deficiency, including hemolytic anemia and cerebellar ataxia.[56]

Pharmacologic doses of tocopherol have been used with apparent success to compensate for genetic defects that limit erythrocyte defense against oxidant injury, even in the absence of overt vitamin E deficiency. Chronic administration of vitamin E 400 to 800 U/day was associated with lengthened red cell life span in some,[57,58] but not all,[59] studies of patients with hereditary hemolytic anemias associated with glutathione synthetase deficiency or glucose-6-phosphate dehydrogenase deficiency.

Administration of vitamin E (450 U/day for 6-36 weeks) to patients with sickle cell anemia significantly reduced the number of irreversibly sickled erythrocytes.[60] Adult patients with sickle cell anemia have significantly lower serum tocopherol values compared with normal control participans,[61,62] and in children with sickle cell anemia, those with vitamin E deficiency had significantly more irreversibly sickled cells than did children without vitamin E deficiency.[63]

●TRACE METAL DEFICIENCY

COPPER DEFICIENCY

Copper is present in a number of metalloproteins. Among the cuproenzymes are cytochrome *c* oxidase, dopamine β-hydroxylase, urate oxidase, tyrosine and lysyl oxidase, ascorbic acid oxidase, and superoxide dismutase (erythrocuprein). More than 90% of the copper in the blood is carried bound to ceruloplasmin, an α_2-globulin with ferroxidase activity. The SLC31 (CTR) family of copper transporters regulates copper transport and acquisition.[64] Copper appears to be required for the absorption and utilization of iron. Copper, in the form of hephaestin,[65] converts iron to the ferric (Fe^{3+}) state for its transport by transferrin.

Copper deficiency has been described in malnourished children[66] and in both infants and adults[67-69] receiving parenteral alimentation. There is increasing recognition of copper deficiency associated with anemia occurring as complication after gastric resection or bariatric gastric reduction surgery.[70,71] Copper deficiency is characterized by an anemia with hypoferremia, that is unresponsive to iron therapy and is often macrocytic, with neutropenia, and usually the presence of vacuolated erythroid and granulocytic precursors in the marrow.[67-70,72] The mechanism of neutropenia remains unknown, but there is some evidence that copper deficiency results in inhibition of differentiation and self-renewal of CD34(+) hematopoietic progenitor cells.[73,74] Iron-containing plasma cells, a decrease in granulocyte precursors, and ring sideroblasts have also been reported.[70,72] Consequently, copper deficiency should enter the differential diagnosis in patients with features of myelodysplastic syndrome, particularly if there is a history of previous gastric surgery.[72] Neurologic findings, most commonly a result of myeloneuropathy, are frequently present so that copper deficiency should be considered in the differential diagnosis of a patient with anemia and associated myeloneuropathy suspected of having cobalamin deficiency with subacute combined degeneration of the spinal cord.[75,76] Radiologic abnormalities generally are present in infants and young children with copper deficiency. These abnormalities include osteoporosis, flaring of the anterior ribs with spontaneous rib fractures, cupping and flaring of long-bone metaphyses with spur formation and submetaphyseal fractures, and epiphyseal separation. These changes have frequently been misinterpreted as signs of scurvy. Copper deficiency with associated microcytic anemia can be produced by chronic ingestion of massive quantities of zinc. This has been reported in patients using excessive quantities of zinc-containing dental fixatives.[71,77] Dietary zinc in large doses leads to copper deficiency by impairing copper absorption.[78,79]

The diagnosis of copper deficiency can be established by demonstrating a low serum ceruloplasmin or serum or 24-hour urine copper level. The serum copper level is thought to be more reliable because ceruloplasmin behaves as an acute phase protein.[70] Adequate normal values for the first 2 to 3 months of age have not been well defined and normally are lower than the levels observed later in life. Despite these limitations, a serum copper level less than 70 mcg/dL (11 μmol/L) or a ceruloplasmin level less than 15 mg/dL after age 1 or 2 months should be regarded as evidence of copper deficiency. In later infancy, childhood, and adulthood, serum copper values should normally exceed 70 mcg/dL. Low serum copper values may be observed in hypoproteinemic states, such as exudative enteropathies and nephrosis, as well as in Wilson disease. In these circumstances, a diagnosis of copper deficiency cannot be established by serum measurements alone but requires analysis of liver copper content or clinical response after a therapeutic trial of copper supplementation.

The anemia and neutropenia are quickly corrected by administration of copper. Treatment of copper-deficient infants consists of administration of approximately 2.5 mg of copper (~80 mcg/kg per day) oral supplementation as a copper sulfate solution.[80] IV bolus injection of copper chloride also has been used.[72] Hematologic manifestations of copper deficiency are fully reversible over a 4- to 12-week period after copper supplementation.[81]

ZINC DEFICIENCY

Zinc is required for a large number of zinc metalloenzymes, zinc-activated enzymes, and "zinc finger" transcription factors. Zinc deficiency occurs in a variety of pathologic states in humans, including hemolytic anemias such as thalassemia[82] and sickle cell anemia.[83] Zinc deficiency with or without an associated copper deficiency has been described in patients with decreased renal reabsorption of trace minerals[84] and in a patient receiving intensive desferrioxamine therapy.[85] Reduced levels of zinc are common in untreated celiac disease patients probably because of loss of brush border proteins and enzymes needed for the absorption of these nutrients. Deficiency of this micronutrient may therefore be seen in conjunction with deficiencies of iron, folate, and vitamin B_{12} in this condition.[86]

Although human zinc deficiency may produce growth retardation, impaired wound healing, impaired taste perception, immunologic abnormalities, and acrodermatitis enteropathica, there is no evidence that isolated zinc deficiency produces anemia.

SELENIUM DEFICIENCY

Selenium deficiency occurs in patients who live in areas where the selenium content of the soil is very low[87] and has been observed in patients receiving total parenteral nutrition.[88,89] Although selenium deficiency results in a striking decrease in the level of red cell glutathione peroxidase, there do not appear to be any adverse hematologic consequences.

An examination of the relationship between serum selenium and hematologic indices found that low serum selenium was independently associated with anemia among older men and women in the United States.[90] A similar association has been reported in adolescent girls living in rural Vietnam.[91] In a study of micronutrient status of adult patients with sickle cell disease, selenium deficiency was found to be the main determinant of hemolysis as assessed by reticulocyte count, hemoglobin, indirect and total bilirubin, and lactate dehydrogenase, suggesting that nutritional supplement protocols for the care of patients with sickle cell disease should include dietary sources of selenium to reduce the risk of hemolysis.[92]

● ANEMIA OF STARVATION

Studies conducted during World War II among prisoners of war and conscientious objectors demonstrated that semistarvation for 24 weeks can result in a mild to moderate normocytic normochromic anemia.[93,94] Marrow cellularity is usually reduced and is accompanied by a decreased erythroid-to-myeloid ratio. Measurements of red cell volume and plasma volume suggest that dilution is a major factor responsible for the reduction in hemoglobin concentration.

In persons subjected to complete starvation either for experimental purposes or as treatment of severe obesity, anemia was not observed during the first 2 to 9 weeks of fasting.[95] Starvation for 9 to 17 weeks produced a decrease in hemoglobin and marrow hypocellularity.[96] Resumption of a normal diet was accompanied by reticulocytosis and disappearance of anemia. It has been suggested that the anemia of starvation is a response to a hypometabolic state with its attendant decrease in oxygen requirements.[97]

● ANEMIA OF PROTEIN DEFICIENCY (KWASHIORKOR)

Even strict vegetarians do not seem to develop hematologic problems related to the absence of animal proteins,[98] except for vegans who have cobalamin deficiency.[99] The deficiency in this situation is caused, however, by cobalamin rather than animal protein insufficiency, and results from the natural occurrence of cobalamin exclusively in foods of animal origin (Chap. 9). Kwashiorkor is largely a disease of the underdeveloped world but occasionally is seen even among the children of educated and well-to-do parents when the children are fed an inappropriate diet.[100,101]

In infants and children with protein-calorie malnutrition, the hemoglobin concentration may fall to 80 g/L of blood,[100,101] but some children with kwashiorkor have normal hemoglobin levels, probably because of a decreased plasma volume. The anemia is typically normocytic and normochromic, but the size and shape of red cells on the blood film vary considerably. The white blood cells and the platelets usually are normal. The marrow is most often normally cellular or slightly hypocellular, with a reduced erythroid-to-myeloid ratio. Erythroblastopenia, reticulocytopenia, and a marrow containing a few giant proerythroblast may be found, particularly if the child has an infection. With treatment of the infection, erythroid precursors may appear in the marrow and the reticulocyte count may rise. In malnourished communities, anemia with erythroblastopenia resulting from parvovirus B-19 infections (Chap. 5) should be distinguished from the similar picture that can arise as a result of protein-calorie malnutrition. When nutrition is improved by giving high-protein diets (powdered milk or essential amino acids), reticulocytosis, a slight fall in hematocrit because of hemodilution, and then a rise in hemoglobin level, hematocrit, and red blood cell count occur. Although the plasma volume is reduced to a variable degree in children with kwashiorkor, the total circulating red cell volume decreases in proportion to the decrease in lean body mass as protein deprivation reduces metabolic demands. During repletion, an increase in plasma volume may occur before an increase in red cell volume, and the anemia may seem to become more severe despite reticulocytosis. Improvement is very slow, however, and during the third or fourth week, when the child has clinically improved and serum protein levels are approaching normal, another episode of erythroid marrow aplasia may develop. An abrupt fall in hemoglobin after protein feeding may be an ominous harbinger of adverse and even fatal outcome and prompt transfusion to restore hemoglobin may be lifesaving.[102] The mechanism of this secondary relapse is not understood but it is not associated with infection, does not respond to antibiotics, and does not remit spontaneously. The erythroblastic aplasia may be a manifestation of riboflavin deficiency.[103] It may respond to either riboflavin or prednisone. In a report from Turkey of patients with protein energy malnutrition, the major cause of anemia was identified as being associated with either deficiency or defective utilization of iron.[104]

The anemia seen in children with protein energy malnutrition is often multifactorial. In studies on two rural populations in Southern Africa, anemia associated with varying severity of protein energy malnutrition was most often caused by coexistent iron deficiency.[105,106] In a study of 131 cases of severe acute malnutrition from India, the most common type of anemia was microcytic (38.6%) followed by megaloblastic (30.5%).[107]

From a study of the anemia of protein deficiency in rats, it was deduced that oxygen consumption and therefore erythropoietin production are reduced.[108] Other studies confirmed this observation but related the reduction to caloric deprivation with its associated decrease in the blood levels of triiodothyronine (T_3) and thyroxine (T_4). As a result, erythropoiesis decreases, and the reticulocyte count falls. The plasma iron turnover and red cell uptake of radioactive iron are markedly reduced, and the red cell volume gradually declines. Protein deficiency also produces a maturation block at the erythroblast level and a slight decrease in the erythropoietin-sensitive progenitor cell pool.[109] If exogenous erythropoietin is provided, normal erythropoiesis is restored despite protein depletion,[110] an observation that explains the successful use of starved rats in the historical bioassay for erythropoietin.

The anemia seen in anorexia nervosa shows some features that resemble protein energy malnutrition. Anemia and leukopenia is found in approximately one-third of patients[111] and 50% of these show marrow atrophy with gelatinous transformation of the marrow stroma.[112]

●ALCOHOLISM

Chronic alcohol ingestion often is associated with anemia. The anemia may result from nutritional deficiencies, chronic gastrointestinal bleeding, hepatic dysfunction, or direct toxic effects of alcohol on erythropoiesis. Quite commonly, all these factors work in concert to produce the anemia. Pyridoxal phosphate and folate deficiency are common in people with alcoholism.[113] Alcohol affects not only the red cells, as described here, but also platelet production.[114,115]

Macrocytosis is common in chronic alcoholism[116] and is often associated with a megaloblastic anemia. Among hospitalized malnourished people with alcoholism, it is the most common type of anemia, occurring alone or in combination with ringed sideroblasts in approximately 40% of patients.[117,118] In contrast, megaloblastic anemia is rarely observed in nonhospitalized people with chronic alcoholism or relatively well-nourished subjects admitted to the hospital for alcohol withdrawal.[119] Anemia, when associated with megaloblastic marrow changes in people with alcoholism, almost always results from folate deficiency. Iron deficiency often is associated with folate deficiency in people with alcoholism.[118] In patients with both nutritional deficiencies, the blood film is "dimorphic," with macrocytes, hypersegmented neutrophils, and hypochromic microcytes. This is also the case when folate deficiency coexists with sideroblastic anemia.[117,120] Consequently, MCV may be normal, but because of marked anisopoikilocytosis, the red cell distribution width (RDW) is elevated.[76] Although liver disease is frequently present in people with alcoholism and megaloblastic anemia, it is not directly responsible for the folate deficiency. Megaloblastic anemia occurs almost exclusively in people with alcoholism who have been eating poorly. The impact of food fortification with folic acid on this association has not been assessed. It is seen more commonly in heavy drinkers of wine and whiskey, which contain little or no folate, than in drinkers of beer, which, depending on its method of preparation, may be a rich source of the vitamin. In addition to folate deficiency, people with chronic alcoholism frequently demonstrate multiple other micronutrient deficiencies, including thiamine, pyridoxine, and vitamin A, which aggravate the risk of anemia.[121] Although decreased dietary folate intake appears to be a necessary factor in the etiology of the megaloblastic anemia, ethanol itself interferes with folate metabolism (Chap. 9).[119,122]

However, macrocytosis does not always indicate the presence of a megaloblastic anemia.[116] A so-called macrocytosis of alcoholism is found in as many as 82% to 96% of people with alcoholism.[123] In these patients, the macrocytosis usually is mild, with MCV in the range of 100 to 110 fl, and anemia is usually absent. In the blood film, the macrocytes are typically round rather than oval, and neutrophil hypersegmentation is not present. The macrocytosis persists until the patient abstains from alcohol. Even then, MCV does not completely return to normal for periods of 2 to 4 months in view of the life span of erythrocytes.[122]

Alcohol ingestion for 5 to 7 days produces vacuolization of early red cell precursors, and formation of vacuoles can be observed in in vitro marrow cell cultures.[117,124] These changes disappear promptly when alcohol ingestion is discontinued. Similar vacuolization occurs in subjects who are fed a phenylalanine-deficient diet, patients treated with chloramphenicol or pyrazinamide, patients in hyperosmolar coma, and individuals deficient in copper or riboflavin.[123]

Two relatively uncommon hematologic complication of alcoholism are Zieve syndrome,[125,126] consisting of alcohol-induced liver disease, often hyperlipidemia, jaundice, and transient spherocytic hemolytic anemia, and hemolytic anemia with acanthocytes, associated with severe alcohol-induced liver disease, often requiring hepatic transplantation for resolution.[127,128] Chap. 23 discusses these syndromes. The ability to metabolize alcohol relating to polymorphisms of alcohol dehydrogenase enzymes affects the degree of rise in acetaldehyde concentrations after alcohol ingestion. Japanese individuals with the inactive genotype show increased susceptibility to macrocytic anemia and leukopenia and have an increased susceptibility to esophageal cancer. Patients with cessation of drinking before surgery or chemoradiation for esophageal cancer showed more rapid recovery from hematologic complications.[129] The association of myelodysplasia with chronic alcohol consumption may result from polymorphisms in alcohol dehydrogenase, which leads to accumulation of reactive aldehydes from ethanol, resulting in genetic damage to hematopoietic stem cells.[130]

ANEMIA IN INFLAMMATORY BOWEL DISEASE

One of the most frequent complications of inflammatory bowel disease (IBD) is anemia, usually caused by malabsorption of hematinic nutrients. The most common cause of anemia in IBD is iron deficiency (Chap. 11), which occurs due to nutritional deficiencies along with anemia of chronic disease (Chap. 6). Discoveries have indicated the role of hepcidin, an acute phase reactant which is increased in the inflammatory milieu, causing defective iron absorption in the duodenum and increased iron retention in the macrophages due to down-regulation of ferroportin[131] (Chap. 6). Studies have also shown that there are a multitude of causes leading to anemia in IBD. These include chronic blood loss due to the disease itself, deficiencies in cobalamin due to surgical resection of the absorptive site for cobalamin in the ileum (Chap. 9), bacterial overgrowth, fistulas, decreased intake, protein losing enteropathies and hepatic dysfunction[132] as well as deficiencies in folate due to the use of immunosuppressive drugs (methotrexate or sulfasalazine)[133,134] (Chap. 9). Moreover, several studies have shown that IBD patients have reduced serum retinol levels,[135] or vitamin A levels[136] and can present with night blindness as reported in a case report, where multiple surgical resections of the small bowel led to the deficiency of Vitamin A which was corrected with reversal of night blindness after parenteral vitamin A therapy.[137] Also, IBD is associated with low mean selenium levels.[138] Another nutrient affected by IBD is zinc and its deficiency has been estimated in 15% of IBD cases.[139] It has been demonstrated that zinc deficiency has been associated with poor clinical outcomes in IBD patients, which can be reversed with zinc supplementation.[140] Although zinc deficiency per se is not a known cause of anemia, its correction may ameliorate the deficiency of other nutrients that may be the cause of anemia.

REFERENCES

1. Blackfan KD, Wolbach SB. Vitamin a deficiency in infants: a clinical and pathological study. *J Pediatr.* 1933;3(5):679-706.
2. Vitamin A and iron deficiency. *Nutr Rev.* 1989;47(4):119-121.
3. Hodges RE, Sauberlich HE, Canham JE, et al. Hematopoietic studies in vitamin A deficiency. *Am J Clin Nutr.* 1978;31(5):876-885.
4. Majia LA, Hodges RE, Arroyave G, et al. Vitamin A deficiency and anemia in Central American children. *Am J Clin Nutr.* 1977;30(7):1175-1184.
5. Lynch S. Influence of infection/inflammation, thalassemia and nutritional status on iron absorption. *Int J Vitam Nutr Res.* 2007;77(3):217-223.
6. Citelli M, Bittencourt LL, da Silva SV, et al. Vitamin A modulates the expression of genes involved in iron bioavailability. *Biol Trace Elem Res.* 2012;149(1):64-70.
7. Kolsteren P, Rahman SR, Hilderbrand K, Diniz A. Treatment for iron deficiency anaemia with a combined supplementation of iron, vitamin A and zinc in women of Dinajpur, Bangladesh. *Eur J Clin Nutr.* 1999;53(2):102-106.
8. Walczyk T, Davidsson L, Rossander-Hulthen L, et al. No enhancing effect of vitamin A on iron absorption in humans. *Am J Clin Nutr.* 2003;77(1):144-149.
9. Mejia LA, Chew F. Hematological effect of supplementing anemic children with vitamin A alone and in combination with iron. *Am J Clin Nutr.* 1988;48(3):595-600.
10. Calis JC, Phiri KS, Faragher EB, et al. Severe anemia in Malawian children. *N Engl J Med.* 2008;358(9):888-899.
11. Tatala SR, Kihamia CM, Kyungu LH, Svanberg U. Risk factors for anaemia in schoolchildren in Tanga Region, Tanzania. *Tanzan J Health Res.* 2008;10(4):189-202.
12. Saraiva BC, Soares MC, Santos LC, et al. Iron deficiency and anemia are associated with low retinol levels in children aged 1 to 5 years. *J Pediatr (Rio J).* 2014;90(6):593-539.
13. Semba RD, Bloem MW. The anemia of vitamin A deficiency: epidemiology and pathogenesis. *Eur J Clin Nutr.* 2002;56(4):271-281.
14. Snyderman SE, Holt LE Jr, Carretero R, Jacobs K. Pyridoxine deficiency in the human infant. *J Clin Nutr.* 1953;1(3):200020-7.
15. Foy H, Kondi A. Hypochromic anemias of the tropics associated with pyridoxine and nicotinic acid deficiency. *Blood.* 1958;13(11):1054-1062.
16. Hisano M, Suzuki R, Sago H, et al. Vitamin B6 deficiency and anemia in pregnancy. *Eur J Clin Nutr.* 2010;64(2):221-223.
17. McCurdy PR, Donohoe RF, Magovern M. Reversible sideroblastic anemia caused by pyrazinoic acid (Pyrazinamide). *Ann Intern Med.* 1966;64(6):1280-1284.
18. Mason DY, Emerson PM. Primary acquired sideroblastic anaemia: response to treatment with pyridoxal-5-phosphate. *Br Med J* 1973;1:389-390.
19. Baumann Kreuziger LM, Wolanskyj AP, et al. Lack of efficacy of pyridoxine (vitamin B6) treatment in acquired idiopathic sideroblastic anaemia, including refractory anaemia with ring sideroblasts. *Eur J Haematol.* 2011;86(6):512-516.
20. Clayton PT. B6-responsive disorders: a model of vitamin dependency. *J Inherit Metab Dis.* 2006;29(2-3):317-326.
21. Yasuda H, Fujiwara N, Ishizaki Y, Komatsu N. Anemia attributed to vitamin B6 deficiency in post-pancreaticoduodenectomy patients. *Pancreatology.* 2015;15(1):81-83.
22. Datta-Mitra A, Vali-Betts E, Green R, et al. Combined Megaloblastic and sideroblastic anemia in an infant fed with goat's milk. *J Pediatr Hematol Oncol.* 2017;39(4):319-320.
23. Anderson BB, Newmark PA, Rawlins M, Green R. Plasma binding of vitamin B6 compounds. *Nature.* 1974;250(5466):502-504.
24. Beutler E, Srivastava SK. Relationship between glutathione reductase activity and drug-induced haemolytic anaemia. *Nature.* 1970;226(5247):759-760.
25. Lane M, Alfrey CP Jr. The anemia of human riboflavin deficiency. *Blood.* 1965;25:432-442.
26. Foy H, Kondi A. A case of true red cell aplastic anaemia successfully treated with riboflavin. *J Pathol Bacteriol.* 1953;65(2):559-564.
27. Aljaadi AM, How RE, Loh SP, et al. Suboptimal biochemical riboflavin status is associated with lower hemoglobin and higher rates of anemia in a sample of Canadian and Malaysian women of reproductive age. *J Nutr.* 2019;149(11):1952-1959.
28. Powers HJ. Riboflavin (vitamin B-2) and health. *Am J Clin Nutr.* 2003;77(6):1352-1360.
29. Hodges RE, Bean WB, Ohlson MA, Bleiler R. Human pantothenic acid deficiency produced by omega-methyl pantothenic acid. *J Clin Invest.* 1959;38(8):1421-1425.
30. Spivak JL, Jackson DL. Pellagra: an analysis of 18 patients and a review of the literature. *Johns Hopkins Med J.* 1977;140(6):295-309.
31. Bay A, Keskin M, Hizli S, et al. Thiamine-responsive megaloblastic anemia syndrome. *Int J Hematol.* 2010;92(3):524-526.
32. Boros LG, Steinkamp MP, Fleming JC, et al. Defective RNA ribose synthesis in fibroblasts from patients with thiamine-responsive megaloblastic anemia (TRMA). *Blood.* 2003;102(10):3556-3361.
33. Beshlawi I, Al Zadjali S, Bashir W, et al. Thiamine responsive megaloblastic anemia: the puzzling phenotype. *Pediatr Blood Cancer.* 2014;61(3):528-531.
34. Zhao R, Goldman ID. Folate and thiamine transporters mediated by facilitative carriers (SLC19A1-3 and SLC46A1) and folate receptors. *Mol Aspects Med.* 2013;34(2-3):373-385.
35. Reuler JB, Broudy VC, Cooney TG. Adult scurvy. *JAMA.* 1985;253(6):805-807.
36. Hodges RE, Baker EM, Hood J, et al. Experimental scurvy in man. *Am J Clin Nutr.* 1969;22(5):535-548.
37. Zalusky R, Herbert V. Megaloblastic anemia in scurvy with response to 50 microgm. of folic acid daily. *N Engl J Med.* 1961;265:1033-1038.
38. Stokes PL, Melikian V, Leeming RL, et al. Folate metabolism in scurvy. *Am J Clin Nutr.* 1975;28(2):126-129.
39. Cox EV, Meynell MJ, Northam BE, Cooke WT. The anaemia of scurvy. *Am J Med.* 1967;42(2):220-227.
40. Clark NG, Sheard NF, Kelleher JF. Treatment of iron-deficiency anemia complicated by scurvy and folic acid deficiency. *Nutr Rev.* 1992;50(5):134-137.
41. Lane DJ, Richardson DR. The active role of vitamin C in mammalian iron metabolism: much more than just enhanced iron absorption! *Free Radic Biol Med.* 2014;75:69-83.
42. Sourabh S, Bhatia P, Jain R. Favourable improvement in haematological parameters in response to oral iron and vitamin C combination in children with iron refractory iron deficiency anemia (IRIDA) phenotype. *Blood Cells Mol Dis.* 2019;75:26-29.
43. Wapnick AA, Lynch SR, Krawitz P, et al. Effects of iron overload on ascorbic acid metabolism. *Br Med J.* 1968;3(5620):704-707.
44. Wapnick AA, Lynch SR, Charlton RW, et al. The effect of ascorbic acid deficiency on desferrioxamine-induced urinary iron excretion. *Br J Haematol.* 1969;17(6):563-568.
45. Chapman RW, Hussain MA, Gorman A, et al. Effect of ascorbic acid deficiency on serum ferritin concentration in patients with beta-thalassaemia major and iron overload. *J Clin Pathol.* 1982;35(5):487-491.
46. Cohen A, Cohen IJ, Schwartz E. Scurvy and altered iron stores in thalassemia major. *N Engl J Med.* 1981;304(3):158-160.
47. Lipschitz DA, Bothwell TH, Seftel HC, et al. The role of ascorbic acid in the metabolism of storage iron. *Br J Haematol.* 1971;20(2):155-163.
48. Bothwell TH, Abrahams C, Bradlow BA, Charlton RW. Idiopathic and Bantu Hemochromatosis. Comparative Histological Study. *Arch Pathol.* 1965;79:163-168.

49. Williams ML, Shoot RJ, O'Neal PL, Oski FA. Role of dietary iron and fat on vitamin E deficiency anemia of infancy. *N Engl J Med.* 1975;292(17):887-890.

50. Oski FA, Barness LA. Hemolytic anemia in vitamin E deficiency. *Am J Clin Nutr.* 1968;21(1):45-50.

51. Ritchie JH, Fish MB, McMasters V, Grossman M. Edema and hemolytic anemia in premature infants. A vitamin E deficiency syndrome. *N Engl J Med.* 1968;279(22):1185-1190.

52. Zipursky A. Vitamin E deficiency anemia in newborn infants. *Clin Perinatol.* 1984;11(2):393-402.

53. Gomez-Pomar E, Hatfield E, Garlitz K, et al. Vitamin E in the preterm infant: a forgotten cause of hemolytic anemia. *Am J Perinatol.* 2018;35(3):305-310.

54. Wilfond BS, Farrell PM, Laxova A, Mischler E. Severe hemolytic anemia associated with vitamin E deficiency in infants with cystic fibrosis. Implications for neonatal screening. *Clin Pediatr (Phila).* 1994;33(1):2-7.

55. Farrell PM, Bieri JG, Fratantoni JF, et al. The occurrence and effects of human vitamin E deficiency. A study in patients with cystic fibrosis. *J Clin Invest.* 1977;60(1):233-241.

56. Okebukola PO, Kansra S, Barrett J. Vitamin E supplementation in people with cystic fibrosis. *Cochrane Database Syst Rev.* 2014;(12):CD009422.

57. Corash L, Spielberg S, Bartsocas C, et al. Reduced chronic hemolysis during high-dose vitamin E administration in Mediterranean-type glucose-6-phosphate dehydrogenase deficiency. *N Engl J Med.* 1980;303(8):416-420.

58. Eldamhougy S, Elhelw Z, Yamamah G, et al. The vitamin E status among glucose-6 phosphate dehydrogenase deficient patients and effectiveness of oral vitamin E. *Int J Vitam Nutr Res.* 1988;58(2):184-188.

59. Johnson GJ, Vatassery GT, Finkel B, Allen DW. High-dose vitamin E does not decrease the rate of chronic hemolysis in glucose-6-phosphate dehydrogenase deficiency. *N Engl J Med.* 1983;308(17):1014-1017.

60. Natta CL, Machlin LJ, Brin M. A decrease in irreversibly sickled erythrocytes in sicle cell anemia patients given vitamin E. *Am J Clin Nutr.* 1980;33(5):968-971.

61. Tangney CC, Phillips G, Bell RA, et al. Selected indices of micronutrient status in adult patients with sickle cell anemia (SCA). *Am J Hematol.* 1989;32(3):161-166.

62. Ren H, Ghebremeskel K, Okpala I, et al. Patients with sickle cell disease have reduced blood antioxidant protection. *Int J Vitam Nutr Res.* 2008;78(3):139-147.

63. Ndombi IO, Kinoti SN. Serum vitamin E and the sickling status in children with sickle cell anaemia. *East Afr Med J.* 1990;67(10):720-725.

64. Kim H, Wu X, Lee J. SLC31 (CTR) family of copper transporters in health and disease. *Mol Aspects Med.* 2013;34(2-3):561-570.

65. Anderson GJ, Frazer DM, McKie AT, Vulpe CD. The ceruloplasmin homolog hephaestin and the control of intestinal iron absorption. *Blood Cells Mol Dis.* 2002;29(3):367-375.

66. Graham GG, Cordano A. Copper depletion and deficiency in the malnourished infant. *Johns Hopkins Med J.* 1969;124(3):139-150.

67. Fuhrman MP, Herrmann V, Masidonski P, Eby C. Pancytopenia after removal of copper from total parenteral nutrition. *JPEN J Parenter Enteral Nutr.* 2000;24(6):361-366.

68. Hirase N, Abe Y, Sadamura S, et al. Anemia and neutropenia in a case of copper deficiency: role of copper in normal hematopoiesis. *Acta Haematol.* 1992;87(4):195-197.

69. Spiegel JE, Willenbucher RF. Rapid development of severe copper deficiency in a patient with Crohn's disease receiving parenteral nutrition. *JPEN J Parenter Enteral Nutr.* 1999;23(3):169-172.

70. Halfdanarson TR, Kumar N, Li CY, et al. Hematological manifestations of copper deficiency: a retrospective review. *Eur J Haematol.* 2008;80(6):523-531.

71. Chen M, Krishnamurthy A, Mohamed AR, Green R. Hematological disorders following gastric bypass surgery: emerging concepts of the interplay between nutritional deficiency and inflammation. *Biomed Res Int.* 2013;2013:205467.

72. Gregg XT, Reddy V, Prchal JT. Copper deficiency masquerading as myelodysplastic syndrome. *Blood.* 2002;100(4):1493-1495.

73. Lazarchick J. Update on anemia and neutropenia in copper deficiency. *Curr Opin Hematol.* 2012;19(1):58-60.

74. Prus E, Peled T, Fibach E. The effect of tetraethylenepentamine, a synthetic copper chelating polyamine, on expression of CD34 and CD38 antigens on normal and leukemic hematopoietic cells. *Leuk Lymphoma.* 2004;45(3):583-589.

75. Kumar N, Gross JB Jr, Ahlskog JE. Copper deficiency myelopathy produces a clinical picture like subacute combined degeneration. *Neurology.* 2004;63(1):33-39.

76. Green R. Anemias beyond B12 and iron deficiency: the buzz about other B's, elementary, and nonelementary problems. *Hematology Am Soc Hematol Educ Program.* 2012;2012:492-498.

77. Gabreyes AA, Abbasi HN, Forbes KP, et al. Hypocupremia associated cytopenia and myelopathy: a national retrospective review. *Eur J Haematol.* 2013;90(1):1-9.

78. Hein MS. Copper deficiency anemia and nephrosis in zinc-toxicity: a case report. *S D J Med.* 2003;56(4):143-147.

79. Igic PG, Lee E, Harper W, Roach KW. Toxic effects associated with consumption of zinc. *Mayo Clin Proc.* 2002;77(7):713-716.

80. Cordano A. Clinical manifestations of nutritional copper deficiency in infants and children. *Am J Clin Nutr.* 1998;67(5 suppl):1012S-1016S.

81. Myint ZW, Oo TH, Thein KZ, et al. Copper deficiency anemia: review article. *Ann Hematol.* 2018;97(9):1527-1534.

82. Fuchs GJ, Tienboon P, Linpisarn S, et al. Nutritional factors and thalassaemia major. *Arch Dis Child.* 1996;74(3):224-227.

83. Prasad AS. Zinc deficiency in patients with sickle cell disease. *Am J Clin Nutr.* 2002;75(2):181-182.

84. Yuzbasiyan-Gurkan VA, Brewer GJ, Vander AJ, et al. Net renal tubular reabsorption of zinc in healthy man and impaired handling in sickle cell anemia. *Am J Hematol.* 1989;31(2):87-90.

85. De Virgiliis S, Congia M, Turco MP, et al. Depletion of trace elements and acute ocular toxicity induced by desferrioxamine in patients with thalassaemia. *Arch Dis Child.* 1988;63(3):250-255.

86. Caruso R, Pallone F, Stasi E, et al. Appropriate nutrient supplementation in celiac disease. *Ann Med.* 2013;45(8):522-531.

87. Thomson CD, Rea HM, Doesburg VM, Robinson MF. Selenium concentrations and glutathione peroxidase activities in whole blood of New Zealand residents. *Br J Nutr.* 1977;37(3):457-460.

88. Cohen HJ, Brown MR, Hamilton D, et al. Glutathione peroxidase and selenium deficiency in patients receiving home parenteral nutrition: time course for development of deficiency and repletion of enzyme activity in plasma and blood cells. *Am J Clin Nutr.* 1989;49(1):132-139.

89. Kien CL, Ganther HE. Manifestations of chronic selenium deficiency in a child receiving total parenteral nutrition. *Am J Clin Nutr.* 1983;37(2):319-328.

90. Semba RD, Ricks MO, Ferrucci L, et al. Low serum selenium is associated with anemia among older adults in the United States. *Eur J Clin Nutr.* 2009;63(1):93-99.

91. Van Nhien N, Yabutani T, Khan NC, et al. Association of low serum selenium with anemia among adolescent girls living in rural Vietnam. *Nutrition.* 2009;25(1):6-10.

92. Delesderrier E, Cople-Rodrigues CS, Omena J, et al. Selenium status and hemolysis in sickle cell disease patients. *Nutrients.* 2019;11(9):2211.

93. Keys A, Brozek J, Henschel A, et al. *The Biology of Human Starvation.* University of Minnesota Press; 1950.

94. Kalm LM, Semba RD. They starved so that others be better fed: remembering Ancel Keys and the Minnesota experiment. *J Nutr.* 2005;135(6):1347-1352.

95. Thomson TJ, Runcie J, Miller V. Treatment of obesity by total fasting for up to 249 days. *Lancet.* 1966;2(7471):992-996.

96. Drenick EJ, Swendseid ME, Blahd WH, Tuttle SG. Prolonged starvation as treatment for severe obesity. *JAMA.* 1964;187:100-105.

97. Caro J, Silver R, Erslev AJ, et al. Erythropoietin production in fasted rats. Effects of thyroid hormones and glucose supplementation. *J Lab Clin Med.* 1981;98(6):860-868.

98. Lowik MR, Schrijver J, Odink J, et al. Long-term effects of a vegetarian diet on the nutritional status of elderly people (Dutch Nutrition Surveillance System). *J Am Coll Nutr.* 1990;9(6):600-609.

99. Chanarin I, Malkowska V, O'Hea AM, et al. Megaloblastic anaemia in a vegetarian Hindu community. *Lancet.* 1985;2(8465):1168-1172.

100. Carvalho NF, Kenney RD, Carrington PH, Hall DE. Severe nutritional deficiencies in toddlers resulting from health food milk alternatives. *Pediatrics.* 2001;107(4):E46.

101. Lunn PG, Morley CJ, Neale G. A case of kwashiorkor in the UK. *Clin Nutr.* 1998;17(3):131-133.

102. Adams EB, Scragg JN, Naidoo BT, et al. Observations on the aetiology and treatment of anaemia in kwashiorkor. *Br Med J.* 1967;3(5563):451-454.

103. Foy H, Kondi A. Comparison between erythroid aplasia in marasmus and kwashiorkor and the experimentally induced erythroid aplasia in baboons by riboflavin deficiency. *Vitam Horm.* 1968;26:653-684.

104. Ozkale M, Sipahi T. Hematologic and bone marrow changes in children with protein-energy malnutrition. *Pediatr Hematol Oncol.* 2014;31(4):349-358.

105. Margo G, Baroni Y, Wells G, et al. Protein energy malnutrition and nutritional anaemia in preschool children in rural KwaZulu. *S Afr Med J.* 1978;53(1):21-26.

106. Margo G, Lipschitz S, Joseph E, et al. Protein calorie malnutrition and nutritional anaemia in Black pre-school children in a South African semirural community. *S Afr Med J.* 1976;50(3):67-74.

107. Thakur N, Chandra J, Pemde H, Singh V. Anemia in severe acute malnutrition. *Nutrition.* 2014;30(4):440-442.

108. Delmonte L, Aschkenasy A, Eyquem A. Studies on the hemolytic nature of protein-deficiency anemia in the rat. *Blood.* 1964;24:49-68.

109. Naets JP, Wittek M. Effect of starvation on the response to erythropoietin in the rat. *Acta Haematol.* 1974;52(3):141-150.

110. Ito K, Reissmann KR. Quantitative and qualitative aspects of steady state erythropoiesis induced in protein-starved rats by long-term erythropoietin injection. *Blood.* 1966;27(3):343-351.

111. Miller KK, Grinspoon SK, Ciampa J, et al. Medical findings in outpatients with anorexia nervosa. *Arch Intern Med.* 2005;165:561-566.

112. Hutter G, Ganepola S, Hofmann WK. The hematology of anorexia nervosa. *Int J Eat Disord.* 2009;42(4):293-300.

113. Gloria L, Cravo M, Camilo ME, et al. Nutritional deficiencies in chronic alcoholics: relation to dietary intake and alcohol consumption. *Am J Gastroenterol.* 1997;92(3):485-489.

114. Savage D, Lindenbaum J. Anemia in alcoholics. *Medicine (Baltimore).* 1986;65(5):322-338.

115. Girard DE, Kumar KL, McAfee JH. Hematologic effects of acute and chronic alcohol abuse. *Hematol Oncol Clin North Am.* 1987;1(2):321-334.

116. Fernando OV, Grimsley EW. Prevalence of folate deficiency and macrocytosis in patients with and without alcohol-related illness. *South Med J.* 1998;91(8):721-725.

117. Sullivan LW, Herbert V. Suppression hematopoiesis by ethanol. *J Clin Invest.* 1964;43:2048-2062.

118. Eichner ER, Hillman RS. Effect of alcohol on serum folate level. *J Clin Invest.* 1973;52(3):584-591.

119. Lindenbaum J. Folate and vitamin B12 deficiencies in alcoholism. *Semin Hematol.* 1980;17(2):119-129.

120. Colman N, Herbert V. Hematologic complications of alcoholism: overview. *Semin Hematol.* 1980;17(3):164-176.

121. Halsted CH. Nutrition and alcoholic liver disease. *Semin Liver Dis.* 2004;24(3):289-304.

122. Seppa K, Laippala P, Saarni M. Macrocytosis as a consequence of alcohol abuse among patients in general practice. *Alcohol Clin Exp Res.* 1991;15(5):871-876.

123. McCurdy PR, Rath CE. Vacuolated nucleated bone marrow cells in alcoholism. *Semin Hematol.* 1980;17(2):100-102.

124. Yeung KY, Klug PP, Lessin LS. Alcohol-induced vacuolization in bone marrow cells: ultrastructure and mechanism of formation. *Blood Cells.* 1988;13(3):487-502.

125. Melrose WD, Bell PA, Jupe DM, Baikie MJ. Alcohol-associated haemolysis in Zieve's syndrome: a clinical and laboratory study of five cases. *Clin Lab Haematol.* 1990;12(2):159-167.

126. Zieve L. Jaundice, hyperlipemia and hemolytic anemia: a heretofore unrecognized syndrome associated with alcoholic fatty liver and cirrhosis. *Ann Intern Med.* 1958;48(3):471-496.

127. Chitale AA, Sterling RK, Post AB, et al. Resolution of spur cell anemia with liver transplantation: a case report and review of the literature. *Transplantation.* 1998;65(7):993-995.

128. Malik P, Bogetti D, Sileri P, et al. Spur cell anemia in alcoholic cirrhosis: cure by orthotopic liver transplantation and recurrence after liver graft failure. *Int Surg.* 2002;87(4):201-204.

129. Yokoyama A, Brooks PJ, Yokoyama T, et al. Recovery from anemia and leukocytopenia after abstinence in Japanese alcoholic men and their genetic polymorphisms of alcohol dehydrogenase-1B and aldehyde dehydrogenase-2. *Jpn J Clin Oncol.* 2017;47(4):306-312.

130. Smith C, Gasparetto M, Jordan C, et al. The effects of alcohol and aldehyde dehydrogenases on disorders of hematopoiesis. *Adv Exp Med Biol.* 2015;815:349-359.

131. Rogler G, Vavricka S. Anemia in inflammatory bowel disease: an under-estimated problem? *Front Med* (Lausanne) 2014;1:58.

132. Battat R, Kopylov U, Szilagyi A, et al. Vitamin B12 deficiency in inflammatory bowel disease: prevalence, risk factors, evaluation, and management. *Inflamm Bowel Dis.* 2014;20:1120-1128.

133. Bermejo F, Algaba A, Guerra I, et al. Should we monitor vitamin B12 and folate levels in Crohn's disease patients? *Scand J Gastroenterol.* 2013;48:1272-1277.

134. Bermejo F, Algaba A, Guerra I, et al. Response to letter: folate deficiency in Crohn's disease. *Scand J Gastroenterol.* 2014;49:255-256.

135. Hashemi J, Asadi J, Amiriani T, et al. Serum vitamins A and E deficiencies in patients with inflammatory bowel disease. *Saudi Med J.* 2013;34:432-434.

136. Alkhouri RH, Hashmi H, Baker RD, et al. Vitamin and mineral status in patients with inflammatory bowel disease. *J Pediatr Gastroenterol Nutr.* 2013;56:89-92.

137. da Rocha Lima B, Pichi F, Lowder CY. Night blindness and Crohn's disease. *Int Ophthalmol.* 2014;34:1141-1144.

138. Geerling BJ, Badart-Smook A, Stockbrugger RW, et al. Comprehensive nutritional status in recently diagnosed patients with inflammatory bowel disease compared with population controls. *Eur J Clin Nutr.* 2000;54:514-521.

139. Vagianos, K, Bector S, McConnell J, Bernstein CN. Nutrition assessment of patients with inflammatory bowel disease. *J Parenter Enteral Nutr.* 2007;31:311-319.

140. Siva S, Rubin DT, Gulotta G, et al. Zinc deficiency is associated with poor clinical outcomes in patients with inflammatory bowel disease. *Inflamm Bowel Dis.* 2017;23:152-157.

CHAPTER 13
ANEMIA ASSOCIATED WITH MARROW INFILTRATION

Vishnu V.B. Reddy and Diana Morlote

SUMMARY

Myelophthisic anemia is caused by marrow infiltration, typically by metastatic cancer but also by any nonhematopoietic conditions such as granulomatous inflammation or fibrosis. It can present with an overt leukoerythroblastic picture or with only a few teardrop-shaped red cells on a blood film. These changes may represent an early spread of the tumor (or other nonhematopoietic entities) to the marrow or may indicate massive replacement of the marrow space. The diagnosis can be made by standard marrow biopsy. Radio-isotope scanning, positron emission tomography/computed tomography (PET/CT), and magnetic resonance imaging (MRI), although not very sensitive, can be helpful in locating the biopsy site and can also help estimating the percentage of involvement of the marrow space.

DEFINITION AND HISTORY

Myelophthisic anemia is the term that has been used to describe diverse pathologic processes, including Fanconi anemia,[1] but currently refers to anemia resulting from the presence of spotty to massive marrow infiltration with abnormal cells or tissue components. Strictly speaking, the blasts of acute leukemia, plasma cells of myeloma, and cells of lymphoma, chronic leukemia, and myeloproliferative neoplasms fit this definition. However, the term *myelophthisic anemia*[2] is best reserved for marrow replacement by nonhematologic tumors and nonhematopoietic entities. Minimal to moderate involvement usually does not cause symptoms or hematologic changes. Such infiltration is clinically significant, however, because in patients with an established diagnosis of cancer, it indicates metastatic dissemination of the tumor and usually an advanced stage. Although extensive infiltration may lead to anemia or even pancytopenia, anemia can be accompanied by an elevated leukocyte count, often with immature myeloid cells in the blood. Platelets can be increased, decreased, or normal (megakaryocytic fragments are seen occasionally in the blood film). The findings accompanied by teardrop-shaped red cells (dacrocytes), nucleated red cells, and immature myeloid cells are referred to as *leukoerythroblastic reaction*, which generally reflect marrow replacement by tumor or extramedullary hematopoiesis.

Acronyms and Abbreviations: ^{99m}Tc, a radioisotope of technetium; ^{99m}Tc sestamibi, a radioisotope of technetium attached to the sestamibi molecule; MAS, macrophage activation syndrome; MRI, magnetic resonance imaging; PET/CT, positron emission tomography-computed tomography; STIM, stromal interaction molecule; TRP, transient receptor potential.

ETIOLOGY AND PATHOGENESIS

Tumor metastasis results from the complex interactions between the tumor cells and the surrounding microenvironment. Invasion is the primary process of metastasis and occurs often as a result of loss of E-cadherin. E-cadherin is a calcium-dependent cell adhesion molecule that likely plays a role in intercellular adhesion and inhibition of invasion by neoplastic cells. The loss of E-cadherin can be caused by several mechanisms, including mutations and gene silencing.[3] Dysregulation of calcium influx pathways through stromal interaction molecule (STIM) and calcium permeable transient receptor potential also play roles in tumor invasive and metastatic behavior.[4] Several members of the family of matrix metalloproteinases can also participate in the process of tumor cell invasion. Ancillary cells, such as tumor-associated macrophages and their secretion of growth factors, such as fibroblast growth factor, can also promote tumor spread.[5]

Table 13-1 lists the most common causes of extensive cellular infiltration of marrow. In myelofibrotic disorders of both primary and secondary origin, the fibrosis or osteosclerosis restricts the available marrow space and disrupts marrow architecture. The disruption may cause cytopenias with production of deformed red cells, especially poikilocytes and teardrop-shaped cells, and premature release of erythroblasts, myelocytes, and giant platelets. The leukocyte count also may be elevated. Similar abnormalities after marrow replacement by calcium oxalate crystals have been reported.[6] Anemia seen in metastatic cancer most frequently results from cytokine release, leading to anemia of chronic inflammation (Chap. 6), iron deficiency as a result of gastrointestinal or uterine bleeding (Chap. 11), or other nutritional deficiencies (Chaps. 9 and 12). However, marrow replacement causing a myelophthisic anemia as the sole cause of anemia also occurs. The marrow microenvironment is susceptible to implantation of bloodborne malignant cells. Almost all cancers can metastasize to the marrow,[7-11] but the most common are cancers of the lung, breast, and prostate. Metastatic foci in the marrow can be found in 20% to 30% of patients with small cell carcinoma of the lung at the time of diagnosis and in more than 50% of patients at autopsy.[12,13] Overt leukoerythroblastic blood picture is less common, and its absence is not a reliable indicator that the marrow is not involved.

The characteristic abnormalities observed in patients with myelophthisic anemia may result partly from an attempt for compensatory extramedullary blood formation that generally reflects extramedullary hematopoiesis predominantly from the spleen. A similar picture can be seen when the marrow is replaced by numerous granulomas,[14,15] for example, those of sarcoidosis, disseminated tuberculosis, fungal infections, or by macrophages containing indigestible lipids, as in Gaucher or Niemann-Pick diseases,[16] and macrophage activation syndrome (MAS).

Marrow necrosis can be an underlying cause of myelophthisic anemia. The morphologic picture, best observed in hematoxylin-and-eosin–stained biopsy of marrow, consists of cell debris and occasional necrotic cells in an eosinophilic amorphus background (Fig. 13-1).[17] Marrow necrosis is generally considered to be very uncommon, observed in fewer than 1% of marrow biopsies. Metastatic tumors, acute lymphoblastic leukemia (children), and septicemia are the most common underlying cause,[17,18] but fat embolism syndrome in sickle cell disease[19] and associated parvovirus B19 infection[20-22] and arsenic therapy in acute promyelocytic leukemia are other causes.[23] Necrotic foci range from small to very extensive (<5%-90% of the biopsy volume). Extensive necrosis often results in inability to perform flow cytometry or molecular analysis satisfactorily. A repeat biopsy at a different site may be needed if that information is required.[17,24,25]

Because myelophthisic anemia is so uncommon, only a few rigorous studies of the pathogenesis of anemia in this entity have been

TABLE 13–1. Causes of Marrow Infiltration

I. Fibroblasts and collagen
   A. Primary myelofibrosis
   B. Fibrosis associated with other myeloproliferative neoplasms
   C. Fibrosis of hairy cell leukemia
   D. Metastatic tumors (eg, breast carcinoma)
   E. Sarcoidosis[14,15]
   F. Secondary myelofibrosis with pulmonary hypertension

II. Other noncellular material
   A. Oxalosis[6]

III. Tumor cells
   A. Carcinomas (breast, lung, prostate, kidney, thyroid, and neuroblastoma)[7,8,11]
   B. Sarcoma[10]

IV. Granulomas[14]
   A. Sarcoidosis
   B. Fungal infections
   C. Miliary tuberculosis

V. Macrophages
   A. Gaucher disease
   B. Niemann-Pick disease[16]
   C. Macrophage activation syndrome[38,39]

VI. Marrow necrosis
   A. Sickle cell anemia[20]
   B. Solid tumor metastasis[18]
   C. Septicemia[18]
   D. Acute lymphoblastic leukemia
   E. Arsenic therapy[23]

VII. Failure of osteoclast development
   A. Osteopetrosis[40]

conducted. In vitro study of hematopoietic progenitors reveals only a moderate decrease of their proportion and proliferative capacity.[26] Similar reports of erythropoiesis quantitation by ferrokinetic studies reveal only a moderate defect (Chap. 2).[27] The following confounding factors contribute to anemia: elevated hepcidin (Chap. 6) and other factors,

including hematopoiesis-inhibiting cytokines released from tumor cells (Chap. 6), and iron (Chap. 11), folate, and cobalamin (Chap. 9) deficiencies. When they are excluded, the finding discussed suggests that only massive marrow replacement leads to anemia.

● CLINICAL FEATURES

Symptoms and signs associated with infiltrative marrow disorders usually are related to the underlying disease. Other symptoms, such as fatigue, often from upregulated cytokines, may also contribute to anemia itself. Some patients are asymptomatic, and the incidental discovery of cytopenias and leukoerythroblastic blood morphology leads to diagnosis of an underlying disorder and initial manifestation of marrow metastasis.[28]

● LABORATORY FEATURES

BLOOD

The anemia usually is mild to moderate, but it can be severe. White cell and platelet counts may vary, but the most characteristic feature is the disturbed morphologic appearance of red cells on the blood film. These cells may show anisocytosis and poikilocytosis, but the presence of teardrop forms and nucleated red cells is particularly suggestive of marrow infiltration (Chap. 1) (Fig. 13–2). The combination of nucleated red cells and immature myeloid precursors constitutes the leukoerythroblastic picture that is characteristic of marrow infiltration and extramedullary hematopoiesis. The presence of cancer cells on the blood film occurs occasionally and always indicates marrow invasion (Fig. 13-3).[29]

MARROW

Marrow biopsy is the most reliable procedure used to diagnose marrow-infiltrative disease and should be performed in all patients with suspected metastatic carcinoma or hematologic features of myelophthisic anemia. Marrow aspiration[25,30] does not provide a reliable yield of tumor cells and is particularly difficult in primary or secondary myelofibrosis. The inability to aspirate marrow (dry tap) leads to a high degree of suspicion of marrow replacement and accompanying myelofibrosis. Because the diagnostic marrow yield from biopsies depends on the amount of tissue examined, bilateral posterior iliac crest marrow biopsies may be necessary. In patients with metastatic cancer involving the marrow, the blood CD34-positive cell count can be up to 50 times higher than in patients with metastatic cancer without marrow involvement.[31]

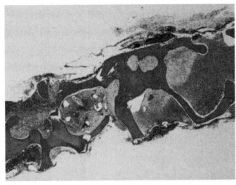
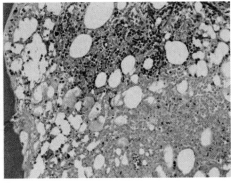

    A   **B**

FIGURE 13–1. Bone marrow necrosis. **A.** Low-magnification view of the biopsy showing mostly necrosis (*pink area*) and focally preserved tumor to the left (*blue area*). **B.** Higher magnification of necrosis with loss of cellular details and granular eosinophilic and pink cell debris.

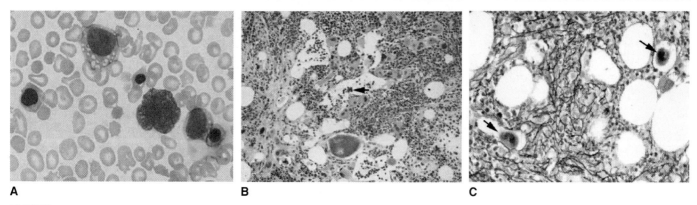

FIGURE 13–2. Leukoerythroblastosis. **A.** Blood film containing several nucleated red blood cells (RBCs), few circulating blasts, and RBCs showing severe anisopoikilocytosis. **B.** Corresponding marrow biopsy with intrasinusoidal hematopoiesis, erythroid precursors (*arrow*). **C.** Marrow biopsy showing reticulin fibrosis (3+) and intrasinusoidal megakaryocytes (*arrows*).

ISOTOPE AND IMAGING PROCEDURES

Technetium-99m (99mTc) sestamibi uptake reliably identifies marrow infiltration by Gaucher cells. Sestamibi is a pharmaceutical agent used in nuclear medicine imaging. Magnetic resonance imaging (MRI) is also helpful for defining the severity of marrow replacement and is being used with increasing frequency. This imaging approach is especially useful for following resolution of marrow infiltration in patients with type 1 Gaucher disease who are treated with enzyme-replacement therapy.[21,32,33] An isotopic bone scan or MRI study showing focal accumulation of radioactive tracers can be helpful in locating a suitable site for biopsy,[21,34] but a negative study of the area does not exclude the possibility of marrow involvement. On MRI, marrow necrosis characteristically has an extensive, diffuse, geographic pattern of signal abnormality consisting of a central area of variable signal intensity surrounded by a distinct peripheral enhancing rim.[22] Positron emission tomography (PET)/computed tomography (CT) evaluation in some cases is more sensitive in detecting marrow infiltration.[35]

● DIFFERENTIAL DIAGNOSIS

A leukoerythroblastic blood picture is known to occur in a patient with metastatic cancer or overt hematologic malignancy. In the absence of a likely cause after clinical evaluation, the initial approach to diagnosis is the marrow biopsy. Although it is not a very sensitive technique, with the help of immunocytochemistry and flow cytometry for tumor-specific antigens, its diagnostic sensitivity and specificity increase. MRI or isotopic scanning before the marrow biopsy may aid in locating the optimal site of the biopsy. Hematologic disorders causing marrow fibrosis, notably primary myelofibrosis, may mimic a myelophthisic disorder, but the distinctions are usually evident. For example, patients with primary myelofibrosis invariably have splenic enlargement, and the patients with metastatic cancer almost never have splenomegaly, unless for another obvious cause (Chap. 25). If the myelophthisis is the result of a storage disease or other infiltrative cause, the appropriate chemical tests, as well as marrow biopsy, are helpful in diagnosis. Nucleated red cells and leukocytosis can be seen in acute conditions, including overwhelming sepsis, acute viral infection (eg, COVID-19),[36] acute severe hypoxia, postcardiac arrest, and chronic conditions such as thalassemia major, congestive heart failure, and severe hemolytic anemia.

● THERAPY, COURSE, AND PROGNOSIS

The goal of treatment is managing the underlying disease. Patients with marrow infiltration caused by cancer should be treated appropriately; however, in some instances, the presence of marrow infiltration may not adversely affect the outcome. If treatment is successful, not only the malignant cells but also the reactive fibrosis surrounding metastatic foci may completely disappear. In hormone-refractory prostate cancer, the presence of a leukoerythroblastic picture does not seem to influence survival.[37] However, in most patients with cancers metastatic to the marrow, only short-term survival is likely.

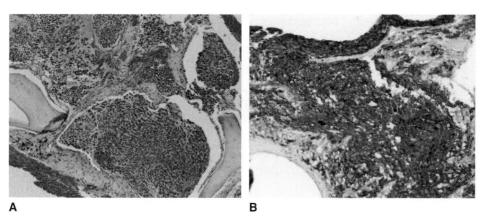

FIGURE 13–3. Metastatic tumor in the marrow. **A.** Marrow packed with neuroblastoma and completely displacing normal marrow elements. Tumor cells have characteristic spindle to round nuclei with minimal or no cytoplasm. **B.** CD56 immunohistochemical stain highlights neuroblastoma infiltrates in the marrow.

REFERENCES

1. Baumann T. Constitutional general myelophthisis with multiple degeneration (Fanconi syndrome). *Ann Paediatr.* 1951;177(2):65-76.
2. Rundles RW, Jonsson U. Metastases in bone marrow and myelophthisic anemia from carcinoma of the prostate. *Am J Med Sci.* 1949;218(3):241-250.
3. Thiery JP. Epithelial-mesenchymal transitions in tumour progression. *Nat Rev Cancer.* 2002;2(6):442-454.
4. Chen YF, Chen YT, Chiu WT, Shen MR. Remodeling of calcium signaling in tumor progression. *J Biomed Sci.* 2013;20:23.
5. Chiang AC, Massague J. Molecular basis of metastasis. *N Engl J Med.* 2008;359(26):2814-2823.
6. Halil O, Farringdon K. Oxalosis: an unusual cause of leucoerythroblastic anaemia. *Br J Haematol.* 2003;122(1):2.
7. Makoni SN, Laber DA. Clinical spectrum of myelophthisis in cancer patients. *Am J Hematol.* 2004;76(1):92-93.
8. Mohanty SK, Dash S. Bone marrow metastasis in solid tumors. *Indian J Pathol Microbiol.* 2003;46(4):613-616.
9. Pham CM, Syed AA, Siddiqui HA, et al. Case of metastatic basal cell carcinoma to bone marrow, resulting in myelophthisic anemia. *Am J Dermatopathol.* 2013;35(2):e34-e36.
10. Shinkoda Y, Nagatoshi Y, Okamura J. Rhabdomyosarcoma masquerading as acute leukemia. *Pediatr Blood Cancer.* 2009;52(2):286-287.
11. Velasco-Rodriguez D, Villarrubia V, Castellonos-Gonzalez C, et al. Metastatic malignant melanoma detected on bone marrow aspiration. *Br J Haematol.* 2013;162(4):432.
12. Hirsch FR, Hansen HH. Bone marrow involvement in small cell anaplastic carcinoma of the lung: prognostic and therapeutic aspects. *Cancer.* 1980;46(1):206-211.
13. Hirsch FR, Osterlind K, Hansen HH, et al. Bone marrow examination in small cell lung cancer. *Ann Intern Med.* 1987;106(6):913.
14. Eid A, Carion W, Nystrom JS. Differential diagnoses of bone marrow granuloma. *West J Med.* 1996;164(6):510-515.
15. Saliba WR, Elias MS. Recurrent severe hypercalcemia caused by bone marrow sarcoidosis. *Am J Med Sci.* 2005;330(3):147-149.
16. Hsu YS, Hwu WL, Huang SF, et al. Niemann-Pick disease type C (a cellular cholesterol lipidosis) treated by bone marrow transplantation. *Bone Marrow Transplant.* 1999;24(1):103-107.
17. Khoshnaw NS, Muhealdeen DN. Bone marrow necrosis in an adult patient with precursor B-cell acute lymphoblastic leukaemia at the time of presentation. *BMJ Case Rep.* 2014;2014.
18. Paydas S, Ergin M, Bolat FA, et al. Bone marrow necrosis: clinicopathologic analysis of 20 cases and review of the literature. *Am J Hematol.* 2002;70(4):300-305.
19. Tsitsikas DA, Gallinella G, Amos RJ, et al. Bone marrow necrosis and fat embolism syndrome in sickle cell disease: increased susceptibility of patients with non-SS genotypes and a possible association with human parvovirus B19 infection. *Blood Rev.* 2014;28(1):23-30.
20. Conrad ME, Studdard H, Anderson LJ. Aplastic crisis in sickle cell disorders: bone marrow necrosis and human parvovirus infection. *Am J Med Sci.* 1988;295(3):212-215.
21. Howe BM, Johnson GB, Wenger DE. Current concepts in MRI of focal and diffuse malignancy of bone marrow. *Semin Musculoskelet Radiol.* 2013;17(2):137-144.
22. Tang YM, Jeavons S, Gill D, et al. MRI features of bone marrow necrosis. *AJR Am J Roentgenol.* 2007;188(2):509-514.
23. Chim CS, Lam CCK, Kwong YL, et al. Atypical blasts and bone marrow necrosis associated with near-triploid relapse of acute promyelocytic leukemia after arsenic trioxide treatment. *Hum Pathol.* 2002;33(8):849-851.
24. Conrad ME. Bone marrow necrosis. *J Intensive Care Med.* 1995;10(4):171-178.
25. Langsteger W, Haim S, Knauer M, et al. Imaging of bone metastases in prostate cancer: an update. *Q J Nucl Med Mol Imaging.* 2012;56(5):447-458.
26. Dainiak DN. Mechanisms of abnormal erythropoiesis in malignancy. *Cancer.* 1983;51(6):1101-1106.
27. Cazzola M, Beramaschi G, Finch CA, et al. Pathophysiological classification of acquired bone marrow failure based on quantitative assessment of erythroid function. *Eur J Haematol.* 1987;38(5):426-432.
28. Fan FS, Yang CF. Leukoerythroblastosis in castration-resistant prostate cancer: A clue to diffuse bone marrow carcinomatosis. *Clin Pract.* 2019;9(2):1124.
29. Gallivan MV, Lokich JJ. Carcinocythemia (carcinoma cell leukemia). Report of two cases with English literature review. *Cancer.* 1984;53(5):1100-1102.
30. Garrett TJ, Gee TS, Clarkson BD, et al. The role of bone marrow aspiration and biopsy in detecting marrow involvement by nonhematologic malignancies. *Cancer.* 1976;38(6):2401-2403.
31. Ciancia R, Martinelli V, Rotoli B, et al. High number of circulating CD34+ cells in patients with myelophthisis. *Haematologica.* 2005;90(7):976-977.
32. Erba PA, Minichilli F, Mariani G, et al. 99mTc-sestamibi scintigraphy to monitor the long-term efficacy of enzyme replacement therapy on bone marrow infiltration in patients with Gaucher disease. *J Nucl Med.* 2013;54(10):1717-1724.
33. Mariani G, Filocamo M, Giona F, et al. Severity of bone marrow involvement in patients with Gaucher's disease evaluated by scintigraphy with 99mTc-sestamibi. *J Nucl Med.* 2003;44(8):1253-1262.
34. Terk MR, Dardashti S, Liebman HA. Bone marrow response in treated patients with Gaucher disease: evaluation by T1-weighted magnetic resonance images and correlation with reduction in liver and spleen volume. *Skeletal Radiol.* 2000;29(10):563-571.
35. Zapata CP, Cuglievan B, De Angulo G, et al. PET/CT versus bone marrow biopsy in the initial evaluation of bone marrow infiltration in various pediatric malignancies. *Pediatr Blood Cancer.* 2018;65(2).
36. Mitra A, DM Denis, S Michael et al. Leukoerythroblastic reaction in a patient with COVID-19 infection. *Am J Hematol.* 2020;95(8):999-1000.
37. Shamdas GJ, Ahmann FR, Ritchie JM, et al. Leukoerythroblastic anemia in metastatic prostate cancer. Clinical and prognostic significance in patients with hormone-refractory disease. *Cancer.* 1993;71(11):3594-3600.
38. George MR. Hemophagocytic lymphohistiocytosis: review of etiologies and management. *J Blood Med.* 2014;5:69-86.
39. Ravelli A, Grom AA, Cron RQ, et al. Macrophage activation syndrome as part of systemic juvenile idiopathic arthritis: diagnosis, genetics, pathophysiology and treatment. *Genes Immun.* 2012;13(4):289-298.
40. Stark Z, Savarirayan R. Osteopetrosis. *Orphanet J Rare Dis.* 2009;4:5.

Part IV Anemias Resulting Principally from Inherited Disorders

CHAPTER 14
THE HEREDITARY DYSERYTHROPOIETIC ANEMIAS

Achille Iolascon, Roberta Russo, and Rami Khoriaty

SUMMARY

The hereditary dyserythropoietic anemias also known as congenital dyserythropoietic anemias (CDAs) are a group of hereditary disorders characterized by (1) anemia caused by ineffective erythropoiesis, (2) erythroid hyperplasia with increased percentage of bi/multinucleated erythroid precursors in the marrow, and often (3) hemochromatosis resulting from increased absorption of iron. The CDAs are classically divided into three types (CDA I, II, and III). CDA I is an autosomal recessive disease resulting from mutations in either *CDAN1* or *CDIN1* and is characterized by a "Swiss cheese" appearance of heterochromatin and internuclear chromatin bridges. CDA II, also an autosomal recessive disease, is the most common CDA type and results from mutations in *SEC23B*. CDA II is characterized by a double-membrane appearance of the red blood cell (RBC) plasma membrane, faster mobility of the RBC membrane protein band 3 by sodium dodecylsulfate polyacrylamide gel electrophoresis (SDS-PAGE), and

lysis of erythrocytes in a subset of acidified human sera, hence its prior designation as hereditary erythroblastic multinuclearity with a positive acidified serum test (commonly known as HEMPAS). CDA III is an autosomal dominant disease resulting from mutations in *KIF23*. CDA III is characterized by giant multinucleated erythroblasts and increased risk of development of angioid streaks and myeloma. Additional CDA variants resulting from mutations in *KLF1, GATA1, ALAS2, LPIN2, CAD, COX4I2,* and *MVK* have been reported. The CDA disease severity is highly variable, ranging from hydrops fetalis to minimal or no anemia. Treatment is largely individualized and depends on the severity of the disease and the specific clinical manifestation. Although allogeneic stem cell transplantation is the only curative modality, it can be justified in only a small subset of patients because of risks associated with the procedure. Other treatment modalities include RBC transfusion support, iron chelation, splenectomy, and interferon-α (for CDA I patients only).

Acronyms and Abbreviations: AE1, band 3 anion transport protein; *ALAS2*, gene encoding 5′-aminolevulinate synthase 2; Arf6 and Asf1b, protein paralogs that are members adenosine diphosphate (ADP)-ribosylation factor 6; Asf1a, a protein that is a member of the H3/H4 family of histone chaperones; ASCT, allogeneic stem cell transplantation; *C15ORF41*, gene encoding a protein with two predicted helix-turn-helix domains of unknown function; *CAD*, gene encoding a trifunctional enzyme (carbamoyl-phosphate synthetase 2, aspartate transcarbamylase, and dihydroorotase); CDA, congenital dyserythropoietic anemia; *CDAN1*, gene encoding codanin-1; COP, cytoplasmic coat protein; *COX4I2*, gene encoding cytochrome c oxidase subunit IV isoform; E2F1, transcription factor 1; ER, endoplasmic reticulum; G6PD, glucose-6-phosphate dehydrogenase; GATA1, transcription factor 1 binding to the DNA sequence GATA; GDF15, growth differentiation factor 15; FLAG-tag, a polypeptide protein tag that can be added to a protein to which specific, high affinity monoclonal antibodies have been developed; HEMPAS, hereditary erythroblastic multinuclearity associated with a positive acidified serum test; HJV, hemojuvelin gene; HLA, human leukocyte antigen; HP1α, heterochromatin protein 1; HS, hereditary spherocytosis; IgM, immunoglobulin M; KIF23, mitotic kinesin-like protein 1; KLF1, a hematopoietic transcription factor; LDH, lactate dehydrogenase; LPIN2 (18p11.31), encoding lipin 2; MCV, mean cell volume; MEL cells, a mouse erythroleukemia cell line; MKD, mevalonate kinase deficiency; *MKLP1*, gene encoding mitotic kinesin-like protein 1; MRI, magnetic resonance imaging; RhAG; Rh-blood group associated glycoprotein; RBC, red blood cell; *SAR1B*, a gene encoding a small guanosine triphosphatase (GTPase) protein; SDS-PAGE, sodium dodecylsulfate polyacrylamide gel electrophoresis; *UGT1A1*, bilirubin uridine diphosphate (UDP)-glucuronosyltransferase 1A1 gene; U-2-OS cells; the human osteosarcoma cell line.

● DEFINITION AND HISTORY

The congenital dyserythropoietic anemias (CDAs) are a group of hereditary disorders characterized by anemia of variable severity resulting from a defect in the later stages of erythroid differentiation (Fig. 14-1A) and distinct morphologic features of the marrow erythroblasts. The abbreviation CDA was used first by Crookston et al[1] and by Heimpel and Wendt.[2] The CDAs are classically divided into three major types (CDA I-CDA III), although additional variants have also been described (Fig. 14-1B).[3] Several marrow features are shared by all of the CDAs, including erythroid hyperplasia and increased percentage of bi-/multinucleated erythroid precursors. However, each CDA type has additional unique characteristics (Fig. 14-2). Except for the *GATA1*-mutated CDA, the nonerythroid hematopoietic lineages are generally unaffected.

Anemia in CDA patients results primarily from ineffective erythropoiesis, defined as death and/or failure of maturation of the erythroid precursors in the marrow (see Fig. 14-2). However, reduced survival of the mature red blood cells (RBCs) might also be a contributing factor. Therefore, it is not uncommon to see elevated lactate dehydrogenase (LDH) and unconjugated bilirubin levels and/or reduced haptoglobin level. Reticulocyte count is normal or mildly elevated, but the reticulocyte response is invariably suboptimal for the degree of anemia, consistent with ineffective erythropoiesis. Splenomegaly is common. In a majority of patients, secondary hemochromatosis develops as a result of increased absorption of iron (Chap. 11), a consequence of ineffective erythropoiesis.

Although most patients present in infancy or childhood with mild or moderate anemia, the degree of anemia and age of presentation are highly variable. Some patients present with very severe disease manifestations (such as hydrops fetalis or severe transfusion-dependent anemia), and others exhibit minimal anemia. Therefore, the term "congenital" could be confusing, because the clinical manifestations of the disease might not be apparent until old age. Consideration should be made to replace "congenital" with "hereditary," as it has been done in diseases such as congenital spherocytosis (now hereditary spherocytosis). In addition, some individuals carrying the disease-causing mutations might exhibit no anemia (incomplete penetrance).

Though abnormal morphology of erythroid progenitors can be seen in other hereditary disorders (such as the thalassemias), certain acquired diseases (such as the myelodysplastic syndromes), or in the setting of rapid regeneration of the erythroid lineage, these latter

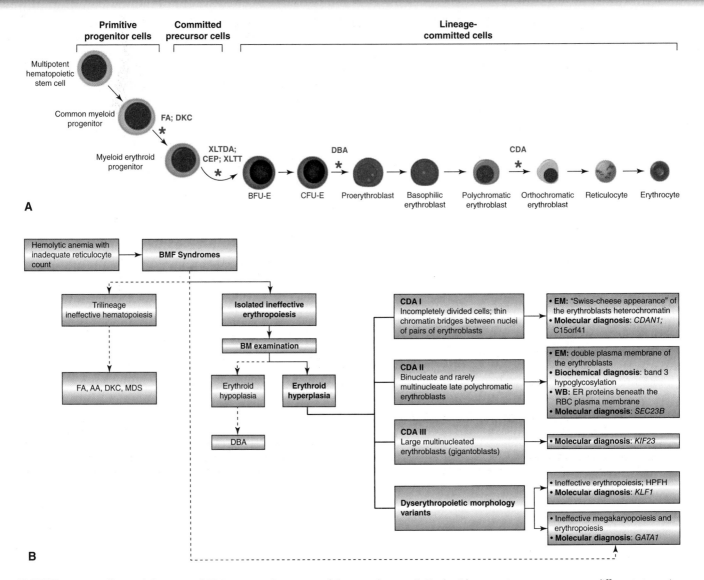

FIGURE 14–1. Differential diagnosis of CDAs versus other marrow failure syndromes. **A.** Erythroid maturation arrest occurs at different stages in various marrow failure syndromes. The CDA marrow is characterized by erythroid hyperplasia because the maturation arrest occurs in the later stages of erythroid development. **B.** Flow diagram for CDA subtypes based on clinical, morphologic, biochemical, and molecular findings. AA, aplastic anemia; BFU-E, burst-forming unit–erythroid; BM, marrow; BMF, marrow failure; CEP, congenital erythropoietic porphyria; CFU-E, colony-forming unit–erythroid; DBA, Diamond-Blackfan anemia; DKC, dyskeratosis congenita; EM, electron microscopy; ER, endoplasmic reticulum; FA, Fanconi anemia; HPFH, hereditary persistence of fetal hemoglobin; MDS, myelodysplastic syndromes; PNH, paroxysmal nocturnal hemoglobinuria; RBC, red blood cell; WB, Western blotting; XLTDA, X-linked thrombocytopenia with dyserythropoietic anemia; XLTT, X-linked thrombocytopenia with β-thalassemia.

disorders are usually readily apparent from the history, clinical scenario, laboratory tests, and additional/specific bone marrow findings. The discovery of the genetic defects underlying the CDAs has not only shed light on the pathophysiology of these disorders, but also allowed for accurate diagnosis and carrier testing for family members.

● EPIDEMIOLOGY

The prevalence of the CDAs is likely underestimated because it is often difficult to make the correct diagnosis. This is particularly true when the disease phenotype is mild. It is therefore not surprising that the CDA diagnosis is often not established until adulthood, sometimes several years after a workup for anemia is initiated.

The prevalence of CDA I and CDA II in Europe is estimated to be approximately 0.24 and 0.71 cases per million, respectively, whereas

CDA III is even less common.[4,5] In 2011, 712 cases (614 families) and 206 cases (183 families) were enrolled in the German and Italian CDA Registries, respectively. In the literature, an additional 169 CDA I patients (143 families) and 454 CDA II patients (356 families) have been reported worldwide. Hence, CDA I is approximately one-third as common as CDA II. Most reported families are from Western European and Middle Eastern countries, but single cases have also been reported in several additional countries, including the United States, India, Japan, and China. The other CDA variants are rare.

The wide variation in the prevalence of CDA throughout Europe could be attributed to the geographic locations of reference centers with expertise in diagnosing and treating these disorders and to genetic factors. Indeed, genetic studies in CDA II have established the presence of a founder effect in Europeans for the two most common mutations in *SEC23B*.[6,7]

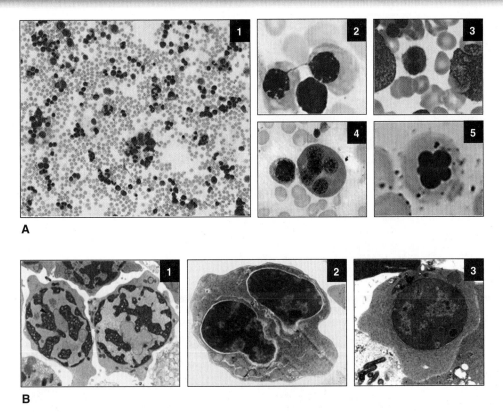

FIGURE 14–2. Morphologic features of the CDA erythroblasts in the marrow. **A.** The CDA marrow invariably shows erythroid hyperplasia on light microscopy *(inset 1)*. However, specific morphologic abnormalities in the erythroid precursors help distinguish the different types of CDAs. The presence of internuclear chromatin bridging is a hallmark of CDA I *(inset 2)*, whereas the presence of high percentage (10%-30%) of bi-/multinucleated late erythroid precursors is a feature of CDA II *(inset 3)*. Giant multinucleated erythroblasts *(inset 4)* and multinucleated erythroblasts *(inset 5)* are typical features of CDA III and CDA IV, respectively. **B.** Electron microscopy of CDA I erythroblasts shows the typical Swiss-cheese heterochromatin pattern in the nucleus *(inset 1)*, whereas CDA II erythroid precursors display the characteristic double plasma membrane appearance *(inset 2)*. CDA IV has non-specific features shared among different CDA types, such as marked heterochromatin, invagination of nuclear membrane, intranuclear precipitated material, and nuclear blebbing *(inset 3)*.

● CONGENITAL DYSERYTHROPOIETIC ANEMIA, TYPE I

CLINICAL FEATURES

CDA I is a disease with a wide spectrum of clinical presentations. Most patients are diagnosed in childhood or early adulthood, exhibit moderate anemia, and do not require transfusion support.[8-10] Some cases, with the most severe forms of the disease, are detected in utero and might require intrauterine transfusion support. These patients typically require lifelong transfusions. On the other end of the spectrum, mild cases might not be apparent until late adulthood.[9]

Anemia is usually macrocytic and frequently associated with intermittent jaundice. Splenomegaly is common, whereas hepatomegaly is rare except in patients diagnosed in the neonatal period. The latter patients with disease manifestations in the neonatal period often have hepatomegaly and prolonged jaundice, may have exhibited intrauterine growth retardation, and may require one or more blood transfusions perinatally. Cholelithiasis is a common complication, and jaundice may be aggravated by the coinheritance of the A[TA]₇TAA polymorphism in the promoter of the *UGT1A1* gene, the main cause of Gilbert syndrome.[11] Increased iron absorption is common; therefore, features of hemochromatosis might be seen, including signs and symptoms of liver cirrhosis, heart failure, diabetes mellitus, and discoloration of the skin (Chap. 11).

The disease is occasionally associated with dysmorphic features (in 4%-14% of affected individuals), mostly involving the bones of the hand and/or foot (syndactyly, hypoplasia of one or several phalanges, presence of supplementary metatarsal bones, and clubfoot) (Fig. 14-3).[12] Small stature, almond-shaped blue eyes, hypertelorism, micrognathism, and other abnormalities have also been reported.

LABORATORY FEATURES

Anemia is usually moderate (hemoglobin 8-10 g/dL) and macrocytic, although approximately 30% of patients have a normal mean corpuscular volume. The blood film demonstrates, in addition to macrocytosis, marked anisocytosis and poikilocytosis as well as occasional nucleated red cells, elliptocytes, ovalocytes, and basophilic stippling. The reticulocyte count is inappropriately low for the degree of anemia.[8-10]

Marrow evaluation demonstrates erythroid hyperplasia and increased percentage of binucleated erythroblasts, comprising approximately 3% to 7% of polychromatic erythroblasts. In addition, internuclear chromatin bridges, a distinguishing feature of CDA I, is identified in 1.4 to .9% of erythroblasts (see Fig. 14-2A).[13] Electron microscopy demonstrates a "spongy heterochromatin" (or "Swiss cheese appearance") in up to 60% of early and late polychromatic erythroblasts, referring to the presence of electron lucent areas within an abnormally dense heterochromatin (see Fig. 14-2B).[10,12]

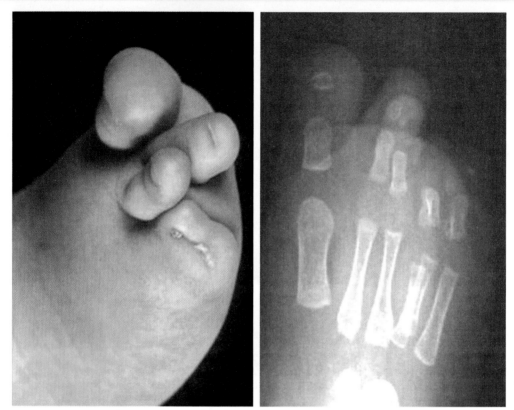

FIGURE 14–3. Foot dysmorphology in CDA I. *Left*, Photograph showing hypoplastic nails, a broad first toe, hypoplastic third toe, and brachysyndac-tyly of the fourth and the fifth toes. *Right*, Radiograph showing a duplication of the fourth metatarsal bone (both bones being hypoplastic), a dupli-cation of the fourth proximal phalanx, a single middle phalanx for the fourth and fifth toe, and the absence of the fourth distal phalanx. *(Reproduced with permission from Tamary H, Dgany O, Proust A, et al: Clinical and molecular variability in congenital dyserythropoietic anemia type I.* Br J Haematol. *2005 Aug;130[4]:628-634.)*

GENETICS

CDA I is inherited as an autosomal recessive disease. The majority (~80%) of cases result from homozygous or compound heterozygous mutations in *CDAN1* (chr 15q15.1–15.3), a gene that spans 15 kb and contains 28 exons.[14,15] The encoded protein, codanin-1, contains 1227 amino acids and is ubiquitously expressed. More than 50 unique disease-causing mutations in *CDAN1* have been reported,[16] and one founder mutation (R1042W) was observed in Bedouins.[3,8,17] Patients with bial-lelic null *CDAN1* mutations have not been reported, suggesting that complete absence of codanin-1 is lethal. Mice with germline deficiency for codanin-1 die at embryonic day 6.5, before the onset of erythropoie-sis, likely caused by a critical role of this protein in development.[18]

In approximately 20% of patients, CDA I is unexplained by muta-tions in *CDAN1*.[19] A subset of these cases (~10% of CDA I patients) result from biallelic mutations in *CDIN1* (CDAN1-interacting nucle-ase 1, previously named *C15ORF41*),[20] a gene which contains 11 exons and encodes a 281-amino-acid protein belonging to a family of endo-nucleases. At least six disease-causing mutations in *CDIN1* have been reported.[16,20-22] The remaining nearly 10% of CDA I patients are unac-counted for by mutations in the coding sequences of either *CDAN1* or *CDIN1*. These patients might have mutations in novel unidentified CDA I genes or in noncoding regulatory elements that affect the expres-sion of *CDAN1* or *CDIN1*.

Despite the identification of the genetic defects underlying 90% of CDA I patients, the pathophysiology of the disease remains unknown. The absence of appropriate models faithfully recapitulating the CDA I phenotype is one of the main obstacles to studying the pathogenesis of

the disease. Most of our knowledge about the function of codanin-1 stems from studies using a cervical cancer cell line (HeLa) and an osteosar-coma cell line (U-2-OS). It is unknown whether findings observed in these immortalized, aneuploid, nonhematopoietic cell lines would be relevant to erythroid cells. However, recently developed induced pluripotent stem cells derived from CDA I patients, as well as optimized strategies for differentiation of patient-derived CD34+ hematopoietic stem and progenitor cells into erythroid cells and generation of human erythroid cell lines with engineered *CDAN1* mutations, are expected to result in improved understanding of the pathophysiology of the disease.[23-27]

Another shortcoming in the study of CDA I is the lack of validated antibodies, as demonstrated by the discrepant intracellular localization of codanin-1 (nuclear vs cytoplasmic) described in various reports (see details further). Based on the drawbacks summarized here, the biologic insights described in this chapter need to be interpreted cautiously.

In one study, codanin-1 was found to be localized to the het-erochromatin of CDA I erythroblasts, with a similar localization pattern observed in HeLa cells, U-2-OS cells, and the human K562 erythroid cell line.[28] Additional experiments in the same study demonstrated that codanin-1 localizes with DNA specifically during interphase and cytoki-nesis, but not during mitosis (HeLa cells). The exclusion of codanin-1 from condensed chromosomes during mitosis was associated with phos-phorylation of the protein. Further studies (U-2-OS cells) demonstrated that codanin-1 is a direct target of the transcription factor E2F1, possi-bly explaining the increased codanin-1 protein level observed during the S-phase of the cell cycle in HeLa cells.[28]

In striking contrast, several reports demonstrated that codanin-1 was detected primarily in the cytosol.[18,29,30] This finding was confirmed in CDA I erythroblasts, primary human erythroblasts, murine erythroblasts, murine erythroleukemia cells (MEL cell line), HeLa cells, and U-2-OS cells. In one of these two reports, codanin-1 was found to directly bind and sequester the histone chaperone Asf1 in the cytoplasm, preventing Asf1 from delivering histone for chromatin assembly, resulting in impaired S-phase progression and inhibition of DNA replication.[29] In another report, HP1α, a member of the heterochromatin protein family, was found to accumulate in the Golgi apparatus of CDA I intermediate erythroblasts but not control erythroblasts.[18]

To reconcile the disparate findings described earlier, a human erythroid cell line expressing FLAG-tagged codanin-1 at the endogenous locus was recently generated.[31] Future studies using this cell line are expected to accurately determine the subcellular localization of codanin-1 and to define the role of codanin-1 in erythropoiesis.

The cellular function of the restriction endonuclease encoded by *CDIN1* remains poorly understood. This protein localizes either to the cytosol or (mainly) to the nucleus/nucleolus,[22,25,26,30,32] and it interacts with Asf1b, the paralog of Asf1a, which may support the hypothesis that the primary defect in CDA I is confined to DNA replication and chromatin assembly.[33] Recently, *CDIN1* has been shown to interact in a complex with codanin-1,[26,30,32] and that the cellular localization and/or stability of *CDIN1* appears to depend on codanin-1.[29,32] Additional studies are also needed to define the role of *CDIN1* in erythroid development.

TREATMENT, COURSE, AND PROGNOSIS

Management of anemia depends on the disease severity. Some patients never require RBC transfusions, whereas others may require transfusions only perinatally and/or during periods of marrow stress, such as in the setting of infections or pregnancy. Lifelong transfusion dependence is infrequent, estimated at about 4% of cases.[10] Rarely, intrauterine transfusions are warranted to prevent fetal death in patients presenting with hydrops fetalis (Chaps. 17 and 27), in whom the severity of anemia was confirmed by fetal blood sampling.[34]

Iron overload is an invariable complication of this disease, resulting from recurrent transfusions and/or enhanced iron absorption (commonly seen in ineffective erythropoiesis). Hepcidin, a key regulator of iron absorption (Chap. 10), is suppressed in CDA I patients,[35] possibly because of excess erythroferrone production by the expanded pool of erythroblasts or elevated levels of soluble hemojuvelin,[36] ultimately resulting in enhanced iron absorption and iron accumulation in organs (including liver, heart, and pancreas). Growth differentiation factor 15 (GDF15), a marker of ineffective erythropoiesis, is elevated in CDA I patients, correlating with ferritin levels.[35]

Because secondary hemochromatosis is common, transfusions should be avoided whenever possible and systematic monitoring for iron overload should be performed. Although there is no consensus on the frequency of monitoring, one monitoring strategy consists of annual measurement of serum ferritin, as well as annual myocardial T2* magnetic resonance imaging (MRI) and hepatic R2* MRI starting in adolescence (Chap. 11).

To prevent organ damage caused by iron accumulation, iron depletion by phlebotomies or chelation should be instituted when ferritin levels exceed 500 to 1000 mg/L and/or when there is evidence of iron overload seen on MRI. In patients with mild anemia, small-volume regular phlebotomies may be used to decrease body iron (Chap. 11). Conversely, iron chelation may be required for patients with iron overload who cannot tolerate phlebotomies.

Interferon-α was once used in a child with hepatitis C and CDA I and was associated with a robust increase in hemoglobin level. After 9 years of follow-up, the treatment remained effective, and repeated liver biopsies showed that the iron overload was normalized. In this case, the effective dose of interferon-α was 2 million units twice per week[37] and the effective dose of pegylated interferon-α was 30 mcg/week.[37] Since then, additional CDA I patients have been reported to also respond to interferon-α therapy. The mechanism of response to interferon-α is unknown and not all patients respond.[38] The most common side effects of interferon-α are flu-like symptoms, gastrointestinal symptoms, and depression.[39]

At this time, allogeneic hematopoietic stem cell transplantation (ASCT) remains the only curative modality, proven successful in several transfusion-dependent children.[40] However, because of transplant-related mortality and morbidity, ASCT is generally reserved for patients with very severe disease. Splenectomy is usually not beneficial[3,10] and is typically reserved for patients with symptomatic splenomegaly and profound anemia.[41] Administration of recombinant erythropoietin has not been shown to ameliorate the CDA I anemia,[42] and as such is not recommended.

Additional common complications of CDA I include cholelithiasis and osteoporosis. Cholecystectomy for cholelithiasis is commonly performed. For osteoporosis, monitoring with regular bone density testing is recommended, and patients might require calcium, vitamin D, and antiresorptive therapies. Rare complications of the disease include pulmonary hypertension, which has been reported in three Bedouin newborns,[43] and retinal angioid streaks.[44] There are no agreed-upon guidelines for screening and treating pulmonary hypertension for CDA I.

As for every genetic disease, genetic counseling should be offered and performed.

● CONGENITAL DYSERYTHROPOIETIC ANEMIA, TYPE II

CLINICAL AND LABORATORY FEATURES

CDA II is an autosomal recessive disease that, like CDA I, is characterized by dyserythropoiesis and anemia of variable severity, ranging from mild to severe. Approximately 10% to 20% of patients are transfusion-dependent.[3,8,45-47] CDA II presents in most patients in infancy, childhood, or adolescence. Very few cases of hydrops fetalis owing to severe anemia have been reported.[48, 49] More commonly, the anemia is mild, and in several cases, the diagnosis might be delayed into adulthood. In some patients, the diagnosis is made in adults after a workup for iron overload is done.[3,8] Additional clinical manifestations of CDA II include hemolysis, commonly accompanying splenomegaly, hepatomegaly, intermittent jaundice, and cholelithiasis.[46,47]

The blood film demonstrates moderate to marked anisocytosis and anisochromia, polychromatophilic cells, and a variable number of spherocytes. This finding, along with the hemolytic anemia, may lead to misdiagnosing CDA II as hereditary spherocytosis (HS) (Chap. 15). However, there are important clinical and disease features that help distinguish CDA II from HS.[45] First, the ratio of reticulocyte count to hemoglobin concentration is typically higher in HS compared with CDA II, whereas serum transferrin level is lower. Indeed, in CDA II, the reticulocyte count is not appropriately elevated for the degree of anemia. Second, HS is generally an autosomal dominant disease; therefore, a parent is likely to have spherocytosis on peripheral blood film. In contrast, CDA II is inherited in an autosomal recessive manner. Despite these differentiating features, the correct diagnosis of CDA II is occasionally made only after a splenectomy performed for a presumed HS diagnosis fails to normalize the anemia. Additional CDA II characteristics described further, as well as genetic testing, can help differentiate this disease from other disorders.

In the CDA II marrow, erythroid hyperplasia is invariably present and 10% to 30% of the intermediate/late erythroblasts are bi-/multinucleated (see Fig. 14-2A), a percentage higher than that observed in CDA I. Karyorrhexis, which refers to fragmentation of the nucleus, is common. Gaucher-like cells may be seen in approximately 60% of patients,[13] resulting from phagocytosis of erythroblasts by macrophages.

CDA II erythrocytes lyse in a subset of acidified human sera (Ham test; Chap. 8), possibly because of a naturally occurring immunoglobulin (Ig) M class antibody that recognizes an antigen present on CDA II RBCs but not on normal cells. Thus, CDA II is also known as HEMPAS (hereditary erythroblastic multinuclearity with a positive acidified serum test). The technical difficulty of performing this test, and the need to cross-test more than 30 normal human sera to obtain a reliable result, make this test difficult to perform on a regular basis.[50]

Electron microscopy on CDA II RBCs demonstrates a "double membrane" appearance (see Fig. 14-2B), with the inner membrane representing endoplasmic reticulum (ER) cisternae beneath the plasma membrane. This was demonstrated by Western blot on RBC ghosts, immunofluorescence microscopy, and immunogold electron microscopy using antibodies recognizing ER-specific proteins.[51]

Another CDA II characteristic is the finding of narrower band size and faster-than-normal migration of the erythrocyte membrane proteins band 3 (or AE1) and band 4.5 by sodium dodecylsulfate polyacrylamide gel electrophoresis (SDS-PAGE).[52,53] This observation is the result of reduced glycosylation of these proteins. Hypoglycosylation of AE1 has been reported to result in clustering of this protein on the RBC surface, potentially explaining the increased destruction of the CDA II RBC in the spleen.[54] Rarely, patients have been reported without the characteristic band 3 and band 4.5 hypoglycosylation by SDS-PAGE; it is unlikely that these patients have CDA II, and other diseases (including other CDA subtypes) need to be considered.

GENETICS

CDA II is an autosomal recessive disease resulting from homozygous or compound heterozygous loss-of-function mutations in *SEC23B*.[3,8,55] *SEC23B* is one of two paralogous *SEC23* genes (*SEC23A* and *SEC23B*) that encode a core component of COPII (coat protein complex II) vesicles. These vesicles form on the surface of the ER, packaging and trafficking secretory proteins from the ER to the Golgi apparatus,[56] before reaching their final destinations in endosomes, lysosomes, plasma membrane, or extracellular space.[56,57] CDA II is one of many human diseases resulting from mutations in genes encoding COPII components.[58,59] In contrast to *SEC23B*, *SEC23A* mutations in humans result in craniolenticulosutural dysplasia (also known as Boyadjiev–Jabs syndrome), an autosomal recessive disease characterized primarily by bone defects, but with normal erythropoiesis.[58,60]

To date, more than 100 different *SEC23B* mutations have been reported worldwide.[3,8,45,55] As noted earlier, a founder effect for the two most common *SEC23B* mutations in Europeans has been demonstrated.[6,7] Patients with compound heterozygosity for missense and nonsense mutations tend to have more severe clinical phenotypes compared with those homozygous or compound heterozygous for two missense mutations, consistent with a genotype-phenotype correlation. Bi-allelic nonsense *SEC23B* mutations have not been reported, suggesting that complete loss of SEC23B function may be lethal in humans.[58,61]

Unlike humans, hematopoietic deficiency for SEC23B in mice does not result in anemia or other CDA II characteristics.[62] In contrast,

mice with germline deficiency for SEC23B die perinatally, exhibiting massive pancreatic degeneration and additional defects in the salivary glands, nasal glands, stomach, and small intestine.[63] Further studies demonstrated that SEC23B is essential for both pancreatic development[64] and maintenance of pancreatic function[65] in these animals. The SEC23B-deficient phenotype in mice was completely rescued by expression of SEC23A from the endogenous *Sec23b* locus, demonstrating that SEC23A and SEC23B overlap in function.[66] Therefore, the disparate phenotypes of SEC23A and SEC23B deficiency between and across species is likely caused by a shift in the expression programs of the SEC23 paralogs throughout evolution, rather than because of distinct functions of SEC23A and SEC23B.[58,66,67] Consistent with this hypothesis, SEC23B is the predominantly expressed paralog in human erythroid cells.[55,66,68-70] A less likely alternative explanation is the presence of erythroid-specific proteins that might depend specifically on SEC23B for secretion.[59,71] One report showed a milder phenotype in two CDA II patients with higher *SEC23A* levels compared with one CDA II patient with lower *SEC23A* levels.[67] Though this finding should be confirmed in larger cohorts, it is nonetheless consistent with an overlap in function between SEC23A and SEC23B in erythroid cells.

In one study, SEC23B has been shown to colocalize with codanin-1,[18] the protein encoded by the gene most commonly mutated in CDA I, suggesting a possible common pathogenesis for CDA I and CDA II. However, this hypothesis remains unproven and is controversial.

TREATMENT, COURSE, AND PROGNOSIS

The clinical course of CDA II is heterogeneous. Most patients have mild or moderate anemia that does not require medical intervention. Approximately 10% of patients require at least one RBC transfusion in the neonatal period.[8] Although some of these patients become and remain transfusion-independent throughout life,[8,47] others may require rare or intermittent transfusions during periods of erythroid stress, such as during aplastic crises, pregnancy, infections, or major operations. As with CDA I, rare cases of hydrops fetalis have been described. In some cases, severe phenotypes could be the result of coinheritance of glucose-6-phosphate dehydrogenase (G6PD) deficiency or thalassemic trait.[72]

Secondary hemochromatosis is consistently observed even in the absence of RBC transfusions.[3,8,73] In some patients, the diagnosis of CDA II is made in adulthood after a workup for iron overload (Chap. 11). Therefore, ferritin levels should be monitored at least annually, even in patients with only mild anemia, and regardless of transfusion requirement. In addition, as in CDA I, annual myocardial and hepatic MRIs starting in adolescence should be considered. Iron depletion should be instituted when ferritin levels exceed 500 to 1000 mg/L or when iron overload is evident on MRI scan (Chap. 11). When tolerated, a phlebotomy program is the preferred strategy for iron depletion. In patients who cannot tolerate phlebotomies (such as patients with severe anemia), chelating agents may be used. The goal of therapy is to achieve normal ferritin concentrations.[74] Iron overload is associated with high levels of GDF15.[75] However, it is not clear that GDF15 is the primary regulator of iron absorption,[76] and GDF15 concentrations are significantly lower in CDA II compared with CDA I patients despite a similar degree of iron overload in both patient groups, suggesting that additional signals may determine hepatic hepcidin expression and the degree of iron overload in CDA II.[75] Erythroferrone (Chap. 10), an erythroblast-derived hormone, is elevated in CDA II patients.[77,78] It has been shown to inhibit hepcidin production and promote iron absorption[79] and might be the critical regulator of iron absorption in CDA II patients.

Cholelithiasis is frequent in all CDAs. The decision to proceed with cholecystectomy should follow the hereditary spherocytosis guidelines.[80] Coinheritance of the UGT1A (TA)7/(TA)7 genotype could account for an increased rate of gallstones in some patients.[81] Splenomegaly is also common in CDA II; however, splenectomy is not universally recommended. Consensus criteria for splenectomy have not been defined but it should be considered in patients with massive splenomegaly who are transfusion-dependent.[41] In non-transfusion-dependent patients, it is reasonable to follow the guidelines for mild cases of HS.[80] Splenectomy might result in a moderate and sustained increase in hemoglobin concentrations[41] caused by reduced hemolysis. However, splenomegaly does not prevent iron overload, and hemoglobin levels post splenectomy generally do not reach normal values.[6,7]

The only curative modality is ASCT from a human leukocyte antigen (HLA)-identical sibling or a matched unrelated donor. Because of treatment-related morbidity and mortality, ASCT is reserved for patients with severe disease.[48,49,82-84] As for all CDA subtypes, genetic counseling should be offered and performed.

Activin receptor ligand traps (eg, luspatercept, sotatercept) have been shown to improve ineffective erythropoiesis in several clinical settings but have not been studied clinically in CDA patients. A recent study demonstrated that RAP-011, a "murinized" ortholog of sotatercept, appears to restore the expression of erythroid markers in *SEC23B*-silenced K562 cells through inhibition of the phosphorylated SMAD2 pathway, therefore providing support for future clinical studies that aim to define the clinical role of activin receptor ligand traps in human CDAII patients.[85]

● CONGENITAL DYSERYTHROPOIETIC ANEMIA, TYPE III

CLINICAL AND LABORATORY FINDINGS

CDA III is less common than CDA I and CDA II. CDA III is an autosomal dominant disease originally reported in 1951 in a woman and her three children,[86] who all had a distinctive multinuclearity in 16% to 23% of marrow erythroblasts, with up to 12 nuclei per cell. The disease was then named "familial erythroid multinuclearity." Most of our knowledge about CDA III stems from a large family of 26 affected members from the province of Västerbotten in northern Sweden, in whom the disease was coined "hereditary benign erythroreticulosis."[87]

CDA III patients are generally asymptomatic. Anemia is typically mild or moderate or may be absent. Hemolysis is invariably present, as demonstrated by elevated LDH and low or undetectable haptoglobin levels. Jaundice and cholelithiasis are common. In contrast to CDA I and CDA II, splenomegaly and iron overload are not common in CDA III.

In addition to the large Swedish family, a number of sporadic CDA III cases with variable disease severity have been reported.[88] In one particular example, severe presentations with stillbirths and/or hydrops fetalis were reported.[89] The mother, who initially required RBC transfusions, became transfusion-independent after splenectomy.[89]

A typical CDA III blood film demonstrates macrocytosis with sometimes extremely large RBCs (gigantocytes) and poikilocytes. The percent reticulocyte count is typically less than 3%.[86,87] Marrow evaluation shows marked erythroid hyperplasia with large multinucleated erythroblasts containing up to 12 nuclei per cell (see Fig. 14-2A). Additional findings on electron microscopy have been reported, including clefts within heterochromatin, autophagic vacuoles, iron-laden mitochondria, and myelin figures in the cytoplasm.[90]

GENETICS

The large size of the Swedish family made it possible to map the causative gene to 15q22-25.[91] Subsequently, the disease-causing mutation (c.2747C>G) was found in *KIF23* (resulting in p.P916R).[92] The same mutation was also found in CDA III patients from an unrelated US family.[92]

KIF23 encodes kinesin-like protein KIF23, also known as mitotic kinesin-like protein 1 (MKLP1). MKLP1 is a component of central-spindlin, which is required for the formation of the midbody, a structure that maintains cells connected during cytokinesis until abscission occurs. Loss of the midbody before abscission results in inability of the daughter cells to separate. MKLP1 is essential for completion of cytokinesis.[93,94] Depletion of MKLP1 results in cytokinesis failure and binucleated cells[92]; these findings are reversed by expression of wild-type MKLP1 but not p.P916R mutant MKLP1.[92]

Protein 14-3-3 binds the centralspindlin complex, promoting disintegration of the midbody. Arf6 (ADP-ribosylation factor 6) competes with protein 14-3-3 for binding centralspindlin, protecting the midbody from protein 14-3-3–mediated disruption, resulting in enhanced stability of the midbody.[93] Consistent with these findings, Arf6 depletion, similarly to MKLP1 depletion, results in increased percentage of multinucleated cells as a result of failed cytokinesis.[95]

COURSE AND PROGNOSIS

Despite an apparently benign course, CDA III patients are at risk for various long-term complications, including intravascular hemolysis, development of multiple myeloma and other monoclonal gammopathies,[96] and development of angioid streaks.[97]

● OTHER CONGENITAL DYSERYTHROPOIETIC ANEMIAS

The classification of the CDAs is based largely on morphologic evaluation,[98] coupled with genetic analysis. A number of CDA cases that do not fit the diagnosis of CDA types I to III have been reported,[99-104] implicating several additional genes as CDA-causing genes, as summarized further and outlined in Table 14-1.

A unique dominant-negative mutation in the erythroid transcription factor *KLF1* was found to result in CDA IV, an autosomal dominant disease characterized by severe hemolytic anemia, elevated fetal hemoglobin, and deficiency of the erythroid proteins CD44 and aquaporin 1 (see Table 14-1).[105,106] Mutations in another transcription factor, *GATA1*, have been reported to result in X-linked dyserythropoietic anemia with macrothrombocytopenia and hypogranulated platelets.[107] Another X-linked dominant dyserythropoietic anemia has been described in females with mutations in the *ALAS2* gene.[108] This disease is characterized by macrocytic anemia and iron overload, whereas males with mutations in *ALAS2* exhibit sideroblastic anemia.

Moreover, several syndromic forms of CDAs have been described (see Table 14-1). For example, Majeed syndrome is characterized by chronic recurrent multifocal osteomyelitis, inflammatory dermatosis, and CDA. Majeed syndrome is an autosomal recessive disease resulting from mutation in *LPIN2* (18p11.31), which encodes the ER-phosphatidate phosphatase LPIN2.[109] More recently, a syndrome characterized by severe neurodegenerative disease associated with mild CDA-like anemia, marked anisopoikilocytosis, and abnormal glycosylation of the erythrocyte proteins band-3 and RhAG has been reported.[110,111] This disorder, known as *early infantile epileptic encephalopathy-50*, results from bi-allelic mutations in *CAD*, which encodes a trifunctional enzyme that catalyzes the first steps of de novo pyrimidine biosynthesis. Another

TABLE 14–1. Classification of CDA variants

Disease Symbol	Gene Inheritance	Main Clinical Features	Bone Marrow Morphological Features
CDA IV	KLF1 Autosomal dominant	Hemolytic anemia, generally severe, with normal or slightly increased reticulocyte count, and markedly elevated fetal hemoglobin levels	Erythroid hyperplasia with bi- or multi-nucleated erythroblasts; immature erythroid progenitors with atypical cytoplasmic inclusions, invagination of the nuclear membrane, and marked heterochromatin
XLTDA	GATA1 X-linked recessive	Macro-thrombocytopenia, bleeding tendency, and mild-to-severe anemia	Erythroblasts with megaloblastic features, bi- and multi-nucleation, and nuclear irregularities; small dysplastic megakaryocytes with signs of incomplete maturation and reduced number of alpha granules
MJDS	LPIN2 Autosomal recessive	Hypochromic microcytic anemia; chronic recurrent multifocal osteomyelitis and inflammatory dermatosis	Microcytosis and dyserythropoiesis
EIEE50	CAD Autosomal recessive	Autism, developmental delay, and generalized epilepsy; mild CDA II-like anemia with marked anisopoikilocytosis and abnormal glycosylation of the erythrocyte proteins band-3 and RhAG	Erythroid hyperplasia with dyserythropoiesis, bi- and tri-nucleated erythroblasts, prominent cytoplasmic bridging
-	VPS4A De novo autosomal dominant	Microcephaly, hypotonia, global developmental delay, structural brain abnormalities, cataracts; hemolytic anemia	Dyserythropoiesis with bi-nucleated erythroblasts and cytoplasmic bridges
-	ALAS2 X-linked dominant	Macrocytic anemia with iron overload in female individuals	Erythroid hyperplasia with dyserythropoiesis; rare erythroblasts with siderotic granules (no excess iron or sideroblasts)
-	COX4I2 Autosomal recessive	Exocrine pancreatic insufficiency, dyserythropoietic anemia, and calvarial hyperostosis	Erythroid hyperplasia with dyserythropoiesis
MEVA	MVK Autosomal recessive	Mevalonate kinase deficiency associated to CDA II-like anemia	CDA II-like morphological abnormalities of erythroblasts

Abbreviations: CDA IV, CDA type IV; XLTDA, EIEE50, early infantile epileptic encephalopathy-50; MEVA, mevalonic aciduria; MJDS, Majeed syndrome; X-linked thrombocytopenia with or without dyserythropoietic anemia.

form of syndromic CDA is characterized by dyserythropoiesis, exocrine pancreatic insufficiency, and calvarial hyperostosis. This autosomal recessive disease has been described in two Arab families and results from mutations in the *COX4I2* gene.[112] Additionally, mevalonate kinase deficiency resulting from biallelic mutations in *MVK* has also been shown to result in dyserythropoietic anemia associated with recurrent fevers and abdominal pain.[113] Finally, several unrelated individuals have been reported with a syndrome characterized by CDA, structural brain abnormalities, severe neurodevelopmental delay, cataracts, and growth impairment.[114,115] The latter syndrome results from de novo missense mutations in the *VPS4A* gene, which encodes an ATPase that regulates the ESCRT-III machinery in various cellular processes, including cell division and endosomal vesicle trafficking.[114,115]

● DIFFERENTIAL DIAGNOSIS

The differential diagnosis of the CDAs includes thalassemia (Chap. 49) and other hemolytic anemias. Absence of an appropriately elevated reticulocyte count for the degree of anemia, together with marked anisocytosis is consistent with a diagnosis of CDA. In addition, the CDA RBCs are typically either normocytic or macrocytic, in contrast to the microcytic RBCs in thalassemias. However, because of significant overlap between the clinical findings in CDAs and other marrow/RBC disorders, several tests are required to make a definitive diagnosis of a CDA and to rule out other disorders.

The diagnostic workflow for the CDAs includes careful documentation of personal and family history, followed by laboratory tests and blood film evaluation, and subsequently by a marrow biopsy. A marrow biopsy is considered essential to rule out myelodysplastic syndromes and other marrow failure disorders. The marrow biopsy will also demonstrate typical CDA characteristics including an increased percentage of bi-/multinucleated erythroblasts and other findings (discussed earlier). These latter findings are generally not seen in other types of hemolytic anemia or the thalassemias. Genetic testing has become a cornerstone in the diagnosis of the CDAs (see Fig. 14-1). If a patient is suspected to have a particular CDA subtype, the causative gene for that particular subtype can be sequenced. Otherwise, next-generation sequencing using custom panels or whole-exome sequencing is preferred. These tests are currently being used more frequently in the clinic and might help make the correct diagnosis in many patients.[116-118] A genetic-based diagnostic approach led to modifying the original clinical diagnosis in 10% to 40% of patients with other erythroid disorders.[117,118] Furthermore, a recent case series showed that among patients originally classified with CDAs, 45% actually had anemia caused by enzymatic defects (Chap. 48), most commonly the result of pyruvate kinase deficiency resulting from mutations in *PKLR*.[118]

REFERENCES

1. Crookston J, Godwin T, Wightman K, et al. Congenital dyserythropoieic anemia. In: *Abstracts of the 11th Congress of the International Society of Haematology, Sydney.* 1966.

2. Heimpel H, Wendt F. Congenital dyserythropoietic anemia with karyorrhexis and multinuclearity of erythroblasts. *Helv Med Acta.* 1968;34(2):103-115.

3. Iolascon A, Heimpel H, Wahlin A, Tamary H. Congenital dyserythropoietic anemias: molecular insights and diagnostic approach. *Blood.* 2013;122(13):2162-2166.

4. Gulbis B, Eleftheriou A, Angastiniotis M, et al. Epidemiology of rare anaemias in Europe. *Adv Exp Med Biol.* 2010;686:375-396.

5. Heimpel H, Matuschek A, Ahmed M, et al. Frequency of congenital dyserythropoietic anemias in Europe. *Eur J Haematol.* 2010;85(1):20-25.

6. Iolascon A, Servedio V, Carbone R, et al. Geographic distribution of CDA-II: did a founder effect operate in Southern Italy? *Haematologica.* 2000;85(5):470-474.

7. Russo R, Gambale A, Esposito MR, et al. Two founder mutations in the SEC23B gene account for the relatively high frequency of CDA II in the Italian population. *Am J Hematol.* 2011;86(9):727-732.

8. Iolascon A, Andolfo I, Russo R. Congenital dyserythropoietic anemias. *Blood.* 2020;136(11):1274-1283.

9. Tamary H, Shalev H, Luria D, et al. Clinical features and studies of erythropoiesis in Israeli Bedouins with congenital dyserythropoietic anemia type I. *Blood.* 1996;87(5):1763-1770.

10. Heimpel H, Schwarz K, Ebnother M, et al. Congenital dyserythropoietic anemia type I (CDA I): molecular genetics, clinical appearance, and prognosis based on long-term observation. *Blood.* 2006;107(1):334-340.

11. Wickramasinghe SN, Thein SL, Srichairatanakool S, Porter JB. Determinants of iron status and bilirubin levels in congenital dyserythropoietic anaemia type I. *Br J Haematol.* 1999;107(3):522-525.

12. Wickramasinghe SN. Congenital dyserythropoietic anaemias: clinical features, haematological morphology and new biochemical data. *Blood Rev.* 1998;12(3):178-200.

13. Heimpel H, Kellermann K, Neuschwander N, et al. The morphological diagnosis of congenital dyserythropoietic anemia: results of a quantitative analysis of peripheral blood and bone marrow cells. *Haematologica.* 2010;95(6):1034-1036.

14. Tamary H, Shalmon L, Shalev H, et al. Localization of the gene for congenital dyserythropoietic anemia type I to a <1-cM interval on chromosome 15q15.1-15.3. *Am J Hum Genet.* 1998;62(5):1062-1069.

15. Dgany O, Avidan N, Delaunay J, et al. Congenital dyserythropoietic anemia type I is caused by mutations in codanin-1. *Am J Hum Genet.* 2002;71(6):1467-1474.

16. Roy NBA, Babbs C. The pathogenesis, diagnosis and management of congenital dyserythropoietic anaemia type I. *Br J Haematol.* 2019;185(3):436-449.

17. Tamary H, Dgany O, Proust A, et al. Clinical and molecular variability in congenital dyserythropoietic anaemia type I. *Br J Haematol.* 2005;130(4):628-634.

18. Renella R, Roberts NA, Brown JM, et al. Codanin-1 mutations in congenital dyserythropoietic anemia type 1 affect HP1{alpha} localization in erythroblasts. *Blood.* 2011;117(25):6928-6938.

19. Ahmed MR, Chehal A, Zahed L, et al. Linkage and mutational analysis of the CDAN1 gene reveals genetic heterogeneity in congenital dyserythropoietic anemia type I. *Blood.* 2006;107(12):4968-4969.

20. Babbs C, Roberts NA, Sanchez-Pulido L, et al. Homozygous mutations in a predicted endonuclease are a novel cause of congenital dyserythropoietic anemia type I. *Haematologica.* 2013;98(9):1383-1387.

21. Palmblad J, Sander B, Bain B, et al. Congenital dyserythropoietic anemia type 1: a case with novel compound heterozygous mutations in the C15orf41 gene. *Am J Hematol.* 2018.

22. Russo R, Marra R, Andolfo I, et al. Characterization of two cases of congenital dyserythropoietic anemia type i shed light on the uncharacterized C15orf41 protein. *Front Physiol.* 10:621, 2019.

23. Kohara H, Ogura H, Aoki T, et al. Generation and functional analysis of congenital dyserythropoietic anemia patient-specific induced pluripotent stem cells. *Blood.* 2016;128(22):2426. Abstract .

24. Shemer OS, Yao Y, Kupfer G, et al. Modeling congenital dyserythropoietic anemia type I through patient-derived induced pluripotent stem cells. *Blood.* 2012;120(21):3196. Abstract.

25. Scott C, Downes DJ, Brown JM, et al. Recapitulation of erythropoiesis in congenital dyserythropoietic anaemia type I (CDA-I) identifies defects in differentiation and nucleolar abnormalities. *Haematologica.* 2020; doi: 10.3324/haematol.2020.260158. PMID: 33121234.

26. Olijnik A-A, Roy NBA, Scott C, Marsh JA, et al. Genetic and functional insights into CDAI prevalence and pathogenesis. *J Med Genet.* 2020;0:1-11.

27. Murphy ZC, Getman MR, Myers JA, et al. Codanin-1 mutations engineered in human erythroid cells demonstrate role of CDAI in terminal erythroid maturation. *Exp Hematol.* 2020;91:32-38.

28. Noy-Lotan S, Dgany O, Lahmi R, et al. Codanin-1, the protein encoded by the gene mutated in congenital dyserythropoietic anemia type I (CDAN1), is cell cycle-regulated. *Haematologica.* 2009;94(5):629-637.

29. Ask K, Jasencakova Z, Menard P, et al. Codanin-1, mutated in the anaemic disease CDAI, regulates Asf1 function in S-phase histone supply. *EMBO J.* 2012;31(8):2013-2023.

30. Swickley G, Bloch Y, Malka L, et al. Characterization of the interactions between codanin-1 and C15Orf41, two proteins implicated in congenital dyserythropoietic anemia type I disease. *BMC Mol Cell Biol.* 2020;21(1):18.

31. Moir-Meyer G, Cheong PL, Olijnik AA, et al. Robust CRISPR/Cas9 genome editing of the HUDEP-2 erythroid precursor line using plasmids and single-stranded oligonucleotide donors. *Methods Protoc.* 2018;1(3).

32. Shroff M, Knebel A, Toth R, Rouse J. A complex comprising C15ORF41 and Codanin-1-the products of two genes mutated in congenital dyserythropoietic anemia type I (CDA-I). *Biochem J.* 2020;477(10):1893-1905.

33. Ewing RM, Chu P, Elisma F, et al. Large-scale mapping of human protein-protein interactions by mass spectrometry. *Mol Syst Biol.* 2007;3:89.

34. Parez N, Dommergues M, Zupan V, et al. Severe congenital dyserythropoietic anaemia type I. prenatal management, transfusion support and alpha-interferon therapy. *Br J Haematol.* 2000;110(2):420-423.

35. Tamary H, Shalev H, Perez-Avraham G, et al. Elevated growth differentiation factor 15 expression in patients with congenital dyserythropoietic anemia type I. *Blood.* 2008;112(13):5241-5244.

36. Shalev H, Perez-Avraham G, Kapelushnik J, et al. High levels of soluble serum hemojuvelin in patients with congenital dyserythropoietic anemia type I. *Eur J Haematol.* 2013;90(1):31-36.

37. Lavabre-Bertrand T, Ramos J, Delfour C, et al. Long-term alpha interferon treatment is effective on anaemia and significantly reduces iron overload in congenital dyserythropoiesis type I. *Eur J Haematol.* 2004;73(5):380-383.

38. Marwaha RK, Bansal D, Trehan A, Garewal G. Interferon therapy in congenital dyserythropoietic anemia type I/II. *Pediatr Hematol Oncol.* 2005;22(2):133-138.

39. Bader-Meunier B, Leverger G, Tchernia G, et al. Clinical and laboratory manifestations of congenital dyserythropoietic anemia type I in a cohort of French children. *J Pediatr Hematol Oncol.* 2005;27(8):416-419.

40. Ayas M, al-Jefri A, Baothman A, et al. Transfusion-dependent congenital dyserythropoietic anemia type I successfully treated with allogeneic stem cell transplantation. *Bone Marrow Transplant.* 2002;29(8):681-682.

41. Iolascon A, Andolfo I, Barcellini W, et al. Recommendations regarding splenectomy in hereditary hemolytic anemias. *Haematologica.* 2017;102(8):1304-1313.

42. Tamary H, Shalev H, Pinsk V, et al. No response to recombinant human erythropoietin therapy in patients with congenital dyserythropoietic anemia type I. *Pediatr Hematol Oncol.* 1999;16(2):165-168.

43. Shalev H, Moser A, Kapelushnik J, et al. Congenital dyserythropoietic anemia type I presenting as persistent pulmonary hypertension of the newborn. *J Pediatr.* 2000;136(4):553-555.

44. Tamary H, Offret H, Dgany O, et al. Congenital dyserythropoietic anaemia, type I, in a Caucasian patient with retinal angioid streaks (homozygous Arg1042Trp mutation in codanin-1). *Eur J Haematol.* 2008;80(3):271-274.

45. Russo R, Gambale A, Langella C, et al. Retrospective cohort study of 205 cases with congenital dyserythropoietic anemia type II. Definition of clinical and molecular spectrum and identification of new diagnostic scores. *Am J Hematol.* 2014;89(10): E169-E175.

46. Heimpel H, Anselstetter V, Chrobak L, et al. Congenital dyserythropoietic anemia type II. Epidemiology, clinical appearance, and prognosis based on long-term observation. *Blood.* 2003;102(13):4576-4581.

47. Iolascon A, Delaunay J, Wickramasinghe SN, et al. Natural history of congenital dyserythropoietic anemia type II. *Blood.* 2001;98(4):1258-1260.

48. Remacha AF, Badell I, Pujol-Moix N, et al. Hydrops fetalis-associated congenital dyserythropoietic anemia treated with intrauterine transfusions and bone marrow transplantation. *Blood.* 2002;100(1):356-358.

49. Braun M, Wolfl M, Wiegering V, et al. Successful treatment of an infant with CDA type II by intrauterine transfusions and postnatal stem cell transplantation. *Pediatr Blood Cancer.* 2014;61(4):743-745.

50. Crookston JH, Crookston MC, Burnie KL, et al. Hereditary erythroblastic multinuclearity associated with a positive acidified-serum test: a type of congenital dyserythropoietic anaemia. *Br J Haematol.* 1969;17(1):11-26.

51. Alloisio N, Texier P, Denoroy L, et al. The cisternae decorating the red blood cell membrane in congenital dyserythropoietic anaemia (type II) originate from the endoplasmic reticulum. *Blood.* 1996;87(10):4433-4439.

52. Scartezzini P, Forni GL, Baldi M, et al. Decreased glycosylation of band 3 and band 4.5 glycoproteins of erythrocyte membrane in congenital dyserythropoietic anaemia type II. *Br J Haematol.* 1982;51(4):569-576.

53. Fukuda MN, Gaetani GF, Izzo P, et al. Incompletely processed N-glycans of serum glycoproteins in congenital dyserythropoietic anaemia type II (HEMPAS). *Br J Haematol.* 1992;82(4):745-752.

54. De Franceschi L, Turrini F, del Giudice EM, et al. Decreased band 3 anion transport activity and band 3 clusterization in congenital dyserythropoietic anemia type II. *Exp Hematol.* 1998;26(9):869-873.

55. Schwarz K, Iolascon A, Verissimo F, et al. Mutations affecting the secretory COPII coat component SEC23B cause congenital dyserythropoietic anemia type II. *Nat Genet.* 2009;41(8):936-940.

56. Fromme JC, Orci L, Schekman R. Coordination of COPII vesicle trafficking by Sec23. *Trends Cell Biol.* 2008;37(7):330-336.

57. Lee MC, Miller EA, Goldberg J, et al. Bi-directional protein transport between the ER and Golgi. *Annu Rev Cell Dev Biol.* 2004;20:87-123.

58. Khoriaty R, Vasievich MP, Ginsburg D. The COPII pathway and hematologic disease. *Blood.* 2012;120(1):31-38.

59. Russo R, Esposito MR, Iolascon A. Inherited hematological disorders due to defects in coat protein (COP)II complex. *Am J Hematol.* 2013;88(2):135-140.

60. Boyadjiev SA, Fromme JC, Ben J, et al. Cranio-lenticulo-sutural dysplasia is caused by a SEC23A mutation leading to abnormal endoplasmic-reticulum-to-Golgi trafficking. *Nat Genet.* 2006;38(10):1192-1197.

61. Iolascon A, Russo R, Esposito MR, et al. Molecular analysis of 42 patients with congenital dyserythropoietic anemia type II. New mutations in the SEC23B gene and a search for a genotype-phenotype relationship. *Haematologica.* 2010;95(5):708-715.

62. Khoriaty R, Vasievich MP, Jones M, et al. Absence of a red blood cell phenotype in mice with hematopoietic deficiency of SEC23B. *Mol Cell Biol.* 2014;34(19):3721-3734.

63. Tao J, Zhu M, Wang H, et al. SEC23B is required for the maintenance of murine professional secretory tissues. *Proc Natl Acad Sci U S A.* 2012;109(29):E2001-E2009.

64. Khoriaty R, Everett L, Chase J, et al. Pancreatic SEC23B deficiency is sufficient to explain the perinatal lethality of germline SEC23B deficiency in mice. *Sci Rep.* 2016;6:27802.

65. Khoriaty R, Vogel N, Hoenerhoff MJ, et al. SEC23B is required for pancreatic acinar cell function in adult mice. *Mol Biol Cell.* 2017;28(15):2146-2154.

66. Khoriaty R, Hesketh GG, Bernard A, et al. Functions of the COPII gene paralogs SEC23A and SEC23B are interchangeable in vivo. *Proc Natl Acad Sci U S A.* 2018;115(33):E7748-E7757.

67. Russo R, Langella C, Esposito MR, et al. Hypomorphic mutations of SEC23B gene account for mild phenotypes of congenital dyserythropoietic anemia type II. *Blood Cells Mol Dis.* 2013;51(1):17-21.

68. An X, Schulz VP, Li J, et al. Global transcriptome analyses of human and murine terminal erythroid differentiation. *Blood.* 2014;123(22):3466-3477.

69. Pishesha N, Thiru P, Shi J, et al. Transcriptional divergence and conservation of human and mouse erythropoiesis. *Proc Natl Acad Sci U S A.* 2014;111(11):4103-4108.

70. Satchwell TJ, Pellegrin S, Bianchi P, et al. Characteristic phenotypes associated with congenital dyserythropoietic anemia (type II) manifest at different stages of erythropoiesis. *Haematologica.* 2013;98(11):1788-1796.

71. De Matteis MA, Luini A. Mendelian disorders of membrane trafficking. *N Engl J Med.* 2011;365(10):927-938.

72. Gangarossa S, Romano V, Miraglia del Giudice E, et al. Congenital dyserythropoietic anemia type II associated with G6PD Seattle in a Sicilian child. *Acta Haematol.* 1995;93(1):36-39.

73. Fargion S, Valenti L, Fracanzani AL, et al. Hereditary hemochromatosis in a patient with congenital dyserythropoietic anemia. *Blood.* 2000;96(10):3653-3655.

74. Hofmann WK, Kaltwasser JP, Hoelzer D, et al. Successful treatment of iron overload by phlebotomies in a patient with severe congenital dyserythropoietic anemia type II. *Blood.* 1997;89(8):3068-3069.

75. Casanovas G, Swinkels DW, Altamura S, et al. Growth differentiation factor 15 in patients with congenital dyserythropoietic anaemia (CDA) type II. *J Mol Med (Berl).* 2011;89(8):811-816.

76. Casanovas G, Vujic Spasic M, Casu C, et al. The murine growth differentiation factor 15 is not essential for systemic iron homeostasis in phlebotomized mice. *Haematologica.* 2013;98(3):444-447.

77. Andolfo I, Rosato BE, Marra R, et al. The BMP-SMAD pathway mediates the impaired hepatic iron metabolism associated with the ERFE-A260S variant. *Am J Hematol.* 2019;94(11):1227-1235.

78. Russo R, Andolfo I, Manna F, et al. Increased levels of ERFE-encoding FAM132B in patients with congenital dyserythropoietic anemia type II. *Blood.* 2016;128(14):1899-1902.

79. Kautz L, Jung G, Valore EV, et al. Identification of erythroferrone as an erythroid regulator of iron metabolism. *Nat Genet.* 2014;46(7):678-684.

80. Bolton-Maggs PH, Langer JC, Iolascon A, et al. Guidelines for the diagnosis and management of hereditary spherocytosis–2011 update. *Br J Haematol.* 2012;156(1):37-49.

81. Perrotta S, del Giudice EM, Carbone R, et al. Gilbert's syndrome accounts for the phenotypic variability of congenital dyserythropoietic anemia type II (CDA-II). *J Pediatr.* 2000;136(4):556-559.

82. Iolascon A, Sabato V, de Mattia D, Locatelli F. Bone marrow transplantation in a case of severe, type II congenital dyserythropoietic anaemia (CDA II). *Bone Marrow Transplant.* 2001;27(2):213-215.

83. Unal S, Russo R, Gumruk F, et al. Successful hematopoietic stem cell transplantation in a patient with congenital dyserythropoietic anemia type II. *Pediatr Transplant.* 2014;18(4):E130-E133.

84. Uygun V, Russo R, Karasu G, et al. Hematopoietic stem cell transplantation in congenital dyserythropetic anemia type II: a case report and review of the literature. *J Pediatr Hematol Oncol.* 2019. doi: 10.1097/MPH.0000000000001612.

85. De Rosa G, Andolfo I, Marra R, et al. RAP-011 Rescues the disease phenotype in a cellular model of congenital dyserythropoietic anemia type ii by inhibiting the SMAD2-3 pathway. *Int J Mol Sci.* 2020;2:5577.

86. Wolff JA, Von Hofe FH. Familial erythroid multinuclearity. *Blood.* 1951;6(12):1274-1283.

87. Bergstrom I, Jacobsson L. Hereditary benign erythroreticulosis. *Blood.* 19:296-303, 1962.

88. Accame EA, de Tezanos Pinto M. [Congenital dyserythropoiesis with erythroblastic polyploidy. Report of a variety found in Argentinian Mesopotamia (author's transl)]. *Sangre (Barc).* 1981;26(5-A):545-555.

89. Jijina F, Ghosh K, Yavagal D, et al. A patient with congenital dyserythropoietic anaemia type III presenting with stillbirths. *Acta Haematol.* 1998;99(1):31-33.

90. Sandstrom H, Wahlin A. Congenital dyserythropoietic anemia type III. *Haematologica.* 2000;85(7):753-757.

91. Lind L, Sandstrom H, Wahlin A, et al. Localization of the gene for congenital dyserythropoietic anemia type III, CDAN3, to chromosome 15q21-q25. *Hum Mol Genet.* 1995;4(1):109-112.

92. Liljeholm M, Irvine AF, Vikberg AL, et al. Congenital dyserythropoietic anemia type III (CDA III) is caused by a mutation in kinesin family member, KIF23. *Blood.* 2013;121(23):4791-4799.

93. Boman AL, Kuai J, Zhu X, et al. Arf proteins bind to mitotic kinesin-like protein 1 (MKLP1) in a GTP-dependent fashion. *Cell Motil Cytoskeleton.* 1999;44(2):119-132.

94. Joseph N, Hutterer A, Poser I, Mishima M. ARF6 GTPase protects the post-mitotic midbody from 14-3-3-mediated disintegration. *EMBO J.* 2012;31(11):2604-2614.

95. Makyio H, Ohgi M, Takei T, et al. Structural basis for Arf6-MKLP1 complex formation on the Flemming body responsible for cytokinesis. *EMBO J.* 2012;31(11):2590-2603.

96. Sandstrom H, Wahlin A, Eriksson M, et al. Intravascular haemolysis and increased prevalence of myeloma and monoclonal gammopathy in congenital dyserythropoietic anemia, type III. *Eur J Haematol.* 1994;52(1):42-46.

97. Sandstrom H, Wahlin A, Eriksson M, et al. Angioid streaks are part of a familial syndrome of dyserythropoietic anaemia (CDA III). *Br J Haematol.* 1997;98(4):845-849.

98. Wickramasinghe SN, Wood WG. Advances in the understanding of the congenital dyserythropoietic anaemias. *Br J Haematol.* 2005;131(4):431-446.

99. David G, van Dorpe A. Aberrant congenital dyserythropoietic anaemias. In: SM Lewis Verwilghen RL, eds. *Dyserythropoiesis.* Academic Press; 1977:93.

100. Bethlenfalvay NC, Hadnagy C, Heimpel H. Unclassified type of congenital dyserythropoietic anaemia (CDA) with prominent peripheral erythroblastosis. *Br J Haematol.* 1985;60(3):541-550.

101. Brien WF, Mant MJ, Etches WS. Variant congenital dyserythropoietic anaemia with ringed sideroblasts. *Clin Lab Haematol.* 1985;7(3):231-237.

102. Pothier B, Morle L, Alloisio N, et al. Aberrant pattern of red cell membrane and cytosolic proteins in a case of congenital dyserythropoietic anaemia. *Br J Haematol.* 1987;66(3):393-400.

103. Ohisalo JJ, Viitala J, Lintula R, Ruutu T. A new congenital dyserythropoietic anaemia. *Br J Haematol.* 1988;68(1):111-114.

104. Woessner S, Trujillo M, Florensa L, et al. Congenital dyserthropoietic anaemia other than type I to III with a peculiar erythroblastic morphology. *Eur J Haematol.* 2003;71(3):211-214.

105. Arnaud L, Saison C, Helias V, et al. A dominant mutation in the gene encoding the erythroid transcription factor KLF1 causes a congenital dyserythropoietic anemia. *Am J Hum Genet.* 2010;87(5):721-727.

106. Jaffray JA, Mitchell WB, Gnanapragasam MN, et al. Erythroid transcription factor EKLF/KLF1 mutation causing congenital dyserythropoietic anemia type IV in a patient of Taiwanese origin: review of all reported cases and development of a clinical diagnostic paradigm. *Blood Cells Mol Dis.* 2013;51(2):71-75.

107. Ciovacco WA, Raskind WH, Kacena MA. Human phenotypes associated with GATA-1 mutations. *Gene.* 2008;427(1-2):1-6.

108. Sankaran VG, Ulirsch JC, Tchaikovskii V, et al. X-linked macrocytic dyserythropoietic anemia in females with an ALAS2 mutation. *J Clin Invest.* 2015;125(4):1665-1669.

109. Ferguson PJ, Chen S, Tayeh MK, et al. Homozygous mutations in LPIN2 are responsible for the syndrome of chronic recurrent multifocal osteomyelitis and congenital dyserythropoietic anaemia (Majeed syndrome). *J Med Genet.* 2005;42(7):551-557.

110. Koch J, Mayr JA, Alhaddad B, et al. CAD mutations and uridine-responsive epileptic encephalopathy. *Brain.* 2017;140(2):279-286.

111. Ng BG, Wolfe LA, Ichikawa M, et al. Biallelic mutations in CAD, impair de novo pyrimidine biosynthesis and decrease glycosylation precursors. *Hum Mol Genet.* 2015;24(11):3050-3057.

112. Shteyer E, Saada A, Shaag A, et al. Exocrine pancreatic insufficiency, dyserythropoeitic anemia, and calvarial hyperostosis are caused by a mutation in the COX4I2 gene. *Am J Hum Genet.* 2009;84(3):412-417.

113. Samkari A, Borzutzky A, Fermo E, et al. A novel missense mutation in MVK associated with MK deficiency and dyserythropoietic anemia. *Pediatrics.* 2010;125(4):e964-e968.

114. Rodger C, Flex E, Allison RJ, et al. De novo VPS4A mutations cause multisystem disease with abnormal neurodevelopment. *Am J Hum Genet.* 2020;107(6):1129-1148. doi: 10.1016/j.ajhg.2020.10.012. PMID: 33186545.

115. Seu KG, Trump LR, Emberesh S, et al. VPS4A mutations in humans cause syndromic congenital dyserythropoietic anemia due to cytokinesis and trafficking defects. *Am J Hum Genet.* 2020;107(6):1149-1156. doi: 10.1016/j.ajhg.2020.10.013. PMID: 33186543.

116. Hamada M, Doisaki S, Okuno Y, et al. Whole-exome analysis to detect congenital hemolytic anemia mimicking congenital dyserythropoietic anemia. *Int J Hematol.* 2018;108(3):306-311.

117. Roy NB, Wilson EA, Henderson S, et al. A novel 33-Gene targeted resequencing panel provides accurate, clinical-grade diagnosis and improves patient management for rare inherited anaemias. *Br J Haematol.* 2016;175(2):318-330.

118. Russo R, Andolfo I, Manna F, et al. Multi-gene panel testing improves diagnosis and management of patients with hereditary anemias. *Am J Hematol.* 2018;93(5):672-682.

CHAPTER 15
ERYTHROCYTE MEMBRANE DISORDERS

Theresa L. Coetzer

SUMMARY

The human erythrocyte membrane consists of a lipid bilayer containing transmembrane proteins and an underlying membrane skeleton that is attached to the bilayer by linker protein complexes. The membrane is critical in maintaining the unique biconcave disk shape of the erythrocyte and enabling it to withstand circulatory shear stress. The integrity of the membrane is ensured by vertical interactions between the skeleton and the transmembrane proteins, as well as by horizontal interactions between skeletal proteins. Inherited defects of membrane proteins compromise these interactions and alter the shape and deformability of the cells, which ultimately results in their premature destruction, seen clinically as hemolytic anemia. The disorders are typically inherited in an autosomal dominant manner and exhibit significant clinical, laboratory, biochemical and genetic heterogeneity.

Hereditary spherocytosis (HS) is a common condition characterized by spherically shaped erythrocytes on the blood film, reticulocytosis, and splenomegaly. The underlying defect is a deficiency of one of the membrane proteins, including ankyrin, anion exchanger-1 (AE1, formerly band 3), α-spectrin, β-spectrin, or protein 4.2. These defects weaken vertical membrane interactions, resulting in loss of membrane and surface area. Spherocytes have diminished deformability, which predisposes them to entrapment and destruction

in the spleen. *Hereditary elliptocytosis* (HE) is characterized by the presence of elliptical erythrocytes on the blood film. The principal abnormality affects horizontal membrane protein interactions and typically involves α-spectrin, β-spectrin, protein 4.1R, or glycophorin C. The membrane skeleton is destabilized and unable to maintain the biconcave disk shape, which manifests as an elliptical distortion of the cells in the circulation. *Hereditary pyropoikilocytosis* (HPP) is a rare, severe hemolytic anemia characterized by markedly abnormal erythrocyte morphology resulting from defective spectrin. *South East Asian Ovalocytosis* (SAO) is largely asymptomatic and is caused by a defect in AE1. The blood film shows large oval red cells with a transverse ridge across the central area. *Acanthocytosis* is typified by contracted, dense erythrocytes with irregular projections, which may be seen in patients with severe liver disease, abetalipoproteinemia, various neurologic disorders, certain aberrant red cell antigens, and postsplenectomy. *Stomatocytosis* is a rare group of inherited disorders associated with abnormal membrane permeability and red cell cation content, which either cause overhydration or dehydration of the cells.

● INTRODUCTION

The erythrocyte membrane plays a critical role in the function and structure of the red cell. It is a key determinant of the unique biconcave disk shape and provides the cell with a finely tuned combination of flexibility and durability. These properties enable the erythrocyte to withstand the shear forces experienced in the circulation and allow it to undergo extensive and repeated deformation while negotiating the microvasculature and the spleen, thus ensuring survival during its average 120-day life span. The red cell membrane maintains a nonreactive surface so that erythrocytes do not adhere to the endothelium or aggregate and occlude capillaries. It provides a barrier with selective permeability, which retains vital components inside the cell and permits the efflux of metabolic waste. To facilitate the transfer of carbon dioxide and to maintain pH homeostasis, the membrane exchanges chloride and bicarbonate anions, and it also actively controls the cation and water content of the erythrocyte. The membrane acts to retain reducing agents required to prevent oxidative damage to hemoglobin and other cellular components, and it plays a role in regulating metabolism by reversibly binding and inactivating selected glycolytic enzymes.

Abnormalities of the erythrocyte membrane alter the shape of the cell and compromise its integrity and ability to survive the rigors of circulation, which leads to premature destruction and hemolysis. Erythrocyte membrane disorders comprise an important group of hereditary hemolytic anemias, which are classified according to the altered red cell morphology and include hereditary spherocytosis (HS); hereditary elliptocytosis (HE) and related disorders; acanthocytosis; and disorders of red cell hydration, including hereditary stomatocytosis (HSt) syndromes. This chapter summarizes our current understanding of the erythrocyte membrane in normal cells followed by a discussion of the underlying molecular defects and their role in the pathophysiology and clinical manifestations of these disorders. The main emphasis is on spherocytosis and elliptocytosis, the most common and best characterized diseases.

● OVERVIEW OF THE ERYTHROCYTE MEMBRANE

The erythrocyte membrane is the most studied plasma membrane and serves as a paradigm for all cellular membranes. Mature erythrocytes are readily accessible; they contain no intracellular organelles, which

Acronyms and Abbreviations: αLELY, α-spectrin low-expression Lyon; αLEPRA, α-spectrin low-expression Prague; AE1, anion exchanger-1 (formerly band 3); AGLT, acidified glycerol lysis test; *ANK1*, ankyrin gene; ANK, ankyrin; apo-B, apolipoprotein B; ATP11C, P-IV ATPase (flippase); AQP1, aquaporin-1; BPG, bisphosphoglycerate; CDAII, congenital dyserythropoietic anemia type II; DAT, direct antiglobulin test; DI, deformability index; EMA, eosin 5′maleimide; G3PD, glyceraldehyde 3-phosphate dehydrogenase; GLT, glycerol lysis test; GLUT-1, glucose transporter-1; GP, glycophorin; GP A-B-C-D-E, various members of glycophorin family; GSSG, oxidized glutathione; HAc, hereditary acanthocytosis; HDL2, Huntington Disease-Like 2; HE, hereditary elliptocytosis; HPP, hereditary pyropoikilocytosis; HS, hereditary spherocytosis; HSt, hereditary stomatocytosis; ICSH, International Council on Standardization in Haematology; *JPH3*, Junctophilin-3 gene; *KCNN4*, Potassium Calcium-activated channel subfamily N member 4 gene; MAGUK, membrane-associated guanylate kinase; MARCKS, myristylated alanine-rich C kinase substrate; MCHC, mean corpuscular hemoglobin concentration; MCV, mean corpuscular volume; MTTP, microsomal triglyceride transfer protein; NGS, next-generation DNA sequencing technology; OF, osmotic fragility; PKAN, pantothenate kinase-associated neurodegeneration; PLSCR1, phospholipid scramblase 1; 4.1R, erythrocyte isoform of protein 4.1; RhAG, Rh-associated glycoprotein; SAO, South East Asian Ovalocytosis; SDS PAGE, sodium dodecyl sulfate polyacrylamide gel electrophoresis; *SLC4A1*, AE1 gene; *SPTA1*, α spectrin gene; *SPTB*, β spectrin gene; *VPS13A*, vacuolar protein sorting 13 homolog A gene; UGT1, uridine diphosphate glucuronosyl transferase 1.

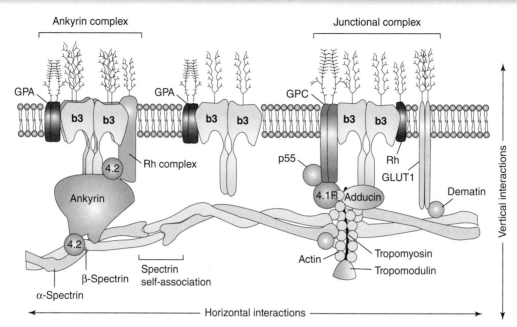

Figure 15–1. Simplified schematic model of the human erythrocyte membrane. The molecular assembly of the major proteins is indicated. *Vertical* interactions are perpendicular to the plane of the membrane and are represented by the ankyrin and junctional protein complexes that connect the membrane spectrin skeleton to the integral proteins embedded in the lipid bilayer. *Horizontal* interactions occur parallel to the plane of the membrane and involve spectrin tetramers and protein 4.1R. The proteins and lipids are not drawn to scale. b3, band 3 (AE1); GPA/GPC, glycophorin A/C; GLUT-1, glucose transporter-1.

facilitates the isolation of pure erythrocyte membranes; and "experiments of nature" resulting in abnormal erythrocyte morphology have provided unique opportunities to investigate the function of membrane components. These studies revealed the primary structure and several important functions of the red cell membrane. Ongoing research, using the latest molecular technologies, continues to yield important insights into our understanding of membrane structure–function relationships, as well as genotype–phenotype correlations.

The erythrocyte membrane is a complex structure consisting of a relatively fluid lipid bilayer stabilized by an underlying two-dimensional membrane skeleton, which maintains the integrity of the biconcave disk shape of the erythrocyte (Fig. 15-1). The skeleton provides the cell with the strength and flexibility to deform rapidly and repeatedly and thus endure the shear stress encountered in the capillaries of the microcirculation and in the sinuses of the spleen. The lipid bilayer separates the erythrocyte cytoplasm from the external plasma environment and contains phospholipids and cholesterol, as well as integral transmembrane proteins, which are tethered to the skeleton by interactions with linker proteins.

● COMPONENTS OF THE ERYTHROCYTE MEMBRANE

MEMBRANE LIPIDS

The lipid bilayer comprises approximately 50% of the membrane mass and contains unesterified cholesterol and phospholipids in approximately equal amounts, with small amounts of glycolipids and phosphoinositides (Chap. 1).[1] Mature erythrocytes are unable to synthesize fatty acids, phospholipids, or cholesterol de novo, and they depend on lipid exchange and limited phospholipid repair.

Cholesterol regulates the fluidity of the membrane and is present in both leaflets, whereas the phospholipids are asymmetrically distributed.[1] The choline phospholipids, phosphatidylcholine, and sphingomyelin,

are predominantly located in the outer leaflet and play a role in plasma lipid exchange and renewal of membrane phospholipids. Glycolipids carry several important red cell antigens, including A, B, H, and P, and are only found in the external leaflet with their carbohydrate moieties extending into the plasma. The aminophospholipids, phosphatidylserine and phosphatidylethanolamine, as well as phosphatidylinositol are located in the inner leaflet of the lipid bilayer.[1]

This asymmetric distribution of phospholipids is maintained by a dynamic process involving flippase (ATP11C) and floppase enzymes that translocate the aminophospholipids to the inner and outer leaflets, respectively.[1,2] A missense mutation in the *ATP11C* gene on the X chromosome causes mild hemolytic anemia.[2] A calcium-dependent phospholipid scramblase (PLSCR1) mediates ATP-independent bidirectional movement of phospholipids down their concentration gradient and contributes to the maintenance of phosphatidylserine on the inner leaflet of the membrane. Scramblase activity is suppressed by cholesterol.[2] Asymmetry of the phospholipids is important for the survival of the erythrocyte because exposure of phosphatidylserine on the cell surface, as found in sickle cell disease and thalassemia, has several deleterious consequences. It activates the coagulation cascade and may contribute to thromboses; it facilitates adhesion to the vascular endothelium; it provides a recognition signal for macrophages to phagocytose these cells; and it decreases the interaction of skeletal proteins with the bilayer, which destabilizes the membrane.[1,2]

Lipid rafts have been identified in erythrocytes. They form detergent-resistant membrane microdomains, enriched in cholesterol and sphingolipids, and are associated with several proteins, including stomatin, flotillin-1 and flotillin-2.[1] These rafts are anchored to spectrin and play a role in signaling and invasion of malaria parasites.

MEMBRANE PROTEINS

Pioneering studies resolved the major proteins of the red cell membrane by sodium dodecyl sulfate polyacrylamide gel electrophoresis

(SDS-PAGE) and numbers from 1 to 8 were assigned to each protein starting with the largest protein, which migrated the slowest (Chap. 1).[3] Subsequent research revealed minor bands between the major proteins and these were designated with decimals. Analysis of the individual proteins led to the renaming of some of them, such as band 1 and band 2, which are now known as α-spectrin and β-spectrin, respectively. Technological advances have enabled an in-depth analysis of the erythrocyte proteome by sophisticated purification techniques and multienzyme cleavage strategies followed by mass spectrometry revealing a total of ~480 membrane proteins.[4,5] Table 15-1 summarizes the properties of the major components of the erythrocyte proteome.

The membrane proteins are classified as either integral or peripheral based on the ease with which they can be removed from whole red cell membrane preparations in the laboratory. Integral or transmembrane proteins are embedded in the lipid bilayer by hydrophobic interactions and require detergents to extract them. They often protrude from the bilayer and extend into the plasma and/or the interior of the erythrocyte and these structural features correlate with their functions as transport proteins, receptors, signaling molecules, and carriers of red cell antigens.

Peripheral proteins constitute the membrane skeleton and are loosely attached to the cytoplasmic face of the lipid bilayer and can be extracted by high or low salt concentrations or by high pH. Attachment is mediated indirectly by covalent or noncovalent interactions with the cytoplasmic domains of the transmembrane proteins, as well as by direct interactions with the inner leaflet of the lipid bilayer. These associations are dynamic and the affinity of binding is regulated by posttranslational modifications of the proteins, including phosphorylation, methylation, glycosylation, and lipid modification (myristoylation, palmitoylation, or farnesylation). Peripheral proteins typically function

TABLE 15–1. Major Red Cell Membrane Proteins

SDS-PAGE band	Protein	Mr kDa (gel)	Mr kDa (calc)	Copies Per Cell[a] (×10³)	Percentage of Total Protein[b]	Gene Symbol	Gene Size (kb)	Exons	Chromosome	Amino Acids
1	α-Spectrin	240	280	242	16	SPTA1	80	52	1q21-1q23	2429
2	β-Spectrin	220	246	242	14	SPTB	>100	32	14q23-q24.1	2137
2.1	Ankyrin	210	206	120	4.5	ANK1	>100	42	8p11.21	1881
2.9	α-Adducin	103	81	30	2	ADD1	85	16	4p16.3	737
2.9	β-Adducin	97	80	30	2	ADD2	~100	17	2p13.3	726
3	Anion exchanger-1	90-100	102	1200	27	SLC4A1	17	20	17q21.31	911
4.1	Protein 4.1R	80	66	200	5	EPB41	>100	23	1p33-p34.2	588
4.2	Protein 4.2	72	77	250	5	EPB42	20	13	15q15-q21	691
4.9	Dematin[c]	48 + 52[d]	43	40[d]	1	DMTN	>33	21	8p21.3	383
4.9	p55[c]	55	53	180	—	MPP1	>42	13	Xq28	466
5	β-Actin	43	42	400-500	5.5	ACTB	>4	6	7p22	375
5	Tropomodulin	43	41	30	—	TMOD1	>70	9	9q22.33	359
6	G3PD	35	37	500	3.5[e]	GAPD	5	9	12p13	335
7	Stomatin	31	32	643	2.5	STOM	12	7	9q33.2	288
7	Tropomyosin	27 + 29[f]	28	70	1	TPM3	42	13	1q21.3	239
PAS-1	Glycophorin A[g]	36	14	500-1000	85	GYPA	>40	7	4q31.21	131
PAS-2	Glycophorin C[g]	32	14	50-100	4	GYPC	14	4	2q14-q21	128
PAS-3	Glycophorin B[g]	20	8	100-300	10	GYPB	>30	5	4q31.21	72
	Glycophorin D[g]	23	11	20	1	GYPD	14	4	2q14-q21	107
	Glycophorin E[g]	—	—	—	—	GYPE	>30	4	4q31.21	59

Abbreviations: —, information not available; G3PD, glyceraldehyde 3-phosphate dehydrogenase; PAS, periodic acid Schiff stain.

[a]The number of monomer copies/red cell of each protein is approximate.

[b]Quantitation is based on densitometry of SDS polyacrylamide gels of red cell membranes prepared from normal individuals. For glycophorins, values indicate the fraction of PAS-positive material.

[c]Both dematin and p55 migrate within the 4.9 band.

[d]Dematin has 2 isoforms and approximately 40,000 dematin heterotrimers (two 48-kDa subunits and one 52-kDa subunit) are present per red cell.

[e]Variable amounts of band 6 are detected in red cell membranes.

[f]Tropomyosin exists in 2 isoforms of 27 kDa and 29 kDa, which form a heterodimer.

[g]Detectable on PAS-stained gels only.

either as structural proteins and form part of the membrane skeleton or they serve as linker proteins attaching the skeleton to the bilayer.

Many erythrocyte proteins belong to superfamilies and have homologues in nonerythroid cells that are structurally related but are encoded by different genes. This genetic diversity explains why the clinical expression of most (but not all) red cell membrane protein mutations is confined to the erythroid lineage. Several proteins exist in different isoforms, created by tissue-specific and developmental stage–specific alternative splicing or by the use of alternative initiation codons or promoters. Many of the membrane proteins are large, multifunctional proteins; consequently, the position of a mutation determines the functional abnormality and clinical phenotype.

Integral Membrane Proteins

The most abundant and important erythrocyte transmembrane proteins are the anion exchanger-1 (AE1, encoded by the *SLC4A1* gene and previously known as band 3) and the glycophorins (GPs).

Anion Exchanger-1 The red cell contains approximately 1.2 million copies of AE1, a multifunctional and major integral membrane protein (see Table 15-1). It has a molecular mass of 102 kDa, but migrates as a diffuse band on SDS polyacrylamide gels because of heterogeneous N-glycosylation. The 911 amino acid protein consists of 2 functional domains: an N-terminal 43-kDa cytoplasmic domain (amino acids 1-360) and a 52-kDa transmembrane channel (amino acids 361-911), including a short 33-amino-acid C-terminal cytoplasmic tail (Fig. 15-2).[6] The anion exchange domain encompasses 13 α-helical transmembrane segments and 1 nonhelical segment, all connected by hydrophilic loops.[7-9] The short cytoplasmic tail binds cytosolic carbonic anhydrase II to form a metabolon with the transmembrane domain, enabling the exchange of HCO_3^- and Cl^- anions, which is a critical function of the red cell.[10] Cell surface-linked carbonic anhydrase IV interacts with external loop 4 of AE1 and constitutes the extracellular component of the transport metabolon.[11] The external surface of the transmembrane domain of AE1 carries several antigens, including Diego, I/i, and Wright blood groups.[7]

The N-terminal phosphorylated cytoplasmic domain serves as a major hub for protein-protein interactions, which perform key functions (see Figs. 15-1 and 15-2).[12] It regulates metabolic pathways by sequestering key glycolytic enzymes such as glyceraldehyde-3-phosphate dehydrogenase, phosphofructokinase, and aldolase, which are inactive when bound. Phosphorylation at tyrosine residues 8 and 21 or deoxygenation of the red blood cell prevents binding, which liberates the active enzymes.[13] In addition to the binding site at the N-terminus, a new binding site for lactate dehydrogenase and pyruvate kinase (Chap. 16) has been identified at residues 356 to 384, which are adjacent to the N-terminus in the crystal structure of the cytoplasmic domain of AE1. Some enzymes of this pathway are also bound to proteins associated with AE1 and it thus serves as the primary anchor of the glycolytic enzyme metabolon.[13] The cytoplasmic domain interacts with hemoglobin and hemichromes, and plays a role in red cell aging[14]; it associates with several peripheral membrane proteins, including protein 4.1R,[14] protein 4.2,[15] and adducin,[16] as well as phosphatases and kinases. This domain also serves as the major attachment site of the membrane to the underlying skeleton through its interaction with ankyrin, which binds to spectrin (see Figs. 15-1 and 15-2).[17,18]

Erythroid AE1 associates with other transmembrane proteins to form macromolecular complexes (see Fig. 15-1).[19] This includes the major GP, GPA,[20] and the Rh protein complex, consisting of Rh-associated glycoprotein (RhAG), Rh, CD47, LW (Landsteiner-Wiener antigens), and GPB (Chap. 29).[19] In addition, AE1 participates in the protein 4.1–based junctional complex of proteins.[6,14]

AE1 is encoded by the *SLC4A1* gene, which produces different tissue-specific isoforms.[6,21] The erythroid isoform is controlled by a promoter upstream of exon 1, whereas transcription of the kidney isoform is initiated from a promoter in intron 3, resulting in a protein lacking the first N-terminal 65 amino acids.

Glycophorins GPs are integral membrane glycoproteins comprising an extracellular hydrophilic N-terminal domain, a single α-helical membrane-spanning domain, and a C-terminal cytoplasmic tail. GPA, GPB, and GPE are homologous and are encoded by closely linked genes that arose by duplication of the ancestral GPA gene.[22] GPC and GPD are encoded by the same gene but make use of alternate initiation codons.[23]

GPs have a very high sialic acid content and are responsible for most of the external negative charge of red cells, which prevents the adherence of cells to each other and the vascular endothelium since all mammalian cells have a net negative charge. The GPs carry a large number of blood group antigens, including MN, SsU, Miltenberger, En(a–), M[K], and Gerbich (Chap. 29). They also function as receptors for *Plasmodium falciparum*, the most virulent malaria parasite. Within the lipid bilayer of the membrane, GPA interacts with AE1 as part of a macromolecular complex, and may serve as a chaperone to support protein targeting to the membrane (see Fig. 15-1).[6,7,20] GPC associates with protein 4.1R and p55, thereby providing an additional contact site between the membrane and the skeleton (see Fig. 15-1).[14] These interactions play a role in stabilizing the membrane.

Other Integral Membrane Proteins The Rh-RhAG group of proteins is part of a macromolecular AE1 complex, which stabilizes the membrane.[19] RhAG belongs to the ammonium transporter family of proteins, but its function is controversial. Numerous other proteins are

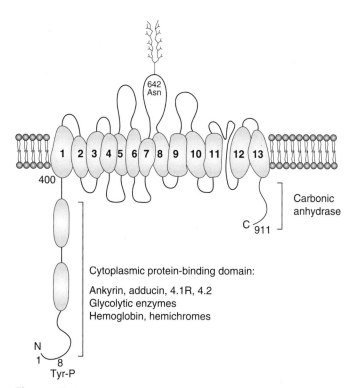

Figure 15–2. Schematic model of human erythrocyte AE1 (band 3). The N- and C-terminal regions of the protein extend into the cytoplasm and provide binding sites for several red cell proteins and enzymes. The transmembrane domain forms an anion exchange channel and consists of 13 α-helical segments embedded in the lipid bilayer and 1 nonhelical segment. Asparagine 642 is linked to complex carbohydrates that protrude on the exterior of the red cell. Tyrosine 8 is phosphorylated. The domains are not drawn to scale.

embedded in the lipid bilayer, many of which are implicated in clinical immunohematology and membrane disorders, such as the XK, Kell, Kidd, Duffy, and Lutheran glycoproteins (see Fig. 15-1).[6,14] Additional integral membrane proteins include ion pumps and channels, such as stomatin, aquaporin, glucose transporter-1 (GLUT-1), and various cation and anion transporters.[14]

Peripheral Membrane Proteins

Underlying the lipid bilayer is the peripheral membrane skeleton, an interlocking network of structural proteins, which plays a critical role in maintaining the shape and integrity of the red cell. The major proteins of the erythrocyte membrane skeleton are spectrin, actin, proteins 4.1R, 4.2, 4.9, p55, and the adducins, which interact in a horizontal plane. Linker proteins mediate the vertical attachment of the skeleton to integral membrane proteins in the lipid bilayer (see Fig. 15-1). The primary connecting protein is ankyrin, which links spectrin to the cytoplasmic domain of AE1, as well as to the Rh/RhAG complex. Protein 4.1R provides an additional link with GPC and AE1.

Spectrin Spectrin is the major constituent of the erythrocyte membrane skeleton and is present at approximately 242,000 molecules per cell.[14] It is a multifunctional protein comprising two homologous, but structurally distinct, subunits, α and β, encoded by separate genes, *SPTA1* and *SPTB*, respectively, which may have evolved from duplication of a single ancestral gene (see Table 15-1 and Fig. 15-3).[24] Both α-spectrin and β-spectrin contain tandem homologous spectrin repeats that are approximately 106 amino acids long and are folded into 3 antiparallel helices, A, B, and C. Each repeat is connected to the adjacent repeat by short-ordered α-helical linkers (see Fig. 15-3).[25,26] Erythrocyte α-spectrin is a 280-kDa protein comprising 20 complete homologous repeats, an N-terminal partial repeat, a central Src homology 3 (SH3) domain (nonhomologous repeat 10), and a C-terminal calcium-binding EF hand. The β-spectrin subunit is a 247-kDa polypeptide consisting of 16 complete repeats, an N-terminal actin-binding domain, a partial repeat near the C-terminus, and a nonhomologous phosphorylated C-terminus. Mild trypsin treatment of spectrin cleaves the two subunits into distinct structural domains: αI–αV and βI–βIV. The triple helical structure of the spectrin repeats renders the molecule highly flexible and enables it to extend and condense reversibly, which provides the red cell with elasticity and durability to withstand the shear stress encountered in the circulation.[14,25]

The core structure of the erythrocyte skeleton consists of spectrin heterotetramers, which are strong but flexible filaments. Tetramers are assembled from the monomers in a series of events. For initial heterodimer formation, the α-spectrin and β-spectrin chains align in an antiparallel fashion and interact with high affinity through long-range electrostatic interactions at a nucleation site, comprising repeats α20–α21

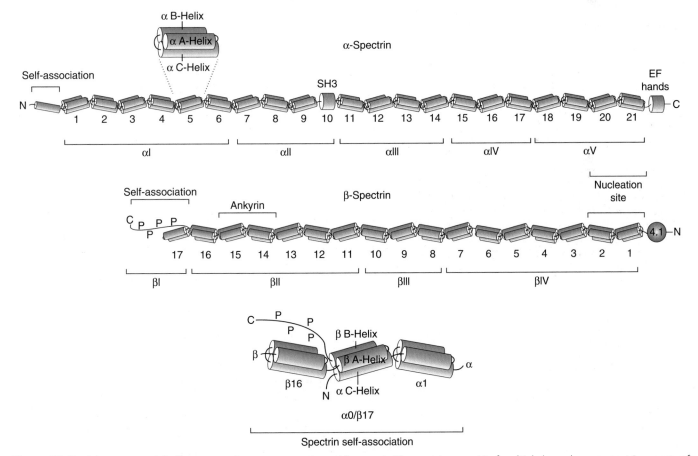

Figure 15–3. Schematic model of human erythrocyte α-spectrin and β-spectrin. The proteins consist of multiple homologous spectrin repeats of approximately 106 amino acids numbered from the N-terminal. Each repeat is composed of 3 α-helices. Nonhomologous regions include an SH3 (Src homology 3) domain and calcium-binding EF hands in α-spectrin, a protein 4.1R binding domain, and a C-terminal phosphorylated tail in β-spectrin. The nucleation site indicates the initial region of interaction between α and β monomers to form an antiparallel heterodimer. Spectrin heterodimer self-association into tetramers involves helix C of the α0 partial repeat of α-spectrin and helices A and B of the partial β17 repeat of β-spectrin to form a complete triple helical repeat. Ankyrin binds to repeats 14 and 15 of β-spectrin. Limited tryptic digestion of spectrin cleaves the proteins into discrete αI-αV and βI-βIV domains.

and β1-β2.[27] This triggers the association of the remaining repeats in the two subunits in a zipper-like fashion. Repeats at the N-terminus of α-spectrin (αI domain) and the C-terminus of β-spectrin (βI domain) are the regions involved in heterodimer self-association to form tetramers. Partial repeat β17 consists of two helices (A and B) that interact with the single helix C of partial repeat α0 to form a complete triple helical repeat (see Fig. 15-3). The interface of this tetramerization site is dominated by hydrophobic contacts supplemented by electrostatic interactions.[28] Phosphorylation of the C-terminal region of β-spectrin beyond the self-association site decreases the mechanical stability of the membrane.

At the opposite tail end of the spectrin tetramers, the N-terminus of β-spectrin binds to short F-actin filaments, which is potentiated by protein 4.1R, to form the core of a junctional complex,[29] which links six tetramers together into a hexagonal skeletal network (Fig. 15-4).[30] The C-terminal EF hand of α-spectrin enhances this spectrin–actin–protein 4.1R interaction.[31] Numerous other proteins participate in the junctional complex, including adducin, protein 4.9, p55, tropomodulin, and tropomyosin (see Fig. 15-1).[6,14] Protein 4.1R binds to GPC and AE1, which serves as a secondary attachment site of the skeleton to integral membrane proteins. The main interaction tethering the skeleton to the lipid bilayer is accomplished by ankyrin, which links β-spectrin

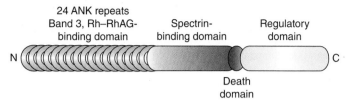

Figure 15–5. Schematic model of human erythrocyte ankyrin. The N-terminal domain consists of 24 ANK repeats, which bind to AE1 (band 3) and the Rh–RhAg complex. The central domain attaches to spectrin. The C-terminal domain varies in different isoforms of ankyrin, which are produced by alternative splicing of the gene. This domain also contains a conserved death domain of unknown function. AE1, anion exchanger-1; ANK, ankyrin; RhAG, Rh-associated glycoprotein.

to AE1 (see Fig. 15-1). The ankyrin binding site is a flexible pocket formed by repeats 14 and 15 of β-spectrin near the C-terminal end of the molecule.[32,33] Spectrin also interacts with phosphatidylserine on the inner leaflet of the lipid bilayer.

Nonrepeat sequences in spectrin provide the recognition sites for binding to modifiers, including kinases and calmodulin. The functions of spectrin are to maintain the biconcave disk shape of the red cell, regulate the lateral mobility of integral membrane proteins, and provide structural support for the lipid bilayer.

Ankyrin Erythrocyte ankyrin is encoded by the *ANK1* gene, which contains 3 separate tissue-specific promoters and first exons that are spliced to a common exon 2.[34] The 206-kDa protein is a versatile binding partner and has 3 functional domains: an N-terminal 89-kDa membrane-binding domain that contains sites for AE1 and other ligands; a central 62-kDa spectrin-binding domain; and a C-terminal 55-kDa regulatory domain that is responsible for the different isoforms of the protein, which influence ankyrin–protein interactions (Fig. 15-5).[14]

The membrane-binding domain contains 24 tandem ANK repeats, which are stacked into a superhelical array that is coiled into a solenoid. This structure behaves like a reversible spring, which may contribute to the elasticity of the membrane.[17] Each 33-amino-acid ANK repeat is highly conserved and forms an L-shaped structure composed of 2 antiparallel α-helices separated by a β-hairpin.[35] The ANK repeats are connected by unstructured loops and provide an interface for numerous protein–protein interactions. Erythrocyte ANK repeats specifically bind to AE1 and the Rh–RhAG macromolecular complex.[6,14]

The spectrin-binding domain contains a small unique subdomain termed ZU5-ANK, which has a β-strand core with several surface loops and binds to β-spectrin at the junction between repeats 14 and 15 through hydrophobic and electrostatic interactions.[36] The regulatory domain contains a highly conserved death domain of unknown function in the red cell. The C-terminal section of the regulatory domain varies in the different isoforms of ankyrin, proteins 2.1-2.6, which are created by alternative splicing,[37] and which exhibit different binding affinities for AE1 and spectrin. Phosphorylation of ankyrin reduces binding to AE1 and spectrin tetramers.

Protein 4.1R The gene encoding protein 4.1 (*EPB41*) produces diverse isoforms in different tissues and different developmental stages. This diversity is accomplished by the use of alternate first exons under the control of different promoters, and alternate initiation codons. This transcriptional regulation is coupled to complex pre-mRNA splicing events.[38] The erythrocyte isoform, protein 4.1R, is produced from the downstream initiation codon and contains exon 16, which encodes an essential part of the spectrin-actin–binding domain.

Protein 4.1R is a globular phosphoprotein that contains 4 structural and functional domains of 30 kDa, 16 kDa, 10 kDa, and 22-24 kDa

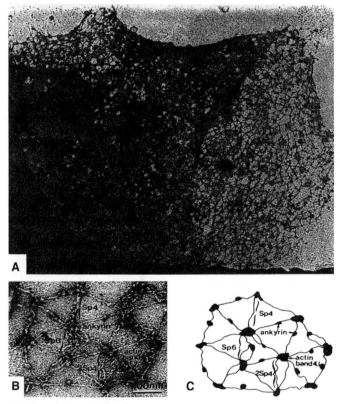

Figure 15–4. Electron micrograph of the human erythrocyte membrane skeleton. Membrane lipids and transmembrane proteins have been removed and the skeletons were extended during preparation and negative staining to reveal the structure. **A.** Low-magnification image reveals an ordered network of proteins. **B, C.** High-magnification image and schematic diagram of the hexagonal lattice showing spectrin tetramers (Sp4) and hexamers (Sp6) or double tetramers (2Sp4). Junctional complexes contain actin filaments and protein 4.1R. Globular ankyrin molecules are bound to spectrin tetramers. *(Reproduced with permission from Liu SC, Derick LH, Palek J. Visualisation of the hexagonal lattice in the erythrocyte membrane skeleton. J Cell Biol. 1987 Mar;104[3]:527-536.)*

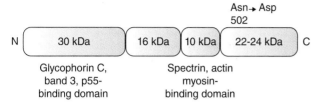

Figure 15–6. Schematic model of human erythrocyte protein 4.1R. The protein consists of 4 domains, with the 30-kDa and the 10-kDa domains involved in binding to other red cell membrane proteins. The C-terminal domain has an asparagine residue at position 502 in isoform 4.1a, which is deamidated in older red cells to form aspartic acid and isoform 4.1b.

(Fig. 15-6). The N-terminal 30-kDa domain is responsible for binding to the cytoplasmic domains of AE1 and GPC, as well as to p55, thereby linking the skeleton to the lipid bilayer (see Fig. 15-1).[14] The 10-kDa domain enhances the interaction between spectrin and actin in the junctional complex, which connects spectrin tetramers to each other. The functions of the other two domains are not characterized. Phosphorylation of protein 4.1R inhibits spectrin–actin–protein 4.1R complex formation and also decreases binding to AE1. Protein 4.1R binds weakly to phosphatidylserine in the lipid bilayer.

Two forms of protein 4.1R, a and b, are present in red cells, with protein 4.1b predominating in young erythrocytes. The difference between the 2 isoforms relates to the gradual deamidation of asparagine 502 to aspartic acid in a nonenzymatic, age-dependent manner, which influences the mobility of the protein on SDS polyacrylamide gels.[39]

Protein 4.2 Protein 4.2 is a member of the transglutaminase family of proteins,[40] but it has no enzyme activity because it lacks the critical triad of residues that form the active transglutaminase site. The exact role of protein 4.2 has not been elucidated, but it stabilizes the link between the skeleton and the lipid bilayer. Protein 4.2 interacts with several proteins, including the cytoplasmic domain of AE1 and this binding site has been identified as a hairpin region toward the center of the protein 4.2 molecule.[6,40] Interactions with the ANK repeats in the membrane-binding domain of ankyrin[40] and CD47, a component of the Rh complex, have been documented (see Fig. 15-1).[14,40] In vitro binding studies revealed an association of protein 4.2 with protein 4.1R and spectrin. Protein 4.2 binds calcium adjacent to the spectrin-binding loop, suggesting that calcium may regulate this interaction. The protein undergoes posttranslational palmitoylation and myristoylation, which suggests an interaction with the lipid bilayer.[40]

p55 The p55 molecule is a phosphoprotein member of the membrane-associated guanylate kinase (MAGUK) family of proteins. In the red cell it is found as part of a ternary complex with GPC and protein 4.1R, and it strengthens the link between the skeleton and the bilayer (see Fig. 15-1).[14] p55 contains 5 domains, including an N-terminal PDZ domain, which binds to GPC; an SH3 domain; a central HOOK domain interacting with the 30-kDa domain of protein 4.1R; a region

with tyrosine phosphorylation sites; and a C-terminal guanylate kinase domain (Fig. 15-7).[41] The protein is extensively palmitoylated, reflecting an interaction with the membrane bilayer.[14]

Adducin Adducin, a calcium/calmodulin-binding phosphoprotein located at the spectrin–actin junctional complex, is composed of αβ-adducin heterodimers, which are structurally similar proteins encoded by separate genes. Adducins contain a 39-kDa globular head region, a small neck region of 9 kDa implicated in oligomerization to form $\alpha_2\beta_2$ heterotetramers, and a 30-kDa cytoplasmic tail with a myristoylated alanine-rich C kinase substrate (MARCKS) phosphorylation domain at the C terminus (Fig. 15-8). The adducin tails cap actin filaments and promote interaction of spectrin and actin.[42] They also bind AE1 and GLUT-1, and thus form part of the macromolecular junctional complex linking the spectrin skeleton to the lipid bilayer (see Fig. 15-1).[14,16,43] The function of adducin is regulated by calcium-dependent calmodulin binding and differential phosphorylation. Although a primary deficiency of adducin in human disease has not been described, mice with targeted inactivation of α-adducin or β-adducin suffer from compensated spherocytic anemia, suggesting that the adducin mutations may be candidates for recessively inherited hemolytic anemia.[44]

Actin and Actin-Binding Proteins The erythrocyte contains β-type actin assembled into dynamic short F-actin protofilaments of 14 to 16 monomers with a uniform length of ~37nm (see Fig. 15-1). The length of the filaments is regulated by a "molecular ruler" of two rod-shaped tropomyosin molecules, which are bound along the filament, as well as by two tropomodulin molecules, which cap the filaments at the pointed ends.[14,45] At the barbed end, actin is capped by an adducin heterodimer. Dematin or protein 4.9 is a trimeric phosphoprotein, consisting of a core domain and a compact headpiece, which bundles the actin filaments[46] and also acts as a linker molecule by binding to the transmembrane GLUT-1 (see Fig. 15-1).[16,43] In a knockout mouse model in which full-length dematin was deleted, the mice developed severe anemia and exhibited striking changes in red blood cell morphology and a profound decrease in membrane stability.[47] The levels of adducin, actin, and spectrin were markedly reduced. These findings indicate that dematin plays a critical role as an anchor of the junctional complex and is a major determinant of membrane integrity.

● MEMBRANE ORGANIZATION

The structure of the erythrocyte membrane is determined by multiple protein–protein interactions among (1) integral membrane proteins within the lipid bilayer, (2) peripheral proteins in the skeleton, and (3) linker proteins, which tether the skeleton to the transmembrane proteins (see Fig. 15-1). Protein–lipid interactions within the bilayer or between the anionic phospholipids and the underlying membrane skeleton also play a role in cohesion of the membrane components. By using the cytoplasmic domains of embedded proteins as attachment points, the membrane skeleton not only affixes itself to the lipid bilayer but also

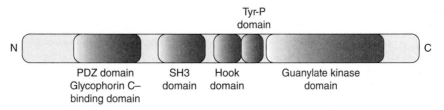

Figure 15–7. Schematic model of human erythrocyte p55. The protein is part of the membrane-associated guanylate kinase family and the kinase domain is close to the C-terminus. Adjacent is a tyrosine phosphorylation zone. The central HOOK domain binds protein 4.1R.

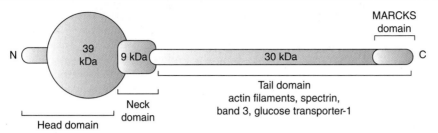

Figure 15–8. Schematic model of human erythrocyte adducin. The domain structures for α-adducin and β-adducin are similar. The neck domain is responsible for oligomerization and the tail represents the major binding site for other red cell membrane proteins. MARCKS, myristoylated alanine-rich C-kinase substrate.

influences the topology of the transmembrane proteins and constrains their lateral and rotational mobility.

The membrane skeleton resembles a lattice-like network, with approximately 60% of the lipid bilayer directly laminated to the underlying skeleton.[30] Electron microscopy of stretched membrane skeletons indicate that the individual proteins can be visualized as a highly ordered meshwork of hexagons (see Fig. 15-4).[30] The corners of each hexagon consist of a globular macromolecular junctional complex of proteins, including protein 4.1R, actin, and dematin, which interact with spectrin tetramers, as well as adducin, tropomyosin, tropomodulin, and p55.[14,16,43] Spectrin tetramers form the arms of the hexagons, crossbridging individual junctional complexes. These *horizontal* protein interactions are important in the maintenance of the structural integrity of the cell, accounting for the high tensile strength of the erythrocyte (see Fig. 15-1).

The spectrin–actin skeleton is anchored to the phospholipid bilayer by two major membrane protein complexes: (1) an ankyrin complex that contains transmembrane proteins, AE1, GPA, Rh, and RhAG complex proteins, as well as peripheral proteins ankyrin, protein 4.2, and several glycolytic enzymes, and (2) a distal junctional complex that contains the membrane-spanning proteins AE1, GPC, GLUT-1, Rh, Kell, and XK proteins, in addition to peripheral proteins 4.1R, actin, dematin, adducin, tropomyosin, tropomodulin, and p55.[6,14] These *vertical* protein–protein interactions are critical in the stabilization of the lipid bilayer, preventing loss of microvesicles from the cells (see Fig. 15-1).

The avidity of these horizontal and vertical interactions is modulated by posttranslational modifications of the participating proteins, especially phosphorylation. The erythrocyte contains multiple protein kinases and phosphatases that constantly phosphorylate and dephosphorylate specific serine, threonine, and tyrosine residues on AE1, β-spectrin, ankyrin, protein 4.1R, adducin, and dematin, in a dynamic manner, thereby tightly regulating the structural properties of the membrane. Additionally, membrane protein associations are also influenced by a variety of intracellular factors, including calcium, calmodulin, phosphoinositides, and polyanions such as 2,3-bisphosphoglycerate (BPG). Red cell membrane proteins are also subject to a variety of other posttranslational modifications, including myristoylation, palmitoylation, glycosylation, methylation, deamidation, oxidation, and limited proteolytic cleavage, but the functional effects of these alterations are generally not known.

CELLULAR DEFORMABILITY AND MEMBRANE STABILITY

In performing its primary function of oxygen delivery to the tissues the erythrocyte has to repeatedly negotiate capillaries in the microvasculature, as well as narrow slits in the splenic sinuses, which are much smaller than the diameter of the cell. It therefore has to undergo extensive deformation without fragmentation or loss of integrity and this property of deformability is critical for survival during its average 120-day life span. The structure of the red cell membrane endows the cell with unique material properties, which makes it highly flexible, yet incredibly resilient, and enables a very rapid response to circulatory shear stress.

Elegant biophysical studies have identified three features that regulate the deformability of the cell: (1) the biconcave disk shape which reflects the cell surface area to volume ratio; (2) the viscoelastic properties of the membrane, which depend on the structural and functional integrity of the membrane skeleton; and (3) the cytoplasmic viscosity, which is determined primarily by the intracellular hemoglobin concentration.[1]

The unique biconcave disk shape of the erythrocyte provides a high ratio of surface area to cellular volume and this excess of membrane is critical for survival of the cell. It is the major determinant that enables the red cell to deform when it passes through the microcirculation and protects it from premature destruction.[48] To maintain the shape of the cell and to prevent loss of membrane microvesicles, the lipid bilayer and the skeleton have to be in direct contact with each other. The cohesion between the two sections of the membrane depends on protein–protein interactions between transmembrane proteins and peripheral proteins in the vertical plane of the membrane. These contacts are represented by the two macromolecular complexes (ankyrin-AE1 complex and the junctional complex) anchoring the skeleton to the integral proteins. To prevent fragmentation of the membrane and loss of the biconcave disk shape, the structural integrity of the membrane skeleton is critical. In this regard, the horizontal interactions of the peripheral proteins of the junctional complex, mainly protein 4.1R and actin, which link the tail ends of the spectrin tetramers together, is a major determinant of membrane stability. Spectrin heterodimer self-association, which links the head regions of the spectrin tetramers, is also of paramount importance.

The viscoelastic properties of the membrane are intrinsic features of the spectrin skeleton. The enormous distortion imposed on the cell during passage through the microvasculature is accommodated by the dynamic dissociation of spectrin tetramers into dimers, and subsequent reassociation to restore the original shape once the shear stress is removed.[1,14] The lattice structure of the skeleton facilitates this flexibility, as the individual hexagons are either in a compact configuration, with the junctional complexes close to each other and the spectrin tetramers coiled between them, or in an extended configuration, which allows large unidirectional deformation without disruption of the skeleton (see Fig. 15-4). The structure of the spectrin repeats also play a major role in the elasticity of the skeleton. Each triple helical repeat behaves partly as an independently folding unit and has a different thermal stability.[1,14] Cysteine-labeling studies indicated that shear stress forced the unfolding of the least stable repeats.[1] These studies highlight the flexibility of

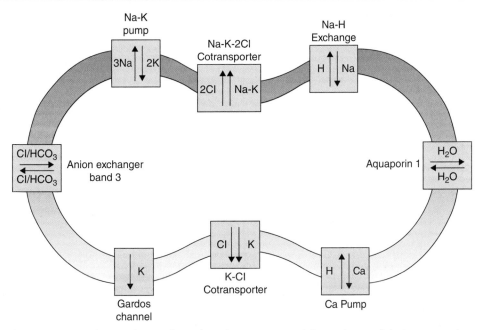

Figure 15–9. Principal ion transport and ion exchange channels and passive permeability pathways of the human erythrocyte.

the spectrin repeats and support the concept that their unfolding and refolding contributes to the deformability of the membrane. In addition, the elasticity of the ANK repeats may also facilitate the dynamic changes in the membrane during circulatory shear stress.[17]

Red cell viscosity is largely determined by the concentration of intracellular hemoglobin, which is tightly regulated to minimize cytoplasmic viscous dissipation during cellular deformation. As the mean cell hemoglobin concentration rises above 370 g/L, the viscosity increases exponentially, and this compromises the deformability of the cell under increased circulatory shear stress.[1] The hemoglobin concentration is critically dependent on red cell volume, which is primarily determined by the total cation content of the cell. Numerous membrane pumps and ion channels regulate the transport of sodium and potassium across the membrane (Fig. 15-9).

MEMBRANE PERMEABILITY

The red cell membrane displays selective permeability to cations and anions and it maintains a high potassium, low sodium, and very-low calcium content within the cell.[49] Ion transport pathways in the red cell membrane (see Fig. 15-9) include energy-driven membrane pumps, gradient-driven systems, and various channels. Several transport mechanisms exist for cations, including two energy-driven pumps.[49] The sodium pump is a Na$^+$K$^+$ ATPase that extrudes three sodium ions in exchange for two potassium ions entering the red cell. Calcium is pumped out of the cell by a calmodulin-activated Ca^{2+} ATPase, which protects the cell from deleterious effects of calcium, such as echinocytosis, membrane vesiculation, calpain activation, membrane proteolysis, and cellular dehydration.[49] The Ca^{2+}-activated K$^+$ channel, also called the Gardos channel, causes selective loss of K$^+$ in response to increased intracellular Ca^{2+}. The Na$^+$K$^+$ gradient established by the sodium pump is used by several passive, gradient-driven systems to move ions across the red cell membrane.[49] The systems include the K$^+$Cl$^-$ cotransporter, the Na$^+$K$^+$2Cl$^-$ cotransporter, and the Na$^+$H$^+$ exchanger.

Chloride and bicarbonate anions are readily exchanged through AE1. The red cell is highly permeable to water, which is transported by aquaporin-1 (AQP1),[50] and glucose is taken up by the glucose transporter.[51] The membrane also contains an ATP-driven oxidized glutathione (GSSG) transporter and amino acid transport systems.[49] Larger charged molecules such as ATP do not cross the membrane.

ERYTHROCYTE MEMBRANE DISORDERS

Hemolytic anemias resulting from structural defects in the erythrocyte membrane comprise an important group of hereditary anemias. The disorders are characterized by altered red cell morphology, which is reflected in the nomenclature of hereditary spherocytosis (HS), hereditary elliptocytosis (HE), hereditary pyropoikilocytosis (HPP) and South-East Asian ovalocytosis (SAO), which are the most common disorders in this group. Protein studies have identified the underlying membrane abnormalities and advances in molecular biology have enabled further characterization of these disorders as well as, in many cases, identification of the causative mutations. These molecular analyses have provided additional information on the pathogenesis of these disorders and important insights into the structure–function relationships of erythrocyte membrane proteins.

As postulated in 1984 by Jiri Palek[52] and confirmed by subsequent studies, structural protein defects that compromise *vertical* interactions between the membrane skeleton and the lipid bilayer result in destabilization of the bilayer, loss of membrane microvesicles and spherocyte formation; whereas mutations affecting *horizontal* protein interactions within the membrane skeletal network disrupt the skeleton resulting in defective shape recovery and elliptocytes (Table 15-2). These red cell membrane disorders exhibit significant heterogeneity in their clinical, morphologic, laboratory, and molecular characteristics.

HEREDITARY SPHEROCYTOSIS
Definition and History

Hereditary spherocytosis is characterized by the presence of osmotically fragile spherical red blood cells that are evident on the blood film

TABLE 15–2. Erythrocyte Membrane Protein Defects in Inherited Disorders of Red Cell Shape

Protein	Disorder	Comment
α-Spectrin	HS, HE, HPP	Functional self-association defect is the most common cause of HE and HPP
		Position of mutation determines clinical severity
		Deficiency is a rare cause of severe HS
β-Spectrin	HS, HE, HPP	Deficiency causes HS
		"Acanthocytic" spherocytes present on blood film presplenectomy
		Functional self-association defect causes HE and HPP
Ankyrin	HS	Deficiency is the most common cause of HS in North America
AE1	HS, SAO, HAc	Deficiency is the most common cause of HS in parts of Europe and South Africa
		"Pincered" spherocytes are common on blood film presplenectomy
		SAO is caused by a deletion of 9 amino acids
Protein 4.1R	HE	Deficiency found in certain European, African, and Arab populations
Protein 4.2	HS	Deficiency primarily found in Japanese patients
GPC	HE	Concomitant protein 4.1 deficiency is the basis of HE

Abbreviations: AE1, anion exchanger-1 (band 3); GPC, glycophorin C; HAc, hereditary acanthocytosis; HE, hereditary elliptocytosis; HPP, hereditary pyropoikilocytosis; HS, hereditary spherocytosis; SAO, South East Asian Ovalocytosis.

(Fig. 15-10B). The disorder was first described in 1871 as microcythemia in a case history by two Belgian physicians.[53]

Epidemiology

HS occurs in all racial and ethnic groups. It is the most common inherited hemolytic anemia in individuals of northern European ancestry, affecting approximately 1 in 2000 individuals in North America and Europe.[54] It is also common in Japan and in Africans from southern Africa. Men and women are affected equally.

Etiology and Pathogenesis

The hallmark of HS erythrocytes is loss of membrane surface area relative to intracellular volume, which accounts for the spherical shape and marked diminution or loss of central pallor of the cell (see Fig. 15-10B). Spherocytes exhibit decreased deformability and are thus selectively retained, damaged and ultimately destroyed in the spleen, which causes the hemolysis experienced by HS patients. The HS red cell membrane is destabilized by a deficiency of a critical membrane protein, including spectrin, ankyrin, AE1, and protein 4.2, which decreases the vertical interactions between the skeleton and the bilayer, resulting in the release of microvesicles and loss of surface area (Fig. 15-11C). It is hypothesized that two mechanisms underlie the membrane loss: (1) in cells with spectrin/ankyrin deficiency, sections of the lipid bilayer and AE1 are not in contact with the skeleton, which will increase the lateral and rotational mobility of AE1, allowing lipid microvesicles containing AE1 to be generated; and (2) in cells with decreased amounts of AE1/protein 4.2, the stabilizing effect of the transmembrane section of AE1 on the lipid bilayer is lost, facilitating the formation of AE1-free microvesicles.[8,54]

Red Cell Membrane Protein Defects

Analysis of HS red cell membrane proteins by several research groups has revealed quantitative abnormalities of spectrin, ankyrin, AE1, and protein 4.2 in 70% to 97% of the cases.[7,54-56] This spectrum of defects is found worldwide in all the HS cohorts that have been studied; however, the relative frequency of each defect varies with the geographical area and ethnic group. In the United States, Canada, parts of Europe, Argentina, and India, the most common defect is ankyrin deficiency (30%-60%).[54,56,57,58-60] In Korea, the number of patients with ankyrin mutations is similar to the number of patients with spectrin defects.[60,61] Spectrin mutations are common in Brazil, Mexico, and the Netherlands.[55,62] In Portugal and parts of Italy,[55,63,64] as well as in South Africa (unpublished), AE1 deficiency is the main defect. In Japan, almost half of the HS cases are the result of a decreased amount of protein 4.2; in South Africa, this is the second most common defect; in other populations, protein 4.2 deficiency is rare (<6%).[54,55,65] The underlying gene mutations have not been investigated in all HS subjects, but research that has been conducted on the defective genes has identified more than 200 different mutations, many of which are unique to a family.

Ankyrin Concomitant ankyrin and spectrin deficiency was first described in two patients with severe atypical HS and the primary defect was identified as an ankyrin abnormality.[66] Subsequent DNA analysis of the *ANK1* gene in patients with typical HS identified several mutations[67] and numerous other additional studies have shown that ankyrin–spectrin deficiency is a common cause of HS. Ankyrin binds to spectrin with high affinity and attaches it to the membrane, which stabilizes the molecule. Because ankyrin is present in limiting amounts, a deficiency of ankyrin causes an equivalent loss of spectrin.

Different types of ankyrin mutations have been identified throughout the gene, indicating that there are several mechanisms that ultimately result in a decreased amount of ankyrin in the membrane. The majority of these mutations are frameshift and nonsense mutations that either result in unstable transcripts that are destroyed by nonsense-mediated mRNA decay or else produce a truncated defective ankyrin molecule.[56,57,59-62] More than 100 mutations have been documented. Although they are typically family-specific, a few recurrent mutations have been described[54,56,61,67] and 15% to 30% of mutations are de novo.[54,56,59,61] Some mutations have been documented in all the ankyrin domains, although most of them occur in the membrane-binding domain, and are thought to disrupt normal ankyrin–protein interactions.[60-62] A few splicing mutations have been identified,[56,59,61,67] including a mutation in intron 16, which created a new splice acceptor site and a complex pattern of aberrant splicing.[68] Both parents were heterozygous for this mutation and the proband was homozygous, indicating that homozygosity for an ankyrin mutation is compatible with life.

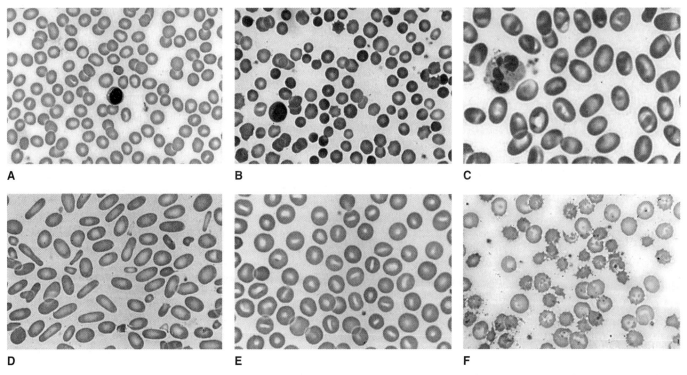

Figure 15–10. Blood films from patients with erythrocyte membrane disorders. **A.** Normal blood film. **B.** Hereditary spherocytosis with dense spherocytes. **C.** South East Asian ovalocytosis with large ovalocytes exhibiting a transverse ridge. **D.** Hereditary elliptocytosis with elongated elliptocytes and some poikilocytes. **E.** Hereditary stomatocytosis with cup-shaped stomatocytes. **F.** Hereditary abetalipoproteinemia with acanthocytes. *(Reproduced with permission from Lichtman MA, Shafer MS, Felgar RE, et al: Lichtman's Atlas of Hematology 2016. New York, NY: McGraw Hill; 2017.)*

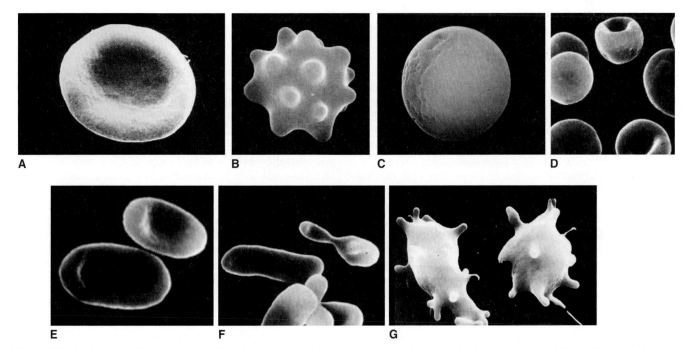

Figure 15–11. Scanning electron micrographs of erythrocytes with abnormal morphology resulting from membrane defects. **A.** Normal discocyte. **B.** Echinocyte. **C.** Spherocyte. **D.** Stomatocytes. **E.** Ovalocytes. **F.** Elliptocytes. **G.** Acanthocytes. *(Reproduced with permission from Lichtman MA, Shafer MS, Felgar RE, et al: Lichtman's Atlas of Hematology 2016. New York, NY: McGraw Hill; 2017.)*

Mutations in the erythroid-specific promoter of the *ANK1* gene are common in recessive HS.[63] A dinucleotide deletion impairs the binding of a transcription factor complex, which leads to a reduced number of ankyrin transcripts.[69] Point mutations in a barrier insulator element of the promoter also decrease transcription of the gene.[70]

Cytogenetic studies and DNA sequencing have identified a few ankyrin-deficient HS patients with a contiguous gene syndrome that includes deletion of the ankyrin gene locus at 8p11.2.[54,56] These patients additionally suffer from dysmorphic features, psychomotor retardation, and hypogonadism.[71]

Anion Exchanger-1 A subset of HS patients presents with AE1 deficiency, typically accompanied by a secondary decrease in protein 4.2, a consequence of the reduction in protein 4.2 binding sites in the cytoplasmic domain of AE1. The extent of the protein deficiency in heterozygous patients ranges between 20% and 50%, depending on the severity of the mutation, and the compensatory effect of the *in trans* normal allele. Mushroom-shaped "pincered" cells are commonly seen on the blood film of HS patients with an AE1 abnormality.

More than 60 underlying mutations, which are variable and occur throughout the *SLC4A1* gene, have been described.[8,54,56,60,62,65] Null mutations are typically family-specific and are caused by frameshift or nonsense mutations, or in a few cases by abnormal splicing, all of which result in truncated nonfunctional proteins or in unstable transcripts that are not translated into protein. Missense mutations are common and often occur in several kindred. Highly conserved arginine residues at the internal boundaries of the transmembrane segments of the protein (see Fig. 15-2) are frequently mutated, including residues 490, 518, 760, 808, and 870.[7,72] These mutations likely interfere with the cotranslational insertion of AE1 into the endoplasmic reticulum, and ultimately into the red cell membrane. Short in-frame insertions or deletions have been documented and presumably also impair insertion of the mutant protein into the lipid bilayer.

Mutations in the cytoplasmic domain of AE1 impact on its interaction with proteins in the membrane skeleton, or may alter the conformation of the protein rendering it unstable and prone to degradation prior to insertion into the membrane. Some cytoplasmic mutations, such as Cape Town (E90K) and Mondega (E40K and P147S), are silent in the heterozygous state but exacerbate the clinical presentation when inherited *in trans* to another mutation.[73,74]

Several HS patients with homozygous AE1 mutations have been described who are severely affected. One patient was described as having a missense mutation (Coimbra V488M) and a second patient was described as having a nonsense mutation (Vienna S477X). The Coimbra and Vienna missense mutations are null mutations that result in a complete absence of the protein in the homozygous state.[75,76] These two patients are transfusion dependent, although the Coimbra patient was free of transfusion for several years after splenectomy. They demonstrate that long-term survival without AE1 is possible, as in 2017 the Vienna patient was 5 years old and the Coimbra patient was 19 years old. Some homozygous mutations are associated with very-low levels of AE1. These include Courcouronnes (S667F), Punjab (S725R), and the A858D mutation found in several kindred in Oman and India.[77-80] These mutations compromise anion transport activity and thus also result in distal renal tubular acidosis (see "Nonerythroid Manifestations" further). An exception is homozygosity for Neapolis, a splicing mutation upstream of the start of the kidney AE1 isoform, resulting in a mutant protein lacking the first 11 amino acids, including the tyrosine 8 phosphorylation site and the aldolase binding site.[81]

Spectrin Erythrocytes from HS patients with defects in spectrin or ankyrin are deficient in spectrin. The degree of deficiency correlates with the severity of hemolysis, the response to splenectomy and the ability to withstand mechanical shear stress.[82,83] Visualization of the membrane skeleton of these red cells revealed a decreased density of the spectrin filaments connecting the junctional complexes.[84] The causative mutations occur in either α-spectrin or β-spectrin genes.

α-Spectrin Defects in α-spectrin are rare and are associated with severe recessive HS, caused mainly by nonsense or frameshift mutations.[54,85,86] However, in a cohort of 95 Dutch patients, defects in the *SPTA1* gene were the most common abnormality and three patients were identified with apparent autosomal dominant inheritance, although an unidentified mutation may be present in the other allele.[62] During erythropoiesis α-spectrin is synthesized in a two- to four-fold excess over β-spectrin,[87] and heterozygotes still produce sufficient α-spectrin to form heterodimers with all the β-spectrin molecules, which should not result in spectrin deficiency. The defect only manifests in individuals who are homozygous or doubly heterozygous for mutations in the *SPTA1* gene. The mechanism underlying spectrin deficiency has not been fully elucidated, but a low-expression allele or a polymorphism inherited *in trans* to a causative null mutation may play a role.[62] An example of a low-expression allele is αLEPRA (low-expression Prague), which produces less than 20% of the normal amount of α-spectrin transcripts owing to a splicing and mRNA processing defect, whereby the new termination codon in the elongated transcript triggers nonsense-mediated mRNA decay.[86] In combination with a null mutation on the other *SPTA1* allele, which produces a nonfunctional truncated protein, it causes severe spectrin deficiency and anemia.[86,88,89] A polymorphic missense mutation in the αII domain in spectrin Bug Hill has been identified in several patients who also carry αLEPRA *in trans* and present with spectrin-deficient, recessive HS.[86,91] In contrast, inheritance of an *SPTA1* null mutation *in trans* with the low-expression allele αLELY (low-expression Lyon),[90] causes no disease as sufficient α-spectrin is still produced.[89] Extensive analysis of the α-spectrin gene in a proband with severe nondominant HS revealed a partial maternal isodisomy of chromosome 1, resulting in homozygosity of the 1q23 region containing the maternal *SPTA1* gene, which carried an R891X nonsense mutation.[92] Uniparental disomy therefore unmasked a recessive mutation in the mother, which caused severe clinical symptoms in the child.

β-Spectrin The production of β-spectrin polypeptides is the limiting factor in spectrin heterodimer formation and one mutant allele is sufficient to cause spectrin deficiency in autosomal dominant HS. The blood films of these patients typically show a subpopulation of spiculated cells (acanthocytes and echinocytes) in addition to spherocytes.[54] Mutations in β-spectrin are found throughout the gene and are mainly null mutations caused by frameshift, nonsense, splicing, and initiator codon defects, which silence the mutant allele.[56,59-62,93] With a few exceptions the mutations are all kindred-specific. Truncated β-spectrin proteins also have been described and are caused by frameshift mutations, in-frame deletions, or exon skipping. These mutations lead to, for example, reduced synthesis of an unstable protein,[94] or impairment of the interaction with ankyrin, which prevents the insertion of spectrin into the membrane.[95] A few missense mutations clustering at the N-terminal actin-binding domain of the protein have been identified,[61,62] including β-spectrin Kissimmee caused by a W202R mutation.[96] The mutant protein is unstable and does not bind to protein 4.1R and thus it only interacts weakly with actin, which may explain why these red cells are deficient in spectrin.[96]

Protein 4.2 Protein 4.2 deficiency is common in Japanese patients with recessively inherited HS who exhibit almost a complete absence of the protein.[54,65] A small number of recurrent causative mutations have been described in Japanese patients, including three missense mutations (protein 4.2 Nippon [A142T]; protein 4.2 Shiga [R317C]; protein 4.2 Komatsu [D175Y]), one nonsense mutation (protein 4.2 Fukuoka [W119X]), and a splicing mutation in intron 6 leading to a frameshift (protein 4.2 Notame).[40,65,97] The most common mutation is protein 4.2

Nippon, and patients may be homozygous for this mutation or compound heterozygotes with a second mutation on the other allele.[40]

Protein 4.2 deficiency also occurs sporadically in whites and other population groups from Europe, Tunisia, and Pakistan with autosomal recessive HS,[40,98] and is common in South African kindred with autosomal dominant HS. Several mutations have been described in the *EPB42* gene of non-Japanese kindred, including a missense mutation[98] and predominantly in-frame deletion and insertion of nucleotides, which lead to frameshift mutations. These frameshifts cause premature termination of translation and these mutant truncated proteins are not detected on the membrane, indicating that they are unstable and presumably degraded. Amino acids 306 to 320 are highly conserved and 5 of the known mutations occur in this region, which is adjacent to the hairpin that binds to AE1 in the predicted tertiary structure of protein 4.2.[40]

Secondary Membrane Defects

The decreased membrane surface area in hereditary spherocytes involves a symmetrical loss of each species of membrane lipid. The relative proportions of cholesterol and phospholipids are therefore normal and the asymmetrical distribution of phospholipids is maintained.

HS red cells exhibit increased cation permeability, presumably secondary to the underlying membrane defect.[99] The excessive sodium influx activates the Na^+-K^+ ATPase cation pump, which increases ATP turnover and glycolysis. Spherocytes are dehydrated, especially cells obtained from the splenic pulp, but the underlying mechanism has not been clearly defined. The acidic environment of the spleen and oxidative damage by splenic macrophages increase the activity of the K^+Cl^- cotransporter, which may play a role in dehydration. The hyperactive Na^+-K^+ ATPase pump may also contribute as three sodium ions are extruded in exchange for two potassium ions, and this loss of monovalent cations is accompanied by the loss of water. Dehydration also may be related to loss of surface area.

Molecular Determinants of Clinical Severity

Affected individuals of the same kindred typically experience similar degrees of hemolysis. However, in some families the clinical expression is variable, and this may be influenced by several factors. Low-expression alleles decrease transcription of the gene or influence the expression or incorporation of the protein into the membrane, but there is no phenotypic effect in the heterozygous state as the normal allele compensates for the deleterious effect. However, when inherited with a mutant allele that causes HS, it exacerbates the clinical expression of the disease. Examples of low-expression alleles that influence HS include AE1 Genas and Mondego, as well as two α-spectrin alleles, αLELY and αLEPRA.[62,74,75,88-91,100]

Variable penetrance of the defective gene, a de novo mutation or a mild form of recessively inherited HS may also influence the clinical severity. Double heterozygosity for two mild AE1 mutations can have an additive effect,[73] and rare cases caused by homozygous defects in AE1 result in severe transfusion-dependent hemolytic anemia or fetal death.[75-81] Coinheritance of other hematologic disorders or Gilbert syndrome, caused by homozygosity for a polymorphism in the promoter of the uridine diphosphate-glucuronosyltransferase (*UGT1*) gene, can also alter the clinical symptoms.[54,59-61,101,102]

Role of the Spleen

The spleen plays a secondary, but important, role in the pathophysiology of HS. Spherocytes are retained and ultimately destroyed in the spleen (Chap. 25) and this is the primary cause of the chronic hemolysis experienced by HS patients (Fig. 15-12). The reduced deformability of spherocytes impedes their passage through the interendothelial slits separating the splenic cords of the red pulp from the splenic sinuses. The decrease in red cell deformability is primarily related to a loss of surface area, and to a lesser extent, to an increase in internal viscosity resulting from mild cellular dehydration. Ex vivo experiments using perfused human spleens and red cells treated with lysophosphatidylcholine to induce spherocytosis revealed that the degree of splenic retention correlated with the reduction in the surface-area-to-volume ratio.[103]

The spleen is a metabolically hostile environment with a decreased pH, low concentrations of glucose and ATP, and increased oxidants, all of which are detrimental to the red cell. Spherocytes are "conditioned" during erythrostasis in the spleen and become more osmotically fragile and increasingly spherocytic.[104] Exposure to macrophages in the spleen eventually leads to erythrophagocytosis and destruction.

Inheritance

In approximately 75% of HS patients, inheritance is autosomal dominant. In the remaining patients, the disorder may be

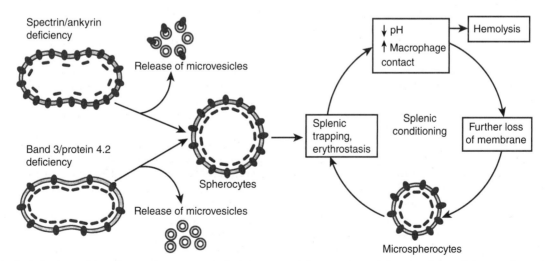

Figure 15-12. Pathobiology of hereditary spherocytosis (HS). The primary defect in HS is a deficiency of one of the membrane proteins, which destabilizes the lipid bilayer and leads to a loss of membrane in the form of microvesicles. This reduces the surface area of the cell and leads to spherocyte formation. Red cells with a deficiency of spectrin or ankyrin produce microvesicles containing AE1 (band 3), whereas a reduced amount of AE1 or protein 4.1R gives rise to AE1-free microvesicles. Spherocytes have decreased deformability and are trapped in the spleen where the membrane is further damaged by splenic conditioning, which ultimately results in hemolysis. ↓, Decreased; ↑, increased.

TABLE 15–3. Clinical Classification of Hereditary Spherocytosis

	Carrier	Mild	Moderate	Moderately Severe[a]	Severe[b]
Hemoglobin (g/L)	Normal	110-150	80-120	60-80	<60
Reticulocytes (%)	1.5%-3%	<6%	>6%	≥10	≥10
Bilirubin (mg/dL)	0-1	1-2	± 2	2-3	≥3
Blood film	Normal	Few spherocytes	Spherocytes	Spherocytes	Spherocytes, poikilocytes
Inheritance	Autosomal dominant	Autosomal dominant	Autosomal dominant; de novo mutations	Autosomal dominant; de novo mutations	Autosomal recessive

[a]Values in nontransfused patients.

[b]Values prior to transfusion.

autosomal recessive or result from de novo mutations, which is relatively common.[54,61] Mutations in α-spectrin or protein 4.2 are often associated with recessive HS.[52]

Clinical Features

The clinical manifestations of HS vary widely. The typical clinical picture combines evidence of hemolysis (anemia, jaundice, reticulocytosis, gallstones, splenomegaly) with spherocytosis (spherocytes on the blood film and increased osmotic fragility [OF]) and a positive family history. Mild, moderate, and severe forms of HS have been defined according to differences in hemoglobin, bilirubin, and reticulocyte counts (Table 15-3), which can be correlated with the degree of compensation for hemolysis. Initial assessment of a patient with suspected HS should include a family history and questions about history of anemia, jaundice, gallstones, and splenectomy. Physical examination should seek signs such as scleral icterus, jaundice and splenomegaly.

Typical Hereditary Spherocytosis Approximately 60% to 70% of HS patients have moderate disease, which typically presents in infancy or childhood but may present at any age. In children, anemia is the most frequent finding (50% of cases), followed by splenomegaly, jaundice, or a positive family history.[8,54] No comparable data exist for adults. Hemolysis may be incompletely compensated with mild to moderate anemia (see Table 15-3). The moderate anemia may often be asymptomatic; however, fatigue and mild pallor or both may be present. Jaundice may be intermittent and is seen in approximately half of patients, usually in association with viral infections. When present, jaundice is acholuric, characterized by unconjugated hyperbilirubinemia without detectable bilirubinuria. Palpable splenomegaly is evident in most (>75%) older children and adults. Typically, the spleen is modestly enlarged (2-6 cm below the costal margin), but it may be massive. No proven correlation exists between the spleen size and the severity of HS. However, given the pathophysiology and response of the disease to splenectomy, such a correlation probably exists.

Mild Hereditary Spherocytosis Approximately 20% to 30% of HS patients have mild disease with "compensated hemolysis," that is, red blood cell production and destruction are balanced, and the hemoglobin concentration of the blood is normal (see Table 15-3).[54,105] The life span of spherocytes is decreased, but patients adequately compensate for hemolysis with increased marrow erythropoiesis. These patients are usually asymptomatic. Splenomegaly is mild, reticulocyte counts are generally less than 6%, and spherocytes on the blood film may be minimal, which complicates the diagnosis. Many of these individuals escape detection until adulthood when they are being evaluated for unrelated disorders or when complications related to anemia or chronic hemolysis occur. Hemolysis may become severe with illnesses that further increase splenomegaly, such as infectious mononucleosis, or may be exacerbated by other factors, such as pregnancy or sustained, vigorous exercise. Because of the asymptomatic course of HS in these patients, diagnosis of HS should be considered during evaluation of incidentally noted splenomegaly, gallstones at a young age, or anemia resulting from parvovirus infection or other viral infections.

Moderately Severe and Severe Hereditary Spherocytosis Approximately 5% to 10% of HS patients have moderately severe disease, as evidenced by indicators of anemia that are more pronounced than in typical moderate HS, and an intermittent requirement for transfusions (see Table 15-3). This category includes patients with dominant and recessive HS. A small number (<5%) of patients have severe disease with life-threatening anemia and are transfusion-dependent. They almost always have recessive HS. Most have severe spectrin deficiency, which is thought to result from a defect in α-spectrin,[82,83,86] but defects in ankyrin or AE1 have also been identified.[75,81] Patients with severe HS often have irregularly contoured or budding spherocytes or bizarre poikilocytes in addition to typical spherocytes and microspherocytes on the blood film. Added to the risks of recurrent transfusions, patients often suffer from hemolytic and aplastic crises and may develop complications of severe uncompensated anemia, including growth retardation, delayed sexual maturation, and aspects of thalassemic facies.

Asymptomatic Carriers Parents of patients with recessive HS are clinically asymptomatic and do not have anemia, splenomegaly, hyperbilirubinemia, or spherocytosis on the blood films. However, most have subtle laboratory signs of HS (see Table 15-3), including slight reticulocytosis, diminished haptoglobin levels, and slightly elevated incubated OF, particularly the 100% red cell lysis point, which occurs at a higher sodium chloride concentration in carriers compared to normal subjects.[105] The acidified glycerol lysis test (AGLT) also may be useful to detect carriers. Approximately 1% of the population in North America and parts of Europe is estimated to be silent carriers.[54]

Pregnancy and Hereditary Spherocytosis

Most patients do well during pregnancy[106] although anemia may be exacerbated due to plasma volume expansion and increased hemolysis. A few patients are symptomatic only during pregnancy. Transfusions are rarely required.

Hereditary Spherocytosis in the Neonate

Jaundice is the most common finding in neonates with HS, present in approximately 90% of cases. It may be accentuated by coinheritance of Gilbert syndrome, caused by homozygosity for a polymorphism in the promoter of the *UGT1* gene (Chaps. 2 and 16).[54,101,102] Fewer than half of infants are anemic and severe anemia is rare. A few cases of hydrops fetalis resulting from homozygosity or compound heterozygosity for AE1 or spectrin defects have been reported.[75,107,108]

Complications

Gallbladder Disease Chronic hemolysis leads to formation of bilirubinate gallstones, the most frequently reported complication in as many as half of HS patients. Coinheritance of Gilbert syndrome markedly increases the risk of gallstone formation. Although gallstones have been detected in children, they mainly occur in adolescents and young adults.[8,54] Routine management should include interval ultrasonography to detect gallstones because many patients with cholelithiasis and HS are asymptomatic. Interval ultrasonography allows prompt diagnosis and treatment and prevents complications of symptomatic biliary tract disease, including biliary obstruction, cholecystitis, and cholangitis.

Hemolytic, Aplastic, and Megaloblastic Crises Hemolytic crises are the most common, are usually associated with viral illnesses, and typically occur in childhood.[8,54] They are generally mild and characterized by jaundice, splenomegaly, anemia, and reticulocytosis. Medical intervention is seldom necessary. During rare severe hemolytic crises, red cell transfusion may be required.

Aplastic crises following virally induced marrow suppression are uncommon but may result in severe anemia, requiring hospitalization and transfusion with serious complications, including congestive heart failure or death.[8,54] The most common etiologic agent in these cases is parvovirus (Chap. 5). The virus selectively infects erythropoietic progenitor cells and inhibits their growth leading to the characteristic finding of a low number of reticulocytes despite severe anemia. Aplastic crises usually last for 10 to 14 days and may bring asymptomatic, undiagnosed HS patients with compensated hemolysis to medical attention.[54]

Megaloblastic crises may occur in HS patients with increased folate demands, such as pregnant patients, growing children, or patients recovering from an aplastic crisis. This complication can be prevented with appropriate folate supplementation.

Other Complications Leg ulcers, chronic dermatitis on the legs and gout are rare manifestations of HS, which usually heal rapidly after splenectomy. In severe cases, skeletal abnormalities resulting from expansion of the marrow can occur. Extramedullary hematopoiesis can lead to tumors, particularly along the thoracic and lumbar spine or in the kidney hila, in nonsplenectomized patients with mild to moderate HS.[8,54] Postsplenectomy, the masses involute and undergo fatty metamorphosis.

HS has been suggested to predispose patients to hematologic malignancies, including myeloproliferative neoplasms and myeloma, but cause and effect are not proven. Thrombosis has been reported in several HS patients, usually postsplenectomy. Untreated HS may aggravate other underlying diseases, such as congestive heart disease and hemochromatosis.[8,54]

Nonerythroid Manifestations

Clinical manifestations are confined to the erythroid lineage in the majority of patients with HS, but a few exceptions have been observed. Several HS kindred have been reported with cosegregating nonerythroid manifestations, particularly neuromuscular abnormalities, including cardiomyopathy, slowly progressive spinocerebellar degenerative disease, spinal cord dysfunction, and movement disorders. Erythrocyte ankyrin and β-spectrin are also expressed in muscle, brain, and spinal cord, which raise the possibility that these HS patients suffer from defects of one of these proteins.[8]

An isoform of AE1 is expressed in the kidney and heterozygous defects of the protein have been described in patients with inherited distal renal tubular acidosis and normal erythrocytes. This finding is in contrast to most patients with heterozygous mutations of AE1, who have normal renal acidification and abnormal erythrocytes. Kindred with HS

and renal acidification defects resulting from AE1 mRNA processing mutations, Pribram and Campinas, have been described.[109,110] Homozygosity for AE1 mutations resulted in the absence of the erythroid and kidney proteins, causing renal tubular acidosis and severe HS.[75-79]

Laboratory Features

Laboratory findings in HS are variable, which correlate with the heterogeneous clinical presentation. Several tests are available in routine diagnostic laboratories, whereas more sophisticated technologies to identify the defective protein and gene mutations are only performed in specialized research-oriented laboratories. Guidelines from the International Council on Standardization in Hematology (ICSH) outline clinical criteria, as well as current diagnostic tests and their limitations.[111]

Blood Film Erythrocyte morphology in HS is not uniform. Typical HS patients have blood films with easily identifiable spherocytes lacking central pallor (see Figs. 15-10B and 15-11C). Patients with mild HS may present with only a few spherocytes, whereas at the other end of the spectrum, severely affected patients exhibit numerous dense microspherocytes and bizarre erythrocyte morphology with anisocytosis and poikilocytosis. Blood films from patients with AE1 defects often exhibit "pincered" or mushroom-shaped red cells, whereas spherocytic acanthocytes are associated with β-spectrin mutations.[112] When examining blood from a patient with suspected spherocytosis, a high-quality film with the erythrocytes properly separated and some cells with central pallor in the field of examination are important because spherocytes can be an artifact.

Erythrocyte Indices Most patients have mild to moderate anemia with hemoglobin in the 90 to 120 g/L range (see Table 15-3). Mean corpuscular hemoglobin concentration (MCHC) is increased (>36 g/dL) because of relative cellular dehydration in approximately half of patients, but all HS patients have some dehydrated cells. Mean corpuscular volume (MCV) is usually normal except in cases of severe HS, when MCV is slightly decreased. Some automated hematology analyzers measure the hemoglobin concentration of individual red cells and a demonstration of a population of hyperdense erythrocytes can be useful as a screening test for HS, especially when combined with an increased red cell distribution width.

Markers of Hemolysis Other laboratory features of HS are markers of ongoing hemolysis. Reticulocytosis, variably increased lactate dehydrogenase, increased urinary and fecal urobilinogen, unconjugated hyperbilirubinemia, and decreased serum haptoglobin reflect hemolysis and increased erythropoiesis (Chap. 2). The reticulocyte count may appear to be elevated disproportionately relative to the degree of anemia. A decreased mean reticulocyte volume and a low percentage of immature reticulocytes are additional parameters of value in differentiating HS from other conditions.[113,114]

Erythrocyte Fragility Tests Spherocytes have a decreased surface area relative to cell volume and this renders them osmotically fragile. Several laboratory tests exploit this characteristic and are used to diagnose HS. The most common OF test measures lysis of red cells, either from freshly drawn blood or after incubation of the sample at 37°C for 24 hours, in a range of hypotonic concentrations of sodium chloride. Spherocytes typically swell and burst at higher sodium chloride concentrations than do normal biconcave disk-shaped red cells. Other tests based on the same principle measure the rate and extent of cell lysis in buffered glycerol solutions and include the glycerol lysis test (GLT) and the AGLT. These tests, however, have relatively poor sensitivity and do not detect all cases of mild HS or those with small numbers of spherocytes, including patients who had recent blood transfusions.[54,64,111,115] These tests also may be unreliable and give normal results in the presence of iron deficiency, obstructive jaundice, or, during the recovery phase, of an aplastic crisis.[54] In addition, these tests do not differentiate

HS from other disorders with secondary spherocytosis, such as the autoimmune hemolytic anemias (Chap. 26). Other fragility tests include the cryohemolysis test, which is based on the sensitivity of HS red cells to cooling at 0°C in hypertonic conditions,[52] and the autohemolysis test, but these tests also do not detect all cases of HS.[8]

Eosin 5′-Maleimide Flow Cytometry Test Eosin 5′-maleimide (EMA) is a fluorescent dye that binds to the transmembrane proteins, AE1, Rh protein, Rh glycoprotein, and CD47.[116] Patients with HS, including neonates, exhibit decreased fluorescence compared to controls, irrespective of the underlying defective membrane protein, although not all patients with HS are detected.[111,115,117] In addition, lower fluorescence values also may be observed in patients with HE, HPP, some red cell enzymopathies, and other abnormalities of AE1, such as congenital dyserythropoietic anemia type II (CDAII) (Chap. 14). This test is commonly used, but flow cytometers from different manufacturers give different values for the mean fluorescence intensity; consequently, there are no universal reference ranges. The cutoff value to distinguish HS from normal samples is still being debated and varies between different laboratories, yielding different sensitivities and specificities of the test. There is also a "gray area" where control and HS values overlap and interpretation of these results requires consideration of clinical and other laboratory features.[111,115,118-120]

Osmotic Gradient Ektacytometry This useful test monitors red cell deformability under a continuous osmotic gradient and a known shear stress, which generates a deformability index (DI) profile.[111,112,121] HS red cells show a decreased maximum DI combined with an increased minimum osmotic (Omin) gradient, indicative of OF, and a decreased hyperosmolality corresponding to half the maximum deformability (Ohyper), reflecting dehydration of the cells. Highly specialized equipment is required for this procedure, which limits its availability.

Sodium Dodecyl Sulfate Polyacrylamide Gel Electrophoresis This highly informative test identifies the underlying defective protein after separation of the red cell membrane proteins by SDS-PAGE, followed by densitometric scanning of the stained protein bands to quantify the amounts of each protein.[111] A deficiency in one of the proteins is easily detected. Patients with clinically identified HS and normal SDS-PAGE results may have a slight decrease of 10% to 15% in one of the membrane proteins, which may be missed by the densitometric analysis, or they may have an abnormality in a protein that is currently not quantified, for example, adducin. The sensitivity of this test varies between laboratories and different patient populations, but typically an abnormality is defined in 72% to 93% of cases.[54,58,64,67,111] Knowledge of the defective protein facilitates subsequent DNA/RNA investigations to characterize the gene defect. However, SDS-PAGE is a specialized, labor-intensive test and thus it is only available in a few laboratories.

Molecular Genetic Diagnostics The laboratory tests for HS described earlier exploit the abnormal morphologic and biochemical characteristics of the defective red cells, which, in combination with clinical data and family history, are usually sufficient to diagnose the disorder. However, the results may be inconclusive or the patient may have had recent transfusions, which present a diagnostic challenge. Neonates with unexplained hemolytic anemia also may be difficult to diagnose. Advances in next-generation DNA sequencing technology (NGS) and the availability of new computational programs have facilitated the use of targeted NGS to detect the underlying gene mutations in such cases. Unlike whole-genome sequencing or whole-exome sequencing, the targeted NGS approach is much simpler and less costly and involves the use of customized gene panels encompassing relevant coding and noncoding regions of genes known to be involved in the pathogenesis of hemolytic anemia.[122,123] Identifying the causative mutation enables a definitive diagnosis, which guides the management and treatment of patients.

Targeted NGS is also increasingly being used in research-oriented laboratories to analyze large cohorts of HS patients to establish genotype–phenotype correlations and to identify the heterogeneous spectrum of HS mutations in distinct population groups.[56,59,60,62] Targeted NGS improved the diagnostic rate to a variable degree depending on the gene panels used, but in approximately 10% to 36% of HS patients, no pathogenic mutation could be detected.[59,60,62] A large number of novel mutations have been identified with targeted NGS, but the interpretation of results is challenging and care should be taken in assigning pathogenic mutations, especially in ethnic groups with poor or no sequence coverage in international databases. The quality of the sequencing reads should be assessed and the data should be subjected to a thorough and rigorous analysis. The sequences should be processed through various filters to remove irrelevant variants using the numerous software programs and databases that are available. Programs to predict pathogenicity of mutations and to model these changes on the three-dimensional structure of the defective proteins have been developed to assist the analysis. Potential pathogenic mutations should be validated by Sanger sequencing and family studies, if possible, and the results should correlate with biochemical and clinical data on the patient.[59,60,62,122,123]

Several clinical laboratories are now offering a targeted NGS service and in view of the increasing complexity of the data, the American College of Medical Genetics and Genomics, the Association for Molecular Pathology, and the College of American Pathologists have developed consensus recommendations and guidelines for the interpretation of sequence variants.[124] They recommend the use of specific standard terminology whereby "mutations" and "polymorphisms" are replaced by "variant" with the following categories: (1) pathogenic, (2) likely pathogenic, (3) uncertain significance, (4) likely benign, or (5) benign. Criteria to classify the variants are described and a standard gene nomenclature is also recommended to enable unambiguous designation of a variant.[124]

Differential Diagnosis

International diagnostic guidelines and flowcharts for the differential diagnosis of HS and other red cell membranopathies have been outlined.[111,112,121] Clinical features and family history should accompany an initial, first-line laboratory investigation comprising a complete blood count with a blood film, reticulocyte count, direct antiglobulin test (Coombs test), and serum bilirubin. Other causes of anemia should be excluded, particularly autoimmune hemolytic anemia, CDAII, and HSt.[54,111,112] Further routine diagnostic tests or second-line investigations (discussed in "Laboratory Features" earlier), are not standardized as reflected by a European survey of 25 centers.[125] A consistent finding was that all the laboratories used at least two tests to make a final diagnosis, as none of the currently available methods have 100% sensitivity. The EMA test was the most commonly used test and a combination of the EMA and AGLTs identified all cases in a series of 150 HS patients.[115,125] Third-line investigations are highly specialized tests with limited availability that provide insight into the molecular defects and pathogenesis of HS and are useful in refining the diagnosis and management of the disorder.[121] These tests, discussed earlier, include SDS-PAGE of membrane proteins and DNA sequencing of either the defective gene or whole-exome sequencing or targeted NGS, with NGS becoming the most common approach.[122,123]

In neonates, the characteristic triad of jaundice, anemia, and splenomegaly is rare; jaundice is the most common presenting feature.[126] Examination of the blood film is useful, but not all neonates with HS will exhibit spherocytes. Family history is important and a neonatal HS ratio (MCHC divided by MCV) of greater than 0.36 has a very high sensitivity and specificity. ABO incompatibility should be ruled out and the EMA flow cytometry test can be helpful.[126] Other causes of spherocytic hemolytic anemia, such as autoimmune hemolysis, clostridial sepsis, transfusion reactions, severe burns, and bites from snakes, spiders, bees, and wasps (Chaps. 23, 24, and 26), should be viewed in the appropriate clinical context.

Occasional spherocytes are seen in patients with a large spleen (eg, in cirrhosis or myelofibrosis) or in patients with microangiopathic anemias (Chap. 22), but differentiation of these conditions from HS does not usually present diagnostic difficulties. HS may be obscured in disorders that increase the surface-to-volume ratio of erythrocytes, such as obstructive jaundice, iron deficiency (Chap. 11), β-thalassemia trait or hemoglobin SC disease (Chaps. 17 and 18), and vitamin B_{12} or folate deficiency (Chap. 9).

Therapy and Prognosis

Splenectomy Splenic sequestration is the primary determinant of erythrocyte survival in HS patients. Thus, splenectomy cures or alleviates the anemia in the overwhelming majority of patients, reducing or eliminating the need for red cell transfusions, which has obvious implications for future iron overload and hemochromatosis-related end-organ damage. The incidence of cholelithiasis is decreased. Postsplenectomy, spherocytosis, and altered OF persist, but the "tail" of the OF curve, created by conditioning of a subpopulation of spherocytes by the spleen, disappears. Erythrocyte life span nearly normalizes, and reticulocyte counts fall to normal or near-normal levels. Changes typical of the postsplenectomy state, including Howell-Jolly bodies, target cells, Pappenheimer bodies (siderocytes), and acanthocytes (Chaps. 1 and 25), become evident on the blood film. Postsplenectomy, patients with the severest forms of HS still suffer from shortened erythrocyte survival and hemolysis, but their clinical improvement is striking.[83]

Complications of Splenectomy Early complications of splenectomy include local infection, thrombotic complications (especially hepatic and mesenteric thrombosis), bleeding, and pancreatitis, presumably resulting from injury to the tail of the pancreas incurred during spleen removal. In general, the morbidity of splenectomy for HS is lower than the morbidity of other hematologic disorders. The complications of splenectomy are discussed in chapter 25.

Indications for Splenectomy In the past, splenectomy, which has a low operative mortality, was considered routine in HS patients. However, the risk of overwhelming postsplenectomy infection and the emergence of penicillin-resistant pneumococci have led to reevaluation of the role of splenectomy in the treatment of HS.[127] Considering the risks and benefits, a reasonable approach is to splenectomize all patients with transfusion-dependent severe spherocytosis and all patients suffering from significant signs or symptoms of anemia, including growth failure, skeletal changes, leg ulcers, and extramedullary hematopoietic tumors. Other candidates for splenectomy are HS patients suffering from vascular compromise of vital organs.

Whether patients with moderate HS and compensated, asymptomatic anemia should undergo splenectomy is controversial. Patients with mild HS and compensated hemolysis can be followed and referred to for splenectomy if clinically indicated. Splenectomy of patients with mild to moderate HS and gallstones is debatable, particularly because new treatments for cholelithiasis, including laparoscopic cholecystectomy, and endoscopic sphincterotomy, lower the risk of this complication. If such patients have symptomatic gallstones, a combined cholecystectomy and splenectomy can be performed, particularly if acute cholecystitis or biliary obstruction has occurred. There is no evidence to indicate any benefit to performing cholecystectomy and splenectomy separately, as done in the past.

Because the risk of postsplenectomy sepsis is very high during infancy and early childhood, splenectomy should be delayed until age 5 to 9 years if possible and to at least 3 years if feasible, even if chronic transfusions are required in the interim. There is no evidence to indicate that further delay is useful. In fact, a delay may be harmful because the risk of cholelithiasis increases dramatically in children older than 10 years.

When splenectomy is warranted, laparoscopic splenectomy has become the method of choice in centers with surgeons experienced in the technique.[120] If desired, the procedure can be combined with laparoscopic cholecystectomy. Laparoscopic splenectomy results in less postoperative discomfort, a quicker return to preoperative diet and activities, shorter hospitalization, decreased costs, and smaller scars. The risk of bleeding increases during the operation and approximately 10% of laparoscopic operations (for all causes) must be converted to standard splenectomies. Even very large spleens (>600 g) can be removed laparoscopically because the spleen is placed in a large bag, diced, and eliminated via suction catheters.

Partial splenectomy via laparotomy has been advocated for infants and young children with significant anemia associated with erythrocyte membrane disorders.[129] The goals of this procedure are to allow for palliation of hemolysis and anemia while maintaining some residual splenic immune function. In a cohort of 79 HS patients followed for 3 to 23 years after partial splenectomy, the benefits of the procedure depended on the initial severity of the disease.[130] In children younger than 6 years with severe anemia and/or transfusion dependence, the procedure induced a sustained increase in hemoglobin levels and reduced the need for transfusions, although approximately half of these patients eventually required a total splenectomy.[130]

Prior to splenectomy, patients should be immunized with vaccines against pneumococcus, *Haemophilus influenzae* type B, and meningococcus, preferably several weeks preoperatively. Use of prophylactic antibiotics postsplenectomy for prevention of pneumococcal sepsis is controversial. Postsplenectomy, prophylactic antibiotics (penicillin V 125 mg orally twice daily for patients younger than 7 years or 250 mg orally twice daily for those older than 7 years, including adults), are recommended for at least 5 years postsplenectomy by some and for life by others. The optimal duration of prophylactic antibiotic therapy postsplenectomy is unknown. Presplenectomy and, in severe cases, post-splenectomy, HS patients should take folic acid (1 mg/day orally) to prevent folate deficiency.

Splenectomy Failure Splenectomy failure is uncommon. Failure may result from an accessory spleen missed during splenectomy, from development of splenunculi as a consequence of autotransplantation of splenic tissue during surgery, or from another intrinsic red cell defect, such as pyruvate kinase deficiency (Chap. 16). Accessory spleens occur in 15% to 40% of patients and must always be sought. Recurrence of hemolytic anemia years or even decades following splenectomy should raise suspicion of an accessory spleen particularly if Howell-Jolly bodies are no longer found on blood film (Chap. 1). Definitive confirmation of ectopic splenic tissue can be achieved by a radiocolloid liver–spleen scan or a scan using ^{51}Cr-labeled, heat-damaged red cells.

Genetic Counseling

After a patient is diagnosed with HS, family members should be examined for the presence of HS. A history, physical examination for splenomegaly, complete blood count, examination of the blood film for spherocytes, and a reticulocyte count should be obtained for parents, children, and siblings, if available.

HEREDITARY ELLIPTOCYTOSIS AND PYROPOIKILOCYTOSIS

Definition and History

HE is characterized by the presence of elliptical or oval erythrocytes on the blood films of affected individuals (see Figs. 15-10D and 15-11F).

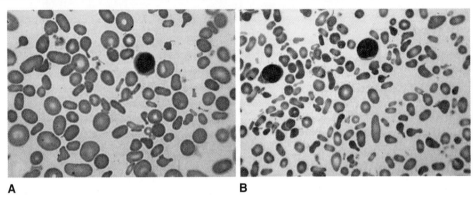

Figure 15–13. Blood films from a patient with hereditary pyropoikilocytosis (HPP). **A.** Presplenectomy. **B.** Postsplenectomy. Note the prominent micropoikilocytosis, microspherocytosis, and fragmentation especially after splenectomy. *(Reproduced with permission from Lichtman MA, Shafer MS, Felgar RE, et al: Lichtman's Atlas of Hematology 2016. New York, NY: McGraw Hill; 2017.)*

In 1904, Dresbach, a physiologist at Ohio State University in Columbus, Ohio, published the first description of elliptical red blood cells in one of his students, which were noticed during a laboratory exercise in which the students were examining their own blood.[131] The report elicited controversy because the student died soon thereafter, leading to speculation that he had actually suffered from pernicious anemia. The demonstration of elliptocytosis in three generations of one family established the hereditary nature of this disorder.[132] HPP, a related disorder, is a rare disease that was first described in 1975 in children with severe neonatal anemia with abnormal poikilocytic red cell morphology reminiscent of that seen in patients suffering from severe burns (Fig. 15-13).[133] The erythrocytes from these patients exhibited increased thermal sensitivity.

Epidemiology and Inheritance

HE has a worldwide distribution but the true incidence is unknown because the disease is heterogeneous and many patients are asymptomatic. In the United States, the incidence is estimated to be 1 in 2000 to 4000 individuals.[8,134] HE occurs in all racial groups but is more prevalent in individuals of West African descent, possibly because elliptocytes may confer some resistance to malaria.[135,136] HPP is typically found in patients of African descent, but it also has been diagnosed in persons of European and Arabic descent and seems to be particularly common in Thailand.[134,137-140]

Etiology and Pathogenesis

The primary abnormality in HE and HPP erythrocytes is defective horizontal interactions between components of the membrane skeleton, which weakens the skeleton and compromises its ability to maintain the biconcave disk shape of the red cell during circulatory shear stress. Investigations of erythrocyte membrane proteins in these disorders have identified abnormalities in α-spectrin, β-spectrin, protein 4.1R, and GPC.[134] The most common defects occur in spectrin, the main structural protein of the erythrocyte membrane skeleton, and these defects impair the ability of spectrin dimers to self-associate into tetramers and oligomers, thereby disrupting the skeletal lattice. Abnormalities in protein 4.1R diminish the interaction between the tail ends of spectrin tetramers in the junctional complex, destabilizing the skeleton. Deficiency of GPC and/or GPD is associated with reduced levels of protein 4.1R, which presumably is responsible for the elliptocytosis.

When the integrity of the skeleton is compromised, the capacity of the erythrocyte to undergo flow-induced deformation and rearrangement of the skeleton is reduced. Disruption of the dynamic dissociation

and reassociation of spectrin tetramers causes mechanical instability of the membrane, which precludes the recovery of the normal biconcave disk shape of the cell after prolonged and repeated unidirectional axial distortion in the microcirculation.[1] HE reticulocytes have a normal shape when released into the circulation, but the mature red cells become progressively more elliptical as they age and, ultimately, the abnormal shape becomes permanent.[8,134] As the severity of the defect increases, poikilocytes are formed and the cells become prone to fragmentation. HPP patients exhibit a combination of horizontal (impaired spectrin tetramer formation) and vertical (spectrin deficiency) defects, with the vertical defects causing microspherocytes and exacerbating the hemolytic anemia.[141,142]

Red Cell Membrane Protein Defects

Spectrin Mutations that affect spectrin heterodimer self-association are found in the majority of HE patients and in all patients with HPP. This functional defect results in an increased percentage of spectrin dimers relative to tetramers,[143] which is reflected on a structural level by an abnormal tryptic digest pattern of the protein, whereby the normal peptide is decreased with a concomitant increase in an abnormal peptide of lower molecular weight. Most of the defects affect the 80-kDa αI domain of α-spectrin and of the nine structural variants the most common are Spα$^{I/74}$, Spα$^{I/65}$, and Spα$^{I/46\ or\ 50a}$.[141]

More than 70 mutations have been identified in either α-spectrin or β-spectrin genes. The majority of the mutations are missense mutations that substitute highly conserved amino acids or those in close proximity. The abnormal amino acids typically have a different charge, or in the case of glycine or proline substitutions, they disrupt the helical structure of the spectrin repeats, which alter the interactions between α and β subunits. Interestingly, mutations in α-spectrin primarily occur in helix C of the repeats, which highlights the importance of this helix in the triple helical bundle (see Fig. 15-3). Several mechanisms have been identified by which the mutations impair spectrin tetramer formation.

Spα$^{I/74}$ mutations are mostly missense mutations that cluster in exon 2 of the *SPTA1* gene. At the protein level, these mutations are found at the self-association site, which consists of helix C of the α0 partial spectrin repeat that interacts with helices B and C of β-spectrin partial repeat 17 to form a complete triple helical bundle (see Fig 15-3).[28] In vitro studies on missense mutations in α0 revealed that the mutant peptides were stable folded structures, similar to wild-type, but their binding affinities to β-spectrin peptides were variable. This suggested that their effect on tetramer formation was exerted through defective molecular recognition and disruption of protein–protein interactions at the contact site, rather than an altered structure.[144] These findings contrasted with mutations in the β17 repeat of β-spectrin, which perturbed the structural conformation of this partial repeat and the adjacent β16 repeat.[145] Codon 28 in helix C of α0 has been identified as a mutation "hotspot" because 4 different point mutations occur in this position, resulting in different amino acid substitutions, and the mutations also have been found in several unrelated kindred.[146-148] Arginine 28 is a highly conserved amino acid and any changes in this position are typically associated with severe HE or HPP.[146,148] A case of HE Spα[I/74] involving an intragenic crossover in the α-spectrin gene and uniparental disomy, together with an underlying R34P mutation, was described in a Utah family.[138]

Spα[I/74] defects are also caused by mutations in β-spectrin, predominantly in exon 29 of the *SPTB* gene, which codes for partial repeat 17 that interacts with the αI domain of spectrin and presumably exposes it to increased tryptic digestion. Missense mutations are found in both helices A and B of the β17 repeat,[139,140,149-152] but some in helix A are particularly severe, causing extreme fetal or neonatal anemia and nonimmune hydrops fetalis when inherited in the homozygous state.[107,108,140,153] These include spectrin Providence (S2019P), spectrin Cagliari (A2018G), and a A2053P mutation, where the mutated glycine or proline residues disrupt the α-helical structure of the spectrin repeats.[107,153-155] In the case of spectrin Buffalo (L2025R) there is a charge shift from a hydrophobic amino acid to a positively charged residue at a highly conserved site.[108] Nonsense mutations, frameshift mutations and splicing defects, resulting in truncated spectrin molecules lacking the self-association site also have been described.[134,140,155,156]

Spα[I/65] is a mild defect, even in the homozygous state, which results from a duplication of leucine 154 in helix C of the α1 repeat.[157] It is very common in Africans from West and Central Africa, as well as Arabs in North Africa, suggesting genetic selection, possibly by protecting carriers against *P. falciparum* malaria.[8,134,135]

Spα[I/46 or 50a] mutations are distal from the self-association site and usually occur close to the helical linker regions between individual repeats and often involve the substitution of an amino acid with a proline residue (eg, L207P, L260P), which is a helix breaker.[8,134] In vitro studies on Q471P between repeats 4 and 5 of α-spectrin showed that the mutation uncoupled the repeats and caused cooperative unfolding, which abolished the stabilizing influence of the helical linker on adjacent repeats.[158] Because β-spectrin has fewer repeats than α-spectrin, the alignment of the heterodimers places α4 and α5 in contact with β16 and β17, suggesting that unfolding of the mutant spectrin repeats interferes with the self-association site and prevents tetramer formation.[159] The L260P mutation is in a similar position to Q471P, but is between repeats α2 and α3 of spectrin. When heterodimers are aligned, repeats α0 to α3 are not in contact with β-spectrin, and they represent an open dimer configuration, which facilitates tetramer formation. Open dimers are in equilibrium with closed dimers whereby α0 to α3 are folded onto β16 and β17 of the same dimer, thus preventing bivalent tetramer formation.[159] In vitro experiments on the L260P mutation revealed a conformational change, which stabilized the mutant spectrin in the closed dimer configuration and reduced tetramer assembly.[160]

Mutations in the αII domain of spectrin implicated in HE are rare.[134] Spectrin St Claude is caused by a single point mutation in intron 19 of α-spectrin,[161,162] which creates complex splicing events that ultimately impair the function of both α-spectrin and β-spectrin, resulting in decreased binding to ankyrin, defective spectrin self-association, and spectrin deficiency.[161] These membrane abnormalities have profound effects on red blood cell morphology and survival, manifesting as severe HE. Spectrin Jendouba (Spα[II/31]) is caused by a D791E mutation located in repeat α8, which is far from the self-association site and it is thus asymptomatic in the heterozygous state.[163]

Protein 4.1R Defects in the erythrocyte isoform of protein 4.1 associated with HE are relatively common in some Arab and European populations.[8,134] Heterozygotes exhibit partial deficiency of protein 4.1R, manifesting as mild or asymptomatic HE, whereas rare homozygotes lack protein 4.1R and p55, have a reduced content of GPC, and present with severe HE. These red blood cells are mechanically unstable and fragment at moderate shear stress, but the stability can be restored by reconstituting the deficient red cells with protein 4.1R or the protein 4.1R spectrin–actin binding domain.[164] The protein 4.1R null erythrocytes demonstrate decreased invasion and growth of *P. falciparum* parasites in vitro.[165]

Mutations in the *EPB41* gene often affect the erythroid-specific initiation codon, which abolishes transcription, or else they tend to cluster in the spectrin-actin binding domain where exon deletions or duplications result in mutant proteins that are smaller or larger than normal.[134] A homozygous genomic deletion of 50 kb encompassing the *EPB41* gene of a patient with severe HE and an absence of protein 4.1, resulted in multiple splicing defects and degradation of the abnormal transcripts by nonsense-mediated mRNA decay.[166]

Glycophorin C GPC and GPD carry the Gerbich antigens and rare patients with the Leach phenotype are Gerbich negative and lack both GPs. The underlying mutations are either a 7-kb deletion of genomic DNA or a frameshift mutation.[167] Heterozygous carriers are asymptomatic, with normal red blood cell morphology, whereas homozygous subjects exhibit elliptocytes on the blood film and present with mild HE, presumably caused by the concomitant partial deficiency of protein 4.1R.[8,167]

Molecular Determinants of Clinical Severity

HE patients exhibit marked clinical heterogeneity ranging from asymptomatic carrier to severe, transfusion-dependent anemia. In patients with spectrin heterodimer self-association defects, the resultant increase in spectrin dimers and concomitant decrease in spectrin tetramers, weakens the membrane skeleton and facilitates the formation of elliptocytes under circulatory shear stress. The most important determinants of the severity of hemolysis in these patients are the percentage of spectrin dimers and the spectrin content of the membrane skeleton. These parameters are influenced by the degree of dysfunction of the mutant spectrin, and the gene dose (heterozygote vs homozygote or compound heterozygote).[141] Genotype–phenotype correlations indicate that the order of clinical severity of αI domain defects is Spα[I/74] > Spα[I/46-50a] > Spα[I/65], and it depends on the position of the mutations within the proteins, as well as the type of mutation. Defects in the spectrin dimer self-association contact site leading to Spα[I/74] mutants are the most severe[141] and, for example, codon 28 mutations, which affect a highly conserved and critical arginine residue, are generally associated with phenotypically severe HE or HPP.[146-148] A more distal mutation, such as the duplication of leucine 154, which causes Spα[I/65], is phenotypically very mild, even in the homozygous state.[157] Proline or glycine helix-breaking mutations resulting in Spα[I/46 or 50a] are more severe even though they are further away from the self-association site.[158,160]

The clinical expression of HE often varies within the same kindred, despite all the affected individuals carrying the same causative mutation. This heterogeneity is a result of the inheritance of modifier alleles or additional defects. αLELY, the low-expression Lyon α-spectrin allele, is the most common polymorphism affecting spectrin content and clinical severity. The allele is characterized by an L1857V amino acid substitution, and partial skipping of exon 47 in 50% of the α-spectrin mRNA.[90] The 6 amino acids encoded by exon 47 are essential for spectrin heterodimer assembly. Consequently, αLELY results in a reduced amount of spectrin as monomers are rapidly degraded.[168] The αLELY allele is clinically silent, even when homozygous, because α-spectrin is normally synthesized in three- to four-fold excess.[87] Inheritance of αLELY *in cis* to an elliptocytogenic α-spectrin mutation ameliorates symptoms,[169,170] whereas inheritance *in trans* causes a relative increase in the mutant spectrin, exacerbating the disease manifesting as either severe HE or HPP.[91,151] Rare cases of more than one variant in the *SPTA1* gene have been described.[121,123,171]

Coinheritance of defects in both *SPTA1* and *SPTAB* genes has been identified.[123,151,152,170,172] The phenotypic effect of the double heterozygous mutations varied, depending on the presence or absence of αLELY and whether it was inherited *in cis* or *in trans* to the pathogenic mutation.

Coinheritance of other molecular defects also plays a role in modifying the clinical expression. HPP patients are severely affected because they are homozygous or doubly heterozygous for spectrin self-association mutations and are also deficient in spectrin.[142] Several molecular mechanisms have been identified that underlie the spectrin deficiency, including an RNA processing defect[173]; reduced α-spectrin mRNA and protein synthesis[174]; abnormal splicing resulting in a premature stop codon[175]; degradation of α-spectrin[174]; and nonsense mutations.[176] Complex genotype–phenotype interactions in two large Utah families of Northern European descent in whom a novel R34P mutation in α-spectrin was associated with three morphologic phenotypes have been described.[138] This heterogeneity was caused by an intricate interplay and coinheritance of other factors, including αLELY *in trans*, reduced transcription from the α-spectrin gene, and intragenic crossover.[138]

In neonates the clinical severity of HE can be affected by the weak binding of BPG to fetal hemoglobin leading to an increase in free BPG, which, in turn, destabilizes the spectrin–actin–protein 4.1 interaction.[177] Finally, hemolytic anemia can be exacerbated by several acquired conditions, including those that alter microcirculatory stress to the cells.

Inheritance

HE is typically inherited as an autosomal dominant disorder. De novo mutations are rare.[121] The severity of clinical symptoms is highly variable reflecting heterogeneous molecular abnormalities, as well as the coinheritance of other genetic defects or polymorphisms that modify disease. HPP is an autosomal recessive disorder and a strong genetic relationship exists between HE and HPP, whereby parents or siblings of patients with HPP often have typical HE.

Clinical Features

The clinical presentation of HE is heterogeneous, ranging from asymptomatic carriers to patients with severe, life-threatening anemia. The overwhelming majority of patients with HE are asymptomatic and are diagnosed incidentally during testing for unrelated conditions. HPP patients present in infancy or early childhood with severe hemolytic anemia.

Asymptomatic carriers who possess the same molecular defect as an affected HE relative but who have normal or near-normal blood films have been identified. The erythrocyte life span is normal, and the patients are not anemic. Asymptomatic HE patients may experience hemolysis in association with infections, hypersplenism, vitamin B$_{12}$ deficiency, or microangiopathic hemolysis such as disseminated intravascular coagulation or thrombotic thrombocytopenic purpura. In disseminated intravascular coagulation and thrombotic thrombocytopenic purpura, increased hemolysis may result from microcirculatory damage superimposed on the underlying mechanical instability of red cells.

HE patients with chronic hemolysis experience moderate to severe hemolytic anemia with elliptocytes and poikilocytes on the blood film (see Figs. 15-10D and 15-11F). Red cell life span is decreased and patients may develop complications of chronic hemolysis, such as gallbladder disease. In some kindreds, the hemolytic HE has been transmitted through several generations. In other kindreds, not all HE subjects have chronic hemolysis; some have only mild hemolysis, presumably

because another genetic factor modifies disease expression. The blood films of the most severe HE patients with chronic hemolysis exhibit elliptocytes, poikilocytes, fragments, and small microspherocytes, reminiscent of HPP (see Fig. 15-13).

HPP represents a subtype of common HE, as evidenced by the coexistence of HE and HPP in the same family and the presence of the same molecular defects of spectrin.[143] HE relatives are heterozygous for an elliptocytogenic spectrin mutation, whereas HPP patients are homozygous or doubly heterozygous and are also partially deficient in spectrin.[141,142]

Hereditary Elliptocytosis and Pyropoikilocytosis in Infancy Clinical symptoms of elliptocytosis are uncommon in the neonatal period. Typically, elliptocytes do not appear on the blood film until the patient is 4 to 6 months old. Occasionally, severe forms of HE present in the neonatal period with severe, hemolytic anemia with marked poikilocytosis and jaundice. These patients may require red cell transfusion, phototherapy, or exchange transfusion. Usually, even in severely affected patients, the hemolysis abates between 9 and 12 months of age, and the patient progresses to typical HE with mild anemia. Infrequently, patients remain transfusion-dependent beyond the first year of life and require early splenectomy (see "Indications for splenectomy" earlier for a discussion of splenectomy in a child). In cases of suspected neonatal HE or HPP, review of family history and analysis of blood films from the parents usually are of greater diagnostic benefit than other available studies.

A few cases of hydrops fetalis accompanied by fetal or early neonatal death as a result of unusually severe forms of HE or HPP have been described.[107,140] Some of these hydropic infants survive, but are transfusion-dependent and require splenectomy.[108,140]

Laboratory Features

The hallmark of HE is the presence of cigar-shaped elliptocytes on blood films (see Figs. 15-10D and 15-11F). These normochromic, normocytic elliptocytes may number from a few to all (100%). The degree of hemolysis does not correlate with the number of elliptocytes present. Spherocytes, stomatocytes, and fragmented cells may be seen. OF is increased in severe HE and in HPP.[111,121] The reticulocyte count generally is less than 5% but may be higher when hemolysis is severe. Other laboratory findings in HE are similar to those of other hemolytic anemias and are nonspecific markers of increased erythrocyte production and destruction. For example, increased serum bilirubin, increased urinary urobilinogen, and decreased serum haptoglobin reflect increased erythrocyte destruction.

HPP blood films exhibit similar features to severe HE, but in addition, they reveal extreme poikilocytosis, some bizarre-shaped cells with fragmentation or budding, and often only very few or no elliptocytes (see Fig. 15-13). Microspherocytosis is common and MCV is usually low, ranging between 50 fL and 70 fL. Pyknocytes are prominent on blood films of neonates with HPP. The thermal instability of erythrocytes, originally reported as diagnostic of HPP, is not unique to this disorder as it is also commonly found in HE erythrocytes.

Specialized testing may be required in difficult cases when family history and routine laboratory tests are uninformative or in cases requiring a molecular diagnosis.[111,121,122] Tests on isolated membrane proteins include analysis and quantitation of the proteins by SDS-PAGE; extraction of spectrin from the membranes to evaluate the spectrin dimer/tetramer ratio on nondenaturing gels; and limited tryptic digestion of spectrin followed by SDS-PAGE or 2-dimensional gel electrophoresis to identify the defective domain.[111] Ektacytometry may be used to measure membrane stability and deformability, and the profile exhibits a decreased maximum DI, which is more severe in HPP patients.[111,112,121,151] The EMA test shows a marked reduction in fluorescence in patients with

HPP.[111] Genomic DNA and/or complementary DNA analyses of the defective genes are used to determine the underlying mutation. Targeted NGS[139,151,171,172] and, less frequently, whole-exome sequencing[140] are increasingly being used to identify mutations in HE and HPP patients. Sequencing results of novel mutations should be thoroughly interrogated and should correlate with biochemical features and, where applicable, with *in silico* modeling of the putative mutations on the three-dimensional structure of the proposed defective protein.[124,151]

Differential Diagnosis

Elliptocytes may be seen in association with several disorders, including megaloblastic anemias, hypochromic microcytic anemias (iron-deficiency anemia and thalassemia), myelodysplastic syndromes, and myelofibrosis. In these conditions, elliptocytosis is acquired and generally represents less than 25% of red cells seen on the blood film. History and additional laboratory testing usually clarify the diagnosis of these disorders. Targeted NGS to investigate and diagnose patients with hemolytic anemia has become more affordable and is thus increasingly being used in research-oriented laboratories.[111,121-123] Pseudoelliptocytosis is an artifact of blood film preparation and these cells are found only in certain areas of the film, usually near its tail. The long axes of pseudoelliptocytes are parallel, whereas the axes of true elliptocytes are distributed randomly.

Therapy and Prognosis

Therapy is rarely needed in patients with HE. In rare cases, occasional red blood cell transfusions may be required. In cases of severe HE and HPP, splenectomy has been palliative, as the spleen is the site of erythrocyte sequestration and destruction. The same indications for splenectomy in HS can be applied to patients with symptomatic HE or HPP. Postsplenectomy, patients with HE or HPP exhibit increased hematocrit, decreased reticulocyte counts, and improved clinical symptoms.

Patients should be followed for signs of decompensation during acute illnesses, characterized by acute decrease of hematocrit from nonspecific suppression of erythropoiesis by a concurrent acute event. HE, and particularly HPP patients, are at increased risk for parvovirus infection generally requiring short-lasting transfusion support (Chap. 5).[178] Interval ultrasonography to detect gallstones should be performed. Patients with significant hemolysis should receive daily folate supplementation.

SOUTH EAST ASIAN OVALOCYTOSIS

SAO, also known as Melanesian elliptocytosis or stomatocytic elliptocytosis, is widespread in certain ethnic groups of South-East Asia and the South Pacific, including Malaysia, Papua New Guinea, the Philippines, southern Thailand, and Indonesia,[135] but is also common in the Cape population of mixed-race ancestry in South Africa.[179] It is characterized by the presence of large oval red cells, many of which contain one or two transverse ridges or a longitudinal slit (see Figs. 15-10C and 15-11E).

SAO erythrocytes are rigid and hyperstable because of a structurally and functionally abnormal AE1. SAO AE1 binds tightly to ankyrin, forms oligomers, exhibits restricted lateral and rotational mobility[180] and is unable to transport anions.[181] The underlying molecular abnormality is an in-frame deletion of 27 base pairs (bp) in the *SLC4A1* gene resulting in the loss of amino acids 400 to 408 located at the boundary of the cytoplasmic and the first transmembrane domain of AE1.[182] The first transmembrane domain is a signal anchor that mediates cotranslational insertion of the polypeptide into the membrane. The sequence N-terminal to the domain is an amphipathic helix containing a proline at position 403, which produces a bend that joins the helix to the transmembrane domain. The SAO deletion removes this critical proline and

disrupts the proper folding of the protein.[183] The defective *SLC4A1* allele also carries a linked AE1 Memphis polymorphism, L56E.

SAO is a dominantly inherited trait and homozygosity is postulated to be lethal during embryonic development.[184] A unique case of homozygous SAO has been described where the fetus was kept alive by two intrauterine transfusions and since birth the child has been on a monthly transfusion program.[185] Distal renal tubular acidosis was diagnosed at 3 months caused by the inability of the SAO AE1 to transport anions.

A remarkable feature of SAO erythrocytes is their resistance to infection by several species of malaria parasites, including *P. falciparum* and *P. vivax*. This has been demonstrated by numerous in vitro studies, as well as by in vivo evidence indicating that SAO provides protection against severe malaria and cerebral malaria.[135,186] Epidemiologic data and the increased prevalence of SAO in populations challenged by malaria suggest a selective advantage of the gene.[135] Numerous factors have been implicated in the protective effect,[187] but the precise mechanism of malaria resistance of SAO red cells has not been fully elucidated.

Clinically, the presence on the blood film of at least 20% ovalocytic red cells, some containing a central slit or a transverse ridge, and the notable absence of clinical and laboratory evidence of hemolysis are highly suggestive of SAO. However, a study in Thailand found that babies who were heterozygous for the SAO deletion exhibited significant neonatal hemolysis and anemia, which resolved within a few months.[188] Rapid genetic diagnosis can be made by amplifying the defective region of the *SLC4A1* gene and demonstrating heterozygosity for the SAO allele containing the 27-bp deletion.

ACANTHOCYTOSIS

Spiculated red cells are classified into two types: acanthocytes and echinocytes. *Acanthocytes* are contracted, dense cells with irregular projections from the red cell surface that vary in width and length (see Figs. 15-10F and 15-11G). *Echinocytes* have small, uniform projections spread evenly over the circumference of the red cell (see Fig. 15-11B). Diagnostically, the distinction is not critical, and disorders of spiculated red cells are generally classified together. Normal adults may have as many as 3% of spiculated erythrocytes, but care should be taken when preparing and examining the blood film, because spiculated cells, particularly echinocytes, are common artifacts of blood film preparation and blood storage.

Acanthocytes/echinocytes are found in various inherited disorders and acquired conditions. Spiculated cells can occur transiently in several instances, such as after transfusion with stored blood, ingestion of alcohol and certain drugs, exposure to ionizing radiation or certain venoms, and during hemodialysis.[8] Spiculated cells are commonly seen on the blood films of patients with functional or actual splenectomy, severe liver disease, severe uremia, abetalipoproteinemia, certain inherited neurologic disorders, and abnormalities of the Kell blood group. Occasionally acanthocytes and/or echinocytes may be present in patients with glycolytic enzyme defects, myelodysplasia, hypothyroidism, anorexia nervosa, and vitamin E deficiency, and in premature infants.[8] Individuals with suppressed expression of Lu[a] and Lu[b], the major antigens of the Lutheran blood group system, may also exhibit acanthocytes.[8]

The molecular mechanisms whereby acanthocytes are generated have not been fully elucidated. However, alterations in the conformation of AE1 have emerged as a pivotal causative factor. The abnormal red cell membrane lipid composition and altered lipid distribution between the inner and outer leaflets of the bilayer are only found in some, but not all, of these disorders, implying that they may play a secondary role.[189] The altered morphology and fluidity of acanthocytes render them vulnerable to entrapment and destruction in the spleen, which leads to hemolytic anemia.

ACANTHOCYTOSIS IN SEVERE LIVER DISEASE

Definition

The anemia in patients with liver disease is often called "spur-cell anemia," owing to the projections on the red cells. Although only a small number of patients with end-stage liver disease acquire spur-cell anemia, these individuals typically account for the majority of cases of acanthocytosis seen in clinical practice.

Etiology and Pathogenesis

The anemia in patients with liver disease is of complex etiology. Common causes include blood loss, iron or folate deficiency, hypersplenism, and marrow suppression from alcohol, malnutrition, hepatitis infection, or other factors. Acquired abnormalities of the red cell membrane may contribute to the anemia in some patients.[190]

In vivo acanthocyte formation in spur-cell anemia is a two-step process involving accumulation of free (nonesterified) cholesterol in the red cell membrane and remodeling of abnormally shaped red cells by the spleen.[8,190] The diseased liver of the patient produces abnormal lipoproteins with excess cholesterol, which is acquired by circulating erythrocytes, increasing their cholesterol content. The cholesterol preferentially partitions into the outer leaflet, increasing the surface-area-to-volume ratio and forming scalloped edges. In the spleen, membrane fragments are lost and the cells develop the characteristic projections of acanthocytes. Cholesterol interacts with AE1 and changes its conformation, which may affect the membrane skeleton and reduce the deformability of the cell,[189] causing it to be trapped and eventually destroyed in the narrow sinusoids of the spleen.

Clinical Features

Spur-cell anemia is characterized by rapidly progressive hemolytic anemia with large numbers of acanthocytes on the blood film. Splenomegaly and jaundice become more prominent and are accompanied by severe ascites, bleeding diatheses, and hepatic encephalopathy. Spur-cell anemia is most common in patients with alcoholic liver disease, but similar clinical syndromes have been described in association with advanced metastatic liver disease, cardiac cirrhosis, Wilson disease, fulminant hepatitis, and infantile cholestatic liver disease.[8]

Laboratory Features

Most patients have moderate anemia with a hematocrit of 20% to 30%, marked indirect hyperbilirubinemia, and laboratory evidence of severe hepatocellular disease. Blood films reveal significant acanthocytosis and in some patients, echinocytes, target cells, and microspherocytes, many with very fine spicules, are visible.

Differential Diagnosis

Spur-cell hemolytic anemia should be distinguished from other hemolytic syndromes associated with liver disease, including congestive splenomegaly, in which patients exhibit chronic, mild hemolysis and occasional spherocytes, and patients with transient hemolytic episodes.

Therapy, Course, and Prognosis

The anemia of spur cell anemia usually is not a significant clinical problem, but it can aggravate preexisting anemia resulting from, for example, gastrointestinal bleeding, to the point that erythrocyte transfusion is required. The life span of spur cells is markedly decreased because of splenic sequestration, and, as expected, hemolysis abates after splenectomy. However, splenectomy is a dangerous and potentially fatal procedure in these critically ill patients and is not recommended. The prognosis for patients with alcoholic liver disease and more than 5% spur cells is very poor. A liver transplant is currently the only effective treatment option, combined with alcohol abstinence.[191]

NEUROACANTHOCYTOSIS

Neuroacanthocytosis describes a heterogeneous group of rare disorders with variable clinical phenotypes and inheritance.[192] The common features are a degeneration of neurons and abnormal acanthocytic erythrocyte morphology. These syndromes may be divided into: (1) lipoprotein abnormalities, which cause peripheral neuropathy, such as abetalipoproteinemia and hypobetalipoproteinemia; (2) neural degeneration of the basal ganglia resulting in movement disorders with normal lipoproteins, such as chorea-acanthocytosis and McLeod syndrome; and (3) movement abnormalities in which acanthocytes are occasionally seen, such as Huntington disease-like 2 (HDL2) and pantothenate kinase-associated neurodegeneration (PKAN).

Abetalipoproteinemia

Definition Abetalipoproteinemia or Bassen-Kornzweig syndrome is a very rare autosomal recessive disorder characterized by progressive ataxic neurologic disease, malabsorption of dietary fat and lipid-soluble vitamins (A, D, E, and K), retinal degradation, and acanthocytosis found in people of diverse ethnic backgrounds.[193]

Etiology and Pathogenesis The primary molecular defect in abetalipoproteinemia is a lack of the microsomal triglyceride transfer protein (MTTP), which is an essential cofactor for the assembly and secretion of lipoprotein particles that contain apolipoprotein B (apoB) from enterocytes (chylomicrons) and hepatocytes (very low-density lipoproteins).[194] The absence of apoB-containing lipoproteins leads to malabsorption of lipids and lipid-soluble vitamins, which underlie the clinical manifestations.[192,194] More than 60 MTTP pathogenic variants, which are dispersed throughout the gene, have been identified.[193,195] The majority of these are nonsense mutations, splicing defects, or small indels causing a frameshift, but several pathogenic missense variants that affect MTTP function have been described.[193,195]

The altered plasma lipid profile affects the relative distribution of erythrocyte membrane phospholipids whereby the phosphatidylcholine content is decreased with a corresponding increase in sphingomyelin. The excess sphingomyelin is preferentially confined to the outer leaflet of the membrane bilayer, where it presumably causes an expansion of this layer and modifies the conformation of AE1, which contributes to acanthocyte formation.[189] Red cell precursors and reticulocytes have a normal shape and acanthocytosis only becomes apparent as the red cells mature in the circulation, worsening with increasing red cell age.

Clinical Features The disorder manifests in infancy by failure to thrive, severe diarrhea, vomiting, and steatorrhea.[193] Untreated individuals may develop atypical pigmentation of the retina, which often results in blindness, and progressive neurologic abnormalities characterized by ataxia and intention tremors develop between the first and second decade of life and progress to death in the second or third decade.[193]

Laboratory Features Patients usually have mild anemia with normal red cell indices and normal or slightly increased reticulocyte counts.[193] Acanthocytosis is prominent, ranging from approximately 50% to 90% of red cells. Patients manifest with absent or extremely low low-density lipoprotein cholesterol, triglyceride, and apoB levels.[193] Despite the red cell lipid abnormalities, the hemolysis is mild and the spleen is normal in patients with abetalipoproteinemia, in contrast to spur-cell anemia. There is marked vitamin E deficiency (Chap. 12), which is thought to be a primary cause of the neuropathy. Coagulopathy related to vitamin K deficiency may be observed.[193] Targeted NGS using a multigene panel or single-gene testing is used to identify biallelic mutations in the MTTP gene.[193,195]

Differential Diagnosis Diagnosis of abetalipoproteinemia may be difficult because of its similarity to related conditions hypobetalipoproteinemia, normotriglyceridemic abetalipoproteinemia, and chylomicron retention disease. These disorders are associated with partial production of apoB-containing lipoproteins or with secretion of lipoproteins containing truncated forms of apoB, and patients may experience neurologic disease and acanthocytosis, depending on the severity of the underlying defect. Definitive diagnosis of abetalipoproteinemia involves identifying the mutations in both alleles of the MTTP gene.[193,195]

Therapy, Course, and Prognosis Untreated patients develop severe symptoms with a poor prognosis and typically do not survive beyond the third decade of life. However, lifelong treatment with a low-fat diet and supplementation with high oral doses of vitamins A, K, D, and E, extends the life span considerably with minimal symptoms.[193]

Chorea-Acanthocytosis Syndrome

Chorea-acanthocytosis is a rare autosomal-recessive movement disorder characterized by atrophy of the basal ganglia and progressive neurodegenerative disease with onset in adolescence or early adult life.[196] It has been reported in diverse ethnic groups from many countries. The red blood cells exhibit marked acanthocytosis, which may precede the onset of neurologic symptoms. The lipoproteins are normal.

Two research groups independently identified the causative gene as *VPS13A* (vacuolar protein sorting 13 homolog A), which consists of 73 exons spanning approximately 250 kb of chromosome 9q21. The gene codes for a 360-kDa protein, named chorein, ubiquitously expressed in the brain and also found in mature red cells.[197,198] It is a member of a conserved protein family involved in trafficking of membrane proteins between cellular compartments, but its role in red cells and the pathogenesis of the disorder and acanthocytes is unknown. More than 120 mutations have been identified, which occur throughout the gene and are mainly nonsense or frameshift mutations, as well as splice-site defects and deletions/insertions.[192,196,199] There is no clear genotype–phenotype correlation and the clinical presentation can differ between members of a family.[196] The mutations result in the absence or markedly reduced levels of chorein, and founder mutations have been identified in Japanese and French-Canadian families.[196,199]

Patients are not anemic, and red cell survival is only slightly decreased. Plasma and erythrocyte membrane lipids, as well as membrane protein composition and content, are normal, but electron microscopy studies revealed structural abnormalities in the skeleton and an uneven distribution of intramembrane particles.[192,200] Red cell membrane fluidity is decreased. Increased serine-threonine and tyrosine phosphorylation of AE1, as well as several other membrane proteins, has been documented.[192] In particular, abnormal accumulation of active Lyn kinase, a Src family tyrosine kinase, a consequence of delayed proteasomal degradation and dysregulated autophagy, results in increased tyrosine phosphorylation of AE1.[192,200] This alters the association of AE1 with β-adducin and the junctional complex of the skeleton, which may lead to localized disruption of the skeleton–membrane interaction, facilitating the formation of protrusions.[192] In addition to these posttranslational modifications of membrane proteins, chorein interacts with β-actin and β-adducin, and the loss of chorein may destabilize the skeleton. Interestingly, expression of β-adducin is restricted to the brain and hematopoietic tissues, which corresponds to the main areas of pathology in chorea-acanthocytosis patients.[200]

McLeod Syndrome

The McLeod phenotype is a rare X-linked disorder of the Kell blood group system (Chap. 29), whereby cells react poorly with Kell antisera.[196]

The XK protein is a 50-kDa integral membrane transport channel protein that is covalently linked to the Kell antigen by a single disulfide bond, and is associated with the protein 4.1-based junctional complex in the red cell membrane.[192,201] More than 50 mutations throughout the *XK* gene have been described and are mainly large deletions, nonsense or frameshift mutations that result in the absence of the XK protein, or a dysfunctional truncated protein.[192,201] Some missense mutations produce a milder phenotype. Large deletions involving not only the XK locus at Xp21.1, but also contiguous genes, result in the McLeod syndrome associated with other diseases, such as chronic granulomatous disease of childhood, retinitis pigmentosa, or Duchenne muscular dystrophy.[201]

Male hemizygotes who lack XK exhibit marked acanthocytosis on the blood film with mild, compensated hemolysis.[192] They develop neurologic symptoms during middle age and the clinical features overlap significantly with those of chorea-acanthocytosis.[196,201] The major distinguishing features are the mode of inheritance, the red blood cell immunophenotype and cardiomyopathy. Patients with McLeod syndrome also show a much broader spectrum of phenotypic variability and severity, even within families.[196,201] Female heterozygous carriers with mild symptoms from mosaicism in X chromosome inactivation have occasionally been reported.[196,201]

Red cell membrane protein and lipid composition are normal, but the distribution of intramembrane particles is heterogeneous. Increased tyrosine phosphorylation of membrane proteins, notably ankyrin, protein 4.1R, and AE1, has been noted, which may account for the decreased red cell deformability as measured by ektacytometry.[192] In a Japanese study of several McLeod syndrome patients, reduced levels of chorein were noted and molecular analysis demonstrated a noncovalent interaction of chorein with the XK protein.[202] It is thus likely that multiple factors are involved in destabilizing the membrane and generating acanthocytes in these patients.

Other Neuroacanthocytosis Syndromes

HDL2 is a very rare disorder caused by expanded CGT/CAG trinucleotide repeats in exon 2A of the Junctophilin-3 *(JPH3)* gene on chromosome 16q24.3.[196,203] Normal individuals have between 6 and 27 repeats, whereas HDL2 patients have between 39 and 59 repeats. The age of onset is mainly 40 years and older and correlates inversely with the length of the repeats. The clinical features encompass involuntary movements, neuropsychiatric symptoms, and cognitive defects. The disease is autosomal dominant and has only been reported in individuals of African ancestry. The majority of cases are found in South Africa and the United States.[196,203]

The *JPH3* gene codes for junctophilin-3, a junctional phosphoprotein expressed specifically in the brain where it links the endoplasmic reticulum membrane to the plasma membrane in neurons.[203] Patients have no anemia and acanthocytes (>30%) have only been noted in a small minority of patients.[192,203] Proteolysis of AE1 was noted in only 1 case but this was not verified in a prospective study of 12 HDL2 patients where red cell membrane proteins were normal on SDS-PAGE analysis and no acanthocytes were present. This raises the question of whether HDL2 should be classified as a neuroacanthocytosis.[204]

Acanthocytes have been noted in approximately 10% of patients with PKAN (formerly known as Hallervorden-Spatz syndrome) with features including progressive dystonia, and cognitive impairment in childhood, but no anemia.[192,196] This autosomal recessive disorder is caused by mutations in the *PANK2* gene on chromosome 20p.13 coding for pantothenate kinase 2, an enzyme involved in synthesis of coenzyme A, which is an important component of many biochemical pathways, including phospholipid synthesis.[192,196]

Differential Diagnosis of Neuroacanthocytosis with Normal Lipoproteins Chorea-acanthocytosis, McLeod syndrome, HDL2, and pantothenate kinase disorders present with overlapping neurologic symptoms and clinical phenotypes and also resemble Huntington disease, which renders the clinical diagnosis difficult. Identification of the underlying gene defects and the availability of molecular tests have markedly improved the diagnostic accuracy. This also provides insight into the underlying pathogenesis and suggests that the affected proteins, which are all linked to membrane structure, may participate in a common pathway that ultimately causes degeneration of the basal ganglia.

ERYTHROCYTE HYDRATION DISORDERS

Water and solute homeostasis in the red blood cell is critical for its survival. Several pathways mediate this dynamic process (see Fig. 15-9), but regulation of the intracellular concentration of the monovalent cations, Na^+ and K^+, plays a key role in the maintenance of erythrocyte volume and hydration status. A net increase in these cations causes water to enter the cells resulting in overhydrated cells or stomatocytes, which are cup-shaped red cells characterized by a central hemoglobin-free area (see Figs. 15-10E and 15-11D). The molecular mechanism of stomatocyte formation has not been elucidated. A net loss of cations dehydrates the cells and forms xerocytes.

There is marked clinical, biochemical, and genetic heterogeneity in these disorders (Table 15-4). In over-hydration syndromes the causative genes are *RHAG*, *SLC4A1*, and *GLUT1*, whereas *PIEZO1* and *KCNN4* have been implicated in dehydration syndromes.[205-207] Despite these advances, the underlying molecular defect in several of these patients is still unknown.

Disorders of red cell cation permeability are rare conditions that are typically inherited in an autosomal dominant fashion but de novo mutations have been reported.[205] Diagnosis may be challenging and thus these syndromes may be underdiagnosed.[206] A bioinformatics study described a gain-of-function *PIEZO1* E756del mutation with a predicted allele frequency of ~18% in African populations. Red blood cells from E756del carriers are dehydrated and are less susceptible to invasion by *P. falciparum* in vitro. These findings imply an association of this *PIEZO1* allele with resistance to malaria.[208]

HEREDITARY XEROCYTOSIS

Definition and History

Hereditary xerocytosis, also known as dehydrated HSt, is the most common form of the cation permeability defects. The disorder was first described in 1971, but the defective *PIEZO1* gene was first identified more than 30 years later by three independent research groups.[209] It is an autosomal dominant hemolytic anemia characterized by an efflux of K^+ leading to red cell dehydration. Hereditary xerocytosis is part of a pleiotropic syndrome and patients may also exhibit pseudohyperkalemia and perinatal edema.[207,209]

Etiology and Pathogenesis

The underlying membrane permeability defect is complex and involves a net loss of potassium from the red cells that is not accompanied by a proportional gain of sodium. Consequently, the net intracellular cation content and cell water content are decreased.

The majority of hereditary xerocytosis patients harbor mutations in the *PIEZO1* gene.[205-207,210] The PIEZO1 protein is a large integral membrane protein that assembles into a trimer and serves as a cation selective channel that is activated by mechanical stimuli encountered by red cells as they navigate narrow capillaries and splenic sinusoids.[205,207,210] Most of the mutations are missense, gain-of-function defects, that are spread throughout the gene. Three mutations, R2456H, T2127M, and a duplication of L2495 and E2496, cluster in the C-terminal portion of the protein that forms the pore and accounts for more than 50% of all the mutations in hereditary xerocytosis patients.[205-207] The defective PIEZO1 protein typically displays enhanced activation and a slower rate of inactivation, which increases cation efflux.[205-207] PIEZO1 is expressed in early erythroid progenitor cells and plays a role in erythropoiesis, which correlates with in vitro studies on primary cells from patients with PIEZO1 mutations that demonstrated a delay in erythroid differentiation.[211] Delayed maturation of reticulocytes has also been documented.[212] Several mechanisms have been proposed to cause dehydration of the cells, but the exact molecular sequence of events remains to be fully clarified.

A minority of hereditary xerocytosis patients have mutations in the *KCNN4* gene, which codes for the Gardos channel, a calcium-activated

TABLE 15-4. Hereditary Stomatocytosis Syndromes

| | Hydrocytosis | | Cryohydrocytosis | Xerocytosis |
	Severe Hemolysis	Mild Hemolysis		
Hemolysis	Severe	Mild to moderate	Mild to moderate	Mild to moderate
Anemia	Severe	Mild to moderate	Mild to moderate	Mild to moderate
Blood film	Stomatocytes	Stomatocytes	Stomatocytes	Target cells, echinocytes
MCV (80-100 fL)[a]	110-150	95-130	90-105	90-110
MCHC (32%-36%)	24-30	26-29	34-40	34-38
Unincubated osmotic fragility	Markedly increased	Increased	Normal	Markedly decreased
RBC Na^+ (5-12 mEq/L)	60-150	30-60	40-50	10-20
RBC K^+ (90-103 mEq/L)	20-55	40-85	55-65	60-80
RBC $Na^+ + K^+$ (95-110 mEq/L)	110-170	115-145	100-105	75-90
Effect of splenectomy[b]	Good	Good	Little or no effect	Poor
Gene defects	*RHAG*	*SLC4A1*	*GLUT1*	*PIEZO1/KCNN4*

[a]Values in parentheses are the reference range.
[b]Splenectomy may be contraindicated in these syndromes.

K+ channel.[206,207] and it has been suggested to refer to these cases as Gardos channelopathy.[213,214] The protein is inactive in normal mature red cells and its role has not been clearly elucidated. The *KCNN4* mutations are predominantly missense, including a recurrent p.Arg352His mutation, but an 18 bp deletion has also been reported.[213] The mutant proteins display altered kinetics and cation transport.[205,206]

Clinical Features

Patients may present with symptoms of compensated hemolytic anemia, including jaundice, splenomegaly, and gallstones. Some patients may also exhibit pseudohyperkalemia and perinatal edema, and even hydrops fetalis that usually resolves spontaneously.[8,205,207,209] Patients display a strong tendency to iron overload regardless of transfusion history (Chap. 11).[205,209,213] There is significant variation in clinical symptoms not only between unrelated kindred, but even between individuals in the same family, implying that other, as yet unknown, modifying factors influence disease severity.

Laboratory Features

The hematologic picture is that of mild to moderate compensated hemolytic anemia (see Table 15-4) with an elevated reticulocyte count. The K+ content is decreased and the Na+ content is increased, but the total monovalent cation content may be slightly reduced. The MCHC is increased reflecting cellular dehydration and the MCV is frequently mildly increased.[205,209] Studies on the metabolome of red cells from patients with *PIEZO1* mutations revealed impaired glycolysis and an increased affinity of hemoglobin for oxygen.[215]

Erythrocytes are resistant to osmotic lysis and the osmotic gradient ektacytometry curve is shifted to the left reflecting cellular dehydration and reduced deformability,[112,205,207,214] but in some patients with Gardos channelopathy, the ektacytometry curve is normal.[214] NGS with appropriate gene panels is recommended to identify underlying mutations and to prevent misdiagnosis.[112]

Stomatocytes are not a prominent feature on blood films, but occasional target cells are seen.[205,206,209,210] In some cells, hemoglobin is concentrated ("puddled") in discrete areas on the cell periphery.[205]

Therapy, Course, and Prognosis

Most patients experience only mild anemia and therapy is generally not required, but transfusions may be administered in patients with symptomatic moderate anemia.[209] The patients should receive folate supplementation and be monitored for complications of hemolysis and iron overload.[112] Splenectomy does not significantly improve the anemia, which suggests that xerocytes are detected and eliminated in other areas of the mononuclear phagocyte system. Because of a markedly high risk of hypercoagulability and life-threatening thrombotic episodes after splenectomy, the procedure is contraindicated.[8,112,205,209]

OVERHYDRATED HEREDITARY STOMATOCYTOSIS

Definition and History

Overhydrated HSt, also known as hereditary hydrocytosis, is a very rare heterogeneous disorder characterized by a marked passive sodium leak, which increases the water content of the cell and causes macrocytosis. It is inherited in an autosomal dominant manner and was first described in a girl with hemolytic anemia whose blood film contained stomatocytes.[207]

Etiology and Pathogenesis

The red cell membrane of stomatocytes has greatly enhanced permeability toward monovalent cations, especially sodium ions. This marked passive sodium leak into the cell represents the principal lesion in this disorder. The Na+-K+ ATPase pump, which normally maintains low intracellular sodium and high potassium concentrations, is stimulated but this increase in active transport, coupled to enhanced glycolysis to provide ATP, is insufficient to overcome the leak.[205,207]

In most patients there is either a lack of stomatin or, less often, very low levels of this 31-kDa integral membrane protein. However, no gene mutations have been found, which implies that the absence of the protein is a secondary phenomenon. Its role in the pathogenesis of the disorder is unknown.[205,207]

In some overhydrated stomatocytosis patients, heterozygous missense mutations causing amino acid substitutions of highly conserved residues in the transmembrane domain of the RhAG protein, have been described.[207] RhAG is a component of the AE1 macromolecular protein complex in the membrane and is a transport protein that may function as a CO_2 and/or ammonium channel. The mutations are thought to dilate the channel allowing cations to leak through the membrane.[205-207] Several missense mutations in the corresponding *SLC4A1* gene have been identified in some overhydrated stomatocytosis patients. These do not alter the AE1 protein content of the membrane, but they affect the transmembrane domain and it is proposed that they change the conformation of the protein, which stimulates cation transport through the multiprotein anion exchanger complex.[206,207]

Clinical Features

Moderate to severe anemia is present, but patients with AE1 mutations are less severely affected.[205,206] Jaundice and splenomegaly are common, as are complications of chronic hemolysis such as cholelithiasis. Patients exhibit a tendency for iron overload, independent of transfusion status or splenectomy. No other organ system abnormalities have been noted.[8]

Laboratory Features

The blood film reveals striking stomatocytosis and as much as 50% of red cells may have abnormal morphology (see Figs. 15-10E and 15-11D).[205,206] In addition to the anemia, red cell indices show decreased MCHC and marked macrocytosis, as reflected by an elevated MCV, which can reach 150 fL in some severely affected patients (see Table 15-4). The K+ content is decreased and the Na+ content is markedly increased, leading to elevated total monovalent cation content. The OF of stomatocytes is markedly increased because many of the swollen red cells approach their critical hemolytic volume, which causes a shift of the osmotic gradient ektacytometer curve to the right.[205] Red cell deformability is decreased.

Therapy, Course, and Prognosis

The majority of hydrocytosis patients suffer from significant lifelong anemia. They should be monitored for complications of hemolysis, such as cholelithiasis and parvovirus infection, and iron overload, and should receive folate supplementation. The outcome of splenectomy has been variable, but typically it has been beneficial and improved the hemolytic anemia in severely affected patients.[8] This is expected because stomatocytes expend large amounts of ATP to pump cations in an attempt to avoid osmotic lysis, which makes the stomatocytes vulnerable in the metabolically challenging environment of the spleen. However, splenectomy should be carefully considered in patients with this disorder, because they are at high risk of developing chronic pulmonary hypertension, as well as hypercoagulability after splenectomy, leading to catastrophic thrombotic episodes.[8,205]

CRYOHYDROCYTOSIS

Cryohydrocytosis patients exhibit a mild cation leak that is markedly enhanced at low temperatures. It is a very rare condition associated with mild to moderate hemolytic anemia, and splenectomy appears to have little or no effect.[205] Missense mutations have been found in the transmembrane section of AE1 and in vitro studies indicate that the mutant proteins lose their anion exchange capability and are converted to a nonselective cation channel.[205,210]

A few cases of cryohydrocytosis and stomatin deficiency have been described with mutations in the *GLUT1* gene.[205] These alter the folding of the GLUT1 protein, which impedes glucose transport and creates a cation leak.[206,207,210]

OTHER STOMATOCYTIC DISORDERS

Intermediate syndromes are very rare cases where the clinical phenotype and biochemical features of some patients with stomatocytes are intermediate between the extremes of hereditary hydrocytosis and hereditary xerocytosis. In some patients, red cells exhibit an increase in phosphatidylcholine.[8] Mutations have been noted in the *PIEZO1* gene, but the defect is unknown in other instances.[205]

Familial deficiency of high-density lipoproteins is a rare condition that leads to accumulation of cholesteryl esters in many tissues, resulting in clinical findings of large orange tonsils and hepatosplenomegaly. Hematologic manifestations include moderately severe hemolytic anemia with stomatocytosis. Red cell membrane lipid analyses revealed a low cholesterol content and a relative increase in phosphatidylcholine at the expense of sphingomyelin.[8]

ACQUIRED STOMATOCYTOSIS

Acquired stomatocytosis is common in alcoholics, particularly in acute alcoholism.[210] Vinca alkaloids, such as vincristine and vinblastine, may induce hemolysis with increased sodium permeability and stomatocytosis at the doses used for chemotherapy of leukemias and lymphomas. Transient stomatocytosis has been observed in long-distance runners immediately after a race.[210] The molecular basis of acquired stomatocytosis is unknown.

REFERENCES

1. Mohandas N, Gallagher PG. Red cell membrane: past, present, and future. *Blood.* 2008;112:3939.
2. Arashiki N, Takakuwa Y. Maintenance and regulation of asymmetric phospholipid distribution in human erythrocyte membranes: implications for erythrocyte functions. *Curr Opin Hematol.* 2017;24:167.
3. Fairbanks G, Steck TL, Wallach DF. Electrophoretic analysis of the major polypeptides of the human erythrocyte membrane. *Biochemistry.* 1971;10:2606.
4. Bryk AH, Wisniewski JR. Quantitative analysis of human red cell proteome. *J Proteome Res.* 2017;16:2752.
5. Gautier E, Leduc M, Cochet S, et al. Absolute proteome quantification of highly purified populations of circulating reticulocytes and mature erythrocytes. *Blood Adv.* 2018;2:2646.
6. van den Akker E, Satchwell TJ, Williamson RC, et al. Band 3 multiprotein complexes in the red cell membrane; of mice and men. *Blood Cells Mol Dis.* 2010;45:1.
7. Reithmeier RA, Casey JR, Kalli AC, et al. Band 3, the human red cell chloride/bicarbonate anion exchanger (AE1, SLC4A1), in a structural context. *Biochim Biophys Acta.* 2016;1858:1507.
8. Walensky LD, Narla M, Lux SE. Disorders of the red blood cell membrane. In: Handin RI, Lux SE, Stossel TP, eds. *Blood: Principles and Practice of Hematology.* 2nd ed. Lippincott Williams & Wilkins; 2003:1709.
9. Arakawa T, Kobayashi-Yurugi T, Alguel Y, et al. Crystal structure of the anion exchanger domain of human erythrocyte band 3. *Science.* 2015;350:680.
10. Sterling D, Reithmeier RA, Casey JR. A transport metabolon. Functional interaction of carbonic anhydrase II and chloride/bicarbonate exchangers. *J Biol Chem.* 2001;276:47886.
11. Sterling D, Alvarez BV, Casey JR. The extracellular component of a transport metabolon. Extracellular loop 4 of the human AE1 Cl–/HCO3– exchanger binds carbonic anhydrase IV. *J Biol Chem.* 2002;277:25239.
12. Zhang D, Kiyatkin A, Bolin JT, et al. Crystallographic structure and functional interpretation of the cytoplasmic domain of erythrocyte membrane band 3. *Blood.* 2000;96:2925.
13. Puchulu-Campanella E, Chu H, Anstee DJ, et al. Identification of the components of a glycolytic enzyme metabolon on the human red blood cell membrane. *J Biol Chem.* 2013;288:848.
14. Lux SE. Anatomy of the red cell membrane skeleton: unanswered questions. *Blood.* 2016;127:187.
15. Rybicki AC, Musto S, Schwartz RS. Identification of a band-3 binding site near the N-terminus of erythrocyte membrane protein 4.2. *Biochem J.* 1995;309:677.
16. Anong WA, Franco T, Chu H, et al. Adducin forms a bridge between the erythrocyte membrane and its cytoskeleton and regulates membrane cohesion. *Blood.* 2009;114:1904.
17. Lee G, Abdi K, Jiang Y, et al. Nanospring behaviour of ankyrin repeats. *Nature.* 2006;440:247.
18. Michaely P, Bennett V. The ANK repeats of erythrocyte ankyrin form two distinct but cooperative binding sites for the erythrocyte anion exchanger. *J Biol Chem.* 1995;270:22050.
19. Bruce LJ, Beckmann R, Ribeiro ML, et al. A band 3–based macrocomplex of integral and peripheral proteins in the RBC membrane. *Blood.* 2003;101:4180.
20. Williamson RC, Toye AM. Glycophorin A: band 3 aid. *Blood Cells Mol Dis.* 2008;41:35.
21. Schofield A, Martin P, Spillett D, et al. The structure of the human red blood cell anion exchanger (EPB3, AE1, band 3) gene. *Blood.* 1994;84:2000.
22. Rearden A, Magnet A, Kudo S, et al. Glycophorin B and glycophorin E genes arose from the glycophorin A ancestral gene via two duplications during primate evolution. *J Biol Chem.* 1993;268:2260.
23. Cartron JP, Le Van Kim C, Colin Y. Glycophorin C and related glycoproteins: structure, function, and regulation. *Semin Hematol.* 1993;30:152.
24. Thomas GH, Newbern EC, Korte CC, et al. Intragenic duplication and divergence in the spectrin superfamily of proteins. *Mol Biol Evol.* 1997;14:1285.
25. Grum VL, Li D, MacDonald RI, et al. Structures of two repeats of spectrin suggest models of flexibility. *Cell.* 1999;98:523.
26. Speicher DW, Marchesi VT. Erythrocyte spectrin is comprised of many homologous triple helical segments. *Nature.* 1984;311:177.
27. Li D, Tang H-Y, Speicher DW. A structural model of the erythrocyte spectrin heterodimer initiation site determined using homology modeling and chemical cross-linking. *J Biol Chem.* 2008;283:1553.
28. Ipsaro JJ, Harper SL, Messick TE, et al. Crystal structure and functional interpretation of the erythrocyte spectrin tetramerization domain complex. *Blood.* 2010;115:4843.
29. Becker PS, Schwartz MA, Morrow JS, et al. Radiolabel-transfer cross-linking demonstrates that protein 4.1 binds to the N-terminal region of β spectrin and to actin in binary interactions. *Eur J Biochem.* 1990;193:827.
30. Liu SC, Derick LH, Palek J. Visualization of the hexagonal lattice in the erythrocyte membrane skeleton. *J Cell Biol.* 1987;104:527.
31. Korsgren C, Lux SE. The carboxyterminal EF domain of erythroid α-spectrin is necessary for optimal spectrin-actin binding. *Blood.* 2010;116:2600.
32. Ipsaro JJ, Huang L, Mondragón A. Structures of the spectrin-ankyrin interaction binding domains. *Blood.* 2009;113:5385.
33. Stabach PR, Simonović I, Ranieri MA, et al. The structure of the ankyrin-binding site of β-spectrin reveals how tandem spectrin-repeats generate unique ligand-binding properties. *Blood.* 2009;113:5377.
34. Yocum AO, Steiner LA, Seidel NE, et al. A tissue-specific chromatin loop activates the erythroid ankyrin-1 promoter. *Blood.* 2012;120:3586.
35. Michaely P, Tomchick DR, Machius M, et al. Crystal structure of a 12 ANK repeat stack from human ankyrinR. *EMBO J.* 2002;21:6387.
36. Ipsaro JJ, Mondragón A. Structural basis for spectrin recognition by ankyrin. *Blood.* 2010;115:4093.
37. Gallagher PG, Tse WT, Scarpa AL, et al. Structure and organization of the human ankyrin-1 gene: basis for complexity of pre-mRNA processing. *J Biol Chem.* 1997;272:19220.
38. Parra MK, Gee SL, Koury MJ, et al. Alternative 5′ exons and differential splicing regulate expression of protein 4.1R isoforms with distinct N-termini. *Blood.* 2003;101:4164.
39. Inaba M, Gupta K, Kuwabara M, et al. Deamidation of human erythrocyte protein 4.1: possible role in aging. *Blood.* 1992;79:3355.
40. Satchwell TJ, Shoemark DK, Sessions RB, et al. Protein 4.2: a complex linker. *Blood Cells Mol Dis.* 2009;42:201.
41. Chishti AH. Function of p55 and its nonerythroid homologues. *Curr Opin Hematol.* 1998;5:116.
42. Li X, Matsuoka Y, Bennett V. Adducin preferentially recruits spectrin to the fast growing ends of actin filaments in a complex requiring the MARCKS-related domain and a newly defined oligomerization domain. *J Biol Chem.* 1998;273:19329.
43. Khan AA, Hanada T, Mohseni M, et al. Dematin and adducin provide a novel link between the spectrin cytoskeleton and human erythrocyte membrane by directly interacting with glucose transporter-1. *J Biol Chem.* 2008;283:14600.
44. Robledo RF, Ciciotte SL, Gwynn B, et al. Targeted deletion of α-adducin results in absent β- and γ-adducin, compensated hemolytic anemia, and lethal hydrocephalus in mice. *Blood.* 2008;112:4298.
45. Gokhin DS, Fowler VM. Feisty filaments: actin dynamics in the red blood cell membrane skeleton. *Curr Opin Hematol.* 2016;23:206.
46. Azim AC, Knoll JH, Beggs AH, Chishti AH. Isoform cloning, actin binding, and chromosomal localization of human erythroid dematin, a member of the villin superfamily. *J Biol Chem.* 1995;270:17407.
47. Lu Y, Hanada T, Fujiwara Y, et al. Gene disruption of dematin causes precipitous loss of erythrocyte membrane stability and severe hemolytic anemia. *Blood.* 2016;128:93.

48. Namvar A, Blanch AJ, Dixon MW, et al. Surface area-to-volume ratio, not cellular viscoelasticity, is the major determinant of red blood cell traversal through small channels. *Cellular Microbiol.* 2021;23:e13270.

49. Brugnara C. Erythrocyte membrane transport physiology. *Curr Opin Hematol.* 1997;4:122.

50. Agre P, King LS, Yasui M, et al. Aquaporin water channels—from atomic structure to clinical medicine. *J Physiol.* 2002;542:3.

51. Mueckler M, Caruso C, Baldwin S, et al. Sequence and structure of a human glucose transporter. *Science.* 1985;229:941.

52. Palek J. Disorders of the red cell membrane skeleton: an overview. Erythrocyte membranes 3: recent clinical and experimental advances, edited by WL Kruckeberg, EJ W, GJ Brewer and AR Liss. p. 177. Liss, New York, 1984.

53. Vanlair C, Masius J. De la microcythemie. *Bull Acad R Med Belg.* 1871;5:515.

54. Perrotta S, Gallagher PG, Mohandas N. Hereditary spherocytosis. *Lancet.* 2008; 372:1411.

55. Iolascon A, Avvisati RA. Genotype/phenotype correlation in hereditary spherocytosis. *Haematologica.* 2008;93:1283.

56. Tole S, Dhir P, Pugi J, et al. Genotype-phenotype correlation in children with hereditary spherocytosis. *Br J Haematol.* 2020;191:486.

57. Hao L, Li S, Ma D, et al. Two novel *ANK1* loss-of-function mutations in Chinese families with hereditary spherocytosis. *J Cell Mol Med.* 2019;23:4454.

58. Crisp RL, Solari L, Vota D, et al. A prospective study to assess the predictive value for hereditary spherocytosis using five laboratory tests (cryohemolysis test, eosin-5'-maleimide flow cytometry, osmotic fragility test, autohemolysis test, and SDS-PAGE) on 50 hereditary spherocytosis families in Argentina. *Ann Hematol.* 2011; 90:625.

59. Aggarwal A, Jamwal M, Sharma P, et al. Deciphering molecular heterogeneity of Indian families with hereditary spherocytosis using targeted next-generation sequencing: First South Asian study. *Br J Haematol.* 2020;188:784.

60. Choi HS, Choi Q, Kim JA, et al. Molecular diagnosis of hereditary spherocytosis by multi-gene target sequencing in Korea: matching with osmotic fragility test and presence of spherocyte. *Orphanet J Rare Dis.* 2019;14:114.

61. Park J, Jeong DC, Yoo J, et al. Mutational characteristics of ANK1 and SPTB genes in hereditary spherocytosis. *Clin Genet.* 2016;90:69.

62. van Vuren A, van der Zwaag B, Huisjes R, et al. The complexity of genotype-phenotype correlations in hereditary spherocytosis: a cohort of 95 patients: genotype-phenotype correlation in hereditary spherocytosis. *Hemasphere.* 2019;3:e276.

63. Rocha S, Rebelo I, Costa E, et al. Protein deficiency balance as a predictor of clinical outcome in hereditary spherocytosis. *Eur J Haematol.* 2005;74:374.

64. Mariani M, Barcellini W, Vercellati C, et al. Clinical and hematologic features of 300 patients affected by hereditary spherocytosis grouped according to the type of the membrane protein defect. *Haematologica.* 2008;93:1310.

65. Yawata Y, Kanzaki A, Yawata A, et al. Characteristic features of the genotype and phenotype of hereditary spherocytosis in the Japanese population. *Int J Hematol.* 2000;71:118.

66. Coetzer TL, Lawler J, Liu S-C, et al. Partial ankyrin and spectrin deficiency in severe, atypical hereditary spherocytosis. *N Engl J Med.* 1988;318:230.

67. Eber SW, Gonzalez JM, Lux ML, et al. Ankyrin-1 mutations are a major cause of dominant and recessive hereditary spherocytosis. *Nat Genet.* 1996;13:214.

68. Edelman EJ, Maksimova Y, Duru F, et al. A complex splicing defect associated with homozygous ankyrin-deficient hereditary spherocytosis. *Blood.* 2007;109:5491.

69. Gallagher PG, Nilson DG, Wong C, et al. A dinucleotide deletion in the ankyrin promoter alters gene expression, transcription initiation and TFIID complex formation in hereditary spherocytosis. *Hum Mol Genet.* 2005;14:2501.

70. Gallagher PG, Steiner LA, Liem RI, et al. Mutation of a barrier insulator in the human ankyrin-1 gene is associated with hereditary spherocytosis. *J Clin Invest.* 2010;120:4453.

71. Lux SE, Tse WT, Menninger JC, et al. Hereditary spherocytosis associated with deletion of human erythrocyte ankyrin gene on chromosome 8. *Nature.* 1990;345:736.

72. Jarolim P, Rubin H, Brabec V, et al. Mutations of conserved arginines in the membrane domain of erythroid band 3 lead to a decrease in membrane-associated band 3 and to the phenotype of hereditary spherocytosis. *Blood.* 1995;85:634.

73. Bracher NA, Lyons CA, Wessels G, et al. Band 3 Cape Town (E90K) causes severe hereditary spherocytosis in combination with band 3 Prague III. *Br J Haematol.* 2001;113:689.

74. Alloisio N, Texier P, Vallier A, et al. Modulation of clinical expression and band 3 deficiency in hereditary spherocytosis. *Blood.* 1997;90:414.

75. Ribeiro ML, Alloisio N, Almeida H, et al. Severe hereditary spherocytosis and distal renal tubular acidosis associated with the total absence of band 3. *Blood.* 2000;96:1602.

76. Kager L, Bruce LJ, Zeitlhofer P, et al. Band 3 null(VIENNA), a novel homozygous SLC4A1 p.Ser477X variant causing severe hemolytic anemia, dyserythropoiesis and complete distal renal tubular acidosis. *Pediatr Blood Cancer.* 2017;64:10.1002/pbc.26227. doi:10.1002/pbc.26227.

77. Yang E, Seo-Mayer P, Lezon-Geyda K, et al. A Ser725Arg mutation in band 3 abolishes transport function and leads to anemia and renal tubular acidosis. *Blood.* 2018;131:1759.

78. Fawaz NA, Beshlawi IO, Al Zadjali S, et al. dRTA and hemolytic anemia: first detailed description of SLC4A1 A858D mutation in homozygous state. *Eur J Haematol.* 2012;88:350.

79. Shmukler BE, Kedar PS, Warang P, et al. Hemolytic anemia and distal renal tubular acidosis in two Indian patients homozygous for SLC4A1/AE1 mutation A858D. *Am J Hematol.* 2010;85:824.

80. Toye AM, Williamson RC, Khanfar M, et al. Band 3 Courcouronnes (Ser667Phe): a trafficking mutant differentially rescued by wild-type band 3 and glycophorin A. *Blood.* 2008;111:5380.

81. Perrotta S, Borriello A, Scaloni A, et al. The N-terminal 11 amino acids of human erythrocyte band 3 are critical for aldolase binding and protein phosphorylation: implications for band 3 function. *Blood.* 2005;106:4359.

82. Agre P, Casella JF, Zinkham WH, et al. Partial deficiency of erythrocyte spectrin in hereditary spherocytosis. *Nature.* 1985;314:380.

83. Agre P, Asimos A, Casella JF, et al. Inheritance pattern and clinical response to splenectomy as a reflection of erythrocyte spectrin deficiency in hereditary spherocytosis. *N Engl J Med.* 1986;315:1579.

84. Liu S, Derick L, Agre P, et al. Alteration of the erythrocyte membrane skeletal ultrastructure in hereditary spherocytosis, hereditary elliptocytosis, and pyropoikilocytosis. *Blood.* 1990;76:198.

85. Chonat S, Risinger M, Sakthivel H, et al. The spectrum of SPTA1-associated hereditary spherocytosis. *Front Physiol.* 2019;10:815.

86. Gallagher PG, Maksimova Y, Lezon-Geyda K, et al. Aberrant splicing contributes to severe α-spectrin-linked congenital hemolytic anemia. *J Clin Invest.* 2019;129:2878.

87. Hanspal M, Palek J. Biogenesis of normal and abnormal red blood cell membrane skeleton. *Semin Hematol.* 1992;29:305.

88. Wichterle H, Hanspal M, Palek J, et al. Combination of two mutant alpha spectrin alleles underlies a severe spherocytic hemolytic anemia. *J Clin Invest.* 1996; 98:2300.

89. Delaunay J, Nouyrigat V, Proust A, et al. Different impacts of alleles αLEPRA and αLELY as assessed versus a novel, virtually null allele of the SPTA1 gene in trans. *Br J Haematol.* 2004;127:118.

90. Wilmotte R, Maréchal J, Morlé L, et al. Low expression allele alpha LELY of red cell spectrin is associated with mutations in exon 40 (alpha V/41 polymorphism) and intron 45 and with partial skipping of exon 46. *J Clin Invest.* 1993;91:2091.

91. Tse WT, Gallagher PG, Jenkins PB, et al. Amino-acid substitution in α-spectrin commonly coinherited with nondominant hereditary spherocytosis. *Am J Hematol.* 1997;54:233.

92. Bogardus H, Schulz VP, Maksimova Y, et al. Severe nondominant hereditary spherocytosis due to uniparental isodisomy at the SPTA1 locus. *Haematologica.* 2014;99:e168.

93. Hassoun H, Vassiliadis JN, Murray J, et al. Characterization of the underlying molecular defect in hereditary spherocytosis associated with spectrin deficiency. *Blood.* 1997;90:398.

94. Hassoun H, Vassiliadis J, Murray J, et al. Hereditary spherocytosis with spectrin deficiency due to an unstable truncated beta spectrin. *Blood.* 1996;87:2538.

95. Hassoun H, Vassiliadis JN, Murray J, et al. Molecular basis of spectrin deficiency in beta spectrin Durham. A deletion within beta spectrin adjacent to the ankyrin-binding site precludes spectrin attachment to the membrane in hereditary spherocytosis. *J Clin Invest.* 1995;96:2623.

96. Becker PS, Tse WT, Lux SE, et al. Beta spectrin kissimmee: a spectrin variant associated with autosomal dominant hereditary spherocytosis and defective binding to protein 4.1. *J Clin Invest.* 1993;92:612.

97. Bouhassira E, Schwartz R, Yawata Y, et al. An alanine-to-threonine substitution in protein 4.2 cDNA is associated with a Japanese form of hereditary hemolytic anemia (protein 4.2NIPPON). *Blood.* 1992;79:1847.

98. Hammill AM, Risinger MA, Joiner CH, et al. Compound heterozygosity for two novel mutations in the erythrocyte protein 4.2 gene causing spherocytosis in a Caucasian patient. *Br J Haematol.* 2011;152:780.

99. De Franceschi L, Olivieri O, del Giudice EM, et al. Membrane cation and anion transport activities in erythrocytes of hereditary spherocytosis: effects of different membrane protein defects. *Am J Hematol.* 1997;55:121.

100. Alloisio N, Maillet P, Carre G, et al. Hereditary spherocytosis with band 3 deficiency. Association with a nonsense mutation of the band 3 gene (allele Lyon), and aggravation by a low-expression allele occurring in trans (allele Genas). *Blood.* 1996;88:1062.

101. Delhommeau F, Cynober T, Schischmanoff PO, et al. Natural history of hereditary spherocytosis during the first year of life. *Blood.* 2000;95:393.

102. Iolascon A, Faienza MF, Moretti A, et al. UGT1 promoter polymorphism accounts for increased neonatal appearance of hereditary spherocytosis. *Blood.* 1998;91:1093.

103. Safeukui I, Buffet PA, Deplaine G, et al. Quantitative assessment of sensing and sequestration of spherocytic erythrocytes by the human spleen. *Blood.* 2012;120:424.

104. Emerson CP Jr, Shen SC, Ham TH, et al. Studies on the destruction of red blood cells: IX. Quantitative methods for determining the osmotic and mechanical fragility of red cells in the peripheral blood and splenic pulp; the mechanism of increased hemolysis in hereditary spherocytosis (congenital hemolytic jaundice) as related to the functions of the spleen. *AMA Arch Intern Med.* 1956;97:1.

105. Eber SW, Armbrust R, Schröter W. Variable clinical severity of hereditary spherocytosis: relation to erythrocytic spectrin concentration, osmotic fragility, and autohemolysis. *J Pediatr.* 1990;117:409.

106. Pajor A, Lehoczky D, Szakács Z. Pregnancy and hereditary spherocytosis. *Arch Gynecol Obstet.* 1993;253:37.

107. Gallagher PG, Weed SA, Tse WT, et al. Recurrent fatal hydrops fetalis associated with a nucleotide substitution in the erythrocyte beta-spectrin gene. *J Clin Invest.* 1995;95:1174.

108. Gallagher PG, Petruzzi MJ, Weed SA, et al. Mutation of a highly conserved residue of betaI spectrin associated with fatal and near-fatal neonatal hemolytic anemia. *J Clin Invest.* 1997;99:267.

109. Lima PR, Gontijo JA, Lopes de Faria JB, et al. Band 3 Campinas: a novel splicing mutation in the band 3 gene (AE1) associated with hereditary spherocytosis, hyperactivity of Na+/Li+ countertransport and an abnormal renal bicarbonate handling. *Blood.* 1997;90:2810.

110. Rysavá R, Tesar V, Jirsa M Jr, et al. Incomplete distal renal tubular acidosis coinherited with a mutation in the band 3 (AE1) gene. *Nephrol Dial Transplant.* 1997;12:1869.

111. King MJ, Garcon L, Hoyer JD, et al. ICSH guidelines for the laboratory diagnosis of nonimmune hereditary red cell membrane disorders. *Int J Lab Hematol.* 2015;37:304.

112. Risinger M, Kalfa TA. Red Cell Membrane disorders: structure meets function. *Blood.*2020;136:1250.

113. Sottiaux J, Favresse J, Chevalier C, et al. Evaluation of a hereditary spherocytosis screening algorithm by automated blood count using reticulocytes and erythrocytic parameters on the Sysmex XN-series. *Int J Lab Hematol.* 2020;42:e88.

114. Liao L, Xu Y, Wei H, et al. Blood cell parameters for screening and diagnosis of hereditary spherocytosis. *J Clin Lab Anal.* 2019;33:e22844.

115. Bianchi P, Fermo E, Vercellati C, et al. Diagnostic power of laboratory tests for hereditary spherocytosis: a comparison study in 150 patients grouped according to molecular and clinical characteristics. *Haematologica.* 2012;97:516.

116. King M-J, Smythe JS, Mushens R. Eosin-5-maleimide binding to band 3 and Rh-related proteins forms the basis of a screening test for hereditary spherocytosis. *Br J Haematol.* 2004;124:106.

117. Christensen RD, Agarwal AM, Nussenzveig RH, et al. Evaluating eosin-5-maleimide binding as a diagnostic test for hereditary spherocytosis in newborn infants. *J Perinatol.* 2015;35:357.

118. Bianchi P, Fermo E, Zanella A. Reply to "Testing for hereditary spherocytosis: a French experience." *Haematologica.* 2012;97(12):e48-9. *Haematologica.* 2012;97:e52.

119. Mackiewicz G, Bailly F, Favre B, et al. Flow cytometry test for hereditary spherocytosis. *Haematologica.* 2012;97:e47.

120. Mayeur-Rousse C, Gentil M, Botton J, et al. Testing for hereditary spherocytosis: a French experience. *Haematologica.* 2012;97:e48.

121. Andolfo I, Russo R, Gambale A, et al. New insights on hereditary erythrocyte membrane defects. *Haematologica.* 2016;101:1284.

122. Agarwal AM, Nussenzveig RH, Reading NS, et al. Clinical utility of next-generation sequencing in the diagnosis of hereditary haemolytic anaemias. *Br J Haematol.* 2016;174:806.

123. Russo R, Andolfo I, Manna F, et al. Multi-gene panel testing improves diagnosis and management of patients with hereditary anemias. *Am J Hematol.* 2018;93:672.

124. Richards S, Aziz N, Bale S, et al. Standards and guidelines for the interpretation of sequence variants: a joint consensus recommendation of the American College of Medical Genetics and Genomics and the Association for Molecular Pathology. *Genet Med.* 2015;17:405.

125. Bianchi P. Current diagnostic approach and screening methods for hereditary spherocytosis. *Thalassemia Rep.* 2013;3:e32.

126. Christensen RD, Yaish HM, Gallagher PG. A pediatrician's practical guide to diagnosing and treating hereditary spherocytosis in neonates. *Pediatrics.* 2015;135:1107.

127. Schilling RF. Risks and benefits of splenectomy versus no splenectomy for hereditary spherocytosis—a personal view. *Br J Haematol.* 2009;145:728.

128. Rescorla FJ, West KW, Engum SA, et al. Laparoscopic splenic procedures in children: experience in 231 children. *Ann Surg.* 2007;246:683.

129. Tracy ET, Rice HE. Partial splenectomy for hereditary spherocytosis. *Pediatr Clin North Am.* 2008;55:503.

130. Pincez T, Guitton C, Gauthier F, et al. Long-term follow-up of subtotal splenectomy for hereditary spherocytosis: a single-center study. *Blood.* 2016;127:1616.

131. Dresbach M. Elliptical human red corpuscles. *Science.* 1904;19:469.

132. Hunter WC, Adams RB. Hematologic study of three generations of a white family showing elliptical erythrocytes. *Ann Intern Med.* 1929;2:1162.

133. Zarkowsky HS, Mohandas N, Speaker CB, et al. A congenital haemolytic anaemia with thermal sensitivity of the erythrocyte membrane. *Br J Haematol.* 1975;29:537.

134. Gallagher PG. Hereditary elliptocytosis: spectrin and protein 4.1R. *Semin Hematol.* 2004;41:142.

135. Nurse GT, Coetzer TL, Palek J. The elliptocytoses, ovalocytosis and related disorders. *Baillieres Clin Haematol.* 1992;5:187.

136. Glele-Kakai C, Garbarz M, Lecomte M-C, et al. Epidemiological studies of spectrin mutations related to hereditary elliptocytosis and spectrin polymorphisms in Benin. *Br J Haematol.* 1996;95:57.

137. Garbarz M, Lecomte M, Feo C, et al. Hereditary pyropoikilocytosis and elliptocytosis in a white French family with the spectrin alpha I/74 variant related to a CGT to CAT codon change (Arg to His) at position 22 of the spectrin alpha I domain. *Blood.* 1990;75:1691.

138. Swierczek S, Agarwal AM, Naidoo K, et al. Novel exon 2 α spectrin mutation and intragenic crossover: three morphological phenotypes associated with four distinct α spectrin defects. *Haematologica.* 2013;98:1972.

139. Al-Riyami AZ, Iolascon A, Al-Zadjali S, et al. Targeted next generation sequencing identifies a novel beta-spectrin gene mutation A2059P in two Omani children with hereditary pyropoikilocytosis. *Am J Hematol.* 2017;92:E607.

140. Ittiwut C, Natesirinilkul R, Tongprasert F, et al. Novel mutations in SPTA1 and SPTB identified by whole exome sequencing in eight Thai families with hereditary pyropoikilocytosis presenting with severe fetal and neonatal anaemia. *Br J Haematol.* 2019;185:578.

141. Coetzer T, Palek J, Lawler J, et al. Structural and functional heterogeneity of alpha spectrin mutations involving the spectrin heterodimer self-association site: relationships to hematologic expression of homozygous hereditary elliptocytosis and hereditary pyropoikilocytosis. *Blood.* 1990;75:2235.

142. Coetzer T, Palek J. Partial spectrin deficiency in hereditary pyropoikilocytosis. *Blood.* 1986;67:919.

143. Coetzer T, Lawler J, Prchal J, et al. Molecular determinants of clinical expression of hereditary elliptocytosis and pyropoikilocytosis. *Blood.* 1987;70:766.

144. Gaetani M, Mootien S, Harper S, et al. Structural and functional effects of hereditary hemolytic anemia-associated point mutations in the alpha spectrin tetramer site. *Blood.* 2008;111:5712.

145. Lecomte MC, Nicolas G, Dhermy D, et al. Properties of normal and mutant polypeptide fragments from the dimer self-association sites of human red cell spectrin. *Eur Biophys J.* 1999;28:208.

146. Coetzer TL, Sahr K, Prchal J, et al. Four different mutations in codon 28 of alpha spectrin are associated with structurally and functionally abnormal spectrin alpha I/74 in hereditary elliptocytosis. *J Clin Invest.* 1991;88:743.

147. Franck P, Postma C, Spaans A, et al. Hereditary elliptocytosis: variable clinical severity caused by 3 variants in the alpha-spectrin gene. *Int J Lab Hematol.* 2018;40:e66.

148. Lorenzo F, del Giudice EM, Alloisio N, et al. Severe poikilocytosis is associated with a de novo alpha 28 Arg→Cys mutation in spectrin. *Br J Haematol.* 1993;83:152.

149. Nicolas G, Pedroni S, Fournier C, et al. Spectrin self-association site: characterization and study of β-spectrin mutations associated with hereditary elliptocytosis. *Biochem J.* 1998;332:81.

150. Qualtieri A, Pasqua A, Bisconte MG, et al. Spectrin Cosenza: a novel beta chain variant associated with Sp alphaI/74 hereditary elliptocytosis. *Br J Haematol.* 1997;97:273.

151. Niss O, Chonat S, Dagaonkar N, et al. Genotype-phenotype correlations in hereditary elliptocytosis and hereditary pyropoikilocytosis. *Blood Cells Mol Dis.* 2016;61:4.

152. Lin PC, Chiou SS, Lin CY, et al. Whole-exome sequencing for the genetic diagnosis of congenital red blood cell membrane disorders in Taiwan. *Clin Chim Acta.* 2018;487:311.

153. Sahr KE, Coetzer TL, Moy LS, et al. Spectrin Cagliari. An Ala—>Gly substitution in helix 1 of beta spectrin repeat 17 that severely disrupts the structure and self-association of the erythrocyte spectrin heterodimer. *J Biol Chem.* 1993;268:22656.

154. Tse WT, Lecomte MC, Costa FF, et al. Point mutation in the beta-spectrin gene associated with alpha I/74 hereditary elliptocytosis. Implications for the mechanism of spectrin dimer self-association. *J Clin Invest.* 1990;86:909.

155. Yoon SH, Yu H, Eber S, et al. Molecular defect of truncated beta-spectrin associated with hereditary elliptocytosis. Beta-spectrin Gottingen. *J Biol Chem.* 1991;266:8490.

156. Garbarz M, Boulanger L, Pedroni S, et al. Spectrin beta Tandil, a novel shortened beta-chain variant associated with hereditary elliptocytosis is due to a deletional frameshift mutation in the beta-spectrin gene. *Blood.* 1992;80:1066.

157. Roux A, Morle F, Guetarni D, et al. Molecular basis of Sp alpha I/65 hereditary elliptocytosis in North Africa: insertion of a TTG triplet between codons 147 and 149 in the alpha-spectrin gene from five unrelated families. *Blood.* 1989;73:2196.

158. Johnson CP, Gaetani M, Ortiz V, et al. Pathogenic proline mutation in the linker between spectrin repeats: disease caused by spectrin unfolding. *Blood.* 2006;109:3538.

159. Harper SL, Li D, Maksimova Y, et al. A fused alpha-beta "mini-spectrin" mimics the intact erythrocyte spectrin head-to-head tetramer. *J Biol Chem.* 2010;285:11003.

160. Harper SL, Sriswasdi S, Tang H-Y, et al. The common hereditary elliptocytosis-associated α-spectrin L260P mutation perturbs erythrocyte membranes by stabilizing spectrin in the closed dimer conformation. *Blood.* 2013;122:3045.

161. Burke JP, Van Zyl D, Zail SS, Coetzer TL. Reduced spectrin-ankyrin binding in a South African hereditary elliptocytosis kindred homozygous for spectrin St Claude. *Blood.* 1998;92:2591.

162. Fournier CM, Nicolas G, Gallagher PG, et al. Spectrin St Claude, a splicing mutation of the human alpha-spectrin gene associated with severe poikilocytic anemia. *Blood.* 1997;89:4584.

163. Alloisio N, Wilmotte R, Morlé L, et al. Spectrin Jendouba: an alpha II/31 spectrin variant that is associated with elliptocytosis and carries a mutation distant from the dimer self- association site. *Blood.* 1992;80:809.

164. Takakuwa Y, Tchernia G, Rossi M, et al. Restoration of normal membrane stability to unstable protein 4.1-deficient erythrocyte membranes by incorporation of purified protein 4.1. *J Clin Invest.* 1986;78:80.

165. Chishti A, Palek J, Fisher D, et al. Reduced invasion and growth of *Plasmodium falciparum* into elliptocytic red blood cells with a combined deficiency of protein 4.1, glycophorin C, and p55. *Blood.* 1996;87:3462.

166. Baklouti F, Moriniere M, Haj-Khelil A, et al. Homozygous deletion of EPB41 genuine AUG-containing exons results in mRNA splicing defects, NMD activation and protein 4.1R complete deficiency in hereditary elliptocytosis. *Blood Cells Mol Dis.* 2011;47:158.

167. Winardi R, Reid M, Conboy J, et al. Molecular analysis of glycophorin C deficiency in human erythrocytes. *Blood.* 1993;81:2799.

168. Wilmotte R, Harper SL, Ursitti JA, et al. The exon 46-encoded sequence is essential for stability of human erythroid alpha-spectrin and heterodimer formation. *Blood.* 1997;90:4188.

169. Randon J, Boulanger L, Marechal J, et al. A variant of spectrin low-expression allele alpha LELY carrying a hereditary elliptocytosis mutation in codon 28. *Br J Haematol.* 1994;88:534.

170. Dhermy D, Galand C, Bournier O, et al. Coinheritance of alpha- and beta-spectrin gene mutations in a case of hereditary elliptocytosis. *Blood.* 1998;92:4481.

171. Christensen RD, Agarwal AM, Yaish HM, et al. Three novel spectrin variants in jaundiced neonates. *Clin Pediatr (Phila)*. 2018;57:19.

172. Christensen RD, Nussenzveig RH, Reading NS, et al. Variations in both alpha-spectrin (SPTA1) and beta-spectrin (SPTB) in a neonate with prolonged jaundice in a family where nine individuals had hereditary elliptocytosis. *Neonatology*. 2014;105:1.

173. Gallagher PG, Tse WT, Marchesi SL, et al. A defect in alpha-spectrin mRNA accumulation in hereditary pyropoikilocytosis. *Trans Assoc Am Physicians*. 1991;104:32.

174. Hanspal M, Hanspal J, Sahr K, et al. Molecular basis of spectrin deficiency in hereditary pyropoikilocytosis. *Blood*. 1993;82:1652.

175. Costa DB, Lozovatsky L, Gallagher PG, et al. A novel splicing mutation of the α-spectrin gene in the original hereditary pyropoikilocytosis kindred. *Blood*. 2005;106:4367.

176. Tolpinrud W, Maksimova YD, Forget BG, et al. Nonsense mutations of the alpha-spectrin gene in hereditary pyropoikilocytosis. *Haematologica*. 2008;93:1752.

177. Mentzer WC Jr, Iarocci TA, Mohandas N, et al. Modulation of erythrocyte membrane mechanical stability by 2,3-diphosphoglycerate in the neonatal poikilocytosis/elliptocytosis syndrome. *J Clin Invest*. 1987;79:943.

178. Lowenthal E, Prchal J. Parvovirus B19 induced red blood cell aplasia in a patient with hereditary pyropoikilocytosis [letter]. *Blood*. 1995;86:411.

179. Coetzer T, Beeton L, van Zyl D, et al. Southeast Asian ovalocytosis in a South African kindred with hemolytic anemia [letter]. *Blood*. 1996;87:1656.

180. Liu S-C, Zhai S, Palek J, et al. Molecular defect of the band 3 protein in Southeast Asian ovalocytosis. *N Engl J Med*. 1990;323:1530.

181. Schofield AE, Reardon DM, Tanner MJ. Defective anion transport activity of the abnormal band 3 in hereditary ovalocytic red blood cells. *Nature*. 1992;355:836.

182. Jarolim P, Palek J, Amato D, et al. Deletion in erythrocyte band 3 gene in malaria-resistant Southeast Asian ovalocytosis. *Proc Natl Acad Sci U S A*. 1991;88:11022.

183. Fowler PW, Sansom MS, Reithmeier RA. Effect of the Southeast Asian ovalocytosis deletion on the conformational dynamics of signal-anchor transmembrane segment 1 of red cell anion exchanger 1 (AE1, band 3, or SLC4A1). *Biochemistry*. 2017;56:712.

184. Liu S, Jarolim P, Rubin H, et al. The homozygous state for the band 3 protein mutation in Southeast Asian ovalocytosis may be lethal [letter]. *Blood*. 1994;84:3590.

185. Picard V, Proust A, Eveillard M, et al. Homozygous Southeast Asian ovalocytosis is a severe dyserythropoietic anemia associated with distal renal tubular acidosis. *Blood*. 2014;123:1963.

186. Genton B, Ai-Yaman F, Mgone CS, et al. Ovalocytosis and cerebral malaria. *Nature*. 1995;378:564.

187. Williams TN. Human red blood cell polymorphisms and malaria. *Curr Opin Microbiol*. 2006;9:388.

188. Laosombat V, Viprakasit V, Dissaneevate S, et al. Natural history of Southeast Asian ovalocytosis during the first 3 years of life. *Blood Cells Mol Dis*. 2010;45:29.

189. Wong P. A basis of the acanthocytosis in inherited and acquired disorders. *Med Hypotheses*. 2004;62:966.

190. Cooper RA. Hemolytic syndromes and red cell membrane abnormalities in liver disease. *Semin Hematol*. 1980;17:103.

191. Marks EI, Ollila TA. Acanthocytosis causing chronic hemolysis in a patient with advanced cirrhosis. *Blood*. 2019;133:1518.

192. De Franceschi L, Bosman GJ, Mohandas N. Abnormal red cell features associated with hereditary neurodegenerative disorders: the neuroacanthocytosis syndromes. *Curr Opin Hematol*. 2014;21:201.

193. Burnett JR, Hooper AJ, Hegele RA. Abetalipoproteinemia. In: Adam MP, Ardinger HH, Pagon RA, et al., eds. *GeneReviews*. Seattle (WA): University of Washington, Seattle; 2018.

194. Wetterau JR, Aggerbeck LP. Absence of microsomal triglyceride transfer protein in individuals with abetalipoproteinemia. *Science*. 1992;258:999.

195. Aers X-P, Leroy BP, Defesche JC, et al. Abetalipoproteinemia from previously unreported gene mutations. *Ann Intern Med*. 2019;170:211.

196. Walker RH. Untangling the thorns: advances in the neuroacanthocytosis syndromes. *J Mov Disord*. 2015;8:41.

197. Rampoldi L, Dobson-Stone C, Rubio JP, et al. A conserved sorting-associated protein is mutant in chorea-acanthocytosis. *Nat Genet*. 2001;28:119.

198. Ueno S-i, Maruki Y, Nakamura M, et al. The gene encoding a newly discovered protein, chorein, is mutated in chorea-acanthocytosis. *Nat Genet*. 2001;28:121.

199. Nishida Y, Nakamura M, Urata Y, et al. Novel pathogenic VPS13A gene mutations in Japanese patients with chorea-acanthocytosis. *Neurol Genet*. 2019;5:e332.

200. Peikert K, Danek A, Hermann A. Current state of knowledge in chorea-acanthocytosis as core neuroacanthocytosis syndrome. *Eur J Med Genet*. 2018;61:699.

201. Roulis E, Hyland C, Flower R, et al. Molecular basis and clinical overview of McLeod syndrome compared with other neuroacanthocytosis syndromes: a review. *JAMA Neurol*. 2018;75:1554.

202. Urata Y, Nakamura M, Sasaki N, et al. Novel pathogenic XK mutations in McLeod syndrome and interaction between XK protein and chorein. *Neurol Genet*. 2019;5:e328.

203. Anderson DG, Walker RH, Connor M, et al. A systematic review of the Huntington disease-like 2 phenotype. *J Huntingtons Dis*. 2017;6:37.

204. Anderson DG, Carmona S, Naidoo K, et al. Absence of acanthocytosis in Huntington's disease-like 2: a prospective comparison with Huntington's disease. *Tremor Other Hyperkinet Mov (N Y)*. 2017;7:512.

205. Gallagher PG. Disorders of erythrocyte hydration. *Blood*. 2017;130:2699.

206. Andolfo I, Russo R, Gambale A, et al. Hereditary stomatocytosis: an underdiagnosed condition. *Am J Hematol*. 2018;93:107.

207. Badens C, Guizouarn H. Advances in understanding the pathogenesis of the red cell volume disorders. *Br J Haematol*. 2016;174:674.

208. Ma S, Cahalan S, LaMonte G, et al. Common PIEZO1 allele in African populations causes dehydration and attenuates *Plasmodium* infection. *Cell*. 2018;173:443.

209. Frederiksen H. Dehydrated hereditary stomatocytosis: clinical perspectives. *J Blood Med*. 2019;10:183.

210. Iolascon A, Andolfo I, Russo R. Advances in understanding the pathogenesis of red cell membrane disorders. *Br J Haematol*. 2019;187:13.

211. Caulier A, Jankovsky N, Demont Y, et al. PIEZO1 activation delays erythroid differentiation of normal and hereditary xerocytosis-derived human progenitor cells. *Haematologica*. 2020;105:610.

212. Moura PL, Hawley BR, Dobbe, JGG, et al. PIEZO1 gain-of-function mutations delay reticulocyte maturation in hereditary xerocytosis. *Haematologica*. 2020;105:e271.

213. Picard V, Guitton C, Thuret I, et al. Clinical and biological features in PIEZO1-reditary xerocytosis and Gardos channelopathy: a retrospective series of 126 patients. *Haematologica*. 2019;104:1554.

214. Fermo E, Monedero-Alonso D, Petkova-Kirova P, et al. Gardos Channelopathy: functional analysis of a novel *KCCN4* variant. *Blood Adv*. 2020;4:6336.

215. Kiger L, Oliveira L, Guitton C, et al. Piezo1-xerocytosis red cell metabolome shows impaired glycolysis and increased hemoglobin oxygen affinity. *Blood Adv*. 2021;5:84.

CHAPTER 16
ERYTHROCYTE ENZYME DISORDERS

Marije Bartels, Eduard J. van Beers, and Richard van Wijk

SUMMARY

Red cells possess an active metabolic machinery that provides energy to pump ions against electrochemical gradients, to maintain red cell shape, to keep hemoglobin iron in the reduced form, and to maintain enzyme and hemoglobin sulfhydryl groups. The main source of metabolic energy comes from glucose. Glucose is metabolized through the glycolytic pathway and through the hexose monophosphate shunt. Glycolysis catabolizes glucose to pyruvate and lactate, which represent the end products of glucose metabolism in the erythrocyte, because it lacks the mitochondria required for further oxidation of pyruvate. Adenosine diphosphate (ADP) is phosphorylated to adenosine triphosphate (ATP), and nicotinamide adenine dinucleotide (NAD)$^+$ is reduced to its reduced form, nicotinamide adenine dinucleotide (NADH), during glycolysis. 2,3-Bisphosphoglycerate, an important regulator of the oxygen affinity of hemoglobin, is generated during glycolysis. The hexose monophosphate shunt oxidizes glucose-6-phosphate, reducing nicotinamide adenine dinucleotide phosphate (NADP$^+$) to reduced nicotinamide adenine dinucleotide phosphate (NADPH). In addition to glucose, the red cell has the capacity to use some other sugars and nucleosides as a source of energy. The red cell lacks the capacity for de novo purine synthesis, but has a salvage pathway that permits synthesis of purine nucleotides from purine bases. The red cell contains high concentrations of glutathione, which is maintained almost entirely in the reduced state by NADPH through the catalytic activity of glutathione reductase. Glutathione is synthesized from glycine, cysteine, and glutamic acid in a two-step process that requires ATP as a source of energy. Catalase and glutathione peroxidase serve to protect the red cell from oxidative damage. The maturation of reticulocytes into erythrocytes is associated with a rapid decrease in the activity of several enzymes. However, the decrease in activities of other enzymes occurs much more slowly or not at all with aging.

Erythrocyte enzyme deficiencies may lead to hemolytic anemia; expression of the defect in other cell lines may lead to pathologic changes such as neuromuscular abnormalities. Glucose-6-phosphate dehydrogenase (G6PD) deficiency is the most common erythrocyte enzyme defect. In some populations, more than 20% of people may be affected by this enzyme deficiency. In the common polymorphic forms, such as G6PD A−, G6PD Mediterranean, or G6PD Canton, hemolysis occurs only during the stress imposed by infection or administration of "oxidative" drugs, and in some individuals upon ingestion of fava beans (favism). Neonatal icterus, which appears largely as a result of an interaction with an independent defect in bilirubin conjugation, is the clinically most serious complication of G6PD deficiency, but can be the presenting symptom of other enzyme deficiencies as well. Patients with uncommon, functionally very severe, genetic variants of G6PD experience chronic hemolysis, a disorder designated hereditary nonspherocytic hemolytic anemia.

Hereditary nonspherocytic hemolytic anemia also occurs as a consequence of other enzyme deficiencies, the most common of which is pyruvate kinase deficiency. Glucosephosphate isomerase, hexokinase, and pyrimidine 5'-nucleotidase deficiency are included among the rare causes of hereditary nonspherocytic hemolytic anemia. In the case of some deficiencies, notably those of glutathione synthetase, triosephosphate isomerase, and phosphoglycerate kinase, the defect is expressed throughout the body, and neurologic and other defects may be a prominent part of the clinical syndrome.

Diagnosis is best achieved by determining red cell enzyme activity either with a quantitative assay or a screening test. Except for the basophilic stippling of erythrocytes that is characteristic, but not specific, of pyrimidine 5'-nucleotidase deficiency, red cell morphology is of little or no help in differentiating one red cell enzyme deficiency from another. A variety of molecular lesions have been defined in most of these enzyme deficiencies. Confirmation of the diagnosis by DNA analysis is recommended: it is necessary for genetic counseling and is helpful in recommendations for treatment, as patients with some enzyme deficiencies (eg, glucosephosphate isomerase deficiency) tend to respond more favorably to splenectomy than do others (eg, G6PD deficiency). Some of the defects, such as pyruvate kinase and glucosephosphate isomerase deficiencies, are transmitted as autosomal recessive disorders, whereas G6PD and phosphoglycerate kinase deficiencies are X linked.

Acronyms and Abbreviations: 2,3-BPG, 2,3-bisphosphoglycerate; 2,3-DPG, 2,3-diphosphoglycerate; ADA, adenosine deaminase; ADP, adenosine diphosphate; AIDS, acquired immunodeficiency disease; AK, adenylate kinase; *ALDOA*, gene encoding aldolase A; AP-1, a transcription factor; ATP, adenosine triphosphate; BPG, bisphosphoglycerate; BPGM, bisphosphoglycerate mutase enzyme; CDP, cytidine diphosphate; DPG, diphosphoglycerate; EDTA, ethylenediaminetetraacetic acid; EMP, Embden-Meyerhof direct glycolytic pathway; *ENO1*, gene encoding enolase; FAD, flavin adenine dinucleotide; GAPDH, glyceraldehyde-3-phosphate dehydrogenase; G-6-PD, glucose-6-phosphate dehydrogenase; GCL, glutamate cysteine ligase; *GCLC*, gene encoding the catalytic subunit of GCL; *GCLM*, gene encoding the modifier subunit of GCL; GLUT1, glucose transporter 1, GPI, glucose phosphate isomerase; GR, glutathione reductase; GS, glutathione synthetase; GSH, reduced glutathione; *GSR*, gene encoding glutathione reductase; GSSG, oxidized glutathione; *HFE*, the gene associated with hereditary hemochromatosis; HK, hexokinase; HNSHA, hereditary nonspherocytic hemolytic anemia; kDa, the standard unit that is used for indicating mass; KLF1, key erythroid transcription factor; LDH, lactate dehydrogenase; miR, micro RNA; mRNA, messenger ribonucleic acid; MRP1, multidrug resistance protein 1; NAD, nicotinamide adenine dinucleotide; NADPH, nicotinamide adenine dinucleotide phosphate (reduced form); nt, nucleotide; P5'N1, pyrimidine-5'-nucleotidase-1; PFK, phosphofructose kinase; *PFKM*, gene encoding muscle subunit of PFK; PGK, phosphoglycerate kinase; PK, pyruvate kinase; *PKLR*, gene encoding PK enzyme activity in red cells and liver; SNP, single nucleotide polymorphism; SOD1, superoxide dismutase; TPI, triose-phosphate isomerase; UDPG, uridine diphosphoglucose; UDPGT, uridine diphosphoglucuronate glucuronosyltransferase; WHO, World Health Organization.

● DEFINITION AND HISTORY

Deficiencies in the activities of a number of erythrocyte enzymes may lead to shortening of the red cell life span. Glucose-6-phosphate dehydrogenase (G6PD) deficiency was the first to be recognized and is the most common.

The recognition of G6PD deficiency was the result of investigations performed in the 1950s of the hemolytic effect of the antimalarial drug primaquine; the investigations are described in detail elsewhere.[1-3] These early studies defined G6PD deficiency as a hereditary sex-linked enzyme deficiency that affected primarily the erythrocytes, older cells being more severely affected than newly formed ones because of age-dependent decline of mutant enzyme activity. The studies showed that this enzyme deficiency was very prevalent in individuals of African, Mediterranean, and Asian ethnic origins, but that it could be found in virtually any population. The common (polymorphic) forms of G6PD deficiency were found to be associated with anemia only under conditions of stress, such as the administration of oxidative drugs, infection, and the neonatal period.

Chronic hemolysis in the absence of a stress occurs in uncommon, functionally severe forms of G6PD deficiency and in patients with a variety of other red cell enzyme deficiencies. Such patients suffer from *hereditary nonspherocytic hemolytic anemia*. Although patients fitting the description of hereditary nonspherocytic hemolytic anemia had been documented earlier, the designation was first introduced by Crosby in 1950.[4] Dacie and colleagues[5] subsequently reported on several families in which affected members manifested hemolytic anemia from an early age and in whom the osmotic fragility of the red cells was normal. The finding of osmotic fragility was the main feature that distinguished this disorder from hereditary spherocytosis. Thus, defined essentially by exclusion as a hereditary hemolytic anemia that is not hereditary spherocytosis (or without any other major aberration of red cell morphology), it is not at all surprising that hereditary nonspherocytic hemolytic anemia has proven to be extremely heterogeneous both in etiology and in clinical manifestations. Sometimes, this disorder is also designated *congenital nonspherocytic hemolytic anemia*, but *hereditary* is more accurate than *congenital*, and is therefore preferable. Although hereditary ovalocytosis, pyropoikilocytosis, stomatocytosis (Chap. 15), thalassemia major (Chap. 17), and sickle cell disease (Chap. 18) are hereditary hemolytic anemias that are also nonspherocytic, they are not included in this category.

Although a deficiency of G6PD was found to be responsible for hemolysis in a few patients with hereditary nonspherocytic hemolytic anemia, in the overwhelming majority of cases the cause remained obscure. In 1954, Selwyn and Dacie[6] studied autohemolysis (spontaneous lysis of red cells after sterile incubation for 24-48 hours at 37°C) in four patients with hereditary nonspherocytic hemolytic anemia and found that in two of the patients, lysis was only slightly increased and was prevented by glucose; these patients were designated as type 1, whereas the others, in whom glucose failed to correct autohemolysis, were classified as type 2. Autohemolysis of the erythrocytes of type 2 patients was modified by the addition of ATP. ATP does not penetrate the red cell membrane. Instead, its modifying influence was probably exerted chiefly by virtue of its effect on the osmolarity and pH of the suspending solution. However, these findings suggested to DeGruchy and associates[7] that patients with type 2 autohemolysis suffered from a defect in ATP generation. This proposal, born of a misunderstanding of red cell biochemistry, turned out to be correct, as a major cause of hereditary nonspherocytic hemolytic anemia proved to be a deficiency of the ATP-generating enzyme pyruvate kinase (PK).[8] PK deficiency was the first of a large number of enzyme defects that have been shown to cause this heterogeneous syndrome.

● EPIDEMIOLOGY

The prevalence of most red blood cell enzyme deficiencies is unknown. The most common red cell enzyme abnormality is deficiency of G6PD. Its prevalence among white populations ranges from less than 1 in 1000

among northern European populations to 50% of the males among Kurdish Jews. The lowest frequencies of G6PD deficiency are found in both North and South America (≤1%), and highest rates are predicted across the tropical belt of sub-Saharan Africa (15%–30%) (Fig. 16–1). The distribution across Asia and Asia Pacific is generally heterogeneous, ranging from virtually absent to relatively high.[9,10] Although many of the highest frequencies are predicted from sub-Saharan African countries, the very high population densities across Asia infers that the overall population burden is largely focused here. Based on a Bayesian geostatistical model, using results of large community surveys, the overall allele frequency of G6PD deficiency across all malaria endemic countries is predicted to be 8%, reflected by 220 million affected males and an estimated 133 million females.[9] However, because diagnosing female carriers, who express two populations of red blood cells (see "Laboratory Features" fruther), based on enzyme activity level alone is challenging, these data should be interpreted with caution. Details on the distribution of G6PD deficiency among various population groups are presented elsewhere.[10-12]

The high frequency of G6PD-deficient genes in many populations implies that G6PD deficiency confers a selective advantage. The suggestion that resistance to malaria accounts for the high frequency of G6PD deficiency paralleling the worldwide distribution of malaria is supported by the sheer diversity of variants in the *G6PD* gene. Many of these are found at polymorphic frequencies in genetically isolated populations, suggesting independent selection of each variant.[13,14] Important supporting evidence was obtained from studies in heterozygotes for G6PD A−that showed a higher degree of infestation of G6PD-sufficient cells than of G6PD-deficient cells.[15] Deficient cells infested with malaria parasites may be phagocytosed more efficiently than normal cells.[16] The issue of which G6PD genotypes confers[17] protection from malarial infection remains subject to debate.[17,18] The majority of studies conclude that G6PD deficiency in hemizygous males, and probably also homozygous females, confers significant protection against malarial infection. The nature of protection from the mosaic state of G6PD deficiency in heterozygous females remains to be established.[18]

Although it has been suggested that a higher prevalence of G6PD deficiency in individuals with sickle cell disease than in the general African population reflects a favorable effect of the enzyme deficiency on the clinical course of the sickling disorders,[19] newer studies have found no evidence for this effect.[20,21]

In addition to common G6PD mutations, there are mutations in other enzyme-coding genes that are repeatedly encountered in the population. PK deficiency is the most common cause of hereditary nonspherocytic hemolytic anemia. Based on large-scale mutation analysis, it is estimated that the population prevalence of PK deficiency among whites is approximately 50 cases per 1 million population.[22] More than 260 mutations in the *PKLR* gene have been reported so far, distributed throughout the entire gene, and occurring in patients with various ethnic backgrounds. The c.1529G>A, p.(Arg510Gln) mutation is the most common mutation in the United States and in northern and central Europe, whereas the c.1456C>T, p.(Arg486Trp) mutation is prevalent in southern Europe and the c.1468C>T (p.Arg490Trp) mutation is frequently found in Asia.[23] Similarly, the c.315G>C, p.(Glu104Asp) mutation is recurrently encountered in triose phosphate isomerase (TPI) deficiency.[24] Although the exact prevalence is not known, glucose-6-phosphate isomerase deficiency is considered the second most common glycolytic erythrocyte enzyme disorder, reported in approximately 60 families worldwide and with more than 50 causative mutations identified (see "Other Enzyme Deficiencies—Glucosephosphate Isomerase Deficiency" further). Pyrimidine 5′ nucleotidase (P5′N) deficiency is a rare cause of nonspherocytic hemolytic anemia but it is the most common enzyme abnormality affecting nucleotide metabolism (more than

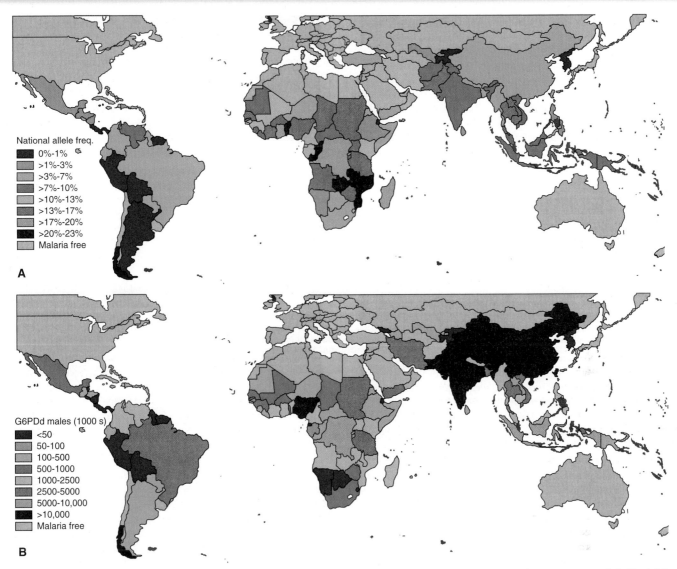

Figure 16–1. Estimated prevalence of G6PD deficiency. **A.** National-level allele frequencies. **B.** National-level population estimates of G6PD-deficient (G6PDd) males. *(Reproduced with permission from Howes RE, Piel FB, Patil AP, et al. G6PD deficiency prevalence and estimates of affected populations in malaria endemic countries: a geostatistical model-based map. PLoS Med. 2012;9[11]:e1001339.)*

100 patients reported, see "Other Enzyme Deficiencies—Pyrimidine 5′-Nucleotidase Deficiency" further). In phosphofructose kinase (PFK) deficiency, one-third of the reported patients are of Jewish origin and in this population an intronic splice site mutation, c.237+1G>A and a single base-pair deletion, c.2003delC, are among the most frequently encountered mutations.[25] In a number of these instances, the existence of each mutation in the context of the same haplotype implies that there has been a *founder effect*, that is, the mutation occurred only once, and all individuals now carrying it are descendants of the person who sustained the original mutation. The expansion of the mutation could represent a selective advantage for heterozygotes, but also may result from random factors or from a selective advantage provided by one or more tightly linked genes.

Estimates of frequencies of other deficiency alleles, such as those for adenylate kinase, diphosphoglycerate mutase, enolase, TPI, and phosphoglycerate kinase (PGK), have been made on large numbers of cord bloods.[26] A particularly high incidence of heterozygous TPI deficiency (>4%) in Americans of African descent is supported by family

studies.[27] As this is not reflected in a correspondingly high birth incidence, the allele might be lethal in the homozygous state.

● ETIOLOGY AND PATHOGENESIS

RED CELL METABOLISM

Although the binding, transport, and delivery of oxygen do not require the expenditure of metabolic energy by the red cell, a source of energy is required if the red cell is to perform its function efficiently and to survive in the circulation for its full life span of approximately 120 days. This energy is needed to maintain (a) the iron of hemoglobin in the divalent form; (b) the high potassium and low calcium and sodium levels within the cell against a gradient imposed by the high plasma calcium and sodium and low plasma potassium levels; (c) the sulfhydryl groups of red cell enzymes, hemoglobin, and membranes in the active, reduced form; and (d) the biconcave shape of the cell. If the red cell is deprived of a source of energy, it becomes sodium and calcium logged and potassium depleted, and the red cell shape changes from a flexible biconcave disk. Such a cell is quickly removed from the circulation by the filtering action of the spleen and the monocyte–macrophage system. Even if it survived, such an energy-deprived cell would gradually turn brown as hemoglobin is oxidized to methemoglobin by the very high concentrations of oxygen within the erythrocyte. The cell would then be unable to perform its function of transporting oxygen and carbon dioxide.

The process of extracting energy from a substrate, such as glucose, and of using this energy is carried out by a large number of enzymes (Table 16–1). Because the red cell loses its nucleus before it enters the circulation and most of its RNA within 1 or 2 days of its release into the circulation, it does not have the capacity to synthesize new proteins to replace those that may become degraded during its life span. The enzymes present in the red cells were formed largely by the nucleated cell in the marrow and, to a lesser extent, the reticulocyte.

Glucose Metabolism

Glucose is the normal energy source of the red cell. It is metabolized by the erythrocyte along 2 major routes: the glycolytic pathway and the hexose monophosphate shunt. The steps in these pathways are essentially the same as those found in other tissues. Unlike most other cells, however, the red cell lacks a citric acid cycle. Only the reticulocytes maintain some capacity for the breakdown of pyruvate to CO_2, with the attendant highly efficient production of ATP. The mature red cell extracts energy from glucose almost solely by anaerobic glycolysis. Before glucose can be metabolized by the red cell, it must pass through the membrane. Transport into the interior of the cell is facilitated by glucose receptor GLUT1 (glucose transporter 1), and regulated by the abundantly expressed membrane protein stomatin.[28] In humans, and other mammals that have lost the ability to synthesize ascorbic acid from glucose, GLUT1 also facilitates transport of L-dehydroascorbic acid.[28] The red cell membrane contains insulin receptors, but the transport of glucose into red cells is independent of insulin.

Pathways of Glucose Metabolism

Direct Glycolytic Pathway In the Embden-Meyerhof direct glycolytic pathway (Fig. 16–2), glucose is catabolized anaerobically to pyruvate or lactate. Although 2 moles of high-energy phosphate in the form of ATP are used in preparing glucose for its further metabolism, up to 4 moles of adenosine diphosphate (ADP) may be phosphorylated to ATP during the metabolism of each mole of glucose, giving a net yield of 2 moles of ATP per mole of glucose metabolized. The rate of glucose use is limited largely by the hexokinase and PFK reactions. Both of the enzymes catalyzing these reactions have a relatively high pH optimum and have very little activity at pH levels lower than 7. For this reason, red cell glycolysis is very pH sensitive, being stimulated by a rise in pH.

Branching of the metabolic stream after the formation of 1,3-bisphosphoglycerate (1,3-BPG) provides the red cell with flexibility in regard to the amount of ATP formed in the metabolism of each mole of glucose. 1,3-BPG may be metabolized to 2,3-bisphosphoglycerate (2,3-BPG), thus "wasting" the high-energy phosphate bond in position 1 of the glycerate. Removing the phosphate group at position 2 by bisphosphoglycerate phosphatase results in the formation of 3-phosphoglycerate. Both reactions in this unique glycolytic bypass, known as the *Rapoport-Luebering shunt*, are catalyzed by the erythroid-specific multifunctional enzyme bisphosphoglycerate mutase.[29] In mammalian erythrocytes, a separate 2,3-BPG phosphatase activity has been ascribed to multiple inositol polyphosphate phosphatase.[30] In contrast to bisphosphoglycerate mutase, multiple inositol polyphosphate phosphatase-1 is able to remove the phosphate at position 3, thereby bypassing the formation of 3-phosphoglycerate. The precise functional significance

TABLE 16–1. Activities of Some Red Cell Enzymes

Enzyme	Activity at 37 °C IU/g Hb (mean ± SD)
Acetylcholinesterase	36.93 ± 3.83
Adenosine deaminase	1.11 ± 0.23
Adenylate kinase	258 ± 29.3
Aldolase	3.19 ± 0.86
Bisphosphoglyceromutase	4.78 ± 0.65
Catalase	153,117 ± 2390
Enolase	5.39 ± 0.83
Galactokinase	0.0291 ± 0.004
Galactose-4-epimerase	0.231 ± 0.061
Glucose phosphate isomerase	60.8 ± 11.0
Glucose-6-phosphate dehydrogenase	8.34 ± 1.59
γ-Glutamylcysteine synthetase	1.05 ± 0.19
Glutathione peroxidase[a]	30.82 ± 4.65
Glutathione reductase without FAD	7.18 ± 1.09
Glutathione reductase with FAD	10.4 ± 1.50
Glutathione-S-transferase	6.66 ± 1.81
Glutathione synthetase	0.34 ± 0.06
Glyceraldehyde phosphate dehydrogenase	226 ± 41.9
Hexokinase	1.78 ± 0.38
Lactate dehydrogenase	200 ± 26.5
Monophosphoglyceromutase	37.71 ± 5.56
NADH-methemoglobin reductase	19.2 ± 3.85(30°)
NADPH diaphorase	2.26 ± 0.16
Nucleoside phosphorylase	359 ± 32
Phosphofructokinase	11.01 ± 2.33
Phosphoglucomutase	5.50 ± 0.62
Phosphoglycerate kinase	320 ± 36.1
Phosphoglycolate phosphatase	1.23 ± 0.10
Phosphomannose isomerase	0.054 ± 0.026
Pyrimidine 5′-nucleotidase	0.138 ± 0.018
Pyruvate kinase	15.0 ± 1.99
6-Phosphogluconate dehydrogenase	8.78 ± 0.78
6-Phosphogluconolactonase	50.6 ± 5.9
Ribosephosphate isomerase	200
Superoxide dismutase	2225 ± 303
Transaldolase	1.21 ± 0.24
Transketolase	0.725 ± 0.17
Triose phosphate isomerase	2111 ± 397

FAD, flavin adenine dinucleotide; Hb, hemoglobin; NADH, reduced form of nicotinamide adenine dinucleotide; NADPH, nicotinamide adenine dinucleotide phosphate.

[a]For United States and European subjects.

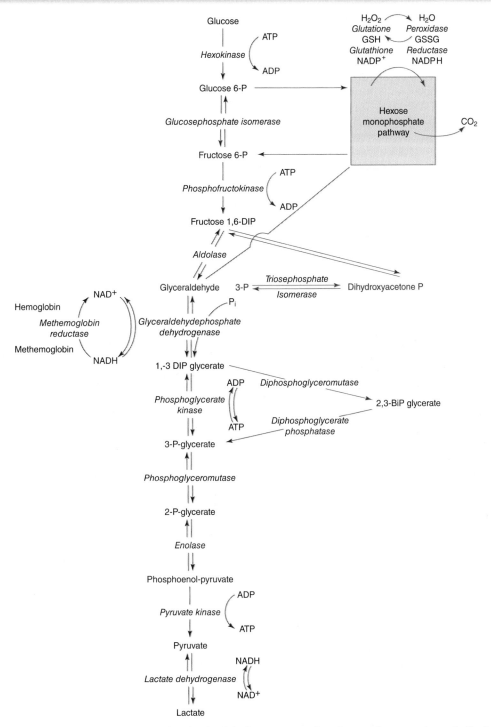

Figure 16–2. Glucose metabolism of the erythrocyte. The details of the hexose monophosphate pathway are shown in Fig. 16–3.

of multiple inositol polyphosphate phosphatase-1 for human red cell physiology and regulation of 2,3-BPG levels remains to be established.

3-Phosphoglycerate also may be formed directly from 1,3-BPG through the PGK step, resulting in phosphorylation of 1 mole of ADP to ATP. Although metabolism of glucose through the 2,3-BPG step occurs without any net gain of high-energy phosphate bonds in the form of ATP, metabolism through the PGK step results in the formation of two such bonds per mole of glucose metabolized. This portion of the direct glycolytic pathway has been called the *energy clutch*. Regulation of metabolism at this branch point determines not only the rate of

ADP phosphorylation to ATP but also the concentration of 2,3-BPG, an important regulator of the oxygen affinity of hemoglobin (Chaps. 19 and 28). The concentration of 2,3-BPG depends on the balance between its rate of formation and degradation by bisphosphoglycerate mutase. Hydrogen ions inhibit the bisphosphoglycerate mutase reaction and stimulate the phosphatase reaction. Thus, red cell 2,3-BPG levels are exquisitely sensitive to pH: a rise in pH causes a rise in 2,3-BPG levels, whereas acidosis results in 2,3-BPG depletion. It may be that the ratio of oxyhemoglobin to deoxyhemoglobin also influences 2,3-BPG synthesis by virtue of the fact that only deoxyhemoglobin binds this compound, thus affecting the concentration of free 2,3-BPG that is available for feedback inhibition of the enzymes that lead to its formation. However, the available evidence suggests that the pH is the primary controlling factor.

Metabolism of glucose by way of the Embden-Meyerhof pathway may also yield reducing energy in the form of the reduced form of nicotinamide adenine dinucleotide (NAD); that is, NADH. The reduction of NAD⁺ to NADH occurs in the glyceraldehyde-3-phosphate dehydrogenase (GAPDH) step. If NADH is reoxidized in reducing methemoglobin to hemoglobin, the end product of glucose metabolism is pyruvate. If NADH is not reoxidized by methemoglobin, however, pyruvate is reduced in the lactate dehydrogenase (LDH) step, forming lactate as the final end product of glucose metabolism. The lactate or pyruvate formed is transported from the red cell and is metabolized elsewhere in the body. Thus, the erythrocyte has a flexible Embden-Meyerhof pathway that can adjust the amount of ADP phosphorylated per mole of glucose according to the requirement of the cell.

The regulation of red cell glycolytic metabolism is very complex. Products of some reactions may stimulate others. For example, the PK reaction is exquisitely sensitive to fructose 1,6-diphosphate, the product of PFK. Conversely, other metabolic products may serve as strong enzyme inhibitors. In addition, there is increasing evidence that glycolytic enzymes assemble into enzyme complexes to the interior of the red cell membrane.[31] The assembly of these complexes seems to be regulated by the oxygen status of hemoglobin and the phosphorylation status of band 3,[31,32] suggesting they play a direct role in the regulation of oxygen-dependent changes in glycolytic and pentose shunt fluxes.[33]

Notably, a number of glycolytic enzymes show additional functional activities. For instance, in addition to its role in glycolysis, glucosephosphate isomerase also functions as a neuroleukin or autocrine motility factor. Another example is enolase, which is reported to also function as a plasminogen receptor.[34,35] The additional functional activities of these moonlighting enzymes could contribute to the complexity of the phenotype of the associated disorder.[36]

Hexose Monophosphate Shunt   Not all the glucose metabolized by the red cell passes through the direct glycolytic pathway. A direct oxidative pathway of metabolism, the hexose monophosphate shunt, also functions. In this pathway, glucose-6-phosphate is oxidized at position 1, yielding CO_2. In the process of glucose oxidation, NADP⁺ is reduced to NADPH. The pentose phosphate formed when glucose is decarboxylated undergoes a series of molecular rearrangements, eventuating in the formation of a triose, glyceraldehyde-3-phosphate, and a hexose, fructose-6-phosphate (Fig. 16–3). These are normal intermediates in anaerobic glycolysis and thus can rejoin that metabolic stream. Because the glucose phosphate isomerase reaction is freely reversible, allowing fructose-6-phosphate to be converted to glucose-6-phosphate, recycling through the hexose monophosphate pathway is also possible. Unlike the anaerobic glycolytic pathway, the hexose monophosphate pathway does not generate any high-energy phosphate bonds. Its primary function is the formation of NADPH, and, indeed, the amount of glucose passing through this pathway is regulated by the amount of NADP⁺ that has been made available by the oxidation of NADPH. NADPH functions primarily as a substrate for the reduction of glutathione-containing disulfides in the erythrocyte through mediation of the enzyme glutathione reductase, which catalyzes the conversion of oxidized glutathione (GSSG) to reduced glutathione (GSH) and the reduction of mixed disulfides of hemoglobin and GSH.[37]

Enzymes of Glucose Metabolism

Hexokinase   Hexokinase catalyzes the phosphorylation of glucose in position 6 by ATP. It thus serves as the first step in the utilization of glucose, whether by the anaerobic or the hexose monophosphate pathway. Mannose or fructose may also serve as a substrate for this enzyme.

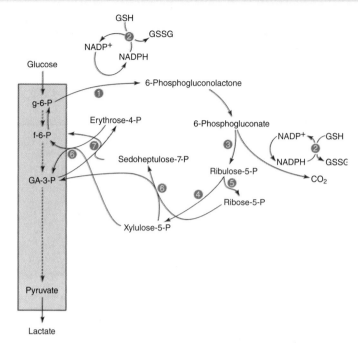

Figure 16–3. Hexose monophosphate pathway of the erythrocyte: (1) glucose-6-phosphate dehydrogenase, (2) glutathione reductase, (3) phosphogluconate dehydrogenase, (4) ribulose-phosphate epimerase, (5) ribosephosphate isomerase, (6) transketolase, and (7) transaldolase.

Hexokinase is the glycolytic enzyme with the lowest activity. Reticulocytes have much higher levels of hexokinase activity than do mature red cells.[38,39]

Hexokinase has an absolute requirement for magnesium. It is strongly inhibited by its product, glucose-6-phosphate, and is released from this inhibition by the inorganic phosphate ion[40,41] and by high concentrations of glucose.[42] Inorganic phosphate enhances the rate of glucose use by red cells. This effect is not exerted through hexokinase but through stimulation of the PFK reaction, resulting in a lowered glucose-6-phosphate concentration within the cell, which releases hexokinase from inhibition.[43] GSSG[44] and other disulfides, as well as 2,3-BPG,[45] inhibit hexokinase. The determination of the structures of the human and rat hexokinase isozymes have provided substantial insight into ligand-binding sites and subsequent modes of interaction of these ligands.[46,47]

The 2 major fractions of red cell hexokinase (HK) are designated HK$_I$ and HK$_R$, with HK$_R$ being unique to erythrocytes and particularly to reticulocytes.[48] Both red cell isozymes are monomers and produced from the hexokinase I gene (HK1)[49] with an apparent molecular weight of 112 kDa.[50] The HK1 gene is localized on chromosome 10q22 and spans more than 100 kb. It contains 29 exons,[51,52] which, by tissue-specific transcription, generate multiple transcripts by alternative use of the 5′ exons.[52,53] Erythroid-specific transcriptional control results in a unique red blood cell–specific mRNA that differs from HK$_I$ transcripts at the 5′ end. Consequently, HK$_R$ lacks the porin-binding domain that mediates HK$_I$ binding to mitochondria.[54] A single-nucleotide polymorphism in the first intron of HK$_R$ was found to be strongly associated with reduced hemoglobin and hematocrit levels in the European population.[55] Hexokinase deficiency is a rare cause of hereditary nonspherocytic hemolytic anemia.

Glucose Phosphate Isomerase   Glucose-6-phosphate isomerase (GPI) catalyzes the interconversion of glucose-6-phosphate and fructose-6-phosphate, the second step of the Embden-Meyerhof pathway. The crystal structure of human GPI has been resolved. The enzyme is a homodimer, composed of 2 subunits of 63 kDa each. The enzyme's active site is composed of polypeptide chains from both subunits, making the dimeric form essential for catalytic activity.[56] Residues that are not in direct contact with the reacting substrate molecule also have been implicated as important for catalytic function of GPI.[57] The gene encoding GPI (*GPI*) is located on chromosome 19q13.1 and consists of 18 exons, spanning at least 50 kb, with a complementary DNA (cDNA) of 1.9 kb in length.[58] GPI deficiency is considered one of the (relatively) more common causes of hereditary nonspherocytic hemolytic anemia.

Phosphofructokinase PFK catalyzes the rate-limiting phosphorylation of fructose-6-phosphate by ATP to fructose-1,6-diphosphate. Under intracellular conditions this reaction is nearly irreversible, making PFK an important regulator of glycolytic flux. The enzyme has a molecular mass of approximately 340 kDa. Red cell phosphofructokinase exists as five different homotetramers or heterotetramers comprised of muscle (M) and liver (L) subunits. Each tetramer displays unique properties with respect to catalytic function and regulation. The enzyme requires magnesium for activity. PFK activity is tightly controlled and subject to regulation by many metabolic effectors. Among the most important activators are ADP, cyclic adenosine monophosphate, and fructose-2,6-diphosphate, whereas PFK is inhibited by its substrate ATP, citrate, and lactate.[59,60] These metabolic effectors exert their effects probably by stabilizing either the minimally active dimeric or the fully active tetrameric form of PFK.[61] PFK activity is also regulated by its binding to calmodulin.[62] Association of the enzyme with the red cell membrane,[63] in particular binding to band 3[64,65] and actin,[66] inhibits and stimulates PFK activity, respectively.

A preliminary crystallographic analysis of dimeric wild-type human muscle PFK has been presented.[67] The gene encoding the 85-kDa M subunit (*PFKM*) is located on chromosome 12q13.3 and spans 30 kb. It contains 27 exons and at least 3 promoter regions.[68] The 80-kDa L-subunit encoding gene (*PFKL*) is located on chromosome 21q22.3, contains 22 exons, and spans more than 28 kb.[69] Deficiency of PFK is associated with mild hemolytic anemia and type VII glycogen storage disease (Tarui disease).[70]

Aldolase Aldolase reversibly cleaves fructose-1,6-diphosphate into two trioses. The "upper" half of the fructose-1,6-diphosphate molecule becomes dihydroxyacetone phosphate and the "lower" half becomes glyceraldehyde-3-phosphate. Aldolase is a 159-kDa homotetrameric enzyme comprised of subunits of 40 kDa each.[71] Three distinct isoenzymes have been identified: aldolase A, B, and C. The 364-amino-acids-long aldolase A subunits are primarily expressed in erythrocytes and muscle cells.[72] The structure of human aldolase A is known.[73] Red cell aldolase binds to F-actin[74] and the N-terminal part of band 3,[75] which inhibits its activity.[65] The gene for aldolase A (*ALDOA*) is located on chromosome 16q22-24. It spans 7.5 kb and consists of 12 exons. Several transcription-initiation sites have been identified and *ALDOA* pre-mRNA is spliced in a tissue-specific manner.[76] Aldolase deficiency is a very rare cause of hereditary nonspherocytic hemolytic anemia.

Triosephosphate Isomerase Triosephosphate isomerase is the enzyme of the anaerobic glycolytic pathway that has the highest activity. Its metabolic role is to catalyze interconversion of the two trioses formed by the action of aldolase: dihydroxyacetone phosphate and glyceraldehyde-3-phosphate.[77] Although equilibrium is in favor of dihydroxyacetone phosphate, glyceraldehyde-3-phosphate undergoes continued oxidation through the action of glyceraldehyde phosphate dehydrogenase and is thus removed from the equilibrium. Triosephosphate isomerase is a dimer consisting of two identical 27-kDa subunits of 248 amino acids.[78] Several crystal structures have been resolved.[79,80] These show that the active site is at the dimer interface and a number of critical residues have been identified. There are no isoenzymes known, but three distinct electrophoretic forms can be distinguished

as a result of posttranslational modifications.[81] Red blood cell triosephosphate isomerase activity is not red-cell-age dependent. Triosephosphate isomerase is transcribed from a single gene (*TPI1*), located on chromosome 12p13. The gene spans 3.5 kb and contains 7 exons. Three processed pseudogenes have been identified.[82] A deficiency of triosephosphate isomerase causes hereditary nonspherocytic hemolytic anemia and a severe neuromuscular disorder.

Glyceraldehyde-3-Phosphate Dehydrogenase GAPDH performs the dual functions of oxidizing and phosphorylating glyceraldehyde-3-phosphate, producing 1,3-BPG. In the process, NAD+ is reduced to NADH. This enzyme is closely associated with the red cell membrane[83] where it binds to the N-terminal part of band 3.[65] Membrane binding influences the activity of GAPDH[84] thereby regulating glycolytic flux[85] and antioxidant capacity.[86] Human red blood cell GAPDH is a homotetramer of approximately 150 kDa, composed of 36-kDa subunits and shows an absolute specificity for NAD+.[87] One of the many nonglycolytic functions of GAPDH[34,35] may include its role in iron metabolism[88] (Chap. 10). The crystal structure of human liver GAPDH reveals a homotetramer, each subunit of which is bound to a NAD+ molecule.[89] Deficiency of GAPDH seems a rare occurrence without functional consequences.[90]

Phosphoglycerate Kinase PGK effects the transfer to ADP of the high-energy phosphate from the 1-carbon of 1,3-diphosphoglycerate to form ATP. The reaction is readily reversible and can be bypassed by the Rapoport-Luebering shunt. The isoenzyme PGK-1 is ubiquitously expressed in all somatic cells and is a 48-kDa monomeric enzyme of 417 amino acids.[91] Expression of isozyme PGK-2 has been found in testis.[92] PGK is composed of two domains. The N-terminal domain binds 3-phosphoglycerate and 1,3-diphosphoglycerate, whereas ADP and ATP bind to the C-terminal domain. For catalysis to occur, the protein needs to undergo a large conformational change ("hinge bending").[93-95] The gene encoding PGK (*PGK1*) is located on the long arm of the X-chromosome (Xq13), spans 23 kb, and is composed of 11 exons. Nonfunctional pseudogenes have been located on chromosome 19 and the X-chromosome.[92] Deficiency of PGK is a rare cause of nonspherocytic hemolytic anemia, often associated with neuromuscular abnormalities.

Bisphosphoglycerate Mutase The same protein molecule is responsible for both bisphosphoglycerate mutase and bisphosphoglycerate phosphatase activities in the erythrocyte.[29,96] This enzyme is particularly important because it regulates the concentration of 2,3-BPG of erythrocytes. In its role as a bisphosphoglyceromutase, the enzyme competes with PGK for 1,3-BPG as a substrate. It changes 1,3-BPG to 2,3-BPG, thereby dissipating the energy of the high-energy acylphosphate bond.[97] It is inhibited by its product 2,3-BPG and by inorganic phosphate, and it is activated by 2-phosphoglycerate and by increased pH levels. It requires 3-phosphoglycerate for activity. In its role as bisphosphoglycerate phosphatase, it catalyzes the removal of the phosphate group from carbon 2 of 2,3-BPG.[97] It is inhibited by its product 3-phosphoglycerate and by sulfhydryl reagents. It is most active at a slightly acid pH and is strongly stimulated by bisulfite and phosphoglycolate. Phosphoglycolate, the most potent activator of phosphatase activity, is present in erythrocytes at very low concentrations, but the source of this substance in red cells is unknown.[98,99] Phosphoglycolate phosphatase, the enzyme that hydrolyzes phosphoglycolate, also has been identified in erythrocytes.[100]

Bisphosphoglycerate mutase is a homodimer, with 30-kDa subunits consisting of 258 amino acids. The crystal structure of human bisphosphoglycerate mutase has been determined, providing a rationale for the specific residues that are crucial for synthase, mutase, and phosphatase activity.[101,102] The gene for bisphosphoglycerate mutase (*BPGM*) has been mapped to chromosome 7q31-34 and it consists of three exons, spanning more than 22 kb.

A deficiency of bisphosphoglycerate mutase results in a marked decrease in red cell 2,3-BPG levels. The consequent left shift of the oxygen dissociation curve leads to erythrocytosis (Chap. 28).

Phosphoglycerate Mutase An equilibrium is established between 3-phosphoglycerate and 2-phosphoglycerate by phosphoglycerate mutase.[103] 2,3-BPG acts as an essential cofactor for the transformation. Red blood cell phosphoglycerate mutase is a heterodimer consisting of M and B subunits, encoded by separate genes.[104] Only one case of partial red blood cell monophosphoglycerate mutase deficiency has been described in a patient with hereditary spherocytosis. The patient showed homozygosity for a p.Met230Ile amino acid change in the B subunit.[105] The mutant enzyme showed increased instability.[106] Unexpectedly, all glycolytic intermediates were decreased, possibly from lactate accumulation.[107] The exact clinical consequences of this red blood cell enzymopathy remain to be established.

Enolase Enolase is homodimeric enzyme that establishes an equilibrium between 2-phosphoglycerate and phosphoenolpyruvate. The reaction is facilitated by the presence of metal ions.[108] Aside from its enzymatic function in the glycolytic pathway, α-enolase (ENO1) has been implicated in numerous diseases, including glycogen storage disease, metastatic cancer, autoimmune disorders, ischemia, and bacterial infection.[109] The *ENO1* gene is located on chromosome 1p36.23. Enolase deficiency is extremely rare. It has been reported in association with hereditary nonspherocytic hemolytic anemia[110,111] but also in a patient with Diamond-Blackfan anemia.[112] A clear cause-and-effect relationship for enolase deficiency has not yet been firmly established.

Pyruvate Kinase The transfer of phosphate from phosphoenolpyruvate to ADP, forming ATP and pyruvate, is catalyzed by PK. This is the second energy-yielding step of glycolysis. PK is allosterically activated by fructose 1,6-bisphosphate. Four PK isoenzymes are present in mammalian tissues: PK-M1 (in skeletal muscle), PK-M2 (in leukocytes, kidney, adipose tissue, and lungs), PK-L (in liver), and PK-R (in red blood cells). The four PK isoenzymes are products of only two genes (*PKLR* and *PKM2*). The PK-M1 and PK-M2 enzymes are formed from the *PKM2* gene by alternative splicing.[113] PK-L (the liver enzyme) and PK-R (the erythrocyte enzyme) are products of the other gene (*PKLR*), transcribed from two different, tissue-specific promoters.[114,115] Notably, mutations in other genes, that is, *KLF1*, have been associated with severe transfusion-dependent hemolytic anemia and PK deficiency,[116] and there is evidence that other yet unknown, regulatory elements are involved in *PKLR* gene expression.[117] *PKLR* consists of 12 exons and spans more than 10 kb. Exon 2, but not exon 1, is present in the processed liver transcript; in the red cell enzyme, exon 1, but not exon 2, is represented.[115] The red blood cell–specific mRNA is 2 kb in length and codes for a full-length 63-kDa PK-R subunit of 574 amino acids.[118] Red blood cell PK is a heterotetramer comprised of two 62-63-kDa and two 57-58-kDa subunits, with the 57-58-kDa subunits resulting from limited proteolytic cleavage of the full-length subunit.[119,120] Each subunit of PK-R contains an N domain, A domain, B domain, and C domain (Fig. 16–4).[121] Domain A is the most highly conserved, whereas the B and C domains are more variable.[122] The functional role of the N domain is unknown, but it may play a role in enzyme regulation.[123,124] The active site of PK lies in a cleft between the A domain and the flexible B domain. The C domain contains the binding site for fructose-1,6-diphosphate. Both intrasubunit and intersubunit interactions are considered to be key determinants of the allosteric response, which involves

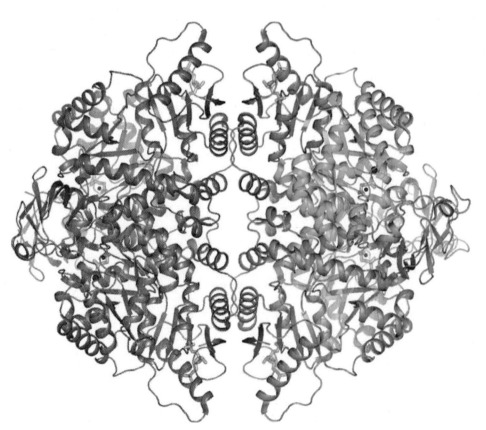

Figure 16–4. Ribbon representation of the human erythrocyte pyruvate kinase monomer tetramer. The substrate phosphoglycolate and fructose-1,6-diphosphate are shown in ball-and-stick representation, and colored yellow and gray, respectively. Metal ions in the active site are shown as blue (potassium) and pink (manganese) spheres. Individual subunits are colored lime, cyan, violet, and orange.

switching of the PK tetramer from the low-affinity T-state to the high-affinity R-state.[125-129] Red cell PK manifests sigmoid kinetics with respect to phosphoenolpyruvate in the absence of fructose-1,6-diphosphate. Hyperbolic kinetics are observed in the presence of even minute amounts of fructose-1,6-diphosphate,[119,130] so that at low concentrations of phosphoenolpyruvate the enzyme activity is greatly increased by fructose diphosphate. PK deficiency is the most common disorder of red blood cell glycolysis and the second most common cause of nonspherocytic hemolytic anemia.

Lactate Dehydrogenase LDH catalyzes the reversible reduction of pyruvate to lactate by NADH, the last step in the Embden-Meyerhof pathway. The enzyme is composed of H (heart) and M (muscle) subunits. In red cells, the predominant subunit is H. Hereditary absence of the H subunit seems to be a benign condition, usually without clinical manifestations,[131,132] although 1 case with hemolysis has been reported.[133] Absence of the M subunit has been reported as well,[134] and was unaccompanied by hematologic manifestations. Judging from the origin of the reports, LDH deficiency is most common in Japan, where population surveys show a gene frequency of approximately 0.05 for each deficiency, and several mutations have been identified.[135]

Glucose-6-Phosphate Dehydrogenase G6PD is the most extensively studied erythrocyte enzyme. It catalyzes the oxidation of glucose-6-phosphate to 6-phosphogluconolactone, which is rapidly hydrolyzed to 6-phosphogluconic acid, in the first and rate-limiting step of the hexose monophosphate pathway. $NADP^+$ is reduced to NADPH in this reaction, generating 1 mole of NADPH. In the erythrocyte, the hexose monophosphate pathway is the only source of NADPH, which is crucial in maintaining high cellular levels of GSH to protect the cell from oxidative stress-induced damage.

The G6PD monomer is composed of 515 amino acids with a calculated molecular weight of approximately 59 kDa.[136] Aggregation of these inactive monomers into catalytically active dimers and higher forms requires the presence of $NADP^+$ (Fig. 16–5).[137] Hence, $NADP^+$ is bound to the enzyme both as a structural component, in the subunit interface, and as one of the substrates of the reaction.[138-140] Under physiologic conditions, the active human enzyme exists in a dimer–tetramer equilibrium. Lowering the pH causes a shift toward the tetrameric form.[138,141,142]

G6PD is strongly inhibited by physiologic amounts of NADPH[143] and, to a lesser extent, by physiologic concentrations of ATP.[144] It has much higher enzyme activity in reticulocytes than in mature red cells, especially for the mutant forms of the enzyme.[38,145,146]

The three-dimensional model of the crystal structure of human G6PD shows that the G6PD monomer is built up by two domains, a N-terminal domain and a large β+α domain with an antiparallel 9-stranded sheet. The extensive interface between the two monomers is of crucial importance for enzymatic stability and activity.[140] The fully conserved amino acids 198-205 (Arg-Ile-Asp-His-Tyr-Leu-Gly-Lys) are essential for substrate binding and catalysis.[140,147-149]

The gene for G6PD (*G6PD*) is located on the X-chromosome (Xq28). It spans 18 kb and consists of 13 exons of which exon 1 is noncoding. G6PD deficiency is one of the world's most common hereditary disorders, and many mutations and variants have been reported and studied.[2,150-152]

Phosphogluconolactonase Although 6-phosphogluconolactone, the direct product of the oxidation of glucose-6-phosphate by G6PD, hydrolyzes spontaneously at a relatively rapid rate at a physiologic pH, enzymatic hydrolysis is much more rapid and is required for normal metabolic flow through the stimulated hexose monophosphate pathway.[153,154] Partial deficiency of the enzyme has been observed[155] and is probably benign.

Phosphogluconate Dehydrogenase Phosphogluconate dehydrogenase catalyzes the oxidation of phosphogluconate to ribulose-5-phosphate and CO_2 and the reduction of $NADP^+$ to NADPH. Variability of electrophoretic mobility of the enzyme is common in humans and in several animal species.[156] Deficiency of the enzyme has been observed rarely and is essentially innocuous or possibly associated with mild hemolysis.[157-159]

Ribosephosphate Isomerase Ribosephosphate isomerase catalyzes the interconversion of ribulose-5-phosphate and ribose-5-phosphate. Deficiency of the enzyme has been described as one of the rarest human disorders.[160] It manifests with progressive leukoencephalopathy and neuropathy. No dysfunction of red cells is reported.[161]

Ribulose-Phosphate Epimerase Ribulose-phosphate epimerase converts ribulose-5-phosphate to xylulose-5-phosphate. The exact activity of this enzyme in human hemolysates has not been reported but seems to be less than that of ribosephosphate isomerase.

Transketolase Transketolase effects the transfer of 2 carbon atoms from xylulose-5-phosphate to ribose-5-phosphate, resulting in the formation of the 7-carbon sugar sedoheptulose-7-phosphate and the 3-carbon sugar glyceraldehyde-3-phosphate.[162] It can also catalyze the reaction between xylulose-5-phosphate and erythrose-4-phosphate, producing fructose-6-phosphate and glyceraldehyde-3-phosphate.

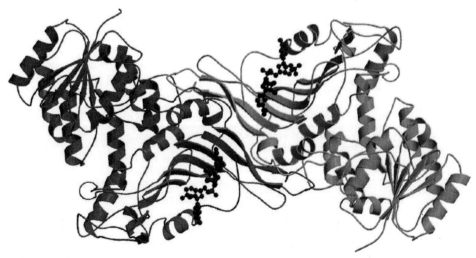

Figure 16–5. A dimer of human glucose-6-phosphate dehydrogenase. Subunits A and B are colored red and blue. Structural $NADP^+$ molecules are drawn in ball-and-stick mode and colored dark blue.

Thiamine pyrophosphate is a coenzyme for transketolase, and the activity of erythrocyte transketolase is used as an index of the adequacy of thiamine nutrition.[163] Red cell transketolase was found to be downregulated in patients with pyrimidine-5'-nucleotidase (P5'N) deficiency, and may represent a biomarker for this enzyme deficiency.[164]

Transaldolase The conversion of seduhepulose-7-phosphate and glyceraldehyde-3-phosphate into erythrose-4-phosphate and fructose-6-phosphate is catalyzed by transaldolase.[165] This is another in the series of molecular rearrangements that leads in the conversion of the five-carbon sugar formed in the phosphogluconate dehydrogenase step to metabolic intermediates of the Embden-Meyerhof direct glycolytic pathway. Transaldolase deficiency is a very rare disorder and first reported in 2001 as a new inborn error of the pentose phosphate pathway.[166] It is a pleiotropic metabolic disorder, and patients present in the neonatal or antenatal period with dysmorphic features, hepatosplenomegaly, abnormal liver function, cardiac defects, thrombocytopenia, bleeding tendencies, and anemia. The anemia is hemolytic in nature, possibly as a consequence of decreased levels of NADPH.[167]

L-Hexonate Dehydrogenase Red cells contain L-hexonate dehydrogenase, an enzyme that has the capacity to reduce aldoses, such as glucose, galactose, and glyceraldehyde, to their corresponding polyol (ie, glucose to sorbitol, galactose to dulcitol, and glyceraldehyde to glycerol). NADPH serves as a hydrogen donor for this reaction.[168] Aldose reductase is another enzyme that can catalyze this reaction. It is present in red cells,[169] and increased levels have been implicated in diabetic complications, such as retinopathy[170] and autonomic neuropathy.[171]

Use of Substrates Other Than Glucose as Energy Sources

The red cell has the capacity to use several other substrates in addition to glucose as a source of energy. Among these other substrates are adenosine, inosine, fructose, mannose, galactose, dihydroxyacetone, and lactate.[172] Although in the circulation red cells normally rely on glucose as their energy source, the use of other substrates, particularly during blood storage (Chap. 30) and in certain experimental situations, is of interest.

Glutathione Metabolism of the Erythrocyte

The red cell contains a high concentration of the sulfhydryl-containing tripeptide GSH. It serves a major role in antioxidant defense, detoxification, and maintenance of thiol status. Reported concentrations range between 0.4 and 3.0 mM, with a terminal half-life of approximately 4 days.[173] The wide interindividual range suggests that GSH levels are, at least in part, genetically determined.[174] In its role of defense against oxidative stress GSH is oxidized to GSSG, which can be reverted back to GSH by mediation of GSH reductase. In addition, GSSG can be transported out of the cell.[175]

GSH biosynthesis occurs in two ATP-dependent steps:

$$\text{Glutamate} + \text{Cysteine} + \text{ATP} \rightarrow \gamma\text{-Glutamylcysteine} + \text{ADP}$$

$$+ \text{P}_i\,\gamma\text{-Glutamylcysteine} + \text{Glycine} + \text{ATP} \rightarrow \text{GSH} + \text{ADP} + \text{P}_i$$

The first step is rate limiting and catalyzed by glutamate cysteine ligase (GCL; γ-glutamylcysteine synthetase). Feedback inhibition of GCL by GSH is commonly considered a key regulatory step in GSH homeostasis, but other pathways are likely to play a role in maintaining GSH levels.[176] GCL is a heterodimer composed of a 73-kDa catalytic subunit (GCLC) and a 31-kDa modifier subunit (GCLM).[177,178] An intersubunit disulfide bond has been implicated in stabilization and catalytic efficiency of the heterodimer, acting as a cellular reduction–oxidation (redox) switch to couple enzyme activity, and consequently GSH levels, with the redox state of the cell.[179,180] An alternative model suggests that increased levels of oxidative stress induce the formation of

high activity heterodimer complexes from low activity monomeric and holoenzyme forms of the enzyme.[181] GCL subunits are encoded by separate genes, located on chromosome 6p12 (*GCLC*) and 1p22.1 (*GCLM*), respectively. *GCLC* contains 16 exons that encode the 637 amino acids of the catalytic subunit, whereas *GCLM* contains 7 exons that encode the 274 amino acids of the modifier subunit. GCL deficiency is a very rare cause of hemolytic anemia.

The second step in GSH synthesis is irreversible and mediated by glutathione synthetase (GS). This enzyme is a homodimer composed of 52-kDa subunits,[182] and the crystal structure of human GS has been resolved.[183] There is 1 gene coding for GS. This 23-kb gene (*GSS*) is located on chromosome 20q11.2 and contains 13 exons, of which the first is noncoding, that code for the 474-amino-acids-long protein. Deficiency of GS is the most common disorder of GSH synthesis and is associated with hemolytic anemia.

One important function of GSH in the erythrocyte is the detoxification of low levels of hydrogen peroxide that may form spontaneously, enzymatically, or as a result of drug administration. Hydrogen peroxide is reduced to water through mediation of the enzyme GSH peroxidase,[184] thereby oxidizing GSH to GSSG (Fig. 16–6). Several GSH peroxidases exist but only type 1 is expressed in red blood cells.[185]

GSH peroxidase is a selenium-containing tetrameric enzyme consisting of 21-kDa subunits. A polymorphism affecting the activity of this enzyme, which is most common in persons of Mediterranean descent,[186] has been described. The consequent decreases in enzyme activity are without clinical effect.[187] In agreement with this, complete loss of GSH peroxidase activity in mice was found to be without any consequences, even at high levels of oxidative stress, thus suggesting that GSH peroxidase is of minor significance for red cell function.[185]

GSH also functions in maintaining integrity of the erythrocyte by reducing sulfhydryl groups of membrane proteins,[188] and glycolytic

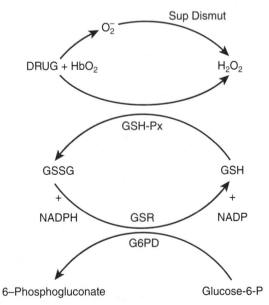

Figure 16–6. Reactions through which hydrogen peroxide (H_2O_2) is generated and detoxified in the erythrocyte. In glucose-6-phosphate dehydrogenase (G6PD) deficiency and related disorders, inadequate generation of nicotinamide adenine dinucleotide phosphate (NADPH) results in accumulation of GSSG and probably of H_2O_2. The accumulation of these substances leads to hemoglobin denaturation, Heinz body formation, and, consequently, to decreased red cell survival. GSR, glutathione reductase; GSH-Px, glutathione peroxidase; GSSG, glutathione disulfide (oxidized glutathione); HbO₂, oxyhemoglobin; Sup Dismut, superoxide dismutase.

enzymes,[189] for example, PK.[190] In the process of reducing peroxides or oxidized protein sulfhydryl groups, GSH is converted to GSSG, or may form mixed disulfides. Thus, for instance, GSSG has the capacity to inhibit red cell hexokinase,[44] although greater than physiologic levels may be needed for this effect. It may also complex with hemoglobin A to form hemoglobin A$_3$.[191]

Glutathione reductase (GSR) provides an efficient mechanism for the reduction of GSSG to regenerate GSH, and thus maintaining high intracellular levels of GSH. A mitochondrial and a cytoplasmic isozyme are both produced from the same mRNA, most likely by alternative initiation of translation.[192] GSR is a homodimer, linked by a disulfide bridge. Each 56-kDa subunit contains 4 domains, of which domains 1 and 2 bind flavin adenine dinucleotide and NADPH, respectively. Domain 4 constitutes the interface.[193] The subunit is encoded by the *GSR* gene, located on chromosome 8p21.1. *GSR* spans 50 kb, contains 13 exons and encodes a 522-amino-acids-long protein. GSR is a flavin enzyme, and either NADPH or NADH may serve as a hydrogen donor although in the intact cell, only the NADPH system functions.[194] The same enzyme system has the capacity to reduce mixed disulfides of GSH and proteins.[37] The activity of red cell GSR is strongly influenced by the riboflavin content of the diet[195] and its activity is used as a biomarker for riboflavin status. Correction of partial GSR deficiency by riboflavin administration has been reported to ameliorate hemolysis in a case of unstable hemoglobin.[196] Hereditary deficiency of GSR is a very rare disorder that is associated with hemolytic anemia.

Red cells also contain glutaredoxin (thioltransferase) that can catalyze GSH-dependent reduction of some disulfides.[197]

GSSG is actively extruded from the erythrocyte.[198] GSSG efflux is likely an important regulator of GSH turnover in red blood cells.[199] The system consists of at least 2 GSSG-activated ATPs that serve as an enzymatic basis for this transport process.[200] In addition to transporting GSSG, the system has the capacity to transport thioether conjugates of GSH and electrophiles formed by the action of glutathione-*S*-transferase.[201] Preliminary evidence indicates that multidrug resistance protein 1 may be the exporter protein of both glutathione-S conjugates and GSSG.[176]

Erythrocytes contain glutathione-*S*-transferases rho, sigma, and theta.[202-204] The major isoform, however, is GSH transferase phi.[205] Glutathione-*S*-transferase catalyzes the formation of a thioether bond between GSH and a variety of xenobiotics. The role of glutathione-*S*-transferase in the erythrocyte has not been established. It may be that it serves to cleanse the blood of xenobiotics to which the red cell membrane is permeable. Glutathione-*S*-transferase could conjugate such substances to GSH, and the detoxified product of conjugation would be transported out of the red cell for subsequent disposal. The enzyme has the capacity to reversibly bind heme, and a possible role in heme transport has been postulated.[206] Fairly severe deficiency of this enzyme is associated with hemolytic anemia, but a cause-and-effect relationship has not been established.[207]

Other Antioxidant Enzymes

Superoxide radicals that are formed are converted to hydrogen peroxide by the action of the copper-containing enzyme superoxide dismutase (SOD1). Red blood cells contain SOD type 1 (encoded by the *SOD1* gene). Mutations in *SOD1* are associated with the dominant disorder familial amyotrophic lateral sclerosis.[208] Patients display no hematologic phenotype, even in complete absence of SOD1 activity.[209] SOD1 null mice are viable, but show elevated levels of oxidative stress that causes regenerative anemia and triggers autoantibody production.[210]

Apart from GSH peroxidase, hydrogen peroxide can be decomposed to water and oxygen by catalase and peroxiredoxin. Both enzymes are abundantly present in the red blood cell, suggesting an important role in the cell's oxidative defense.[211] Nevertheless, acatalasemia, or catalase deficiency, is a rare benign condition without hematologic consequences.[212] Deficiencies of peroxiredoxin 2, the major red cell peroxiredoxin have not been reported in humans. Peroxiredoxin 2 null mice, however, develop severe hemolytic anemia with Heinz body formation,[213] and show signs of abnormal erythropoiesis.[214] Based on mouse models, it has been postulated that GSH peroxidase, catalase, and peroxiredoxin each have distinct roles in the scavenging of hydrogen peroxide and antioxidative defense.[215-217]

Nucleotide Metabolism of the Erythrocyte

Approximately 97% of the total nucleotide content of the mature red blood cell consists of interconvertible adenosine phosphates (Chaps. 1 and 2). Less than 3% of total nucleotides are guanosine phosphates. ATP is the most abundant adenosine phosphate (comprising roughly 84% of total adenosine ribonucleotides), whereas ADP (14%) and adenosine monophosphate (AMP, 1%) are present in considerably lower amounts. The interconversion of adenine nucleotides is modulated by adenylate kinase (AK):

$$Mg^{2+} + ATP + AMP \rightarrow Mg^{2+} + ADP + ADP$$

By catalyzing the reversible phosphoryl transfer among ATP, ADP, and AMP, AK contributes to cellular adenine nucleotide homeostasis. Red cells contain the AK1 isozyme, which is present in the cytosol as a monomeric enzyme composed of 194 amino acids. The recombinant purified enzyme has a molecular mass of approximately 22 kDa.[218] The gene (*AK1*) is localized on chromosome 9q34.1, and consists of 7 exons of which exon 1 is noncoding. AK activity depends on the presence of Mg^{2+}.

ATP serves as a cofactor in a number of reactions, such as the phosphorylation steps mediated by HK and PFK in glycolysis, the synthesis of GSH, and ATPase-dependent function of membrane pumps. Therefore, ATP is crucial in maintenance of the red cell's structure and function. Because the mature red cell is unable to synthesize adenosine phosphates from precursor molecules it relies on salvage pathways to preserve adenosine ribonucleotides. This is of particular importance for AMP because this adenosine ribonucleotide is at risk of being lost from the adenine pool by dephosphorylation to adenosine and, subsequent, irreversible deamination to inosine by the enzyme adenosine deaminase (ADA). ADA thus plays a regulatory role in the concentration of adenosine ribonucleotides in the red cell. At the same time, mouse models suggest that AMP uptake and ATP release may also contribute to recycling and maintaining the adenine nucleotide pool.[219] The gene encoding ADA (*ADA*) is located on chromosome 20q13.12. It comprises 12 exons that encode a 363-amino-acid protein.

Deficiency of AK and, even more, hyperactivity of ADA are both very rare causes of hereditary nonspherocytic hemolytic anemia.

Additional enzymes of purine metabolism are also present in the red cell. Although disorders of these enzymes are associated with a number of metabolic diseases, their function does not appear to be relevant for the red blood cell as these disorders are without hematologic consequences.[220]

Pyrimidine ribonucleotides are found only in trace amounts in the mature red blood cell. They are lost from the cell together with the degradation of ribosomes and RNA during reticulocyte maturation. P5′N1 mediates this loss by catalyzing the dephosphorylation of pyrimidine nucleoside monophosphates into the corresponding nucleosides (cytidine and uridine), which are freely diffusible across the membrane.[221] P5′N1 is specific for pyrimidine nucleotides and does not use purine nucleotides as substrate.[222] The enzyme requires Mg^{2+} for it activity, and is inhibited by a number of heavy metals, including Pb^{2+}.[223] Like other red blood cell enzymes, P5′N1 activity is much higher in reticulocytes.

The enzyme, however, displays a unique pattern of decline in activity during red cell aging.[224] P5′N1 also has phosphotransferase properties, suggesting an additional role of this enzyme in nucleotide metabolism.[225] The crystal structure of mouse P5′N1 has been published, providing a framework for understanding the kinetics of both nucleotidase and phosphotransferase activities of human P5′N1.[226]

P5′N1 is encoded by the *NT5C3* gene on chromosome 7p14.3. It comprises 11 exons, and produces 3 distinct mRNAs by alternative splicing. Red cell P5′N1 is translated from the mRNA lacking exons 2 and R.[227,228] It is a 286-amino-acids-long monomeric protein with an apparent molecular weight of 34 kDa.[227]

A second P5′N enzyme, P5′N2, is present in red blood cells and its activity is generally measured together with that of P5′N1. P5′N2 is encoded by a separate gene, shows little homology to P5′N1, and is not strictly pyrimidine-specific. It is unable to compensate for deficient function of P5′N1.[225,229] P5′N1 deficiency is one of the most common causes of hereditary nonspherocytic hemolytic anemia.

Human red blood cells have been found to express low NAD synthesis activity, mediated by nicotinamide mononucleotide adenylyltransferase.[230] The predominant isozyme in red blood cells is nicotinamide mononucleotide adenylyltransferase-3.[231] Human dysfunction of this enzyme has not been reported but the deficiency in mice blocks glycolysis at the GAPDH step and is associated with hemolytic anemia.[232]

GENETICS

The great majority of red cell enzyme deficiencies that cause hemolytic anemia are hereditary. Most are inherited as autosomal recessive disorders, but G6PD deficiency and PGK deficiency are X-chromosome-linked. The vast majority of the genes encoding for the red cell enzymes have been identified, making the molecular diagnosis of hereditary red cell enzyme deficiency possible. Occasionally, acquired forms of enzyme deficiencies, particularly PK deficiency, have been encountered, usually in patients with hematologic neoplasia.[233-237] PK levels are also pathologically reduced in patients with red blood cell disorders caused by mutations in *KLF1*.[116]

ENZYME DEFICIENCIES: BIOCHEMICAL GENETICS AND MOLECULAR BIOLOGY

Table 16–2 lists the erythrocyte enzyme deficiencies that have been shown to cause hemolytic disease. Other red cell enzyme deficiencies (Table 16–3) do not appear to cause hemolysis.[187] For example, acatalasemia, the state in which there is a virtually total absence of red cell catalase, is devoid of hematologic manifestations.[238] Similarly, red cells without acetylcholinesterase survive normally in most cases.[239] Other red cell enzyme deficiencies may be associated with hereditary hematologic diseases, such as erythrocytosis caused by bisphosphoglycerate mutase deficiency (see "Bisphosphoglycerate Mutase Deficiency" further) or methemoglobinemia caused by cytochrome-b5-reductase deficiency (Chap. 19).

The lack of clinical manifestations is not always clear-cut. In some instances, hemolytic anemia is reported in some individuals with a given deficiency, but not in others. For example, most subjects with LDH deficiency have no anemia, but cases with hemolysis have been reported.[133] Such ambiguity could result from differences in environmental and genetic factors or from bias of ascertainment. Erythrocyte enzyme assays are usually carried out on patients with hemolytic anemia. Thus, a benign enzyme defect may be thought, mistakenly, to cause hemolysis because it is found in a patient with hemolytic anemia. Table 16–3 includes deficiencies that may cause hemolytic anemia but for which a cause-and-effect relationship has not been clearly

established, such as those of phosphogluconolactonase,[155] enolase,[110,111] and glutathione-*S*-transferase.[207]

Patients with unstable hemoglobins (Chap. 18) may present with the clinical picture of hereditary nonspherocytic hemolytic anemia. Hemolytic anemia resulting from abnormalities in the lipid composition of the red cell membrane, particularly increased phosphatidyl choline, occurs rarely (Chap. 15).

Glucose-6-Phosphate Dehydrogenase

The "normal" or wild-type enzyme is designated as G6PD B. Many variants of G6PD have been detected all over the world, associated with a wide range of biochemical characteristics and phenotypes. Accordingly, five classes of G6PD variants can be distinguished based on enzymatic activity and clinical manifestations (Table 16–4).[240] Before it became possible to characterize G6PD variants at the DNA level, they were distinguished from each other on the basis of biochemical characteristics, such as electrophoretic mobility, K_m (Michaelis constant) for NADP and glucose-6-P, ability to use substrate analogues, pH activity profile, and thermal stability. The amount of enzyme antigen in the red cells declines concurrently with enzyme activity.[241] This suggests that the mutant protein in these variants is rendered unusually sensitive to proteolysis in the environment of the erythrocyte.[242] By far the majority of mutations (85%) are missense mutations causing the substitution of a single amino acid. More severe mutations causing a complete loss of activity are absent, indicating that some residual activity is required for survival. In agreement with this, targeted deletion of G6PD in the mouse causes embryonic lethality.[243]

Detailed biochemical and genetic characteristics of some 400 putatively distinct G6PD variants and more than 200 different mutations have been tabulated.[244,245] Table 16–4 lists the common G6PD variants that have reached polymorphic frequencies in certain populations.

African Variants Among persons of African descent, a mutant enzyme G6PD A+, with normal activity is polymorphic. It migrates electrophoretically more rapidly than the normal B enzyme, has substitution of Asn to Asp at codon 126, resulting from nucleotide change c.376A>G.[246] G6PD A– is the principal deficient variant found among people of African origin. The red cells contain only 5% to 15% of the normal amount of enzyme activity; however, because of the instability of the enzyme, the age-dependent decline of the activity renders old red cells severely deficient and susceptible to hemolysis. These two electrophoretically rapid variants are common in African populations have in common a nucleotide substitution at cDNA nucleotide 376 that produces the amino acid substitution responsible for the rapid electrophoretic mobility. Most samples with G6PD A– manifest an additional in *cis* G>A mutation at cDNA nucleotide 202 (c.202G>A; p.Val68Met), which accounts for its in vivo instability.[247] Less commonly, the additional mutation is at a different site [c.680G>T p.(Arg227Leu) or c.968T>C p.(Leu323Pro)].[247] Thus G6PD A– arose in an individual who already had the G6PD A+ mutation. Although it has been suggested that only the interaction of p.Val68Met and p.Asn126Asp results in G6PD deficiency,[248] the c.202G>A mutation has been found in a G6PD-deficient patient with acute hemolysis without the presence of the mutation at cDNA nt 376.[249]

Variants in the Mediterranean Region Among white populations, G6PD deficiency is most common in Mediterranean countries. The most common enzyme variant in this region is G6PD Mediterranean. The enzyme activity of the red cells of individuals with this mutation is hardly detectable. Other variants are also prevalent in the Mediterranean region, including G6PD A– and G6PD Seattle (see Table 16–4).

Variants in Asia A great many different variants have been described in Asian populations. Some of these proved to be identical

TABLE 16–2. Red Cell Enzyme Abnormalities Leading to Hemolytic Disease

Enzyme	Clinical Features	Inheritance	Red Cell Morphology	Diagnosis (Reference) Screening Test	Diagnosis (Reference) Assay	Response to Splenectomy[a]	Approximate Frequency[b]
Hexokinase	HNSHA	AR	Unremarkable	—	541	+ +	Rare
Glucose phosphate isomerase	HNSHA; neurologic abnormalities	AR	Unremarkable	541	541	+ + +	Unusual
Phosphofructokinase	HNSHA and/or muscle glycogen storage disease	AR	Unremarkable	—	541	0	Rare
Aldolase	HNSHA and mild liver glycogen storage; myopathy, mental retardation	AR	Unremarkable	—	541	?	Very rare
Triosephosphate isomerase	HNSHA and severe neuromuscular disease	AR	Unremarkable	541	541	?	Rare
Phosphoglycerate kinase	HNSHA; myopathy neuromuscular disorder	SL	Unremarkable	—	541	+ +	Rare
Pyruvate kinase	HNSHA	AR	Usually unremarkable; occasionally contracted echinocytes	541	541	+ +	Unusual
Glucose-6-phosphate dehydrogenase	HNSHA; drug- or infection-induced hemolysis; favism	SL	Usually unremarkable; rarely "bite cells"	541	541	±	Very common
Glutathione reductase	Drug-sensitive hemolytic anemia and favism	AR	Unremarkable	541	541	?	Very rare
Glutamate cysteine ligase	HNSHA, drug- or infection-induced hemolysis, neurologic abnormalities	AR	Unremarkable	194	596	?	Very rare
Glutathione synthetase	HNSHA; drug- or infection-induced hemolysis; neurologic defect and 5-oxoprolinuria in some cases	AR	Usually unremarkable	194	596	0	Rare
Pyrimidine 5′-nucleotidase	HNSHA; mental retardation in some cases	AR	Prominent stippling	222	597	0	Unusual
Adenylate kinase	HNSHA; neurologic abnormalities	AR	Unremarkable	—	541	?	Rare
Adenosine deaminase (increased activity)	HNSHA	AD	Unremarkable	—	541	?	Very rare

AD, autosomal dominant; AR, autosomal recessive; HNSHA, hereditary nonspherocytic hemolytic anemia; NA, not applicable; SL, sex linked

[a]On a scale of 0 to 4+, where 4+ is a complete response. In many cases, data are meager.

[b]Very common if incidence is >5%. Unusual if more than 100 cases reported. Rare if 10-100 cases reported. Very rare if fewer than 10 cases reported.

TABLE 16-3. Red Cell Enzyme Abnormalities Not Leading to Hemolytic Disease

Enzyme	Clinical Features	Inheritance	Diagnosis Reference Assay	Estimated Frequency[a]	Reference
6-Phosphogluconate dehydrogenase (complete deficiency)	None, HNSHA?	AR	541	Unusual	157-159
6-Phosphogluconolactonase (partial defect)	Probably none	AD	598	Unusual	155
δ-ALA dehydrase	None	AD	599		
Acetylcholinesterase	None	AR	541	Very rare	239
Adenine phosphoribosyl transferase	Kidney stones, nephropathy	AR	600	Rare	601
Adenosine deaminase (decreased activity)	Severe immunodeficiency (SCID)	AR	541	Rare	602
AMP deaminase	None	AR	603	Unusual	604
Bisphosphoglycerate mutase	Erythrocytosis	AR	541	Very rare	343, 346
Carbonic anhydrase I	None	AR	605	Rare	606
Carbonic anhydrase II	Osteoporosis	AR		Rare	607
Catalase	Oral ulcers in some types	AR	541	Rare	608
Cytochrome-b5-reductase	Methemoglobinemia; mental retardation	AR	541	Unusual	609, 610
Enolase	HNSHA?	AD?	541	Rare	110, 111
Galactokinase	Cataracts, galactosemia type 2	AR	541	Rare	611, 612
Galactose-1-P-uridyltransferase	Galactosemia type 1 (cataracts; mental retardation; infertility)	AR	541	Rare	613, 614
Glutathione peroxidase (partial deficiency)	None, HNSHA?	AR and AD	541	Very common	187, 541, 615
Glutathione reductase (partial deficiency)	None	Usually not inherited	541	Very common	187, 195
Glutathione-S-transferase	HNSHA?	?	541	Very rare	207
Glyceraldehyde-3-phosphate dehydrogenase (partial defect)	None	AD	541	Unusual	90
Glyoxalase I	None	AR		Rare	616
Hypoxanthine-guanine phosphoribosyl transferase (HGPRT)	Lesch-Nyhan syndrome (neurologic symptoms, gout, nephropathy); Kelley-Seegmuller syndrome (partial defect)	SL	617	Rare	618, 619
Inosine triphosphatase	None	AR	606	Rare	620, 621
Lactate dehydrogenase (H-subunit)	None, HNSHA?	AR	541	Rare	132, 133
NADPH diaphorase	None	AR	541	Rare	622
Phosphoglucomutase	None	AR	541	Rare	623, 624
Transaldolase	Congenital heart disease, intra uterine growth retardation, hepatosplenomegaly, pancytopenia, HNSHA?	AR	625	Rare	165, 167
Uroporphyrinogen 1 synthase	Porphyria	AR	626	Unusual (common in selected populations)	627, 628

AD, autosomal dominant; ALA, aminolevulinic acid; AMP, adenosine monophosphate; AR, autosomal recessive; HNSHA, hereditary nonspherocytic hemolytic anemia; SL, sex linked.

[a]Very common if incidence is >5%, common if 1%-5%, unusual if 0.01%-1%, rare if <0.01%.

TABLE 16–4. Major Polymorphic Glucose-6-Phosphate Dehydrogenase Variants

Variant	Nucleotide Substitution	Amino Acid Substitution	WHO Class[a]	Distribution	Reference
Gaohe	c.95A>G	p.(His32Arg)	III	China	[629]
Honiara	c.99A>G	p.(Ile33Met)	I	Solomon Islands	[630]
	c.1360C>T	p.(Arg454Cys)			
Orissa	c.131C>G	p.(Ala44Gly)	III	India, Italy	[631, 632]
Aures	c.143T>C	p.(Ile48Thr)	III	Algeria, Tunisia	[633, 634]
Metaponto	c.172G>A	p.(Asp58Asn)	III	Italy	[635]
A–	c.202G>A	p.(Val68Met)	III	Africa	[636]
	c.376A>G	p.(Asn126Asp)			
Namoru	c.208T>C	p.(Tyr70His)	II	Vanuatu Archipelago	[637]
Ube-Konan	c.241C>T	p.(Arg81Cys)	III	Japan, Italy	[632, 638]
A+	c.376A>G	p.(Asn126Asp)	III-IV	Africa, Mediterranean	[246]
Vanua Lava	c.383T>C	p.(Leu128Pro)	II	Southwestern Pacific	[637]
Quing Yan	c.392G>T	p.(Gly131Val)	III	China	[639]
Mahidol	c.487G>A	p.(Gly163Ser)	III	Southeast Asia	[640]
Santamaria	c.542A>T	p.(Asp181Val)	II	Costa Rica, Italy	[641, 642]
	c.376A>G	p.(Asn126Asp)			
Mediterranean, Dallas, Panama, Sassari	c.563C>T	p.(Ser188Phe)	II	Mediterranean	[636, 643]
Coimbra	c.592C>T	p.(Arg198Cys)	II	India, Portugal	[644]
A–	c.680G>T	p.(Arg227Leu)	III	Africa	[645]
	c.376A>G	p.(Asn126Asp)			
Seattle, Lodi, Modena, Ferrara II, Athens-like,		p.(Asp282His)	III	USA, Italy	[646-648]
Montalbano	c.854G>A	p.(Arg285His)	III	Italy	[649]
Viangchan, Jammu	c.871G>A	p.(Val291Met)	II	China	[650, 651]
Kalyan, Kerala, Jamnaga, Rohini	c.949G>A	p.(Glu317Lys)	III	India	[652, 653]
A–, Betica, Selma, Guantanamo	c.968T>C	p.(Leu323Pro)	III	Africa, Spain	[645]
	c.376A>G	p.(Asn126Asp)			
Chatham	c.1003G>A	p.(Ala335Thr)	II	Italy, Asia, Africa	[636]
Chinese-5	c.1024C>T	p.(Leu342Phe)	III	China	[639]
Ierapetra	c.1057C>T	p.(Pro353Ser)	II	Greece	[654]
Cassano	c.1347G>C	p.(Gln449His)	II	Italy, Greece	[655, 656]
Union, Maewo, Chinese-2, Kalo	c.1360C>T	p.(Arg454Cys)	II	Italy, Spain, China, Japan	[655, 657, 658]
Canton, Taiwan-Hakka, Gifu-like, Agrigento-like	c.1376G>T	p.(Arg459Leu)	II	Japan, Italy	[659, 660]
Cosenza	c.1376G>C	p.(Arg459Pro)	II	Italy	[655]
Kaiping, Anant, Dhon, Sapporo-like, Wosera	c.1388G>A	p.(Arg463His)	II	China	[658, 660]

See A Minucci, K Moradkhani, MJ Hwang, et al,[244] for complete tabulation of glucose-6-phosphate dehydrogenase (G6PD) variants.

[a]Class 1, severely deficient, associated with nonspherocytic hemolytic anemia; class 2, severe deficiency (1%-10% residual activity), associated with acute hemolytic anemia; class 3, moderate deficiency (10%-60% residual activity); class 4, not deficient (60%-150% activity); class 5, increased activity (>150%).

Data from Mason PJ, Bautista JM, Gilsanz F. G6PD deficiency: the genotype-phenotype association. *Blood Rev.* 2007;21:267-283. Minucci A, Moradkhani K, Hwang MJ, et al. Glucose-6-phosphate dehydrogenase (G6PD) mutations database: review of the "old" and update of the new mutations. *Blood Cells Mol Dis.* 2012;48:154-165.

at a molecular level (eg, G6PD Gifu-like, Canton, Agrigento-like, and Taiwan-Hakka all have the same mutation at cDNA nucleotide 1376) (see Table 16–4). DNA analysis has shown that more than 100 different mutations are found in various Asian populations.[244,245]

Variants Producing Hereditary Nonspherocytic Hemolytic Anemia Some mutations of G6PD result in chronic hemolysis, which is exacerbated by precipitating causes. These variants are class I mutants (World Health Organization [WHO] class 1).[240] From a functional point of view, these mutations are more severe than the more commonly occurring polymorphic forms of the enzyme, such as G6PD Mediterranean and G6PD A–. On a molecular level, these variants are often caused by mutations located in exon 10 or 11, encoding the subunit interface, or affect residues that bind the structural NADP molecule.[140,150] There are, however, exceptions to this rule[250,251] and the clinical severity of these variants can be quite variable.[252]

Cunninghamella elegans, mouse, and zebrafish animal models of G6PD deficiency have been produced and may become validated for preclinical testing of new drugs in G6PD deficiency.[152] G6PD deficiency in mice has been rescued by stable in vivo expression of the human *G6PD* gene in hematopoietic tissues by a gene transfer approach.[253]

Pyruvate Kinase

PK deficiency is the most common enzyme disorder in glycolysis and the most common cause of nonspherocytic hemolytic anemia.[254] Like G6PD deficiency, the disease is genetically heterogeneous, with many different mutations causing different kinetic changes in the enzyme that is formed. There are even cases in which the activity of PK as measured in vitro is higher than normal, but a kinetically abnormal enzyme is responsible for the occurrence of hemolytic anemia.[255] Kinetic characterization and analysis of PK mutants is considerably more complex than analysis of G6PD mutants. Most PK-deficient patients are compound heterozygous for two different (missense) mutations, rather than homozygous for one mutation. Assuming that stable mutant monomers are synthesized, up to seven different tetrameric forms of PK may be present in compound heterozygous individuals, each with distinct structural and kinetic properties. This complicates genotype-to-phenotype correlations in these individuals, as it is difficult to infer which mutation is primarily responsible for deficient enzyme function and the clinical phenotype.[256,257] More than 260 mutations in the *PKLR* gene encoding the red cell PK have been identified.[23] Two-thirds of these mutations are missense mutations affecting conserved residues in structurally and functionally important domains of PK. There is no direct relationship between the nature and location of the substituted amino acid and the type of molecular perturbation.[121] Hence, the nature of the mutation has relatively little predictive value with respect to the severity of the clinical course and the phenotypic expression of identical mutations can be strikingly different in patients.[256-259] A limited genotype–phenotype correlation was identified in a large cohort, in which patients with two missense mutations had a lower likelihood of splenectomy, fewer transfusions, and a lower rate of iron overload. Patients with two nonmissense mutations were less likely to have a complete or partial response to splenectomy.[260]

Apart from decreased red blood cell survival, ineffective erythropoiesis resulting from increased numbers of apoptotic cells has been implicated as one of the pathophysiologic features of PK deficiency. In particular, glycolytic inhibition by mutation of PK-R has been suggested to augment oxidative stress, leading to proapoptotic gene expression.[261]

A deficiency of PK was a key feature of severe congenital hemolytic anemia caused by mutations in the key erythroid transcription factor KLF1.[116]

There is evidence that PK deficiency provides protection against infection and replication of *Plasmodium falciparum* in human erythrocytes,[262] an effect possibly mediated by reduced ATP levels in PK-deficient red blood cells.[263] This indicates that PK deficiency may confer a protective advantage against malaria in human populations in areas where this disease is endemic. In agreement with this, population studies on sub-Saharan African populations indicate that malaria is acting as a selective force in the *PKLR* genomic region.[264,265]

PK deficiency also has been recognized in mice, dogs, and multiple breeds of domestic cats.[266] In all these animals, the deficiency causes severe anemia and marked reticulocytosis, closely resembling human PK deficiency. Basenji dogs with PK deficiency completely lack PK-R enzymatic activity and, instead, only the PK-M2 isozyme is expressed in their red blood cells.[267] A unique feature of PK deficiency in dogs is the progressive development of myelofibrosis and osteosclerosis. Marrow fibrosis may occur in response to damage caused by iron overload.[268] PK-deficient mice show delayed switching from PK-M2 to PK-R, resulting in delayed onset of the hemolytic anemia.[269] PK deficiency in mice has been rescued by expression of the human PK-R isozyme in murine hematopoietic stem cells.[270]

Other Enzyme Deficiencies

Hexokinase Deficiency Approximately 30 patients with HK deficiency have been described as of this writing.[271-277] Most mutations associated with HK deficiency identified as of this writing are missense mutations, and most patients are compound heterozygous. Homozygosity for a premature stop codon at position 12 was identified in a 9-month-old child, whereas an out of frame deletion of exons 5-8 was found to be lethal.[272,277] In three patients from two families, a regulatory mutation was identified in the putative erythroid-specific promoter. In vitro, this mutation disrupted binding of the AP-1 transcription factor complex, leading to strongly decreased gene expression.[273]

In mice, a mutation designated *downeast anemia* causes severe hemolytic anemia with extensive tissue iron deposition and marked reticulocytosis, representing a mouse model of generalized HK deficiency.[278]

Glucosephosphate Isomerase Deficiency Glucosephosphate isomerase deficiency is considered to be second to PK deficiency in frequency, with respect to glycolytic enzymopathies. As of this writing, approximately 60 families with glucosephosphate isomerase deficiency have been described worldwide.[279-282] Most of these patients are compound heterozygous for mutations that partially inactivate the enzyme. Most of the 50 *GPI* mutations reported as of this writing are missense mutations, some of which may be recurrent (Arg347His, Arg347Cys, Thr195Ile, and Val101Met).[279,282] Mapping of missense mutations to the crystal structure of the human enzyme and recombinant expression of genetic variants has provided considerable insight in the molecular mechanisms causing hemolytic anemia in this disorder.[56,283] The majority of the mutations disrupt key interactions that contribute directly or indirectly to the architecture of the enzyme's active site.[56] In rare cases, GPI deficiency also affects nonerythroid tissues, causing severe neuromuscular symptoms and granulocyte dysfunction.[284-289] The finding that GPI also functions as a neuroleukin,[290] an autocrine motility factor,[27] a nerve growth factor,[291] and a differentiation and maturation mediator[292] has led to the hypothesis that the mutation-dependent loss of cytokine function of GPI could account for the neuromuscular symptoms.[293] An alternative explanation involves disturbed glycerolipid biosynthesis in GPI deficiency, which could have significant effects on membrane formation, membrane function, and axonal migration.[294]

Homozygous GPI-deficient mice exhibit hematologic features resembling that of the human enzymopathy. In addition, other tissues are also affected, indicating a reduced glycolytic capability of the whole organism.[295] Complete loss of GPI in mice is an embryonic lethal.[296]

Phosphofructokinase Deficiency Because red cells contain both PFK M and L subunits, mutations affecting either gene will lead to a partially reduced red cell enzyme activity in PFK deficiency. Mutations in the *PFKM* gene cause PFKM deficiency or glycogen storage disease VII (Tarui disease).[297] The disease is characterized predominantly by mild to severe myopathy, in particular exercise intolerance, cramps, and myoglobinuria. The associated hemolysis is usually mild but may be absent. As of this writing, there has been only one reported case in which an unstable L subunit was identified. This patient exhibited no signs of myopathy or hemolysis.[70] Approximately 100 cases of PFK deficiency and 23 mutant *PFKM* alleles have been reported as of this writing. Approximately 60% of the reported mutations are missense mutations; the remaining mutations mostly affect splicing. Intriguingly, PFK-deficient Ashkenazi Jews share two common mutations: a G>A base change affecting the donor splice site of intron 5 (c.237+1G>A) and a single base deletion in exon 2 (c.2003delC).[25,298] The mode of action by which missense mutations cause disease is largely unknown.[25,299-306]

PFK deficiency in dogs[266] is characterized by the association of hemolytic crises with strenuous exercise.[307] *Pfkm* null mice show exercise intolerance, reduced life span, and progressive cardiac hypertrophy, suggesting that Tarui disease should be considered as a complex systemic disorder rather than a muscle glycogenosis.[308,309]

Aldolase Deficiency As of this writing only seven patients with red cell aldolase deficiency have been described, four of whom have been characterized at the DNA level. Six of the seven patients displayed moderate chronic hemolytic anemia, either by itself[310] or accompanied by myopathy,[311,312] rhabdomyolysis,[313] psychomotor retardation,[311] or mental retardation.[72,311] One patient presented with fever-induced rhabdomyolysis without hemolytic anemia, possibly caused by tissue-specific behavior of a thermolabile mutant aldolase.[314]

Triosephosphate Isomerase Deficiency Triosephosphate isomerase deficiency is characterized by hemolytic anemia, often accompanied by neonatal hyperbilirubinemia requiring exchange transfusion. In addition, patients display progressive neurologic dysfunction, increased susceptibility to infection, and cardiomyopathy.[315] Most affected individuals die in childhood before the age of 6 years, but there are remarkable exceptions.[316] Triosephosphate isomerase deficiency is the severest disorder of glycolysis. Key in the pathophysiology of the severe neuromuscular disease is the formation of toxic protein aggregates: accumulation of the substrate dihydroxyacetone phosphate results in elevated levels of the toxic methylglyoxal, leading to the formation of advanced glycation end products, whereas mutation-induced changes in the quaternary structure of triosephosphate isomerase lead to the formation of an aggregation-prone protein.[317,318] As a result, it has been suggested that triosephosphate isomerase deficiency represents a conformational rather than a metabolic disease.[317]

Approximately 50 patients and more than 20 different mutations have been reported in triosephosphate isomerase deficiency.[315,318-325] Most patients are compound heterozygous for missense mutations that alter the stability of the protein with consequent effects on dimerization and catalysis.[326] The most common mutation is the p.(Glu104Asp) amino acid change which is detected in approximately 80% of patients, all descendants from a common ancestor.[24] Studies on recombinant mutant triosephosphate isomerase show that the p.(Glu104Asp) does not affect catalysis. Instead, the mutation disrupts a conserved network of buried water molecules, which prevents efficient formation of the active triosephosphate isomerase dimer, causing its dissociation in inactive monomers.[80] Triosephosphate isomerase–null mice die at an early stage of development.[327] Other studies on TPI-deficient mouse models show that without the stability defect a strong decline in TPI activity is not sufficient to explain TPI-deficient pathology.[328] This finding is confirmed by studies on a *Drosophila* model recapitulating the neurologic phenotype of TPI deficiency, suggesting that impairment of TPI dimerization is sufficient to elicit neurologic dysfunction by impeding vesicle dynamics at the synapse.[329]

Phosphoglycerate Kinase Deficiency PGK deficiency is one of the relatively uncommon causes of hereditary nonspherocytic hemolytic anemia. Mutations in the X chromosome-linked gene may cause mild to severe chronic hemolysis, neurologic dysfunction, and myopathy.[330] More than 50 patients with PGK deficiency have been reported.[331-333] Most patients manifest either hemolytic anemia in combination with neurologic symptoms, including mental retardation, seizures, progressive decline of motor function, and developmental delay, or isolated myopathy.[334-336] The combination of all clinical manifestations is a rare event, described in only a few patients.[337,338] A case series study showed that multisystem involvement is associated with a lower residual enzyme activity than patients displaying only myopathy.[339] Splenectomy is reported to be beneficial but does not correct the hemolytic process.[300,330] Marrow transplantation has been performed to prevent the manifestation of severe neurologic symptoms.[340]

Approximately 35 unique mutations have been identified.[331-333] Of these mutations, 80% are missense mutations. Most of the encoded amino acid changes heavily affect the protein's thermal stability and to a different extent catalytic efficiency.[335,341] The most deleterious mutants show a reduced stability, supporting a pivotal role of thermodynamic stability in the propensity toward aggregation and proteolysis of pathogenic variants in vitro and intracellularly.[342] In an attempt to correlate the genotype to the phenotype, it was found that amino acid changes grossly impairing protein stability but moderately affecting kinetic properties were associated mostly with hemolytic anemia and neurologic symptoms. Mutations perturbing both catalysis and heat stability were associated with myopathy alone, whereas mutations faintly affecting molecular properties of PGK correlated with a wide range of clinical symptoms.[341] That there is still no explanation for the wide range of clinical manifestations following mutations in the same gene, suggests that other, yet unknown environmental, metabolic, genetic, and/or epigenetic factors are involved.[336,341]

Bisphosphoglycerate Mutase Deficiency Bisphosphoglycerate mutase deficiency is a very rare disorder. Only three affected families have been characterized. Bisphosphoglycerate mutase deficiency is inherited as an autosomal recessive disorder. However, some heterozygous relatives have had a borderline-high hemoglobin concentration,[343,344] and in one affected patient only one mutation was identified.[345] Erythrocytosis was the predominant feature of the clinically normal probands, likely resulting from reduced 2,3-BPG levels[346] and, consequently, the increased oxygen affinity of hemoglobin (Chap. 28).

Glutamate Cysteine Ligase Deficiency GCL deficiency is associated with mild hereditary nonspherocytic hemolytic anemia that may be fully compensated. Drug-induced and infection-induced hemolytic crises can occur as a consequence of strongly reduced GSH levels. As of this writing, 12 cases of GCL deficiency have been described.[347] In approximately 33% of the patients with GCL deficiency, the hemolytic anemia was accompanied by impaired neurologic function.[347] Six different mutations have been reported.[347] In all these cases, the causative mutation affected the GCLC. Clinically observed mutations have been mapped to a homology model of the human enzyme, based on the crystal structure of GCL of *Saccharomyces cerevisiae*, thus explaining the molecular basis of GSH depletion as a result of GCL deficiency.[179] Complementary expression studies in mice showed that these GCLC mutations impair GSH production by reducing the activity of the GCLC. Addition of the modifier subunit was able to largely restore enzymatic activity, thereby underscoring the critical role of GCLM.[348] Complete deficiency of GCLC has shown to be lethal in mice,[349,350] whereas GCLM null mice are viable and show no overt phenotype despite strongly reduced GSH levels, including a reduction of more than 90% in red blood cells.[351] Upon exposure to oxidative stress, however, red blood cells from such mice undergo massive hemolysis with fatal outcome.[352]

Glutathione Synthetase Deficiency GS deficiency is the most common abnormality of red cell GSH metabolism. Three distinct clinical forms of GS deficiency can be distinguished,[353] most likely reflecting different mutations or epigenetic modifications in the *GSS* gene.[354] Patients with mild GS deficiency display mild hemolytic anemia as their only symptom. In contrast, patients with a moderate deficiency usually present in the neonatal period with metabolic acidosis, 5-oxoprolinuria, and mild-to-moderate hemolytic anemia. In addition to these symptoms, patients with the third and severest type develop progressive neurologic symptoms such as psychomotor retardation, mental retardation, seizures, ataxia, and spasticity. 5-Oxoprolinuria results from accumulation of γ-glutamylcysteine because of decreased feedback inhibition of GCL by the decreased levels of GSH.[355] 5-Oxoprolinuria may have other causes.[356] Experiments in rats have shown that acute administration of 5-oxoproline induces oxidative damage in the brain, a mechanism that may be involved in the neurologic symptoms of severe GS deficiency.[357]

The diagnosis of GS deficiency has been established in more than 75 patients,[354,355,358-364] of whom 18 (approximately 24%) died in childhood.[358] More than 40 mutations have been identified as being associated with GS deficiency. Based on the nature of the mutation, and taking into account GS activity and GSH levels, it seems possible to predict a mild versus a more severe phenotype.[354] The structural effects of a number of missense mutations have been determined.[183,365]

A long-term followup study showed that early diagnosis, correction of acidosis, and early supplementation with antioxidants vitamins C and E improve survival and long-term outcome.[353]

Complete deficiency of GS is lethal in mice, whereas heterozygous animals survive with no distinct phenotype.[366]

Glutathione Reductase Deficiency Only two families with hereditary GSR deficiency have been described and characterized.[367,368] The complete absence of GSR in the red cells of members of one family was associated with only rare episodes of hemolysis, possibly caused by fava beans. GSR deficiency was caused by homozygosity for a large genomic deletion. GSR deficiency in the other family was caused by compound heterozygosity for a nonsense mutation, and a missense mutation affecting a highly conserved residue. GSR in red cells was undetectable, but some residual activity was found in the patient's leucocytes.[367]

In vitro studies on members of one of the GSR-deficient families has provided experimental evidence that GSR deficiency may protect from malarial infection by enhancing phagocytosis of ring-infected red blood cells.[369]

Adenylate Kinase Deficiency AK deficiency has been reported in more than 10 patients, in whom 10 different mutations have been identified,[370,371] mostly missense ones. The deficiency was associated with moderate to severe hemolytic anemia, which could be resolved by splenectomy.[370] In some of the patients, mental retardation and psychomotor impairment was also observed.[370] Studies on a number of recombinant proteins revealed strongly altered catalytic properties or protein stability resulting from mutation.[218] In contrast, patient's cells sometimes displayed considerable residual enzymatic activity. The activation of expression of other isozymes, that is, AK2 and AK3, has been proposed as one of the factors contributing to this apparent discrepancy.[372]

Adenosine Deaminase Hyperactivity An increased activity of ADA is associated with hereditary nonspherocytic hemolytic anemia. It is the only red cell disorder that is inherited in an autosomal dominant disorder.[373] ADA hyperactivity results in depletion of red cell ATP.[373,374] Few cases with a 30-fold to 70-fold increase in activity have been described. The molecular mechanism of this disorder has not

been identified but the markedly increased amounts of ADA mRNA in affected individuals indicate that the red blood cell–specific overexpression occurs at the mRNA level,[375] causing an overproduction of a structurally normal enzyme.[376] ADA hyperactivity probably results from a *cis*-acting mutation in the vicinity of the *ADA* gene.[377]

For reasons that are not understood, milder elevations of red cell ADA activity (twofold to sixfold) are also increased in most, but not all, patients with Diamond-Blackfan anemia.[378] Deficiency of ADA is associated with severe combined immunodeficiency. In this disorder, large quantities of deoxyadenine nucleotides, not normally present in erythrocytes, accumulate.

Pyrimidine 5′-Nucleotidase Deficiency P5′N deficiency is the most frequent disorder of red cell nucleotide metabolism and a relatively common cause of mild-to-moderate hemolytic anemia.[379-381] More than 100 patients have been reported, but because of the relatively mild phenotype, many patients may remain undetected. Deficient enzyme function leads to the accumulation of pyrimidine nucleotides. This effect results in prominent stippling on the blood film, the hallmark of this disorder (Fig. 16–7).[222] Hence, P5′N1 deficiency is the only red cell enzyme deficiency in which red cell morphology is helpful in establishing the diagnosis. The precise mechanism leading to premature destruction of P5′N1-deficient red cells is unknown. Some proposed pathophysiologic mechanisms have related the accumulation of pyrimidine nucleotide to alterations of the red cell membrane causing increased levels of cytidine diphosphate choline and cytidine diphosphate ethanolamide,[382] decreased pentose phosphate shunt activity,[383-385] chelation of Mg^{2+} ions that serves as a cofactor for a number of enzymes,[386] decreased phosphoribosyl pyrophosphate synthetase activity,[387,388] increased activity of pyrimidine nucleoside monophosphate kinase,[389] increased levels of GSH,[390] and competition with reactions that require ADP or ATP.[391] However, clear cause-and-effect relationships have not been established.

As of this writing, more than 100 different patients with P5′N deficiency have been described, and approximately 30 different mutations have been reported in *NT5C3A*.[379,392-396] Most patients were found to be homozygous for a specific mutation. The majority of mutations concern frameshift or nonsense mutations, deletions, or mutations that affect splicing. Functional analysis of reported missense mutations was

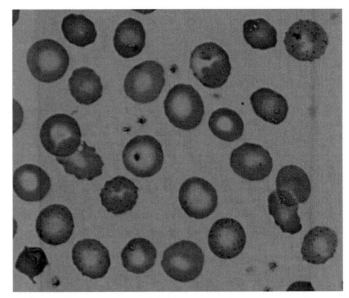

Figure 16–7. Prominent basophilic stippling in pyrimidine 5′-nucleotidase 1 (P5′N1) deficiency.

studied using recombinant mutant proteins. These rendered contrasting results between the substantial changes in kinetic behavior and thermostability and the actual residual enzymatic activity in patient's red cells, probably from compensation by upregulation of other nucleotidases.[397] Of interest is the observation that none of the reported missense mutations affect residues of the catalytic site, suggesting that the reduced catalytic efficiency and/or instability result from secondary effects related to conformational changes.[226]

Acquired deficiency of P5′N1 may result from lead poisoning. Structural studies show that Pb^{2+} specifically binds within the active site, in a different position than Mg^{2+} but with much higher affinity.[226] Because simultaneous binding of Mg^{2+} and Pb^{2+} is not possible, Pb^{2+} outcompetes Mg^{2+}, thereby preventing this essential cofactor from binding, thus abolishing catalytic activity. P5′N1 activity is also inhibited in β-thalassemia and related disorders that result in excess α-globin chains, such as hemoglobin E, probably as a consequence of oxidative damage induced by excess α-globin chains.[398,399]

Intriguingly, a large number of unrelated patients with chronic hemolytic anemia have been reported in which red cell P5′N1 activity was normal but an accumulation of pyrimidine nucleotide metabolites was observed, in particular cytidine diphosphate choline. It remains to be determined whether this is based on a yet unidentified enzymatic defect.[400]

MECHANISM OF HEMOLYSIS

Glucose-6-Phosphate Dehydrogenase Deficiency
The life span of G6PD–deficient red cells is not usually shortened but under many circumstances, particularly during drug administration and infection, it is.

Drug-Induced Hemolysis Drug-induced hemolysis in G6PD-deficient cells is generally accompanied by the formation of Heinz bodies, particles of denatured hemoglobin, and stromal protein (Chap. 18), formed only in the presence of oxidants. Together with the inability to protect their GSH against drug challenge, this suggests that a major component of the hemolytic process is the inability of G6PD-deficient cells to protect sulfhydryl groups against oxidative damage.[2] The mechanism by which Heinz bodies are formed and become attached to red cell stroma has been the subject of considerable investigation and speculation. Exposure of red cells to certain drugs results in the formation of low levels of hydrogen peroxide as the drug interacts with hemoglobin.[401] In addition, some drugs may form free radicals that oxidize GSH without the formation of peroxide as an intermediate.[402] The formation of free radicals of GSH through the action of peroxide or by the direct action of drugs may be followed either by oxidation of GSH to the disulfide form (GSSG) or complexing of the GSH with hemoglobin to form a mixed disulfide. Such mixed disulfides are believed to form initially with the sulfhydryl group of the β-93 position of hemoglobin.[403] The mixed disulfide of GSH and hemoglobin is probably unstable and undergoes conformational changes exposing interior sulfhydryl groups to oxidation and mixed disulfide formation. Globin chain separation into free α and β chains also occurs.[404] Once such oxidation has occurred, hemoglobin is denatured irreversibly and will precipitate as Heinz bodies. Normal red cells can defend themselves to a considerable extent against such changes by reducing GSSG to GSH and by reducing the mixed disulfides of GSH and hemoglobin through the GSR reaction.[37] However, the reduction of these disulfide bonds requires a source of NADPH. Because G6PD-deficient red cells are unable to reduce $NADP^+$ to NADPH at a normal rate, they are unable to reduce hydrogen peroxide or the mixed disulfides of hemoglobin and GSH. Moreover, because catalase contains tightly bound NADPH[405] that is required for activity, the lack of freely available NADPH generation may, in addition, impede disposal of hydrogen peroxide by the catalase-dependent pathway.[406] When such cells are challenged by drugs, they form Heinz bodies more readily than do normal cells. Cells containing Heinz bodies encounter difficulty in traversing the splenic pulp[407] (Chap. 25) and are eliminated relatively rapidly from the circulation. Figure 16–6 summarizes a plausible scenario of the metabolic events that lead to red cell damage and, eventually, destruction. However, in mice, targeted disruption of the gene encoding GSH peroxidase has little effect on oxidation of hemoglobin of murine red cells challenged with peroxides.[185] In addition, catalase null mice show negligible antioxidant function of catalase in oxidant injury.[408] If such murine models reflect the situation in humans, then different pathways requiring GSH, such as the thioredoxin, and/or peroxiredoxin reactions, may be important.[408,409]

The formation of methemoglobin (Chap. 19) frequently accompanies the administration of drugs that have the capacity to produce hemolysis of G6PD-deficient cells.[410] The heme groups of methemoglobin become detached from the globin more readily than do the heme groups of oxyhemoglobin.[411] It is not clear whether methemoglobin formation plays an important role in the oxidative degradation of hemoglobin to Heinz bodies or whether formation of methemoglobin is merely an incidental side effect of oxidative drugs.[412]

Infection-Induced Hemolysis The mechanism of hemolysis induced by infection or occurring spontaneously in G6PD-deficient subjects is not well understood. The generation of hydrogen peroxide by phagocytizing leukocytes may play a role in this type of hemolytic reaction.[412]

Favism Substances capable of depleting red cell GSH content (ie, divicine and isouramil)[413] have been isolated from fava beans and the mechanism of action leading to red cell destruction has been reported in detail.[414,415] Favism occurs only in G6PD-deficient subjects, but not all individuals in a particular family may be sensitive to the hemolytic effect of the beans. Nonetheless, some tendency toward familial occurrence has suggested that an additional genetic factor may be important.[416] Increased levels of red cell calcium[417] and consequent "cross-bonding" of membranes may occur. Other membrane alterations that have been described are oxidation and clustering of membrane proteins, hemichrome binding to the internal face of the membrane, destabilization of the membrane, impairment of the proteolytic system, and the release of microvesicles.[418–422]

Icterus Neonatorum G6PD-deficient neonates are at increased risk of developing severe icterus neonatorum. The icterus is frequently unaccompanied by changes in hematologic indices reflective of a hemolytic proces.[423,424] The reason for this discrepancy is unclear. Moderate icterus probably results from inadequate processing of bilirubin by the immature liver of G6PD–deficient infants. The demonstrated increase in carboxyhemoglobin levels, indicative of increased heme catabolism, suggests however that shortening of red cell life span also plays a role,[425] particularly in extreme hyperbilirubinemia.[426] A predisposing factor for severe jaundice in G6PD deficiency is mutation of the uridine diphosphoglucuronate glucuronosyltransferase-1 gene (*UGT1A1*) promoter[427] or, in Asia, the c.211G>A coding mutation.[428] In adults, these mutations are associated with Gilbert syndrome. The limited data available on liver G6PD in deficient adults[429] suggest that a considerable degree of deficiency may be present in that organ. If such a deficiency also is present in infants, it may play a role in impairing the borderline ability of infant livers with the *UGT1A1* promoter defect to catabolize bilirubin, in particular when a hemolytic process is set off by contact with environmental factors (eg, certain drugs, naphthalene-containing mothballs). However, modulation of bilirubin metabolism and serum bilirubin levels is under complex genetic control, and coexpressing of mutations in other genes, for example, *SLCO1B3*,[430] may contribute further to the bilirubin production–conjugation imbalance in G6PD-deficient individuals.[431]

Deficiencies of Other Enzymes of the Hexose Monophosphate Shunt and of Glutathione Metabolism

Deficiencies of glutamate cysteine synthetase, GS, and GSR are associated with a decrease in red cell GSH levels. The generally mild hemolysis that occurs in these disorders probably has a pathogenesis similar to the hemolysis that occurs in G6PD deficiency. Other defects of the hexose monophosphate shunt and associated metabolic pathways are not associated with hemolysis (see Table 16–3).

Other Enzyme Deficiencies How deficiencies of enzymes other than those of the hexose monophosphate pathway result in shortening of red cell life span remains unknown, although it has been the object of much experimental work and of speculation. It is often believed that ATP depletion is a common pathway in producing damage to the cell leading to its destruction,[432] but the evidence that this is the case is not always compelling. Nevertheless, it seems reasonable to assume that a red cell, deprived of a source of energy becomes sodium and calcium logged and potassium depleted, and the red cell shape changes from a flexible biconcave disk. Such a cell is quickly removed from the circulation by the filtering action of the spleen (Chap. 25) and the monocyte-macrophage system. Even if it survived, such an energy-deprived cell would gradually turn brown as hemoglobin is oxidized to methemoglobin by the very high concentrations of oxygen within the erythrocyte. Calcium has been proposed to play a central role. In particular, malfunction of ATP-dependent calcium transporters could lead to increased intracellular calcium levels that could affect red cell membrane proteins (ie, protein 4.1; Chap. 15), the lipid bilayer, volume regulation, metabolism, and redox state preservation, consequently leading to proteolysis, oxidation, irreversible cellular shrinkage, phosphatidyl exposure, and premature clearance.[433] In agreement with this, PFK deficiency has been shown to result in increased calcium levels, accompanied by volume loss and metabolic dysregulation.[434,435]

It is possible that, at least in some cases, alteration of the levels of red cell intermediate metabolites interferes with synthesis of cell components in early stages of development of the cell. In agreement with this, the lack of pyruvate has been implicated in the ineffective maturation of erythroid progenitors in PK-deficient mice.[261]

● CLINICAL FEATURES

COMMON FORMS OF GLUCOSE-6-PHOSPHATE DEHYDROGENASE DEFICIENCY

The major clinical consequence of G6PD deficiency is hemolytic anemia in adults and neonatal icterus in infants. Usually the anemia is episodic, but some of the unusual variants of G6PD may cause nonspherocytic congenital hemolytic disease (see "Variants Producing Hereditary Nonspherocytic Hemolytic Anemia" earlier). In general, hemolysis is associated with stress, most notably drug administration, infection, and, in certain individuals, exposure to fava beans.

G6PD deficiency is an X-linked disease but this does not imply its expression is strictly sex-linked. As a result of lyonization (X chromosome inactivation) heterozygous females are genetic mosaics, displaying a broad range of enzyme activities ranging from normal to G6PD-deficient as seen in homozygotes. Thus, extremely skewed X-inactivation can result in a phenotype resembling the hemizygous male. Indeed, a small minority (1.3%-5.1%) of heterozygous women have a G6PD-deficient phenotype identical to hemizygous males with the same mutation.[436]

Drug-Induced Hemolytic Anemia

Table 16–5 is an evidence-based[152,437] list of drugs and other chemicals that are predicted to precipitate hemolytic reactions in G6PD-deficient

TABLE 16–5. Drugs That Can Trigger Hemolysis in G6PD-Deficient Individuals

Category of Drug	Predictable Hemolysis	Possible Hemolysis
Antimalarials	Dapsone-containing combinations	Chloroquine
	Primaquine	Quinine
	Pamaquine	Quinidine
	Methylene blue	Mepacrine
Analgesics/ Antipyretics	Phenazopyridine	Aspirin (Acetylsalicylic acid, high doses)
		Paracetamol (Acetaminophen)
Antibacterials	Cotrimoxazole	Sulfasalazine
	Niridazole	Sulfadiazine
	Quinolones (including nalidixic acid, ciprofloxacin, ofloxacin, movifloxacin, norfloxacin)	Sulfonylureas
	Nitrofurantoin	
Other	Rasburicase	Chloramphenicol
	Toluidine blue	Isoniazid
		Ascorbic acid
		Glibenclamide
		Vitamin K analogues
		Isosorbide dinitrate
		Sulfonylureas
		Dimercaptosuccinic acid

Reproduced with pemission from Luzzatto L, Seneca E. G6PD deficiency: a classic example of pharmacogenetics with on-going clinical implications. *Br J Haematol*. 2014 Feb;164(4):469-480.

individuals, and drugs that are innocuous when given in normal doses, but may be hemolytic when given in excessive doses. A case in point is ascorbic acid, which does not cause hemolytic anemia in normal doses, but which can produce severe, even fatal, hemolysis at doses of 80 g or more intravenously.[438-440] Specific guidelines have been developed for rasburicase therapy in the context of G6PD deficiency.[441] Some drugs, such as chloramphenicol, may induce mild hemolysis in a person with severe, Mediterranean-type G6PD deficiency,[442] but not in those with the milder A− or Canton[443] types of deficiency. Furthermore, there appears to be a difference in the severity of the reaction to the same drug of different individuals with the same G6PD variant. For example, red cells from a single G6PD-deficient individual were hemolyzed in the circulation of some recipients who were given thiazolsulfone, but their survival was normal in the circulation of others.[444] Sulfamethoxazole, which was clearly hemolytic in experimental studies, does not appear to be a common cause of hemolysis in a clinical setting.[445] Undoubtedly, individual differences in the metabolism and excretion of drugs influence the extent to which G6PD-deficient red cells are destroyed.[446,447]

Typically, an episode of drug-induced hemolysis in G6PD-deficient individuals begins 1- to 3 days after drug administration is initiated.[448] Heinz bodies appear in the red cells, and the hemoglobin concentration begins to decline rapidly.[449] As hemolysis progresses, Heinz bodies disappear from the circulation, presumably as they or the erythrocytes that contain them are removed by the spleen. In severe cases, abdominal or back pain may occur. The urine may turn dark or even black. Within 4- to 6 days, there is generally an increase in the reticulocyte count, except in instances in which the patient has received the offending drug for treatment of an active infection as infection depresses erythropoiesis (Chaps. 2, 6, and 24). Because of the tendency of infections and certain other stressful situations to precipitate hemolysis in G6PD-deficient individuals, many drugs have been incorrectly implicated as a cause. Other drugs, such as aspirin, have appeared on many lists of proscribed medications because large doses could slightly reduce the red cell life span. Such drugs do not produce clinically significant hemolytic anemia. Advising patients not to ingest these drugs may not only deprive patients of potentially helpful medications, but will also weaken their confidence in the advice that they have received. Most G6PD-deficient patients, after all, have taken aspirin without untoward effect and are likely to distrust an advisor who counsels them that the ingestion of aspirin will have catastrophic effects.

In the A− type of G6PD deficiency, the hemolytic anemia is self-limited[448] because the young red cells produced in response to hemolysis have nearly normal G6PD levels and are relatively resistant to hemolysis.[449] The hemoglobin level may return to normal even while the same dose of drug that initially precipitated hemolysis is administered. In contrast, hemolysis is not self-limited with continuing hemolysis precipitating agent in the more severe Mediterranean type of deficiency.[450]

Hemolytic Anemia Occurring During Infection

Anemia often develops rather suddenly in G6PD-deficient individuals within a few days of onset of a febrile illness. The anemia is usually relatively mild, with a decline in the hemoglobin concentration of 30 or 40 g/L. Hemolysis has been noted particularly in patients suffering from hepatitis A and B, cytomegalovirus, pneumonia, and in those with typhoid fever.[451-453] The fulminating form of the disease occurs particularly frequently among G6PD-deficient patients who are infected with Rocky Mountain spotted fever.[454] Jaundice is not a prominent part of the clinical picture, except where hemolysis occurs in association with infectious hepatitis.[455,456] In that case, it can be quite intense. Presumably because of the effect of the infection, reticulocytosis is usually absent, and recovery from the anemia is generally delayed until after the active infection has abated. In rare cases, G6PD deficiency may present as transient aplastic crisis due to viral infection.[457,458]

Favism

Favism is potentially one of the gravest clinical consequences of G6PD deficiency.[415] It occurs much more commonly in unknowing or undiagnosed children than in adults, and occurs almost exclusively in persons who have inherited variants of G6PD that cause severe deficiency (most frequently associated with the Mediterranean variant[459]), but may be also present in patients with G6PD A−.[460] The onset of hemolysis may be quite sudden, having been reported to occur within the first hours after exposure to fava beans. More commonly, the onset is gradual, hemolysis being noticed 1- to 2 days after ingestion of the beans.[461] The urine becomes red or quite dark, and in severe cases, shock may develop within a short time. Care should be taken to avoid acute renal failure. The oxidative stress causes membrane changes in erythrocytes, leading to extravascular hemolysis (in addition to the intravascular destruction).[415] Sometimes the patient or parent does not realize that fava beans have been ingested, as they may be incorporated into foods such as Yew Dow, eaten by the Chinese,[462] or falafel, eaten in the Middle East. Occasionally ingestion of other foodstuffs, such as unripe peaches[463] or a spiced Nigerian barbecued meat known as red suya,[464] has been reported to precipitate hemolysis. The toxic constituents of the fava beans are transmitted into the milk of breastfeeding mothers, putting affected babies at risk.[465]

Neonatal Icterus

Although serious, the clinical consequences of drug-induced hemolysis, favism, or chronic hemolytic anemia are usually not devastating, and nowadays death from favism is a very rare event. The most serious consequence of G6PD deficiency is severe icterus neonatorum.[466] G6PD-deficient neonates are an estimated three to four-times more at risk for hyperbilirubinemia and phototherapy than G6PD-adequate neonates,[467] depending on population groups and geographic area.[468] Jaundice commences in the immediate perinatal period, and is usually evident by 1- to 4 days of age, similar to physiologic jaundice, but is seen at a later time than in blood group alloimmunization.[469] The peak bilirubin level is usually on day 3.[415] The jaundice may be quite severe and, if untreated, may result in kernicterus: bilirubin-induced brain damage. Reports indicate an overrepresentation of G6PD deficiency among cases of kernicterus relative to the frequency of in the background population, also in countries with a low overall frequency of G6PD deficiency.[431] Thus, kernicterus in the context of G6PD deficiency is a preventable cause of mental retardation[415,466] and this aspect of the disorder has considerable public health significance. Neonatal screening for G6PD deficiency has been associated with a decrease in the number of cases of kernicterus.[431]

Nonspherocytic Hemolytic Anemia

The anemia in G6PD deficiency is usually episodic and acute, but some sporadic variants of G6PD may cause nonspherocytic congenital hemolytic disease, exacerbated by oxidative stress. Affected individuals have a history of severe neonatal jaundice, and features of chronic hemolysis (see "Hereditary Nonspherocytic Hemolytic Anemia" further). The hemolysis is mainly extravascular.

Effects on Other Tissues

In the common variants of G6PD, such as G6PD A− and Mediterranean, and even in most of the severely deficient variants, there is usually no demonstrated defect in leukocyte number or function.[470] However, there are reports of isolated instances of leukocyte dysfunction associated with rare, severely deficient variants of G6PD.[250,251,471-475] Patients with G6PD deficiency do not have a bleeding tendency, and studies of platelet function have yielded conflicting results.[476,477] Occasionally, cataracts have been observed in patients with variants of G6PD that produce nonspherocytic hemolytic anemia,[478-480] or in neonatal patients.[481] The incidence of senile cataracts may be increased in G6PD deficiency,[482,483] but this remains controversial.[484,485] Small studies from the Middle East are suggestive that decreased G6PD activity may predispose to the development of diabetes.[486-488]

A number of studies reported on acute rhabdomyolysis in patients with G6PD deficiency, suggesting that this condition could predispose to muscle damage,[488-493] probably through the depletion of NADPH.[494] Others however, have demonstrated that G6PD-deficient individuals can participate in various physical activities, even high-intensity muscle-damaging activities,[495] without a negative impact on muscle function and redox status.[496,497]

Although claims have been made that an association exists between various kinds of G6PD deficiency and cancer,[498,499] the relationship between G6PD status and cancer is not clear as epidemiologic studies have not demonstrated any difference in risk for cancers between G6PD-deficient and normal patients.[500-502] Some role for G6PD in carcinogenesis is conceivable though, given the finding that mutation of p53 abolishes the direct binding of this major tumor-suppressor gene to G6PD, thereby enhancing hexose monophosphate shunt flux and tumor cell biosynthesis.[503]

Population studies are needed to better elucidate the postulated effects of G6PD deficiency on the development of cardiovascular disease.[504,505]

HEREDITARY NONSPHEROCYTIC HEMOLYTIC ANEMIA

Most patients with hereditary nonspherocytic hemolytic anemia manifest only the usual clinical signs and symptoms of chronic hemolysis. The degree of anemia in this group of disorders varies widely. In some cases of very severe PK deficiency, scarcely any deficient cells survive in the circulation, and only transfused cells are found or steady-state hemoglobin levels as low as 50 g/L are encountered. Other patients with hereditary nonspherocytic hemolytic anemia may manifest compensated hemolysis with a normal steady-state hemoglobin concentration. Chronic jaundice is a common finding, and splenomegaly is often present. Gallstones are common. As in other forms of chronic hemolytic anemia, ankle ulcers and pulmonary hypertension may be present.[260,506,507] Regardless of transfusion status, many patients with PK deficiency, as any patients with augmented compensatory erythropoiesis, suffer from iron overload.[508] This is mediated by high erythroferrone that downregulates hepcidin (Chap. 10). Hence, complications related to iron overload, such as liver cirrhosis, osteoporosis, and hormonal disfunction (Chap. 7), are prevalent as well.[509] Pregnancy has been thought to precipitate hemolysis in patients with PK deficiency, perhaps even in heterozygotes.[510-512] In PK deficiency, the increased 2,3-BPG levels may ameliorate the anemia by lowering the oxygen-affinity of hemoglobin.[513,514] Some PK-deficient patients present with hydrops fetalis.[515]

In the case of some enzyme defects, characteristic nonhematologic systemic manifestations may be present, and these may be the only sign of the enzyme deficiency. For example, patients with PFK deficiency may have type VII muscle glycogen storage disease. In some patients with this defect, hemolysis is present without muscle manifestations, but in others both muscle abnormalities and hemolysis occur.[70] GS deficiency may be associated with 5-oxoprolinuria and neuromuscular disturbances, and such abnormalities may occur either with[516] or without[517] hematologic abnormalities. On the other hand, some patients with GS deficiency manifest only the hematologic abnormalities.[518] Spinocerebellar degeneration was documented in the first case of glutamate cysteine synthetase described,[519,520] but was not present in subsequently investigated patients.[518,521] Patients with TPI deficiency nearly always manifest serious neuromuscular disease, and most of the patients who inherit this abnormality die in the first decade of life,[522,523] but there are exceptions, as only one of two brothers with the same genotype manifested neurologic disease (see "Genetic Modifiers of the Phenotypes" further).[524,525] Neurologic symptoms also have been noted in patients with deficiencies of glucosephosphate isomerase and PGK.[293,526] Myoglobinuria has been encountered in patients with PGK,[527,528] aldolase,[311] and G6PD deficiency.[492] Table 16–2 summarizes the clinical features of enzyme deficiencies causing nonspherocytic hemolytic anemia.

GENETIC MODIFIERS OF THE PHENOTYPES

The clinical phenotype of both acute and chronic hemolysis can be modified by coinherited (although unrelated) other defects of the red

cells. Combined deficiencies of, for example, GPI and G6PD,[529] of PK and band 3,[530-532] of PK and α-thalassemia,[533] and of PK and G6PD[534] have been documented.

The inheritance of polymorphic *UGT1A1* promoter alleles exacerbates the icterus both in neonates and in adults with G6PD deficiency (see also "Mechanism of Hemolysis" earlier).[431] Overt iron overload and iron-related morbidity in PK deficiency has been attributed to coinheritance of mutations in *HFE*, the gene associated with hereditary hemochromatosis.[535]

A striking example of complex interplay defining the differences between the genotype and the phenotype was described in a Hungarian family with TPI deficiency. Two adult germline-identical compound heterozygous brothers displayed strikingly different phenotypes. Both had the same severe decrease in TPI activity and congenital hemolytic anemia, but only one suffered from severe neurologic disorder. Studies aimed at the pathogenesis of this differing phenotype indicated functional differences between the two brothers in lipid environment of the red cell membrane proteins influencing the enzyme activities,[524] as well as differences in *TPI1* mRNA expression, and protein expression levels of prolyl oligopeptidase, the activity decrease of which has been reported in well-characterized neurodegenerative diseases.[536]

The variety of clinical features associated with the various enzymopathies, regardless of the underlying molecular mechanism, do unequivocally demonstrate that the phenotype of hereditary red blood cell enzymopathies, is not solely dependent on the molecular properties of mutant proteins but rather reflects a complex interplay between physiologic, environmental, and other (genetic) factors. Putative phenotypic modifiers include differences in genetic background, concomitant functional polymorphisms of other glycolytic enzymes (many enzymes are regulated by their product or other metabolites), posttranslational modification, ineffective erythropoiesis, and different splenic function. As an example, persistent expression of the PK-M2 isozyme has been reported in the red blood cells of patients (and animals) with severe PK deficiency.[135,258] The survival of these patients, though not in all cases, may be enabled by this compensatory increase in PK activity.[537]

●LABORATORY FEATURES

Varying degrees of anemia and reticulocytosis are the main hematologic laboratory features of patients with hereditary nonspherocytic hemolytic anemia. Heinz bodies often are found in the erythrocytes of G6PD-deficient patients undergoing drug-induced hemolysis. In the absence of hemolysis, the light-microscopic morphology of G6PD–deficient red cells is normal. When a hemolytic drug is administered to a G6PD-deficient patient, Heinz bodies (Chap. 2) develop in the erythrocytes immediately preceding and in the early phases of the hemolytic episode. Despite the fact that "bite cells" may be noted in the blood of a G6PD-deficient patient undergoing drug-induced hemolysis, the association with G6PD deficiency is doubtful as such cells are usually absent in acute hemolytic states of patients with common G6PD variants or in G6PD-deficient patients with chronic hemolysis. Moreover, "bite cells" have been noted in G6PD-replete patients.[538,539]

The presence of small, densely staining cells has often been noted in the blood films of patients with hereditary nonspherocytic hemolytic anemia with defects other than G6PD deficiency. Particularly when manifesting an echinocytic appearance, such cells have been thought to be common in PK deficiency. However, cells of this type are seen in many blood films both from patients with glycolytic enzyme deficiencies and from those with other disorders, and it is hazardous to attempt to make an enzymatic diagnosis on the basis of such findings. Basophilic stippling of the erythrocytes is prominent in most patients with P5′N deficiency but is on itself an unspecific finding. Leukopenia occasionally is observed in patients with hereditary nonspherocytic hemolytic anemia, possibly secondary to splenic enlargement. Other laboratory stigmata of increased hemolysis may include increased levels of serum bilirubin, decreased haptoglobin levels, and increased serum LDH activity. Reticulocytosis is frequently observed, which may result in increased mean corpuscular volume of erythrocytes. In PK deficiency, splenectomy increases reticulocyte counts even further to levels greater than 50%. This is not seen in other disorders and results mainly because the younger PK-deficient red blood cells are preferentially sequestered by the spleen.[540] Also in P5′N1 and GPI deficiency, reticulocytes tend to be higher in splenectomized patients than in nonsplenectomized patients.[279,379]

Diagnosis of red cell enzyme deficiencies usually depends on the demonstration of decreased enzyme activity either through a quantitative assay or a screening test.[541] Assay of most of the enzymes generally is carried out by measuring the rate of reduction or oxidation of nicotinamide adenine nucleotides in an ultraviolet spectrophotometer.

However, difficulties arise when the patient has been transfused so that the blood drawn represents a mixture of the patient's own cells and those obtained from the blood bank. Under the circumstances, DNA analysis may prove invaluable, because the DNA is extracted from blood leukocytes and transfused leukocytes do not persist in the circulation. Alternatively, density fractionation has been applied to isolate fractions of patient's red cells, in which an enzyme deficiency can be detected.[542]

Although detection of G6PD deficiency in the healthy, fully affected (hemizygous) male can be achieved readily through either assay or screening tests, difficulties arise when a patient with G6PD deficiency of the A− type has undergone a hemolytic episode. As the older, more enzyme-deficient cells are removed from the circulation and are replaced by young cells, the level of the enzyme begins to increase toward normal. Under such circumstances, suspicion that the patient may be G6PD deficient should be raised by the fact that enzyme activity is not increased, even though the reticulocyte count is elevated. Centrifugation of the blood followed by testing of the most dense, reticulocyte-depleted red cells has been employed as a means for the detection of G6PD deficiency in persons with the A− defect who recently underwent hemolysis.[543] It is helpful to carry out family studies or to wait until the circulating red cells have aged sufficiently to betray their lack of enzyme.

Even greater difficulties are encountered in attempting to diagnose heterozygotes for G6PD deficiency. Because the gene is X linked, a population of normal red cells coexists with the deficient cells. This may mask the enzyme deficiency when screening tests are used. Even enzyme assays carried out on erythrocytes of heterozygous females frequently may be in the reference range. Here cytochemical or flow cytometry-based methods may be useful,[544,545] or DNA analysis.

Guidelines and consensus recommendations have been published for the laboratory diagnosis of G6PD deficiency and PK deficiency, respectively.[546,547] Testing for red cell enzyme deficiencies is best done in specialized laboratories. Specimens can be shipped by mail to reference laboratories. As a rule, whole-blood specimens anticoagulated with ethylenediaminetetraacetic acid (EDTA) are suitable and the specimens can best be sent at 4°C as some enzymes, notably PFK, are relatively unstable.[541] Blood from healthy volunteers should be shipped together with blood from the patient to serve as a shipping control. Exceptions are assays for phosphorylated sugar intermediates, 2,3-BPG, and nucleotide intermediates, which are unstable in freshly drawn blood and require immediate deproteinization in perchloric acid. Several aspects should be kept in mind when interpreting test results. First, care must be taken to remove leukocytes and platelets in assays such as for PK, as these cells do contain PK activity, obscuring a deficiency in the red

cells.[547] Second, one should be aware of the already mentioned red cell age dependency of, for example, PK, HK, and G6PD. The measurement of these enzymes simultaneously can give an idea about red cell age and relative deficiencies. If patients received blood transfusions, interpreting results from red cell enzyme assays is generally not possible because the presence of donor erythrocytes will obscure any deficiencies. Some mutant enzymes also display a normal activity in vitro, whereas in vivo severe hemolysis can occur, reflecting the differences between optimal circumstances in vitro and the in vivo cellular environment. More sophisticated assays to measure, for example, heat instability and kinetics, have to be used in those cases. Interpretation can be particularly challenging in newborn patients given the differences in red cell energy metabolism and enzymatic activities between adults and newborn infants.[548-552] Molecular diagnosis is highly recommended to confirm a suspected red cell enzyme deficiency.

● DIFFERENTIAL DIAGNOSIS

Drug-induced hemolytic anemia resulting from G6PD deficiency is similar in its clinical features and in certain laboratory features, to drug-induced hemolytic anemia associated with unstable hemoglobins (Chap. 18). Other enzyme defects affecting the pentose–phosphate shunt, such as a deficiency of GS, also may mimic G6PD deficiency. The diagnosis of hemoglobinopathies can be excluded by performing high-performance liquid chromatography (HPLC) analysis for the detection of hemoglobin variants or DNA sequence analysis. These are normal in G6PD deficiency. Some of the screening tests, particularly the ascorbate cyanide test,[553] may give positive results in the abovenamed disorders, but a G6PD assay or the fluorescent screening test will be positive only in G6PD deficiency. In addition, defects of the erythrocyte membrane should be excluded (Chap. 15), but these cytoskeletal and other membrane defects are generally associated with characteristic morphologic abnormalities, and specific patterns in osmotic gradient ektacytometry testing, which discriminates them from hemolysis as a result of enzyme defects.

Physicians often attempt to establish the cause of hereditary nonspherocytic hemolytic anemia on the basis of the appearance of red cells on a blood film. In reality, red cell morphology is helpful only in the diagnosis of P5′N deficiency because of the characteristic stippling of the red cells that is observed in that disorder. The appearance of Heinz bodies suggests the possible presence of an unstable hemoglobin, or defective GSH metabolism. They are more likely to be present after splenectomy.

Because the laboratory diagnosis of these disorders may entail considerable expenditure of time and effort, it is prudent to perform the simplest tests for the most common causes of hereditary nonspherocytic hemolytic anemia first. Accordingly, it is useful to carry out screening[554] tests for G6PD and PK activity and HPLC analysis or an isopropanol test to detect an abnormal or unstable hemoglobin. If prominent basophilic stippling of erythrocytes is present, examination of the ultraviolet spectrum of a perchloric acid extract of the erythrocytes, reflecting the ratio between pyrimidine and purine nucleotide content, may help to establish the diagnosis of P5′N deficiency.[555] Beyond these relatively simple procedures it is probably rarely useful to pick and choose individual enzyme assays on the basis of family history or clinical manifestations. Rather, it is usually appropriate to submit a blood sample to a reference laboratory that has the capability of performing all the enzyme assays listed in Table 16–3. Preferably, the suspicion of a specific enzyme disorder causing hereditary nonspherocytic hemolytic anemia is confirmed by DNA sequence analysis. This also enables prenatal diagnosis which has already been achieved for some of enzymatic defects.

Notably, in an estimated 70% of cases of suspected hereditary nonspherocytic hemolytic anemia, no enzymatic abnormality is found.[556,557] Current promising approaches such as red cell proteome analysis,[558-560] the use of next-generation sequencing technologies[561] and potentially metabolomics[562,563] may aid in a better and more comprehensive understanding of the etiology of this disorder.

●THERAPY

GLUCOSE-6-PHOSPHATE DEHYDROGENASE DEFICIENCY

G6PD-deficient individuals should avoid drugs that are predicted to induce hemolytic episodes (see Table 16–5). However, it is important to realize that such patients are able to tolerate most drugs. Unfortunately, in the past, a number of case reports incorrectly suggested that some drugs had hemolytic potential that subsequently were shown to be safe (see Table 16–5, possible hemolysis). Although it is possible that some of these may be hemolytic in some patients or under some circumstances, this is unlikely, and G6PD-deficient patients should not be deprived of the possible benefit of these drugs.

If hemolysis occurs as a result of drug ingestion or infection, particularly in the milder A− type of deficiency, transfusion usually is not required. If, however, the rate of hemolysis is very rapid, as may occur, for example, in favism, transfusions of packed cells may be useful. Good urine flow should be maintained in patients with hemoglobinuria to avert renal damage. Infants with neonatal jaundice resulting from G6PD deficiency may require phototherapy or exchange transfusion; in areas in which G6PD deficiency is prevalent, care must be taken not to give G6PD–deficient blood to such newborns.[564] A single dose of Sn-mesoporphyrin, a potent inhibitor of heme oxygenase, has been advocated to reduce bilirubin production and eliminate the need for phototherapy.[565] Patients with HNSHA resulting from G6PD deficiency usually do not require any therapy. In most cases, the anemia is not severe; in some instances, however, frequent transfusions may be necessary.[566,567] Whereas the reported effect of splenectomy varies, experts suggest that splenectomy is a therapeutic option when splenomegaly becomes a physical encumbrance, or when there is evidence of hypersplenism and/or severe anemia (see Table 16–2).[568,569] The antioxidant properties of vitamin E have been tested in G6PD-deficient subjects but didn't show clear benefit.[570-573] It has been reported that deferoxamine slightly reduces transfusion burden during acute hemolysis in G6PD-deficient subjects.[574,575]

OTHER ENZYME DEFICIENCIES

Most patients with hereditary nonspherocytic hemolytic anemia secondary to red cell enzymopathies do not require therapy, other than blood transfusion during hemolytic periods, if the anemia needs clinically to be corrected. There are patients with HK, PK, GPI, and P5′N deficiency that are transfusion dependent. Chronic transfusion therapy always requires concomitant treatment with iron chelation, while even in non–transfusion-dependent patients it could be argued that some patients possibly will develop iron overload as a result of the increased erythropoiesis. Although there is no consensus whether erythropoiesis in enzymopathies should be regarded as ineffective, at least for PK deficiency it was shown that patients who never received blood transfusion have an increased risk of developing iron overload. In addition, other complications, such as aplastic crises, osteopenia/bone fragility, extramedullary hematopoiesis, postsplenectomy sepsis, pulmonary hypertension, and leg ulcers, are not rare in PK deficiency.[260] Most experts regard these complications as not intrinsically related to the

glycolytic defect, but as a consequence of chronic hemolysis, anemia, and side effects of splenectomy and/or transfusions. Consequently, it can be speculated that patients with other enzymopathies have an increased prevalence of these complications as well.[508] While guidelines on screening patients with enzymopathies for secondary organ damage are not available yet, experts have suggested to consider screening for these complications similar to screening for complications in thalassemia.[576] Table 16–6 provides a list of prevalent organ damage in patients with hereditary nonspherocytic anemia caused by enzymopathies that could be considered to screen for.

The principal decision that the physician must make regarding patients with HNSHA is whether they require a splenectomy. This decision is not made easily as the response is unpredictable, and some patients who fail to respond may develop serious thrombotic complications resulting from postsplenectomy thrombocytosis that is often exaggerated when splenectomy does not ameliorate the hemolysis. The recommendation that is made should be based upon the following considerations: (a) severity of the disease, (b) family history of response

TABLE 16–6. Prevalent Forms of Organ Damage in Patients with Hereditary Nonspherocytic Anemia

	General Population[a]	HNSHA[b] (screened for organ damage)	PK deficiency[c] (nonscreened for organ damage)
N	NA	30	254
Pulmonary hypertension[d]	3%	17%	3%
Thrombotic event	<1%	10%	11%
Iron overload (liver)	<1%	68%	48%
Microalbuminuria	7%	39%	NR
Renal failure	4%	3%	NR
Cholecystectomy	<1%	73%	40%
Osteoporosis	3%	15%	NR
Fractures	7%	0%	17%
Leg ulceration	<1%	7%	2%
Low testosterone	2%	14%	0%
Vitamin D deficiency	49%	50%	NR
IGF-1 deficiency	2%	43%	3%

HNSHA, hereditary nonspherocytic hemolytic anemia; IGF, insulin-like growth factor deficiency was defined as ≥2 SD from healthy controls; NA, Not applicable; NR, not reported; PK, pyruvate kinase.

[a]Disease prevalence in the general Dutch population.

[b]Number of patients: 23 patients with PK deficiency; 4 glucose-6-phosphate dehydrogenase (G6PD) deficiency; 2 hexokinase (HK) deficiency; 1 glutamate cysteine ligase (GCL) deficiency; Data from van Straaten S, Verhoeven J, Hagens S, et al. Organ involvement occurs in all forms of hereditary haemolytic anaemia. *Br J Haematol.* 2019 May;185(3):602-605.

[c]Data from Grace RF, Bianchi P, van Beers EJ, et al. Clinical spectrum of pyruvate kinase deficiency: data from the Pyruvate Kinase Deficiency Natural History Study. *Blood.* 2018 May 17;131(20):2183-2192.

[d]Defined as tricuspid regurgitant jet flow velocity >2.5 m/s by cardiac ultrasound.

to splenectomy, (c) the underlying defect, and (d) (perhaps) the need for cholecystectomy. Because it is unusual to obtain more than a partial response to splenectomy, this procedure should probably be reserved for patients whose quality of life is impaired by their anemia. The operation needs to be particularly considered for patients who need frequent transfusion and for those who require gallbladder surgery, in which splenectomy might be carried out as part of the same procedure. The best guide to the likely efficacy of splenectomy is probably the response to splenectomy of other affected family members. Unfortunately, such information is only occasionally available. The physician must therefore rely upon the experience of other patients with HNSHA of similar etiology to serve as a guide. However, even as the large group of patients with HNSHA represents a heterogeneous population, so individuals with a single enzymatic lesion, such as PK deficiency, are heterogeneous. Each family is likely to be afflicted with a distinct mutant enzyme, and the various mutants may differ both with respect to clinical manifestations and with respect to response to splenectomy. Yet, splenectomy is a well-accepted treatment option in PK deficiency.[568] In the PK deficiency Natural History Study, splenectomy was associated with a median increase in hemoglobin of 16 g/L and a decreased transfusion burden in 90% of patients.[260] However, it is associated with a number of side effects that are comparable to those described in thalassemia, most importantly, a high risk of postsplenectomy infection and an increased risk of thrombosis. For GPI deficiency, it has been reported that four of five patients with GPI deficiency significantly improved following splenectomy (data available before and after splenectomy).[279] For other enzymopathies, the effect of splenectomy has not been well described. Some of the available information regarding response to splenectomy of patients with HNSHA has been reviewed[569] and is summarized in Table 16–2.

Jaundice in GPI deficiency has been treated by the administration of phenobarbital but has been employed in other enzymopathies as well.[577] Glucocorticoids are of no known value in enzymopathies. Folic acid is often given, as in other patients with increased marrow activity, but without proven hematologic benefit. In the absence of iron deficiency, iron is contraindicated (unless iron deficiency is present), because of above described risk of iron overload.

New developments in therapy for enzymopathies have been reported for PK deficiency. Successful allogeneic stem cell transplantation has been reported in PK deficiency,[578,579] PGK deficiency,[340] and in a case with HK deficiency.[580] A small case series of patients with PK deficiency suggest that transplantation very early in life yields better results and that graft-versus-host disease is a more important problem than engraftment.[579] A clinical trial for gene therapy in PK deficiency was launched in 2020. Although the results are pending at the time of writing this chapter, gene therapy holds promise for severely affected patients with PK deficiency. The method that is used in the current PK deficiency gene therapy study has been successfully used for Fanconi anemia.[581] Unfortunately, conditioning of the patients before gene therapy still includes a myeloablative regimen that includes busulfan, an alkylating antineoplastic agent that comes with acute cytotoxic, teratogenic, and mutagenic side effects.

Preliminary evidence indicates that small-molecule activation of mutant PK may be able to restore glycolytic pathway activity and normalize red cell metabolism in PK deficiency.[582] A clinical trial using an oral, small-molecule allosteric activator of PK in red cells has been reported.[583] The administration of the PK activator was associated with a rapid increase in the hemoglobin level in about half of the patients. Adverse effects were mainly low grade and transient.[583] At the time of writing, the phase III placebo-controlled, randomized clinical trial is ongoing.

Besides the abovementioned developments, the new chemotherapy-free conditioning regimens that are developed for allogeneic stem

cell transplantation in sickle cell disease holds promise for red cell enzymopathies as well.[584,585] As long as stem cell transplantation harbors significant long-term risks and toxicity, physicians and patients will be reluctant to employ this treatment option for very rare hematologic diseases where ample data is available to support treatment decisions.

● COURSE AND PROGNOSIS

Hemolytic episodes in the A– type of deficiency are usually self-limited, even if drug administration is continued. This is not the case in the more severe Mediterranean type of deficiency.[586] In patients with HNSHA resulting from G6PD deficiency, gallstones may occur, and the incidence of cholelithiasis may even be increased in patients with polymorphic forms of G6PD deficiency in Sardinia.[587] During periods of infections or drug administration, anemia may increase in severity. Otherwise, the hemoglobin level of affected subjects remains relatively stable.

Nearly all patients with drug-induced or infection-induced hemolysis recover uneventfully. Favism must be considered, by comparison, a relatively dangerous disease. The most serious complication of G6PD deficiency is neonatal icterus. If not recognized early and properly treated, it can lead to kernicterus (see "Clinical Features" earlier).

In one large population study, a decreasing incidence of G6PD deficiency was noted with increasing age of the population,[588] but no such change was observed in another.[589] Although age stratification might represent evidence of a shorter life span for individuals with the A– deficiency, other factors are more likely explanations. Examination of the health records of more than 65,000 U.S. Veterans Administration males failed to reveal any higher frequency of any illness in G6PD-deficient compared to nondeficient participants.[590] Furthermore, it appears that there are no indications that G6PD-deficient individuals should systematically be excluded from serving as blood donors,[591] or hematopoietic stem cell donors.[592] In view of the benign nature of the common types of G6PD deficiency, community-based population screening is not recommended. However, screening for G6PD deficiency of all patients admitted to the hospital may be useful in anticipating hemolytic reactions and in understanding them if they occur; however, this recommendation has not been submitted to rigorous analysis and is controversial because of low likelihood of any preventable hemolysis. Screening is particularly prudent if a drug such as dapsone or rasburicase, known to cause hemolysis in G6PD-deficient individuals, is to be given.[441,593] Study of family members of patients with this X-chromosome–linked enzyme deficiency can be helpful in providing appropriate counseling to affected individuals.

The diagnosis of HNSHA has been made as late as the seventh decade,[187] and the disease can be fatal in the first few years of life. TPI deficiency has the worst prognosis of all of the known defects that cause this disorder. With few exceptions, patients with this deficiency have died by the fifth or sixth year of life, usually of cardiopulmonary failure. PK deficiency, too, can be fatal in early childhood; the gene prevalent among the Amish of Pennsylvania produces particularly severe disease.[594] Unless the affected homozygous children have their spleens removed, the disorder is commonly lethal. In PK deficiency, compound heterozygotes and homozygotes can suffer of major side effects as a result of the chronic hemolysis and the burden of repeated transfusions and iron chelation. In general, most physicians regard HNSHA as a relatively mild disease with a relatively good prognosis. However, a recent small case series of PK deficiency showed that even in nontransfused, so-called mild patients, the subjective burden of disease is considerable.[595] In addition, as discussed earlier ("Therapy") the majority of patients have an increased risk of developing secondary organ damage (eg, osteoporosis, iron overload, pulmonary hypertension) initially without clinical symptoms, and therefore often not recognized, suggesting that the prognosis may not be that good as generally considered. In other words, the burden of disease of patients with HNSHA can only become clear when the right questions are asked and adequate screening for complications is performed.

REFERENCES

1. Beutler E. G6PD deficiency. *Blood.* 1994;84:3613.
2. Beutler E. Glucose-6-phosphate dehydrogenase deficiency: a historical perspective. *Blood.* 2008;111:16.
3. Luzzatto L, Seneca E. G6PD deficiency: a classic example of pharmacogenetics with on-going clinical implications. *Br J Haematol.* 2014;164:469.
4. Crosby WH. Hereditary nonspherocytic hemolytic anemia. *Blood.* 1950;5:233.
5. Dacie JV. The congenital anaemias. In: *The Haemolytic Anaemias: Congenital and Acquired.* 2nd ed. Grune & Stratton; 1960:171.
6. Selwyn JG, Dacie JV. Autohemolysis and other changes resulting from the incubation in vitro of red cells from patients with congenital hemolytic anemia. *Blood.* 1954;9:414.
7. Robinson MA, Loder PB, De Gruchy GC. Red-cell metabolism in non-spherocytic congenital haemolytic anaemia. *Br J Haematol.* 1961;7:327.
8. Valentine WN, Tanaka KR, Miwa S. A specific erythrocyte glycolytic enzyme defect (pyruvate kinase) in three subjects with congenital non-spherocytic hemolytic anemia. *Trans Assoc Am Physicians.* 1961;74:100.
9. Howes RE, Piel FB, Patil AP, et al. G6PD deficiency prevalence and estimates of affected populations in malaria endemic countries: a geostatistical model-based map. *PLoS Med.* 2012;9:e1001339.
10. Howes RE, Dewi M, Piel FB, et al. Spatial distribution of G6PD deficiency variants across malaria-endemic regions. *Malar J.* 2013;12:418.
11. Nkhoma ET, Poole C, Vannappagari V, et al. The global prevalence of glucose-6-phosphate dehydrogenase deficiency: a systematic review and meta-analysis. *Blood Cells Mol Dis.* 2009;42:267.
12. Lippi G, Mattiuzzi C. Updated worldwide epidemiology of inherited erythrocyte disorders. *Acta Haematol.* Preprint. Posted online September 24, 2019. doi: 10.1159/000502434.
13. Tishkoff SA, Varkonyi R, Cahinhinan N, et al. Haplotype diversity and linkage disequilibrium at human G6PD: recent origin of alleles that confer malarial resistance. *Science.* 2001;293:455.
14. Howes RE, Battle KE, Satyagraha AW, et al. G6PD deficiency: global distribution, genetic variants and primaquine therapy. *Adv Parasitol.* 2013;81:133.
15. Luzzatto L, Usanga FA, Reddy S. Glucose-6-phosphate dehydrogenase deficient red cells: resistance to infection by malarial parasites. *Science.* 1969;164:839.
16. Cappadoro M, Giribaldi G, O'Brien E, et al. Early phagocytosis of glucose-6-phosphate dehydrogenase (G6PD)-deficient erythrocytes parasitized by *Plasmodium falciparum* may explain malaria protection in G6PD deficiency. *Blood.* 1998;92:2527.
17. Luzzatto L. G6PD deficiency and malaria selection. *Heredity (Edinb).* 2012;108:456.
18. Guindo A, Fairhurst RM, Doumbo OK, et al. X-linked G6PD deficiency protects hemizygous males but not heterozygous females against severe malaria. *PLoS Med.* 2007;4:e66.
19. Piomelli S, Reindorf CA, Arzanian MT, et al. Clinical and biochemical interactions of glucose-6-phosphate dehydrogenase deficiency and sickle-cell anemia. *N Engl J Med.* 1972;287:213.
20. Benkerrou M, Alberti C, Couque N, et al. Impact of glucose-6-phosphate dehydrogenase deficiency on sickle cell anaemia expression in infancy and early childhood: a prospective study. *Br J Haematol.* 2013;163:646.
21. Karafin MS, Fu X, D'Alessandro A, et al. The clinical impact of glucose-6-phosphate dehydrogenase deficiency in patients with sickle cell disease. *Curr Opin Hematol.* 2018;25:494.
22. Beutler E, Gelbart T. Estimating the prevalence of pyruvate kinase deficiency from the gene frequency in the general white population. *Blood.* 2000;95:3585.
23. Canu G, De Bonis M, Minucci A, et al. Red blood cell PK deficiency: an update of PK-LR gene mutation database. *Blood Cells Mol Dis.* 2016;57:100.
24. Schneider A, Westwood B, Yim C, et al. The 1591C mutation in triosephosphate isomerase (TPI) deficiency. Tightly linked polymorphisms and a common haplotype in all known families. *Blood Cells Mol Dis.* 1996;22:115.
25. Sherman JB, Raben N, Nicastri C, et al. Common mutations in the phosphofructokinase-M gene in Ashkenazi Jewish patients with glycogenesis VII—and their population frequency. *Am J Hum Genet.* 1994;55:305.
26. Mohrenweiser HW. Functional hemizygosity in the human genome: direct estimate from twelve erythrocyte enzyme loci. *Hum Genet.* 1987;77:241.
27. Watanabe M, Zingg BC, Mohrenweiser HW. Molecular analysis of a series of alleles in humans with reduced activity at the triosephosphate isomerase locus. *Am J Hum Genet.* 1996;58:308.
28. Montel-Hagen A, Kinet S, Manel N, et al. Erythrocyte Glut1 triggers dehydroascorbic acid uptake in mammals unable to synthesize vitamin C. *Cell.* 2008;132:1039.
29. Rosa R, Gaillardon J, Rosa J. Diphosphoglycerate mutase and 2,3-diphosphoglycerate phosphatase activities of red cells: comparative electrophoretic study. *Biochem Biophys Res Commun.* 1973;51:536.
30. Cho J, King JS, Qian X, et al. Dephosphorylation of 2,3-bisphosphoglycerate by MIPP expands the regulatory capacity of the Rapoport-Luebering glycolytic shunt. *Proc Natl Acad Sci U S A.* 2008;105:5998.
31. Puchulu-Campanella E, Chu H, Anstee DJ, et al. Identification of the components of a glycolytic enzyme metabolon on the human red blood cell membrane. *J Biol Chem.* 2013;288:848.
32. Campanella ME, Chu H, Low PS. Assembly and regulation of a glycolytic enzyme complex on the human erythrocyte membrane. *Proc Natl Acad Sci U S A.* 2005;102:2402.
33. Lewis IA, Campanella ME, Markley JL, et al. Role of band 3 in regulating metabolic flux of red blood cells. *Proc Natl Acad Sci U S A.* 2009;106:18515.
34. Sriram G, Martinez JA, McCabe ERB, et al. Single-gene disorders: what role could moonlighting enzymes play? *Am J Hum Genet.* 2005;76:911.
35. Kim J-W, Dang CV. Multifaceted roles of glycolytic enzymes. *Trends Biochem Sci.* 2005;30:142.
36. Henderson B, Martin AC. Protein moonlighting: a new factor in biology and medicine. *Biochem Soc Trans.* 2014;42:1671.
37. Srivastava SK, Beutler E. Glutathione metabolism of the erythrocyte. The enzymic cleavage of glutathione-haemoglobin preparations by glutathione reductase. *Biochem J.* 1970;119:353.
38. Jansen G, Koenderman L, Rijksen G, et al. Age dependent behaviour of red cell glycolytic enzymes in haematological disorders. *Br J Haematol.* 1985;61:51.
39. Lakomek M, Schröter W, De Maeyer G, et al. On the diagnosis of erythrocyte enzyme defects in the presence of high reticulocyte counts. *Br J Haematol.* 1989;72:445.
40. Wilson JE. Isozymes of mammalian hexokinase: structure, subcellular localization and metabolic function. *J Exp Biol.* 2003;206:2049.
41. Cárdenas ML, Cornish-Bowden A, Ureta T. Evolution and regulatory role of the hexokinases. *Biochim Biophys Acta.* 1998;1401:242.
42. Fujii S, Beutler E. High glucose concentrations partially release hexokinase from inhibition by glucose 6-phosphate. *Proc Natl Acad Sci U S A.* 1985;82:1552.
43. Gerber G, Kloppick E, Rapoport S. On the influence of inorganic phosphates on glycolysis; its ineffectiveness on the hexokinase of human erythrocytes. Article in German. *Acta Biol Med Ger.* 1967;18:305.
44. Beutler E, Teeple L. The effect of oxidized glutathione (GSSG) on human erythrocyte hexokinase activity. *Acta Biol Med Ger.* 1969;22:707.
45. Beutler E. 2,3-Diphosphoglycerate affects enzymes of glucose metabolism in red blood cells. *Nat New Biol.* 1971;232:20.
46. Mulichak AM, Wilson JE, Padmanabhan K, et al. The structure of mammalian hexokinase-1. *Nat Struct Biol.* 1998;5:555.
47. Aleshin AE, Kirby C, Liu X, et al. Crystal structures of mutant monomeric hexokinase I reveal multiple ADP binding sites and conformational changes relevant to allosteric regulation. *J Mol Biol.* 2000;296:1001.
48. Murakami K, Blei F, Tilton W, et al. An isozyme of hexokinase specific for the human red blood cell (HK$_R$). *Blood.* 1990;75:770.
49. Ruzzo A, Andreoni F, Magnani M. Structure of the human hexokinase type I gene and nucleotide sequence of the 5′ flanking region. *Biochem J.* 1998;331:607.
50. Magnani M, Serafini G, Stocchi V. Hexokinase type I multiplicity in human erythrocytes. *Biochem J.* 1988;254:617.
51. Andreoni F, Ruzzo A, Magnani M. Structure of the 5′ region of the human hexokinase type I (HKI) gene and identification of an additional testis-specific HKI mRNA. *Biochim Biophys Acta.* 2000;1493:19.
52. Hantke J, Chandler D, King R, et al. A mutation in an alternative untranslated exon of hexokinase 1 associated with hereditary motor and sensory neuropathy—Russe (HMSNR). *Eur J Hum Genet.* 2009;17:1606.
53. Murakami K, Kanno H, Miwa S, et al. Human HK$_R$ isozyme: organization of the hexokinase I gene, the erythroid-specific promoter, and transcription initiation site. *Mol Genet Metab.* 1999;67:118.
54. Murakami K, Piomelli S. Identification of the cDNA for human red blood cell-specific hexokinase isozyme [see comments]. *Blood.* 1997;89:762.
55. Bonnefond A, Vaxillaire M, Labrune Y, et al. Genetic variant in HK1 is associated with a proanemic state and A1C but not other glycemic control-related traits. *Diabetes.* 2009;58:2687.
56. Read J, Pearce J, Li X, et al. The crystal structure of human phosphoglucose isomerase at 1.6 A resolution: implications for catalytic mechanism, cytokine activity and haemolytic anaemia. *J Mol Biol.* 2001;309:447.
57. Somarowthu S, Brodkin HR, D'Aquino JA, et al. A tale of two isomerases: compact versus extended active sites in ketosteroid isomerase and phosphoglucose isomerase. *Biochemistry.* 2011;50:9283.
58. Xu W, Lee P, Beutler E. Human glucose phosphate isomerase: exon mapping and gene structure. *Genomics.* 1995;29:732.
59. Sola-Penna M, Da Silva D, Coelho WS, et al. Regulation of mammalian muscle type 6-phosphofructo-1-kinase and its implication for the control of the metabolism. *IUBMB Life.* 2010;62:791.
60. Schöneberg T, Kloos M, Brüser A, et al. Structure and allosteric regulation of eukaryotic 6-phosphofructokinases. *Biol Chem.* 2013;394:977.
61. Costa Leite T, Da Silva D, Guimaraes Coelho R, et al. Lactate favours the dissociation of skeletal muscle 6-phosphofructo-1-kinase tetramers down-regulating the enzyme and muscle glycolysis. *Biochem J.* 2007;408:123.
62. Marinho-Carvalho MM, Costa-Mattos PV, Spitz GA, et al. Calmodulin upregulates skeletal muscle 6-phosphofructo-1-kinase reversing the inhibitory effects of allosteric modulators. *Biochim Biophys Acta.* 2009;1794:1175.

63. Higashi T, Richards CS, Uyeda K. The interaction of phosphofructokinase with erythrocyte membranes. *J Biol Chem.* 1979;254:9542.

64. Jenkins JD, Kezdy FJ, Steck TL. Mode of interaction of phosphofructokinase with the erythrocyte membrane. *J Biol Chem.* 1985;260:10426.

65. Chu H, Low PS. Mapping of glycolytic enzyme binding sites on human erythrocyte band 3. *Biochem J.* 2006;400:143.

66. Real-Hohn A, Zancan P, Da Silva D, et al. Filamentous actin and its associated binding proteins are the stimulatory site for 6-phosphofructo-1-kinase association within the membrane of human erythrocytes. *Biochimie.* 2010;92:538.

67. Kloos M, Bruser A, Kirchberger J, et al. Crystallization and preliminary crystallographic analysis of human muscle phosphofructokinase, the main regulator of glycolysis. *Acta Crystallogr F Struct Biol Commun.* 2014;70:578.

68. Yamada S, Nakajima H, Kuehn MR. Novel testis- and embryo-specific isoforms of the phosphofructokinase-1 muscle type gene. *Biochem Biophys Res Commun.* 2004;316:580.

69. Elson A, Levanon D, Brandeis M, et al. The structure of the human liver-type phosphofructokinase gene. *Genomics.* 1990;7:47.

70. Vora S, Davidson M, Seaman C, et al. Heterogeneity of the molecular lesions in inherited phosphofructokinase deficiency. *J Clin Invest.* 1983;72:1995.

71. Yeltman DR, Harris BG. Fructose-bisphosphate aldolase from human erythrocytes. *Methods Enzymol.* 1982;90(pt E):251.

72. Beutler E, Scott S, Bishop A, et al. Red cell aldolase deficiency and hemolytic anemia: a new syndrome. *Trans Assoc Am Physicians.* 1973;86:154.

73. Dalby A, Dauter Z, Littlechild JA. Crystal structure of human muscle aldolase complexed with fructose 1,6-bisphosphate: mechanistic implications. *Protein Sci.* 1999;8:291.

74. Yeltman DR, Harris BG. Localization and membrane association of aldolase in human erythrocytes. *Arch Biochem Biophys.* 1980;199:186.

75. Perrotta S, Borriello A, Scaloni A, et al. The N-terminal 11 amino acids of human erythrocyte band 3 are critical for aldolase binding and protein phosphorylation: implications for band 3 function. *Blood.* 2005;106:4359.

76. Izzo P, Costanzo P, Lupo A, et al. Human aldolase A gene. Structural organization and tissue-specific expression by multiple promoters and alternate mRNA processing. *Eur J Biochem.* 1988;174:569.

77. Wierenga RK, Kapetaniou EG, Venkatesan R. Triosephosphate isomerase: a highly evolved biocatalyst. *Cell Mol Life Sci.* 2010;67:3961.

78. Lu HS, Yuan PM, Gracy RW. Primary structure of human triosephosphate isomerase. *J Biol Chem.* 1984;259:11958.

79. Mande SC, Mainfroid V, Kalk KH, et al. Crystal structure of recombinant human triosephosphate isomerase at 2.8 A resolution. Triosephosphate isomerase-related human genetic disorders and comparison with the trypanosomal enzyme. *Protein Sci.* 1994;3:810.

80. Rodríguez-Almazán C, Arreola R, Rodríguez-Larrea D, et al. Structural basis of human triosephosphate isomerase deficiency: mutation E104D is related to alterations of a conserved water network at the dimer interface. *J Biol Chem.* 2008;283:23254.

81. Peters J, Hopkinson DA, Harris H. Genetic and non-genetic variation of triose phosphate isomerase isozymes in human tissues. *Ann Hum Genet.* 1973;36:297.

82. Brown JR, Daar IO, Krug JR, et al. Characterization of the functional gene and several processed pseudogenes in the human triosephosphate isomerase gene family. *Mol Cell Biol.* 1985;5:1694.

83. Rogalski AA, Steck TL, Waseem A. Association of glyceraldehyde-3-phosphate dehydrogenase with the plasma membrane of the intact human red blood cell. *J Biol Chem.* 1989;264:6438.

84. Tsai IH, Murthy SN, Steck TL. Effect of red cell membrane binding on the catalytic activity of glyceraldehyde-3-phosphate dehydrogenase. *J Biol Chem.* 1982;257:1438.

85. Low PS, Rathinavelu P, Harrison ML. Regulation of glycolysis via reversible enzyme binding to the membrane protein, band 3. *J Biol Chem.* 1993;268:14627.

86. Rogers SC, Ross JG, d'Avignon A, et al. Sickle hemoglobin disturbs normal coupling among erythrocyte O2 content, glycolysis, and antioxidant capacity. *Blood.* 2013;121:1651.

87. Mountassif D, Baibai T, Fourrat L, et al. Immunoaffinity purification and characterization of glyceraldehyde-3-phosphate dehydrogenase from human erythrocytes. *Acta Biochim Biophys Sin (Shanghai).* 2009;41:399.

88. Boradia VM, Raje M, Raje CI. Protein moonlighting in iron metabolism: glyceraldehyde-3-phosphate dehydrogenase (GAPDH). *Biochem Soc Trans.* 2014;42:1796.

89. Ismail SA, Park HW. Structural analysis of human liver glyceraldehyde-3-phosphate dehydrogenase. *Acta Crystallogr D Biol Crystallogr.* 2005;61:1508.

90. McCann SR, Finkel B, Cadman S, et al. Study of a kindred with hereditary spherocytosis and glyceraldehyde-3-phosphate dehydrogenase deficiency. *Blood.* 1976;47:171.

91. Huang IY, Welch CD, Yoshida A. Complete amino acid sequence of human phosphoglycerate kinase. Cyanogen bromide peptides and complete amino acid sequence. *J Biol Chem.* 1980;255:6412.

92. McCarrey JR, Thomas K. Human testis-specific PGK gene lacks introns and possesses characteristics of a processed gene. *Nature.* 1987;326:501.

93. Banks RD, Blake CC, Evans PR, et al. Sequence, structure and activity of phosphoglycerate kinase: a possible hinge-bending enzyme. *Nature.* 1979;279:773.

94. Szabo J, Varga A, Flachner B, et al. Communication between the nucleotide site and the main molecular hinge of 3-phosphoglycerate kinase. *Biochemistry.* 2008;47:6735.

95. Palmai Z, Chaloin L, Lionne C, et al. Substrate binding modifies the hinge bending characteristics of human 3-phosphoglycerate kinase: a molecular dynamics study. *Proteins.* 2009;77:319.

96. Ikura K, Sasaki R, Narita H, et al. Multifunctional enzyme, bisphosphoglyceromutase/2,3-bisphosphoglycerate phosphatase/phosphoglyceromutase, from human erythrocytes. Evidence for a common active site. *Eur J Biochem.* 1976;66:515.

97. Rose ZB. The enzymology of 2,3-bisphosphoglycerate. *Adv Enzymol Relat Areas Mol Biol.* 1980;51:211.

98. Fujii S, Beutler E. Where does phosphoglycolate come from in red cells? *Acta Haematol.* 1985;73:26.

99. Sasaki H, Fujii S, Yoshizaki Y, et al. Phosphoglycolate synthesis by human erythrocyte pyruvate kinase. *Acta Haematol.* 1987;77:83.

100. Beutler E, West C. An improved assay and some properties of phosphoglycolate phosphatase. *Anal Biochem.* 1980;106:163.

101. Wang Y, Wei Z, Bian Q, et al. Crystal structure of human bisphosphoglycerate mutase. *J Biol Chem.* 2004;279:39132.

102. Patterson A, Price NC, Nairn J. Unliganded structure of human bisphosphoglycerate mutase reveals side-chain movements induced by ligand binding. *Acta Crystallogr Sect F Struct Biol Cryst Commun.* 2010;66:1415.

103. Hass LF, Kappel WK, Miller KB, et al. Evidence for structural homology between human red cell phosphoglycerate mutase and 2,3-bisphosphoglycerate synthase. *J Biol Chem.* 1978;253:77.

104. Climent F, Roset F, Repiso A, et al. Red cell glycolytic enzyme disorders caused by mutations: an update. *Cardiovasc Hematol Disord Drug Targets.* 2009;9:95.

105. Repiso A, Pérez de la Ossa P, Avilés X, et al. Red blood cell phosphoglycerate mutase. Description of the first human BB isoenzyme mutation. *Haematologica.* 2003;88:ECR07.

106. de Atauri P, Repiso A, Oliva B, et al. Characterization of the first described mutation of human red blood cell phosphoglycerate mutase. *Biochim Biophys Acta.* 2005;1740:403.

107. Repiso A, Ramirez Bajo MJ, Corrons JL, et al. Phosphoglycerate mutase BB isoenzyme deficiency in a patient with non-spherocytic anemia: familial and metabolic studies. *Haematologica.* 2005;90:257.

108. Hoorn RKJ, Flikweert JP, Staal GEJ. Purification and properties of enolase of human erythrocytes. *Int J Biochem.* 1974;5:845.

109. Kang HJ, Jung SK, Kim SJ, et al. Structure of human alpha-enolase (hENO1), a multifunctional glycolytic enzyme. *Acta Crystallogr D Biol Crystallogr.* 2008;64:651.

110. Stefanini M. Chronic hemolytic anemia associated with erythrocyte enolase deficiency exacerbated by ingestion of nitrofurantoin. *Am J Clin Pathol.* 1972;58:408.

111. Boulard-Heitzmann P, Boulard M, Tallineau C, et al. Decreased red cell enolase activity in a 40-year-old woman with compensated haemolysis. *Scand J Haematol.* 1984;33:401.

112. Park JA, Lim YJ, Park HJ, et al. Normalization of red cell enolase level following allogeneic bone marrow transplantation in a child with Diamond-Blackfan anemia. *J Korean Med Sci.* 2010;25:626.

113. Noguchi T, Inoue H, Tanaka T. The M1- and M2-type isozymes of rat pyruvate kinase are produced from the same gene by alternative RNA splicing. *J Biol Chem.* 1986;261:13807.

114. Kanno H, Fujii H, Miwa S. Structural analysis of human pyruvate kinase L-gene and identification of the promoter activity in erythroid cells. *Biochem Biophys Res Commun.* 1992;188:516.

115. Noguchi T, Yamada K, Inoue H, et al. The L- and R-type isozymes of rat pyruvate kinase are produced from a single gene by use of different promoters. *J Biol Chem.* 1987;262:14366.

116. Viprakasit V, Ekwattanakit S, Riolueang S, et al. Mutations in Krüppel-like factor 1 cause transfusion-dependent hemolytic anemia and persistence of embryonic globin gene expression. *Blood.* 2014;123:1586.

117. van Oirschot BA, Francois JJ, van Solinge WW, et al. Novel type of red blood cell pyruvate kinase hyperactivity predicts a remote regulatory locus involved in PKLR gene expression. *Am J Hematol.* 2014;89:380.

118. Kanno H, Fujii H, Hirono A, et al. cDNA cloning of human R-type pyruvate kinase and identification of a single amino acid substitution (Thr384→Met) affecting enzymatic stability in a pyruvate kinase variant (PK Tokyo) associated with hereditary hemolytic anemia. *Proc Natl Acad Sci U S A.* 1991;88:8218.

119. Kahn A, Marie J, Garreau H, et al. The genetic system of the L-type pyruvate kinase forms in man. Subunit structure, interrelation and kinetic characteristics of the pyruvate kinase enzymes from erythrocytes and liver. *Biochim Biophys Acta.* 1978;523:59.

120. Kahn A, Marie J. Pyruvate kinases from human erythrocytes and liver. *Methods Enzymol.* 1982;90:131.

121. Valentini G, Chiarelli LR, Fortin R, et al. Structure and function of human erythrocyte pyruvate kinase. Molecular basis of nonspherocytic hemolytic anemia. *J Biol Chem.* 2002;277:23807.

122. Enriqueta Muñoz M, Ponce E. Pyruvate kinase: current status of regulatory and functional properties. *Comp Biochem Physiol B Biochem Mol Biol.* 2003;135:197.

123. Wang C, Chiarelli LR, Bianchi P, et al. Human erythrocyte pyruvate kinase: characterization of the recombinant enzyme and a mutant form (R510Q) causing nonspherocytic hemolytic anemia. *Blood.* 2001;98:3113.

124. Fenton AW, Tang Q. An activating interaction between the unphosphorylated n-terminus of human liver pyruvate kinase and the main body of the protein is interrupted by phosphorylation. *Biochemistry.* 2009;48:3816.

125. Jurica MS, Mesecar A, Heath PJ, et al. The allosteric regulation of pyruvate kinase by fructose-1,6-bisphosphate. *Structure.* 1998;6:195.

126. Rigden DJ, Phillips SE, Michels PA, et al. The structure of pyruvate kinase from *Leishmania mexicana* reveals details of the allosteric transition and unusual effector specificity. *J Mol Biol.* 1999;291:615.

127. Valentini G, Chiarelli L, Fortin R, et al. The allosteric regulation of pyruvate kinase. *J Biol Chem.* 2000;275:18145.

128. Wooll JO, Friesen RHE, White MA, et al. Structural and functional linkages between subunit interfaces in mammalian pyruvate kinase. *J Mol Biol.* 2001;312:525.

129. Fenton AW, Blair JB. Kinetic and allosteric consequences of mutations in the subunit and domain interfaces and the allosteric site of yeast pyruvate kinase. *Arch Biochem Biophys.* 2002;397:28.

130. Blume KG, Hoffbauer RW, Busch D, et al. Purification and properties of pyruvate kinase in normal and in pyruvate kinase deficient human red blood cells. *Biochim Biophys Acta.* 1971;227:364.

131. Kitamura M, Iijima N, Hashimoto F, et al. Hereditary deficiency of subunit H of lactate dehydrogenase. *Clin Chim Acta.* 1971;34:419.

132. Joukyuu R, Mizuno S, Amakawa T, et al. Hereditary complete deficiency of lactate dehydrogenase H-subunit. *Clin Chem.* 1989;35:687.

133. Wakabayashi H, Tsuchiya M, Yoshino K, et al. Hereditary deficiency of lactate dehydrogenase H-subunit. *Intern Med.* 1996;35:550.

134. Kanno T, Maekawa M. Lactate dehydrogenase M-subunit deficiencies: clinical features, metabolic background, and genetic heterogeneities. *Muscle Nerve Suppl.* 1995;3:S54.

135. Maekawa M, Sudo K, Nagura K, et al. Population screening of lactate dehydrogenase deficiencies in Fukuoka Prefecture in Japan and molecular characterization of three independent mutations in the lactate dehydrogenase-B(H) gene. *Hum Genet.* 1994;93:74.

136. Persico MG, Viglietto G, Martini G, et al. Isolation of human glucose-6-phosphate dehydrogenase (G6PD) cDNA clones: primary structure of the protein and unusual 5' non-coding region. *Nucleic Acids Res.* 1986;14:2511.

137. Kirkman HN, Hendrickson EM. Glucose 6-phosphate dehydrogenase from human erythrocytes. II. Subactive states of the enzyme from normal persons. *J Biol Chem.* 1962;237:2371.

138. Bonsignore A, Cancedda R, Nicolini A, et al. Metabolism of human erythrocyte glucose-6-phosphate dehydrogenase. VI. Interconversion of multiple molecular forms. *Arch Biochem Biophys.* 1971;147:493.

139. Canepa L, Ferraris AM, Miglino M, et al. Bound and unbound pyridine dinucleotides in normal and glucose-6-phosphate dehydrogenase-deficient erythrocytes. *Biochim Biophys Acta.* 1991;1074:101.

140. Au SW, Gover S, Lam VM, Adams MJ. Human glucose-6-phosphate dehydrogenase: the crystal structure reveals a structural NADP(+) molecule and provides insights into enzyme deficiency. *Structure.* 2000;8:293.

141. Cohen P, Rosemeyer MA. Subunit interactions of glucose-6-phosphate dehydrogenase from human erythrocytes. *Eur J Biochem.* 1969;8:8.

142. Wrigley NG, Heather JV, Bonsignore A, et al. Human erythrocyte glucose 6-phosphate dehydrogenase: electron microscope studies on structure and interconversion of tetramers, dimers and monomers. *J Mol Biol.* 1972;68:483.

143. Yoshida A. Hemolytic anemia and G6PD deficiency. *Science.* 1973;179:532.

144. Ben-Bassat I, Beutler E. Inhibition by ATP of erythrocyte glucose-6-phosphate dehydrogenase variants. *Proc Soc Exp Biol Med.* 1973;142:410.

145. Zimran A, Torem S, Beutler E. The in vivo ageing of red cell enzymes: direct evidence of biphasic decay from polycythaemic rabbits with reticulocytosis. *Br J Haematol.* 1988;69:67.

146. Morelli A, Benatti U, Gaetani GF, et al. Biochemical mechanisms of glucose-6-phosphate dehydrogenase deficiency. *Proc Natl Acad Sci U S A.* 1978;75:1979.

147. Cosgrove MS, Naylor C, Paludan S, et al. On the mechanism of the reaction catalyzed by glucose 6-phosphate dehydrogenase. *Biochemistry.* 1998;37:2759.

148. Lee WT, Levy HR. Lysine-21 of Leuconostoc mesenteroides glucose 6-phosphate dehydrogenase participates in substrate binding through charge-charge interaction. *Protein Sci.* 1992;1:329.

149. Bautista JM, Mason PJ, Luzzatto L. Human glucose-6-phosphate dehydrogenase. Lysine 205 is dispensable for substrate binding but essential for catalysis. *FEBS Lett.* 1995;366:61.

150. Mason PJ, Bautista JM, Gilsanz F. G6PD deficiency: the genotype-phenotype association. *Blood Rev.* 2007;21:267.

151. Cappellini MD, Fiorelli G. Glucose-6-phosphate dehydrogenase deficiency. *Lancet.* 2008;371:64.

152. Luzzatto L, Nannelli C, Notaro R. Glucose-6-phosphate dehydrogenase deficiency. *Hematol Oncol Clin North Am.* 2016;30:373.

153. Beutler E, Kuhl W. Limiting role of 6-phosphogluconolactonase in erythrocyte hexose monophosphate pathway metabolism. *J Lab Clin Med.* 1985;106:573.

154. Rakitzis ET, Papandreou P. Kinetic analysis of 6-phosphogluconolactone hydrolysis in hemolysates. *Biochem Mol Biol Int.* 1995;37:747.

155. Beutler E, Kuhl W, Gelbart T. 6-Phosphogluconolactonase deficiency, a hereditary erythrocyte enzyme deficiency: possible interaction with glucose-6-phosphate dehydrogenase deficiency. *Proc Natl Acad Sci U S A.* 1985;82:3876.

156. Shih LY, Justice P, Hsia DY. Purification and characterization of genetic variants of 6-phosphogluconate dehydrogenase. *Biochem Genet.* 1968;1:359.

157. Parr CW, Fitch LI. Inherited quantitative variations of human phosphogluconate dehydrogenase. *Ann Hum Genet.* 1967;30:339.

158. Caprari P, Caforio MP, Cianciulli P, et al. 6-Phosphogluconate dehydrogenase deficiency in an Italian family. *Ann Hematol.* 2001;80:41.

159. Vives Corrons JL, Colomer D, Pujades A, et al. Congenital 6-phosphogluconate dehydrogenase (6PGD) deficiency associated with chronic hemolytic anemia in a Spanish family. *Am J Hematol.* 1996;53:221.

160. Wamelink MM, Gruning NM, Jansen EE, et al. The difference between rare and exceptionally rare: molecular characterization of ribose 5-phosphate isomerase deficiency. *J Mol Med (Berl).* 2010;88:931.

161. Huck JH, Verhoeven NM, Struys EA, et al. Ribose-5-phosphate isomerase deficiency: new inborn error in the pentose phosphate pathway associated with a slowly progressive leukoencephalopathy. *Am J Hum Genet.* 2004;74:745.

162. Kochetov GA, Solovjeva ON. Structure and functioning mechanism of transketolase. *Biochim Biophys Acta.* 2014;1844:1608.

163. Soukaloun D, Lee SJ, Chamberlain K, et al. Erythrocyte transketolase activity, markers of cardiac dysfunction and the diagnosis of infantile beriberi. *PLoS Negl Trop Dis.* 2011;5:e971.

164. Barasa BA, van Oirschot BA, Bianchi P, et al. Proteomics reveals reduced expression of transketolase in pyrimidine 5'-nucleotidase deficient patients. *Proteomics Clin Appl.* 2016;10:859.

165. Wamelink MM, Struys EA, Jakobs C. The biochemistry, metabolism and inherited defects of the pentose phosphate pathway: a review. *J Inherit Metab Dis.* 2008;31:703.

166. Verhoeven NM, Huck JH, Roos B, et al. Transaldolase deficiency: liver cirrhosis associated with a new inborn error in the pentose phosphate pathway. *Am J Hum Genet.* 2001;68:1086.

167. Williams M, Valayannopoulos V, Altassan R, et al. Clinical, biochemical, and molecular overview of transaldolase deficiency and evaluation of the endocrine function: update of 34 patients. *J Inherit Metab Dis.* 2019;42:147.

168. Beutler E, Guinto E. The reduction of glyceraldehyde by human erythrocytes. L-hexonate dehydrogenase activity. *J Clin Invest.* 1974;53:1258.

169. Das B, Srivastava SK. Purification and properties of aldose reductase and aldehyde reductase II from human erythrocyte. *Arch Biochem Biophys.* 1985;238:670.

170. Reddy GB, Satyanarayana A, Balakrishna N, et al. Erythrocyte aldose reductase activity and sorbitol levels in diabetic retinopathy. *Mol Vis.* 2008;14:593.

171. Gupta V, Verma N, Bhattacharya S, et al. Association of diabetic autonomic neuropathy with red blood cell aldose reductase activity. *Can J Diabetes.* 2014;38:22.

172. van Solinge WW, van Wijk R. Disorders of red cells resulting from enzyme abnormalities. In: Kaushansky KJ, Lichtman MA, Beutler E, et al, eds. *Williams Hematology.* 8th ed. McGraw-Hill; 2010:647.

173. Dimant E, Landsberg E, London IM. The metabolic behavior of reduced glutathione in human and avian erythrocytes. *J Biol Chem.* 1955;213:769.

174. van 't Erve TJ, Wagner BA, Ryckman KK, et al. The concentration of glutathione in human erythrocytes is a heritable trait. *Free Radic Biol Med.* 2013;65:742.

175. Kondo T, Dale GL, Beutler E. Thiol transport from human red blood cells. *Methods Enzymol.* 1995;252:72.

176. Ellison I, Richie JP Jr. Mechanisms of glutathione disulfide efflux from erythrocytes. *Biochem Pharmacol.* 2012;83:164.

177. Gipp JJ, Chang C, Mulcahy RT. Cloning and nucleotide sequence of a full-length cDNA for human liver gamma-glutamylcysteine synthetase. *Biochem Biophys Res Commun.* 1992;185:29.

178. Gipp JJ, Bailey HH, Mulcahy RT. Cloning and sequencing of the cDNA for the light subunit of human liver gamma-glutamylcysteine synthetase and relative mRNA levels for heavy and light subunits in human normal tissues. *Biochem Biophys Res Commun.* 1995;206:584.

179. Biterova EI, Barycki JJ. Mechanistic details of glutathione biosynthesis revealed by crystal structures of *Saccharomyces cerevisiae* glutamate cysteine ligase. *J Biol Chem.* 2009;284:32700.

180. Kumar S, Kasturia N, Sharma A, et al. Redox-dependent stability of the gamma-glutamylcysteine synthetase enzyme of *Escherichia coli*: a novel means of redox regulation. *Biochem J.* 2013;449:783.

181. Krejsa CM, Franklin CC, White CC, et al. Rapid activation of glutamate cysteine ligase following oxidative stress. *J Biol Chem.* 2010;285:16116.

182. Gali RR, Board PG. Sequencing and expression of a cDNA for human glutathione synthetase. *Biochem J.* 1995;310(pt 1):353.

183. Polekhina G, Board PG, Gali RR, et al. Molecular basis of glutathione synthetase deficiency and a rare gene permutation event. *EMBO J.* 1999;18:3204.

184. Cohen G, Hochstein P. Glutathione peroxidase: the primary agent for the elimination of hydrogen peroxide in erythrocytes. *Biochemistry.* 1963;2:1420.

185. Johnson RM, Goyette G Jr, Ravindranath Y, et al. Red cells from glutathione peroxidase-1-deficient mice have nearly normal defenses against exogenous peroxides. *Blood.* 2000;96:1985.

186. Beutler E, Matsumoto F. Ethnic variation in red cell glutathione peroxidase activity. *Blood.* 1975;46:103.

187. Beutler E. Red cell enzyme defects as nondiseases and as diseases. *Blood.* 1979;54:1.

188. Jacob HS, Jandl JH. Effects of sulfhydryl inhibition on red blood cells. I. Mechanism of hemolysis. *J Clin Invest.* 1962;41:779.

189. Valentine WN, Toohey JI, Paglia DE, et al. Modification of erythrocyte enzyme activities by persulfides and methanethiol: possible regulatory role. *Proc Natl Acad Sci U S A.* 1987;84:1394.

190. Ogasawara Y, Funakoshi M, Ishii K. Pyruvate kinase is protected by glutathione-dependent redox balance in human red blood cells exposed to reactive oxygen species. *Biol Pharm Bull.* 2008;31:1875.

191. Huisman TH, Dozy AM. Studies on the heterogeneity of hemoglobin. V. Binding of hemoglobin with oxidized glutathione. *J Lab Clin Med.* 1962;60:302.

192. Kelner MJ, Montoya MA. Structural organization of the human glutathione reductase gene: determination of correct cDNA sequence and identification of a mitochondrial leader sequence. *Biochem Biophys Res Commun.* 2000;269:366.

193. Karplus PA, Schulz GE. Refined structure of glutathione reductase at 1.54 A resolution. *J Mol Biol.* 1987;195:701.

194. Beutler E, Duron O, Kelly BM. Improved method for the determination of blood glutathione. *J Lab Clin Med.* 1963;61:882.

195. Beutler E. Effect of flavin compounds on glutathione reductase activity: in vivo and in vitro studies. *J Clin Invest.* 1969;48:1957.

196. Mojzikova R, Dolezel P, Pavlicek J, et al. Partial glutathione reductase deficiency as a cause of diverse clinical manifestations in a family with unstable hemoglobin (Hemoglobin Haná, β63(E7) His-Asn). *Blood Cells Mol Dis.* 2010;45:219.

197. Mieyal JJ, Starke DW, Gravina SA, et al. Thioltransferase in human red blood cells: purification and properties. *Biochemistry.* 1991;30:6088.

198. Srivastava SK, Beutler E. The transport of oxidized glutathione from human erythrocytes. *J Biol Chem.* 1969;244:9.

199. Lunn G, Dale GL, Beutler E. Transport accounts for glutathione turnover in human erythrocytes. *Blood.* 1979;54:238.

200. Kondo T, Kawakami Y, Taniguchi N, et al. Glutathione disulfide-stimulated Mg2+-ATPase of human erythrocyte membranes. *Proc Natl Acad Sci U S A.* 1987;84:7373.

201. Kondo T, Murao M, Taniguchi N. Glutathione S-conjugate transport using inside-out vesicles from human erythrocytes. *Eur J Biochem.* 1982;125:551.

202. Marcus CJ, Habig WH, Jakoby WB. Glutathione transferase from human erythrocytes. Nonidentity with the enzymes from liver. *Arch Biochem Biophys.* 1978;188:287.

203. Awasthi YC, Singh SV. Purification and characterization of a new form of glutathione S-transferase from human erythrocytes. *Biochem Biophys Res Commun.* 1984;125:1053.

204. Schroder KR, Hallier E, Meyer DJ, et al. Purification and characterization of a new glutathione S-transferase, class theta, from human erythrocytes. *Arch Toxicol.* 1996;70:559.

205. Awasthi YC, Sharma R, Singhal SS. Human glutathione S-transferases. *Int J Biochem.* 1994;26:295.

206. Harvey JW, Beutler E. Binding of heme by glutathione S-transferase: a possible role of the erythrocyte enzyme. *Blood.* 1982;60:1227.

207. Beutler E, Dunning D, Dabe IB, et al. Erythrocyte glutathione S-transferase deficiency and hemolytic anemia. *Blood.* 1988;72:73.

208. Andersen PM, Al-Chalabi A. Clinical genetics of amyotrophic lateral sclerosis: what do we really know? *Nat Rev Neurol.* 2011;7:603.

209. Andersen PM, Nordstrom U, Tsiakas K, et al. Phenotype in an infant with SOD1 homozygous truncating mutation. *N Engl J Med.* 2019;381:486.

210. Homma T, Kurahashi T, Lee J, et al. SOD1 deficiency decreases proteasomal function, leading to the accumulation of ubiquitinated proteins in erythrocytes. *Arch Biochem Biophys.* 2015;583:65.

211. Rocha S, Gomes D, Lima M, et al. Peroxiredoxin 2, glutathione peroxidase, and catalase in the cytosol and membrane of erythrocytes under H2O2-induced oxidative stress. *Free Radic Res.* 2015;49:990.

212. Goth L, Nagy T. Inherited catalase deficiency: is it benign or a factor in various age related disorders? *Mutat Res.* 2013;753:147.

213. Lee T-H, Kim S-U, Yu S-L, et al. Peroxiredoxin II is essential for sustaining life span of erythrocytes in mice. *Blood.* 2003;101:5033.

214. Kwon TH, Han YH, Hong SG, et al. Reactive oxygen species mediated DNA damage is essential for abnormal erythropoiesis in peroxiredoxin II(-/-) mice. *Biochem Biophys Res Commun.* 2012;424:189.

215. Johnson RM, Ho Y-S, Yu D-Y, et al. The effects of disruption of genes for peroxiredoxin-2, glutathione peroxidase-1, and catalase on erythrocyte oxidative metabolism. *Free Radic Biol Med.* 2010;48:519.

216. Nagababu E, Mohanty JG, Friedman JS, et al. Role of peroxiredoxin-2 in protecting RBCs from hydrogen peroxide-induced oxidative stress. *Free Radic Res.* 2013;47:164.

217. van Zwieten R, Verhoeven AJ, Roos D. Inborn defects in the antioxidant systems of human red blood cells. *Free Radic Biol Med.* 2014;67:377.

218. Abrusci P, Chiarelli LR, Galizzi A, et al. Erythrocyte adenylate kinase deficiency: characterization of recombinant mutant forms and relationship with nonspherocytic hemolytic anemia. *Exp Hematol.* 2007;35:1182.

219. O'Brien WG 3rd, Ling HS, Zhao Z, et al. New insights on the regulation of the adenine nucleotide pool of erythrocytes in mouse models. *PLoS One.* 2017;12:e0180948.

220. Jurecka A. Inborn errors of purine and pyrimidine metabolism. *J Inherit Metab Dis.* 2009;32:24.

221. Valentine WN, Paglia DE. Erythrocyte disorders of purine and pyrimidine metabolism. *Hemoglobin.* 1980;4:669.

222. Valentine WN, Fink K, Paglia DE. Hereditary hemolytic anemia with human erythrocyte pyrimidine 5′-nucleotidase deficiency. *J Clin Invest.* 1974;54:866.

223. Paglia DE, Valentine WN. Characteristics of a pyrimidine-specific 5′-nucleotidase in human erythrocytes. *J Biol Chem.* 1975;250:7973.

224. Beutler E, Hartman G. Age-related red cell enzymes in children with transient erythroblastopenia of childhood and with hemolytic anemia. *Pediatr Res.* 1985;19:44.

225. Amici A, Emanuelli M, Magni G, et al. Pyrimidine nucleotidases from human erythrocyte possess phosphotransferase activities specific for pyrimidine nucleotides. *FEBS Lett.* 1997;419:263.

226. Bitto E, Bingman CA, Wesenberg GE, et al. Structure of pyrimidine 5′-nucleotidase type I. Insight into mechanism of action and inhibition during lead poisoning. *J Biol Chem.* 2006;281:20521.

227. Marinaki AM, Escuredo E, Duley JA, et al. Genetic basis of hemolytic anemia caused by pyrimidine 5′ nucleotidase deficiency. *Blood.* 2001;97:3327.

228. Kanno H, Takizawa T, Miwa S, et al. Molecular basis of Japanese variants of pyrimidine 5′-nucleotidase deficiency. *Br J Haematol.* 2004;126:265.

229. Hirono A, Fujii H, Natori H, et al. Chromatographic analysis of human erythrocyte pyrimidine 5′-nucleotidase from five patients with pyrimidine 5′-nucleotidase deficiency. *Br J Haematol.* 1987;65:35.

230. Sestini S, Ricci C, Micheli V, et al. Nicotinamide mononucleotide adenylyltransferase activity in human erythrocytes. *Arch Biochem Biophys.* 1993;302:206.

231. Di Stefano M, Galassi L, Magni G. Unique expression pattern of human nicotinamide mononucleotide adenylyltransferase isozymes in red blood cells. *Blood Cells Mol Dis.* 2010;45:33.

232. Hikosaka K, Ikutani M, Shito M, et al. Deficiency of nicotinamide mononucleotide adenylyltransferase 3 (Nmnat3) causes hemolytic anemia by altering the glycolytic flow in mature erythrocytes. *J Biol Chem.* 2014;289:14796.

233. Arnold H, Blume KG, Lohr GW, et al. "Acquired" red cell enzyme defects in hematological diseases. *Clin Chim Acta.* 1974;57:187.

234. Boivin P, Galand C, Hakim J, et al. Acquired erythroenzymopathies in blood disorders: study of 200 cases. *Br J Haematol.* 1975;31:531.

235. Kahn A, Marie J, Bernard J-F, et al. Mechanisms of the acquired erythrocyte enzyme deficiencies in blood diseases. *Clin Chim Acta.* 1976;71:379.

236. Kahn A. Abnormalities of erythrocyte enzymes in dyserythropoiesis and malignancies. *Clin Haematol.* 1981;10:123.

237. Kornberg A, Goldfarb A. Preleukemia manifested by hemolytic anemia with pyruvate-kinase deficiency. *Arch Intern Med.* 1986;146:785.

238. Nandi A, Yan LJ, Jana CK, et al. Role of catalase in oxidative stress- and age-associated degenerative diseases. *Oxid Med Cell Longev.* 2019;2019:9613090.

239. Shinohara K, Tanaka KR. Hereditary deficiency of erythrocyte acetylcholinesterase. *Am J Hematol.* 1979;7:313.

240. Glucose-6-phosphate dehydrogenase deficiency. WHO Working Group. *Bull World Health Organ.* 1989;67:601.

241. Kahn A, Cottreau D, Boivin P. Molecular mechanism of glucose-6-phosphate dehydrogenase deficiency. *Humangenetik.* 1974;25:101.

242. Beutler E. Selectivity of proteases as a basis for tissue distribution of enzymes in hereditary deficiencies. *Proc Natl Acad Sci U S A.* 1983;80:3767.

243. Longo L, Vanegas OC, Patel M, et al. Maternally transmitted severe glucose 6-phosphate dehydrogenase deficiency is an embryonic lethal. *EMBO J.* 2002;21:4229.

244. Minucci A, Moradkhani K, Hwang MJ, et al. Glucose-6-phosphate dehydrogenase (G6PD) mutations database: review of the "old" and update of the new mutations. *Blood Cells Mol Dis.* 2012;48:154.

245. Gomez-Manzo S, Marcial-Quino J, Vanoye-Carlo A, et al. Glucose-6-phosphate dehydrogenase: update and analysis of new mutations around the world. *Int J Mol Sci.* 17:2016.

246. Takizawa T, Yoneyama Y, Miwa S, et al. A single nucleotide base transition is the basis of the common human glucose-6-phosphate dehydrogenase variant A (+). *Genomics.* 1987;1:228.

247. Hirono A, Beutler E. Molecular cloning and nucleotide sequence of cDNA for human glucose-6-phosphate dehydrogenase variant A(−). *Proc Natl Acad Sci U S A.* 1988;85:3951.

248. Town M, Bautista JM, Mason PJ, et al. Both mutations in G6PD A− are necessary to produce the G6PD deficient phenotype. *Hum Mol Genet.* 1992;1:171.

249. Hirono A, Kawate K, Honda A, et al. A single mutation 202G>A in the human glucose-6-phosphate dehydrogenase gene (*G6PD*) can cause acute hemolysis by itself. *Blood.* 2002;99:1498.

250. Roos D, van Zwieten R, Wijnen JT, et al. Molecular basis and enzymatic properties of glucose 6-phosphate dehydrogenase volendam, leading to chronic nonspherocytic anemia, granulocyte dysfunction, and increased susceptibility to infections. *Blood.* 1999;94:2955.

251. van Bruggen R, Bautista JM, Petropoulou T, et al. Deletion of leucine 61 in glucose-6-phosphate dehydrogenase leads to chronic nonspherocytic anemia, granulocyte dysfunction, and increased susceptibility to infections. *Blood.* 2002;100:1026.

252. van Wijk R, Huizinga EG, Prins I, et al. Distinct phenotypic expression of two de novo missense mutations affecting the dimer interface of glucose-6-phosphate dehydrogenase. *Blood Cells Mol Dis.* 2004;32:112.

253. Rovira A, De Angioletti M, Camacho-Vanegas O, et al. Stable in vivo expression of glucose-6-phosphate dehydrogenase (G6PD) and rescue of G6PD deficiency in stem cells by gene transfer. *Blood.* 2000;96:4111.

254. Grace RF, Zanella A, Neufeld EJ, et al. Erythrocyte pyruvate kinase deficiency: 2015 status report. *Am J Hematol.* 2015;90:825.

255. Beutler E, Forman L, Rios-Larrain E. Elevated pyruvate kinase activity in patients with hemolytic anemia due to red cell pyruvate kinase "deficiency." *Am J Med.* 1987;83:899.

256. Zanella A, Fermo E, Bianchi P, et al. Pyruvate kinase deficiency: the genotype-phenotype association. *Blood Rev.* 2007;21:217.

257. Van Wijk R, Huizinga EG, Van Wesel ACW, et al. Fifteen novel mutations in *PKLR* associated with pyruvate kinase (PK) deficiency: structural implications of amino acid substitutions in PK. *Hum Mutat.* 2009;30:446.

258. Lenzner C, Nurnberg P, Jacobasch G, et al. Molecular analysis of 29 pyruvate kinase-deficient patients from Central Europe with hereditary hemolytic anemia. *Blood.* 1997;89:1793.

259. Demina A, Varughese KI, Barbot J, et al. Six previously undescribed pyruvate kinase mutations causing enzyme deficiency. *Blood.* 1998;92:647.

260. Grace RF, Bianchi P, van Beers EJ, et al. Clinical spectrum of pyruvate kinase deficiency: data from the Pyruvate Kinase Deficiency Natural History Study. *Blood.* 2018;131:2183.

261. Aisaki K, Aizawa S, Fujii H, et al. Glycolytic inhibition by mutation of pyruvate kinase gene increases oxidative stress and causes apoptosis of a pyruvate kinase deficient cell line. *Exp Hematol.* 2007;35:1190.

262. Ayi K, Min-Oo G, Serghides L, et al. Pyruvate kinase deficiency and malaria. *N Engl J Med.* 2008;358:1805.

263. Ayi K, Liles WC, Gros P, et al. Adenosine triphosphate depletion of erythrocytes simulates the phenotype associated with pyruvate kinase deficiency and confers protection against *Plasmodium falciparum* in vitro. *J Infect Dis.* 2009;200:1289.

264. Berghout J, Higgins S, Loucoubar C, et al. Genetic diversity in human erythrocyte pyruvate kinase. *Genes Immun.* 2011;13:98.

265. Machado P, Manco L, Gomes C, et al. Pyruvate kinase deficiency in sub-Saharan Africa: identification of a highly frequent missense mutation (G829A;Glu277Lys) and association with malaria. *PLoS One.* 2012;7:e47071.

266. Owen JL, Harvey JW. Hemolytic anemia in dogs and cats due to erythrocyte enzyme deficiencies. *Vet Clin North Am Small Anim Pract.* 2012;42:73.

267. Whitney KM, Goodman SA, Bailey EM, et al. The molecular basis of canine pyruvate kinase deficiency. *Exp Hematol.* 1994;22:866.

268. Zaucha JA, Yu C, Lothrop CD Jr, et al. Severe canine hereditary hemolytic anemia treated by nonmyeloablative marrow transplantation. *Biol Blood Marrow Transplant.* 2001;7:14.

269. Tsujino K, Kanno H, Hashimoto K, et al. Delayed onset of hemolytic anemia in CBA-*Pk-1*slk/*Pk-1*slk mice with a point mutation of the gene encoding red blood cell type pyruvate kinase. *Blood.* 1998;91:2169.

270. Meza NW, Alonso-Ferrero ME, Navarro S, et al. Rescue of pyruvate kinase deficiency in mice by gene therapy using the human isoenzyme. *Mol Ther.* 2009;17:2000.

271. Kanno H. Hexokinase: gene structure and mutations. *Baillieres Best Pract Res Clin Haematol.* 2000;13:83.

272. Kanno H, Murakami K, Hariyama Y, et al. Homozygous intragenic deletion of type I hexokinase gene causes lethal hemolytic anemia of the affected fetus. *Blood.* 2002;100:1930.

273. de Vooght KMK, van Solinge WW, van Wesel AC, et al. First mutation in the red blood cell-specific promoter of hexokinase combined with a novel missense mutation causes hexokinase deficiency and mild chronic hemolysis. *Haematologica.* 2009;94:1203.

274. Bianchi M, Magnani M. Hexokinase mutations that produce nonspherocytic hemolytic anemia. *Blood Cells Mol Dis.* 1995;21:2.

275. van Wijk R, Rijksen G, Huizinga EG, et al. HK Utrecht: missense mutation in the active site of human hexokinase associated with hexokinase deficiency and severe nonspherocytic hemolytic anemia. *Blood.* 2003;101:345.

276. Koralkova P, Mojzikova R, van Oirschot B, et al. Molecular characterization of six new cases of red blood cell hexokinase deficiency yields four novel mutations in *HK1. Blood Cells Mol Dis.* 2016;59:71.

277. Jamwal M, Aggarwal A, Palodi A, et al. A nonsense variant in the hexokinase 1 gene (HK1) causing severe non-spherocytic haemolytic anaemia: genetic analysis exemplifies ambiguity due to multiple isoforms. *Br J Haematol.* 2019;186:e142.

278. Peters LL, Lane PW, Andersen SG, et al. Downeast anemia (*dea*), a new mouse model of severe nonspherocytic hemolytic anemia caused by hexokinase (HKₗ) deficiency. *Blood Cells Mol Dis.* 2001;27:850.

279. Fermo E, Vercellati C, Marcello AP, et al. Clinical and molecular spectrum of glucose-6-phosphate isomerase deficiency. Report of 12 new cases. *Front Physiol.* 2019;10:467.

280. Burger NCM, van Wijk R, Bresters D, et al. A novel mutation of glucose phosphate isomerase (GPI) causing severe neonatal anemia due to GPI deficiency. *J Pediatr Hematol Oncol.* 2019;41:e186.

281. See WQ, So CJ, Cheuk DK, et al. Congenital hemolytic anemia because of glucose phosphate isomerase deficiency: identification of 2 novel missense mutations in the GPI gene. *J Pediatr Hematol Oncol.* Preprint. Posted online August 14, 2019. doi: 10.1097/MPH.0000000000001582.

282. Kedar PS, Dongerdiye R, Chilwirwar P, et al. Glucose phosphate isomerase deficiency: high prevalence of p.Arg347His mutation in Indian population associated with severe hereditary non-spherocytic hemolytic anemia coupled with neurological dysfunction. *Indian J Pediatr.* 2019;86:692.

283. Lin H-Y, Kao Y-H, Chen S-T, et al. Effects of inherited mutations on catalytic activity and structural stability of human glucose-6-phosphate isomerase expressed in *Escherichia coli. Biochim Biophys Acta.* 2009;1794:315.

284. Helleman PW, Van Biervliet JP. Haematological studies in a new variant of glucose-phosphate isomerase deficiency (GPI Utrecht). *Helv Paediatr Acta.* 1976;30:525.

285. Kahn A, Buc HA, Girot R, et al. Molecular and functional anomalies in two new mutant glucose-phosphate-insomerase variants with enzyme deficiency and chronic hemolysis. *Hum Genet.* 1978;40:293.

286. Schröter W, Eber SW, Bardosi A, et al. Generalised glucosephosphate isomerase (GPI) deficiency causing haemolytic anaemia, neuromuscular symptoms and impairment of granulocytic function: a new syndrome due to a new stable GPI variant with diminished specific activity (GPI Homburg). *Eur J Pediatr.* 1985;144:301.

287. Beutler E, West C, Britton HA, et al. Glucosephosphate isomerase (GPI) deficiency mutations associated with hereditary nonspherocytic hemolytic anemia (HNSHA). *Blood Cells Mol Dis.* 1997;23:402.

288. Zanella A, Izzo C, Rebulla P, et al. The first stable variant of erythrocyte glucose-phosphate isomerase associated with severe hemolytic anemia. *Am J Hematol.* 1980;9:1.

289. Shalev O, Shalev RS, Forman L, et al. GPI Mount Scopus—a variant of glucosephosphate isomerase deficiency. *Ann Hematol.* 1993;67:197.

290. Chaput M, Claes V, Portetelle D, et al. The neurotrophic factor neuroleukin is 90% homologous with phosphohexose isomerase. *Nature.* 1988;332:454.

291. Gurney ME, Heinrich SP, Lee MR, et al. Molecular cloning and expression of neuroleukin, a neurotrophic factor for spinal and sensory neurons. *Science.* 1986;234:566.

292. Xu W, Seiter K, Feldman E, et al. The differentiation and maturation mediator for human myeloid leukemia cells shares homology with neuroleukin or phosphoglucose isomerase. *Blood.* 1996;87:4502.

293. Kugler W, Breme K, Laspe P, et al. Molecular basis of neurological dysfunction coupled with haemolytic anaemia in human glucose-6-phosphate isomerase (GPI) deficiency. *Hum Genet.* 1998;103:450.

294. Haller JF, Krawczyk SA, Gostilovitch L, et al. Glucose-6-phosphate isomerase deficiency results in mTOR activation, failed translocation of lipin 1α to the nucleus and hypersensitivity to glucose: implications for the inherited glycolytic disease. *Biochim Biophys Acta.* 2011;1812:1393.

295. Merkle S, Pretsch W. Glucose-6-phosphate isomerase deficiency associated with nonspherocytic hemolytic anemia in the mouse: an animal model for the human disease. *Blood.* 1993;81:206.

296. West JD. A genetically defined animal model of anembryonic pregnancy. *Hum Reprod.* 1993;8:1316.

297. Nakajima H, Raben N, Hamaguchi T, et al. Phosphofructokinase deficiency; past, present and future. *Curr Mol Med.* 2002;2:197.

298. Raben N, Sherman J, Miller F, et al. A 5′ splice junction mutation leading to exon deletion in an Ashkenazic Jewish family with phosphofructokinase deficiency (Tarui disease). *J Biol Chem.* 1993;268:4963.

299. Tsujino S, Servidei S, Tonin P, et al. Identification of three novel mutations in non-Ashkenazi Italian patients with muscle phosphofructokinase deficiency. *Am J Hum Genet.* 1994;54:812.

300. Fujii H, Miwa S. Other erythrocyte enzyme deficiencies associated with non-haematological symptoms: phosphoglycerate kinase and phosphofructokinase deficiency. *Baillieres Best Pract Res Clin Haematol.* 2000;13:141.

301. Raben N, Exelbert R, Spiegel R, et al. Functional expression of human mutant phosphofructokinase in yeast: genetic defects in French Canadian and Swiss patients with phosphofructokinase deficiency. *Am J Hum Genet.* 1995;56:131.

302. Musumeci O, Bruno C, Mongini T, et al. Clinical features and new molecular findings in muscle phosphofructokinase deficiency (GSD type VII). *Neuromuscul Disord.* 2012;22:325.

303. Vives Corrons J-L, Koralkova P, Grau JM, et al. First identification of phosphofructokinase deficiency in Spain: identification of a novel homozygous missense mutation in the PFKM gene. *Front Physiol.* 2013;4:393.

304. Brüser A, Kirchberger J, Schöneberg T. Altered allosteric regulation of muscle 6-phosphofructokinase causes Tarui disease. *Biochem Biophys Res Commun.* 2012;427:133.

305. Nichols RC, Rudolphi O, Ek B, et al. Glycogenosis type VII (Tarui disease) in a Swedish family: two novel mutations in muscle phosphofructokinase gene (PFK-M) resulting in intron retentions. *Am J Hum Genet.* 1996;59:59.

306. Hamaguchi T, Nakajima H, Noguchi T, et al. Novel missense mutation (W686C) of the phosphofructokinase-M gene in a Japanese patient with a mild form of glycogenosis VII. *Hum Mutat.* 1996;8:273.

307. Inal Gultekin G, Raj K, Lehman S, et al. Missense mutation in *PFKM* associated with muscle-type phosphofructokinase deficiency in the Wachtelhund dog. *Mol Cell Probes.* 2012;26:243.

308. Garcia M, Pujol A, Ruzo A, et al. Phosphofructo-1-kinase deficiency leads to a severe cardiac and hematological disorder in addition to skeletal muscle glycogenosis. *PLoS Genet.* 2009;5:e1000465.

309. Gerber K, Harvey JW, D'Agorne S, et al. Hemolysis, myopathy, and cardiac disease associated with hereditary phosphofructokinase deficiency in two Whippets. *Vet Clin Pathol.* 2009;38:46.

310. Miwa S, Fujii H, Tani K, et al. Two cases of red cell aldolase deficiency associated with hereditary hemolytic anemia in a Japanese family. *Am J Hematol.* 1981;11:425.

311. Kreuder J, Borkhardt A, Repp R, et al. Brief report: inherited metabolic myopathy and hemolysis due to a mutation in aldolase A. *N Engl J Med.* 1996;334:1100.

312. Esposito G, Vitagliano L, Costanzo P, et al. Human aldolase A natural mutants: relationship between flexibility of the C-terminal region and enzyme function. *Biochem J.* 2004;380:51.

313. Yao DC, Tolan DR, Murray MF, et al. Hemolytic anemia and severe rhabdomyolysis caused by compound heterozygous mutations of the gene for erythrocyte/muscle isozyme of aldolase, ALDOA(Arg303X/Cys338Tyr). *Blood.* 2004;103:2401.

314. Mamoune A, Bahuau M, Hamel Y, et al. A Thermolabile aldolase A mutant causes fever-induced recurrent rhabdomyolysis without hemolytic anemia. *PLoS Genet.* 2014;10:e1004711.

315. Schneider AS. Triosephosphate isomerase deficiency: historical perspectives and molecular aspects. *Baillieres Best Pract Res Clin Haematol.* 2000;13:119.

316. Orosz F, Oláh J, Alvarez M, et al. Distinct behavior of mutant triosephosphate isomerase in hemolysate and in isolated form: molecular basis of enzyme deficiency. *Blood.* 2001;98:3106.

317. Orosz F, Oláh J, Ovádi J. Triosephosphate isomerase deficiency: new insights into an enigmatic disease. *Biochim Biophys Acta.* 2009;1792:1168.

318. Orosz F, Oláh J, Ovádi J. Triosephosphate isomerase deficiency: facts and doubts. *IUBMB Life.* 2006;58:703.

319. Serdaroglu G, Aydinok Y, Yilmaz S, et al. Triosephosphate isomerase deficiency: a patient with Val231Met mutation. *Pediatr Neurol.* 2011;44:139.

320. Fermo E, Bianchi P, Vercellati C, et al. Triose phosphate isomerase deficiency associated with two novel mutations in TPI gene. *Eur J Haematol.* 2010;85:170.

321. Aissa K, Kamoun F, Sfaihi L, et al. Hemolytic anemia and progressive neurologic impairment: think about triosephosphate isomerase deficiency. *Fetal Pediatr Pathol.* 2014;33:234.

322. Manco L, Ribeiro ML. Novel human pathological mutations. Gene symbol: TPI1. Disease: triosephosphate isomerase deficiency. *Hum Genet.* 2007;121:650.

323. Sarper N, Zengin E, Jakobs C, et al. Mild hemolytic anemia, progressive neuromotor retardation and fatal outcome: a disorder of glycolysis, triose–phosphate isomerase deficiency. *Turk J Pediatr.* 2013;55:198.

324. Nolan D, Carlson M. Whole exome sequencing in pediatric neurology patients: clinical implications and estimated cost analysis. *J Child Neurol.* 2016;31:887.

325. Roland BP, Richards KR, Hrizo SL, et al. Missense variant in TPI1 (Arg189Gln) causes neurologic deficits through structural changes in the triosephosphate isomerase catalytic site and reduced enzyme levels in vivo. *Biochim Biophys Acta Mol Basis Dis.* 2019;1865:2257.

326. Oliver C, Timson DJ. In silico prediction of the effects of mutations in the human triose phosphate isomerase gene: towards a predictive framework for TPI deficiency. *Eur J Med Genet.* 2017;60:289.

327. Zingg BC, Pretsch W, Mohrenweiser HW. Molecular analysis of four ENU induced triosephosphate isomerase null mutants in Mus musculus. *Mutat Res.* 1995;328:163.

328. Segal J, Mulleder M, Kruger A, et al. Low catalytic activity is insufficient to induce disease pathology in triosephosphate isomerase deficiency. *J Inherit Metab Dis.* 2019;42:839.

329. Roland BP, Zeccola AM, Larsen SB, et al. Structural and genetic studies demonstrate neurologic dysfunction in triosephosphate isomerase deficiency is associated with impaired synaptic vesicle dynamics. *PLoS Genet.* 2016;12:e1005941.

330. Beutler E. PGK deficiency. *Br J Haematol.* 2007;136:3.

331. Garcia-Solaesa V, Serrano-Lorenzo P, Ramos-Arroyo MA, et al. A novel missense variant associated with a splicing defect in a myopathic form of PGK1 deficiency in the Spanish population. *Genes (Basel).* 2019;10:785.

332. Zaidi AU, Bagla S, Ravindranath Y. Identification of a novel variant in phosphoglycerate kinase-1 (PGK1) in an African-American child (PGK1 Detroit). *Pediatr Hematol Oncol.* 2019;36:302.

333. Echaniz-Laguna A, Nadjar Y, Behin A, et al. Phosphoglycerate kinase deficiency: a nationwide multicenter retrospective study. *J Inherit Metab Dis.* 2019;42:803.

334. Tamai M, Kawano T, Saito R, et al. Phosphoglycerate kinase deficiency due to a novel mutation (c. 1180A>G) manifesting as chronic hemolytic anemia in a Japanese boy. *Int J Hematol.* 2014;100:393.

335. Valentini G, Maggi M, Pey AL. Protein stability, folding and misfolding in human PGK1 deficiency. *Biomolecules.* 2013;3:1030.

336. Spiegel R, Gomez EA, Akman HO, et al. Myopathic form of phosphoglycerate kinase (PGK) deficiency: a new case and pathogenic considerations. *Neuromuscul Disord.* 2009;19:207.

337. Morimoto A, Ueda I, Hirashima Y, et al. A novel missense mutation (1060G → C) in the phosphoglycerate kinase gene in a Japanese boy with chronic haemolytic anaemia, developmental delay and rhabdomyolysis. *Br J Haematol.* 2003;122:1009.

338. Fermo E, Bianchi P, Chiarelli LR, et al. A new variant of phosphoglycerate kinase deficiency (p.I371K) with multiple tissue involvement: molecular and functional characterization. *Mol Genet Metab.* 2012;106:455.

339. Vissing J, Akman HO, Aasly J, et al. Level of residual enzyme activity modulates the phenotype in phosphoglycerate kinase deficiency. *Neurology.* 2018;91:e1077.

340. Rhodes M, Ashford L, Manes B, et al. Bone marrow transplantation in phosphoglycerate kinase (PGK) deficiency. *Br J Haematol.* 2011;152:500.

341. Chiarelli LR, Morera SM, Bianchi P, et al. Molecular insights on pathogenic effects of mutations causing phosphoglycerate kinase deficiency. *PLoS One.* 2012;7:e32065.

342. Pey AL, Maggi M, Valentini G. Insights into human phosphoglycerate kinase 1 deficiency as a conformational disease from biochemical, biophysical, and in vitro expression analyses. *J Inherit Metab Dis.* 2014;37:909.

343. Lemarchandel V, Joulin V, Valentin C, et al. Compound heterozygosity in a complete erythrocyte bisphosphoglycerate mutase deficiency. *Blood.* 1992;80:2643.

344. Hoyer JD, Allen SL, Beutler E, et al. Erythrocytosis due to bisphosphoglycerate mutase deficiency with concurrent glucose-6-phosphate dehydrogenase (G-6-PD) deficiency. *Am J Hematol.* 2004;75:205.

345. Petousi N, Copley RR, Lappin TR, et al. Erythrocytosis associated with a novel missense mutation in the BPGM gene. *Haematologica.* 2014;99:e201.

346. Rosa R, Prehu M-O, Beuzard Y, et al. The first case of a complete deficiency of diphosphoglycerate mutase in human erythrocytes. *J Clin Invest.* 1978;62:907.

347. Almusafri F, Elamin HE, Khalaf TE, et al. Clinical and molecular characterization of 6 children with glutamate-cysteine ligase deficiency causing hemolytic anemia. *Blood Cells Mol Dis.* 2017;65:73.

348. Willis MN, Liu Y, Biterova EI, et al. Enzymatic defects underlying hereditary glutamate cysteine ligase deficiency are mitigated by association of the catalytic and regulatory subunits. *Biochemistry.* 2011;50:6508.

349. Shi ZZ, Osei-Frimpong J, Kala G, et al. Glutathione synthesis is essential for mouse development but not for cell growth in culture. *Proc Natl Acad Sci U S A.* 2000;97:5101.

350. Dalton TP, Dieter MZ, Yang Y, et al. Knockout of the mouse glutamate cysteine ligase catalytic subunit (Gclc) gene: embryonic lethal when homozygous, and proposed model for moderate glutathione deficiency when heterozygous. *Biochem Biophys Res Commun.* 2000;279:324.

351. Yang Y, Dieter MZ, Chen Y, et al. Initial characterization of the glutamate-cysteine ligase modifier subunit Gclm(–/–) knockout mouse. Novel model system for a severely compromised oxidative stress response. *J Biol Chem.* 2002;277:49446.

352. Foller M, Harris IS, Elia A, et al. Functional significance of glutamate-cysteine ligase modifier for erythrocyte survival in vitro and in vivo. *Cell Death Differ.* 2013;20:1350.

353. Ristoff E, Mayatepek E, Larsson A. Long-term clinical outcome in patients with glutathione synthetase deficiency. *J Pediatr.* 2001;139:79.

354. Njålsson R, Ristoff E, Carlsson K, et al. Genotype, enzyme activity, glutathione level, and clinical phenotype in patients with glutathione synthetase deficiency. *Hum Genet.* 2005;116:384.

355. Ristoff E. Inborn errors of GSH metabolism. In: Masella R, Mazza G, eds. *Glutathione and Sulfur Amino Acids in Human Health and Disease.*, John Wiley & Sons; 2009:343.

356. Riudor E, Arranz JA, Alvarez R, et al. Massive 5-oxoprolinuria with normal 5-oxoprolinase and glutathione synthetase activities. *J Inherit Metab Dis.* 2001;24:404.

357. Pederzolli CD, Mescka CP, Zandona BR, et al. Acute administration of 5-oxoproline induces oxidative damage to lipids and proteins and impairs antioxidant defenses in cerebral cortex and cerebellum of young rats. *Metab Brain Dis.* 2010;25:145.

358. Simon E, Vogel M, Fingerhut R, et al. Diagnosis of glutathione synthetase deficiency in newborn screening. *J Inherit Metab Dis.* 2009;32(suppl 1):S269.

359. Burstedt MS, Ristoff E, Larsson A, et al. Rod-cone dystrophy with maculopathy in genetic glutathione synthetase deficiency: a morphologic and electrophysiologic study. *Ophthalmology.* 2009;116:324.

360. Xia H, Ye J, Wang L, et al. A case of severe glutathione synthetase deficiency with novel GSS mutations. *Braz J Med Biol Res.* 2018;51:e6853.

361. Guney Varal I, Dogan P, Gorukmez O, et al. Glutathione synthetase deficiency: a novel mutation with femur agenesis. *Fetal Pediatr Pathol.* 2020;39:38.

362. Soylu Ustkoyuncu P, Mutlu FT, Kiraz A, et al. A rare cause of neonatal hemolytic anemia: glutathione synthetase deficiency. *J Pediatr Hematol Oncol.* 2018;40:e45.

363. Ameur SB, Aloulou H, Nasrallah F, et al. Hemolytic anemia and metabolic acidosis: think about glutathione synthetase deficiency. *Fetal Pediatr Pathol.* 2015;34:18.

364. Signolet I, Chenouard R, Oca F, et al. Recurrent isolated neonatal hemolytic anemia: think about glutathione synthetase deficiency. *Pediatrics.* 2016;138:111.

365. Ingle BL, Shrestha B, De Jesus MC, et al. Genetic mutations in the S-loop of human glutathione synthetase: links between substrate binding, active site structure and allostery. *Comput Struct Biotechnol J.* 2019;17:31.

366. Winkler A, Njalsson R, Carlsson K, et al. Glutathione is essential for early embryogenesis—analysis of a glutathione synthetase knockout mouse. *Biochem Biophys Res Commun.* 2011;412:121.

367. Kamerbeek NM, van Zwieten R, de Boer M, et al. Molecular basis of glutathione reductase deficiency in human blood cells. *Blood.* 2007;109:3560.

368. Loos H, Roos D, Weening R, et al. Familial deficiency of glutathione reductase in human blood cells. *Blood.* 1976;48:53.

369. Gallo V, Schwarzer E, Rahlfs S, et al. Inherited glutathione reductase deficiency and Plasmodium falciparum malaria—a case study. *PLoS One.* 2009;4:e7303.

370. Niizuma H, Kanno H, Sato A, et al. Splenectomy resolves hemolytic anemia caused by adenylate kinase deficiency. *Pediatr Int.* 2017;59:228.

371. Dongerdiye R, Kamat P, Jain P, et al. Red cell adenylate kinase deficiency in India: identification of two novel missense mutations (c.71A>G and c.413G>A). *J Clin Pathol.* 2019;72:393.

372. Fermo E, Bianchi P, Vercellati C, et al. A new variant of adenylate kinase (delG138) associated with severe hemolytic anemia. *Blood Cells Mol Dis.* 2004;33:146.

373. Valentine WN, Paglia DE, Tartaglia AP, et al. Hereditary hemolytic anemia with increased red cell adenosine deaminase (45- to 70-fold) and decreased adenosine triphosphate. *Science.* 1977;195:783.

374. Perignon JL, Hamet M, Buc HA, et al. Biochemical study of a case of hemolytic anemia with increased (85 fold) red cell adenosine deaminase. *Clin Chim Acta.* 1982;124:205.

375. Chottiner EG, Ginsburg D, Tartaglia AP, et al. Erythrocyte adenosine deaminase overproduction in hereditary hemolytic anemia. *Blood.* 1989;74:448.

376. Fujii H, Miwa S, Suzuki K. Purification and properties of adenosine deaminase in normal and hereditary hemolytic anemia with increased red cell activity. *Hemoglobin.* 1980;4:693.

377. Chen EH, Tartaglia AP, Mitchell BS. Hereditary overexpression of adenosine deaminase in erythrocytes: evidence for a *cis*-acting mutation. *Am J Hum Genet.* 1993;53:889.

378. Fargo JH, Kratz CP, Giri N, et al. Erythrocyte adenosine deaminase: diagnostic value for Diamond-Blackfan anaemia. *Br J Haematol.* 2013;160:547.

379. Zanella A, Bianchi P, Fermo E, et al. Hereditary pyrimidine 5′-nucleotidase deficiency: from genetics to clinical manifestations. *Br J Haematol.* 2006;133:113.

380. Rees DC, Duley JA, Marinaki AM. Pyrimidine 5′ nucleotidase deficiency. *Br J Haematol.* 2003;120:375.

381. Vives i Corrons JL. Chronic non-spherocytic haemolytic anaemia due to congenital pyrimidine 5′ nucleotidase deficiency: 25 years later. *Baillieres Best Pract Res Clin Haematol.* 2000;13:103.

382. Swanson MS, Markin RS, Stohs SJ, et al. Identification of cytidine diphosphodiesters in erythrocytes from a patient with pyrimidine nucleotidase deficiency. *Blood.* 1984;63:665.

383. Tomoda A, Noble NA, Lachant NA, et al. Hemolytic anemia in hereditary pyrimidine 5′-nucleotidase deficiency: nucleotide inhibition of G6PD and the pentose phosphate shunt. *Blood.* 1982;60:1212.

384. David O, Ramenghi U, Camaschella C, et al. Inhibition of hexose monophosphate shunt in young erythrocytes by pyrimidine nucleotides in hereditary pyrimidine 5′ nucleotidase deficiency. *Eur J Haematol.* 1991;47:48.

385. Rees DC, Duley J, Simmonds HA, et al. Interaction of hemoglobin E and pyrimidine 5′ nucleotidase deficiency. *Blood.* 1996;88:2761.

386. Lachant NA, Tanaka KR. Red cell metabolism in hereditary pyrimidine 5′-nucleotidase deficiency: effect of magnesium. *Br J Haematol.* 1986;63:615.

387. Lachant NA, Zerez CR, Tanaka KR. Pyrimidine nucleotides impair phosphoribosylpyrophosphate (PRPP) synthetase subunit aggregation by sequestering magnesium. A mechanism for the decreased PRPP synthetase activity in hereditary erythrocyte pyrimidine 5'-nucleotidase deficiency. *Biochim Biophys Acta.* 1989;994:81.

388. Zerez CR, Lachant NA, Tanaka KR. Decrease in subunit aggregation of phosphoribosylpyrophosphate synthetase: a mechanism for decreased nucleotide concentrations in pyruvate kinase-deficient human erythrocytes. *Blood.* 1986;68:1024.

389. Lachant NA, Zerez CR, Tanaka KR. Pyrimidine nucleoside monophosphate kinase hyperactivity in hereditary erythrocyte pyrimidine 5'-nucleotidase deficiency. *Br J Haematol.* 1987;66:91.

390. Valentine WN, Anderson HM, Paglia DE, et al. Studies on human erythrocyte nucleotide metabolism. II. Nonspherocytic hemolytic anemia, high red cell ATP, and ribose-phosphate pyrophosphokinase (RPK, E.C.2.7.6.1) deficiency. *Blood.* 1972;39:674.

391. Oda E, Oda S, Tomoda A, et al. Hemolytic anemia in hereditary pyrimidine 5'-nucleotidase deficiency. II. Effect of pyrimidine nucleotides and their derivatives on glycolytic and pentose phosphate shunt enzyme activity. *Clin Chim Acta.* 1984;141:93.

392. Chiarelli LR, Morera SM, Galizzi A, et al. Molecular basis of pyrimidine 5'-nucleotidase deficiency caused by 3 newly identified missense mutations (c.187T>C, c.469G>C and c.740T>C) and a tabulation of known mutations. *Blood Cells Mol Dis.* 2008;40:295.

393. Warang P, Kedar P, Kar R, et al. New missense homozygous mutation (Q270Ter) in the pyrimidine 5' nucleotidase type I-related gene in two Indian families with hereditary non-spherocytic hemolytic anemia. *Ann Hematol.* 2013;92:715.

394. Koker SA, Oymak Y, Bianchi P, et al. A new homozygous mutation (c.393-394del TA/c.393-394del TA) in the NT5C3 gene associated with pyrimidine-5'-nucleotidase deficiency: a case report. *J Pediatr Hematol Oncol.* 2019;41:e484.

395. Santos A, Dantas LE, Traina F, et al. Pyrimidine-5'-nucleotidase Campinas, a new mutation (p.R56G) in the NT5C3 gene associated with pyrimidine-5'-nucleotidase type I deficiency and influence of Gilbert's syndrome on clinical expression. *Blood Cells Mol Dis.* 2014;53:246.

396. Warang P, Devendra R, Chiddarwar A, et al. Does novel P5'N-1 mutation in combination with G6PD Asahi in an Indian male contribute to Budd Chiari syndrome? *Blood Cells Mol Dis.* 2017;66:8.

397. Chiarelli LR, Bianchi P, Fermo E, et al. Functional analysis of pyrimidine 5'-nucleotidase mutants causing nonspherocytic hemolytic anemia. *Blood.* 2005;105:3340.

398. David O, Vota MG, Piga A, et al. Pyrimidine 5'-nucleotidase acquired deficiency in beta-thalassemia: involvement of enzyme-SH groups in the inactivation process. *Acta Haematol.* 1989;82:69.

399. Vives Corrons JL, Pujades MA, Aguilar i Bascompte JL, et al. Pyrimidine 5'nucleotidase and several other red cell enzyme activities in beta-thalassaemia trait. *Br J Haematol.* 1984;56:483.

400. Karadsheh NS, Simmonds HA. Chronic hemolytic anemia and accumulation of pyrimidine nucleotide metabolites. *Int J Lab Hematol.* 2015;37:e72.

401. Cohen G, Hochstein P. Generation of hydrogen peroxide in erythrocytes by hemolytic agents. *Biochemistry.* 1964;3:895.

402. Kosower NS, Song KR, Kosower EM, et al. Glutathione. II. Chemical aspects of azoester procedure for oxidation to disulfide. *Biochim Biophys Acta.* 1969;192:8.

403. Birchmeier W, Tuchschmid PE, Winterhalter KH. Comparison of human hemoglobin A carrying glutathione as a mixed disulfide with the naturally occurring human hemoglobin A. *Biochemistry.* 1973;12:3667.

404. Rachmilewitz EA, Harari E, Winterhalter KH. Separation of alpha- and beta-chains of hemoglobin A by acetylphenylhydrazine. *Biochim Biophys Acta.* 1974;371:402.

405. Kirkman HN, Gaetani GF. Catalase: a tetrameric enzyme with four tightly bound molecules of NADPH. *Proc Natl Acad Sci U S A.* 1984;81:4343.

406. Gaetani GF, Rolfo M, Arena S, et al. Active involvement of catalase during hemolytic crises of favism. *Blood.* 1996;88:1084.

407. Rifkind RA. Heinz body anemia: an ultrastructural study. II. Red cell sequestration and destruction. *Blood.* 1965;26:433.

408. Ho YS, Xiong Y, Ma W, et al. Mice lacking catalase develop normally but show differential sensitivity to oxidant tissue injury. *J Biol Chem.* 2004;279:32804.

409. Cheah FC, Peskin AV, Wong FL, et al. Increased basal oxidation of peroxiredoxin 2 and limited peroxiredoxin recycling in glucose-6-phosphate dehydrogenase-deficient erythrocytes from newborn infants. *FASEB J.* 2014;28:3205.

410. Bunn HF, Jandl JH. Exchange of heme among hemoglobin molecules. *Proc Natl Acad Sci U S A.* 1966;56:974.

411. Jandl JH. The Heinz body hemolytic anemias. *Ann Intern Med.* 1963;58:702.

412. Baehner RL, Nathan DG, Castle WB. Oxidant injury of Caucasian glucose-6-phosphate dehydrogenase-deficient red blood cells by phagocytosing leukocytes during infection. *J Clin Invest.* 1971;50:2466.

413. Chevion M, Navok T, Glaser G, et al. The chemistry of favism-inducing compounds. The properties of isouramil and divicine and their reaction with glutathione. *Eur J Biochem.* 1982;127:405.

414. Arese P, De Flora A. Pathophysiology of hemolysis in glucose-6-phosphate dehydrogenase deficiency. *Semin Hematol.* 1990;27:1.

415. Luzzatto L, Arese P. Favism and glucose-6-phosphate dehydrogenase deficiency. *N Engl J Med.* 2018;378:60.

416. Stamatoyannopoulos G, Fraser GR, Motulsky AC, et al. On the familial predisposition to favism. *Am J Hum Genet.* 1966;18:253.

417. Damonte G, Guida L, Sdraffa A, et al. Mechanisms of perturbation of erythrocyte calcium homeostasis in favism. *Cell Calcium.* 1992;13:649.

418. Fischer TM, Meloni T, Pescarmona GP, et al. Membrane cross bonding in red cells in favic crisis: a missing link in the mechanism of extravascular haemolysis. *Br J Haematol.* 1985;59:159.

419. Caprari P, Bozzi A, Ferroni L, et al. Membrane alterations in G6PD- and PK-deficient erythrocytes exposed to oxidizing agents. *Biochem Med Metab Biol.* 1991;45:16.

420. Johnson RM, Ravindranath Y, ElAlfy MS, et al. Oxidant damage to erythrocyte membrane in glucose-6-phosphate dehydrogenase deficiency: correlation with in vivo reduced glutathione concentration and membrane protein oxidation. *Blood.* 1994;83:1117.

421. Pantaleo A, Ferru E, Carta F, et al. Irreversible AE1 tyrosine phosphorylation leads to membrane vesiculation in G6PD deficient red cells. *PLoS One.* 2011;6:e15847.

422. Morelli A, Grasso M, Meloni T, et al. Favism: impairment of proteolytic systems in red blood cells. *Blood.* 1987;69:1753.

423. Mukthapuram S, Dewar D, Maisels MJ. Extreme hyperbilirubinemia and G6PD deficiency with no laboratory evidence of hemolysis. *Clin Pediatr (Phila).* 2016;55:686.

424. Kaplan M, Hammerman C, Vreman HJ, et al. Severe hemolysis with normal blood count in a glucose-6-phosphate dehydrogenase deficient neonate. *J Perinatol.* 2008;28:306.

425. Kaplan M, Herschel M, Hammerman C, et al. Studies in hemolysis in glucose-6-phosphate dehydrogenase-deficient African American neonates. *Clin Chim Acta.* 2006;365:177.

426. Kaplan M, Wong RJ, Stevenson DK. Hemolysis and glucose-6-phosphate dehydrogenase deficiency-related neonatal hyperbilirubinemia. *Neonatology.* 2018;114:223.

427. Kaplan M, Renbaum P, Levy-Lahad E, et al. Gilbert syndrome and glucose-6-phosphate dehydrogenase deficiency: a dose-dependent genetic interaction crucial to neonatal hyperbilirubinemia. *Proc Natl Acad Sci U S A.* 1997;94:12128.

428. Huang CS, Chang PF, Huang MJ, et al. Glucose-6-phosphate dehydrogenase deficiency, the UDP-glucuronosyl transferase 1A1 gene, and neonatal hyperbilirubinemia. *Gastroenterology.* 2002;123:127.

429. Oluboyede OA, Esan GJ, Francis TI, et al. Genetically determined deficiency of glucose 6-phosphate dehydrogenase (type-A-) is expressed in the liver. *J Lab Clin Med.* 1979;93:783.

430. Sanna S, Busonero F, Maschio A, et al. Common variants in the SLCO1B3 locus are associated with bilirubin levels and unconjugated hyperbilirubinemia. *Hum Mol Genet.* 2009;18:2711.

431. Kaplan M, Hammerman C. Glucose-6-phosphate dehydrogenase deficiency and severe neonatal hyperbilirubinemia: a complexity of interactions between genes and environment. *Semin Fetal Neonatal Med.* 2010;15:148.

432. Valentine WN, Paglia DE. The primary cause of hemolysis in enzymopathies of anaerobic glycolysis: a viewpoint. *Blood Cells.* 1980;6:819.

433. Bogdanova A, Makhro A, Wang J, et al. Calcium in red blood cells-a perilous balance. *Int J Mol Sci.* 2013;14:9848.

434. Ronquist G, Rudolphi O, Engström I, et al. Familial phosphofructokinase deficiency is associated with a disturbed calcium homeostasis in erythrocytes. *J Intern Med.* 2001;249:85.

435. Sabina RL, Waldenström A, Ronquist G. The contribution of Ca+ calmodulin activation of human erythrocyte AMP deaminase (isoform E) to the erythrocyte metabolic dysregulation of familial phosphofructokinase deficiency. *Haematologica.* 2006;91:652.

436. Rinaldi A, Filippi G, Siniscalco M. Variability of red cell phenotypes between and within individuals in an unbiased sample of 77 heterozygotes for G6PD deficiency in Sardinia. *Am J Hum Genet.* 1976;28:496.

437. Youngster I, Arcavi L, Schechmaster R, et al. Medications and glucose-6-phosphate dehydrogenase deficiency: an evidence-based review. *Drug Saf.* 2010;33:713.

438. Campbell GD Jr, Steinberg MH, Bower JD. Letter: ascorbic acid-induced hemolysis in G-6-PD deficiency. *Ann Intern Med.* 1975;82:810.

439. Rees DC, Kelsey H, Richards JD. Acute haemolysis induced by high dose ascorbic acid in glucose-6-phosphate dehydrogenase deficiency. *BMJ.* 1993;306:841.

440. Mehta JB, Singhal SB, Mehta BC. Ascorbic-acid-induced haemolysis in G-6-PD deficiency. *Lancet.* 1990;336:944.

441. Relling MV, McDonagh EM, Chang T, et al. Clinical Pharmacogenetics Implementation Consortium (CPIC) guidelines for rasburicase therapy in the context of G6PD deficiency genotype. *Clin Pharmacol Ther.* 2014;96:169.

442. McCaffrey RP, Halsted CH, Wahab MF, et al. Chloramphenicol-induced hemolysis in Caucasian glucose-6-phosphate dehydrogenase deficiency. *Ann Intern Med.* 1971;74:722.

443. Chan TK, Chesterman CN, McFadzean AJ, et al. The survival of glucose-6-phosphate dehydrogenase—deficient erythrocytes in patients with typhoid fever on chloramphenicol therapy. *J Lab Clin Med.* 1971;77:177.

444. Dern RJ, Beutler E, Alving AS. The hemolytic effect of primaquine. V. Primaquine sensitivity as a manifestation of a multiple drug sensitivity. *J Lab Clin Med.* 1955;45:30.

445. Markowitz N, Saravolatz LD. Use of trimethoprim-sulfamethoxazole in a glucose-6-phosphate dehydrogenase-deficient population. *Rev Infect Dis.* 1987;9(suppl 2):S218.

446. Magon AM, Leipzig RM, Zannoni VG, et al. Interactions of glucose-6-phosphate dehydrogenase deficiency with drug acetylation and hydroxylation reactions. *J Lab Clin Med.* 1981;97:764.

447. Woolhouse NM, Atu-Taylor LC. Influence of double genetic polymorphism on response to sulfamethazine. *Clin Pharmacol Ther.* 1982;31:377.

448. Dern RJ, Beutler E, Alving AS. The hemolytic effect of primaquine. II. The natural course of the hemolytic anemia and the mechanism of its self-limited character. *J Lab Clin Med.* 1954;44:171.

449. Beutler E, Dern RJ, Alving AS. The hemolytic effect of primaquine. III. A study of primaquine-sensitive erythrocytes. *J Lab Clin Med.* 1954;44:177.

450. George JN, Sears DA, McCurdy P, et al. Primaquine sensitivity in Caucasians: hemolytic reactions induced by primaquine in G-6-PD deficient subjects. *J Lab Clin Med.* 1967;70:80.

451. Siddiqui T, Khan AH. Hepatitis A and cytomegalovirus infection precipitating acute hemolysis in glucose-6-phosphate dehydrogenase deficiency. *Mil Med.* 1998;163:434.

452. Tugwell P. Glucose-6-phosphate-dehydrogenase deficiency in Nigerians with jaundice associated with lobar pneumonia. *Lancet.* 1973;1:968.

453. Choremis C, Kattamis CA, Kyriazakou M, et al. Viral hepatitis in G.-6-P.D. deficiency. *Lancet.* 1966;1:269.

454. Walker DH, Hawkins HK, Hudson P. Fulminant Rocky Mountain spotted fever. Its pathologic characteristics associated with glucose-6-phosphate dehydrogenase deficiency. *Arch Pathol Lab Med.* 1983;107:121.

455. Huo TI, Wu JC, Chiu CF, et al. Severe hyperbilirubinemia due to acute hepatitis A superimposed on a chronic hepatitis B carrier with glucose-6-phosphate dehydrogenase deficiency. *Am J Gastroenterol.* 1996;91:158.

456. Chau TN, Lai ST, Lai JY, et al. Haemolysis complicating acute viral hepatitis in patients with normal or deficient glucose-6-phosphate dehydrogenase activity. *Scand J Infect Dis.* 1997;29:551.

457. Green L, De Lord C, Clark B, et al. Transient aplastic crisis as presentation of a previously unknown G6PD deficiency with iron overload. *Br J Haematol.* 2011;154:288.

458. Garcia S, Linares M, Colomina P, et al. Cytomegalovirus infection and aplastic crisis in glucose-6-phosphate dehydrogenase deficiency. *Lancet.* 1987;2:105.

459. Reading NS, Sirdah MM, Shubair ME, et al. Favism, the commonest form of severe hemolytic anemia in Palestinian children, varies in severity with three different variants of G6PD deficiency within the same community. *Blood Cells Mol Dis.* 2016;60:58.

460. Pietrapertosa A, Palma A, Campanale D, et al. Genotype and phenotype correlation in glucose-6-phosphate dehydrogenase deficiency. *Haematologica.* 2001;86:30.

461. Kattamis CA, Kyriazakou M, Chaidas S. Favism: clinical and biochemical data. *J Med Genet.* 1969;6:34.

462. Wong WY, Powars D, Williams WD. 'Yewdow'-induced anemia. *West J Med.* 1989;151:459.

463. Globerman H, Navok T, Chevion M. Haemolysis in a G6PD-deficient child induced by eating unripe peaches. *Scand J Haematol.* 1984;33:337.

464. Williams CK, Osotimehin BO, Ogunmola GB, et al. Haemolytic anaemia associated with Nigerian barbecued meat (red suya). *Afr J Med Med Sci.* 1988;17:71.

465. Schiliro G, Russo A, Curreri R, et al. Glucose-6-phosphate dehydrogenase deficiency in Sicily. Incidence, biochemical characteristics and clinical implications. *Clin Genet.* 1979;15:183.

466. Kaplan M, Hammerman C, Bhutani VK. The preterm infant: a high-risk situation for neonatal hyperbilirubinemia due to glucose-6-phosphate dehydrogenase deficiency. *Clin Perinatol.* 2016;43:325.

467. Liu H, Liu W, Tang X, et al. Association between G6PD deficiency and hyperbilirubinemia in neonates: a meta-analysis. *Pediatr Hematol Oncol.* 2015;32:92.

468. Valaes T. Severe neonatal jaundice associated with glucose-6-phosphate dehydrogenase deficiency: pathogenesis and global epidemiology. *Acta Paediatr Suppl.* 1994;394:58.

469. Kaplan M, Hammerman C, Vreman HJ, et al. Acute hemolysis and severe neonatal hyperbilirubinemia in glucose-6-phosphate dehydrogenase-deficient heterozygotes. *J Pediatr.* 2001;139:137.

470. Ardati KO, Bajakian KM, Tabbara KS. Effect of glucose-6-phosphate dehydrogenase deficiency on neutrophil function. *Acta Haematol.* 1997;97:211.

471. Cooper MR, DeChatelet LR, McCall CE, et al. Complete deficiency of leukocyte glucose-6-phosphate dehydrogenase with defective bactericidal activity. *J Clin Invest.* 1972;51:769.

472. Gray GR, Stamatoyannopoulos G, Naiman SC, et al. Neutrophil dysfunction, chronic granulomatous disease, and non-spherocytic haemolytic anaemia caused by complete deficiency of glucose-6-phosphate dehydrogenase. *Lancet.* 1973;2:530.

473. Vives-Corrons JL, Feliu E, Pujades MA, et al. Severe glucose-6-phosphate dehydrogenase (G6PD) deficiency associated with chronic hemolytic anemia, granulocyte dysfunction and increased susceptibility to infections. Description of a new molecular variant (G6PD Barcelona). *Blood.* 1982;59:428.

474. Rosa-Borges A, Sampaio MG, Condino-Neto A, et al. Glucose-6-phosphate dehydrogenase deficiency with recurrent infections: case report. *J Pediatr (Rio J).* 2001;77:331.

475. Chao YC, Huang CS, Lee CN, et al. Higher infection of dengue virus serotype 2 in human monocytes of patients with G6PD deficiency. *PLoS One.* 2008;3:e1557.

476. Gray GR, Naiman SC, Robinson GC. Letter: platelet function and G.-6-P.D. deficiency. *Lancet.* 1974;1:997.

477. Schwartz JP, Cooperberg AA, Rosenberg A. Platelet-function studies in patients with glucose-6-phosphate dehydrogenase deficiency. *Br J Haematol.* 1974;27:273.

478. Westring DW, Pisciotta AV. Anemia, cataracts, and seizures in patient with glucose-6-phosphate dehydrogenase deficiency. *Arch Intern Med.* 1966;118:385.

479. Harley JD, Agar NS, Gruca MA, et al. Letter: cataracts with a glucose-6-phosphate dehydrogenase variant. *Br Med J.* 1975;2:86.

480. Harley JD, Agar NS, Yoshida A. Glucose-6-phosphate dehydrogenase variants: Gd (+) Alexandra associated with neonatal jaundice and Gd (−) Camperdown in a young man with lamellar cataracts. *J Lab Clin Med.* 1978;91:295.

481. Nair V, Hasan SU, Romanchuk K, et al. Bilateral cataracts associated with glucose-6-phosphate dehydrogenase deficiency. *J Perinatol.* 2013;33:574.

482. Panich V, Na-Nakorn S. G6PD deficiency in senile cataracts. *Hum Genet.* 1980;55:123.

483. Orzalesi N, Sorcinelli R, Guiso G. Increased incidence of cataracts in male subjects deficient in glucose-6-phosphate dehydrogenase. *Arch Ophthalmol.* 1981;99:69.

484. Bhatia RP, Patel R, Dubey B. Senile cataract and glucose-6-phosphate dehydrogenase deficiency in Indians. *Trop Geogr Med.* 1990;42:349.

485. Assaf AA, Tabbara KF, el-Hazmi MA. Cataracts in male subjects with glucose-6-phosphate dehydrogenase deficiency. *Ophthalmic Paediatr Genet.* 1993;14:81.

486. Niazi GA. Glucose-6-phosphate dehydrogenase deficiency and diabetes mellitus. *Int J Hematol.* 1991;54:295.

487. Saeed TK, Hamamy HA, Alwan AA. Association of glucose-6-phosphate dehydrogenase deficiency with diabetes mellitus. *Diabet Med.* 1985;2:110.

488. Heymann AD, Cohen Y, Chodick G. Glucose-6-phosphate dehydrogenase deficiency and type 2 diabetes. *Diabetes Care.* 2012;35:e58.

489. Ninfali P, Bresolin N, Baronciani L, et al. Glucose-6-phosphate dehydrogenase Lodi[844C]: a study on its expression in blood cells and muscle. *Enzyme.* 1991;45:180.

490. Ninfali P, Baronciani L, Bardoni A, et al. Muscle expression of glucose-6-phosphate dehydrogenase deficiency in different variants. *Clin Genet.* 1995;48:232.

491. Bresolin N, Bet L, Moggio M, et al. Muscle G6PD deficiency. *Lancet.* 1987;2:212.

492. Bresolin N, Bet L, Moggio M, et al. Muscle glucose-6-phosphate dehydrogenase deficiency. *J Neurol.* 1989;236:193.

493. Liguori R, Giannoccaro MP, Pasini E, et al. Acute rhabdomyolysis induced by tonic-clonic epileptic seizures in a patient with glucose-6-phosphate dehydrogenase deficiency. *J Neurol.* 2013;260:2669.

494. Mailloux RJ, Harper ME. Glucose regulates enzymatic sources of mitochondrial NADPH in skeletal muscle cells; a novel role for glucose-6-phosphate dehydrogenase. *FASEB J.* 2010;24:2495.

495. Demir AY, van Solinge WW, van Oirschot B, et al. Glucose 6-phosphate dehydrogenase deficiency in an elite long-distance runner. *Blood.* 2009;113:2118.

496. Theodorou AA, Nikolaidis MG, Paschalis V, et al. Comparison between glucose-6-phosphate dehydrogenase-deficient and normal individuals after eccentric exercise. *Med Sci Sports Exerc.* 2010;42:1113.

497. Jamurtas AZ, Fatouros IG, Koukosias N, et al. Effect of exercise on oxidative stress in individuals with glucose-6-phosphate dehydrogenase deficiency. *In Vivo.* 2006;20:875.

498. Sulis E. G.-6-PD deficiency and cancer. *Lancet.* 1972;1:1185.

499. Zampella EJ, Bradley EL, Pretlow TG. Glucose-6-phosphate dehydrogenase: a possible clinical indicator for prostatic carcinoma. *Cancer.* 1982;49:384.

500. Ferraris AM, Broccia G, Meloni T, et al. Glucose-6-phosphate dehydrogenase deficiency and incidence of hematologic malignancy. *Am J Hum Genet.* 1988;42:516.

501. Forteleoni G, Argiolas L, Farris A, et al. G6PD deficiency and breast cancer. *Tumori.* 1988;74:665.

502. Pisano M, Cocco P, Cherchi R, et al. Glucose-6-phosphate dehydrogenase deficiency and lung cancer: a hospital based case-control study. *Tumori.* 1991;77:12.

503. Jiang P, Du W, Wang X, et al. p53 regulates biosynthesis through direct inactivation of glucose-6-phosphate dehydrogenase. *Nat Cell Biol.* 2011;13:310.

504. Ho HY, Cheng ML, Chiu DT. Glucose-6-phosphate dehydrogenase-beyond the realm of red cell biology. *Free Radic Res.* 2014;48:1028.

505. Hecker PA, Leopold JA, Gupte SA, et al. Impact of glucose-6-phosphate dehydrogenase deficiency on the pathophysiology of cardiovascular disease. *Am J Physiol Heart Circ Physiol.* 2013;304:H491.

506. Müller-Soyano A, Tovar de Roura E, Duke PR, et al. Pyruvate kinase deficiency and leg ulcers. *Blood.* 1976;47:807.

507. Curiel CD, Velasquez GA, Papa R. Hemolytic anemia and leg ulcers due to pyruvate kinase deficiency. Report of the second Venezuelan family. *Sangre (Barc).* 1977;22:64.

508. van Straaten S, Verhoeven J, Hagens S, et al. Organ involvement occurs in all forms of hereditary haemolytic anaemia. *Br J Haematol.* 2019;185:602.

509. van Beers EJ, van Straaten S, Morton DH, et al. Prevalence and management of iron overload in pyruvate kinase deficiency: report from the Pyruvate Kinase Deficiency Natural History Study. *Haematologica.* 2019;104:e51.

510. Dolan LM, Ryan M, Moohan J. Pyruvate kinase deficiency in pregnancy complicated by iron overload. *BJOG.* 2002;109:844.

511. Wax JR, Pinette MG, Cartin A, et al. Pyruvate kinase deficiency complicating pregnancy. *Obstet Gynecol.* 2007;109:553.

512. Fanning J, Hinkle RS. Pyruvate kinase deficiency hemolytic anemia: two successful pregnancy outcomes. *Am J Obstet Gynecol.* 1985;153:313.

513. Delivoria-Papadopoulos M, Oski FA, Gottlieb AJ. Oxygen-hemoglobin dissociation curves: effect of inherited enzyme defects of the red cell. *Science.* 1969;165:601.

514. Gordon-Smith EC. Erythrocyte enzyme deficiencies. Pyruvate kinase deficiency. *J Clin Pathol Suppl (R Coll Pathol).* 1974;8:128.

515. Ferreira P, Morais I, Costa R, et al. Hydrops fetalis associated with erythrocyte pyruvate kinase deficiency. *Eur J Pediatr.* 2000;159:481.

516. Wellner VP, Sekura R, Meister A, et al. Glutathione synthetase deficiency, an inborn error of metabolism involving the gamma-glutamyl cycle in patients with 5-oxoprolinuria (pyroglutamic aciduria). *Proc Natl Acad Sci U S A.* 1974;71:2505.

517. Marstein S, Jellum E, Halpern B, et al. Biochemical studies of erythrocytes in a patient with pyroglutamic acidemia (5-oxoprolinemia). *N Engl J Med.* 1976;295:406.

518. Hirono A, Iyori H, Sekine I, et al. Three cases of hereditary nonspherocytic hemolytic anemia associated with red blood cell glutathione deficiency. *Blood.* 1996;87:2071.

519. Konrad PN, Richards F, Valentine WN, et al. Gamma-glutamyl-cysteine synthetase deficiency. *N Engl J Med.* 1972;286:557.

520. Richards F 2nd, Cooper MR, Pearce LA, et al. Familial spinocerebellar degeneration, hemolytic anemia, and glutathione deficiency. *Arch Intern Med.* 1974;134:534.

521. Beutler E, Moroose R, Kramer L, et al. Gamma-glutamylcysteine synthetase deficiency and hemolytic anemia. *Blood.* 1990;75:271.

522. Skala H, Dreyfus JC, Vives-Corrons JL, et al. Triose phosphate isomerase deficiency. *Biochem Med.* 1977;18:226.

523. Valentine WN, Schneider AS, Baughan MA, et al. Hereditary hemolytic anemia with triosephosphate isomerase deficiency. *Am J Med.* 1966;41:27.

524. Hollán S, Magócsi M, Fodor E, et al. Search for the pathogenesis of the differing phenotype in two compound heterozygote Hungarian brothers with the same genotypic triosephosphate isomerase deficiency. *Proc Natl Acad Sci U S A.* 1997;94:10362.

525. Hollán S, Fujii H, Hirono A, et al. Hereditary triosephosphate isomerase (TPI) deficiency: two severely affected brothers one with and one without neurological symptoms. *Hum Genet.* 1993;92:486.

526. Noel N, Flanagan JM, Ramirez Bajo MJ, et al. Two new phosphoglycerate kinase mutations associated with chronic haemolytic anaemia and neurological dysfunction in two patients from Spain. *Br J Haematol.* 2006;132:523.

527. Rosa R, George C, Fardeau M, et al. A new case of phosphoglycerate kinase deficiency: PGK Creteil associated with rhabdomyolysis and lacking hemolytic anemia. *Blood.* 1982;60:84.

528. DiMauro S, Dalakas M, Miranda AF. Phosphoglycerate kinase deficiency: another cause of recurrent myoglobinuria. *Ann Neurol.* 1983;13:11.

529. Clarke JL, Vulliamy TJ, Roper D, et al. Combined glucose-6-phosphate dehydrogenase and glucosephosphate isomerase deficiency can alter clinical outcome. *Blood Cells Mol Dis.* 2003;30:258.

530. Branca R, Costa E, Rocha S, et al. Coexistence of congenital red cell pyruvate kinase and band 3 deficiency. *Clin Lab Haematol.* 2004;26:297.

531. Zarza R, Moscardó M, Alvarez R, et al. Co-existence of hereditary spherocytosis and a new red cell pyruvate kinase variant: PK Mallorca. *Haematologica.* 2000;85:227.

532. Vercellati C, Marcello AP, Fermo E, et al. A case of hereditary spherocytosis misdiagnosed as pyruvate kinase deficient hemolytic anemia. *Clin Lab.* 2013;59:421.

533. Beutler E, Forman L. Coexistence of α-thalassemia and a new pyruvate kinase variant: PK Fukien. *Acta Haematol.* 1983;69:3.

534. Vives Corrons J-L, García AM, Sosa AM, et al. Heterozygous pyruvate kinase deficiency and severe hemolytic anemia in a pregnant woman with concomitant, glucose-6-phosphate dehydrogenase deficiency. *Ann Hematol.* 1991;62:190.

535. Zanella A, Bianchi P, Iurlo A, et al. Iron status and *HFE* genotype in erythrocyte pyruvate kinase deficiency: study of Italian cases. *Blood Cells Mol Dis.* 2001;27:653.

536. Olah J, Orosz F, Puskas LG, et al. Triosephosphate isomerase deficiency: consequences of an inherited mutation at mRNA, protein and metabolic levels. *Biochem J.* 2005;392:675.

537. Diez A, Gilsanz F, Martinez J, et al. Life-threatening nonspherocytic hemolytic anemia in a patient with a null mutation in the PKLR gene and no compensatory PKM gene expression. *Blood.* 2005;106:1851.

538. Greenberg MS. Heinz body hemolytic anemia. *Arch Intern Med.* 1976;136:153.

539. Nathan DM, Siegel AJ, Bunn HF. Acute methemoglobinemia and hemolytic anemia with phenazopyridine. *Arch Intern Med.* 1977;137:1636.

540. Mentzer WC Jr, Baehner RL, Schmidt-Schönbein H, et al. Selective reticulocyte destruction in erythrocyte pyruvate kinase deficiency. *J Clin Invest.* 1971;50:688.

541. Beutler E. *Red Cell Metabolism. A Manual of Biochemical Methods.* Grune & Stratton; 1984.

542. Rijksen G, Veerman AJ, Schipper-Kester GP, et al. Diagnosis of pyruvate kinase deficiency in a transfusion-dependent patient with severe hemolytic anemia. *Am J Hematol.* 1990;35:187.

543. Herz F, Kaplan E, Scheye ES. Diagnosis of erythrocyte glucose-6-phosphate dehydrogenase deficiency in the negro male despite hemolytic crisis. *Blood.* 1970;35:90.

544. Vogels IM, Van Noorden CJ, Wolf BH, et al. Cytochemical determination of heterozygous glucose-6-phosphate dehydrogenase deficiency in erythrocytes. *Br J Haematol.* 1986;63:402.

545. Bancone G, Kalnoky M, Chu CS, et al. The G6PD flow-cytometric assay is a reliable tool for diagnosis of G6PD deficiency in women and anaemic subjects. *Sci Rep.* 2017;7:9822.

546. Roper D, Layton M, Rees D, et al. Laboratory diagnosis of G6PD deficiency. A British Society for Haematology Guideline. *Br J Haematol.* 2020;189:24.

547. Bianchi P, Fermo E, Glader B, et al. Addressing the diagnostic gaps in pyruvate kinase deficiency: consensus recommendations on the diagnosis of pyruvate kinase deficiency. *Am J Hematol.* 2019;94:149.

548. Oski FA. Red cell metabolism in the newborn infant. V. Glycolytic intermediates and glycolytic enzymes. *Pediatrics.* 1969;44:84.

549. Travis SF, Kumar SP, Paez PC, et al. Red cell metabolic alterations in postnatal life in term infants: glycolytic enzymes and glucose-6-phosphate dehydrogenase. *Pediatr Res.* 1980;14:1349.

550. Gross RT, Schroeder EA, Brounstein SA. Energy metabolism in the erythrocytes of premature infants compared to full term newborn infants and adults. *Blood.* 1963;21:755.

551. Lestas AN, Rodeck CH, White JM. Normal activities of glycolytic enzymes in the fetal erythrocytes. *Br J Haematol.* 1982;50:439.

552. Konrad PN, Valentine WN, Paglia DE. Enzymatic activities and glutathione content of erythrocytes in the newborn: comparison with red cells of older normal subjects and those with comparable reticulocytosis. *Acta Haematol.* 1972;48:193.

553. Jacob HS, Jandl JH. A simple visual screening test for glucose-6-phosphate dehydrogenase deficiency employing ascorbate and cyanide. *N Engl J Med.* 1966;274:1162.

554. Koralkova P, van Solinge WW, van Wijk R. Rare hereditary red blood cell enzymopathies associated with hemolytic anemia-pathophysiology, clinical aspects, and laboratory diagnosis. *Int J Lab Hematol.* 2014;36:388.

555. Valentine WN, Paglia DE, Fink K, et al. Lead poisoning: association with hemolytic anemia, basophilic stippling, erythrocyte pyrimidine 5′-nucleotidase deficiency, and intraerythrocytic accumulation of pyrimidines. *J Clin Invest.* 1976;58:926.

556. Hirono A, Forman L, Beutler E. Enzymatic diagnosis in non-spherocytic hemolytic anemia. *Medicine (Baltimore).* 1988;67:110.

557. Beutler E, Luzzatto L. Hemolytic anemia. *Semin Hematol.* 1999;36:38.

558. Barasa B, Slijper M. Challenges for red blood cell biomarker discovery through proteomics. *Biochim Biophys Acta.* 2014;1844:1003.

559. Bordbar A, Jamshidi N, Palsson BO. iAB-RBC-283: a proteomically derived knowledge-base of erythrocyte metabolism that can be used to simulate its physiological and patho-physiological states. *BMC Syst Biol.* 2011;5:110.

560. von Lohneysen K, Scott TM, Soldau K, et al. Assessment of the red cell proteome of young patients with unexplained hemolytic anemia by two-dimensional differential in-gel electrophoresis (DIGE). *PLoS One.* 2012;7:e34237.

561. Lyon GJ, Jiang T, Van Wijk R, et al. Exome sequencing and unrelated findings in the context of complex disease research: ethical and clinical implications. *Discov Med.* 2011;12:41.

562. Yurkovich JT, Yang L, Palsson BO. Biomarkers are used to predict quantitative metabolite concentration profiles in human red blood cells. *PLoS Comput Biol.* 2017;13:e1005424.

563. D'Alessandro A, Nemkov T, Reisz J, et al. Omics markers of the red cell storage lesion and metabolic linkage. *Blood Transfus.* 2017;15:137.

564. Mimouni F, Shohat S, Reisner SH. G6PD-deficiency donor blood as a cause of hemolysis in two preterm infants. *Isr J Med Sci.* 1986;22:120.

565. Kappas A, Drummond GS, Valaes T. A single dose of Sn-mesoporphyrin prevents development of severe hyperbilirubinemia in glucose-6-phosphate dehydrogenase-deficient newborns. *Pediatrics.* 2001;108:25.

566. Baronciani L, Tricta F, Beutler E. G6PD "Campinas:" a deficient enzyme with a mutation at the far 3′ end of the gene. *Hum Mutat.* 1993;2:77.

567. Beutler E, Mathai CK, Smith JE. Biochemical variants of glucose-6-phosphate dehydrogenase giving rise to congenital nonspherocytic hemolytic disease. *Blood.* 1968;31:131.

568. Iolascon A, Andolfo I, Barcellini W, et al. Recommendations for splenectomy in hereditary hemolytic anemias. *Haematologica.* 2017;102:1304.

569. Beutler E. *Hemolytic Anemia in Disorders of Red Cell Metabolism.* Plenum Press; 1978.

570. Corash L, Spielberg S, Bartsocas C, et al. Reduced chronic hemolysis during high-dose vitamin E administration in Mediterranean-type glucose-6-phosphate dehydrogenase deficiency. *N Engl J Med.* 1980;303:416.

571. Spielberg SP, Boxer LA, Corash LM, et al. Improved erythrocyte survival with high dose vitamin E in chronic hemolyzing G6PD and glutathione synthetase deficiencies. *Ann Intern Med.* 1978;90:53.

572. Johnson GJ, Vatassery GT, Finkel B, et al. High-dose vitamin E does not decrease the rate of chronic hemolysis in glucose-6-phosphate dehydrogenase deficiency. *N Engl J Med.* 1983;308:1014.

573. Newman JG, Newman TB, Bowie LJ, et al. An examination of the role of vitamin E in glucose-6-phosphate dehydrogenase deficiency. *Clin Biochem.* 1979;12:149.

574. Al Rimawi HS, Al Sheyyab M, Batieha A, et al. Effect of desferrioxamine in acute haemolytic anaemia of glucose-6-phosphate dehydrogenase deficiency. *Acta Haematol.* 1999;101:145.

575. Ekert H, Rawlinson I. Deferoxamine and favism. *N Engl J Med.* 1985;312:1260.

576. Grace RF, Mark Layton D, Barcellini W. How we manage patients with pyruvate kinase deficiency. *Br J Haematol.* 2019;184:721.

577. Schroter W. Successful long-term phenobarbital therapy of hyperbilirubinemia in congenital hemolytic anemia due to glucose phosphate isomerase deficiency. *Eur J Pediatr.* 1980;135:41.

578. Tanphaichitr VS, Suvatte V, Issaragrisil S, et al. Successful bone marrow transplantation in a child with red blood cell pyruvate kinase deficiency. *Bone Marrow Transplant.* 2000;26:689.

579. van Straaten S, Bierings MB, Bianchi P, et al. Worldwide study of hematopoietic allogeneic stem cell transplantation in pyruvate kinase deficiency. *Haematologica.* 2018;103:e82.

580. Khazal S, Polishchuk V, Manwani D, et al. Allogeneic bone marrow transplantation for treatment of severe hemolytic anemia attributable to hexokinase deficiency. *Blood.* 2016;128:735.

581. Rio P, Navarro S, Wang W, et al. Successful engraftment of gene-corrected hematopoietic stem cells in non-conditioned patients with Fanconi anemia. *Nat Med.* 2019;25:1396.

582. Kung C, Hixon J, Kosinski PA, et al. AG-348 enhances pyruvate kinase activity in red blood cells from patients with pyruvate kinase deficiency. *Blood.* 2017;130:1347.

583. Grace RF, Rose C, Layton DM, et al. Safety and efficacy of mitapivat in pyruvate kinase deficiency. *N Engl J Med.* 2019;381:933.

584. Hsieh MM, Fitzhugh CD, Weitzel RP, et al. Nonmyeloablative HLA-matched sibling allogeneic hematopoietic stem cell transplantation for severe sickle cell phenotype. *JAMA.* 2014;312:48.

585. Limerick E, Fitzhugh C. Choice of donor source and conditioning regimen for hematopoietic stem cell transplantation in sickle cell disease. *J Clin Med.* 2019;8:1997.

586. Pannacciulli I, Tizianello A, Ajmar F, et al. The course of experimentally-induced hemolytic anemia in a primaquine- sensitive Caucasian. A case study. *Blood.* 1965;25:92.

587. Meloni T, Forteleoni G, Noja G, et al. Increased prevalence of glucose-6-phosphate dehydrogenase deficiency in patients with cholelithiasis. *Acta Haematol.* 1991;85:76.

588. Petrakis NL, Wiesenfeld SL, Sams BJ, et al. Prevalence of sickle-cell trait and glucose-6-phosphate dehydrogenase deficiency. *N Engl J Med.* 1970;282:767.

589. Steinberg MH, West MS, Gallagher D, et al. Effects of glucose-6-phosphate dehydrogenase deficiency upon sickle cell anemia. *Blood.* 1988;71:748.

590. Heller P, Best WR, Nelson RB, et al. Clinical implications of sickle-cell trait and glucose-6-phosphate dehydrogenase deficiency in hospitalized black male patients. *N Engl J Med.* 1979;300:1001.

591. Renzaho AM, Husser E, Polonsky M. Should blood donors be routinely screened for glucose-6-phosphate dehydrogenase deficiency? A systematic review of clinical studies focusing on patients transfused with glucose-6-phosphate dehydrogenase-deficient red cells. *Transfus Med Rev.* 2014;28:7.

592. Pilo F, Baronciani D, Depau C, et al. Safety of hematopoietic stem cell donation in glucose 6 phosphate dehydrogenase-deficient donors. *Bone Marrow Transplant.* 2013;48:36.

593. Pamba A, Richardson ND, Carter N, et al. Clinical spectrum and severity of hemolytic anemia in glucose 6-phosphate dehydrogenase-deficient children receiving dapsone. *Blood.* 2012;120:4123.

594. Bowman HS, McKusick VA, Dronamraju KR. Pyruvate kinase deficient hemolytic anemia in an Amish isolate. *Am J Hum Genet.* 1965;17:1.

595. Grace RF, Cohen J, Egan S, et al. The burden of disease in pyruvate kinase deficiency: patients' perception of the impact on health-related quality of life. *Eur J Haematol.* 2018;101:758.

596. Beutler E, Gelbart T. Improved assay of the enzymes of glutathione synthesis: γ-glutamylcysteine synthetase and glutathione synthetase. *Clin Chim Acta.* 1986;158:115.

597. Torrance J, West C, Beutler E. A simple rapid radiometric assay for pyrimidine-5′-nucleotidase. *J Lab Clin Med.* 1977;90:563.

598. Beutler E, Kuhl W, Gelbart T. Blood cell phosphogluconolactonase: assay and properties. *Br J Haematol.* 1986;62:577.

599. Bird TD, Hamernyik P, Nutter JY, et al. Inherited deficiency of delta-aminolevulinic acid dehydratase. *Am J Hum Genet.* 1979;31:662.

600. Kamatani N, Hakoda M, Otsuka S, et al. Only three mutations account for almost all defective alleles causing adenine phosphoribosyltransferase deficiency in Japanese patients. *J Clin Invest.* 1992;90:130.

601. Runolfsdottir HL, Palsson R, Agustsdottir IM, et al. Kidney disease in adenine phosphoribosyltransferase deficiency. *Am J Kidney Dis.* 2016;67:431.

602. Flinn AM, Gennery AR. Adenosine deaminase deficiency: a review. *Orphanet J Rare Dis.* 2018;13:65.

603. Ogasawara N, Goto H, Yamada Y, et al. Distribution of AMP-deaminase isozymes in rat tissues. *Eur J Biochem.* 1978;87:297.

604. Yamada Y, Goto H, Wakamatsu N, et al. A rare case of complete human erythrocyte AMP deaminase deficiency due to two novel missense mutations in AMPD3. *Hum Mutat.* 2001;17:78.

605. Armstrong JM, Myers DV, Verpoorte JA, et al. Purification and properties of human erythrocyte carbonic anhydrases. *J Biol Chem.* 1966;241:5137.

606. Kendall AG, Tashian RE. Erythrocyte carbonic anhydrase I. inherited deficiency in humans. *Science.* 1977;197:471.

607. Roth DE, Venta PJ, Tashian RE, et al. Molecular basis of human carbonic anhydrase II deficiency. *Proc Natl Acad Sci U S A.* 1992;89:1804.

608. Goth L, Rass P, Pay A. Catalase enzyme mutations and their association with diseases. *Mol Diagn.* 2004;8:141.

609. Percy MJ, Lappin TR. Recessive congenital methaemoglobinaemia: cytochrome b(5) reductase deficiency. *Br J Haematol.* 2008;141:298.

610. Gupta V, Kulkarni A, Warang P, et al. Mutation update: variants of the CYB5R3 gene in recessive congenital methemoglobinemia. *Hum Mutat.* 2020;41:737.

611. Simonelli F, Giovane A, Frunzio S, et al. Galactokinase activity in patients with idiopathic presenile and senile cataract. *Metab Pediatr Syst Ophthalmol (1985).* 1992;15:53.

612. P S, Ebrahimi EA, Ghazala SA, et al. Structural analysis of missense mutations in galactokinase 1 (GALK1) leading to galactosemia type-2. *J Cell Biochem.* 2018;119:7585.

613. Karas N, Gobec L, Pfeifer V, et al. Mutations in galactose-1-phosphate uridyltransferase gene in patients with idiopathic presenile cataract. *J Inherit Metab Dis.* 2003;26:699.

614. Coelho AI, Rubio-Gozalbo ME, Vicente JB, et al. Sweet and sour: an update on classic galactosemia. *J Inherit Metab Dis.* 2017;40:325.

615. Necheles TF, Steinberg MH, Cameron D. Erythrocyte glutathione-peroxidase deficiency. *Br J Haematol.* 1970;19:605.

616. Valentine WN, Paglia DE, Neerhout RC, et al. Erythrocyte glyoxalase II deficiency with coincidental hereditary elliptocytosis. *Blood.* 1970;36:797.

617. Johnson LA, Gordon RB, Emmerson BT. Hypoxanthine-guanine phosphoribosyltransferase: a simple spectrophotometric assay. *Clin Chim Acta.* 1977;80:203.

618. Larovere LE, Romero N, Fairbanks LD, et al. A novel missense mutation, c.584A > C (Y195S), in two unrelated Argentine patients with hypoxanthine-guanine phosphoribosyl-transferase deficiency, neurological variant. *Mol Genet Metab.* 2004;81:352.

619. van Dael CM, Pierik LJ, Reijngoud DJ, et al. Partial hypoxanthine-guanine phosphoribosyl transferase deficiency without elevated urinary hypoxanthine excretion. *Mol Genet Metab.* 2007;90:221.

620. Sumi S, Marinaki AM, Arenas M, et al. Genetic basis of inosine triphosphate pyrophosphohydrolase deficiency. *Hum Genet.* 2002;111:360.

621. Handley MT, Reddy K, Wills J, et al. ITPase deficiency causes a Martsolf-like syndrome with a lethal infantile dilated cardiomyopathy. *PLoS Genet.* 2019;15:e1007605.

622. Sass MD, Caruso CJ, Farhangi M. TPNH-methemoglobin reductase deficiency: a new red-cell enzyme defect. *J Lab Clin Med.* 1967;70:760.

623. Ferrell RE, Escallon M, Aguilar L, et al. Erythrocyte phosphoglucomutase: a family study of a PGM1 deficient allele. *Hum Genet.* 1984;67:306.

624. Lukka M, Ehnholm C, Kuusi T. Phosphoglucomutase (PGM1) subtypes in a Finnish population determined by isoelectric focusing in agarose gel. *Hum Hered.* 1985;35:95.

625. Banki K, Hutter E, Colombo E, et al. Glutathione levels and sensitivity to apoptosis are regulated by changes in transaldolase expression. *J Biol Chem.* 1996;271:32994.

626. Chamberlain BR, Buttery JE. Reappraisal of the uroporphyrinogen I synthase assay, and a proposed modified method. *Clin Chem.* 1980;26:1346.

627. Strand LJ, Meyer UA, Felsher BF, et al. Decreased red cell uroporphyrinogen I synthetase activity in intermittent acute porphyria. *J Clin Invest.* 1972;51:2530.

628. Stein PE, Badminton MN, Rees DC. Update review of the acute porphyrias. *Br J Haematol.* 2017;176:527.

629. Chao LT, Du CS, Louie E, et al. A to G substitution identified in exon 2 of the G6PD gene among G6PD deficient Chinese. *Nucleic Acids Res.* 1991;19:6056.

630. Hirono A, Ishii A, Kere N, et al. Molecular analysis of glucose-6-phosphate dehydrogenase variants in the Solomon Islands. *Am J Hum Genet.* 1995;56:1243.

631. Kaeda JS, Chhotray GP, Ranjit MR, et al. A new glucose-6-phosphate dehydrogenase variant, G6PD Orissa (44 Ala→Gly), is the major polymorphic variant in tribal populations in India. *Am J Hum Genet.* 1995;57:1335.

632. Minucci A, Antenucci M, Giardina B, et al. G6PD Murcia, G6PD Ube and G6PD Orissa: report of three G6PD mutations unusual for Italian population. *Clin Biochem.* 2010;43:1180.

633. Nafa K, Reghis A, Osmani N, et al. G6PD Aures: a new mutation (48 Ile→Thr) causing mild G6PD deficiency is associated with favism. *Hum Mol Genet.* 1993;2:81.

634. Daoud BB, Mosbehi I, Prehu C, et al. Molecular characterization of erythrocyte glucose-6-phosphate dehydrogenase deficiency in Tunisia. *Pathol Biol (Paris).* 2008;56:260.

635. Calabro V, Giacobbe A, Vallone D, et al. Genetic heterogeneity at the glucose-6-phosphate dehydrogenase locus in southern Italy: a study on a population from the Matera district. *Hum Genet.* 1990;86:49.

636. Vulliamy TJ, D'Urso M, Battistuzzi G, et al. Diverse point mutations in the human glucose-6-phosphate dehydrogenase gene cause enzyme deficiency and mild or severe hemolytic anemia. *Proc Natl Acad Sci U S A.* 1988;85:5171.

637. Ganczakowski M, Town M, Bowden DK, et al. Multiple glucose 6-phosphate dehydrogenase-deficient variants correlate with malaria endemicity in the Vanuatu archipelago (southwestern Pacific). *Am J Hum Genet.* 1995;56:294.

638. Nakatsuji T, Miwa S. Incidence and characteristics of glucose-6-phosphate dehydrogenase variants in Japan. *Hum Genet.* 1979;51:297.

639. Chiu DT, Zuo L, Chao L, et al. Molecular characterization of glucose-6-phosphate dehydrogenase (G6PD) deficiency in patients of Chinese descent and identification of new base substitutions in the human G6PD gene. *Blood.* 1993;81:2150.

640. Vulliamy TJ, Wanachiwanawin W, Mason PJ, et al. G6PD Mahidol, a common deficient variant in South East Asia is caused by a (163)glycine- - -serine mutation. *Nucleic Acids Res.* 1989;17:5868.

641. Beutler E, Kuhl W, Saenz GF, et al. Mutation analysis of glucose-6-phosphate dehydrogenase (G6PD) variants in Costa Rica. *Hum Genet.* 1991;87:462.

642. Cittadella R, Civitelli D, Manna I, et al. Genetic heterogeneity of glucose-6-phosphate dehydrogenase deficiency in south-east Sicily. *Ann Hum Genet.* 1997;61:229.

643. De Vita G, Alcalay M, Sampietro M, et al. Two point mutations are responsible for G6PD polymorphism in Sardinia. *Am J Hum Genet.* 1989;44:233.

644. Corcoran CM, Calabro V, Tamagnini G, et al. Molecular heterogeneity underlying the G6PD Mediterranean phenotype. *Hum Genet.* 1992;88:688.

645. Beutler E, Kuhl W, Vives-Corrons JL, et al. Molecular heterogeneity of glucose-6-phosphate dehydrogenase A. *Blood.* 1989;74:2550.

646. Kirkman HN, Simon ER, Pickard BM. Seattle variant of glucose-6-phosphate dehydrogenase. *J Lab Clin Med.* 1965;66:834.

647. Cappellini MD, Sampietro M, Toniolo D, et al. Biochemical and molecular characterization of a new sporadic glucose-6-phosphate dehydrogenase variant described in Italy: G6PD Modena. *Br J Haematol.* 1994;87:209.

648. Cappellini MD, Martinez di Montemuros F, Dotti C, et al. Molecular characterisation of the glucose-6-phosphate dehydrogenase (G6PD) Ferrara II variant. *Hum Genet.* 1995;95:440.

649. Viglietto G, Montanaro V, Calabro V, et al. Common glucose-6-phosphate dehydrogenase (G6PD) variants from the Italian population: biochemical and molecular characterization. *Ann Hum Genet.* 1990;54:1.

650. Poon MC, Hall K, Scott CW, et al. G6PD Viangchan: a new glucose 6-phosphate dehydrogenase variant from Laos. *Hum Genet.* 1988;78:98.

651. Beutler E, Westwood B, Kuhl W. Definition of the mutations of G6PD Wayne, G6PD Viangchan, G6PD Jammu, and G6PD 'LeJeune'. *Acta Haematol.* 1991;86:179.

652. Ahluwalia A, Corcoran CM, Vulliamy TJ, et al. G6PD Kalyan and G6PD Kerala; two deficient variants in India caused by the same 317 Glu→Lys mutation. *Hum Mol Genet.* 1992;1:209.

653. Sukumar S, Mukherjee MB, Colah RB, et al. Two distinct Indian G6PD variants G6PD Jamnagar and G6PD Rohini caused by the same 949 G→A mutation. *Blood Cells Mol Dis.* 2005;35:193.

654. Beutler E, Westwood B, Prchal JT, et al. New glucose-6-phosphate dehydrogenase mutations from various ethnic groups. *Blood.* 1992;80:255.

655. Calabro V, Mason PJ, Filosa S, et al. Genetic heterogeneity of glucose-6-phosphate dehydrogenase deficiency revealed by single-strand conformation and sequence analysis. *Am J Hum Genet.* 1993;52:527.

656. Menounos P, Zervas C, Garinis G, et al. Molecular heterogeneity of the glucose-6-phosphate dehydrogenase deficiency in the Hellenic population. *Hum Hered.* 2000;50:237.

657. Perng LI, Chiou SS, Liu TC, et al. A novel C to T substitution at nucleotide 1360 of cDNA which abolishes a natural Hha I site accounts for a new G6PD deficiency gene in Chinese. *Hum Mol Genet.* 1992;1:205.

658. Wagner G, Bhatia K, Board P. Glucose-6-phosphate dehydrogenase deficiency mutations in Papua New Guinea. *Hum Biol.* 1996;68:383.

659. Stevens DJ, Wanachiwanawin W, Mason PJ, et al. G6PD Canton a common deficient variant in South East Asia caused by a 459 Arg—Leu mutation. *Nucleic Acids Res.* 1990;18:7190.

660. Chiu DT, Zuo L, Chen E, et al. Two commonly occurring nucleotide base substitutions in Chinese G6PD variants. *Biochem Biophys Res Commun.* 1991;180:988.

CHAPTER 17
THALASSEMIA: A DISORDER OF GLOBIN SYNTHESIS

Sujit Sheth and Swee Lay Thein

SUMMARY

The thalassemia syndromes are the commonest monogenic diseases in humans; they result from mutations in the genes regulating globin expression. The two main classes of thalassemia, α and β, involve the α-globin and β-globin genes; rarer forms are caused by abnormalities of the other globin genes, γ and δ, which are expressed in smaller amounts in adults. Thalassemia is found predominantly in populations originating around the Mediterranean, through the Middle East, the Indian subcontinent, and throughout Southeast Asia, including Myanmar, Thailand, Cambodia, Laos, Vietnam, the Malay peninsula, and extending to southern China and the Pacific islands, areas historically endemic for falciparum malaria. With migration, patients with thalassemia syndromes now live all over the world, including Europe and the Americas. The high frequency and genetic diversity of thalassemia is related to past or present heterozygote resistance to malaria.

Normal hemoglobin A is a heterodimer of α-globin and β-globin chains. The common theme in α-thalassemia and β-thalassemia is the decreased production of α-globin and β-globin chains, respectively, resulting in imbalanced globin and decreased hemoglobin production, and anemia. Hundreds of mutations at the α-globin and β-globin loci have been defined as the cause

of the reduced or absent synthesis of α-globin or β-globin chains. Rarer forms of thalassemia include γ-thalassemia, δ-thalassemia, or combinations, such as γδ-thalassemia or γδβ-thalassemia that are associated with hereditary persistence of fetal hemoglobin. Other rare forms of thalassemia, εγδβ, lead to absent production of ε-globin, γ-globin, δ-globin, and β-globin chains, and are lethal in the homozygous condition.

Throughout human development, production of the α-like and β-like globin chains are balanced, such that β-thalassemia will lead to excess α-globin chains, and α-thalassemia, to excess β-globin chains. The pathophysiology and clinical manifestations of thalassemia result from the effects of this chain imbalance between the globin chain subunits. In β-thalassemia, excess α-globin chains cause damage to intramedullary red cell precursors and red cells, leading to apoptosis, impaired red cell production, and anemia. This signature of ineffective erythropoiesis leads to marrow expansion and extramedullary hematopoiesis, which causes many of the manifestations of the disease when not treated optimally. Complications of treatment and inadequate treatment lead to significant morbidity and mortality. Iron overload results from increased intestinal iron absorption relating to ineffective erythropoiesis, and from transfusional loading; they account for the majority of complications in transfused thalassemia patients, whereas extramedullary hematopoiesis and iron toxicity account for the major manifestations in nontransfused or undertransfused patients. α-Thalassemia leads to an excess of β-globin chains that form $β_4$ molecules (β tetramers or hemoglobin H), which is soluble and does not precipitate in the precursors in the marrow, but hemoglobin H is unstable and precipitates in circulating red cells. Hence, the anemia of α-thalassemia tends to be more hemolytic rather than dyserythropoietic.

The clinical presentation and course of α-thalassemia and β-thalassemia vary widely based on the causative mutations, coinherited genetic variants, and other disease modifying factors, such as access to treatment, and therapy-related complications, including iron overload, infections, and alloimmunization. Transfusion therapy is the mainstay of the more severe forms of the disease, and the resulting iron overload must be managed optimally to minimize the risk of tissue iron toxicity. The only curative treatment currently is hematopoietic stem cell transplantation, but gene therapy is in the late stages of clinical trials and is expected to become part of the routine management repertoire in due course.

Acronyms and Abbreviations: AATAAA, the polyadenylation signal site; ATP, adenosine triphosphate; ATR-16, *a*-thalassemia chromosome 16-linked mental retardation syndrome; ATR-X, *a*-thalassemia X-linked mental retardation syndrome; bp, base pair; *BCL11A*, B-cell lymphoma/leukemia oncogene important for γ to β globin switching; CAP site, a DNA site located in or near a promoter; DAT, direct antiglobulin test; DNase I, an enzyme used to detect DNA-protein interaction; ERFE, erythroferrone; GATA-1, an erythroid specific transcription factor; Hb, hemoglobin; HS, nuclease-hypersensitive sites; HPFH, hereditary persistence of fetal hemoglobin; HPLC, high performance liquid chromatography; HSCT, hematopoietic stem cell transplantation; IVS, intervening sequence of a gene (ie, an intron); KLF1, Kruppel-like factor 1, previously known as EKLF, erythroid Kruppel-like factor; LCR, locus control region; MCS, multispecies conserved sequences; MCH, mean corpuscular hemoglobin; MCV, mean corpuscular volume; MRI, magnetic resonance imaging; mRNA, messenger RNA; NTDT, non-transfusion dependent thalassemia; NMD, nonsense mediated RNA decay; NFE-2, "nuclear factor, erythroid 2", a transcription factor essential for productive erythropoiesis; PHD region, known as plant homeodomain is a DNA region with zinc finger motif commonly deleted in ATR-X *a*-thalassemia; QTL, quantitative trait locus; RFLP, restriction fragment length polymorphism; ROS, reactive oxygen species; TATA box, a DNA sequence (cis-regulatory element) found in the promoter region of genes; TDT, transfusion dependent thalassemia; TTD, trichodystrophy—caused by mutation of *XPD* gene; VCN, vector copy number; XPD, xeroderma pigmentosa.

● DEFINITIONS AND HISTORY

Thalassemia is a group of disorders, each resulting from an inherited abnormality of production of the globin moiety of hemoglobin.[1-3] Initially called Cooley's anemia, thalassemia was first described in 1925 by Cooley and Lee[4] as a form of severe anemia associated with splenomegaly and bone changes that occurred early in life. As is usual, the first description was of the severest form of the disease. A comprehensive description of the disease and its pathology was published in 1932 by George H. Whipple, a pathologist, and William L. Bradford, a pediatrician.[5] It was Whipple who coined the phrase thalassic anemia,[6,7] later condensing it to thalassemia, from Thalassa (θαλασσα), or "the sea," because all of the patients described to that point were from around the Mediterranean Sea. The inheritance pattern of the disease, and its wide spectrum of severity was not fully appreciated until later. Discovered to be inherited in an autosomal recessive manner, the homozygous condition was the most severe, termed *thalassemia major*; the heterozygous condition, mild, termed *thalassemia minor*; and *thalassemia intermedia*, a clinical state of severity in between major and minor.[1,6,8,9] Occasionally, these three degrees of severity were amplified by the term *thalassemia minima* in those who were heterozygotes and did not have anemia (also referred to as *silent carriers*).

Thalassemia results from mutations in the globin genes and are part of the spectrum of diseases known collectively as the hemoglobinopathies. This group may be subdivided into qualitative disorders in which structural hemoglobin (Hb) variants are produced, such as sickle cell anemia, unstable Hbs, and methemoglobins (Chaps. 18 and 19), and quantitative disorders in which normal globin production is diminished or absent. The clinical manifestations of the two groups are quite different. Manifestations of the structural Hb variants depend on the nature and site of the structural change in the Hb molecule. The A-to-T substitution in codon 6 of β-globin of the Hb molecule in sickle cell disease leads to changes in red cell shape, rheology, and adhesiveness, and multisystemic clinical complications (Chap. 18). The majority of qualitative mutations, however, cause no significant change in Hb properties or clinical problems. However, some mutations lead to a Hb variant that is also produced in reduced amounts, for example, HbE (β26 Glu→Lys), the most common β-thalassemia mutation in Southeast Asia. Other Hb variants lead to a thalassemia phenotype as a result of the globin chain being highly unstable and causing a functional deficiency. In β-thalassemia major and intermedia, the manifestations are mostly related to the ineffective erythropoiesis and its consequences, variably severe anemia, iron overload, bone disease, and intramedullary hemolysis, and these diseases are more aptly termed *syndromes of ineffective erythropoiesis*.

Several monographs describe the historical aspects of thalassemia in greater detail.[1,9]

FORMS OF THALASSEMIA

Thalassemias are classified into α-, β-, δ-, γ-, δβ-, γδβ-, and εγδβ-thalassemia, according to the type of globin chain(s) that is produced in reduced amounts (Table 17-1). The two major forms are α- and β-thalassemia and the rare forms include γ-, δ-, and εγδβ-thalassemia. The mutations that cause a complete absence of globin-chain synthesis are referred to as alpha null- (α⁰-) or beta null- (β⁰-) thalassemia, whereas those that lead to a reduced production are called alpha plus- (α⁺-) or beta plus (β⁺-) thalassemia. δβ-Thalassemia is also subdivided in the same way. In the Lepore Hbs, another form of δβ⁺-thalassemia, an abnormal Hb is produced that has normal α-globin chains combined with non–α-globin chains consisting of the N-terminal residues of the δ-globin chain fused to the C-terminal residues of the β-globin chain. As discussed in more detail later (see "Globin Gene Clusters"), the α-globin gene cluster is found on chromosome 16, consisting of 2 α- and 1 ζ-globin genes, while the β-globin gene cluster is found on chromosome 11 and consists of 1 ε-, 2 γ-, 1 δ-, and 1 β-globin genes.

As a consequence of an overlap in the regions of prevalence of α- and β-thalassemia and some Hb variants (eg, HbS, HbE, and HbC), it is not unusual to encounter individuals who have coinherited α-thalassemia with β-thalassemia and different combinations of structural Hb mutants: for example, HbE/β-thalassemia, HbS/β-thalassemia, and HbS/C-thalassemia, with or without coinheritance of α-thalassemia. These different interactions produce a clinically diverse family of genetic disorders that range in severity from causing death in utero to extremely mild, symptomless microcytic and hypochromic anemias encompassed in the group of disorders known collectively as the thalassemia syndromes.[1] The clinical severity of thalassemia depends largely on the inherited genotype. Being autosomal recessive, homozygotes or compound heterozygotes of β-thalassemia may have severe or moderate anemia, whereas heterozygotes in which one β-globin gene is

TABLE 17–1. Thalassemias and Related Disorders
α-Thalassemia
α⁰
α⁺
Deletion (−α)
Nondeletion (αᵀ)
β-Thalassemia
β⁰
β⁺
Normal hemoglobin A₂
Dominant
Unlinked to β-globin genes
δβ-Thalassemia
(δβ)⁺
(δβ)⁰
(ᴬγ δβ)⁰
γ-Thalassemia
δ-Thalassemia
δ⁰
δ⁺
εγδβ-Thalassemia
Hereditary Persistence of Fetal Hemoglobin
Deletion
(δβ),⁰ (ᴬγ δβ)⁰
Nondeletion
Linked to β-globin genes
ᴳγ β⁺, ᴬγ β⁺
Unlinked to β-globin genes

functioning normally, may have a mild microcytic anemia. Some heterozygotes, such as those with a single α-globin gene deleted, may have no abnormal hematologic parameters (silent carriers). Other rare forms include varieties of β-thalassemia that are inherited in a dominant fashion where heterozygotes may be severely affected (resulting in thalassemia intermedia), and others in which the genetic determinants are not linked to the β-globin gene cluster.[1,10-13]

δ-Thalassemia[1,12] is characterized by reduced output of δ-globin chains and hence reduced HbA₂ levels in heterozygotes and an absence of HbA₂ in homozygotes. They are of no clinical significance except that, when co-inherited with β-thalassemia trait, the level of HbA₂ is reduced to the reference range, making the diagnosis of β-thalassemia trait difficult by Hb characterization alone.

A disorder characterized by defective ε-globin, γ-globin, δ-globin, and β-globin chain synthesis (εγδβ-thalassemia) may result from either a large deletion in chromosome 11 involving all of these genes, or, in some cases, the deletions remove upstream regions, including the β-globin locus control region (LCR) but leaves the β-globin gene itself intact.[1,13] The homozygous state for εγδβ-thalassemia has not been reported and presumably is not compatible with fetal survival; only the heterozygous state has been reported; these persons have normal HbA₂ level.

Hereditary persistence of fetal hemoglobin (HPFH) is a condition in which variably elevated fetal Hb levels persist into adult life. There may or may not be a concomitant absence or reduction in HbA production, and if so, the total Hb is usually reduced.[1,12,14] As a result of the associated increase in fetal Hb, δβ-thalassemia and γδβ-thalassemia have been considered as a type of HPFH. The distinction between conventional HPFH and the (γ)δβ-thalassemias is subtle, and largely based on the degree of compensatory increase in fetal Hb as shown by the total Hb levels and red cell indices, as well as the associated clinical phenotype. HPFH heterozygotes have essentially normal red cell indices, normal HbA$_2$ levels, and HbF levels of 10% to 35%, while heterozygotes for δβ-thalassemia have hypochromic microcytic erythrocytes, HbA$_2$ levels are also normal, but the HbF increases are less (5%-15%). Compound heterozygotes of β-thalassemia and HPFH have a very mild or no anemia in contrast to compound heterozygotes of δβ-thalassemia with β-thalassemia and δβ-thalassemia homozygotes that have disease severity ranging from mild anemia to transfusion dependence. Both rare conditions could be caused by large deletions of the β-globin gene cluster or nucleotide insertions/deletions/substitutions and are generally limited to a geographical region. They are often named according to the population in which they occur, for example, Greek HPFH and British HPFH.[12] Another heterogeneous group of HPFH determinants is associated with very low levels of persistent fetal Hb, the genetic loci of which, at least in some cases, are not linked to the β-globin gene cluster, and are inherited independently of β-thalassemia.[12]

As α-globin is an essential part of normal fetal ($α_2γ_2$) and normal adult ($α_2β_2$) Hb, a deficiency of α-globin chain production affects Hb synthesis in both fetal and adult life. Decreased α-globin chain synthesis in fetal life results in an excess of γ-globin chains, which form $γ_4$ tetramers, given the eponym Hb$_{Bart's}$, as it was first described at St. Bartholomew's Hospital; in adult life, a deficiency of α-globin chains results in an excess of β-globin chains, which form $β_4$ tetramers, given the designation HbH. Normal individuals have four α-globin genes arranged as linked pairs, $α_2$ and $α_1$, at the tip of each chromosome 16, the normal α genotype being represented as αα/αα. α-Thalassemia can be classified as α^0-thalassemia, in which no α-globin chains are produced from the linked pair, and α$^+$-thalassemia in which production of α-globin chain is reduced as a result of the affected genes on that chromosome. α-Thalassemia is most commonly caused by deletions. α^0-Thalassemia is caused by deletion of both α-globin genes on the same chromosome; they vary in size, tend to be geographically isolated, with two particularly common ones, /--^{SEA} in Southeast Asia and /--^{MED} in the Mediterranean region. Two α-globin gene deletions may also occur in *trans* configuration, and the resulting clinical outcome is similar to that of two deletions in *cis* configuration. When all four α genes are defective (homozygous α^0-thalassemia or α-thalassemia major), the result is severe anemia in utero, leading to hydrops fetalis, three gene defects lead to HbH disease, and two gene defects lead to α-thalassemia trait, a mild microcytic anemia similar to β-thalassemia trait.[1,15] Nondeletional mutations have a more heterogenous presentation; some lead to production of a variant that is unstable, such as Hb$^{Constant Spring}$ that has a more severe clinical course then a single α gene deletion. There also may be supernumerary α-globin genes (triplicated or quadruplicated), which in the presence of normal β-globin expression, do not have much clinical significance. However, in the presence of reduced β-globin expression, the extra α-globin genes may exaggerate the α:β-globin chain imbalance, and lead to more severe disease. Similarly, fewer α-globin genes, that is, coinheritance of α-thalassemia in the presence of β-globin abnormalities, may ameliorate severity, as the globin imbalance is less marked.

● EPIDEMIOLOGY AND POPULATION GENETICS

Originally, thalassemia was most prevalent in sub-Saharan African, the Mediterranean, the Middle East, the Indian subcontinent, throughout Southeast Asia and China, and central Asia (Tajikistan, Turkmenistan, Kyrgyzstan) (Fig. 17-1).[1,16] Immigration from these areas to other parts

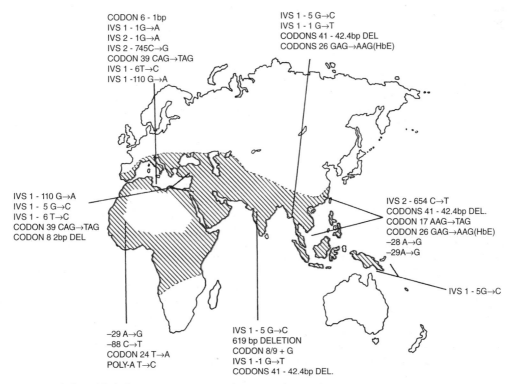

Figure 17–1. Most commonly found β-thalassemia mutations in these prevalent regions.

of the world, including Australia and the Americas, has resulted in the α-thalassemia and β-thalassemia genes and clinical disease being found all over the world. β-Thalassemias in sub-Saharan Africa tend to be of the milder type, and do not pose a major problem. β-Thalassemia also occurs sporadically in all racial groups and has been observed in the homozygous state in persons of apparently pure Anglo-Saxon heritage. A number of these "sporadic" forms have been described in single families and are de novo; unlike the typical autosomal recessive forms that have been coselected by malaria, these de novo variants are dominantly inherited in that individuals with a single copy of the mutation have a thalassemia intermedia phenotype. Thus, while a patient's ethnic background might suggest a decreased predisposition, it does not preclude the diagnosis. New population and immigration studies have provided updated information on the changing epidemiology of thalassemia.[17,18]

δβ-Thalassemia and Hb[Lepore] syndromes have been observed sporadically in many racial groups, although there are few high-frequency populations; the exception is central Italy, Western Europe, and parts of Spain and Portugal, where the Lepore syndromes are more prevalent.

α-Thalassemia also occurs widely throughout the world, including Africa, the Mediterranean countries, the Middle East, and Southeast Asia (Fig. 17-2).[1,16] α-Thalassemia major (α[0]-thalassemia) is found most commonly in Mediterranean and Oriental populations because of the higher prevalence of two-gene deletions in *cis* configuration, but are extremely rare in African and Middle Eastern populations, where two-gene deletions are usually in *trans* configuration. One or two α-gene deletions occur at a high frequency throughout West Africa, the Mediterranean, the Middle East, and Southeast Asia. In the United States, approximately 30% of Americans of African descent carry these defects, predominantly caused by a one-gene deletion. In some parts of Papua New Guinea, up to 80% of the population are carriers. The frequency of nondeletion forms of α[+]-thalassemia in most regions is uncertain; however, they have been reported frequently in some of the Mediterranean island populations and in the Middle Eastern and Southeast Asian populations. The α-globin chain termination mutants, such as Hb[Constant Spring], seem to be particularly common in Southeast Asia. Approximately 4% of the population in Thailand are carriers.

Although more than 300 β-thalassemia alleles have now been described (https://www.ithanet.eu/db/ithagenes; http://globin.bx.psu.edu/hbvar), approximately 40 account for 90% or more of β-thalassemia worldwide.[19] In each of the high-frequency areas for β-thalassemia, a few common mutations and varying numbers of rare mutations are seen (see Fig. 17-1); these are located on the different haplotypes of the β-globin gene cluster.[16,20] Similar observations have been made in α-thalassemia (see Fig. 17-2).[1,16] This indicates that thalassemia arose independently in different populations and then achieved their high frequency by selection. However, with higher resolution haplotyping, some of the notions of "independent" origins are challenged by studies showing that these apparently different haplotypes may have descended from a common ancestral origin as was shown for the sickle cell mutation, challenging Yuet W. Kan's proposal of several independent origins of the sickle mutation.[21,22]

In 1949, J.B.S. Haldane suggested that thalassemia had reached its high frequency in tropical regions because heterozygotes are protected against malaria.[23] In Sardinia, the observation that the β-thalassemia mutation is less common in the mountainous regions and malaria is rare supported Haldane's proposal that β-thalassemia reached its high frequency because of protection against malaria.[24] Other selection factors may co-exist. Malaria endemicity data and globin–gene mapping showed a clear altitude-related effect on the frequency of α-thalassemia in Papua New Guinea. In contrast, gradual change in the frequency of α-thalassemia in the region stretching south from Papua New Guinea through the island populations of Melanesia to New Caledonia is accompanied by a similar gradient in the distribution of malaria.[25] In addition, direct evidence for protection of individuals with mild forms of α[+]-thalassemia against *Plasmodium falciparum* malaria has been provided by a case-control study performed in Papua New Guinea, wherein the homozygous state for α[+]-thalassemia offered approximately 60% protection against hospitalization with coma and severe anemia.[26] Similar levels of protection by α-thalassemia against *P. falciparum* malaria have been found in several different African populations.[27,28] Even though α-thalassemia and the sickle cell trait each offer strong protection against *P. falciparum* malaria, those who inherit both traits are fully susceptible to the disease.[29] Interactions of this type will have an important effect on the gene frequency of protective polymorphisms in countries in which more than 1 polymorphism exists in the same population.

Immune mechanisms contribute to these protective effects against malarial infection. Neonates with α-thalassemia are more prone to *Plasmodium vivax* and *P. falciparum* malaria in the first year of life. Because of cross-immunization between these 2 species, it is likely that early immunization by *P. vivax* may impart greater resistance to *P. falciparum* malaria in those with α-thalassemia later in life.[30] Even though α-thalassemia has no effect on the rates of parasite invasion and growth in red cells, these parasitized red cells are more susceptible to phagocytosis in vitro and have low levels of complement receptor 1.[31] Further details regarding the relationship of thalassemia mutations to malaria may be found in cited sources.[18,28,32]

● ETIOLOGY AND PATHOGENESIS

GENETIC CONTROL AND SYNTHESIS OF HEMOGLOBIN

The structure and ontogeny of the Hbs are reviewed in Chaps. 2 and 18, respectively. Only those aspects with particular relevance to the thalassemia syndromes are discussed here.

Red cells in normal individuals contain a mix of different Hbs, all of which have a similar structure of two separate pairs of identical globin chains (heterodimer) and four heme molecules, each with an atom of iron, the heme molecules being responsible for oxygen binding. Except for some of the embryonic Hbs (see below), all normal human Hbs have one pair of α-globin chains. In adults, HbA (heterodimer of α-globin and β-globin, $\alpha_2\beta_2$) is predominant, with the remainder consisting of

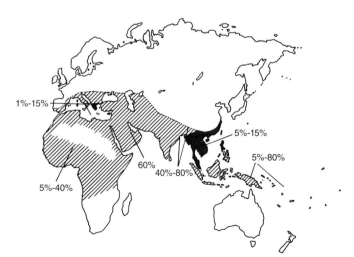

Figure 17–2. Fequency of alpha-thalassemia mutations in the prevalent regions. α[+]-thalassemia *(hatched areas)* and α[0]-thalassemia *(shaded areas)*.

less than 3.5% of HbA$_2$ (heterodimer of α-globin and δ-globin, α$_2$δ$_2$), and less than 2% of fetal Hb or HbF (heterodimer of α-globin and γ-globin, α$_2$γ$_2$). However, there is an adaptive evolution of Hbs from conception through the fetal period, through childhood into adulthood, and knowledge of this progression is important in understanding the pathophysiology and development of the various thalassemia syndromes and for approaches to their prenatal diagnosis.

Red cells are initially made in the yolk sac of the developing embryo and prior to week 8 of intrauterine life, 3 embryonic Hbs—Gower 1 (ξ$_2$ε$_2$), Gower 2 (α$_2$ε$_2$), and Portland (ξ$_2$γ$_2$)—are present. The ξ-globin and ε-globin chains are the embryonic counterparts of the adult α-globin and γ-, β-, and δ- globin chains, respectively. ξ-Globin chain synthesis persists beyond the embryonic stage of development in some forms of α-thalassemia. Persistent ε-globin chain production has not been found in any of the thalassemia syndromes. As the embryo develops into the fetus, erythropoiesis moves to the liver and spleen; there is an orderly switch from ξ-globin to α-globin synthesis and from ε-globin to γ-globin synthesis; and the predominant Hb is HbF or α$_2$γ$_2$. HbF is a mixture of molecular species with the formulas α$_2$γ$_2^{136Gly}$ and α$_2$γ$_2^{136Ala}$ (Chap. 18). The γ–globin chains containing glycine at position 136 are designated ^{G}γ-globin, while those containing alanine are called ^{A}γ-globin chains. At birth, the ratio of molecules containing ^{G}γ-globin chains to those containing ^{A}γ-globin chains is approximately 3:1. Toward the end of the second trimester, the marrow becomes active in erythropoiesis, and red cells produced thereafter contain predominantly adult Hb or HbA-α$_2$β$_2$. At birth, a term infant still has approximately 80% to 90% HbF and the rest is HbA. Postnatally, γ-globin chain production is replaced by β-globin chain production, resulting in the production of mostly HbA, commonly referred to as Hb switching, such that between 6 and 12 months of age, HbA becomes the predominant Hb but residual levels of HbF continue to be produced. From that point on, red cells are produced exclusively in the marrow, and the Hb is predominantly HbA, with less than 1% of HbF still being made; however, production of HbF persists at higher levels in some individuals. The ratio of ^{G}γ-globin chains to ^{A}γ-globin chains in the trace amounts of HbF in normal adults' switches from a ratio of 3:1 to approximately 1:3. HbA$_2$ (α$_2$δ$_2$) is the minor adult Hb, and comprises approximately 2.5% of the total Hb in adults.

During fetal development and at birth, a term infant has a high Hb level as a result of having predominantly high-oxygen-affinity HbF, with relative tissue hypoxemia and an increased erythropoietic drive leading to erythrocytosis. Immediately postnatally, erythropoiesis is switched off given the abundance of oxygen, and the Hb level gradually drops until erythropoietin production resumes at the physiologic nadir

of infancy—at a Hb level of 9–10 g/dL—usually by 8 weeks in a term infant. Erythropoiesis resumes and the Hb level rises again, although not to prenatal levels (Chap. 2).

Figure 17-3 shows the different human Hbs and the arrangements of the α-gene cluster on chromosome 16 and the β-gene cluster on chromosome 11.

GLOBIN GENE CLUSTERS

Although some individual variability exists, the α-gene cluster usually contains one functional ξ gene and two α genes, designated α$_2$ and α$_1$, respectively. It also contains four pseudogenes: ψξ$_1$, ψα$_1$, ψα$_2$, and θ$_1$.[14,15] These four pseudogenes are remarkably conserved among different species. Although they appear to be expressed early in fetal life, their function is unknown. It is likely they do not produce a viable globin chain. Each α gene is located in a region of homology approximately 4 kb long, interrupted by two small nonhomologous regions.[33-35] The homologous regions are believed to result from gene duplication, and the nonhomologous segments are believed to arise subsequently by insertion of DNA into the noncoding regions around one of the two genes. The exons of the two α-globin genes have identical sequences. The first intron in each gene is identical. The second intron of α$_1$ is 9 bases longer and differs by 3 bases from that in the α$_2$ gene.[35-37] Despite their high degree of homology, the sequences of the two α-globin genes diverge in their 3' untranslated regions 13 bases beyond the TAA stop codon. These differences provide an opportunity to assess the relative output of the genes, an important part of the analysis of α-thalassemia.[38,39] Production of α$_2$ mRNA appears to exceed that of α$_1$ by a factor of 1.5-3.0. ψξ$_1$ and ξ genes also are highly homologous and their introns are much larger than those of α-globin genes. In contrast to the latter, their intervening sequence (IVS) of a gene (ie, an intron) differ; IVS-1 is larger than IVS-2. In each ξ gene, IVS-1 contains several copies of a simple repeated 14-base pair (bp) sequence that is similar to sequences located between the two ξ genes and near the human insulin gene. The coding sequence of the first exon of ψξ$_1$ contains three base changes, one of which gives rise to a premature stop codon, thus making ψξ$_1$ an inactive gene, that is, a pseudogene.

The regions separating and surrounding the α-like structural genes have been analyzed in detail. Of particular relevance to thalassemia is the polymorphic nature of this gene cluster.[40] The cluster contains five hypervariable regions: one downstream from the α$_1$ gene, one between the ξ and ψξ genes, one in the first intron of both the ξ and ψξ genes, and one 5' to the cluster. These regions consist of varying numbers of tandem repeats of nucleotide sequences. Taken together with single-base

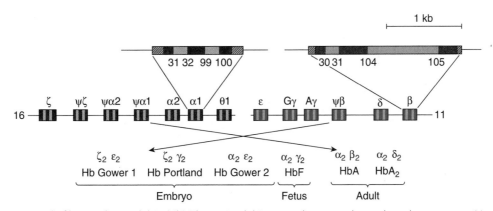

Figure 17–3. Genetic control of human hemoglobin (Hb). The main globin gene clusters are located on chromosomes 11 and 16. At each stage of development, different genes in these clusters are activated or repressed. The different globin chains directed by individual genes are synthesized independently and combine in random fashion as indicated by the arrows.

restriction fragment length polymorphisms (RFLPs), the variability of the α-globin gene cluster reaches a heterozygosity level of approximately 0.95. Thus, each parental α-globin gene cluster can be identified in the majority of persons. This heterogeneity has important implications for tracing the history of the α-thalassemia mutations.

Figure 17-3 shows the arrangement of the β-globin gene cluster on the short arm of chromosome 11. Each of the individual genes and their flanking regions have been sequenced.[41-44] Like the α_1 and α_2 gene pairs, the ^{G}γ and ^{A}γ genes share a similar sequence. In fact, the ^{G}γ and ^{A}γ genes on one chromosome are identical in the region 5′ to the center of the large intron, yet show some divergence 3′ to that position. At the boundary between the conserved and divergent regions, a block of simple sequence may be a "hot spot" for initiation of recombination events that lead to unidirectional gene conversion.

Like the α-globin genes, the β-gene cluster contains multiple single nucleotide variants, some affecting cleavage sites of restriction enzymes, that is, RFLPs. No hypervariable regions have been identified.[45,46] The arrangement of RFLPs, or haplotypes, in the β-globin gene cluster falls into two domains. The 5′ side of the β–globin gene, spanning approximately 32 kb from the ε gene to the 3′ end of the ψβ gene, contains three common patterns of RFLPs. The region encompassing approximately 18 kb to the 3′ side of the β-globin gene also contains three common patterns in different populations. Between these regions is a sequence of approximately 11 kb in which there is randomization of the 5′ and 3′ domains; hence, a relatively higher frequency of recombination can occur, sometimes referred to as "hotspots."[46] The β-globin gene haplotypes are similar in most populations but differ markedly in individuals of African origin. These findings suggest the haplotype arrangements were laid down very early during evolution. The findings are consistent with data obtained from mitochondrial DNA polymorphisms pointing to the early emergence of a relatively small population from Africa with subsequent divergence into other racial groups.[47] Again, they are extremely useful for analyzing the population genetics and history of the thalassemia mutations. Haplotypes based on the RFLPS have very low resolution. Whole-genome sequencing can allow much higher resolution of linkage disequilibrium mapping, and generation of haplotypes based on single nucleotide resolution could provide insights as to whether the mutations share an ancestral origin or arose independently.[21,22]

The regions flanking the coding regions of the globin genes contain a number of conserved sequences essential for their expression.[36,41] The first conserved sequence is in the 5′ (promoter) which encompasses the TATA box (an 8-bp AT-rich sequence in the promoter, and a binding site for the TATA-box binding proteins) that serves accurately to locate the site of transcription initiation at the CAP site (a DNA site located in or near a promoter), usually about 30 bases downstream. It also influences the rate of transcription. In addition, two other upstream promoter elements are present. A second conserved sequence, the CCAAT box, is located 70 bp or 80 bp upstream. The third conserved sequence, the CACCC homology box, is located further 5′, approximately 80-100 bp from the CAP site. It can be either inverted or duplicated. These promoter sequences also are required for optimal transcription. Mutations in this region of the β-globin gene cause its defective expression and these findings provided a foundation for understanding regulation of other human genes. The globin genes also have conserved sequences in their 3′ flanking regions, notably AATAAA, which is the polyadenylation signal site. A sequence important for expression (enhancer) is also found in intron 2 and 600-900 bases downstream of the polyadenylation (AATAAA) site.

REGULATION OF GLOBIN GENE CLUSTERS

Figure 17-4 summarizes the mechanism of globin gene expression. The primary transcript is an mRNA precursor containing both intron and

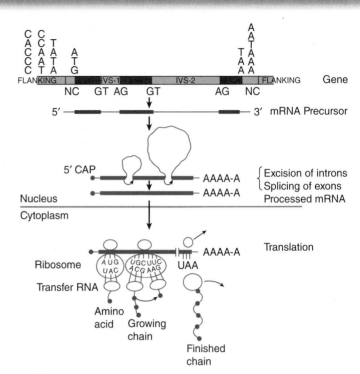

FIGURE 17–4. Expression of a human globin gene.

exon sequences. During its stay in the nucleus, it undergoes processing that entails capping the 5′ end and polyadenylation of the 3′ end, both of which probably serve to stabilize the transcript. The IVSs are removed from the mRNA precursor in a complex two-stage process that relies on certain critical sequences at the intron-exon junctions.

The method by which globin gene clusters are regulated is important for understanding the pathogenesis of thalassemia. Many details remain to be determined, but studies provide at least an outline of some of the major mechanisms of globin gene regulation.[1,10,48-50]

Most of the DNA within cells that is not involved in gene transcription is packaged into a compact form that is inaccessible to transcription factors and RNA polymerase. Transcriptional activity is characterized by a major change in the structure of the chromatin surrounding a particular gene. These alterations in chromatin structure can be identified by enhanced sensitivity to exogenous nucleases. Erythroid lineage-specific nuclease-hypersensitive sites are found at several locations in the β-globin gene cluster, which vary during different stages of development. In fetal life, these sites are associated with the promoter regions of all four globin genes. In adult erythroid cells, the sites associated with the γ genes are absent. The methylation state of the genes plays an important role in their ability to be expressed. In human and other animal tissues, the globin genes are extensively methylated in nonerythroid organs (sites of nonexpression) and are relatively undermethylated in hematopoietic tissues. Changes in chromatin configuration around the globin genes at different stages of development are reflected by alterations in their methylation state.

In addition to the promoter elements, several other important regulatory sequences have been identified in the globin gene clusters. Several enhancer sequences thought to be involved with tissue-specific expression have been identified. Their sequences are similar to the upstream activating sequences of the promoter elements. Both consist of a number of "modules," or motifs, that contain binding sites for transcriptional activators or repressors. The enhancer sequences are thought to act by coming into spatial apposition with the promoter sequences to increase the efficiency of transcription of particular genes.

Transcriptional regulatory proteins may bind to both the promoter region of a gene and to the enhancer. Some of these transcriptional proteins, GATA-1 and NFE-2, for example, are largely restricted to hematopoietic tissues.[49,51] These proteins may bring the promoter and the enhancer into close physical proximity, permitting transcription factors bound to the enhancer to interact with the transcriptional complex that forms near the TATA box. At least some of these hematopoietic gene transcription factors likely will be specific to the developmental stage.

Another set of erythroid-specific nuclease-hypersensitive sites is located upstream from the embryonic globin genes in both the α-globin and β-globin gene clusters. These sites mark the regions of particularly important control elements. In the case of the β-globin gene cluster, the region is marked by five hypersensitive sites to deoxyribonuclease (DNase) I treatment (an enzyme used to detect DNA-protein interaction) and designated HS1 to HS5, distributed between 6 kb and 20 kb upstream of the ε gene.[49] The most 5′ site (HS5) does not show tissue specificity. HS1 through HS4, which together form the β-globin LCR (β-LCR), are largely erythroid specific. Each of the regions of the β-LCR contains a variety of binding sites for erythroid transcription factors. The precise function of the β-LCR is not known, but it is required to establish a transcriptionally active domain spanning the entire globin gene cluster. The α-globin gene cluster also has a major regulatory element of this kind, in this case HS40.[50] This forms part of four highly conserved noncoding sequences, or multispecies conserved sequences (MCSs), called MCS-R1-R4; of these elements only MCS-R2, that is, HS40, is essential for α-globin gene expression. Although deletions of this region inactivate the entire α-globin gene cluster, its action must be fundamentally different from that of the β-LCR because the chromatin structure of the α-gene cluster is in an open conformation in all tissues.

Some forms of α-thalassemia and β-thalassemia result from deletions or single-base mutations involving these regulatory regions. In addition, the phenotypic effects of deletions of these gene clusters are strongly positional, which may reflect the relative distance of particular genes from the β-LCR and HS40.

Developmental Changes in Globin Gene Expression

One particularly important aspect of human globin genes is the switch from fetal to adult Hb production. Because thalassemia and related disorders of the β-globin gene cluster are often associated with persistent γ-globin chain synthesis, a full understanding of their pathophysiology must include an explanation for this important phenomenon, which plays a considerable role in modifying their phenotypic expression.

The complex topic of Hb switching has been the subject of several extensive reviews.[1,48] β-Globin synthesis commences early during fetal life, at approximately 8-10 weeks of gestation. β-Globin synthesis continues at a low level at approximately 10% of the total non–α-globin chain production, up to approximately 36 weeks of gestation, after which it is considerably augmented. At the same time, γ-globin chain synthesis starts to decline so that, at birth, approximately equal amounts of γ-globin and β-globin chains are produced. Over the first year of life, γ-globin chain synthesis gradually declines. By the end of the first year, γ-chain synthesis amounts to less than 1% of the total non–α-globin chain output. The production of γ-globin chain persists at very low levels in adults, and the small amount of HbF is confined to an erythrocyte population called *F cells*.

How this series of developmental switches is regulated is not clear. The process is not organ specific, but is synchronized throughout the developing hematopoietic tissues. Although environmental factors may be involved, the bulk of experimental evidence suggests some form of "time clock" is built into the hematopoietic stem cell. At the chromosomal level, regulation appears to occur in a complex manner involving both developmental stage-specific *trans*-activating factors and the relative proximity of the different genes of the β-globin gene cluster to the β-LCR. A dual mechanism has been proposed for the developmental switch: gene competition for the upstream β-LCR, conferring advantage for the gene closest to the LCR and autonomous silencing (transcriptional repression) of the preceding gene. The ability to compete for the β-LCR and autonomous silencing depends on the change in the abundance and repertoire of various transcription factors that favor promoter-LCR interaction. The ε- and γ-globin genes are autonomously silenced at the appropriate developmental stage, but expression of the adult β-globin gene depends on lack of competition from the upstream γ-gene for the LCR sequences. Concordant with this mechanism, when the γ-gene is upregulated by point mutations in their promoter causing a nondeletion HPFH, expression of the *cis* β-gene is downregulated. BCL11A has been identified as a key repressor of the γ-globin gene and a critical mediator in the switch from fetal to adult Hb expression. KLF1 (erythroid Kruppel-like factor), a developmental stage–enriched protein, activates human β-globin gene expression and also activates BCL11A, thus providing a double advantage for increasing β-globin gene expression in adult life.[52] MYB also has been proposed to modulate HbF expression via activation of KLF1 and other repressors of the γ-globin gene.[48]

Fetal Hb synthesis can be reactivated at low levels in states of hematopoietic stress and at higher levels in certain hematologic malignancies, notably juvenile myelomonocytic leukemia. However, high levels of HbF production are seen consistently in adult life only in the hemoglobinopathies.

● MOLECULAR BASIS OF THE THALASSEMIAS

Once cloning and sequencing of globin genes from patients with many different forms of thalassemia were possible, the wide spectrum of mutations underlying these conditions became clear. A picture of remarkable heterogeneity has emerged. For more extensive coverage of this topic, the reader is referred to several monographs and reviews.[1,10,12,53,54]

β-THALASSEMIA

β-Thalassemia is extremely heterogeneous at the molecular level.[1] More than 300 different mutations have been found in association with the β-thalassemia phenotype (http://www.ithanet.eu/db/ithagenes; http://globin.bx.psu.edu/hbvar).[1] Broadly, they fall into deletions of the β-globin gene and nondeletional mutations that reduce expression of the β-globin gene by affecting transcription, processing, or translation of β-globin messenger RNA (Table 17-2 and Fig. 17-5). In contrast to α-thalassemia, which is mainly caused by deletions, the vast majority of mutations causing β-thalassemia are nondeletional. Each major population group has a different set of β-thalassemia mutations, usually consisting of two or three mutations (possibly reflecting local selection resulting from malaria) forming the bulk and larger numbers of less-common mutations. Consequently, each of these populations has its own spectrum of β-thalassemia alleles. Because of this distribution pattern, approximately 40 alleles account for the majority of all β-thalassemia determinants (see Fig. 17-1).

Gene Deletions

β-Thalassemia is rarely caused by deletions. At least 18 different deletions affecting only the β genes have been described. With one exception, the deletions are rare and appear to be isolated, single events. The 619-bp deletion at the 3′ end of the β-gene is more common,[55] but even that is restricted to the Sind and Gujarati populations of Pakistan and India, where it accounts for approximately 50% of β-thalassemia

TABLE 17–2. Molecular Pathology of the β-Thalassemias

β⁰-Thalassemia or β⁺-thalassemia
  Transcription
    Deletions
    Insertions
    Promoter
    5′-UTR
  Processing of mRNA
    Junctional
    Consensus splicing sequences
    Cryptic splice sites in introns
    Cryptic splice sites in exons
    PolyA addition site
  Translation
    Initiation
    Nonsense
    Frameshift
  Posttranslational stability
    Unstable β-chain variants
Normal hemoglobin A₂ β-thalassemia
    β-Thalassemia and δ-thalassemia, *cis* or *trans*
    "Silent" β-thalassemia
    Some promoter mutations
    CAP +1, CAP +3, etc
    5′ UTR
    Some splice mutations
Dominant β-thalassemia
    Mainly point mutations or rearrangements in exon 3
    Other unstable variants

UTR, untranslated region.
Note: A full list of mutations is given in Refs. 1 and 13.

alleles.[55] The Indian 619-bp deletion removes the 3′ end of the β-gene but leaves the 5′ end intact. A majority of the other deletions, that differ widely in size, remove the 5′ end of the gene that contain the β promoter sequences and leave the δ-gene intact.[56-60] All of these deletions abolish β-globin gene expression, causing β⁰-thalassemia. Even though heterozygotes for the Indian 619-bp deletion have increased HbA₂ and HbF levels identical to those seen in heterozygotes for the other common

forms of β-thalassemia, heterozygotes for the deletions that remove the 5′ end all have much higher HbA₂ and HbF levels. The mechanism underlying the elevated levels of increased δ-globin chain and γ-globin chain production results from increased transcription of these genes in *cis* to the deletion, possibly as a result of reduced competition from the deleted 5′ β-gene for transcription factors and access to the β-LCR. This mechanism may also explain the unusually high HbA₂ and HbF levels that accompany the point mutations in the β promoter region. The increase in HbF appears to be adequate to compensate for the complete absence of HbA in homozygotes for these deletions, of which two cases have been reported and both were reported as having intermediate thalassemia.[61,62]

Nondeletional β-Thalassemia Mutations

Transcriptional Mutations Several different base substitutions involve the conserved sequences upstream from the β-globin gene.[1] In every case, the phenotype is β⁺-thalassemia, although considerable variability exists in the clinical severity associated with different mutations of this type. Several mutations, at positions −88 and −87 relative to the mRNA CAP site,[63,64] are close to the CCAAT box, whereas others lie within the TATA box homology.[65-68]

Some mutations upstream from the β-globin gene are associated with even more subtle alterations in phenotype. For example, a C→T substitution at position −101, which involves one of the upstream promoter elements, is associated with "silent" β-thalassemia, that is, a completely normal ("silent") phenotype that can be identified only by its interaction with more severe forms of β-thalassemia in compound heterozygotes.[69] Another example of a "silent" mutation is an A→C substitution at the CAP site (+1) which was described in an Asian Indian who, despite being homozygous for the mutation, appeared to have a phenotype of the β-thalassemia trait.[70]

Upstream regulatory mutations confirm the importance of the role of conserved sequences in this region as regulators of the transcription of the β-globin genes and provide the basis for some of the mildest forms of β-thalassemia, particularly those in African populations, and for some varieties of "silent" β-thalassemia.

RNA-Processing Mutations One surprise about β-thalassemia has been the remarkable diversity of the single-base mutations that can interfere with the intranuclear processing of mRNA.

The boundaries of exons and introns are marked by invariant dinucleotides, GT at the 5′ (donor) and AG at the 3′ (receptor) sites. Single-base changes that involve either of these splice junctions totally abolish normal RNA splicing and result in the β⁰-thalassemia phenotype.[1,71-75]

Highly conserved sequences involved in mRNA processing surround the invariant dinucleotides at the splice junctions. Different varieties of β-thalassemia involve single-base substitutions within the consensus sequence of the IVS-1 donor site.[64,66,72-78] These mutations are particularly interesting because of the remarkable variability

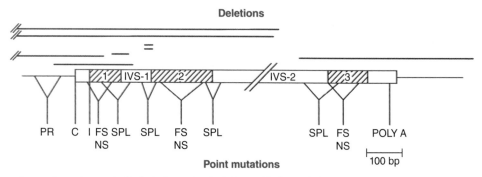

Figure 17–5. Classes of mutations that underlie β-thalassemia. C, CAP site; FS, frameshift; I, initiation site; NS, nonsense mutation; POLY A, polyA addition site mutation; PR, promoter; SPL, splicing mutation. For a complete list, see Ref. 310.

in their associated phenotypes. For example, substitution of the G in position 5 of IVS-1 by C, T, or A, considerably reduces splicing at the mutated donor site compared with the normal β allele, and results in severe β+-thalassemia.[64] On the other hand, a T→C change in the adjacent nucleotide at position 6, found commonly in the Mediterranean region,[79] results in a very mild form of β+-thalassemia. The G→C change at position 5 also has been found in Melanesia and appears to be the most common cause of β-thalassemia in Papua New Guinea.[80]

RNA processing is affected by mutations that create new splice sites within either introns or exons. Again, these lesions are remarkably variable in their phenotypic effect, depending on the degree to which the new site is used compared with the normal splice site. For example, the G→A substitution at position 110 of IVS-1, which is one of the most common forms of β-thalassemia in the Mediterranean region, leads to only approximately 10% splicing at the normal site, which results in a severe β+-thalassemia phenotype.[81,82] Similarly, a mutation that produces a new acceptor site at position 116 in IVS-1 results in little or no β-globin mRNA production and the β0-thalassemia phenotype.[83] Several mutations that generate new donor sites within IVS-2 of the β-globin gene have been described.[64,77]

Another mechanism for abnormal splicing is the activation of donor sites within exons (Fig. 17-6). For example, within exon 1 is a cryptic donor site in the region of codons 24 through 27. This site contains a GT dinucleotide. An adjacent substitution that alters the site so that it more closely resembles the consensus donor splice site results in its activation, even though the normal site is active. Several mutations in this region can activate this site so that it is used during RNA processing, with the production of abnormal mRNAs.[84-87] Three of the substitutions—A→G in codon 19, G→A in codon 26, and G→T in codon 27—result in reduced production of β-globin mRNA and an amino acid substitution so that the mRNA that is spliced normally is translated into protein. The abnormal Hbs produced are Hb[Malay], HbE, and Hb[Knossos], all of which are associated with a β-thalassemia phenotype, presumably as a result of reduced overall output of normal mRNA (Fig. 17-6). A variety of other cryptic splice mutations within introns and exons have been described.[12]

Another class of processing mutation involves the polyadenylation signal site AAUAAA in the 3′ untranslated region of β-globin mRNA.[88-90] For example, a T→C substitution in this sequence leads to only one-tenth the normal amount of β-globin mRNA and hence the severe β+-thalassemia phenotype, while others at this site lead to a mild deficit and are β+-thalassemia alleles.[88]

Mutations Causing Abnormal Translation of mRNA

Base substitutions that change an amino acid codon into a chain termination codon, that is, nonsense mutation, prevent translation of the mRNA and result in β0-thalassemia. Many substitutions of this type have been described.[1,12,13] For example, a codon 17 mutation is common in Southeast Asia,[91,92] and a codon 39 mutation that occurs at a high frequency in the Mediterranean region.[93,94]

The insertion or deletion of 1, 2, or 4 nucleotides in the coding region of the β-globin gene disrupts the normal reading frame and results, upon translation of the mRNA, in the addition of anomalous amino acids until a termination codon is reached in the new reading frame. Several frameshift mutations of this type have been described.[1,12,13] Two mutations—the insertion of 1 nucleotide between codons 8 and 9 and a deletion of 4 nucleotides in codons 41 and 42—are common in Asians.[72] The latter deletions are found frequently in different populations in Southeast Asia.[92] As part of the surveillance mechanism that is active in quality control of the processed mRNA, mRNA harboring a premature termination codon introduced via single-base substitutions or frameshift mutations are destroyed and not transported to the cytoplasm in a phenomenon called *nonsense-mediated RNA decay* to prevent the accumulation of mutant mRNAs coding for truncated peptides.

An unusual β+-thalassemia was described in a patient from the Czech Republic in whom a full-length L1 transposon was inserted into the second intron of β-globin, creating a β+-thalassemia phenotype by an undefined molecular mechanism.[95]

Dominantly Inherited β-Thalassemia

Families indistinguishable from moderately severe β-thalassemia that segregated in a Mendelian dominant fashion have been reported sporadically.[96,97] Because this condition often is characterized by the presence of inclusion bodies in the red cell precursors, it has been called *inclusion-body β-thalassemia*. However, because all severe forms of β-thalassemia have inclusions in the red cell precursors, the term *dominantly inherited β-thalassemia* is preferred to also differentiate such thalassemia mutations from the autosomal recessive forms that are prevalent in malaria-endemic regions.[1,98] Sequence analysis shows that these conditions are heterogeneous at the molecular level, but that many involve mutations in exon 3 of the β-globin gene. The mutations include frameshifts, premature chain-termination mutations, and complex rearrangements that lead to synthesis of truncated or elongated and highly unstable β-globin gene products.[1,99-102] The underlying mechanism of these mutations is that they lead to the production of highly unstable and nonfunctional β-globin variants that are not able to form viable tetramers with α-globin. The most common mutation of this type is a GAA→TAA change at codon 121 that leads to synthesis of a truncated β-globin chain.[103] Although the detection of an abnormal β-globin chain product from loci affected by mutations of this type is unusual because of the chain product's hyperinstability, many of these conditions are designated as Hb variants.

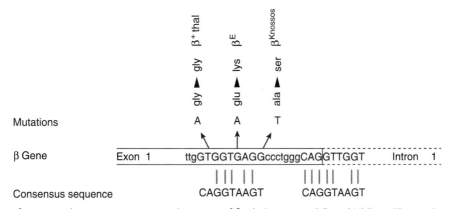

Figure 17–6. Activation of cryptic splice sites in exon 1 as the cause of β+-thalassemia, HbE, and Hb[Knossos]. The similarities between the 5′ splice region of intron 1 and the cryptic splice region in exon 1 are shown in capitals.

Why mutations occurring in exons 1 and 2 produce the classic form of recessive β-thalassemia, whereas the bulk of dominant thalassemia result from mutations in exon 3 has become clearer. In the case of exons 1 and 2, very little abnormal β-globin mRNA is found in the cytoplasm of the red cell precursors, whereas exon 3 mutations are associated with full-length, but abnormal, mRNA accumulations. The different phenotypes of these premature termination codons reflect a nonsense-mediated RNA decay phenomenon, which is a surveillance system to prevent transport of mRNA coding for truncated peptides. Mutations in exon 3 bypass the nonsense-mediated RNA decay surveillance, leading to synthesis of these highly unstable Hb variants.[104-106] A complete list of the mutations that underlie dominant β-thalassemia is given in Ref. 12. The dominantly inherited β-thalassemia variants are rare, and found in dispersed geographical regions where the gene frequency for β-thalassemia is very low. Furthermore, many of these variants are unique to the families described, and occur as de novo mutations.

Silent β-Thalassemia

A number of extremely mild β-thalassemia alleles are either silent or almost unidentifiable in heterozygotes (see Table 17-2). Some alleles are in the region of the promoter boxes of the β-globin gene, but others involve the CAP sites, the 5′ or 3′ untranslated regions.[1,12,13] These alleles are usually identified by finding a form of β-thalassemia intermedia in an individual who has inherited a typical thalassemia mutation from one parent who has a typical thalassemia trait, and another from the other parent who appears to be normal but, in fact, is a carrier of one of the mild β-thalassemia alleles.

β-Thalassemia Mutations Unlinked to the β-Globin Gene Cluster

Rarely, mutations in other genes distinct from the β-globin complex can downregulate β-globin expression.[107] Such cases generally come to light through family studies as in the case of a fourth-generation family with X-linked thrombocytopenia and β-thalassemia, in which the causative mutation was shown to be in the amino finger of erythroid-specific GATA-1, which was affecting DNA binding.[108] Another group affects the xeroderma pigmentosa (XPD) protein, which is part of the general transcription factor TF11H. Eleven patients with trichothiodystrophy with mutations in XPD had hematologic features of β-thalassemia trait.[109]

Variant Forms of β-Thalassemia

In several forms of β-thalassemia, the HbA_2 level is normal in heterozygotes. Some cases result from "silent" β-thalassemia alleles, whereas others reflect the coinheritance of β-thalassemia and δ-thalassemia.[1] Although β-thalassemia is caused by germline mutations inherited from one of the parents, the somatic deletion of the β-globin gene contributes to the unusual severity of the phenotype in unrelated families where the affected were constitutionally heterozygous for β-thalassemia.[110,111]

δβ-THALASSEMIA AND HEREDITARY PERSISTENCE OF FETAL HEMOGLOBIN

δβ-Thalassemia and HPFH are much less common than β-thalassemia. These disorders consist of a range of disorders characterized by decreased or absent HbA production and a variable compensatory increase in HbF synthesis. The distinction between δβ-thalassemia and HPFH is subtle and was originally made on hematologic grounds.[12,112,113] But as more cases became recognized, it became evident that there is considerable overlap between the two groups of disorders. The level of compensatory HbF increase is higher in HPFH compared to δβ-thalassemia. HPFH heterozygotes have essentially normal red cell indices, normal HbA_2 levels, and HbF levels of 10% to 35%, whereas heterozygotes for δβ-thalassemia have hypochromic microcytic erythrocytes, HbA_2 levels that are also normal, but with lower (5%-15%) HbF increases. In the past, a feature that was used to distinguish HPFH from δβ-thalassemia was the intercellular distribution of HbF distribution of HbF. In δβ-thalassaemia, in contrast to a pancellular (or homogeneous) distribution noted in HPFH, the intercellular distribution of HbF is uneven in δβ-thalassemia but this phenomenon maybe a reflection of the magnitude of increase and sensitivity of technique used to stain the F cells.[113]

HPFH is best classified into deletion and nondeletion forms (Table 17-3). The deletion forms of HPFH are heterogeneous (Fig. 17-7). Six deletion forms of HPFH have been described in Africans, Mediterraneans, Indians, and Southeast Asians with deletions ranging from

TABLE 17–3. Hereditary Persistence of Fetal Hemoglobin
Deletion (pancellular[a])
$(\delta\beta)^0$
Black (HPFH 1)
Ghanaian (HPFH 2)
Indian (HPFH 3)
Italian (HPFH 4 and HPFH 5)
Vietnamese (HPFH 6)
$^G\gamma (^A\gamma \beta)^+$ (Hb^{Kenya})
Nondeletion
Linked to β-globin gene cluster (pancellular[a])
$^G\gamma \beta^+$
Black $^G\gamma$-202 C→G
Tunisian$^G\gamma$-200+C
Black/Sardinian$^G\gamma$-175 T→C
Japanese$^G\gamma$-114 C→T
Australian$^G\gamma$-114 C→G
$^A\gamma \beta^+$
Greek/Sardinian/Black $^A\gamma$-117 G→A
British $^A\gamma$-198 T→C
Black $^A\gamma$-202 C→T
Italian/Chinese $^A\gamma$-196 C→T
Brazilian $^A\gamma$-195 C→G
Black $^A\gamma$-175 T→C
Black $^A\gamma$-114 to −102 (del)
Georgia $^A\gamma$-114 C→T
$^G\gamma ^A\gamma \beta^+$
Linked to β-globin gene cluster (heterocellular[a])
Atlanta
Czech
Seattle
Others (including some cases of $^G\gamma$-158 T→C)
Unlinked to β-globin gene cluster (heterocellular[a])
BCL11A Chromosome 6
Others

Hb, hemoglobin; HPFH, hereditary persistence of fetal hemoglobin.
[a]The intercellular distribution of HbF is not always reported, and some inconsistencies are present within groups. Complete details are given in Ref. 1.

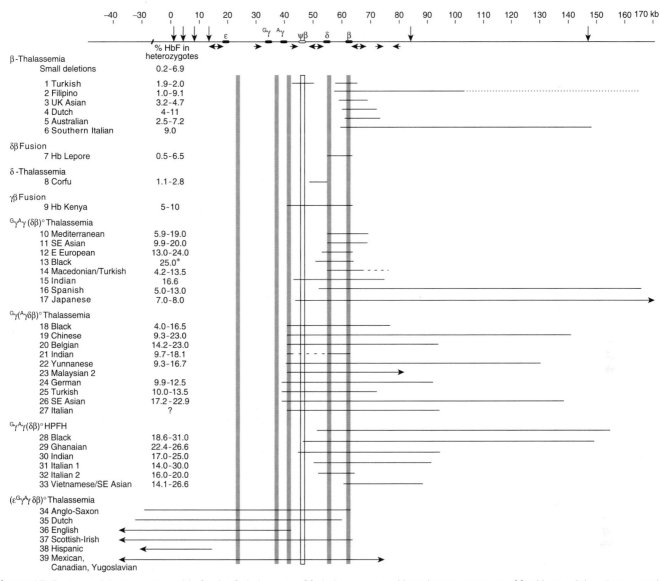

Figure 17–7. Some deletions responsible for the β-thalassemia, δβ-thalassemias, and hereditary persistence of fetal hemoglobin. For a complete list see Ref. 310.

13 kb to 86 kb in size (Fig. 17-7).[12] The commonest forms are the Black HPFH-1 and Black HPFH-2; the latter is also referred to as Ghanaian HPFH. The two African varieties result from extensive deletions of similar length (<70 kb) but with staggered ends, differing phenotypically only in the proportions of $^G\gamma$-globin and $^A\gamma$–globin chains produced.[114] Another type of HPFH results from misalignment during crossing over between the $^A\gamma$-globin and β-globin genes, resulting in production of $^A\gamma\beta$ fusion genes (Fig. 17-8) that combine with α-globin chains to form the Hb variant called Hb$_{Kenya}$.[115,116] Hb$_{Kenya}$ is associated with an increased output of HbF, although at a lower level than in the deletion forms of HPFH. A theory that adequately explains the phenotypic differences between δβ-thalassemia and the deletion forms of HPFH has not been developed.[12]

The nondeletion determinants of HPFH can be classified into those that map within the β-globin gene cluster and those that segregate independently. The former is subdivided into $^G\gamma\beta^+$ and $^A\gamma\beta^+$ varieties, indicating persistent $^G\gamma$-globin or $^A\gamma$-globin chain synthesis in association with β-globin production directed by the β-gene

cis to the HPFH determinant. Analysis of the overexpressed γ-globin genes revealed in each case a single-base substitution or minor deletions in the region immediately upstream from the transcription start site.[1,114,117-119] The mutations are densely clustered in two regions of the promoters, around positions −115 and −200. These regions contain binding sites for ubiquitous and erythroid-specific factors. Altered binding pattern of the transcription factors to the point mutations are thought to be the cause of the elevated HbF levels that vary from 5% to 35% in heterozygotes. The region of DNA at position −115 is involved in binding of the BCL11A repressor protein,[120,121] while the region at position −200 affects binding of ZBTB7A, another γ-globin repressor[120,122] (Fig. 17-9). The most common of these conditions are Greek $^A\gamma\beta^+$ HPFH and a form of $^G\gamma\beta^+$ HPFH that is found in several different African populations. If the upstream point mutations associated with persistent γ-globin chain production occur on the same chromosome as β-globin genes that carry β^0-thalassemia mutations, the clinical phenotype is converted from HPFH to δβ-thalassemia, albeit with different HbA$_2$ levels.

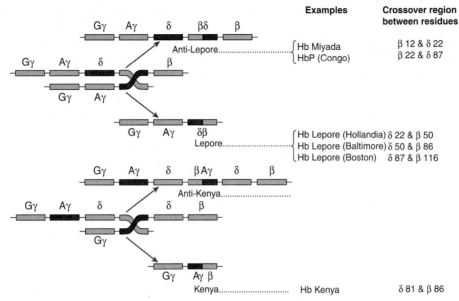

Figure 17–8. Mechanisms for the production of the Lepore and anti-Lepore hemoglobins.

δβ-Thalassemia is classified into δβ+- and δβ0-thalassemia (Table 17-4). δβ0-Thalassemia is further divided into δβ0-thalassemia, in which both the δ-globin and β-globin genes are deleted, and AγδβΒ0-thalassemia, in which the Gγ, δ, and β genes are deleted. Because many different deletion forms of δβ-thalassemia have been described, they are further classified according to the country in which they were first identified (see Table 17-4).

δβ-THALASSEMIA AND AγδβΒ0-THALASSEMIA

Nearly all these conditions result from deletions involving varying lengths of the β-globin gene cluster. Many different varieties have been described in different populations (see Fig. 17-7 and Table 17-4), although their heterozygous and homozygous phenotypes are very similar.[1,12,123] Rare forms of these conditions result from more complex gene rearrangements. For example, one form of AγδβΒ0-thalassemia, found in Indian populations, does not result from a simple linear deletion, but from a complex rearrangement with two deletions, one affecting the Aγ gene and the other the δ-globin and β-globin genes encompassing an intervening region, although intact but is inverted.[124] Figure 17-7 illustrates some of these conditions.

δβ+-THALASSEMIA

δβ+-Thalassemia usually is associated with the production of structural Hb variants called Lepore.[103] HbLepore contains normal α-globin chains and non–α-globin chains that consist of the first 50-80 amino acid residues of the δ-globin chains and the last 60-90 residues of the normal C-terminal amino acid sequence of the β chains. Thus, the Lepore non–α-globin chain is a β-globin fusion chain. Several different varieties of HbLepore have been described—Washington-Boston, Baltimore, and Hollandia—in which the transition from δ to β sequences occurs at different points.[1] The fusion chains probably arose by nonhomologous crossing over between part of the δ-locus on one chromosome and part of the β-locus on the complementary chromosome (see Fig. 17-8). This event results from misalignment of chromosome pairing during meiosis so that a δ-chain gene pairs with a β-globin chain gene instead of with its homologous partner.[125] Figure 17-8 shows such a mechanism giving rise to two abnormal chromosomes: the first, the Lepore chromosome has no normal δ-locus or β-locus but simply a δβ fusion gene. Opposite the homologous pairs of chromosomes is an anti-Lepore (βδ) fusion gene and normal δ-loci and β-loci. A variety of anti–Lepore-like Hbs have been discovered, including HbMiyada, HbP-Congo, HbLincoln Park, and HbP-Nilotic.[1,126] All the HbLepore disorders are characterized by a severe form of δβ-thalassemia. The output of the γ-globin genes on the chromosome with the δβ fusion gene is not increased sufficiently to compensate for the low output of the δβ fusion product. The reduced rate of production of the δβ fusion chains of HbLepore presumably reflects the fact that its genetic determinant has the δ gene promoter region, which is structurally different from the β-globin gene promoter and is associated with a reduced rate of transcription of its gene product.

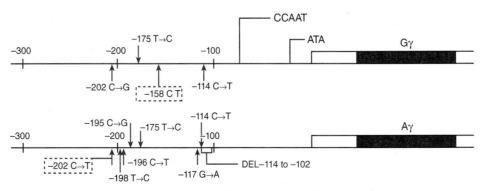

Figure 17–9. Some upstream point mutations associated with hereditary persistence of fetal hemoglobin.

TABLE 17–4. δβ-Thalassemias

(δβ)⁺-Thalassemia

  Hb^Lepore thalassemia

  Hb^Lepore-Washington-Boston

  Hb^Lepore-Hollandia

  Hb^Lepore-Baltimore

  Phenocopies of (δβ)⁺-thalassemia

  Sardinian δβ-thalassemia

  Corfu δβ-thalassemia

  Chinese δβ-thalassemia

  β-Thalassemia with δ-thalassemia

(δβ)⁰-Thalassemia

  Sicilian

  Indian

  Japanese

  Spanish

  Black

  Eastern European

  Macedonian

  Turkish

  Laotian

  Thai

(^Aγδβ)⁰-Thalassemia

  Indian

  German

  Cantonese

  Turkish

  Malay 2

  Belgian

  Black

  Chinese

  Yunnanese

  Thai

  Italian

Hb, hemoglobin.

Note: Details of the molecular pathology of these conditions are given in Refs. 1 and 12.

δβ-Thalassemia-Like Disorders Resulting from Two Mutations in the β-Globin Gene

Cluster A heterogeneous group of nondeletion δβ-thalassemia has been described, most resulting from two mutations, one affecting the β-globin gene, and the other, the γ gene (see Table 17-4). Strictly speaking, they are not all δβ-thalassemia, but they often appear in the literature under this title because their phenotypes resemble the deletion forms of δβ⁰-thalassemia. In the Sardinian form of δβ-thalassemia, the β-globin gene has the common Mediterranean codon 39 nonsense mutation that leads to an absence of β-globin synthesis. The relatively high expression of the ^Aγ gene in *cis* gives this condition the δβ-thalassemia phenotype because of a point mutation at position −196 upstream from the ^Aγ gene (see "Hereditary Persistence of Fetal Hemoglobin" further). The phenotypic picture, in which heterozygotes have 15%

to 20% HbF and normal HbA₂ levels, is identical to that of δβ-thalassemia.[127] Another condition having the β-thalassemia phenotype, with greater than 20% HbF in heterozygotes, has been described in a Chinese patient in whom defective β-globin chain synthesis appears to result from an A→G change in the ATA sequence in the promoter region of the β-globin gene.[128] The increased γ-globin chain synthesis, which appears to involve both ^Gγ and ^Aγ *cis* to this mutation, remains unexplained. A disorder originally called δβ-thalassemia has been described in the Corfu population.[129,130] The condition results from two mutations in the β-globin gene cluster: first, a 7201-bp deletion that starts in the δ-globin gene, IVS-2, position 818-822, and extends upstream to a 5′ breakpoint located 1719-1722 bp 3′ to the ψβ-gene termination codon; and second, a G→A mutation at position 5 in the donor site consensus region of IVS-1 of the β-globin gene. The output from this chromosome consists of relatively high levels of γ-globin chains with very low levels of β-globin chains. The condition resembles δβ-thalassemia in the homozygous state, with almost 100% HbF, traces of HbA, but no HbA₂. Heterozygotes have only slightly elevated HbF levels, with a phenotype similar to "normal HbA₂ β-thalassemia."

Inherited increases in HbF also have been reported in families with β-thalassemia and sickle cell disease; these increases had a modulating effect on the severity of disease. Healthy members of the families may also have slight increases in HbF, and historically these individuals were said to have coinherited heterocellular HPFH, so called because of distribution of HbF among the red blood cells and because the inheritance appeared to segregate independently of the β-globin gene cluster (see Table 17-3). Although this condition originally was called the Swiss form of HPFH because it was first recognized in Swiss army recruits,[131] it is observed in every racial group. It is now clear that HbF in healthy adults is a highly variable quantitative trait, and that heterocellular HPFH represents the upper tail of the natural continuous distribution, including approximately 10% of the population with HbF levels between 0.8% and 5%. Unlike the Mendelian forms of persistent HbF increase that are caused by major deletions or point mutations in the γ globin promoters, the inheritance of heterocellular HPFH is complex with contribution from multiple genetic variants, also referred to as quantitative trait loci (QTL). One QTL for HbF is the sequence variant (T/C) at position −158 of the ^Gγ-globin gene, also referred to Xmn1 ^Gγ site (or *rs74821440*), that was the first HbF QTL to be implicated through family studies. Subsequent genetic association studies confirmed Xmn1 ^Gγ as one of the three major QTLs modulating HbF production in adults, the other two being the *HBS1L-MYB* intergenic region on chromosome 6q and the *BCL11A* oncogene on chromosome 2p. These three QTLs account for a relatively large proportion (20%-50%) of the common variation in HbF levels, not only in healthy adults but also in patients from diverse ethnic groups with β-thalassemia and sickle cell disease. Their coinheritance with these conditions may have an extremely beneficial effect from the associated HbF increase.[132,133]

εγδβ-THALASSEMIA

εγδβ-Thalassemia are rare conditions and result from large deletions of the β-globin gene cluster, which involve the β-LCR.[134-142] The deletions fall into two categories: group I removes all, or a greater part of the complex, including the β-globin gene and the β-LCR, and group II removes extensive upstream regions, including the β-LCR but leaving the β-globin gene itself intact. There is no output from the globin genes of the affected cluster (see Fig. 17-7).[13]

The molecular basis for inactivation of the β-globin gene *cis* to these deletions was clarified by the discovery of the β-LCR approximately 50 kb upstream from the ε-globin gene (see "Genetic Control and Synthesis of Hemoglobin" earlier). Removal of this critical regulatory region seems to completely inactivate the downstream globin gene complex. The Hispanic form of εγδβ-thalassemia[140] results from a deletion that includes most of the LCR, including four of the five DNase-1–hypersensitive sites. These lesions appear to close down the chromatin domain that usually is open in erythroid tissues and delay replication of the β-globin genes in the cell cycle. Thus, although they are rare, the lesions have been of considerable importance because analysis of the Dutch deletion first pointed to the possibility of a major control region upstream from the β-like–globin gene cluster and ultimately led to the discovery of the β-globin LCR. Clearly, the homozygous state would not be compatible with survival. Heterozygotes may have severe hemolytic disease of the newborn, with anemia and hyperbilirubinemia. The severity of anemia and hemolysis is variable, even within a family, and in some cases, blood transfusions are necessary during the neonatal period. If affected individuals survive the neonatal period, they grow and develop normally; in adult life they have the hematologic picture of heterozygous β-thalassemia but HbA_2 levels are normal.

δ-THALASSEMIA

Several point mutations and deletions that reduce δ-globin synthesis have been described. They are summarized in Ref. 1.

α-THALASSEMIA

Table 17-5 summarizes the different classes of α-thalassemia mutations. The α-globin gene haplotype can be written αα, indicating the $α_1$ and $α_2$ genes, respectively. A normal individual has the genotype αα/αα. A deletion involving one (–α) or both (– –) α genes can be further classified based on its size, written as a superscript; thus, $–α^{3.7}$ indicates a deletion of 3.7 kb including one α gene. When the sizes of the deletions are not established, a superscript describing their geographic or family origin is useful; thus, $– –^{MED}$ describes a deletion of both α genes first identified in individuals of Mediterranean origin. In thalassemia haplotypes in which both genes are intact, that is, nondeletion lesions, the nomenclature $α^{ND}α$ is given, with the superscript ND indicating the gene is thalassemic. However, when the precise molecular defect is known, as in Hb Constant Spring, for example, $α^{ND}α$ can be replaced by the more informative $α^{CS}α$. The molecular pathology and population genetics of α-thalassemia have been the subject of several extensive reviews.[1,53,143,144]

α⁰-Thalassemia

Many deletions that involve both α genes, and therefore abolish α-globin chain production from the affected chromosome, have been described (Fig. 17-10).[1] Several of the 3′ breakpoints fall within a 6–8-kb region at the 3′ end of the α-globin complex, suggesting this represents a breakpoint cluster region with a high level of recombination.[145] In at least 5 of the deletions, the 5′ breakpoints also appear to cluster. This gives rise to a situation in which the 5′ breakpoints are located approximately the same distance apart and in the same order along a chromosome as their respective 3′ breakpoints. It is possible that such staggered deletions arise from illegitimate recombination events that delete an integral number of chromatin loops as they pass through their nuclear attachment points during replication. This mechanism also has been suggested to underlie some of the deletion forms of HPFH. One of these deletions ($– –^{MED}$) involves a more complex rearrangement that introduces a new piece of DNA bridging the two breakpoints in the α-gene cluster. This new sequence originates upstream from the α cluster and appears to have been replicated into the junction in a manner suggesting that the upstream segment of DNA also lies at the base of a replication loop. At least some of these deletions seem to have arisen by recombination events between Alu repeat sequences. The Alu repetitive DNA

TABLE 17–5. Classes of Mutations That Cause α-Thalassemia

α⁰-Thalassemia
  Deletions involving both α-globin genes
  Deletions downstream from $α_2$ gene
  Truncations of telomeric region of 16p
  Deletions of HS40 region
α⁺-Thalassemia
  Deletions involving $α_2$ or $α_1$ genes
  Point mutations involving $α_2$ or $α_1$ genes
  mRNA processing
    Splice site
    Poly(A) signal
  mRNA translation
    Initiation
    Nonsense, frameshift
    Termination
  Posttranslational
    Unstable α-globin variants
α-Thalassemia Mental Retardation
  ATR-16
    Deletions or telomeric truncations of 16p
    Translocations
  ATR-X
  Mutations of ATR-X
    Deletions
      Splice site
      Missense
      Nonsense

Note: Complete lists of individual mutations are found in Refs. 1, 15, and 53.

sequences are approximately 300 nucleotides in length and are so called because of the presence of a cleavage site for the restriction enzyme AluI in the center of the repeat sequences. These repetitive sequences facilitate the "illegitimate" recombination events underlying the large DNA sequence rearrangements.[145]

Several other mechanisms for the generation of α⁰-thalassemia have been identified. In a case of unusual genetic interest, a long (>18 kb) deletion that removes the $α_1$ gene and the region downstream was identified in which the $α_2$ gene remains intact but is completely inactivated, giving the α⁰-thalassemia phenotype. Although the inactive $α_2$ gene retains all its local and remote *cis*-regulatory elements, its expression is completely silenced and its CpG island is completely methylated as a result of transcription of antisense RNA expressed from a locus that had been juxtaposed to the $α_2$ gene because of the large deletion.[146,147] Such a mechanism of silencing the α genes can also result from a terminal truncation of the short arm of chromosome 16 to a site 50 kb distal to the α-globin genes.[148] The telomeric consensus sequence (TTAGGGG) n has been added directly to the site of the break. Because this mutation is stably inherited, telomeric DNA alone appears sufficient to stabilize the broken chromosome end. This observation raises the possibility that other genetic diseases could also result from chromosomal truncations.

Several deletions have been identified that appear to downregulate α-globin genes by removing the α-globin regulatory MCS

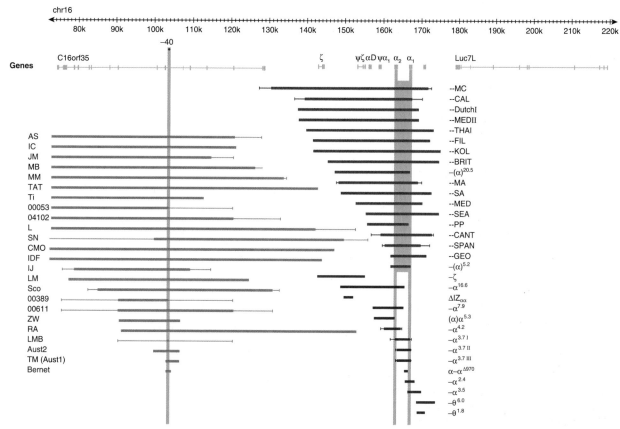

Figure 17–10. Some deletions of the α-globin gene cluster responsible for α⁰-thalassemia. Deletions (listed in order shown in figure): MC, initials of patient; CAL, initials of patient; THAI, Thai; FIL, Filipino; CI, Conway Islands; BRIT, United Kingdom; SA, South Africa; MED, Mediterranean; SEA, Southeast Asian; SPAN, Spanish. The top line indicates the size of the region in kilobases (k). The second line shows the different genes that constitute the α-globin gene cluster, HS40, the major regulatory region of the cluster, and the position of other genes in the region. The lines in *blue* represent the size of the deletions that have been described in α⁰-thalassemia, while those in *red* below them on the right-hand side of the figure show some of the deletions that have now been reported in different forms of α⁺-thalassemia. The lines in *yellow* on the left side of the figure represent some of the deletions that have been reported upstream from the α-globin gene cluster, which, because they remove the major regulatory region, result in the phenotype of α⁰-thalassemia. For a more detailed list of these deletions and references to those marked in this diagram, see Refs. 50 and 53.

elements.[1,149,150] In each case, the α-globin genes are left intact, although in one the 3′ breakpoint is found between the ξ and ψξ genes, thus removing the ξ gene. These deletions appear to completely inactivate the α-globin gene complex, just as deletions of the β-LCR inactivate the entire β-gene complex. Such deletions have not been observed in the homozygous state, presumably because they would be lethal.

α⁺-THALASSEMIA GENE DELETIONS

The most common forms of α⁺-thalassemia (−α^{3.7} and −α^{4.2}) involve deletion of one or the other of the duplicated α-globin genes (see Fig. 17-10 and Fig. 17-11).

Each α-gene is located within a region of homology approximately 4 kb long, interrupted by two nonhomologous regions. The homologous regions are believed to have resulted from an ancient duplication event and to have subsequently subdivided, presumably by insertions and deletions, to give three homologous subsegments referred to as X, Y, and Z (see Fig. 17-11). The duplicated Z boxes are 3.7 kb apart, and the X boxes are 4.2 kb apart. Misalignment and reciprocal crossover between these segments at meiosis can give rise to chromosomes with either single (−α) or triplicated (ααα) α-globin genes. Such an occurrence between homologous Z boxes deletes 3.7 kb of DNA (rightward deletion). A similar crossover between the 2 X blocks deletes 4.2 kb of

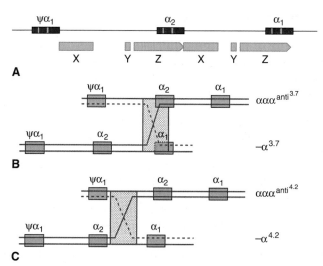

Figure 17–11. Mechanisms for production of the common deletion forms of α⁺-thalassemia. **A.** Normal α-globin gene cluster showing the homology boxes X, Y, and Z. **B.** Rightward crossover through the Z boxes, giving rise to the 3.7-kb deletion and a chromosome with 3 α-globin genes. **C.** Leftward crossover through the X boxes, giving rise to a 4.2-kb deletion and a chromosome containing three α genes.

DNA (leftward deletion −α4.2).[151] The corresponding triplicated α-gene arrangements are referred to as ααα^anti-3.7 and α^anti-4.2.[152-154] More detailed analysis of these crossover events indicates they occur more commonly in the Z box. At least three different −α3.7 deletions have been found, depending on exactly where the crossover occurred.[155] These deletions are designated −α^3.7I, −α^3.7II, and −α^3.7III, respectively. Other rarer deletions of a single α-gene have been observed.[1]

NONDELETION α-THALASSEMIA

Because expression of the α_2 gene is two to three times greater than expression of the α_1 gene, the finding that most of the nondeletion mutants discovered as of this writing, affect predominantly α_2-gene expression is not surprising. Presumably this is ascertainment bias because of the greater phenotypic effect of these lesions. It also is possible that defective expression of the α_2 gene has come under greater selective pressure.

Like the β-thalassemia mutations, α-thalassemia mutations[1] can be classified according to the level of gene expression they affect (see Table 17-5). Several processing mutations have been identified. For example, a pentanucleotide deletion includes the 5′ splice site of IVS-1 of the α_2-globin gene. This mutation involves the invariant GT donor splicing sequence and thus completely inactivates the α_2 gene.[155] A second mutant of this type, found commonly in the Middle East, involves the poly-A addition signal site (AATAAA→AATAAG) and downregulates the α_2 gene by interfering with 3′ end processing.[156,157]

A second group of nondeletion α-thalassemia results from mutations that interfere with translation of mRNA.[7] Several mutations involve the initiation codon.[158-161] In one case, for example, the initiation codon is inactivated by a T→C transition.[158] In another case, efficiency of initiation is reduced by a dinucleotide deletion in the consensus sequence around the start signal.[162] Five mutations that affect termination of translation and give rise to elongated α-globin chains have been identified: Hb^Constant Spring, Hb^Icaria, Hb^Koya Dora, Hb^Seal Rock, and Hb^Pakse.[1] Each mutation specifically changes the termination codon TAA so that an amino acid is inserted instead of the chain terminating (Fig. 17-12). This process is followed by read-through of mRNA that is not normally translated until another "in-phase" stop codon is reached. Thus, each of these variants has an elongated α-globin chain. The "read-through" of α-globin mRNA that usually is not used likely reduces its stability.[152] Several nonsense mutations occur, for example, one in exon 3 of the α_2-globin gene.[153] Finally, several mutations occur that cause α-thalassemia by producing highly unstable α-globin chains, including Hb Quong Sze,[154] Hb Suan Doc,[163] Hb Petah Tikvah,[164] and Hb Evanston.[165] A complete list of nondeletion α-thalassemia alleles is given in reference.[53]

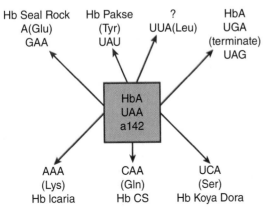

Figure 17-12. Point mutations in the α-globin gene termination codon.

Interactions of α-Thalassemia Haplotypes

Many α-thalassemia phenotypes have been described, and potentially more than 500 interactions are possible.[1] These phenotypes result in four broad categories: (1) normal, (2) conditions characterized by mild hematologic changes but no clinical abnormality, (3) HbH disease, and (4) Hb Bart's hydrops fetalis syndrome. The heterozygous states for deletion or nondeletion forms of α⁺-thalassemia either cause extremely mild hematologic abnormalities or are completely silent. In populations where α-thalassemia is common, the homozygous state for α⁺-thalassemia (−α/−α) can produce a hematologic phenotype identical to that of the heterozygous state for α⁰-thalassemia (− −/αα), that is, mild anemia with reduced mean cell Hb and mean cell volume values.

HbH disease usually results from the compound heterozygous state for α⁰-thalassemia and either deletion or nondeletion α⁺-thalassemia. It occurs most frequently in Southeast Asia (− −^SEA/−α^3.7) and the Mediterranean region (usually − −^MED/−α^3.7).

The Hb Bart's hydrops fetalis syndrome usually results from the homozygous state for α⁰-thalassemia, most commonly − −^SEA/− −^SEA or − −^MED− −^MED. A few infants with this syndrome who synthesized very low levels of α-globin chains at birth have been reported. Gene-mapping studies suggest these cases result from interaction of α⁰-thalassemia with nondeletion mutations (αα^ND).

UNUSUAL FORMS OF α-THALASSEMIA

Some unusual forms of α-thalassemia are completely unrelated to the common forms of the disease that occur in tropical populations. These conditions, which can occur in any racial groups, include α-thalassemia associated with mental retardation or leukemia. Their importance lies with the diagnostic problems they may present and, more importantly, the light that elucidation of the α-thalassemia pathology may shed on broader disease mechanisms.

MOLECULAR PATHOLOGY OF THE α-THALASSEMIA MENTAL RETARDATION SYNDROME

The first descriptions of noninherited forms of α-thalassemia associated with mental retardation suggested the lesions involving the α-globin gene locus were acquired in the paternal germ cells and that their molecular pathology might help elucidate the associated developmental changes.[166] Two separate syndromes of this type now are evident. In one group of patients, long deletions involve the α-globin gene cluster and remove at least 1 Mb.[167] This condition can arise in several ways, including unbalanced translocation involving chromosome 16, truncation of the tip of chromosome 16, and loss of the α-globin gene cluster and parts of its flanking regions by other mechanisms. These findings localize a region of approximately 1.7 Mb in band 16p13.3 proximal to the α-globin genes as being causative of mental handicap.[50]

The second group is characterized by defective α-globin synthesis associated with severe mental retardation and a relatively homogeneous pattern of dysmorphology.[168] Extensive structural studies have shown no abnormalities of the α-globin genes. These chromosomes direct the synthesis of normal amounts of α-globin in mouse erythroleukemia cells, suggesting that α-thalassemia results from deficiency of a *trans*-activating factor involved in regulation of the α-globin genes. This condition is encoded by a locus on the short arm of the X chromosome ATR-X, which because of its mode of inheritance affects boys.[169] ATR-X, the gene involved, is a DNA helicase with many features of a DNA-binding protein. Many different mutations of this gene have been identified in different families with the ATR-X syndrome.[143,170] Studies have identified a plant homeodomain region and an ATPase/helicase domain.[171] Because patients with ATR-X show defective methylation of recombinant DNA arrays and related defects, this condition likely is one of a growing list of disorders that result from disordered chromatin remodeling.[172,173] The product of this gene appears to play an important role in the transcription of the α-globin genes and, undoubtedly, many other genes, during early development. The ATR-X gene also has been reported to be involved in a considerable number of instances of X-linked mental retardation without an α-thalassemia phenotype.

ACQUIRED α-THALASSEMIA AND CLONAL MYELOID DISEASES

The hematologic findings of HbH disease or mild α-thalassemia are occasionally observed in elderly patients with primary myelofibrosis or the myelodysplastic syndrome. Earlier studies suggested this finding resulted from an acquired defect of α-globin synthesis in which the α-globin genes were completely inactivated in the neoplastic hematopoietic cell line.[174] The molecular basis for this observation now is known to reside in a variety of different mutations involving ATR-X.[50,175] The relationship of these somatic mutations of ATR-X to the neoplastic transformation remains to be determined. The molecular defect of other cases of acquired α-thalassemia, such as that seen in variable combined immunodeficiency,[176] also remains to be defined.

● PATHOPHYSIOLOGY

Thalassemias, in general, are syndromes of ineffective erythropoiesis. There is an imbalance in the synthesis of the normal globin chains, and the excess globin either precipitates, as in β-thalassemia, resulting in α-globin chain inclusions, the formation of hemichromes and intramedullary apoptosis, or as in α-thalassemia, forms abnormal Hbs like HbBart's and HbH, which are not able to carry oxygen effectively, resulting in increased red cell turnover. This phenomenon of ineffective erythropoiesis makes thalassemias fundamentally different from all the other genetic and acquired disorders of Hb production, and explains their extreme severity in the homozygous and compound heterozygous states (Fig. 17-13). Whereas ineffective erythropoiesis is present in both α- and β-thalassemia, it is markedly greater in β-thalassemia and contributes much more to the manifestations of the disease as discussed later. In α-thalassemia, whereas there is some ineffective erythropoiesis, it is premature breakdown of cells containing abnormal Hbs, Barts and H, which result in the clinical manifestations.

Ineffective erythropoiesis (IE) is the central pathophysiologic feature of β-thalassemia, which results in anemia. Anemia in β-thalassemia has three major components: (1) most important is ineffective erythropoiesis with intramedullary apoptosis of a variable proportion of the developing red cell precursors; (2) hemolysis resulting from destruction of mature red cells containing α-globin chain inclusions that have shorter life spans because of the formation of hemichromes and iron-related oxidative damage; and (3) the hypochromic and microcytic red cells that result from the overall reduction in Hb synthesis.

Erythropoiesis is essentially a two-phase process, an initial proliferative phase, driven by erythropoietin, which results in stimulation of the erythroid committed progenitor cells fostering formation of the erythroid burst and colony forming units (BFU-E and CFU-E), and a maturation phase leading unipotential precursors to become mature erythrocytes. The precursors, proerythroblasts, mature through several erythroblast phases, into reticulocytes once the nuclei are extruded, and eventually, mature red cells. In β-thalassemia, the defect in the erythropoietic pathway is one of impaired differentiation and maturation of the developing erythroid precursors, beginning at the time globin genes begin expression in the proerythroblast-basophilic erythroblast stages.

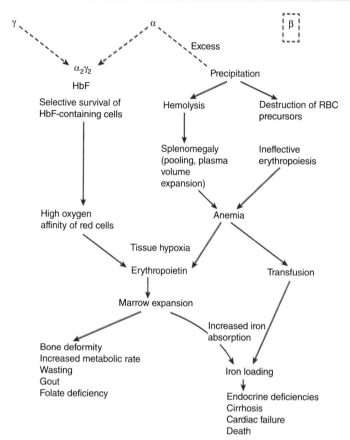

Figure 17–13. Pathophysiology of β-thalassemia. RBC, red blood cell.

As a result of the anemia, there is increased secretion of erythropoietin, and further proliferation of late erythroid progenitors and precursors, with a large fraction of developing erythroid cells failing to reach full maturation. This massive erythroid marrow expansion, as well as stimulation of normally quiescent erythroid progenitors' cells in the liver and spleen, results in extramedullary hematopoiesis. There is also evidence of accumulation of several members of the Transforming Growth Factor-β (TGF-β) superfamily of ligands, notably Growth and Differentiation Factor-11 (GDF-11), which has been used as a therapeutic target in β-thalassemia.[177]

The primary defect in β-thalassemia involves β-globin chain synthesis; consequently, production of HbF and HbA$_2$ are not affected. Fetal development proceeds normally, with normal production of HbF in utero. In the complete absence of β-globin production, as in homozygous β^0-thalassemia, there is no HbA production in utero, and the newborn has a microcytosis and a lower total Hb level, all of it being HbF only. In β$^+$-thalassemia, where there is some but reduced expression of the β-globin gene, there is some HbA but a lower total Hb. However, clinical manifestations appear only when the neonatal switch occurs from predominant γ-globin production to predominant β-globin chain production, which would normally result in a predominance of HbA by 2-3 months of age. In β-thalassemia, there is reduced or absent HbA, and thus anemia. Being born relatively anemic, infants would reach their physiologic nadir earlier and erythropoietin now stimulates red cell production again, with the resulting IE leading to marrow erythroid hyperplasia and extramedullary hematopoiesis. Fetal Hb synthesis persists beyond the neonatal period in nearly all forms of β-thalassemia. Heterozygotes may manifest with some microcytosis at birth, and have a persistence of mild microcytic anemia, but do not have severe manifestations, and have normal Hb proportions at birth. Beyond the neonatal period, there is usually a slight increase in HbF and HbA$_2$ in these individuals, but this may not be the case in some "silent carriers." The elevated level of HbA$_2$ appears to reflect not only a relative decrease in HbA as a result of defective β-globin chain synthesis but also an absolute increase in the output of δ-globin chains both *cis* and *trans* to the mutant β-globin gene.[1]

Anemia is central to the clinical syndrome of α-thalassemia. However, in α-thalassemia, the excess γ-globin and β-globin chains formed as a result of defective α-globin chain production produce soluble homotetramers, HbBart's and HbH, respectively. As described below, these are poor oxygen tranporters and even when present, do not contribute to normal function of red cells. Hence there is less ineffective erythropoiesis than in β-thalassemia and the major cause of anemia is hemolysis and poorly hemoglobinized red cells with normal levels of HbF or HbA$_2$.

IMBALANCED GLOBIN CHAIN SYNTHESIS AND ITS CONSEQUENCES

Studies of in vitro globin chain synthesis in the blood or marrow of thalassemic patients[178,179] and those who also inherited α-globin or β-globin structural variants[1,14] provide the basis for our understanding of the globin chain production imbalance and its consequences. In homozygous β-thalassemia, β-globin synthesis is either absent or markedly reduced. The resulting excessive α-globin chains do not form Hb tetramer, the α-globin chains precipitate in red cell precursors, resulting in inclusion bodies that can be visualized by microscopy in the earliest hemoglobinized precursors and throughout their maturation.[180-181] These large inclusions lead to intramedullary destruction of a large proportion of red cell precursors and result in the ineffective erythropoiesis that characterizes β-thalassemia.[182] Some red cells may still be released, but are prematurely destroyed (see below). β-Thalassemia heterozygotes have a mild imbalance of globin chain synthesis, but the magnitude of α-globin chain excess is partially resolved by the proteolytic enzymes of the red cell precursors.[183] Therefore, ineffective erythropoiesis is mild.

The consequences of excess non–α-globin chain production in α-thalassemia are quite different. α-Globin chains are required for production of both HbF and HbA; therefore, defective α-chain production is manifested in both fetal and adult life. In the fetus, it leads to excess γ-globin chain production, which form γ$_4$-homotetramers or HbBart's[184]; in the adult, it leads to an excess of β-globin chains which form β$_4$-homotetramers or HbH.[185] HbBart's and HbH do not precipitate to any significant degree in the marrow, and therefore α-thalassemia is not characterized by ineffective erythropoiesis.[1,178] The output of the erythroid marrow is, therefore, more effective, and marrow hyperplasia and extramedullary hematopoiesis are not as significant. However, β$_4$ tetramers precipitate as red cells age, with the formation of inclusion bodies, which leads to a shortened survival of red cells mainly taking place in the microvasculature of the spleen. Thus, the anemia of the more severe forms of α-thalassemia in the adult results from hemolysis more than ineffective erythropoiesis. In addition, because of the defect in Hb synthesis, the erythrocytes are hypochromic and microcytic. HbBart's is more stable than HbH and does not form large inclusions. Furthermore, both HbBart's and HbH show no heme-heme cooperative interaction and have almost hyperbolic oxygen dissociation curves with very high oxygen affinities. Thus, they are not able to release oxygen effectively at physiologic tissue tensions making them very poor oxygen carriers (Chap. 19).[1] This exacerbates hypoxia from the anemia. Infants with high levels of HbBart's in α^0-thalassemia have severe intrauterine hypoxia. Deficient fetal oxygenation probably is responsible for (1) the hypertrophied placentas, (2) the severe erythroblastosis, (3) the gross hydropic state of the fetus as a result of increased capillary permeability,

and possibly for (4) the associated developmental abnormalities that occur with the severe forms of intrauterine α-thalassemia.[1] Hence the pathophysiology of anemia is fundamentally different in α-thalassemia compared to β-thalassemia.

MECHANISMS OF DAMAGE TO THE ERYTHROID PRECURSORS AND RED CELLS

Damage to the red cell membrane by the globin-chain precipitation process occurs by two major routes: generation of hemichromes (Chap. 16) from excess α-globin chains with subsequent structural damage to the red cell membrane, and similar damage mediated through the degradation products of excess α-globin chains.[1,186-188] Excess globin chains bind to different membrane proteins and alter their structure and function. Excess iron which is delivered to the erythroid precursors as a result of decreased hepcidin (discussed later in the Abnormal Iron Metabolism and Iron Overload section) generates reactive oxygen species through the Fenton reaction, which damage the red cell membrane and intracellular organelles. The degradation products of free α-globin chains—heme, hemin (oxidized heme), and free iron—also play a role. Heme and its products can catalyze the formation of a variety of reactive oxygen species that also damage the red cell membrane leading to rigid and dehydrated erythrocytes that leak potassium and have increased levels of calcium and low ATP. The rigid inclusion bodies accentuate the damage during passage of the red cells through the spleen. These effects in the red cell precursors lead to an increased rate of apoptosis in the marrow.[189]

In β-thalassemia, excess α-globin chains also result in mechanical instability and oxidative damage to the red cell membrane, primarily to protein 4.1 (Chap. 16). However, in α-thalassemia, while the membranes are stable, there is no evidence of oxidation or dysfunction of protein 4.1. Furthermore, accumulation of excess β-globin chains in α-thalassemia results in increased hydration of the cells. These differences in the pathophysiology of membrane damage between α-thalassemia and β-thalassemia are discussed in detail elsewhere.[1,186-188]

PERSISTENT FETAL HEMOGLOBIN PRODUCTION AND CELLULAR HETEROGENEITY

Normal adults have small quantities of HbF that are heterogeneously distributed among the red cells. In β-thalassemia, ineffective erythropoiesis is central to its pathophysiology. Red cells that produce γ-globin chain will have less of a globin-chain imbalance and will have a selective survival advantage.[1,190-193] Differential centrifugation experiments[191-193] and in vivo labeling studies[190] show that red cells with a greater amount of HbF (called *F cells*) are more efficiently produced and survive longer in the blood. Thus, HbF in the blood of patients with homozygous β-thalassemia is heterogeneously distributed among the red cells.[1,193] As discussed in "Hereditary Persistence of Fetal Hemoglobin" earlier, multiple genetic mechanisms exist for an increase of HbF production in β-thalassemia and sickle cell anemia, resulting in their milder phenotypes.[133,194-197]

INEFFECTIVE ERYTHROPOIESIS, EXTRAMEDULLARY HEMATOPOIESIS, AND BONE DISEASE

Tissue hypoxia is a common feature of all severe forms of thalassemia. In α-thalassemia, circulating HbBart's and HbH are both high-oxygen-affinity Hbs, and in β-thalassemia, HbF also has a higher-oxygen-affinity compared to normal HbA, contributing with anemia to tissue hypoxia. The ensuing increased erythropoietin drives the erythropoiesis, leading to marrow expansion and augmenting the ineffective erythropoiesis. This effect leads to a variety of skeletal defects, including defects of the skull, face, and long bones, as well as increased osteopenia and the frequency of pathologic fractures. Quiescent hematopoietic stem cells (HSCs) in the liver and spleen are activated, resulting in extramedullary hematopoiesis that may result in tumor-like formation in those sites and in other tissue locations, similar to what is seen in primary myelofibrosis. The extramedullary hematopoiesis and bone lesions are particularly prominent in HbE β-thalassemia.[198] Similar changes also may be seen in individuals with HbH disease, though not as severe.

The greatly expanded erythroid mass increases metabolic demands, and accompanied with the tissue hypoxia, leads to failure to thrive, growth and developmental retardation, and tissue wasting, and also may result in hyperuricemia with gout and folate deficiency (Chap. 9).

SPLENOMEGALY

Splenomegaly is commonly seen in the more severe forms of thalassemia because of the extramedullary hematopoiesis and "work hypertrophy" that occurs as a result of the constant exposure of the spleen to the abnormal inclusion of red cells. Hypersplenism (Chap. 25) develops and further contributes to the anemia.[1,15] Splenomegaly expands plasma volume, further augmenting anemia.

ABNORMAL IRON METABOLISM AND IRON OVERLOAD

The iron overload in thalassemia is contributed by the expanded erythropoiesis (Chap. 11). Increased erythroferrone, the product of marrow erythroid precursors, reduces hepcidin production through the bone morphogenetic protein (BMP)/Smad-related and Mad-related protein signaling pathway.[199,200] This effect leads to increased iron absorption and impaired iron sequestration in macrophages,[201] as well as iron overload, even in the absence of transfusional iron loading. As the affected person has no means of excreting excess amounts of iron, iron chelation is an important management tool in thalassemia. When the heart, liver, pancreas, and other endocrine tissues accumulate iron, their organ dysfunction ensues (Chap. 11). These changes are less common in α-thalassemia, since IE is not as severe and thus hepcidin levels are not inappropriately suppressed as much.

Transfusions suppress endogenous erythropoiesis and thus mitigate the ineffective erythropoiesis and the reduced hepcidin production and iron absorption.[1,15] However, secondary iron load from transfusion contributes more to iron loading; each milliliter of red cells contains about 1 mg of iron. Thus, 2 U of packed red cells adds approximately 400 to 500 mg of iron. A proportion of the transfused red cells is rapidly broken down by macrophages, leading to a "bolus" effect, which results in an abrupt increase in free iron. As the body iron increases, the surplus iron is stored in hepatocytes, and macrophages in the liver and other organs.[1,202,203] Iron deposited in the myocardium leads to contractile dysfunction and heart failure, and a variety of arrhythmias. Iron-induced endocrine dysfunction may result in diabetes, growth retardation or failure, delayed puberty and sexual maturity, infertility and decreased sex drive, and bone disease. Noninvasive tissue-iron measurement using magnetic resonance imaging (MRI) technology is a refined method for assessing iron overload, enabling the tailoring of chelation regimens the reduction of morbidity and mortality from iron overload (see details in the treatment section in Iron Chelation). The mechanisms whereby iron mediates tissue damage are discussed in Chaps. 10 and 11.

INFECTION

All forms of severe thalassemia appear to be associated with an increased susceptibility to bacterial infection.[1] The precise pathophysiologic basis for this is not known. Factors that may predispose the patient to bacterial infection include iron overload, blockade of the monocyte-macrophage system, and the asplenic state of those who have been splenectomized. No consistent defects in white cell or immune function have been discovered. Transfusion-dependent patients with thalassemia are at particular risk for bloodborne infections, including hepatitides B and C, HIV/AIDS, parasitic infections such as malaria and babesiosis, and epidemic infections by Zika virus, West Nile virus, and others in locations where the blood supply is not tested meticulously for bloodborne pathogens.

VASCULAR DISEASE AND HYPERCOAGULABLE STATE

The hypercoagulable state in thalassemia has been reviewed in detail.[187-189,205] Damage to the vascular endothelium by fragmented red cells, particularly in the asplenic state, may contribute to the hypercoagulable state making the indication for splenectomy controversial. Although transfusions result in iron overload, effectively transfused patients with β-thalassemia have less vascular disease because IE is suppressed; the nontransfused patients with severe ineffective erythropoiesis and who have undergone splenectomy are at highest risk. The hypercoagulable state results in chronic pulmonary embolism, pulmonary arterial hypertension, silent cerebral infarcts, and persistent leg ulcers. Deep vein thrombosis may also occur more frequently.

Using thalassemic red cells as a source of phospholipids, enhanced thrombin generation has been demonstrated in a prothrombinase assay. The procoagulant effect of thalassemia cells results from increased expression of anionic phospholipids on the red cell surface (Chap. 16). Normally, neutral or negatively charged phospholipids are confined to the inner leaflet of the red cell membrane. In thalassemic red cells these aminophospholipids are moved to the outer leaflet, thus providing a surface on which coagulation can be activated. There is evidence that the hemolytic component of the anemia of β-thalassemia is associated with the release of Hb and arginase, resulting in impaired nitric oxide availability and endothelial dysfunction with progressive pulmonary hypertension.[206]

GENOTYPE-PHENOTYPE CORRELATION AND CLINICAL HETEROGENEITY

The pathophysiologic mechanism forms the basis for the remarkably diverse clinical findings in the thalassemia syndromes.[1,207] The manifestations of β-thalassemia can be related to excess α-globin chain production. Based on the genotype, thalassemia syndromes have been classified as thalassemia minor (including one or two α-globin gene defects and a single β-globin gene defect), thalassemia intermedia (three α-globin gene defects, HbH disease, other nondeletional forms of α-thalassemia such as HbH$^{Constant\ Spring}$, non–β^0/β^0-thalassemia, including β$^+$/β^0, β$^+$/β$^+$, or HbE/β$^+$-thalassemia, and dominant β-thalassemia), and thalassemia major (α^0-thalassemia, severe HbH$^{Constant\ Spring}$, β^0/β^0-thalassemia, E/β^0-thalassemia). While in general, the genotype correlates well with the phenotype, there is heterogeneity, especially if there is coinheritance of mutations in the complementary globin genes. Thus, individuals with severe β-thalassemia mutations with coexistence of α-thalassemia have less severe disease. This confirms that the degree of globin-chain imbalance is the major factor determining the severity of thalassemia.[208,209] However, this effect is much more marked in individuals who are homozygotes or compound heterozygotes for different forms of β$^+$-thalassemia. Coinheritance of α-thalassemia does not appear to have an ameliorating effect in individuals homozygous for β^0-thalassemia.

Severe β-thalassemia can also be modified by the coinheritance of genetic determinants for enhanced production of γ-globin chains. In this situation, the imbalance between α-globin and non–α-globin is ameliorated and more HbF is produced. Several determinants may be involved. For example, inheritance of a particular RFLP haplotype in the region 5′ to the β-globin gene may be an important factor.[210,211] This particular β-globin gene haplotype is associated with a single base change, C→T, at position –158 relative to the ^{G}γ-globin gene, an alteration that creates a cleavage site for the restriction enzyme Xmn I.[212] There is a relatively higher number of individuals homozygous for T (XmnI-^{G}γ) with the phenotype of thalassemia intermedia compared with thalassemia major in different populations.[211,213,214] As discussed under "Hereditary Persistence of Fetal Hemoglobin" earlier, it is now clear that there are two other major loci, the *HBS1L-MYB* intergenic region on chromosome 16 and *BCL11A* on chromosome 2p16, that contribute to the background HbF variation in adults.[198,215-217] It is likely that there are many more loci with relatively small effects and/or rare variants with significant quantitative effects on γ-globin gene expression, and that their coinheritance may significantly modify the phenotype of different forms of β-thalassemia.[217,218]

Some mutations that cause β-thalassemia are associated with a mild phenotype because they result in only modest reduction of β-globin chain production.[1] For example, mutations at positions –29 and –88 are associated with mild β⁺-thalassemia in Africans. Similarly, particularly mild phenotypes are commonly found with a base substitution at position 6 in IVS-1 and at position –87 in the 5′-flanking region of the β-globin gene in Mediterranean populations. The homozygous state for the IVS-1 position 6 mutation usually produces a milder form of β-thalassemia. When these "mild" mutations are coinherited with more-severe β-thalassemia determinants, the compound heterozygous states are characterized by a more-severe form of thalassemia intermedia. Other forms of thalassemia intermedia are associated with the homozygous state for δβ-thalassemia, the various interactions of β-thalassemia with δβ-thalassemia, and heterozygous β-thalassemia of the severe variety or in association with triplicated α-gene loci.[1,15,214] These complex interactions are the subject of several extensive reviews.[201,214,219]

These mechanisms for the phenotypic variability of β-thalassemia represent only the beginning of our understanding of the genetic diversity of these conditions. Hence, defining a series of genetic modifiers that act at different levels is useful.[207] Primary modifiers represent the diversity of mutations at the β-globin gene locus. Secondary modifiers are those, such as α-thalassemia and increased HbF production, that directly modify the relative degree of the imbalanced globin-chain output. However, an increasing number of tertiary modifiers, that is, genetic background, have an important effect on the complications of the disease. These include loci involved in iron, bone, and bilirubin metabolism, and in determining resistance of susceptibility to infection. Furthermore, phenotypic diversity may reflect different degrees of adaptation to anemia and the effect of the environment. These complex issues have been reviewed[207] and are illustrated in Fig. 17-14. Several extensive reviews of the pathophysiology of the intermediate forms of β-thalassemia in different populations are available.[219,220]

α-Thalassemia, particularly HbH disease, shows considerable clinical diversity. Some of this variability can be related to particular genotypes,[1,50] but the reasons for the heterogeneity of these disorders is not clear.

CLINICAL FEATURES

The genotype-phenotype correlation and genetic modifiers are addressed above ("Genotype–Phenotype Correlation and Clinical Heterogeneity"). Syndromes in which the predominant underlying

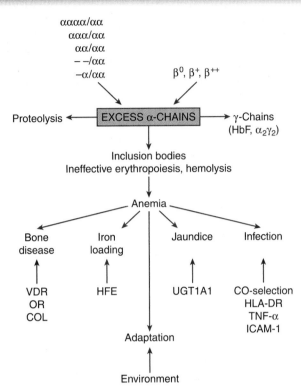

Figure 17–14. Different levels of modification of the β-thalassemia phenotype. COL, various genes involved in collagen metabolism; CO-selection, indicates variable selection of genes involved in susceptibility to infection along with different thalassemia genes; HFE, gene for hereditary hemochromatosis; ICAM, intercellular adhesion molecule; OR, estrogen receptor; TNF, tumor necrosis factor; UGT1A1, uridine diphosphate-glucuronosyltransferase; VDR, vitamin D receptor.

pathophysiology is ineffective erythropoiesis (mostly β-thalassemia) have clinical features related to the ineffective erythropoiesis, and these differ from those in whom ineffective erythropoiesis is only a minor component of the pathophysiology (mostly α-thalassemia). For the purposes of this section, the clinical features are described based on this difference.

SYNDROMES WITH INEFFECTIVE ERYTHROPOIESIS: β-THALASSEMIA AND δβ-THALASSEMIA

β-Thalassemia has been subdivided based on the severity of symptoms and the need for regular transfusions, in descending order of severity, into β-thalassemia major, intermedia, and minor. The most clinically severe form of β-thalassemia is thalassemia major with transfusion dependence. β-Thalassemia intermedia, as the name implies, has intermediate severity with some clinical manifestations and the need for occasional transfusions. β-Thalassemia minor is generally asymptomatic and compatible with a normal life span. This classification is not mutually exclusive for major and intermedia, and individuals with intermedia early in life may begin to need regular transfusions in later life and thus become major. More extensive accounts of the clinical features of these conditions are given in two monographs.[1,14]

β-THALASSEMIA MAJOR

Individuals with the homozygous or compound heterozygous state for β-thalassemia results in the clinical picture first described by Cooley and Lee[4] in 1925. These infants are born without complications and their neonatal course is unremarkable. However, some may be anemic at birth and reach their physiologic anemia nadir earlier than usual. Without the ability to produce β-globin, and therefore HbA, these infants become progressively more anemic over the next few months. Persistent production of HbF is variable and may delay the onset of symptomatic anemia to some degree. However, there is progressive anemia, with increasing ineffective erythropoiesis in the marrow, and extramedullary hematopoiesis develops in the first few months of life. Manifestations include failure to thrive and poor feeding, progressive bone changes, often including frontal and parietal bossing of the skull as the diploic space expands to the suture lines, hepatosplenomegaly, hypotonia, and lethargy. At this point regular transfusions are usually initiated, with resulting amelioration of virtually all symptoms if the Hb level is maintained appropriately.

The goal of the regular transfusion regimen is to suppress the endogenous ineffective erythropoiesis and extramedullary hematopoiesis, and maintain Hb levels adequate for normal growth and development. In the developed world, this is achieved through regularly scheduled transfusions, which, if adequate, lead to reversal of most of the bone changes, and more normal development of skull bones, the maxilla, and the sinuses, as well as regression of the hepatosplenomegaly.[1,14] Transfusion volumes are usually approximately 15 mL/kg of packed red cells in children with the caveat that instead of splitting units when a whole second unit is not indicated, the interval between transfusions may be shortened. With regular transfusions, these children grow and develop normally, and are able to attend school and participate in all the normal activities like their peers. Typically, adults usually receive 2 U of packed red cells each time, with intervals of 2, 3, or 4 weeks, depending on body size. Some centers may transfuse larger volumes at each visit to minimize the frequency of transfusion visits. Complications, such as transfusion reactions and antibody formation, may occur, but their incidence has decreased as a result of leukoreduction. Extended phenotyping limits the development of alloimmunization. After approximately 12-15 transfusions, it is predicted that the liver iron concentration will have more than doubled and iron chelation needs to be initiated to prevent symptoms related to organ dysfunction, which could result from iron overload. Many children will develop splenomegaly over time, usually early in the second decade of life, which may require intervention. If a splenectomy is performed (discussed subsequently in Splenectomy section), the risk of asplenic sepsis is another potential complication.

Unfortunately, in the developing world, where blood supply is limited, and chelation therapy may not be readily available, the course is quite different. This presentation of poorly transfused thalassemia major overlaps considerably with the clinical picture of thalassemia intermedia. Transfusions may not be regularly scheduled and the Hb level is not optimally maintained. In such situations, ineffective erythropoiesis is not suppressed adequately, and the bone disease may progress. The bossing is exaggerated further, the maxilla does not develop normally, and remains filled with the expanded marrow, resulting in nonformation of the normal sinuses. Changes in the maxilla and mandible also result in abnormal dentition and malocclusion, and all of these changes in the skull bones result in the typical "facies" described by Cooley and Lee in 1925. These changes are associated with a characteristic radiologic appearance of the skull, long bones, and hands (Fig. 17-15). The diploe widens, with a "hair on end" or "sunray" appearance and a lacy trabeculation of the long bones and phalanges. Gross skeletal deformities can occur. In addition, growth and development are stunted and these children remain weak and listless as their Hb drops prior to their next transfusion. Many features of a hypermetabolic state, as evidenced by fever, wasting, and hyperuricemia, may develop. The liver and spleen remain enlarged and may progress further as they compensate for the

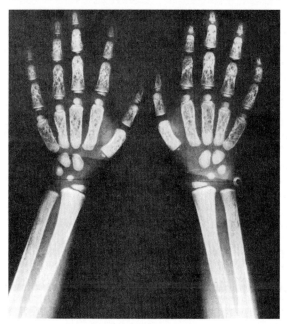

Figure 17–15. Radiologic appearances of the hands in homozygous β-thalassemia. The scattered lucent areas in the bones of the fingers reflect the marked expansion of marrow in distal areas.

anemia. Splenomegaly is often massive and painful, and be susceptible to spontaneous or traumatic rupture, which is often fatal. Hypersplenism may develop early, with leukopenia and thrombocytopenia, and sometimes resulting in bleeding complications, particularly epistaxis. The thinning of the cortices of the long bones may predispose to pathologic fractures that are further exacerbated in later years by the hypogonadism.[221] Extramedullary paraspinal nodules of hematopoietic tissue may cause symptomatic compression of the spinal cord. If iron chelation is not begun appropriately for transfusional iron overload, iron-induced endocrinopathies can develop, usually after approximately 10 years of age. Pituitary dysfunction may result in deficient secretion of growth hormone, leading to an impaired growth spurt, and hypogonadotropic hypogonadism, leading to delayed pubertal development, menarche, and thelarche.[221,222] Diabetes may develop as well, initially not insulin dependent, but eventually may become insulin dependent when the pancreatic islets have been damaged by iron. Hypothyroidism and adrenal insufficiency also occur but are less common.[1,203] Toward the end of the second decade, iron-induced cardiac complications arise, and death usually occurs in the second or third decade as a result of intractable heart failure or ventricular arrhythmias from cardiac siderosis.[204,223,224]

Even the adequately transfused child who has received chelation therapy may suffer a number of complications. Bloodborne infection, notably with hepatitis B or C,[221] HIV,[225] or *Plasmodium* species,[226] is extremely common in some populations, particularly in the developing world, although the frequency is decreasing with the use of widespread blood donor screening programs.

If untreated, the clinical course is characterized by very severe anemia and related complications. If the anemia is not treated, heart failure may develop, resulting in death, usually within the first 2 to 5 years of life.

β-THALASSEMIA INTERMEDIA

Individuals with less-severe genotypes may have a milder course than that described above for thalassemia major, but it is usually symptomatic unlike in individuals with thalassemia minor.[1,219,220] However, the syndrome encompasses disorders with a wide spectrum of manifestations, the severity of which is based on the genotype (described previously in Molecular basis), factors modifying the genotype, and the appropriateness of diagnosis and treatment. Unfortunately, many individuals with these genotypes are inappropriately diagnosed, instead being treated as chronic or refractory iron deficiency. The severity of the presentation is dependent on the degree of ineffective erythropoiesis, those with marked ineffective erythropoiesis are more severely affected with bone changes and pathologic fractures, more severe anemia, with symptoms of fatigue, abnormal facies, and hepatosplenomegaly. If undiagnosed, they may present with these at a variable age, some in the first decade of life, some in the second, and some as late as the third decade of life. Patients do not remain static on the spectrum from thalassemia intermedia to thalassemia major. Those with severe ineffective erythropoiesis and anemia, would benefit from regular transfusion, moving along the spectrum into the major category. However, many such individuals either refuse regular transfusions, or are not able to get them for logistical and economic reasons. These individuals have complications related to underchelation and undertransfusion, including growth retardation, chronic fatigue and malaise, bone pain, and worsening splenomegaly and its downstream effects, as described previously in Pathophysiology. Gallbladder disease from increased red cell turnover and the development of bilirubin gallstones is common. Progressive extramedullary hematopoiesis may result in paraspinal masses as described previously in Pathophysiology. Vascular damage from fragmented and abnormal red cells may lead to clinical manifestations as well. This includes the development of chronic, nonhealing leg ulcers from poor perfusion and the effects of arterial endothelial damage, and, possibly, a hypercoagulable state leading to cerebral infarcts and development of pulmonary hypertension. Others may remain in the intermedia spectrum until adulthood, receiving very few transfusions for stress situations, such as severe infections, pregnancy or surgery, when they may have a decrease of Hb and worsening symptoms related to anemia. Intensive studies of the molecular pathology of this condition have provided some guidelines about genotype-phenotype relationships that are useful for genetic counseling (Table 17-6).

Clinically, significant iron loading as a result of increased absorption is seen even in patients with infrequent transfusions (Chap. 11). Iron overload results in frequent diabetes and endocrine disturbances, typically by the fourth decade of life, although cardiac deposition is relatively rare in individuals with true thalassemia intermedia.[227]

β-THALASSEMIA MINOR

The heterozygous state for β-thalassemia is usually asymptomatic, with individuals being diagnosed either as a result of their family history, a prenatal screen, as part of the workup for refractory iron-deficiency anemia, or by the chance finding of the characteristic hematologic changes during a routine study. They have microcytosis with or without anemia, with no symptoms, no overt evidence of ineffective erythropoiesis or extramedullary hematopoiesis. However, there are some reports in the literature of individuals who have symptoms from anemia and may even have mild splenomegaly, but in the absence of genetic testing, it is not clear that these were all heterozygotes only. A controlled study reported that individuals with the β-thalassemia trait suffer from fatigue and other symptoms at a frequency indistinguishable from those with mild anemias from other causes. There is no difference in the frequency of palpable splenomegaly between those with β-thalassemia minor and unaffected individuals.[228] β-Thalassemia carriers may have some difficulty with endurance activities, such as running marathons,

TABLE 17–6. Genotypes of Patients with β-Thalassemia Intermedia

Mild forms of β-thalassemia
    Homozygosity for mild β⁺-thalassemia alleles
    Compound heterozygosity for two mild β⁺-thalassemia alleles
    Compound heterozygosity for a "silent" or mild and more-severe β-thalassemia allele

Inheritance of α-thalassemia and β-thalassemia
    β⁺-Thalassemia with α⁰-thalassemia ($- -/\alpha\alpha$) or α⁺-thalassemia ($-\alpha/\alpha\alpha$ or $-\alpha/-\alpha$)
    β⁺-Thalassemia with genotype of HbH disease ($- -/-\alpha$)

β-Thalassemia with elevated γ-chain synthesis
    Homozygous β-thalassemia with heterocellular HPFH
    Homozygous β-thalassemia with homozygous $^{G}\gamma$ 158 T→C change (some cases)
    Compound heterozygosity for β-thalassemia and deletion forms of HPFH

Compound heterozygosity for β-thalassemia and β-chain variants
    HbE/β-thalassemia
    Other interactions with rare β-chain variants

Heterozygous β-thalassemia with triplicated or quadruplicated α-chain genes (ααα or αααα)
    Dominant forms of β-thalassemia
    Interactions of β-thalassemia and (δβ)⁺-thalassemia or (δβ)⁰-thalassemia

Hb, hemoglobin; HPFH, hereditary persistence of fetal hemoglobin.

and may not be able to adapt completely to living at high altitudes, both situations in which there is an adaptive increase in Hb normally. Rarely, women may have a moderately severe anemia of pregnancy, in some cases requiring transfusion. Some β-thalassemia carriers have increased iron stores, although this is most often a result of inappropriate long-term iron therapy based on a misdiagnosis. In countries where there is a relatively high frequency of genetic determinants for hemochromatosis, the possibility of their coinheritance should be borne in mind if a patient with β-thalassemia trait with an unusually high plasma iron or serum ferritin level is encountered.

α-THALASSEMIA

As in β-thalassemia, there is heterogeneity in presentation of the more severe forms of α-thalassemia, but this is much less so than in the former. Genotype-phenotype correlation is consistent, and most of these individuals do not have a significant degree of ineffective erythropoiesis.

Hemoglobin Bart's Hydrops Fetalis Syndrome

As discussed in the pathophysiology section above, fetuses with homozygous α⁰-thalassemia (a thalassemia major) will begin to have manifestations of anemia in the second trimester. There is hepatosplenomegaly as these organs are the primary sites of erythropoiesis. With worsening anemia, there is heart failure and anasarca, leading to enlargement of the placenta and to a hydropic fetus, similar to the hydrops fetalis seen in severe Rh incompatibility. A variety of congenital anomalies have been observed. This disorder is a frequent cause of stillbirth in Southeast Asia, usually at 34 to 40 weeks of gestation. Rarely, infants may be born alive but die within the first few hours.[1,229] The new-borns are very pale, have massive edema and hepatosplenomegaly, and poor perfusion. Death results from heart failure. If detected prenatally, intrauterine transfusions may be administered with a good rate of success (Chap. 30). Postnatally, these infants would need to start regular transfusions immediately to ensure survival with normal growth and development.[230,231]

In such pregnancies, there is a high incidence of maternal toxemia and the delivery is often difficult because of the massive placenta.[229] The reason for placental hypertrophy is unknown, although severe intrauterine hypoxia is suspected because a similar phenomenon is observed in hydrops infants with Rh incompatibility.

Hemoglobin H Disease

HbH disease was described independently in the United States in 1956[232] and in Greece in 1955.[233] Although affected individuals have only a single normally functioning α-globin gene, the clinical presentation is somewhat variable. A few patients may have severe anemia, and require regular or intermittent transfusions, but most have a much milder course.[1,234] All patients have anemia, although the degree is variable, based on the expression of the single α-globin gene and any other potential genetic disease modifiers. Chronic microcytic anemia, some symptoms of anemia, such as fatigue and exercise intolerance, may be seen, but these are usually not severe. Splenomegaly is also somewhat variable, but because there is not as much ineffective erythropoiesis, the other clinical manifestations of the thalassemia intermedia syndrome, such as bone disease and iron overload, are not often seen.

As discussed in "Etiology and Pathogenesis" earlier, a few attempts have been made to correlate the genotype with the phenotype of HbH disease. In general, as expected, patients with a nondeletion α mutation on one side and both α deletions on the other, $\alpha^{ND}\alpha/--$, or $\alpha^{Constant Spring}\alpha/--$, tend to have higher HbH levels, a greater degree of anemia, and a more severe clinical course than patients with the $--/-\alpha$ genotype.[235-238] As discussed in preceding text (see "Imbalanced Globin"), HbH does not deliver oxygen efficiently, and the higher the level of this Hb, the more symptomatic individuals may be.

Milder Forms of α-Thalassemia

The carrier states for the deletion and nondeletion forms of α-thalassemia, $-\alpha/\alpha\alpha$ and $\alpha^{ND}\alpha/\alpha\alpha$, are usually completely asymptomatic (silent carrier) as only one gene is not functioning. If two genes are deleted, such as in $-\alpha/-\alpha$, or $--/\alpha\alpha$, individuals have a mild microcytic anemia, but usually are not symptomatic, as in β-thalassemia minor. On the other hand, the nondeletion forms of α-thalassemia, $\alpha^{ND}\alpha/\alpha^{ND}\alpha$, often give rise to an extremely diverse series of phenotypes. Some individuals are more anemic and may have the clinical picture of HbH disease. Others may have only mild hypochromic anemia as in the deletional form.[1] The homozygous states for the chain-termination mutants, notably HbConstant Spring, have the characteristic phenotype of thalassemia intermedia with moderate hemolytic anemia and splenomegaly.[1,239,240]

α-Thalassemia and Mental Retardation

There are two distinct genetic defects that underlie this syndrome, and the clinical picture is different based on the underlying defect. When the syndrome results from a deletion of the tip of chromosome 16 (ATR-16), the clinical manifestations of the defects that are seen will depend on the length of the deletion. Shorter deletions have α-thalassemia and mental retardation but when the deletion is 2000 kb or longer, it may involve genes that, when deleted, are responsible for tuberous sclerosis

and polycystic kidney disease, in which case these will be the dominant cause of symptoms, then α-thalassemia will play a more minor role.[167]

When there are mutations of the ATR-X gene, the syndrome is broader and includes skeletal abnormalities, dysmorphic face, neonatal hypotonus, genital abnormalities, and a variety of less-constant features, in addition to mental retardation and α-thalassemia.[168]

εγδβ-THALASSEMIA

In the heterozygous state, the clinical picture of εγδβ-thalassemia varies with the stage of development, the reasons for which are not clear.[1] Neonates may be significantly anemic and require transfusions, whereas the condition in children and adults is usually asymptomatic with the clinical and laboratory picture of β-thalassemia minor, except for a normal HbA_2 level. The homozygous state is assumed to be lethal and has not been reported.

● LABORATORY FEATURES AND DIFFERENTIAL DIAGNOSIS OF THE THALASSEMIA SYNDROMES

The laboratory diagnosis of the thalassemia syndromes was previously based on careful interpretation of the complete blood count, including the red cell indices, review of the blood film, and characterization of the type of Hb produced. More sophisticated laboratories would perform special staining, measure the α/β-globin chain synthesis ratio or perform other α-globin, β-globin, and γ-globin assessments, and do some DNA studies, especially for known mutations. With the easy availability of sophisticated DNA testing in the developed world, including whole-exome or genome sequencing, it is now possible to characterize the disease more completely, including all of the possible genetic modifiers.[162] This approach forms the basis for a thorough characterization of all of the genotypes described in this section, and offers some predictive insights into the clinical manifestation and future course. Although this is not routinely done for all patients, especially those with mild clinical manifestations, in more complex cases, it may be used to assess the likely clinical course. There also may be some predictive value in genotyping for some of the newer therapies, as is described later in "Novel therapies". Family members should also be tested.

The diagnosis of the more-severe forms of thalassemia, homozygous or compound heterozygous β-thalassemia, and HbH disease is relatively straightforward. However, in milder phenotypes, it may be somewhat more nuanced. The clinician must consider the ethnicity, family history, clinical presentation, physical examination, and laboratory parameters. Figure 17-16 shows a simple flowchart for laboratory investigations of a suspected case.

In early childhood, distinguishing thalassemia from the congenital sideroblastic anemias may be difficult, but the marrow appearances in the latter are quite characteristic. Juvenile myelomonocytic leukemia has a very high HbF level, but the frequent leukocytosis, blood monocytosis, immature myeloid cells in the blood, and a marrow characteristic of myelomonocytic leukemia readily differentiates this disorder from β-thalassemia.

β-THALASSEMIA

Homozygous β⁰-Thalassemia

Patients with the most severe forms of β-thalassemia present in infancy with profound anemia. With better access to medical care, affected infants in developed nations may be diagnosed early with Hb levels of 40–60 g/L, but in the developing world, they may present with

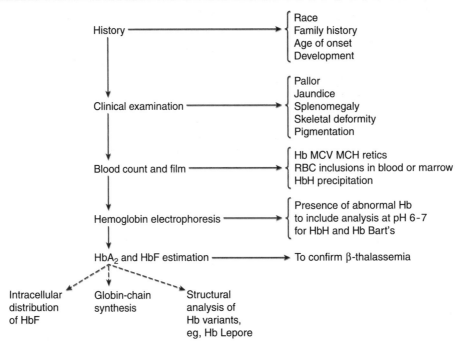

Figure 17–16. Flowchart showing an approach to diagnosis of the thalassemia syndromes. MCH, mean cell hemoglobin (Hb); MCV, mean corpuscular volume; RBC, red blood cell count.

symptoms of heart failure and Hb levels of 20–30 g/L, or even lower. The reticulocyte count is elevated, as are the white cell and platelet count, as a result of the marked marrow hyperplasia. There is microcytosis and anisopoikilocytosis, hypochromia, target cells, nucleated red cells, and basophilic stippling on peripheral film examination (Fig. 17-17). Hypersplenic patients may have low white cell and platelet counts, and after splenectomy, leukocytosis and thrombocytosis are common. Further, asplenic individuals have large, flat macrocytes and small, deformed microcytes, as well as markedly increased nucleated red cell counts, and the white cell count frequently has to be corrected for their presence. Staining of the blood with methyl violet, particularly in splenectomized subjects, reveals basophilic stippling or ragged inclusion bodies in the red cells (Chap. 1).[180] Red cell survival is markedly shortened, but there is some variability with cells containing more fetal Hb, surviving longer.

A marrow examination is not required for diagnosis, but if performed, shows marked erythroid hyperplasia with a maturation arrest, stippling, and inclusions in the red cell precursors, as well as an increased iron content. In vitro Hb synthesis studies using marrow or blood show a marked degree of globin-chain imbalance. Marked excess of α-globin chain over β-globin and γ-globin chain production is always observed.

Characterization of the Hb fractions by high-performance liquid chromatography (HPLC) or Hb electrophoresis shows no HbA in β^0 homozygotes, with HbF comprising the majority of the Hb, and a relative increase in HbA_2 as a proportion of total Hb. If there is compound heterozygosity for HbE, the HbA_2 fraction will be increased as HbE has the same retention time as HbA_2.

At diagnosis, iron studies show the typical picture seen with marked ineffective erythropoiesis, as a result of low hepcidin levels, as described in the pathophysiology section earlier. Serum iron and transferrin saturation are elevated, as is the ferritin level, thus ruling out iron-deficiency anemia as a cause for the microcytic, hypochromic anemia.

With treatment, the Hb level is in the mild to moderate anemia range as a result of the transfusion regimen, being higher in patients on regular transfusions and generally lower in those receiving on-demand transfusions. The mean corpuscular volume (MCV) reflects that of transfused red blood cells, as also the Hb fractions. With continuing transfusions, serum iron and transferrin saturation, as well as ferritin levels, are elevated, and remain so, with the ferritin level declining in response to chelation therapy.

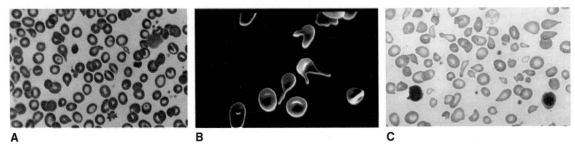

Figure 17–17. Blood films in β-thalassemia. **A.** β-Thalassemia minor. Anisocytosis. poikilocytosis. hypochromia. Occasional spherocytes and stomatocytes. **B.** Scanning electron micrograph of cells in **(A)** showing more detail of the poikilocytes. Note the knizocyte (pinch-bottle cell) at the lower right. **C.** β-Thalassemia major. Marked anisocytosis with many microcytes. Marked poikilocytosis. Anisochromia. Nucleated red cell on the right. Small lymphocyte on the left. *(Reproduced with permission from Lichtman MA, Shafer MS, Felgar RE, et al: Lichtman's Atlas of Hematology 2016. New York, NY: McGraw Hill; 2017.)*

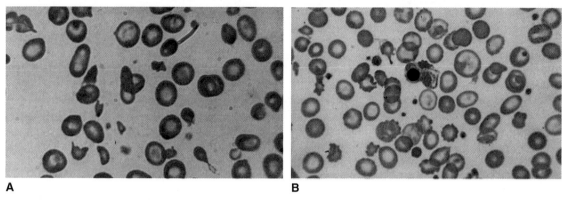

Figure 17–18. A. Thalassemia intermedia. Blood films. Marked anisocytosis, poikilocytosis with elliptical, oval, teardrop-shaped, and fragmented red cells. Target cells. **B.** Postsplenectomy. Morphology similar to that in **(A)** but with a nucleated red cell, coarsely stippled cell in center of field, and large and numerous platelets, indicative of the changes superimposed by splenectomy. *(Reproduced with permission from Lichtman MA, Shafer MS, Felgar RE, et al: Lichtman's Atlas of Hematology 2016. New York, NY: McGraw Hill; 2017.)*

Other laboratory abnormalities as a result of transfusion complications include the development of autoantibodies or alloantibodies with a positive direct antiglobulin test and antibody screen, and iron-related organ dysfunctions. All of these parameters are regularly monitored in transfusion-dependent patients.

Homozygous or Compound Heterozygous β⁺-Thalassemia

In these individuals, the untransfused Hb levels are generally higher than in β⁰ homozygotes, but otherwise, the hematologic changes are similar (Fig. 17-18). In individuals with more-severe anemia, and marked ineffective erythropoiesis, the blood film resembles that of a β-thalassemia major patient prior to starting transfusions. Postsplenectomy, a marked increase in nucleated red cells and the presence of misshapen and fragmented red cells is easily noted on the blood film examination. Examination of the marrow, if performed, would confirm ineffective erythropoiesis to a variable degree, with patients with more-severe anemia having the picture of untreated thalassemia major. HPLC shows a variable amount of HbA depending on the mutation; the rest is HbF and HbA_2. If there is compound heterozygosity for HbE, then the HbA_2 is also increased as HbE has same retention time as HbA_2. In the absence of transfusions, iron studies will show a steady rise in serum iron, transferrin saturation, and ferritin, with the rate of rise determined by the degree of ineffective erythropoiesis and increased intestinal absorption. If transfusions are given intermittently or regularly, the iron levels will rise faster and follow the same course as the rise in individuals with thalassemia major.

Heterozygous β-Thalassemia

The classic picture of β-thalassemia minor is a mild microcytic anemia (see Fig. 17-17), with Hb levels in the range from 90 to 110 g/L. The mean cell Hb (MCH) values are 20 to 22 picograms and MCV values are 50 to 70 fL, both red cell indices being particularly useful in screening for heterozygous carriers of thalassemia in population surveys. The red cell count is usually normal or elevated. The marrow in heterozygous β-thalassemia shows slight erythroid hyperplasia with rare red cell inclusions. Megaloblastic transformation as a result of folic acid deficiency occurs occasionally, particularly during pregnancy. A mild degree of ineffective erythropoiesis is noted, but red cell survival is normal or nearly normal. The HbA_2 level is increased to 3.5% to 7.0%. The level of fetal Hb is elevated in approximately 50% of cases, usually to 2% to 3%, and rarely to greater than 5%. Iron studies are normal, unless concomitant iron deficiency is also present, in which case the transferrin saturation and ferritin are low. In this situation, the Hb is lower, as are the red cell indices and the red cell count.

β-Thalassemia with Normal HbA_2 Levels

Rare forms of β-thalassemia are seen in which heterozygotes have normal HbA_2 levels. The hematologic picture may be completely normal or have a mild microcytic anemia with a completely normal Hb pattern on electrophoresis or HPLC. Thus, they can be confused with the more-severe forms of α-thalassemia in the heterozygous state, causing difficulties in genetic counseling and prenatal diagnosis. Based on hematologic studies, the two main classes of "normal HbA_2 β-thalassemia"—sometimes called types 1 and 2—are seen.[241] Type 1 is the "silent" form of β-thalassemia. Type 2 is heterogeneous, with many cases representing the compound heterozygous state for β-thalassemia and δ-thalassemia.

"Silent" β-thalassemia[1,242] is characterized by no hematologic changes in heterozygotes—there is no anemia—and the MCV is normal. Several mild forms of β-thalassemia that underlie this phenotype are described.[45,46] Although this condition can be partly identified by demonstrating a mild degree of globin-chain imbalance, with α-to-β synthesis ratios of approximately 1.5:1, "silent" β-thalassemia can only be diagnosed with certainty by DNA analysis. Compound heterozygotes for this condition and β⁰-thalassemia have a mild form of β-thalassemia intermedia.

Normal HbA_2 β-thalassemia type 2 in heterozygotes has a hematologic profile of mild microcytic anemia which is indistinguishable from typical β-thalassemia with elevated HbA_2 levels.[241] The homozygous state has not been described. The compound heterozygous state for this gene and for β-thalassemia with raised HbA_2 levels is characterized by a clinical picture of severe transfusion-dependent β-thalassemia. Family data obtained in Italy and Sardinia suggest this condition represents the compound heterozygous state for both β-thalassemia and δ-thalassemia.[243,244] Most cases of δ-thalassemia have been observed *trans* to β-thalassemia. However, the form of δ-thalassemia resulting from loss of an A in codon 59 occurs on the same chromosome as the HbKnossos mutation, which is associated with a mild form of β-thalassemia.[245] This finding explains the normal level of HbA_2 associated with this condition, which is the most common form of normal HbA_2 β-thalassemia in the Mediterranean region.

Several other conditions, mentioned in "Etiology and Pathogenesis" earlier, are associated with a phenotype that is indistinguishable from normal HbA_2 β-thalassemia. These conditions include the heterozygous states for the Corfu form of δβ-thalassemia and εγδβ-thalassemia.

Dominant β-Thalassemia

The clinical features of dominant β-thalassemia resemble the features of thalassemia intermedia.[1] Moderate anemia and splenomegaly are seen, with a blood picture showing thalassemic red cell changes. The marrow shows erythroid hyperplasia with well-marked inclusion bodies in the red cell precursors, which may be seen in the blood after splenectomy. Hb analysis shows HbA and HbA$_2$ are present, and the HbF level is usually elevated much higher than that seen in β-thalassemia trait. HbA$_2$ levels are always raised.[98,99]

Other Unusual Forms of β-Thalassemia

Other unusual varieties of β-thalassemia include those categorized by unusually high HbF or HbA$_2$ levels. Most of these conditions result from deletions involving the β-globin gene and its promoter region. For example, the so-called Dutch[61] form of β-thalassemia is associated with unusually high HbF levels in heterozygotes and high HbA$_2$ levels. Several other conditions of this type, which result from different-size deletions, have been reported.[13,62]

(δβ)⁰-Thalassemia The homozygous state for δβ-thalassemia [(δβ)⁰/(δβ)⁰] is clinically milder and is a form of thalassemia intermedia.[246-248] Only HbF is present; HbA and HbA$_2$ are not produced. Similarly, heterozygosity for both β-thalassemia and δβ-thalassemia [(δβ)⁰/β⁰] or, more rarely, [(δβ)⁰/β⁺], results in an intermedia syndrome clinically. The Hb consists largely of HbF, with a small amount of HbA$_2$, because the associated β-thalassemia mutation is usually a β⁰ mutation.[112]

Heterozygous δβ-thalassemia [(δβ)⁰/β] is hematologically similar to β-thalassemia minor.[1] The fetal Hb level is higher (range: 5%-20%), and the HbA$_2$ value is normal or slightly reduced. As in β-thalassemia, the fetal Hb is heterogeneously distributed among the red cells, thus distinguishing this disorder from HPFH (Fig. 17-19).

δβ-Thalassemia also has been observed in individuals heterozygous for HbS [(δβ)⁰/β^S] or HbC [(δβ)⁰/β^C].[1]

(δβ)⁺-Thalassemia and HbLepore Disorders The HbLepore disorders have been described in the homozygous state [(δβ)^L/(δβ)^L], and in the heterozygous state [β/(δβ)^L], either alone or in association with β⁰ [β⁰/(δβ)^L], β⁺ [β⁺/(δβ)^L], δβ-thalassemia [(δβ)⁺/(δβ)^L], HbS [β^S/(δβ)^L], or HbC [β^C/(δβ)^L].[1,14,249] In the homozygous state, approximately 20% of the Hb is of the Lepore type and 80% is fetal Hb. HbA and HbA$_2$ are absent. The clinical picture is variable. Some cases are identical to transfusion-dependent homozygous β-thalassemia; others are associated with the clinical picture of thalassemia intermedia. Clinically, the heterozygous state is similar to those of β-thalassemia minor but laboratory wise, the Hb consists of approximately 10% HbLepore, with a reduced level of HbA$_2$ and a slight but consistent increase in fetal Hb level. The Lepore Hbs have been found sporadically in most racial groups. In the majority of cases, their analyses have shown that these Hbs are identical to HbLepore-Washington-Boston. HbLepore-Hollandia and HbLepore-Baltimore have been observed in only a few patients.[1,249]

HEREDITARY PERSISTENCE OF FETAL HEMOGLOBIN

The current knowledge about the molecular pathology of HPFH was described in "Etiology and Pathogenesis" earlier. Table 17-3 summarizes the currently accepted classification and nomenclature of this complex group of conditions. The different forms of HPFH are of very little clinical importance except that they may interact with thalassemia or the structural Hb variants.

(δβ)⁰ Hereditary Persistence of Fetal Hemoglobin

Homozygotes for (δβ)⁰ HPFH have 100% HbF. Their blood shows mild thalassemic changes, with reduced MCH and MCV values very similar to those observed in heterozygous β-thalassemia. Similarly, they have imbalanced globin-chain production, with ratios in the range of

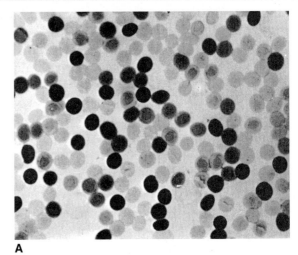

A

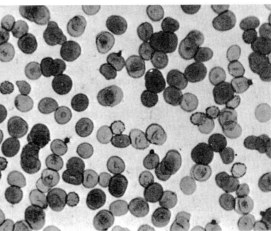

B

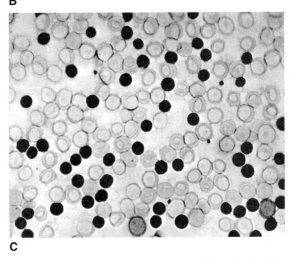

C

Figure 17–19. Acid elution preparations of blood films from **(A)** δβ-thalassemia, **(B)** hereditary persistence of fetal Hb, and **(C)** artificial mixture of fetal and adult red cells. The dark cells contain HbF. HbF is resistant to acid elution. Hb, hemoglobin.

those observed in β-thalassemia heterozygotes.[250] Heterozygotes have approximately 20% to 30% HbF, slightly reduced HbA$_2$ values, and completely normal blood pictures. Thus, this condition appears to be an extremely well-compensated form of δβ-thalassemia in which the output of γ-globin chains almost, but not entirely, compensates for the complete absence of β-globin and δ-globin chains. The different molecular forms of this condition show no difference in phenotype except in the proportion of ^{G}γ-globin chains. The African forms of $(δβ)^0$ HPFH have been found in association with HbS and HbC or with β-thalassemia (Chap. 18). These compound heterozygous states are usually mild and associated with little morbidity.[1]

Nondeletion Types of Hereditary Persistence of Fetal Hemoglobin

Many nondeletion forms of HPFH associated with point mutations upstream from the γ-globin genes have been described (see Table 17-3). ^{G}γβ$^+$ HPFH has been found in the heterozygous and compound heterozygous states with β-globin chain variants in African populations. No associated clinical or hematologic findings have been reported. Compound heterozygotes for ^{G}γβ$^+$ HPFH and HbS or HbC produce 45% of the abnormal Hb, approximately 30% HbA, and approximately 20% HbF containing only ^{G}γ-globin chains.[251,252]

The most common form of nondeletion HPFH is ^{A}γβ$^+$ HPFH, which is found in Greeks.[253-255] In the homozygous state, no clinical or hematologic abnormalities are noted. The Hb findings are characterized by approximately 25% fetal Hb and reduced HbA$_2$ levels of approximately 0.8%.[256] Heterozygotes, who also are hematologically normal, have 10% to 15% HbF, almost all of the ^{A}γ variety. Compound heterozygotes with β-thalassemia have high HbF levels and a clinical picture that is only slightly more severe than the β-thalassemia trait.

In the British form of ^{A}γβ$^+$ HPFH[257], heterozygotes have approximately 5% to 12% HbF, whereas homozygotes have approximately 20%. No associated hematologic abnormalities are seen, although, surprisingly, in this form of nondeletion HPFH, the HbF seems to be unevenly distributed among the red cells.

A heterogeneous group of conditions is associated with persistent production of small amounts of HbF in adult life. They are categorized under the general heading of heterocellular HPFH. Their clinical importance is that, when they are coinherited with different forms of β-thalassemia, they may lead to greater output of HbF and, hence, to a milder phenotype. This type of interaction should be suspected when one parent of a patient with β-thalassemia intermedia has an unusually high level of HbF for the β-thalassemia trait. Similarly, unaffected lateral relatives or other family members with slightly elevated HbF levels may be found.[133,258]

β-THALASSEMIA ASSOCIATED WITH β-GLOBIN CHAIN STRUCTURAL HEMOGLOBIN VARIANTS

The most clinically important associations of β-thalassemia with β structural Hb variants are HbS/β-thalassemia (sickle–β-thalassemia), HbC/β-thalassemia, and HbE/β-thalassemia (Chap. 18). In addition, many interactions of β-thalassemia with rare structural variants have been reported.[1,10,15]

Sickle–β-thalassemia[1,259,260] occurs in parts of Africa and in the Mediterranean, particularly Greece and Italy, as well as the Middle East and parts of India. The clinical consequences of carrying one gene for HbS and one gene for β-thalassemia depend entirely on the type of β-thalassemia mutation. The interaction between the sickle cell gene and β^0-thalassemia is characterized by a clinical disorder that is very similar to sickle cell anemia. Similarly, the interaction of the sickle cell gene with the more severe forms of β$^+$-thalassemia associated with marked reduction in β-globin synthesis yields a similar, but often milder, clinical phenotype. On the other hand, the interaction of the sickle cell gene with very mild forms of β$^+$-thalassemia may be much less severe.[259] HbS/β$^+$-Thalassemia is characterized by mild anemia associated with splenomegaly and a Hb composition of approximately 60% to 70% HbS, 25% HbA, and an elevated level of HbA$_2$. In all these interactions, one parent has the sickle cell trait, and the other parent shows the β-thalassemia trait.

HbC/β-thalassemia is a mild hemolytic disorder associated with splenomegaly.[1,14,15] Again, the Hb pattern varies depending on whether the thalassemia gene is the β$^+$ or β^0 type. This relatively innocuous condition has been recorded mainly in North Africa, but it also is found in West Africa. The blood picture shows a mild microcytic anemia, and the blood film reveals numerous target cells characteristic of all the HbC disorders.

HbE/β-thalassemia, which occurs at a high frequency in the eastern half of the Indian subcontinent and throughout Southeast Asia, is one of the most important hemoglobinopathies in the world population.[1,14,15,261-267] As mentioned in "Etiology and Pathogenesis" earlier, HbE is synthesized at a reduced rate thus producing the clinical phenotype of a mild form of β-thalassemia. Hence, when HbE is inherited with β-thalassemia—and most often this is a β^0-thalassemia or severe β$^+$-thalassemia mutation in Southeast Asia and India—a marked deficit of β-globin chain production results, with the clinical picture of severe β-thalassemia. HbE/β-thalassemia shows a remarkable variability in clinical expression,[263-267] ranging from a mild form of thalassemia intermedia to a transfusion-dependent condition clinically indistinguishable from β-thalassemia major. The reasons for this variability of expression are not understood, although some of the factors involved are identical to those that modify other forms of β-thalassemia.[261,262]

In more-severe cases of HbE/β-thalassemia, the clinical picture of severe thalassemia intermedia with marked ineffective erythropoiesis includes severe anemia with growth retardation, leg ulcers, bone deformity, marked tendency to infection, iron loading, and variable splenomegaly and hypersplenism. Large tumor masses composed of extramedullary erythropoietic tissue may cause a variety of compression syndromes, including a clinical picture that closely mimics a cerebral tumor. Another curious picture that seems to be restricted to splenectomized patients is an obliterative occlusion of the pulmonary vasculature that is believed to result from an extremely high platelet count.[268]

The clinical course and complications in transfusion-dependent patients are similar to those observed in homozygous β-thalassemia. In the milder forms, the main complications are progressive hypersplenism, organ damage as a result of progressive iron loading from an increased rate of absorption, extramedullary erythropoietic tumor masses, bone disease, and infection. The blood picture shows a typical thalassemic pattern. The Hb consists of E, F, and A$_2$ but keep in mind that HbE cannot be distinguished from HbA$_2$ as both Hbs have the same retention time in HPLC. Usually no HbA is present because the β^0-thalassemia is particularly common in the parts of the world where HbE is found.

The complex interactions between genetic factors,[261,262] differences in adaptation to anemia, particularly in early life (see "Pathophysiology" earlier), and the environment, notably proneness to malarial infection, underlie the widely differing and unstable phenotypes of patients with HbE/β-thalassemia.[261,267]

δ^0-THALASSEMIA

δ^0-Thalassemia causes a complete absence of HbA$_2$ in homozygotes and a reduced HbA$_2$ level in heterozygotes.[269] It is of no clinical significance except for its effect of reducing HbA$_2$ levels in β-thalassemia heterozygotes.

εγδβ-THALASSEMIA

This heterogeneous condition has been observed only in the heterozygous state in a few families.[1,135,136,141,142] It is characterized by neonatal hemolysis and, in adult life, by the hematologic picture of heterozygous β-thalassemia with normal HbA$_2$ levels.

β-THALASSEMIA

Hemoglobin Bart's Hydrops Fetalis Syndrome

These infants may be born (if not stillborn) with severe anemia that is microcytic and hypochromic. The blood film shows severe thalassemic changes as described above in the Laboratory features section, with large numbers of nucleated red cells. The Hb is mainly of HbBart's, with persistence of embryonic HbPortland (ζ^{2}γ^2) at 10% to 20%. Usually no HbA, HbA$_2$, or HbF is present because no α-globin chains are synthesized, although rare cases that seem to result from interaction of α^0-thalassemia with a severe nondeletion form of α$^+$-thalassemia may show small amounts of HbA. If these infants survive intrauterine and postnatally with transfusions, they would develop the same laboratory features as individuals with transfusion-dependent β-thalassemia major.

Hemoglobin H Disease

Depending on their underlying genotype and other modifiers, these individuals may have a varying degree of anemia. The blood film shows hypochromia and anisopoikilocytosis. The reticulocyte count is usually elevated. Incubation of the red cells with brilliant cresyl blue results in multiple ragged inclusion bodies in almost all cells resembling golf balls. These bodies form because of precipitation of HbH in vitro as a result of reduction-oxidation action of the dye. After splenectomy, large, single Heinz bodies are observed in some cells (Fig. 17-20). These bodies are formed by in vitro precipitation of the unstable HbH molecule and are seen only after splenectomy. Characterization of the Hb shows 5% to 40% HbH, traces of HbBart's, and a lower than normal HbA$_2$. Iron studies are normal initially but may rise as in β-thalassemia intermedia, but because ineffective erythropoiesis is not a major feature of HbH disease, severe iron loading is not common.

Heterozygous α^0-Thalassemia and Homozygous Deletional α$^+$-Thalassemia

Individuals heterozygous for α^0-thalassemia (– –/αα) or homozygous for deletional α$^+$-thalassemia (–α/–α) have a mild anemia with low MCH and MCV values, similar to those with β-thalassemia trait. In general, the –α$^{4.2}$ deletion is associated with a more-severe phenotype than is the –α$^{3.7}$ deletion.[1] At birth they may have 5% to 15% HbBart's,[7] but this Hb disappears during maturation and is not replaced by a similar amount of HbH; as a result, the HPLC or electrophoretic pattern is normal. An occasional cell with HbH inclusion bodies may appear after incubation with brilliant cresyl blue. Globin-synthesis studies show a deficit of α-globin chain production, with an α-chain–to–β-chain production ratio of approximately 0.7.

Homozygous State for Nondeletion Types of α-Thalassemia

The homozygous state for nondeletion forms of α-thalassemia involving the dominant (α$_2$) globin gene causes a more severe deficit of α-globin chains than do the deletion forms of α$^+$-thalassemia. In some cases, the homozygous state produces HbH disease.

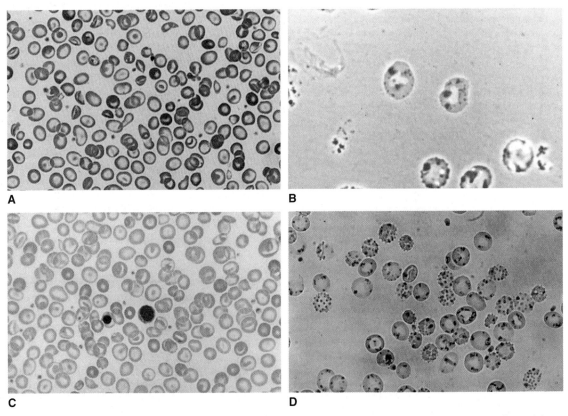

A

B

C

D

Figure 17–20. HbH disease (α-thalassemia). Blood films. **A.** Note hypochromic red cells, anisocytosis, target cells, poikilocytes, including teardrop-shaped red cells. **B.** Wet preparation stained with crystal violet. Inclusions in red cells (Heinz bodies) usually attached to membrane. **C.** Postsplenectomy. Note reduction in poikilocytes and frequency of target cells, a change consistent with HbH disease and enhanced by postsplenectomy effects. A nucleated red cell is in this field, reflecting an increase in their prevalence in the blood after splenectomy. **D.** Blood incubated for 90 minutes with brilliant cresyl blue. Numerous HbH intracellular precipitates (precipitates of excess β-globin chains). The frequent crenation is an artifact of the incubation conditions. Hb, hemoglobin. (*Reproduced with permission from Lichtman MA, Shafer MS, Felgar RE, et al: Lichtman's Atlas of Hematology 2016. New York, NY: McGraw Hill; 2017.*)

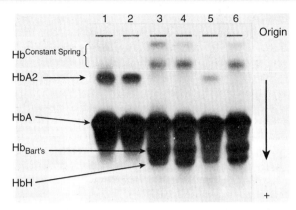

Figure 17–21. Hb^Constant Spring. Starch gel electrophoresis of 1, 2, normal adult; 3, 4, compound heterozygotes for Hb^Constant Spring and α⁰-thalassemia with HbH disease; 5, normal adult; and 6, compound heterozygote for α⁰-thalassemia and Hb^Constant Spring. Hb, hemoglobin.

In the homozygous state for HbConstant Spring or other chain-termination mutations, the blood picture shows mild thalassemic changes with normal-size red cells[239,240] with an associated moderately severe hemolytic anemia. The Hb consists of approximately 5% to 6% HbConstant Spring, normal HbA₂ levels, and trace amounts of HbBart's. The remainder is HbA. For unclear reasons, no HbH is present but small amounts of HbBart's may persist into adult life. The homozygous states for the other nondeletion forms of α⁺-thalassemia are associated with HbH disease.

The heterozygous state for HbConstant Spring shows no hematologic abnormality. The Hb pattern is normal except for the presence of small amounts (approximately 0.5%) of HbConstant Spring. The latter can be observed on alkaline starch-gel electrophoresis as a faint band migrating between HbA₂ and the origin. It is best seen on heavily loaded starch gels and is easily missed if other electrophoretic techniques are used (Fig. 17-21). In the newborn, usually 1% to 3% HbBart's is present in the cord blood.

Heterozygous Deletional α⁺-Thalassemia

The α⁺-thalassemia trait (−α/αα) is characterized by a normal Hb or slight anemia, with a very mild reduction in MCH and MCV values, although in many cases these are also normal. Individuals may have 1% to 2% of HbBart's at birth in some, and a slightly reduced α-chain–to–β-chain production ratio of approximately 0.8. Given the mostly normal hematologic picture, this genotype often is referred to as "silent carrier." Extensive studies comparing the level of HbBart's at birth with DNA analyses demonstrated that there is no detectable HbBart's in a significant number of newborns who are heterozygous for α⁺-thalassemia.[223,224] Globin-gene synthetic ratios can be distinguished from normal only by studying relatively large numbers of samples and comparing the mean α–to–β ratio with that of normal control subjects. This approach is not reliable for diagnosing individual cases of the α⁺-thalassemia trait, and, unfortunately, no reliable method of diagnosis is available except for DNA analysis.

α-THALASSEMIA IN ASSOCIATION WITH α-CHAIN AND β-CHAIN HEMOGLOBIN VARIANTS

Several α-globin structural variants are caused by single-amino-acid substitutions at α-chain loci on chromosomes that carry only a single α-chain gene. Individuals who inherit variants of this type and an

α⁰-thalassemia determinant have a form of HbH disease in which the Hb consists of the α-chain variant Hb and HbH. Well-documented examples include HbQH disease (− −/−α^Q),[270,271] HbG Philadelphia H disease (− −/−α^G),[272,273] and Hb Hasharon H disease (− −/−α^Hash).[274] Many examples of the coexistence of the homozygous or heterozygous states for β-chain Hb variants and different α-thalassemia determinants have been reported.[1,14,15] Particularly well-characterized disorders include the various interactions of α⁰-thalassemia and α⁺-thalassemia with HbE[7,239] and HbS (Chap. 18).[257,258] Carriers for these Hb variants who also have the α⁰-thalassemia or α⁺-thalassemia traits have thalassemic red cell indices and unusually low levels of the abnormal Hb. Individuals with sickle cell anemia who have α-thalassemia show thalassemic red cell changes, more persistent splenomegaly, and lower HbF values than do patients without the thalassemia genes.

●THERAPY, COURSE, AND PROGNOSIS

The goals of treatment for the thalassemia syndromes are to (1) maintain optimal levels of Hb for growth and development in children, and appropriate activity at all ages; (2) minimize the complications related to ineffective erythropoiesis, by adequately suppressing patient's own (endogenous) marrow activity; (3) prevent complications related to the therapy of the disease; and (4) improve longevity while maintaining a good quality of life.

To achieve these goals, the approaches include the judicious use of transfusions, the appropriate use of iron-chelation therapy, regular monitoring for and prompt treatment of complications, and overall good supportive care, including psychosocial support.[1,14] The only currently available curative therapy is HSC transplantation, optimally from a matched related donor. Most patients in the developed world are treated at comprehensive thalassemia centers; a treatment approach is strongly recommended because it incorporates all of the above in an individually tailored programmatic manner. Individuals with thalassemia minor rarely, if ever, require the treatments described herein. It is important to approach management with the idea that there is spectrum of severity between thalassemia major and thalassemia intermedia, and that patients may move on that continuum with increasing severity of clinical disease. Although the management discussed in this section applies mostly to patients with thalassemia major, it also applies to those with thalassemia intermedia as they move toward transfusion dependence.

TRANSFUSION

Transfusions are administered to maintain adequate Hb levels for growth, development, and maintenance of overall well-being. The decision to initiate a regular transfusion regimen is relatively straightforward for patients with homozygous α-thalassemia or β-thalassemia. However, in patients with clinical thalassemia intermedia, it may be more complex and involve patient and family preference, degree of anemia and bone changes related to ineffective erythropoiesis, degree of extramedullary hematopoiesis, and complications such as spinal cord compression, nonhealing leg ulcers, or progressive symptoms related to anemia. Some patients with thalassemia intermedia may only require periodic transfusions at times of stress, such as severe infections, surgery, or pregnancy, whereas others may show a progressive course with more complications and demonstrate a benefit from starting regular transfusions to prevent progression. In general, patients are now also classified as *transfusion-dependent thalassemia* (TDT) and *non–transfusion-dependent thalassemia* (NTDT). In TDT patients, maintaining the pretransfusion Hb in the 95 to 105 g/L range supports near-normal activity, growth and development, and suppression of ineffective erythropoiesis.[275] This is termed a *hypertransfusion* regimen. This allows children with β-thalassemia to grow and develop normally, without the distressing skeletal complications of thalassemia occurring.[1,275] Some patients have greater needs and may be maintained at higher Hb levels, such as active teenagers and those with increased physical activity. A review of transfusion guidelines may be found at the Cooley's Anemia Foundation website (https://www.thalassemia.org/thalassemia-management-checklists-now-available-download/) and the Thalassaemia International Federation website (https://thalassaemia.org.cy/publications/tif-publications/).

In the most sever forms of thalassemia, transfusions are generally begun in the first or second year of life, and continued monthly. It is recommended to have a limited extended phenotype of the recipient red cells, generally including the C, D, E, and Kell red cell antigens (Chap. 29) to minimize alloimmunization. However, practice standards may vary by region, and only involve the standard ABO and Rh antigens in areas where the donor and recipient pools are ethnically similar. There is no evidence that irradiation of the red cells is of benefit to patients with thalassemia. To avoid transfusion reactions, washed, filtered, or frozen red cells should be used so that the majority of the white cells and plasma-protein components are removed (Chaps. 29 and 30). The volume of packed red blood cells transfused at each visit is generally 15 mL/kg in children, to increase to a full unit when the child weighs approximately 15 kg. Split units are not recommended because they do not afford the benefit of the full amount, and yet expose the recipient to another donor. The interval between transfusions may be shortened instead, until the child reaches a weight of approximately 36 to 40 kg, when a second unit may be added. Most adults receive 2 U of packed red blood cells every 2 to 4 weeks. Occasionally, for logistical reasons, more blood may be administered at longer intervals, but this is not recommended because marrow erythropoietic activity may not be suppressed sufficiently with wide swings in Hb levels.

Transfusion reactions range from nonhemolytic complications, such as febrile reactions, allergic reactions including urticarial reactions, and rare anaphylaxis, to hemolytic complications such as acute and delayed hemolysis. The development of antibodies, both autoantibodies and alloantibodies are well known in thalassemia patients. Alloantibodies make it harder to crossmatch blood for patients, although the incidence of development of new alloantibodies is declining with the institution of more standard extended red cell antigen typing.[276] Autoantibodies may also increase transfusion requirements, and should be appropriately treated when clinically significant.

SPLENECTOMY

Splenectomy was a common intervention in both TDT and NTDT patients. In patients with TDT, the development of hypersplenism late in the first decade of life and early in the second, often resulted in increasing transfusion requirements. To minimize the development of hypersplenism and the increased risk of iron overload, as well as to minimize the risk of spontaneous or traumatic rupture of a large spleen, the spleen was surgically removed. Massive splenic enlargement with risk of rupture and pain in the left upper quadrant, as well as a dropping Hb level, were indications for splenectomy in NTDT. Increasing evidence indicates children maintained at a high Hb level do not develop hypersplenism.[1] This is the current practice in much of the developed world, but not so much in the developing world where transfusions are on demand because of logistic and economic reasons. Ongoing ineffective erythropoiesis, extramedullary hematopoiesis, and enlargement of the spleen with increased transfusion requirements occur commonly in patients maintained at a lower Hb level.

There is a move away from splenectomy even when there is an increased transfusion requirement. The proposed rationale for this is that the loss of splenic clearance of deformed and fragmented cells, along with the resulting thrombocytosis, increases the risk of developing chronic pulmonary embolism and pulmonary vascular disease, particularly pulmonary hypertension. This has not been borne out in well-transfused older patients who underwent splenectomy as children; these patients have not developed pulmonary hypertension with greater frequency. If appropriate transfusion is able to maintain suppression of ineffective erythropoiesis, there should not be many misshapen or fragmented cells making it into the circulation. In patients not transfused on a regular basis, this would be a risk factor, and we do see an increased prevalence of vascular disease, including pulmonary hypertension and silent cerebral infarcts in the thalassemia intermedia population.

Splenectomy should not be performed in children younger than 5 years because of the risk of an overwhelming pneumococcal infection. Patients should receive a pneumococcal vaccine prior to the procedure. *Haemophilus influenzae* type B and meningococcal vaccines also are recommended. Vaccinations need to be repeated, mostly after 5 years. Patients should be placed on prophylactic oral penicillin postsplenectomy, and any febrile episode must be treated with caution, with assessment and prompt administration of antibiotics as indicated. Patients with thalassemia and iron overload are predisposed to certain infections other than those expected as a result of splenectomy alone. Presentation with abdominal pain, diarrhea, and vomiting should always suggest an infection with a member of the *Yersinia* class of bacteria, which is an iron-avid organism. Empirical antibiotic treatment should start immediately.

IRON CHELATION

A regular transfusion regimen results in a variety of complications. In the short term, patients may have reactions as discussed in "Transfusion" section on previous page, but long-term complications are more worrisome. With the improved safety of the blood supply and the institution of extended phenotyping of blood in the developed world, the complications of bloodborne infections and alloimmunization have been minimized. The long-term complication that all patients receiving regular transfusions develop is iron overload or secondary hemochromatosis.[227] Irrespective of age, this complication would develop after approximately 15 transfusions because of the body's inability to excrete excess iron. If not treated, iron overload eventually results in deposition in the organs, particularly the heart and endocrine organs, resulting in significant morbidity and even mortality from cardiac complications of myocardial siderosis.[275] The complications have been briefly described in the pathophysiology section earlier. Iron overload and its management in general is described in detail in Chap. 11. Here, the discussion focuses specifically on the nuances related to thalassemia.[277]

The regular measurement of iron stores was almost exclusively done by measuring serum ferritin levels, with liver biopsy and quantitative iron measurement being used in some more advanced centers. The latter is a painful and invasive test, with a significant risk of complications. Since 2000, magnetic resonance techniques have been developed to more accurately assess tissue iron and allow the treatment regimen to be tailored (Chap. 11). There is now strong evidence that, with adequate calibration, the measurement and mapping of liver iron concentrations using MRI is an extremely effective approach for the regular assessment of the effectiveness of chelation therapy.[278] Similarly, there have been advances in the noninvasive estimation of myocardial iron using T2* MRI. Evidence obtained using this approach suggests that there may be a variable correlation between hepatic and cardiac iron concentrations.[279] This technique is able to quantify the liver iron concentration, which is normally less than 1.5 mg/g dry weight, and the myocardial iron level measures as a T2* value, normally longer than 20 milliseconds. Multiple studies have compared ferritin levels with liver iron measurements by both biopsy and MRI, and though the relationship has a significant correlation, there is marked variability between patients, confirming the lower reliability of this measurement. Ferritin is an acute-phase reactant and its level fluctuates markedly even in individual patients. It was standard practice to initiate chelation in thalassemia patients when the serum ferritin reached 1000 mcg/dL. However, this is quite variable, and because we can quantify the rate of iron loading, knowing the volume of blood transfused and its iron content, a serum ferritin of 1000 mcg/dL is not a reasonable starting point. Chelation should be initiated after the patient has received approximately 15 transfusions (by which time the liver iron would be estimated to be approximately 6-8 mg/g dry weight). If possible, an MRI of the liver should be performed to quantify the iron and provide a baseline for monitoring efficacy. Liver MRIs are recommended annually. In children treated with iron chelation, cardiac imaging is usually not performed until the child is older than 10 years. Adults with a longer-standing disease should have cardiac iron assessments along with liver iron assessments. Ferritin levels may still be of use to follow trends and to guide the use of additional MRI assessments or changes in chelation regimens. However, ferritin levels are still used almost exclusively where MRI is not available and they should be used with some caution.[280] In addition, regular monitoring of endocrine functions, including that of the pituitary, endocrine pancreas, thyroid, parathyroid, adrenals, and gonads, as these organs also may be severely affected by iron overload, should begin around 10 years of age.

The excretion of this excess iron must be facilitated by the use of iron chelation. There are three iron chelators in clinical use currently, one administered parenterally and the other two, orally.

Deferoxamine (desferrioxamine) was the first chelating agent of proven long-term value for treatment of iron overload in thalassemia. It is a large molecule that is digested when given orally, and when given parenterally, has a half-life of approximately 30 minutes. To optimize its efficacy it must be given by SQ infusion over 8 to 12 hours, preferably daily, but at least five to six times per week.[281,282] This results in significant discomfort, often resulting in injection-site erythema and irritation, sterile injection abscesses, and, sometimes, cellulitis that requires cessation of chelation and administration of antibiotics. As a result, use compliance is not optimal. With the advent of the new oral chelators, deferoxamine is now used as a second-line agent, mostly when patients are unable to tolerate the oral agents, or in combination with an oral agent, when intensification of chelation is necessary. Individuals who develop siderotic cardiomyopathy-induced heart failure have been successfully treated with continuous IV deferoxamine for prolonged periods of time (years).[283] This necessitates the insertion of a central venous catheter. Long-term side effects of deferoxamine include ototoxicity, with high-frequency hearing loss and tinnitus, and ocular toxicity with visual failure, night and color blindness, and field loss. Ototoxicity and ocular toxicity generally respond to discontinuation of the drug, but in some cases, the effects are irreversible.[284] Careful monitoring for these toxicities is recommended. Deferoxamine can also cause bone changes and growth retardation, and is sometimes associated with bone pain, particularly when used in the absence of significant iron overload. Body measurements characteristically show a reduced crown-pubis–to–pubis-heel ratio.[285] These changes may be associated with radiologic abnormalities of the vertebral column.

Two orally effective iron-chelating agents are currently available, deferasirox and deferiprone. The extensive literature on these agents has been reviewed.[286-288]

Deferasirox is an oral, once-daily iron chelator, with a long half-life. It has become the first-line drug for the management of transfusional iron overload because of its convenience and relatively low toxicity profile. Initially it was available only as a dispersible tablet that had to be taken on an empty stomach, which resulted in some gastrointestinal intolerance. It is now also available as film-coated tablets, as well as sprinkles that can be mixed with yogurt or applesauce, making it palatable to young children. It is effective in removing iron from the heart and other tissues, and with better compliance has changed the landscape of transfusional iron loading in thalassemia considerably. Most children born in the era of oral chelation have very little or no myocardial iron deposition, and thus few cardiac or endocrinal complications. Toxicities include usually nonprogressive elevation of the serum creatinine with some spilling of protein in the urine, and elevation of liver enzymes. Consequently, close monitoring of the blood metabolic profile and urine microalbumin is recommended and dose adjustments should be made accordingly. If a dose-limiting toxicity is observed, the dose may be reduced and a second chelator added.

Deferiprone is also administered orally, but given its short half-life, must be taken three times a day. For this reason alone, it is not used as initial therapy, because compliance is more challenging, particularly for the dose in the middle of the day. Deferiprone has good efficacy at purging iron from the myocardium, and is often used in combination with other chelators in patients with lower cardiac T2* values. It is also used in combination therapy for highly iron-loaded individuals and as a single agent in patients who are not able to tolerate either of the other two agents. In general, it is well tolerated and has low rates of gastrointestinal intolerance or impairment of hepatic or renal function. The most concerning side effect is the development of neutropenia, and occasionally agranulocytosis, making it a high risk for sepsis. For this reason, blood counts should be monitored regularly, and the drug stopped if the neutrophil counts drop. It is also associated with the development of arthropathy and arthralgia, with a variable severity about ethnic groups, being more commonly seen in Asians than in any other ethnic group.

Many different combination regimens of these chelators have been used for patients with severe iron overload, often tailored to whether the overload is more systemic or more cardiac. Deferiprone-containing combinations are more frequently used when cardiac iron overload is present.

A review of chelation guidelines may be found at the Cooley's Anemia Foundation website (https://www.thalassemia.org/thalassemia-management-checklists-now-available-download/) and at the Thalassaemia International Federation website (https://thalassaemia.org.cy/publications/tif-publications/).

STEM CELL TRANSPLANTATION

The only curative treatment available currently is HSC transplantation (HSCT). Outcomes of HSCT in thalassemia are dependent on two critical considerations: (1) the characteristics of the donor and (2) the preexisting morbidities in the recipient. The outcomes are superior when the donor is a fully matched relative, typically a sibling.[289] Although other donor types have been used, mostly in the clinical trial setting, outcomes from matched unrelated donors or any mismatched donor, including a haploidentical donor, are inferior. Thus, current recommendations are to go forward with a matched related donor for the best chance of a cure. Alternative donor sources such as umbilical cord blood have also been used with some success, but this is limited to children under 6 or 8 years of age, to ensure an adequate stem cell dose. Preexisting morbidities such as hepatomegaly, with or without fibrosis, and severe (inadequately treated) iron overload, increase the risk of HSCT failure.[290-292]

The complications related to the procedure are similar to those that would occur in other allogeneic transplants and are related to preparative myeloablative chemotherapy, the risk of infection during the neutropenic period prior to engraftment, the occurrence of graft-versus-host disease, and loss of the graft. In addition, side effects, such as infertility and clonal disease from the conditioning chemotherapy, are sometimes deterrents for patients who are seeking a curative approach. Over the years, results of HSCT have improved quite significantly. Clinical trials of nonmyeloablative and reduced-intensity conditioning regimens, and use of alternative donor sources are ongoing, with some improvement in those outcomes as well, but still quite inferior to the outcomes from myeloablative conditioning and a matched sibling donor.

GENERAL CARE

Management of thalassemia requires a high standard of general supportive care. As patients are living longer, problems related to physiologic ageing add to morbidity of complications related to thalassemia itself and therapy. Comprehensive monitoring for complications related to thalassemia and its treatment should be part of the care regimen. Infection should be treated early, particularly in patients who are iron overloaded and/or have had splenectomy. If the diet is deficient in folate, supplements should be given. Supplementation is unnecessary in patients maintained on a hypertransfusion regimen. In patients who are not hypertransfused, particular attention should be paid to the ear, nose, and throat because of chronic sinus infection and middle-ear diseases resulting from bone deformity of the skull. Similarly, regular dental surveillance is essential because poorly transfused thalassemic children have a variety of deformities of the maxilla and poorly developed teeth. Monitoring for iron overload and its complications is a critical part of comprehensive care. Prompt hormone replacement may, for example, enhance growth before fusion of the growth plates in children, prevent osteoporosis, and prevent complications of diabetes. Monitoring vitamin D levels and supplementing the patient's diet with vitamin D and calcium as needed are also key for bone health.

OTHER CONSIDERATIONS

HbH disease usually requires no specific therapy, although splenectomy may be of value in cases associated with severe anemia and splenomegaly.[1,14,15] Because splenectomy may be followed by a higher incidence of thromboembolic disease the spleen should be removed only in cases of extreme anemia and splenomegaly.[1,3,293] Oxidant drugs should not be given to patients with HbH disease. The management of symptomatic sickle cell thalassemia follows the guidelines described for sickle cell anemia (Chap. 18).

Children with thalassemia intermedia present a particularly complex therapeutic problem. Whether to start transfusions in a child with an "adequate" steady-state Hb level is difficult to determine with certainty. The child should be carefully monitored in all of the hospital visits and important parametrs to be followed closely include growth, development, and normal sexual maturation. If a child grows and develops normally with no evident signs of bone changes, the child could be maintained without transfusion. Bone changes affecting the maxillae and sinuses could also be documented by regular photography of the face. If, however, the child's early growth pattern is retarded or the child's activity is limited because of the child's anemia, the child should be placed on a regular transfusion regimen. Splenomegaly may be reduced once transfusions are initiated but usually does not resolve completely. If hypersplenism plays a role in the child's anemia as the child grows older, splenectomy can be considered. Many of these patients have significant iron loading from the gastrointestinal tract, additionally contributed to by any intermittent transfusions they may receive. Therefore, regular assessments of iron loading should be performed by MRI of the

liver and serial serum ferritin levels to assess the trend of iron loading. Chelation therapy should be instituted when appropriate.

● PROGNOSIS

The overall prognosis for patients with severe forms of β-thalassemia who are adequately treated by transfusion and chelation has improved dramatically. The main factors that have contributed to this are the improved safety of the blood supply, the availability of oral chelation, the improvement of monitoring strategies, particularly MRI for tissue iron assessments, improved treatments for hepatitis C, and improved outcomes for HSCT. A critical factor that affects outcomes is adequacy of iron chelation. This depends not only on the availability of the oral agents but also patients' access to them from the economic standpoint. Compliance is the other main determinant of outcomes related to complications from iron overload.[294-296] Although large longitudinal studies have not been performed in the era of oral chelation and MRI monitoring, if performed they would be expected to show improved compliance as a major factor contributing to increased survival and decreased morbidity from iron-related complications. On the other hand, poor compliance or unavailability of chelating agents are still associated with a poor prospect of survival much beyond the second decade.

● NOVEL THERAPEUTIC APPROACHES

Despite great advances in care, severe thalassemia remains a disease that has a great impact on quality of life. Optimal management requires frequent visits to the hospital for transfusions, monitoring and doctor visits, daily intake of medications with attendant side effects, and despite all of this, the individual has chronic anemia and may develop complications related to the disease itself, or treatment, especially iron overload. All of the hospital visits for care and monitoring result in lost days of school or work, impaired family time, drain on financial resources, and, very importantly, psychosocial impairment. Knowing the inexorable course of the disease, parents and patients with the option of cure by HSCT, most often avail of it, despite the known risk of the described complications. Consequently, there is a need for improved therapies that will affect this course and provide relief from the burden of disease and its management.

Fortunately, significant therapeutic advances have been made thanks to technological developments that have opened a new era of targeted therapies and gene therapy. Several approaches have been advanced, and some are already in advanced stages of clinical trials with impending regulatory approval for clinical application.

Augmentation of Fetal Hemoglobin Production by Editing the BCL11A Gene

In the absence of adequate β-globin production, if the excess α-globin chains could be bound with γ-globin to produce fetal Hb, the Hb level could be increased and ineffective erythropoiesis ameliorated, thus modifying the pathophysiologic course of the disease. Older approaches using butyrate analogues and hydroxyurea[297-300] did not show very positive results, except in homozygotes for HbLepore.[301] Novel approaches based on our better understanding of how BCL11A silences γ-globin gene expression[48] have led to the development of genetic therapy strategies. Two approaches have been used: (1) disrupting the patient's own *BCL11A* gene (a major repressor of γ-globin gene expression) to induce HbF expression using gene-editing approaches. BCL11A also has roles in lymphoid and neurological development but gene-editing exploits the erythroid-specific enhancers in intron 2 of the gene using CRISPR-Cas-9 or zinc finger nucleases, and (2) A gene addition approach that is already in clinical trials (ClinicalTrials.gov Identifier: NCT03282656) for sickle cell disease utilizes a lentiviral mediated erythroid specific short hairpin RNA (shRNA) for BCL11A. This shRNA is modified to target the specific gene and downregulate its expression in erythroid cells. Several of these interventions are already in early phases of development. Early results from the CRISPR trial of CTX001 in thalassemia showed an excellent response, with all subjects becoming transfusion independent with a near normal hemoglobin level, >90% HbF, with a high proportion of edited CD 34+ cells on examination of the bone marrow.[301] The trials are ongoing, and if they show consistent results, could provide another viable curative option.

Targeted Therapies Aimed at Ameliorating Ineffective Erythropoiesis

Several molecules have been/are being developed with the aim of reducing ineffective erythropoiesis, which will not only improve red cell production and reduce anemia but also possibly prevent progressive bone disease.[302] These therapies include luspatercept, ruxolitinib, hepcidin analogues, mitapivat, and correction of the defective globin gene.

Luspatercept Therapy Luspatercept is a recombinant fusion protein containing a modified extracellular domain of ActRIIB, which binds GDF11 and other transforming growth factor-β superfamily ligands, inhibits Smad2/3 signaling, and promotes red cell differentiation/maturation. This allows more of the proliferating erythroid precursors to mature, reduces intramedullary apoptosis, and, thereby, ineffective erythropoiesis. Early studies in normal human volunteers showed a dose-dependent increase in Hb levels and a good tolerability profile.[320] Phase 2 clinical studies confirmed that ineffective erythropoiesis was improved in patients with both TDT and NTDT, with clinically meaningful reductions in transfusion requirements.[304] The phase 3, 48-week BELIEVE study in adults with TDT met all of its primary and secondary end points for significant reduction in transfusion requirements of 33% to 50% compared with baseline.[305,306] Subset analysis of the study showed a response in patients with all different genotypes, and the response seemed to be sustained in the responders. An extension phase is ongoing and will inform as to the durability of this therapy, which is now approved for clinical use.[307]

Ruxolitinib This agent was developed as a JAK2 inhibitor based on the demonstration that JAK2 was a factor mediating ineffective erythropoiesis and that inhibition in the mouse model would improve effective erythropoiesis.[308] However, the phase 2a study in patients with thalassemia did not show a reduction in transfusion requirement, although there was significant shrinkage in spleen size.[309] Further studies using this agent are not planned.

Hepcidin Analogues Better understanding of erythropoiesis in thalassemia and the interaction between erythropoiesis and hepcidin led to the use of hepcidin analogues in the mouse model of thalassemia.[310] The mice showed a reduction in spleen size and improvement of anemia.[311] A further benefit would be to reduce iron absorption and slow the development of iron overload, as well as to prevent release of iron form stores and therefore, and reduce levels transferrin unbound iron and its toxicity to the heart and endocrine organs. Clinical trials of these analogues have been initiated in humans, with reductions in transfusion requirement as the end point. Patients with thalassemia and transfusional iron overload were also given hepcidin to study its effect on myocardial iron. However, this trial was terminated after the interim analysis did not show any effect.

Mitapivat Improving glycolysis and reducing oxidative stress in developing erythroid precursors is another strategy being used to minimize ineffective erythropoiesis in thalassemia. This oral, small-molecule allosteric activator of wild type and a variety of mutated pyruvate kinase-R (PKR) enzymes is in clinical trials in NTDT patients. Early

phase 2 studies conducted in non–transfusion-dependent patients with both alpha (HbH disease) and beta thalassemia showed a good safety profile and a 1 g/dL or greater increase in hemoglobin level in almost all subjects. (abstracts only—presented at EHA and ASH 2020)

Correction of the Defective Globin Gene Perhaps the most advanced and exciting strategy for curing thalassemia is aimed at correction of the defective gene. Currently, the only reliable curative treatment is allogeneic HSCT from a matched sibling, but this is not available to all patients and other donor sources—haplo-identical family members, umbilical cord blood, or matched unrelated donor—have significant risks and morbidities. These limitations can be overcome by autologous transplant, in which the patient receives his/her own HSCs after being modified by genetic therapy.[312-317] Genetic therapy is done either by adding a new copy of the gene or possibly by correcting the defective gene through CRISPR/Cas-9 splicing. The first successful genetic therapy for β-thalassemia was reported in 2010, when a patient with HbE/β⁰-thalassemia was cured with a lentivirus expressing a β-globin variant, T87Q.[318] Gene addition strategies are in advanced stages of clinical trial development. The mechanism by which the new gene is transferred is via an autologous HSC transplant (Fig. 17-22). The patient's stem cells are collected by pheresis after mobilization from the marrow, purified, and taken to the gene transfer facility. A functional copy of the β-globin gene is introduced into the stem cells via transfection by a lentiviral vector. The patient receives myeloablative chemotherapy, and the modified stem cells are reinfused. If these engraft successfully, the patient begins to produce the β-globin variant, HbA^{T87Q}, containing two α-globin chains and two β^{T87Q}-globin chains. The efficacy of the process depends on successful transfection of the stem cells in adequate numbers, the engraftment of these cells, and the maintenance of a high vector copy number (VCN) per cell to ensure adequate β-globin production. An added benefit of this approach is the absence of graft-versus-host disease. Two vectors are currently in trials. The first, BB305 vector (Fig. 17-23), encodes a β-globin gene that produces a β-globin chain with a single amino acid substitution, T87Q, resulting in the production of HbA^{T87Q}, which allows easy measurement of the gene product as different from endogenous production. Conditioning prior to stem cell infusion was myeloablative using a single agent, busulfan. Early clinical trials using this vector demonstrated proof of principle, and a proportion of patients with both non-β⁰/β⁰ and β⁰/β⁰ genotypes showed a response. Patients showed robust production of the HbA^{T87Q}, with transfusion independence, more likely in the non-β⁰/β⁰ patients. Patients who did not respond as well had a reduction in transfusion requirements. There were no deaths or graft failures during the trial, but there were complications similar to those seen from myeloablative conditioning in allogeneic HSCT, including neutropenic fevers, mucositis, and venoocclusive disease. Vector integration was polyclonal, and there was no vector-mediated replication-competent lentivirus detected, which provided reassurance that the risk for insertional mutagenesis was not a concern. In addition, there has been stable transfection, with a VCN in the 0.6-0.7 copies per cell, and stable production of HbA^{T87Q} in most patients.[319]

Currently, clinical trials using the same vector but a refined manufacturing process are underway, in non-β⁰/β⁰ patients and β⁰/β⁰ patients, and preliminary results show improved VCNs in the 2-3 range, with a correspondingly greater production of HbA^{T87Q} and, thus, a greater proportion of patients with transfusion independence. Pediatric patients (over the age of 6 years) have been included and also show excellent preliminary results.

The GLOBE vector, also a lentiviral vector, contains a normal human β-globin gene with no modifications. Differences from the BB305 trials were the use of thiotepa and treosulfan for myeloablative conditioning, and the introduction of modified cells directly into the

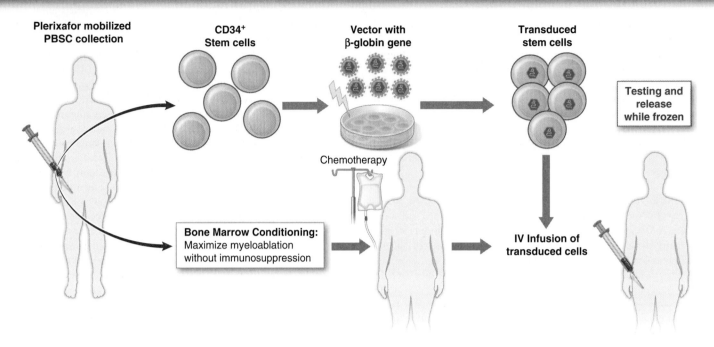

Figure 17–22. Procedure for gene-modified cellular therapy. PBSC, peripheral blood stem cell.

marrow to avoid passage through and possible clearance by the spleen. Although quite early, the preliminary results from this phase 1/2 trial have been positive.[321]

A phase 1 clinical trial to evaluate the safety of in utero HSCT in fetuses with α-thalassemia major is also underway. Maternal marrow is infused at the time of the in utero red cell transfusion. The goal is to take advantage of the maternal-fetal tolerance that exists during pregnancy; thus, no conditioning chemotherapy would be required.

THALASSEMIA AS A GLOBAL HEALTH PROBLEM

The remarkable advances in the diagnosis, prevention, and treatment of thalassemia described in this chapter have mostly affected patients in the developed world.[322] However, the major burden of disease is primarily in the developing world. In many developing countries in which there is a very high frequency of thalassemia, there are very limited facilities for diagnosis and management of thalassemia.[18] Many of these countries are making major strides economically, and provision of resources to the sick and needy are improving dramatically. Survival of patients with thalassemia is also increasing. Children who previously would have perished from the disease for lack of transfusions, or

chelation, or from infectious diseases, are now surviving. While this is a major medical advance, it is also a tremendous financial burden on the economies of these nations.[17,18,323]

Approaches to better control and manage thalassemia in developing countries include the development of partnerships between centers in the developed and developing countries to train workers in managing thalassemia, and, once these partnerships are established, for the partnerships between those developing countries where there is knowledge and expertise of the field to work with those countries that lack the knowledge or facilities to treat and manage thalassemia. In the absence of such cooperative organizations, thalassemia will continue to cause the premature death of hundreds of thousands of infants and children worldwide.

PREVENTION

In parts of the world where the incidence of thalassemia is high, the disease places an immense economic burden on society. For example, if all the thalassemic children born in Cyprus were treated by regular blood transfusions and iron-chelating therapy, it is estimated that within 15 years the total medical budget of the island would be required to treat this single disease.[324] Clearly, this is not feasible, so considerable effort

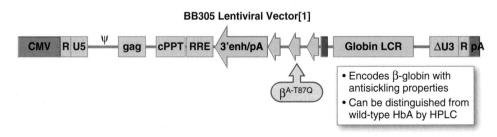

Figure 17–23. Structure of lentiglobin BB305 vector. Hb, hemoglobin; HPLC, high-performance liquid chromatography; LCR, locus control region.

has been directed toward developing programs for prevention of the different forms of thalassemia.[325]

Prevention can be achieved in two ways: genetic counseling and prenatal screening. Prospective (preconceptual) genetic counseling involves screening total populations while the children are in school and warning carriers about the potential risks of having an affected offspring in marriage with another carrier. Few data are available about the value of programs of this type; a pilot study in Greece was unsuccessful.[326] Because it is believed that this approach will not be successful in many populations, considerable effort has been directed toward developing prenatal diagnosis programs.

Prenatal diagnosis for prevention of thalassemia entails screening mothers at the first antenatal visit, screening the father in cases in which the mother is a thalassemia carrier, and offering the couple the possibility of prenatal diagnosis and termination of pregnancy if both mother and father are carriers of a gene for a severe form of thalassemia. Currently, these programs are devoted mainly to prenatal diagnosis of the severe transfusion-dependent forms of homozygous β^+-thalassemia or β^0-thalassemia. Many screening programs concentrate on identifying pregnant women who are thalassemia carriers in the first trimester of pregnancy. This is done by varying combinations of blood tests and the identification of women at high risk of carrying thalassemia based on their ethnic origin. This latter approach is potentially effective in areas with a low prevalence of thalassemia in the native population, such as Northern Europe, although increasing racial admixture is reducing the feasibility of such selective screening, particularly in cities. If a woman is found to be a carrier, screening is then offered to her partner, and if both are carriers, they are counseled about the risk of the fetus inheriting a severe form of thalassemia. Considerable experience also has been gained in prenatal diagnosis of mothers at risk for having a fetus with the Hb Bart's hydrops syndrome, considering the distress caused by a long and difficult pregnancy and the obstetric problems resulting from the birth of a hydropic infant with a massive placenta.

The first efforts at prenatal detection of β-thalassemia used fetal blood sampling and globin-chain synthesis analysis done at approximately week 18 of pregnancy. Despite the technical difficulties involved, the method was applied successfully in many countries and resulted in a reduced birth rate of infants with β-thalassemia.[327] The technique is associated with a low maternal morbidity rate, a fetal mortality rate of approximately 3% to 4%, and an error rate of 1% to 2%. Its main disadvantage is that it must be carried out relatively late in pregnancy. For this reason, efforts turned to first trimester prenatal diagnosis.

DNA technology has enabled diagnosis of important Hb disorders in utero by fetal DNA analysis. Although analysis can be carried out on DNA derived from amniotic fluid, the approach has drawbacks because it must be done relatively late in pregnancy, and often amniotic fluid cells must be grown in culture to obtain a sufficient amount of DNA.[328] However, DNA can be obtained as early as week 9 of pregnancy by chorionic villus sampling. Although the safety of this technique remains to be fully evaluated and limb-reduction deformities may occur when the procedure is performed very early in pregnancy (week 9 or 10), chorionic villus sampling has become the major method for prenatal diagnosis of thalassemia based on subsequent experience with the technique.[1,328-331]

Remarkable advances in DNA technology have provided a variety of methods for the direct identification of mutations in fetal DNA.[1] Even in families with extremely rare mutations, rapid DNA sequencing technology allows a diagnosis to be made quickly. The error rate using these different approaches varies, mainly depending on the experience of the particular laboratory; low rates (<1%) are reported from most centers. Potential sources of error include maternal contamination of fetal DNA and nonpaternity.

The application of this new technology has caused a major reduction in the number of infants born with thalassemia throughout the Mediterranean region and the Middle East, and in parts of the Indian subcontinent and Southeast Asia. Several approaches continue to be explored in an attempt to avoid the use of invasive procedures like chorion villous sampling. A variety of methods are being used to harvest fetal DNA from fetal cells in maternal blood or from maternal plasma.[332,333] Some couples want to avoid having a fetus with thalassemia but find prenatal diagnosis and selective termination unacceptable. Preimplantation genetic diagnosis involves the use of in vitro fertilization to generate 5 to 15 embryos; at the 8-cell stage, one embryonic cell can be removed and tested for thalassemia alleles; it is then possible to only implant embryos without thalassemia. Although appealing, it is currently a difficult, stressful, technically challenging, and expensive procedure, with only 10% to 20% of couples taking home a baby. Advances in reproductive biology and DNA technology are making this technique more accessible, and it is available in an increasing number of countries.[334,335] There is every expectation that some of these approaches will reach the clinic in the near future.[336]

REFERENCES

1. Weatherall DJ, Clegg JB. *The Thalassaemia Syndromes.* 4th ed. Blackwell Science; 2001.
2. Piel FB, Weatherall DJ. The alpha-thalassemias. *N Engl J Med.* 2014;371:1908-1916.
3. Taher AT, Weatherall DJ, Cappellini MD. Thalassaemia. *Lancet.* 2018;391:155-167.
4. Cooley TB, Lee P. A series of cases of splenomegaly in children with anemia and peculiar bone changes. *Trans Am Pediatr Soc.* 1925;37:29.
5. Whipple GH, Bradford WL. Racial or familial anemia of children. Associated with fundamental disturbances of bone and pigment metabolism (Cooley-Von Jaksch). *Am J Dis Child.* 1932;44:336-365.
6. Whipple GH, Bradford WL. Mediterranean disease-thalassemia (erythroblastic anemia of Cooley); associated pigment abnormalities simulating hemochromatosis. *J Pediatr.* 1936;9:279-311.
7. Weatherall DJ. Toward an understanding of the molecular biology of some common inherited anemias: the story of thalassemia In: Wintrobe MM, ed. *Blood, Pure and Eloquent.* McGraw-Hill; 1980:373-414.
8. Chernoff AI. The distribution of the thalassemia gene: a historical review. *Blood.* 1959;14:899-912.
9. Weatherall DJ. *Thalassaemia: The Biography.* Oxford University Press; 2010.
10. Steinberg MH, Forget BG, Higgs DR, Weatherall DJ, eds., *Disorders of Hemoglobin: Genetics, Pathophysiology, and Clinical Management.* 2nd ed. Cambridge University Press; 2009:826.
11. Weatherall DJ. The definition and epidemiology of non-transfusion-dependent thalassemia. *Blood Rev.* 2012;26(suppl 1):S3-S6.
12. Thein SL, Wood WG. The molecular basis of β thalassemia, $\delta\beta$ thalassemia, and hereditary persistence of fetal hemoglobin. In: Steinberg MH, Forget BG, Higgs DR, et al, eds. *Disorders of Hemoglobin: Genetics, Pathophysiology, and Clinical Management.* Cambridge University Press; 2009:323-356.
13. Thein SL. The molecular basis of β-thalassemia. *Cold Spring Harb Perspect Med.* 2013;3:a011700.
14. Steinberg MH, Forget BG, Higgs DR, eds. *Disorders of Hemoglobin.* 2nd ed. Cambridge University Press; 2009.
15. Weatherall DJ, Clegg JB, Higgs DR, et al. The hemoglobinopathies. In: Scriver CR, Beaudet AL, Sly WS, eds. *The Metabolic Basis of Inherited Disease.* 8th ed. McGraw Hill; 2001:4571-4636.
16. Weatherall DJ, Clegg JB. Inherited haemoglobin disorders: an increasing global health problem. *Bull World Health Organ.* 2001;79:704-712.
17. Weatherall DJ. The evolving spectrum of the epidemiology of thalassemia. *Hematol Oncol Clin North Am.* 2018;32:165-175.
18. Williams TN, Weatherall DJ. World distribution, population genetics, and health burden of the hemoglobinopathies. *Cold Spring Harb Perspect Med.* 2012;2:a011692.
19. Kountouris P, Carsten WL, Fanis P, et al. IthaGenes: an interactive database for haemoglobin variations and epidemiology. *PLoS One.* 2014;9:e103020.
20. Orkin SH, Kazazian HH Jr. The mutation and polymorphism of the human beta-globin gene and its surrounding DNA. *Annu Rev Genet.* 1984;18:131-171.
21. Shriner D, Rotimi CN. Whole-genome-sequence-based haplotypes reveal single origin of the sickle allele during the holocene wet phase. *Am J Hum Genet.* 2018;102:547-556.
22. Laval G, Peyregne S, Zidane N, et al. Recent adaptive acquisition by African rainforest hunter-gatherers of the late Pleistocene sickle-cell mutation suggests past differences in malaria exposure. *Am J Hum Genet.* 2019;104:553-561.
23. Haldane JBS. The rate of mutation of human genes. *Proc VIII Int Cong Genetics Hereditas.* 1949;35:267-273.

24. Siniscalco M, Bernini L, Filippi G, et al. Population genetics of haemoglobin variants, thalassaemia and glucose-6-phosphate dehydrogenase deficiency, with particular reference to the malaria hypothesis. *Bull World Health Organ.* 1966;34:379-393.

25. Flint J, Hill AV, Bowden DK, et al. High frequencies of a thalassaemia are the result of natural selection by malaria. *Nature.* 1986;321:744-749.

26. Allen SJ, O'Donnell A, Alexander ND, et al. alpha+-Thalassemia protects children against disease caused by other infections as well as malaria. *Proc Natl Acad Sci U S A.* 1997;94:14736-14741.

27. Williams TN, Wambua S, Uyoga S, et al. Both heterozygous and homozygous alpha+ thalassemias protect against severe and fatal *Plasmodium falciparum* malaria on the coast of Kenya. *Blood.* 2005;106:368-371.

28. Williams TN. Red blood cell defects and malaria. *Mol Biochem Parasitol.* 2006;149:121-127.

29. Williams TN, Mwangi TW, Wambua S, et al. Negative epistasis between the malaria-protective effects of alpha+-thalassemia and the sickle cell trait. *Nat Genet.* 2005;37:1253-1257.

30. Williams TN, Maitland K, Bennett S, et al. High incidence of malaria in alpha-thalassaemic children. *Nature.* 1996;383:522-525.

31. Cockburn IA, Mackinnon MJ, O'Donnell A, et al. A human complement receptor 1 polymorphism that reduces *Plasmodium falciparum* rosetting confers protection against severe malaria. *Proc Natl Acad Sci U S A.* 2004;101:272-277.

32. Weatherall DJ. Genetic variation and susceptibility to infection: the red cell and malaria. *Br J Haematol.* 2008;141:276-286.

33. Lauer J, Shen CK, Maniatis T. The chromosomal arrangement of human alpha-like globin genes: sequence homology and alpha-globin gene deletions. *Cell.* 1980;20:119-130.

34. Orkin SH. The duplicated human alpha globin genes lie close together in cellular DNA. *Proc Natl Acad Sci U S A.* 1978;75:5950-5954.

35. Liebhaber SA, Goossens M, Kan YW. Homology and concerted evolution at the alpha 1 and alpha 2 loci of human alpha-globin. *Nature.* 1981;290:26-29.

36. Liebhaber SA, Goossens MJ, Kan YW. Cloning and complete nucleotide sequence of human 5'-a-globin gene. *Proc Natl Acad Sci U S A.* 1980;77:7054-7058.

37. Proudfoot NJ, Maniatis T. The structure of a human a-globin pseudogene and its relationship to alpha-globin gene duplication. *Cell.* 1980;21:537-544.

38. Liebhaber SA, Kan YW. Differentiation of the mRNA transcripts originating from the alpha1- and alpha2-globin loci in normals and a-thalassemics. *J Clin Invest.* 1981;68:439-446.

39. Orkin SH, Goff SC. The duplicated human a-globin genes: their relative expression as measured by RNA analysis. *Cell.* 1981;24:345-351.

40. Higgs DR, Wainscoat JS, Flint J, et al. Analysis of the human alpha-globin gene cluster reveals a highly informative genetic locus. *Proc Natl Acad Sci U S A.* 1986;83:5165-5169.

41. Fritsch EF, Lawn RM, Maniatis T. Molecular cloning and characterization of the human beta-like globin gene cluster. *Cell.* 1980;19:959-972.

42. Spritz RA, DeRiel JK, Forget BG. Complete nucleotide sequence of the human delta-globin gene. *Cell.* 1980;21:639-646.

43. Baralle FE, Shoulders CC, Proudfoot NJ. The primary structure of the human epsilon-globin gene. *Cell.* 1980;21:621-626.

44. Slightom JL, Blechl AE, Smithies O. Human fetal G gamma- and A gamma-globin genes: complete nucleotide sequences suggest that DNA can be exchanged between these duplicated genes. *Cell.* 1980;21:627-638.

45. Jeffreys AJ. DNA sequence variants in the G gamma-, A gamma-, delta- and beta-globin genes of man. *Cell.* 1979;18:1-10.

46. Antonarakis SE, Boehm CD, Giardinia PJ, Kazazian HH Jr. Nonrandom association of polymorphic restriction sites in the beta-globin gene cluster. *Proc Natl Acad Sci U S A.* 1982;79:137-141.

47. Wainscoat JS, Hill AV, Boyce AL, et al. Evolutionary relationships of human populations from an analysis of nuclear DNA polymorphisms. *Nature.* 1986;319:491-493.

48. Sankaran VG, Orkin SH. The switch from fetal to adult hemoglobin. *Cold Spring Harb Perspect Med.* 2013;3:a011643.

49. Katsumura KR, DeVilbiss AW, Pope NJ, et al. Transcriptional mechanisms underlying hemoglobin synthesis. *Cold Spring Harb Perspect Med.* 2013;3:a015412.

50. Higgs DR, Weatherall DJ. The alpha thalassaemias. *Cell Mol Life Sci.* 2009;66:1154-1162.

51. Katsumura KR, Bresnick EH; GATA Factor Mechanisms Group. The GATA factor revolution in hematology. *Blood.* 2017;129:2092-2102.

52. Donze D, Townes TM, Bieker JJ. Role of erythroid Kruppel-like factor in human gamma- to beta-globin gene switching. *J Biol Chem.* 1995;270:1955-1959.

53. Higgs DR. The molecular basis of alpha-thalassemia. *Cold Spring Harb Perspect Med.* 2013;3:a011718.

54. Giardine B, van Baal S, Kaimakis P, et al. HbVar database of human hemoglobin variants and thalassemia mutations: 2007 update. *Hum Mutat.* 2007;28:206.

55. Thein SL, Old JM, Wainscoat JS, et al. Population and genetic studies suggest a single origin for the Indian deletion beta thalassaemia. *Br J Haematol.* 1984;57:271-278.

56. Anand R, Boehm CD, Kazazian HH Jr, Vanin EF. Molecular characterization of a beta zero-thalassemia resulting from a 1.4 kilobase deletion. *Blood.* 1988;72:636-641.

57. Padanilam BJ, Felice AE, Huisman THJ. Partial deletion of the 5' beta-globin gene region causes beta zero-thalassemia in members of an American black family. *Blood.* 1984;64:941-944.

58. Popovich BW, Rosenblatt DS, Kendall AG, et al. Molecular characterization of an atypical beta-thalassemia caused by a large deletion in the 5' beta-globin gene region. *Am J Hum Genet.* 1986;39:797-810.

59. Diaz-Chico JC, et al. An approximately 300 bp deletion involving part of the 5' beta-globin gene region is observed in members of a Turkish family with beta-thalassemia. *Blood.* 1987;70:583-586.

60. Aulehla-Scholtz C, Spiegelberg R, Horst J. A beta-thalassemia mutant caused by a 300-bp deletion in the human beta-globin gene. *Hum Genet.* 1989;81:298-299.

61. Schokker RC, Went LN, Bok J. A new genetic variant of beta-thalassemia. *Nature.* 1966;209:44-46.

62. Craig JE, Kelly SJ, Barnetson R, et al. Molecular characterization of a novel 10.3 kb deletion causing beta-thalassaemia with unusually high Hb A₂. *Br J Haematol.* 1992;82:735-744.

63. Orkin SH, Antonarakis SE, Kazazian HH Jr. Base substitution at position −88 in a beta-thalassemic globin gene. Further evidence for the role of distal promoter element ACACCC. *J Biol Chem.* 1984;259:8679-8681.

64. Orkin SH, et al. Linkage of beta-thalassaemia mutations and beta-globin gene polymorphisms with DNA polymorphisms in human beta-globin gene cluster. *Nature.* 1982;296:627-631.

65. Poncz M, Ballantine M, Solowiejczyk D, et al. beta-Thalassemia in a Kurdish Jew. Single base changes in the T-A-T-A box. *J Biol Chem.* 1982;257:5994-5996.

66. Antonarakis SE, et al. beta-Thalassemia in American blacks: novel mutations in the "TATA" box and an acceptor splice site. *Proc Natl Acad Sci U S A.* 1984;81:1154-1158.

67. Orkin SH, Sexton JP, Cheng TC, et al. ATA box transcription mutation in beta-thalassemia. *Nucleic Acids Res.* 1983;11:4727-4734.

68. Surrey S, Delgrosso K, Malladi P, et al. Functional analysis of a beta-globin gene containing a TATA box mutation from a Kurdish Jew with beta thalassemia. *J Biol Chem.* 1985;260:6507-6510.

69. Gonzalez-Redondo JM, Stoming TA, Kutlar A, et al. A C->T substitution at nt−101 in a conserved DNA sequence of the promoter region of the beta-globin gene is associated with "silent" beta-thalassemia. *Blood.* 1989;73:1705-1711.

70. Wong C, Dowling CE, Saiki RK, et al. Characterization of beta-thalassaemia mutations using direct genomic sequencing of amplified single copy DNA. *Nature.* 1987;330:384-386.

71. Treisman R, Orkin SH, Maniatis T. Specific transcription and RNA splicing defects in five cloned beta-thalassaemia genes. *Nature.* 1983;302:591-596.

72. Kazazian HH Jr, Orkin SH, Antonarakis SE, et al. Molecular characterization of seven beta-thalassemia mutations in Asian Indians. *EMBO J.* 1984;3:593-596.

73. Padanilam BJ, Huisman TH. The beta zero-thalassemia in an American black family is due to a single nucleotide substitution in the acceptor splice junction of the second intervening sequence. *Am J Hematol.* 1986;22:259-263.

74. Atweh GF, Anagnou NP, Shearin J, et al. Beta-thalassemia resulting from a single nucleotide substitution in an acceptor splice site. *Nucleic Acids Res.* 1985;13:777-790.

75. Orkin SH, Sexton JP, Goff SC, Kazazian HH Jr. Inactivation of an acceptor RNA splice site by a short deletion in beta-thalassemia. *J Biol Chem.* 1983;258:7249-7251.

76. Atweh GF, Wong C, Reed R, et al. A new mutation in IVS-1 of the human beta globin gene causing beta thalassemia due to abnormal splicing. *Blood.* 1987;70:147-151.

77. Cheng TC, Orkin SH, Antonarakis SE, et al. beta-Thalassemia in Chinese: use of in vivo RNA analysis and oligonucleotide hybridization in systematic characterization of molecular defects. *Proc Natl Acad Sci U S A.* 1984;81:2821-2825.

78. Gonzalez-Redondo JM, et al. Clinical and genetic heterogeneity in black patients with homozygous beta-thalassemia from the southeastern United States. *Blood.* 1988;72:1007-1014.

79. Tamagnini GP, Lopes MC, Castanheira ME, et al. Beta + thalassaemia–Portuguese type: clinical, haematological and molecular studies of a newly defined form of beta thalassaemia. *Br J Haematol.* 1983;54:189-200.

80. Hill AVS, Bowden DK, O'Shaughnessey DF, et al. Beta thalassemia in Melanesia: association with malaria and characterization of a common variant (IVS-1 Nt 5 G—C). *Blood.* 1988;72:9-14.

81. Spritz RA, Jagadeeswaran P, Choudary PV, et al. Base substitution in an intervening sequence of a beta+-thalassemic human globin gene. *Proc Natl Acad Sci U S A.* 1981;78:2455-2459.

82. Busslinger M, Moschonas N, Flavell RA. Beta+ thalassemia: aberrant splicing results from a single point mutation in an intron. *Cell.* 1981;27:289-298.

83. Metherall JE, Collins FS, Pan J, et al. Beta zero thalassemia caused by a base substitution that creates an alternative splice acceptor site in an intron. *EMBO J.* 1986;5:2551-2557.

84. Orkin SH, Kazazian HH Jr, Antonarakis SE, et al. Abnormal RNA processing due to the exon mutation of beta E-globin gene. *Nature.* 1982;300:768-769.

85. Goldsmith ME, Humphries RK, Ley T, et al. "Silent" nucleotide substitution in beta+-thalassemia globin gene activates splice site in coding sequence RNA. *Proc Natl Acad Sci U S A.* 1983;80:2318-2322.

86. Orkin SH, Antonarakis S, Loukopoulos D. Abnormal processing of beta Knossos RNA. *Blood.* 1984;64:311-313.

87. Yang KG, Kutlar F, George E, et al. Molecular characterization of beta-globin gene mutations in Malay patients with Hb E-beta-thalassaemia and thalassaemia major. *Br J Haematol.* 1989;72:73-80.

88. Orkin SH, Cheng TC, Antonarakis SE, Kazazian HH Jr. Thalassemia due to a mutation in the cleavage-polyadenylation signal of the human beta-globin gene. *EMBO J.* 1985;4:453-456.

89. Jankovic L, Efremov GD, Petkov G, et al. Two novel polyadenylation mutations leading to beta(+)-thalassaemia. *Br J Haematol.* 1990;75:122-126.

90. Rund D, Filon D, Dowling C, et al. Molecular studies of beta-thalassemia in Israel. Mutational analysis and expression studies. *Ann N Y Acad Sci.* 1990;612:98-105.

91. Chang JC, Kan YW. Beta 0 thalassemia, a nonsense mutation in man. *Proc Natl Acad Sci U S A.* 1979;76:2886-2889.

92. Kazazian HH Jr, Dowling CE, Waber PG, et al. The spectrum of beta-thalassemia genes in China and Southeast Asia. *Blood.* 1986;68:964-966.

93. Trecartin RF, Liebhaber SA, Chang JC, et al. Beta zero thalassemia in Sardinia is caused by a nonsense mutation. *J Clin Invest.* 1981;68:1012-1017.

94. Rosatelli C, Leoni GB, Tuveri T, et al. Beta thalassaemia mutations in Sardinians: implications for prenatal diagnosis. *J Med Genet.* 1987;24:97-100.

95. Kimberland ML, Divoky V, Prchal J, et al. Full-length human L1 insertions retain the capacity for high frequency retrotransposition in cultured cells. *Hum Mol Genet.* 1999;8:1557-1560.

96. Stamatoyannopoulos G, Woodson R, Papayannopoulou T, et al. Inclusion-body beta-thalassemia trait. A form of beta thalassemia producing clinical manifestations in simple heterozygotes. *N Engl J Med.* 1974;290:939-943.

97. Weatherall DJ, Clegg JB, Knox-Macaulay HH, et al. A genetically determined disorder with features both of thalassaemia and congenital dyserythropoietic anaemia. *Br J Haematol.* 1973;24:681-702.

98. Thein SL. Dominant beta thalassaemia: molecular basis and pathophysiology. *Br J Haematol.* 1992;80:273-277.

99. Thein SL, Hesketh C, Taylor P, et al. Molecular basis for dominantly inherited inclusion body beta-thalassemia. *Proc Natl Acad Sci U S A.* 1990;87:3924-3928.

100. Beris P, Miescher PA, Diaz-Chico JC, et al. Inclusion-body beta-thalassemia trait in a Swiss family is caused by an abnormal hemoglobin (Geneva) with an altered and extended beta chain carboxy-terminus due to a modification in codon beta 114. *Blood.* 1988;72:801-805.

101. Kazazian HH Jr, Dowling CE, Hurwitz RL, et al. III. Thalassemia mutations in exon 3 of the β-globin gene often cause a dominant form of thalassemia and show no predilection for malarial-endemic regions of the world. *Am J Hum Genet.* 1989;45:A242.

102. Fei YJ, Stoming TA, Kutlar A, et al. One form of inclusion body beta-thalassemia is due to a GAA->TAA mutation at codon 121 of the beta chain. *Blood.* 1989;73:1075-1077.

103. Kazazian HH Jr, Orkin SH, Boehm CD, et al. Characterisation of a spontaneous mutation to a beta-thalassaemia allele. *Am J Hum Genet.* 1986;38:860-867.

104. Sachs AB. Messenger RNA degradation in eukaryotes. *Cell.* 1993;74:413-421.

105. Thermann R, Neu-Yilik G, Deters A, et al. Binary specification of nonsense codons by splicing and cytoplasmic translation. *EMBO J.* 1998;17:3484-3494.

106. Thein SL. Is it dominantly inherited beta thalassaemia or just a beta-chain variant that is highly unstable? *Br J Haematol.* 1999;107:12-21.

107. Thein SL, Wood WG, Wickramasinghe SN, et al. Beta-thalassemia unlinked to the beta-globin gene in an English family. *Blood.* 1993;82:961-967.

108. Yu C, Niakan KK, Matsushita M, et al. X-linked thrombocytopenia with thalassemia from a mutation in the amino finger of GATA-1 affecting DNA binding rather than FOG-1 interaction. *Blood.* 2002;100:2040-2045.

109. Viprakasit V, Gibbons RJ, Broughton BC, et al. Mutations in the general transcription factor TFIIH result in beta-thalassaemia in individuals with trichothiodystrophy. *Hum Mol Genet.* 2001;10:2797-2802.

110. Badens C, Mattei MG, Imbert AM, et al. A novel mechanism for thalassaemia intermedia. *Lancet.* 2002;359:132-133.

111. Galanello R, Perseu L, Perra C, et al. Somatic deletion of the normal beta-globin gene leading to thalassaemia intermedia in heterozygous beta-thalassaemic patients. *Br J Haematol.* 2004;127:604-606.

112. Rochette J, Craig JE, Thein SL. Fetal hemoglobin levels in adults. *Blood Rev.* 1994;8:213-224.

113. Wood WG, Clegg JB, Weatherall DJ. Hereditary persistence of fetal haemoglobin (HPFH) and delta beta thalassaemia. *Br J Haematol.* 1979;43:509-520.

114. Giglioni B, Casini C, Mantovani R, et al. A molecular study of a family with Greek hereditary persistence of fetal hemoglobin and beta-thalassemia. *EMBO J.* 1984;3:2641-2645.

115. Kendall AG, Ojwang PJ, Schroeder WA, et al. Hemoglobin Kenya, the product of a gamma-beta fusion gene: studies of the family. *Am J Hum Genet.* 1973;25:548-563.

116. Smith DH, Clegg JB, Weatherall DJ, et al. Hereditary persistence of foetal haemoglobin associated with a gamma beta fusion variant, Haemoglobin Kenya. *Nat New Biol.* 1973;246:184-186.

117. Collins FS, Stoeckert CJ Jr, Serjeant GR, et al. G gamma beta+ hereditary persistence of fetal hemoglobin: cosmid cloning and identification of a specific mutation 5' to the G gamma gene. *Proc Natl Acad Sci U S A.* 1984;81:4894-4898.

118. Gelinas R, Endlich B, Pfeiffer C, et al. G to A substitution in the distal CCAAT box of the A gamma-globin gene in Greek hereditary persistence of fetal haemoglobin. *Nature.* 1985;313:323-325.

119. Tate VE, Wood WG, Weatherall DJ. The British form of non-deletion HPFH results from a single base mutation adjacent to an S1 hypersensitive site 5' to the A gamma globin gene. *Blood.* 1986;68:1389-1393.

120. Martyn GE, Wienert B, Yang L, et al. Natural regulatory mutations elevate the fetal globin gene via disruption of BCL11A or ZBTB7A binding. *Nat Genet.* 2018;50:498-503.

121. Liu N, Hargreaves VV, Zhu Q, et al. Direct promoter repression by BCL11A controls the fetal to adult hemoglobin switch. *Cell.* 2018;173:430-442.e417.

122. Masuda T, Wang X, Maeda M, et al. Transcription factors LRF and BCL11A independently repress expression of fetal hemoglobin. *Science.* 2016;351:285-289.

123. Wood WG. Hereditary Persistence of Fetal Hemoglobin and Delta Beta Thalassemia. In: Steinberg MH, Forget BG, Higgs DR, Nagel RL, eds. *Disorders of Hemoglobin: Genetics, Pathophysiology, and Clinical Management.* Cambridge University Press; 2001:356-388.

124. Jones RW, Old JM, Trent RJ, et al. Major rearrangement in the human beta-globin gene cluster. *Nature.* 1981;291:39-44.

125. Baglioni C. The fusion of two peptide chains in hemoglobin Lepore and its interpretation as a genetic deletion. *Proc Natl Acad Sci U S A.* 1962;48:1880-1886.

126. Higgs DR, Thein SL, Wood WG. The biology of the thalassaemias. In: Weatherall DJ, Clegg JB, eds. *The Thalassaemia Syndromes.* Blackwell Science; 2001:65-284.

127. Ottolenghi S, Giglioni B, Pulazzini A, et al. Sardinian delta beta zero-thalassemia: a further example of a C to T substitution at position −196 of the A gamma globin gene promoter. *Blood.* 1987;69:1058-1061.

128. Atweh GF, Zhu XX, Brickner HE, et al. The beta-globin gene on the Chinese delta beta-thalassemia chromosome carries a promoter mutation. *Blood.* 1987;70:1470-1474.

129. Wainscoat JS, Thein SL, Wood WG, et al. A novel deletion in the beta-globin gene complex. *Ann N Y Acad Sci.* 1985;445:20-27.

130. Kulozik A, Yarwood N, Jones RW. The Corfu delta beta zero thalassemia: a small deletion acts at a distance to selectively abolish beta globin gene expression. *Blood.* 1988;71:457-462.

131. Marti HR. *Normale und anormale menschliche Haemoglobine.* Springer Verlag; 1963.

132. Wood WG, Weatherall DJ, Clegg JB. Interaction of heterocellular hereditary persistence of foetal haemoglobin with b thalassaemia and sickle cell anaemia. *Nature.* 1976;264:247-249.

133. Thein SL, Weatherall DJ. A non-deletion hereditary persistence of fetal hemoglobin (HPFH) determinant not linked to the beta-globin gene complex. In: Stamatoyannopoulos G, Nienhuis AW, eds. *Hemoglobin Switching, Part B: Cellular and Molecular Mechanisms.* Alan R Liss; 1989:97-111.

134. Fritsch EF, Lawn RM, Maniatis T. Characterisation of deletions which affect the expression of fetal globin genes in man. *Nature.* 1979;279:598-603.

135. Orkin SH, Goff SC, Nathan DG. Heterogeneity of DNA deletion in gamma delta beta-thalassemia. *J Clin Invest.* 1981;67:878-884.

136. Pirastu M, Kan YW, Lin CC, et al. Hemolytic disease of the newborn caused by a new deletion of the entire beta-globin cluster. *J Clin Invest.* 1983;72:602-609.

137. Fearon ER, et al. The entire beta-globin gene cluster is deleted in a form of gamma delta beta-thalassemia. *Blood.* 1983;61:1269-1274.

138. Van der Ploeg LH, Konings A, Oort M, et al. gamma-beta-Thalassemia studies showing that deletion of the gamma- and delta-genes influences beta-globin gene expression in man. *Nature.* 1980;283:637-642.

139. Curtin P, Pirastu M, Kan YW, et al. A distant gene deletion affects beta-globin gene function in an atypical gamma delta beta-thalassemia. *J Clin Invest.* 1985;76:1554-1558.

140. Driscoll MC, Dobkin CS, Alter BP. Gamma delta beta-thalassemia due to a *de novo* mutation deleting the 5' beta-globin gene activation-region hypersensitive sites. *Proc Natl Acad Sci U S A.* 1989;86:7470-7474.

141. Rooks H, Bergounioux J, Game L, et al. Heterogeneity of the epsilon gamma delta beta-thalassaemias: characterisation of three novel English deletions. *Br J Haematol.* 2005;128:722-729.

142. Rooks H, Clark B, Best S, et al. A novel 506kb deletion causing εγδβ thalassemia. *Blood Cells Mol Dis.* 2012;49:121-127.

143. Gibbons RJ, Wada T, Fisher CA, et al. Mutations in the chromatin-associated protein ATRX. *Hum Mutat.* 2008;29:796-802.

144. Gibbons RJ, Wada T. ATRX and X-linked (alpha)-thalassemia mental retardation syndrome. In: Epstein CJ, Erickson RP, Wynshaw-Boris A, eds. *Inborn Errors of Development.* Oxford University Press; 2004:747-757.

145. Nicholls RD, Fischel-Ghodsian, Higgs DR. Recombination at the human a-globin gene cluster: sequence features and topological constraints. *Cell.* 1987;49:369-378.

146. Barbour VM, Tufarelli C, Sharpe JA, et al. Alpha-thalassemia resulting from a negative chromosomal position effect. *Blood.* 2000;96:800-807.

147. Tufarelli C, Sloane Stanley JA, Garrick D, et al. Transcription of antisense RNA leading to gene silencing and methylation as a novel cause of human genetic disease. *Nat Genet.* 2003;34:157-165.

148. Wilkie AO, Lamb J, Harris PC, et al. A truncated human chromosome 16 associated with a thalassaemia is stabilized by addition of telomeric repeat (TTAGGG). *Nature.* 1990;346:868-871.

149. Hatton CS, Wilkie AO, Drysdale HC, et al. Alpha-thalassaemia caused by a large (62 kb) deletion upstream of the human alpha globin gene cluster. *Blood.* 1990;76:221-227.

150. Liebhaber SA, Griese EU, Weiss I, et al. Inactivation of human alpha-globin gene expression by a de novo deletion located upstream of the alpha-globin gene cluster. *Proc Natl Acad Sci U S A.* 1990;87:9431-9435.

151. Embury SH, Miller JA, Dozy AM, et al. Two different molecular organizations account for the single alpha-globin gene of the alpha-thalassemia-2 genotype. *J Clin Invest.* 1980;66:1319-1325.

152. Higgs DR, Old JM, Pressley L, et al. A novel alpha-globin gene arrangement in man. *Nature.* 1980;284:632-635.

153. Goossens M, Dozy AM, Embury SH, et al. Triplicated alpha-globin loci in humans. *Proc Natl Acad Sci U S A.* 1980;77:518-521.

154. Trent RJ, Higgs DR, Clegg JB, et al. A new triplicated alpha-globin gene arrangement in man. *Br J Haematol.* 1981;49:149-152.

155. Orkin SH, Goff SC, Hechtman RL. Mutation in an intervening sequence splice junction in man. *Proc Natl Acad Sci U S A.* 1981;78:5041-5045.

156. Higgs DR, Goodbourn SE, Lamb J, et al. Alpha-thalassemia caused by a polyadenylation signal mutation. *Nature.* 1983;306:398-400.

157. Thein SL, Wallace RB, Pressley L, et al. The polyadenylation site mutation in the alpha-globin gene cluster. *Blood.* 1988;71:313-319.

158. Pirastu M, Saglio G, Chang JC, et al. Initiation codon mutation as a cause of alpha thalassaemia. *J Biol Chem.* 1984;259:12315-12317.

159. Olivieri NF, Chang LS, Poon AO, et al. An alpha-globin gene initiation codon mutation in a black family with HbH disease. *Blood.* 1987;70:729-732.

160. Paglietti E, Galanello R, Moi P, et al. Molecular pathology of haemoglobin H disease in Sardinians. *Br J Haematol.* 1986;63:485-496.

161. Morlé F, Lopez B, Henni T, et al. alpha-Thalassaemia associated with the deletion of two nucleotides at position -2 and -3 preceding the AUG codon. *EMBO J.* 1985;4:1245-1250.

162. Russo R, Andolfo I, Iolascon A. Next generation research and therapy in red blood cell diseases. *Haematologica.* 2016 May;101(5):515-517. PMID 27132276.

163. Higgs DR, Hill AV, Bowden DK, et al. Independent recombination events between the duplicated human alpha globin genes; implications for their concerted evolution. *Nucleic Acids Res.* 1984;12:6965-6977.

164. Honig GR, Shamsuddin M, Zaizov R, et al. Hemoglobin Peta Tikvah (alpha 110 Ala replaced by Asp): a new unstable variant with alpha-thalassemia-like expression. *Blood.* 1981;57:705-711.

165. Honig GR, et al. Hemoglobin Evanston (alpha 14 Trp—Arg). An unstable alpha-chain variant expressed as alpha-thalassemia. *J Clin Invest.* 1984;73:1740-1749.

166. Weatherall DJ, Higgs DR, Bunch C, et al. Hemoglobin H disease and mental retardation: a new syndrome or a remarkable coincidence? *N Engl J Med.* 1981;305:607-612.

167. Wilkie AO, Buckle VJ, Harris PC, et al. Clinical features and molecular analysis of the alpha thalassemia/mental retardation syndromes. I. Cases due to deletions involving chromosome band 16p13.3. *Am J Hum Genet.* 1990;46:1112-1126.

168. Wilkie AO, Zeitlin HC, Lindenbaum RH, et al. Clinical features and molecular analysis of the alpha thalassemia/mental retardation syndromes. II. Cases without detectable abnormality of the alpha globin complex. *Am J Hum Genet.* 1990;46:1127-1140.

169. Gibbons RJ, Suthers GK, Wilkie AO, et al. X-linked alpha thalassemia/mental retardation (ATR-X) syndrome: localization to Xq12-q21.31 by X inactivation and linkage analysis. *Am J Hum Genet.* 1992;51:1136-1149.

170. Gibbons RJ, Picketts DJ, Villard L, et al. Mutations in a putative global transcriptional regulator cause X-linked mental retardation with a-thalassemia (ATR-X Syndrome). *Cell.* 1995;80:837-845.

171. Gibbons RJ, Bachoo S, Picketts DJ, et al. Mutations in transcriptional regulator *ATRX* establish the functional significance of a PHD-like domain. *Nat Genet.* 1997;17:146-148.

172. Ausio J, Levin DB, De Amorim GV, et al. Syndromes of disordered chromatin remodeling. *Clin Genet.* 2003;64:83-95.

173. Gibbons RJ, McDowell TL, Raman S, et al. Mutations in ATRX, encoding a SWI/SNF-like protein, cause diverse changes in the pattern of DNA methylation. *Nat Genet.* 2000;24:368-371.

174. Weatherall DJ, Old J, Longley J, et al. Acquired haemoglobin H disease in leukaemia: pathophysiology and molecular basis. *Br J Haematol.* 1978;38:305-322.

175. Gibbons RJ. α-Thalassemia, mental retardation, and myelodysplastic syndrome. *Cold Spring Harb Perspect Med.* 2012;2:a011759.

176. Belickova M, Schroeder HW Jr, Guan YL, et al. Clonal hematopoiesis and acquired thalassemia in common variable immunodeficiency. *Mol Med.* 1994;1:56-61.

177. Suragani Rajasekhar NVS, Cadena Samuel M, Cawley Sharon M, et al. Transforming growth factor-β superfamily ligand trap ACE-536 corrects anemia by promoting late-stage erythropoiesis. *Nat Med.* 2014 Apr;20(4):408-414. PMID 24658078.

178. Weatherall DJ, Clegg JB, Naughton DG. Globin synthesis in thalassemia: an in vitro study. *Nature.* 1965;208:1061-1065.

179. Weatherall DJ, Clegg JB, Na-Nakorn S, et al. The pattern of disordered haemoglobin synthesis in homozygous and heterozygous beta-thalassaemia. *Br J Haematol.* 1969;16:251-267.

180. Fessas P. Inclusions of hemoglobin in erythroblasts and erythrocytes of thalassemia. *Blood.* 1963;21:21-32.

181. Wickramasinghe SN, Hughes M. Some features of bone marrow macrophages in patients with homozygous beta-thalassaemia. *Br J Haematol.* 1978;38:23-28.

182. Yataganas X, Fessas P. The pattern of hemoglobin precipitation in thalassemia and its significance. *Ann N Y Acad Sci.* 1969;165:270-287.

183. Finch CA, Deubelbeiss K, Cook JD, et al. Ferrokinetics in man. *Medicine (Baltimore).* 1970;49:17-53.

184. Chalevelakis G, Clegg JB, Weatherall DJ. Imbalanced globin chain synthesis in heterozygous beta-thalassemic bone marrow. *Proc Natl Acad Sci U S A.* 1975;72:3853-3857.

185. Ager JA, Lehmann H. Observations on some fast haemoglobins: K, J, N and Bart's. *Br Med J.* 1958;1:929-931.

186. Rigas DA, Kohler RD, Osgood EE. New hemoglobin possessing a higher electrophoretic mobility than normal adult hemoglobin. *Science.* 1955;121:372-375.

187. Schrier SL. Pathobiology of thalassemic erythrocytes. *Curr Opin Hematol.* 1997;4:75-78.

188. Rund D, Rachmilewitz E. Advances in the pathophysiology and treatment of thalassemia. *Crit Rev Oncol Hematol.* 1995;20:237-254.

189. Fibach E, Rachmilewitz E. The role of oxidative stress in hemolytic anemia. *Curr Mol Med.* 2008;8:609-619.

190. Yuan J, Angelucci E, Lucarelli G, et al. Accelerated programmed cell death (apoptosis) in erythroid precursors of patients with severe beta-thalassemia (Cooley's anemia). *Blood.* 1993;82:374-377.

191. Gabuzda TG, Nathan DG, Gardner FH. The turnover of hemoglobins A, F and A₂ in the peripheral blood of three patients with thalassemia. *J Clin Invest.* 1963;42:1678-1688.

192. Loukopoulos D, Fessas P. The distribution of hemoglobin types in thalassemic erythrocyte. *J Clin Invest.* 1965;44:231-240.

193. Rees DC, Porter JB, Clegg JB, et al. Why are hemoglobin F levels increased in HbE/b thalassemia? *Blood.* 1999;94:3199-3204.

194. Nathan DG, Gunn RB. Thalassemia: the consequences of unbalanced hemoglobin synthesis. *Am J Med.* 1966;41:815-830.

195. Garner C, Silver N, Best S, et al. Quantitative trait locus on chromosome 8q influences the switch from fetal to adult hemoglobin. *Blood.* 2004;104:2184-2186.

196. Menzel S, Garner C, Gut I, et al. A QTL influencing F cell production maps to a gene encoding a zinc-finger protein on chromosome 2p15. *Nat Genet.* 2007;39:1197-1199.

197. Uda M, Galanello R, Sanna S, et al. Genome-wide association study shows BCL11A associated with persistent fetal hemoglobin and amelioration of the phenotype of beta-thalassemia. *Proc Natl Acad Sci U S A.* 2008;105:1620-1625.

198. Menzel S, Thein SL. Genetic architecture of hemoglobin F control. *Curr Opin Hematol.* 2009;16:179-186.

199. O'Donnell A, Premawardhena A, Arambepola M, et al. Age-related changes in adaptation to severe anemia in childhood in developing countries. *Proc Natl Acad Sci U S A.* 2007;104:9440-9444.

200. Kautz L, Jung G, Valore EV, et al. Identification of erythroferrone as an erythroid regulator of iron metabolism. *Nat Genet.* 2014;46:678-684.

201. Kim A, Nemeth E. New insights into iron regulation and erythropoiesis. *Curr Opin Hematol.* 2015;22:199-205.

202. Kautz L, Jung G, Du X, et al. Erythroferrone contributes to hepcidin suppression and iron overload in a mouse model of β-thalassemia. *Blood.* 2015;126:2031-2037.

203. Multicentre study on prevalence of endocrine complications in thalassaemia major. Italian working Group on Endocrine Complications in Non-endocrine Diseases. *Clin Endocrinol (Oxf).* 1995;42:581-586.

204. Wood JC, Enriquez C, Ghugre N, et al. Physiology and pathophysiology of iron cardiomyopathy in thalassemia. *Ann N Y Acad Sci.* 2005;1054:386-395.

205. Singer ST, Ataga KI. Hypercoagulability in sickle cell disease and beta-thalassemia. *Curr Mol Med.* 2008;8:639-645.

206. Morris CR, Kuypers FA, Kato GJ, et al. Hemolysis-associated pulmonary hypertension in thalassemia. *Ann N Y Acad Sci.* 2005;1054:481-485.

207. Weatherall DJ. Phenotype-genotype relationships in monogenic disease: lessons from the thalassaemias. *Nat Rev Genet.* 2001;2:245-255.

208. Weatherall DJ, Pressley L, Wood WG, et al. Molecular basis for mild forms of homozygous beta-thalassemia. *Lancet.* 1981;1:527-529.

209. Wainscoat JS, Old JM, Weatherall DJ, Orkin SH. The molecular basis for the clinical diversity of beta thalassaemia in Cypriots. *Lancet.* 1983;1:1235-1237.

210. Labie D, et al. Common haplotype dependency of high G gamma-globin gene expression and high Hb F levels in beta-thalassemia and sickle cell anemia patients. *Proc Natl Acad Sci U S A.* 1985;82:2111-2114.

211. Thein SL, Wainscoat JS, Sampietro M, et al. Association of thalassaemia intermedia with a beta-globin gene haplotype. *Br J Haematol.* 1987;65:367-373.

212. Gilman JG, Huisman TH. DNA sequence variation associated with elevated fetal G gamma globin production. *Blood.* 1985;66:783-787.

213. Thein SL, Hesketh C, Wallace RB, Weatherall DJ. The molecular basis of thalassaemia major and thalassaemia intermedia in Asian Indians: application to prenatal diagnosis. *Br J Haematol.* 1988;70:225-231.

214. Ho PJ, Hall GW, Luo LY, et al. Beta thalassaemia intermedia: is it possible to consistently predict phenotype from genotype? *Br J Haematol.* 1998;100:70-78.

215. Thein SL, Menzel S, Peng X, et al. Intergenic variants of HBS1L-MYB are responsible for a major quantitative trait locus on chromosome 6q23 influencing fetal hemoglobin levels in adults. *Proc Natl Acad Sci U S A.* 2007;104:11346-11351.

216. Menzel S, Jiang J, Silver N, et al. The HBS1L-MYB intergenic region on chromosome 6q23.3 influences erythrocyte, platelet, and monocyte counts in humans. *Blood.* 2007;110:3624-3626.

217. Thein SL, Menzel S, Lathrop M, Garner C. Control of fetal hemoglobin: new insights emerging from genomics and clinical implications. *Hum Mol Genet.* 2009;18:R216-R223.

218. Liu D, Zhang X, Yu L, et al. *KLF1* mutations are relatively more common in a thalassemia endemic region and ameliorate the severity of β-thalassemia. *Blood.* 2014 Jul 31;124(5):803-811. PMCID 4118488.

219. Rund D, Oron-Karni V, Filon D, et al. Genetic analysis of beta-thalassaemia intermedia in Israel: diversity of mechanisms and unpredictability of phenotype. *Am J Hematol.* 1997;54:16-22.

220. Rund D, Fucharoen S. Genetic modifiers in hemoglobinopathies. *Curr Mol Med.* 2008;8:600-608.

221. Wonke B, Hoffbrand AV, Bouloux P, et al. New approaches to the management of hepatitis and endocrine disorders in Cooley's anemia. *Ann N Y Acad Sci.* 1998;850:232-241.

222. Chatterjee R, Katz M, Cox TF, et al. A prospective study of the hypothalamic-pituitary axis in thalassaemia patients who developed secondary amenorrhoea. *Clin Endocrinol (Oxf).* 1993;39:287-296.

223. Ganz T, Nemeth E. Iron metabolism: interactions with normal and disordered erythropoiesis. *Cold Spring Harb Perspect Med.* 2012;2:a011668.

224. Olivieri NF, Brittenham GM. Iron-chelating therapy and the treatment of thalassemia. *Blood.* 1997;89:739-761.

225. Girot R, Lefrère JJ, Schettini F, et al. HIV infection and AIDS in thalassemia. In: Rebulla P, Fessas P, eds. *Thalassemia 1990. 5th Annual Meeting of the COOLEYCARE Group.* Centro trasfusionale Ospedale Naggiore Policlinico Dio Milano Editore; 1991:69-73.

226. Choudhury NJ, Dubey ML, Jolly JG, et al. Post-transfusion malaria in thalassaemia patients. *Blut.* 1990;61:314-316.

227. Sheth S. Transfusional iron overload. In: Simon TL, McCullough J, Snyder EL, Solheim BG, Strauss, RG, eds. *Rossi's Principles of Transfusion Medicine.* Wiley Blackwell; 2016:685-694.

228. Premawardhena A, Arambepola M, Katugaha N, Weatherall DJ. Is the beta thalassaemia trait of clinical importance? *Br J Haematol.* 2008;141:407-410.

229. Liang ST, Wong VC, So WW, et al. Homozygous alpha-thalassemia: clinical presentation, diagnosis and management. A review of 46 cases. *Br J Obstet Gynaecol.* 1985;92:680-684.

230. Beaudry MA, Ferguson DJ, Pearse K, et al. Survival of a hydropic infant with homozygous alpha-thalassemia-1. *J Pediatr.* 1986;108:713-716.

231. Bianchi DW, Beyer EC, Stark AR, et al. Normal long-term survival with alpha-thalassemia. *J Pediatr.* 1986;108:716-718.

232. Rigas DA, Koler RD, Osgood EE. Hemoglobin H; clinical, laboratory, and genetic studies of a family with a previously undescribed hemoglobin. *J Lab Clin Med.* 1956;47:51-64.

233. Gouttas A, Fessas P, Tsevrenis H, et al. Description d'une nouvelle variété d'anémie hémolytique congenitale. (Etude hematologique, electrophoretique et genetique). *Sang.* 1955;26:911-919.

234. Wasi P. Hemoglobinopathies in Southeast Asia. In: Bowman JE, ed. *Distribution and Evolution of the Hemoglobin and Globin Loci.* Elsevier; 1983:179-209.

235. Kattamis C, Tzotzos S, Kanavakis E, et al. Correlation of clinical phenotype to genotype in haemoglobin H disease. *Lancet.* 1988;1:442-444.

236. Galanello R, Pirastu M, Melis MA, et al. Phenotype-genotype correlation in haemoglobin H disease in childhood. *J Med Genet.* 1983;20:425-429.

237. Fucharoen S, Winichagoon P, Pootrakul P, et al. Differences between two types of Hb H disease, alpha-thalassemia 1/alpha-thalassemia 2 and alpha-thalassemia 1/Hb Constant Spring. *Birth Defects Orig Artic Ser.* 1988;23:309-315.

238. Styles L, Foote DH, Kleman KM, et al. Hemoglobin H-Constant Spring disease: an under-recognized, severe form of alpha thalassemia. *Int J Pediatr Hematol Oncol.* 1997;4:69-74.

239. Lie-Injo LE, Ganesan J, Clegg JB, et al. Homozygous state for Hb Constant Spring (slow moving Hb X components). *Blood.* 1974;43:251-259.

240. Derry S, Wood WG, Pippard M, et al. Hematologic and biosynthetic studies in homozygous hemoglobin Constant Spring. *J Clin Invest.* 1984;73:1673-1682.

241. Kattamis C, Metaxotou-Mavromati A, Wood WG, et al. The heterogeneity of normal Hb A$_2$-beta thalassaemia in Greece. *Br J Haematol.* 1979;42:109-123.

242. Schwartz E. The silent carrier of beta thalassaemia. *N Engl J Med.* 1969;281:1327-1333.

243. Pirastu M, Ristaldi MS, Loudianos G, et al. Molecular analysis of atypical beta-thalassemia heterozygotes. *Ann N Y Acad Sci.* 1990;612:90-97.

244. Bianco I, Graziani B, Carboni C. Genetic patterns in thalassemia intermedia (constitutional microcytic anemia). Familial, hematologic and biosynthetic studies. *Hum Hered.* 1977;27:257.

245. Olds RJ, Sura T, Jackson B, et al. A novel delta o mutation in *cis* with Hb Knossos: a study of different genetic interactions in three Egyptian families. *Br J Haematol.* 1991;78:430-436.

246. Silvestroni E, Bianco I, Reitano G. Three cases of homozygous beta, delta-thalassemia (or microcythaemia) with high haemoglobin F in a Sicilian family. *Acta Haematol.* 1968;40:220-229.

247. Tsistrakis GA, Amarantos SP, Konkouris LL. Homozygous beta delta-thalassaemia. Description of a case and review of the literature. *Acta Haematol.* 1974;51:185-191.

248. Ramot B, Ben-Bassat I, Gafni D, et al. A family with three beta-delta-thalassemia homozygotes. *Blood.* 1970;35:158-165.

249. Efremov GD. Hemoglobion Lepore and anti-Lepore. *Hemoglobin.* 1978;2:197-233.

250. Charache S, Clegg JB, Weatherall DJ. The Negro variety of hereditary persistence of fetal haemoglobin is a mild form of thalassemia. *Br J Haematol.* 1976;34:527-534.

251. Huisman TH, Miller A, Schroeder WA. A G gamma type of the hereditary persistence of fetal hemoglobin with beta chain production in *cis.* *Am J Hum Genet.* 1975;27:765-777.

252. Higgs DR, Clegg JB, Wood WG, et al. G gamma beta + type of hereditary persistence of fetal haemoglobin in association with Hb C. *J Med Genet.* 1979;16:288-295.

253. Fessas P, Stamatoyannopoulos G. Hereditary persistence of fetal hemoglobin in Greece. A study and a comparison. *Blood.* 1964;24:223-240.

254. Sofroniadou K, Wood WG, Nute PE, et al. Globin chain synthesis in the Greek type (A gamma) of hereditary persistence of fetal haemoglobin. *Br J Haematol.* 1975;29:137-148.

255. Clegg JB, Metaxatou-Mavromati A, Kattamis C, et al. Occurrence of G gamma Hb F in Greek HPFH: analysis of heterozygotes and compound heterozygotes with beta thalassaemia. *Br J Haematol.* 1979;43:521-536.

256. Camaschella C, Oggiano L, Sampietro M, et al. The homozygous state of G to A–117A gamma hereditary persistence of fetal hemoglobin. *Blood.* 1989;73:1999-2002.

257. Weatherall DJ, Cartner R, Clegg JB, et al. A form of hereditary persistence of fetal haemoglobin characterized by uneven cellular distribution of haemoglobin F and the production of haemoglobins A and A$_2$ in homozygotes. *Br J Haematol.* 1975;29:205-220.

258. Cappellini MD, Fiorelli G, Bernini LF. Interaction between homozygous beta (o) thalassaemia and the Swiss type of hereditary persistence of fetal haemoglobin. *Br J Haematol.* 1981;48:561-572.

259. Serjeant GR, Serjeant BE. *Sickle Cell Disease.* 3rd ed. Oxford University Press; 2001:772.

260. Silvestroni E, Bianco I. *La Malattia Microdrepanocitica.* Il Pensiero Scientifico, Editore; 1955.

261. Premawardhena A, Fisher CA, Olivieri NF, et al. Haemoglobin E beta thalassaemia in Sri Lanka. *Lancet.* 2005;366:1467-1470.

262. Fisher CA, Premawardhena A, de Silva S, et al. The molecular basis for the thalassaemias in Sri Lanka. *Br J Haematol.* 2003;121:662-671.

263. Fucharoen S, Winichagoon P. Hemoglobinopathies in southeast Asia: molecular biology and clinical medicine. *Hemoglobin.* 1997;21:299-319.

264. Agarwal S, Gulati R, Singh K. Hemoglobin E-beta thalassemia in Uttar Pradesh. *Indian Pediatr.* 1997;34:287-292.

265. Nguyen CK, Le TT, Duong BT, et al. Beta-thalassemia/haemoglobin E disease in Vietnam. *J Trop Pediatr.* 1990;36:43-45.

266. de Silva S, Fisher CA, Premawardhena A, et al. Thalassaemia in Sri Lanka: implications for the future health burden of Asian populations. Sri Lanka Thalassaemia Study Group. *Lancet.* 2000;355:786-791.

267. Olivieri NF, Muraca GM, O'Donnell A, et al. Studies in haemoglobin E beta-thalassaemia. *Br J Haematol.* 2008;141:388-397.

268. Sonakul D, Suwananagool P, Sirivaidyapong P, et al. Distribution of pulmonary thromboembolic lesions in thalassemic patients. *Birth Defects Orig Artic Ser.* 1987;23:375-384.

269. Ota Y, Yamaoka K, Sumida I, et al. Homozygous delta-thalassemia first discovered in Japanese family with hereditary persistence of fetal hemoglobin. *Blood.* 1971;37:706-715.

270. Vella F, Wells RH, Ager JA, et al. A haemoglobinopathy involving haemoglobin H and a new (Q) haemoglobin. *Br Med J.* 1958;1:752-755.

271. Lieinjo LE, Pillay RP, Thuraisingham V. Further cases of Hb Q-H disease (Hb Q-alpha thalassemia). *Blood.* 1966;28:830-839.

272. Milner PF, Huisman TH. Studies on the proportion and synthesis of haemoglobin G Philadelphia in red cells of heterozygotes, a homozygote, and a heterozygote for both haemoglobin G and alpha thalassemia. *Br J Haematol.* 1976;34:207-220.

273. Rieder RF, Woodbury DH, Rucknagel DL. The interaction of alpha-thalassaemia and haemoglobin G Philadelphia. *Br J Haematol.* 1976;32:159-165.

274. Pich P, Saglio G, Camaschella C, et al. Interaction between Hb Hasharon and alpha-thalassaemia: an approach to the problem of the number of human alpha loci. *Blood.* 1978;51:339-346.

275. Olivieri NF, Weatherall DJ. Clinical aspects of beta thalassemia and related disorders. In: Steinberg MH, Forget BG, Higgs DR, Weatherall DJ, eds. *Disorders of Hemoglobin.* Cambridge University Press; 2009:357-416.

276. Vichinsky E, Neumayr L, Trimble S, et al. Transfusion complications in thalassemia patients: a report from the Centers for Disease Control and Prevention (CME). *Transfusion.* 2014;54:972-981; quiz 971.

277. Sheth S. Strategies for managing transfusional iron overload: conventional treatments and novel strategies. *Curr Opin Hematol.* 2019;26:139-144.

278. Wood JC. Use of magnetic resonance imaging to monitor iron overload. *Hematol Oncol Clin North Am.* 2014;28:747-764, vii.

279. Pennell DJ. T2* magnetic resonance and myocardial iron in thalassemia. *Ann N Y Acad Sci.* 2005;1054:373-378.

280. Krittayaphong R, Viprakasit V, Saiviroonporn P, et al. Serum ferritin in the diagnosis of cardiac and liver iron overload in thalassaemia patients real-world practice: a multicentre study. *Br J Haematol.* 2018;182:301-305.

281. Propper RD, Cooper B, Rufo RR, et al. Continuous subcutaneous administration of deferoxamine in patients with iron overload. *N Engl J Med.* 1977;297:418-423.

282. Pippard MJ, Callender ST, Letsky EA, et al. Prevention of iron loading in transfusion-dependent thalassaemia. *Lancet.* 1978;1:1178-1181.

283. Davis BA, Porter JB. Long-term outcome of continuous 24-hour deferoxamine infusion via indwelling intravenous catheters in high-risk beta-thalassemia. *Blood.* 2000;95:1229-1236.

284. Olivieri NF, Buncic JR, Chew E, et al. Visual and auditory neurotoxicity in patients receiving subcutaneous deferoxamine infusions. *N Engl J Med.* 1986;314:869-873.

285. Olivieri NF, Basran RK, Talbot AL, et al. Abnormal growth in thalassemia major associated with deferoxamine-induced destruction of spinal cartilage and compromise of sitting height. *Blood.* 1995;86:482a.

286. Porter JB. Practical management of iron overload. *Br J Haematol.* 2001;115:239-252.

287. Nisbet-Brown E, Olivieri NF, Giardina PJ, et al. Effectiveness and safety of ICL670 in iron-loaded patients with thalassaemia: a randomised, double-blind, placebo-controlled, dose-escalation trial. *Lancet.* 2003;361:1597-1602.

288. Olivieri NF, Brittenham GM. Management of the thalassemias. *Cold Spring Harb Perspect Med.* 2013;3:a011767.

289. Li C, Mathews V, Kim S, et al. Related and unrelated donor transplantation for β-thalassemia major: results of an international survey. *Blood Adv.* 2019;3:2562-2570.

290. Lucarelli G, Giardini C, Baronciani D. Bone marrow transplantation in thalassemia. *Semin Hematol.* 1995;32:297-303.

291. Di Bartolomeo P, Di Girolamo G, Olioso P, et al. The Pescara experience of allogenic bone marrow transplantation in thalassemia. *Bone Marrow Transplant.* 1997;19(suppl 2):48-53.

292. Argiolu F, Sanna MA, Addari MC, et al. Bone marrow transplantation in thalassemia: the experience of Cagliari. *Bone Marrow Transplant.* 1997;19(suppl 2):65-67.

293. Taher AT, Cappellini MD. How I manage medical complications of beta-thalassemia in adults. *Blood.* 2018;132:1781-1791.

294. Olivieri NF, Nathan DG, MacMillan JH, et al. Survival in medically treated patients with homozygous beta-thalassemia. *N Engl J Med.* 1994;331:574-578.

295. Brittenham GM, Griffith PM, Nienhuis AW, et al. Efficacy of deferoxamine in preventing complications of iron overload in patients with thalassemia major. *N Engl J Med.* 1994;331:567-573.

296. Borgna-Pignatti C, Rugolotto S, De Stefano P, et al. Survival and complications in patients with thalassemia major treated with transfusion and deferoxamine. *Haematologica.* 2004;89:1187-1193.

297. Olivieri NF, Weatherall DJ. The therapeutic reactivation of fetal haemoglobin. *Hum Mol Genet.* 1998;7:1655-1658.

298. Swank RA, Stamatoyannopoulos G. Fetal gene reactivation. *Curr Opin Genet Dev.* 1998;8:366-370.

299. Weatherall DJ. Pharmacological treatment of monogenic disease. *Pharmacogenomics J.* 2003;3:264-266.

300. Quek L, Thein SL. Molecular therapies in beta-thalassaemia. *Br J Haematol.* 2007;136:353-365.

301. Olivieri NF, Rees DC, Ginder GD, et al. Treatment of thalassaemia major with phenylbutyrate and hydroxyurea. *Lancet.* 1997;350:491-492.

302. Frangoul H, Altshuler D, Cappellini M. CRISPR-Cas9 gene editing for sickle cell disease and β-thalassemia. *N Engl J Med.* 2021 Jan 21;384(3):252-260.

303. Breda L, Rivella S. Modulators of erythropoiesis: emerging therapies for hemoglobinopathies and disorders of red cell production. *Hematol Oncol Clin North Am.* 2014;28:375-386.

304. Piga A, Perrotta S, Gamberini MR, et al. Luspatercept improves hemoglobin levels and blood transfusion requirements in a study of patients with β-thalassemia. *Blood.* 2019;133:1279-1289.

305. Cappellini M, Viprakasit V, Taher A, et al. A phase 3 trial of luspatercept in patients with transfusion-dependent β-thalassemia. *N Engl J Med.* 2020 Mar 26;382(13):1219-1231. PMID: 32212518.

306. Cappellini M, Taher A. The use of luspatercept for thalassemia in adults. *Blood Adv.* 2021 Jan 12;5(1):326-333. DOI 10.1182/bloodadvances.2020002725.

307. Markham A. Luspatercept: first approval. *Drugs.* 2020;80:85-90.

308. Casu C, Presti VL, Oikonomidou PR, et al. Short-term administration of JAK2 inhibitors reduces splenomegaly in mouse models of β-thalassemia intermedia and major. *Haematologica.* 2018;103:e46-e49.

309. Taher AT, Karakas Z, Cassinerio E, et al. Efficacy and safety of ruxolitinib in regularly transfused patients with thalassemia: results from a phase 2a study. *Blood.* 2018;131:263-265.

310. Casu C, Nemeth E, Rivella S. Hepcidin agonists as therapeutic tools. *Blood.* 2018;131:1790-1794.

311. Casu C, Oikonomidou PR, Chen H, et al. Minihepcidin peptides as disease modifiers in mice affected by β-thalassemia and polycythemia vera. *Blood.* 2016;128:265-276.

312. Dominski Z, Kole R. Restoration of correct splicing in thalassemic pre-mRNA by antisense oligonucleotides. *Proc Natl Acad Sci U S A.* 1993;90:8673-8677.

313. Sadelain M. Genetic treatment of the haemoglobinopathies: recombinations and new combinations. *Br J Haematol.* 1997;98:247-253.

314. Lan N, Howrey RP, Lee SW, et al. Ribozyme-mediated repair of sickle beta-globin mRNAs in erythrocyte precursors. *Science* 1998;280:1593-1596.

315. Rivella S, Sadelain M. Therapeutic globin gene delivery using lentiviral vectors. *Curr Opin Mol Ther.* 2002;4:505-514.

316. Persons DA, Nienhuis AW. Gene therapy for the hemoglobin disorders. *Curr Hematol Rep.* 2003;2:348-355.

317. Nienhuis AW, Persons DA. Development of gene therapy for thalassemia. *Cold Spring Harb Perspect Med.* 2012;2:a011833.

318. Cavazzana-Calvo M, Payen E, Negre O, et al. Transfusion independence and *HMGA2* activation after gene therapy of human β-thalassaemia. *Nature.* 2010;467:318-322.

319. Thompson AA, Walters MC, Kwiatkowski J, et al. Gene therapy in patients with transfusion-dependent β-thalassemia. *N Engl J Med.* 2018;378:1479-1493.

320. Attie KM, Allison MJ, McClure T, et al. A phase 1 study of ACE-536, a regulator of erythroid differentiation, in healthy volunteers. *Am J Hematol.* 2014;89:766-770.

321. Marktel S, Scaramuzza S, Cicalese M, et al. Intrabone hematopoietic stem cell gene therapy for adult and pediatric patients affected by transfusion-dependent β-thalassemia. *Nat Med.* 2019 Feb;25(2):234-241.

322. Weatherall D. Thalassemia: the long road from the bedside through the laboratory to the community. *Nat Med.* 2010;16:1112-1115.

323. Weatherall DJ. The challenge of haemoglobinopathies in resource-poor countries. *Br J Haematol.* 2011;154:736-744.

324. WHO Working Group. Hereditary anaemias: genetic basis, clinical features, diagnosis and treatment. *Bull World Health Organ.* 1982;60:643-653.

325. Weatherall DJ. Thalassemia as a global health problem: recent progress toward its control in the developing countries. *Ann N Y Acad Sci.* 2010;1202:17-23.

326. Stamatoyannopoulos G. Problems of screening and counselling in the hemoglobinopathies. In: Motulsky AG, Lenz W, eds. *IVth International Congress on Birth Defects.* Excerpta Medica; 1973:268-276.

327. Alter BP. Antenatal diagnosis. Summary of results. *Ann N Y Acad Sci.* 1990;612:237-250.

328. Kazazian HH Jr, Phillips JA 3rd, Boehm CD, et al. Prenatal diagnosis of beta-thalassemias by amniocentesis: linkage analysis using multiple polymorphic restriction endonuclease sites. *Blood.* 1980;56:926-930.

329. Old JM, Ward RH, Petrou M, et al. First-trimester fetal diagnosis for haemoglobinopathies: three cases. *Lancet.* 1982;2:1413-1416.

330. Cao A, Galanello R, Rosatelli MC. Prenatal diagnosis and screening of the haemoglobinopathies. In: Rodgers GP, ed. *Baillière's Clinical Haematology.* Vol. 11. Baillière Tindall; 1998:215-238.

331. Modell B, et al. Audit of prenatal diagnosis for haemoglobin disorders in the United Kingdom: the first 20 years. *BMJ.* 1997;315:779-784.

332. Cheung MC, Goldberg JD, Kan YW. Prenatal diagnosis of sickle cell anaemia and thalassaemia by analysis of fetal cells in maternal blood. *Nat Genet.* 1996;14:264-268.

333. Hung EC, Chiu RW, Lo YM. Detection of circulating fetal nucleic acids: a review of methods and applications. *J Clin Pathol.* 2009;62:308-313.

334. Kuliev A, Rechitsky S, Verlinsky O, et al. Preimplantation diagnosis of thalassemias. *J Assist Reprod Genet.* 1998;15:219-225.

335. Kuliev A, Rechitsky S, Verlinsky O, et al. Birth of healthy children after preimplantation diagnosis of thalassemias. *J Assist Reprod Genet.* 1999;16:207-211.

336. Cao A, Kan YW. The prevention of thalassemia. *Cold Spring Harb Perspect Med.* 2013;3:a011775.

CHAPTER 18
DISORDERS OF HEMOGLOBIN STRUCTURE: SICKLE CELL ANEMIA AND OTHER HEMOGLOBINOPATHIES

Vivien A. Sheehan, Victor R. Gordeuk, and Abdullah Kutlar

SUMMARY

Hemoglobinopathies are the most common inherited red blood cell disorders worldwide. Among these disorders, sickle cell disease (SCD) and thalassemias constitute a major public health problem. SCD is caused by a glutamic acid to valine substitution at the sixth amino acid of the β-globin chain. Individuals with SCD may be homozygous for the sickle mutation (HbSS), or be compound heterozygotes, inheriting HbS and β-thalassemia or another β-globin variant such as HbC, HbD, HbE, or HbO$_{Arab}$. The sickle mutation makes the hemoglobin molecule stack and form a polymer when deoxygenated, which makes the red blood cells rigid and have abnormal hemorrheologic properties.

Acronyms and Abbreviations: ACS, acute chest syndrome; ADMA, asymmetric dimethyl arginine; AHSCT, allogeneic hematopoietic stem cell transplantation; AVN, avascular necrosis; 2,3-BPG, 2.3-bisphosphoglycerate; *BCL11A,* B-Cell CLL/Lymphoma 11A; BMP, bone morphogenic protein; CO$_2$, carbon dioxide; CSSCD, Cooperative Study of Sickle Cell Disease; DHTR, delayed hemolytic transfusion reaction; DNA, deoxyribonucleic acid; eNOS, endothelial nitric oxide synthase; FDA, Food and Drug Administration; Hb, hemoglobin; HbAS, sickle cell trait; HbF, fetal hemoglobin; HbS, sickle hemoglobin; *HBSIL,* HBS1 Like Translational GTPase; HbSC, sickle cell-HbC disease; HIF, hypoxia inducible factor; HLA human leukocyte antigen; HPLC, high performance liquid chromatography; HUDEP, human umbilical cord blood-derived erythroid progenitor; IL, interleukin; iNKT cells, invariant natural killer T cells; K$^+$, potassium; KLF1, Kruppel Like Factor 1); LDH, lactate dehydrogenase; MCHC, mean cell hemoglobin concentration; MCV, mean corpuscular volume; MPs, microparticles; MRI, magnetic resonance imaging; NO, nitric oxide; NOS, nitric oxide synthase; NT-pro-BNP, N-terminal pro-brain natriuretic peptide; O$_2$, oxygen; PiSCES, Pain in Sickle Cell Epidemiology Study; PO$_2$, partial pressure of oxygen; P50, point at which hemoglobin is one-half saturated with oxygen; PH, pulmonary hypertension; PCV7, 7 polyvalent conjugate; PIGF, placenta growth factor; R state, relaxed oxy; RNA ribonucleic acid; SCD, sickle cell disease; SCT, stem cell transplantation; sPLA2, secretory phospholipase A2; PPV23, pneumococcal polysaccharide vaccine 23; PSGL-1, P-selectin glycoprotein ligand-1; STOP, Stroke Prevention Trial in Sickle Cell Disease; T state, tense, deoxy; TCD, transcranial Doppler; TF, tissue factor; TGF-β, transforming growth factor, beta; TNF-α, tumor necrosis factor; UDP, uridine diphosphate; UGT1A1, UDP glucuronosyltransferase 1 family; VCAM-1, vascular cell adhesion molecule 1, VOC, vaso-occlusive crisis; VTE, venous thromboembolism; vWF, von Willebrand factor.

The downstream effects of the sickling process include (a) red blood cell membrane changes leading to potassium loss and cellular dehydration; (b) interaction of the red blood cell with neutrophils, monocytes, and the microvascular endothelium; (c) hemolysis and nitric oxide depletion; (d) release of inflammatory proteins from activated immune cells; and (e) activation of coagulation. These processes lead to hemolytic anemia, inflammation, painful vasoocclusive episodes, damage to multiple organ systems, and shortened life expectancy in individuals with SCD.

There is considerable heterogeneity in the severity of SCD; even individuals with the same genotype may have different clinical courses. The best-known modifier of SCD is the level of fetal hemoglobin (HbF), which exerts a potent antisickling effect when present in sufficient amounts in the red blood cell. Coinheritance of α-thalassemia also modifies the disease, reducing hemolysis and ameliorating anemia. Non-globin genetic modifiers of SCD also contribute to clinical variability.

Since the 1980s, advances in supportive care and implementation of disease-modifying therapies, such as hydroxyurea and chronic blood transfusion, have led to an increase in life expectancy, although the average life expectancy is still less than 5 decades for individuals with HbSS. Hydroxyurea is an established and effective disease-modifying agent that has been approved by the FDA for use in children and adults with SCD. Although its main mechanism of action is HbF induction, hydroxyurea also decreases neutrophils, platelets, and adhesion molecule expression, contributing to its efficacy. Newly FDA-approved agents for SCD include L-glutamine, which reduces painful events, crizanlizumab, an anti-adhesive monoclonal antibody that reduces painful events, and voxelotor, which covalently binds to HbS, keeping it in its oxygenated state, and prevents sickling, reduces hemolysis, and increases Hb concentration. Gene-based therapies, which either insert a functional Hb gene similar to HbA or increase HbF via various strategies, are in clinical trials that show early encouraging results. As of this writing, the only curative therapies are allogeneic hematopoietic stem cell transplantation and gene-modification approaches.

Sickle cell trait, the heterozygous state for sickle Hb, affects approximately 8% of Americans of African descent and, with rare exceptions, is asymptomatic. HbC is associated with target cells and spherocytes in the blood film and splenomegaly. HbD disease is essentially asymptomatic. HbE is very common in Southeast Asia, and because of large population movements from this area, has also become a prevalent hemoglobinopathy in other regions of the world. HbE is a thalassemic variant; coinheritance with β-thalassemia mutations can result in thalassemia syndromes of varying severity that are sometimes transfusion-dependent.

Unstable Hb variants appear as rare, sporadic cases and are characterized by hemolytic anemia with Heinz bodies. The latter are Hb precipitates within the erythrocyte that are visible on specially stained blood films. Variants that alter the oxygen affinity of the Hb molecule may lead to erythrocytosis (high oxygen affinity variants) or anemia (low oxygen affinity variants).

●THE STRUCTURE AND FUNCTION OF NORMAL HEMOGLOBIN

Hemoglobin (Hb) is the iron-containing oxygen-transport metalloprotein found in abundance in red blood cells. Hb transports oxygen from the lungs to the tissues and CO$_2$ from the tissues to the lungs.

The oxygen affinity of Hb permits nearly complete saturation with oxygen in the lungs, as well as efficient oxygen unloading in the tissues by an allosteric chemical interaction which is depicted by its sigmoid Hb oxygen dissociation curve. Hb is a 4-subunit molecule; its conformation, and hence the oxygen affinity, changes as each successive molecule of oxygen is bound. Acute acidosis in the tissues of the body is a sign of hypoxia and to achieve more oxygen delivery, the Hb–oxygen affinity decreases, that is, the dissociation curve shifts to the right, enabling more oxygen to be delivered acutely to the tissue. Long-term alkalosis (as occurs at high altitudes) is counteracted by an increase of red cell 2,3-bisphosphoglycerate (2,3-BPG), which also serves to decrease Hb oxygen affinity.

Normal mammalian Hb is made up of two pairs of related globin polypeptide chains: one chain is α or α-like and the other is non-α, or beta-like (β, γ, δ, or ε). The α-globin chains of all human Hb made after early embryogenesis are identical (Chaps. 2 and 17). The non-α globin chains include the β-globin chain of normal adult Hb ($α_2β_2$), the γ-globin chain of HbF ($α_2γ_2$), and the δ-globin chain of the minor adult HbA$_2$ ($α_2δ_2$), which accounts for about 2% of the Hb of normal adults. Chapter 17 discusses the regulation of the production of globin chains.

Approximately 75% of the amino acids in α- and β-globin chains are in an α-helical arrangement. All Hbs studied have a similar helical content (Fig. 18-1A). Eight helical areas, lettered A to H, occur in the β-globin chains. Hb nomenclature specifies that amino acids within helices are designated by the amino acid number and the helix letter, whereas amino acids between helices bear the number of the amino acid and the letters of the preceding and subsequent helices. Thus, residue EF3 is the third residue of the segment connecting the E and F helices, whereas residue F8 is the eighth residue of the F helix. Alignment according to helical designation makes homology evident: residue F8 is the proximal heme linked histidine, and the histidine on the distal side of the heme is E7.

Figures 18-1B and 18-1C show the tertiary structure of the α-globin and β-globin chains. The prosthetic group of Hb is heme (ferroprotoporphyrin IX); Fig. 18-2A shows its structure. The heme group is located in a crevice between the E and F helices in each globin chain (Fig. 18-2B). The highly polar propionate side chains of the heme are on the surface of the globin molecule and are ionized at physiologic pH. The rest of the heme is inside the globin molecule, surrounded by nonpolar residues except for two histidines. The iron atom is linked by a coordinate bond to the imidazole nitrogen (N) of globin histidine F8. The E7 *distal* histidine, on the other side of the heme plane, is not bonded to the iron atom but is very close to the ligand-binding site.

Certain residues in the amino acid sequence of each globin polypeptide chain appear to be critical to protein stability and function; such residues are usually the same (invariant) across species. The NH$_2$-terminal valine residues of the β-globin chains are important in 2,3-BPG interactions. Areas of contact between globin chains and between heme and globin tend to contain invariant residues as well. The non-α (β, γ, δ, or ε)-globin chains are all 146 amino acids in length. The γ-globin chain of fetal hemoglobin (HbF) differs from the β-globin chain by 39 residues. The γ-globin genes are duplicated: one codes for glycine ($^Gγ$) and the other for alanine ($^Aγ$) at residue 136, giving rise to 2 kinds of γ-globin chains. In addition, a common polymorphism, the substitution of threonine for isoleucine, is frequently found at residue 75 of the $^Aγ$-globin chain.

The sigmoid shaped Hb-oxygen dissociation curve is a function of the change of the conformation of the molecule from the liganded to the unliganded state. In the deoxy, or tense state, the Hb tetramer is held together by intersubunit salt bonds (Fig. 18-3) and intersubunit hydrophobic contacts (see Fig. 18-1B), in addition to hydrogen bonds.

2,3-BPG is situated in the central cavity in deoxyhemoglobin, between the two β-globin chains (see Fig. 18-1B). The change in conformation of the Hb molecule is brought about by a complex, coordinated series of changes in the structure of the molecule as heme binds oxygen. The oxygen dissociation curve can be linearized by a transformation known as the Hill plot:

$$\log[y/(1-y)] = \log K + n \log pO_2$$

where K is an empiric overall constant without physicochemical basis. The slope n is taken as a convenient measure of cooperativity. Values of n in noninteracting Hbs that exhibit hyperbolic, not sigmoid, oxygen dissociation curves (eg, myoglobin) are approximately 1. In a tetrameric Hb with 4 oxygen-reactive sites, the maximum value for n is 4.0; however, n values of 2.7 to 3.0 are found in normal Hb.

The point at which the Hb is one-half saturated with oxygen (P_{50}) is the usual measurement of oxygen affinity. It depends upon pH (the Bohr effect), temperature, and 2,3-BPG concentration. In common practice, P_{50} is standardized at 37°C and pH 7.40. P_{50} of freshly drawn blood is approximately 26.7 torr under standard conditions, but the P50 of Hb from which 2,3-BPG has been removed is only approximately 13 torr. Although fetal and newborn red cells have 2,3-BPG levels similar to those of adults, their oxygen dissociation curve is left shifted (increased oxygen affinity) with a P_{50} of approximately 23 torr because HbF does not react as strongly with 2,3-BPG as does HbA.

●NOMENCLATURE OF ABNORMAL HEMOGLOBINS

Following the molecular characterization of HbS by Ingram and colleagues in 1956,[1] there has been a rapid and exponential increase in the number of variant or "abnormal" Hbs described. This number now exceeds 2000. A detailed description of variant Hbs, their chemical and functional properties, and population distribution can be found on the Globin Gene Server website (http://globin.cse.psu.edu/hbvar). Initially, newly described variants were designated by letters of the alphabet (eg, HbC, HbD, HbE, HbJ). When the letters of the alphabet were exhausted, the practice of naming the variant Hbs after the geographic location where they were first described was adapted (eg, Hb$_{Koln}$, Hb$_{Zurich}$). Variants with electrophoretic or functional properties similar to previously described abnormal Hbs were designated with the letter and the geographic location: for example, HbD$_{Punjab}$, HbE$_{Saskatoon}$, HbM$_{Hyde Park}$, and so forth. Some alphabetic designations were also used to indicate electrophoretic properties of certain variants; for example, there are a number of HbDs (HbD$_{Punjab}$, HbD$_{Iran}$, HbD$_{Ibadan}$). All of these variants share the electrophoretic properties of HbS-like mobility on alkaline (cellulose acetate) electrophoresis, while they move with HbA at acidic pH (citrate agar electrophoresis). Similarly, HbEs have HbC-like mobility on alkaline electrophoresis and move with HbA on citrate agar electrophoresis.

The vast majority of Hb variants arose as a result of single nucleotide mutations, leading to an amino acid change in either α-globin, β-globin, δ-globin, or γ-globin subunits of the Hb tetramer. Other mechanisms for producing Hb variants include small deletions or insertions, elongated chains, and fusions (for a description of Hb variants and associated clinical syndromes, see "Other Abnormal Hemoglobins" further).

The coinheritance of HbS and other variant Hbs or β-thalassemia mutations may result in sickle cell disease (SCD), depending on the variant. In the United States, the most common SCD genotype is homozygous HbS (HbSS). Sickle cell anemia specifically refers to HbSS, and is part of the larger category of SCD, which includes

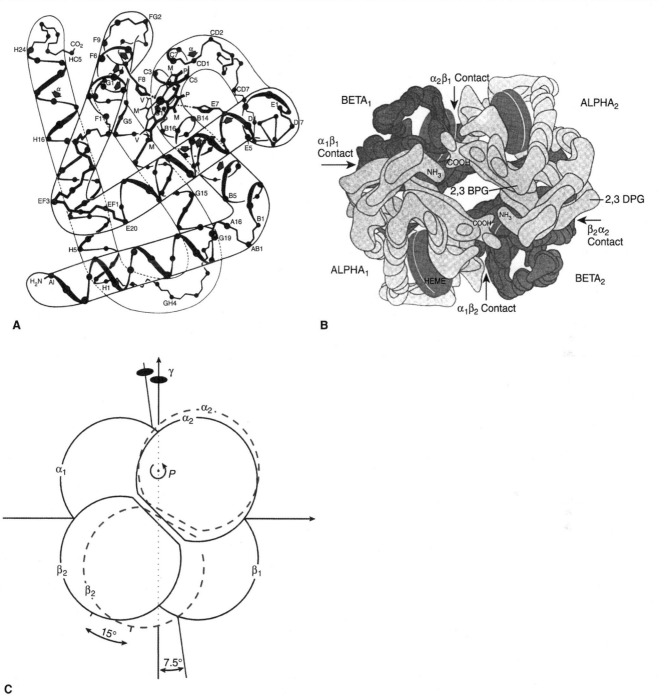

FIGURE 18–1. A. Representation of the structure of β chains. *Arrows* indicate sites of substitutions in a number of unstable hemoglobins. **B.** The hemoglobin molecule, as deduced from x-ray diffraction studies, shown from above. The molecule is composed of four subunits: 2 identical α chains (*light blocks*) and 2 identical β chains (*dark blocks*). 2,3-Bisphosphoglycerate (2,3-BPG) binds to the two β chains in the deoxyhemoglobin molecule. 2,3-DPG, 2,3-diphosphoglycerate. **C.** Schematic of rotation of $\alpha_2\beta_2$ dimer relative to $\alpha_1\beta_1$ in quaternary structure change from deoxyhemoglobin (*solid lines*) to carboxyhemoglobin (*dashed lines*). *(Modified with permission from Baldwin J, Chothia C. Haemoglobin: the structural changes related to ligand binding and its allosteric mechanism. J Mol Biol. 1979 Apr 5;129[2]:175-220.)*

individuals who are compound heterozygotes for HbS and another Hb variant that can result in red blood cell sickling under physiologic conditions. Sickle cell trait is a carrier state; these individuals do not have SCD. Common SCD genotypes include HbSC, HbSβ⁺-thalassemia (HbSβ⁺), and HbSβ⁰-thalassemia (HbSβ⁰) (Chap. 17). Other less-common SCD genotypes include HbSD_Punjab, HbSO_Arab, HbS_Lepore, and HbSE.

In general, HbSS and HbSβ⁰ patients have a greater degree of hemolysis and a more severe anemia than HbSC and HbSβ⁺ patients. Coinheritance of many different, less damaging or abnormal β-globin chain variants with HbS do not result in a symptomatic sickling disorder; rather, they may be clinically and hematologically indistinguishable from sickle cell trait (HbAS).

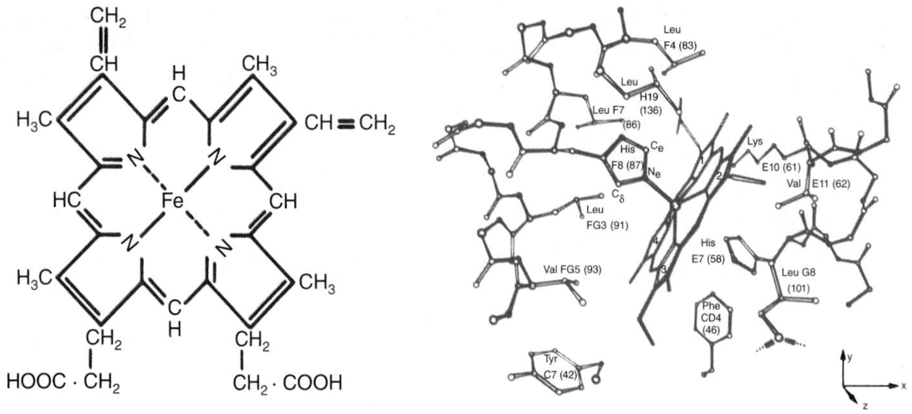

FIGURE 18–2. A. Structure of heme (ferroprotoporphyrin IX). **B.** Heme group and its environment in the unliganded α-chain. Only selected side chains are shown; the heme 4-propionate is omitted. *(Reproduced from Gelin BR, Lee AW, Karplus M. Hemoglobin tertiary structural change on ligand binding. Its role in the co-operative mechanism. J Mol Biol. 1983 Dec 25;171[4]:489-559.)*

HbC is found in 17% to 28% of West Africans, particularly east of the Niger River in the vicinity of North Ghana. HbC confers some resistance to malaria, but to a lesser degree than HbS.[2] The homozygous state, HbCC, is relatively asymptomatic. The prevalence of HbC among Americans of African descent is 2% to 3%. Sporadic cases also have been reported in other populations, including Italians. HbD_{Punjab}, now recognized to be identical to $HbD_{Los\ Angeles}$ because both have the structure $\alpha_2\beta_2$ [121]Glu→Gln, also interacts with HbS in forming aggregates or polymers of Hb when in the deoxy conformation. This HbD variant is found in many parts of the world, including Africa, northern Europe, and India.

HbE prevalence is second only to HbS, and found principally in Burma, Thailand, Laos, Cambodia, Vietnam, Malaysia, and Indonesia, but not in China. In some areas of Southeast Asia, the population has an HbE carrier rate of 30%. Studies of restriction length polymorphisms in the β-globin cluster suggest that the HbE mutation has arisen several times independently. As with HbS and HbC, HbE appears to confer some resistance to infection with malaria.[3]

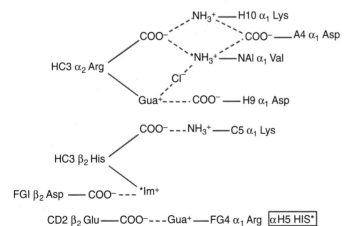

FIGURE 18–3. Salt bridges in deoxyhemoglobin (* = ionizable group less protonated at pH 9.0 than at pH 7.0). These groups account for 60% of the alkaline Bohr effect. The remainder is a result of αH5 His. *(Data from Perutz MF, Wilkinson AJ, Paoli M, et al. The stereochemical mechanism of the cooperative effects in hemoglobin revisited. Annu Rev Biophys Biomol Struct. 1998;27:1-34.)*

● SICKLE CELL DISEASE

DEFINITION AND HISTORY

The first case of SCD reported in the Western medical literature appeared in 1910, describing the case of a dental student from Grenada, Walter Clement-Noel. Dr. James Herrick and his intern, Dr. Ernest Irons, provided medical care for Mr. Noel between 1904 and 1907, during which he experienced several bouts of fever and cough, leg ulcers, jaundice, and exercise intolerance.[4] Herrick and Irons prepared blood films and photomicrographs showing nucleated red blood cells and red cells with a "slender sickle shape" (Fig. 18-4).[4] During the period 1908-1917, two more cases of this unusual anemia were reported. In 1915, Cook and Meyer raised the question of a genetic basis for the disorder based on the family history of the third reported case.[5] In 1917, Victor Emmel used in vitro culture to show that sickle red blood cells represent a physical alteration of morphologically normal-appearing red cells and that they were not released from the marrow as sickle cells.[6] He also demonstrated that morphologically normal red cells of the father with HbAS of a patient with SCD became sickle shaped after in vitro culture. Vernon Mason, who reported the fourth case in 1922, coined the term *sickle cell anemia* after observing the similarities between all the cases reported up to that time.[7] In 1923, Sydenstricker[8] and Huck[9,10] noted "latent-sicklers" among relatives of the diagnosed patients, confirming and expanding on Emmel's finding. In 1927, Hahn and Gillespie showed that sickling was related to low oxygen tension and low pH.[11] In 1933, Diggs distinguished between symptomatic cases called sickle cell anemia and asymptomatic cases that were termed *sickle cell trait*, and found that approximately 8% of Americans of African descent had sickle cell trait.[12]

Irving Sherman, while a medical student at Johns Hopkins, showed that sickled red blood cells were birefringent under a polarizing microscope and that this finding was reversible with oxygenation of the cells. This observation ultimately led Linus Pauling to study sickle Hb after being advised of this property of sickle cells by William Castle, a noted research hematologist. In 1949, Pauling and his colleagues demonstrated electrophoretic differences between Hbs from normal, sickle cell trait, and sickle cell anemia people and hypothesized that there must be chemical differences, thus establishing SCD as the first disease for which a molecular basis was described.[13] In the late 1950s, Hunt and Ingram sequenced the globin peptide and linked the abnormality to a change

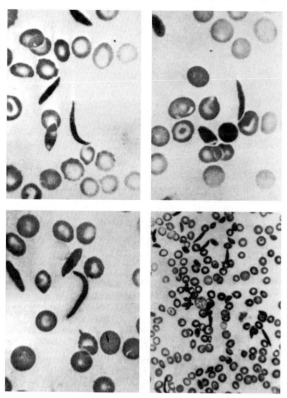

FIGURE 18–4. Peculiar elongated and sickle-shaped red cells from the first report of sickle cell anemia with depiction of sickle cells. *(Reproduced with permission from Herrick JB. Peculiar elongated and sickle-shaped red corpuscles in a case of severe anemia. Arch Intern Med. 1910:517:6.)*

in the amino acid composition of the β-globin chain (replacement of glutamic acid by valine at residue 6). Marotta and coworkers showed in 1977 that the corresponding change in codon 6 of the β-globin gene was GAG→GTG.[14] The discovery of a variant fragment in HbS versus HbA during restriction endonuclease mapping of amniotic fluid cells by Y.W. Kan paved the way for antenatal diagnosis of SCD and opened the way for modern genetics using recombinant DNA technology.[15] The history of SCD serves as an inspiring reminder of the power of clinical and laboratory observations, and in an era of mechanistic basic science research, serves to highlight the importance of bedside to bench and bench to bedside research integration.[16-19]

EPIDEMIOLOGY

The idea that individuals with sickle cell trait might have a survival advantage against environmental factors was first suggested by Dr. Alan Raper in East Africa in 1949.[20] Drs. Mackey and Vivarelli postulated that the environmental influence was likely malaria, given the striking geographical overlap between falciparum malaria prevalence and that of sickle cell trait.[21] Blood from individuals with sickle cell trait often contained fewer malarial parasites.[22] Sickle trait confers some protection against malaria in early childhood, and is maximally protective against severe malaria as opposed to asymptomatic parasitemia or mild disease.[23] The mechanism of such a protection has been the matter of much debate. Plausible mechanisms include selective sickling of parasitized red blood cells, resulting in more effective removal by the monocyte–macrophage system, and inhibitory effect on parasite growth by increased red cell potassium loss, decreased red cell pH, and increased endothelial adherence of parasitized sickle red cells.[24]

The World Health Organization estimates that 5% of the world population carries a gene for a hemoglobinopathy.[25] SCD is highly prevalent in sub-Saharan and equatorial Africa, with lesser but significant prevalence in the Middle East, India, and the Mediterranean. The incidence of SCD in sub-Saharan African countries ranges between 1% and 2%. It is estimated that 300,000 infants with SCD are born annually, two-thirds of them in Africa.[26] In the Jamaican cohort study, newborn screening in 100,000 consecutive vaginal deliveries resulted in the finding of sickle cell trait in 10% of newborns.[27]

In the United States, the Centers for Disease Control and Prevention estimates that SCD is present in 1 in 500 live births among Americans of African descent; 1 in 12 Americans of African descent have the trait, and approximately 100,000 Americans, largely Americans of African descent, live with the disease. In Americans of Hispanic descent, the rate of SCD is 1 in 36,000 live births.[28] Accurate population statistics of SCD are difficult to obtain in the United States because of a lack of standardized data collection and central reporting.

As of 2002, in the United States, more than 1 billion dollars are spent per year on hospitalizations for SCD.[29] Data from a single state Medicaid program estimated a lifetime cost of care of $500,000 per patient with SCD. In this patient population, costs increased with increasing age, including costs of non-SCD health issues. The majority of the costs were for inpatient health care utilization.[30]

There has been speculation regarding the origin of the sickle mutation for decades: Did it arise once and then gain worldwide distribution or did it arise multiple times, independently in different regions of the world? The nonrandom association of restriction endonuclease polymorphisms in the β-globin cluster were used to define the β-globin haplotype, yielding five distinct haplotypes associated with sickle cell mutations, and associated with varying clinical severity and HbF levels.[31-33] Four of the five patterns occur in Africa and are designated as the Senegal, Benin, Bantu, and Cameroon haplotypes, whereas the fifth arose on the Indian subcontinent.[34] These findings were used to support the theory that the sickle mutation arose five different times in five different locations. The origin of the sickle mutation was investigated using whole-genome sequencing data from 2932 individuals, 156 carrying the sickle mutation. A combination of forward time simulation, phylogenetic network analysis, and coalescent analysis suggests a single origin of the sickle allele approximately 7300 years ago, during the Holocene Wet Phase.[35]

PATHOPHYSIOLOGY

The sine qua non of sickle cell anemia is a Glu→Val substitution in the sixth amino acid of the β-globin molecule. This substitution results in replacement of negatively charged, hydrophilic glutamic acid by hydrophobic valine at position 6 (*HBB*; glu(E)6val(A); GAG-GTG; rs334), with devastating consequences to the individual who is homozygous for the mutation. Homozygotes for the sickle mutation produce defective Hb tetramers that polymerize and aggregate upon deoxygenation, changing the flexible, soft, discoid red blood cells into stiff, sickle-shaped cells. The pathophysiologic processes that result in the clinical phenotype extend beyond the red blood cell (Fig. 18-5). We now understand that the pathophysiology of SCD is more complex than hypoxia-induced microvascular occlusion mediated by a rigid red blood cell. SCD is a chronic inflammatory state punctuated by acute increases in inflammation wherein the endothelium, neutrophils and monocytes, platelets, coagulation pathways, several plasma proteins, adhesion molecules, and derangements in nitric oxide metabolism interact in concert with the abnormality in Hb polymerization described several decades ago (Fig. 18-6).

Variation in several genes other than the β-globin gene that modify the milieu in which organ damage occurs may play a role. While the

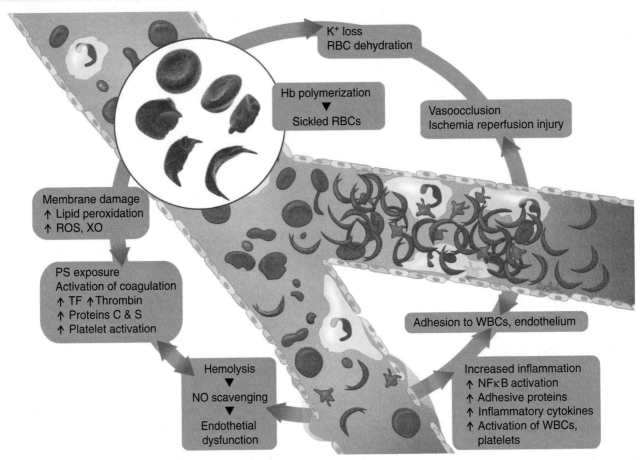

FIGURE 18–5. Schema summarizing the pathophysiology of sickle cell anemia. K+, potassium; NFκB, nuclear factor κB; NO, nitric oxide; PS, phosphatidylserine; RBC, red blood cell; ROS, reactive oxygen species; TF, tissue factor; WBC, white blood cell; XO, xanthine oxidase.

effects of HbF levels, α-thalassemia, UDP glucuronosyltransferase family 1 member A1 (*UGTA1A*) polymorphisms, and glucose-6-phosphate dehydrogenase deficiency on SCD have been extensively studied, these variables do not explain all of the clinical heterogeneity of SCD. For example, it was reported that non-G6PD-deficient HbSS patients with a common African-specific cytochrome b5 reductase 3 polymorphism (*CYB5R3*[c.350C>G]) have lower red blood cell CYB5R 3 activity, higher red blood cell NADH/NAD+ ratios, and less severe anemia.[36] It is not known why some patients develop certain complications, and it is difficult to predict which complications a particular patient will experience. Much work has been done to identify genetic variants associated with these disease complications; many associations remain unvalidated. As the field continues to move beyond small sample collections and candidate gene approaches into whole-genome sequencing and merging of samples from all over the world, it will be possible to identify more genetic variants associated with development of specific SCD related complications, and, hopefully, to leverage this knowledge into targeted therapies.

Hemoglobin Polymerization

Aggregation of deoxy HbS molecules into polymers occurs when aggregates reach a thermodynamically critical size. This process is termed *homogenous nucleation*, and the smallest aggregate formed that favors polymer growth is called the *critical nucleus*.[37-42] Addition of subsequent deoxy HbS molecules to already formed polymers is termed *heterogenous nucleation*, which results in polymer branching. Polymer growth is an exponential process wherein there is a delay

time between the presence of deoxy HbS molecules and polymer formation. This delay time is inversely proportional to the concentration of HbS molecules. Polymer formation alters the rheologic properties of the red blood cell.

The quaternary structure of oxy HbS cannot maintain axial and lateral hydrophobic contacts necessary for polymerization unlike deoxy HbS, thus explaining the unsickling phenomenon upon reoxygenation.[43-46] The sickling process is initially reversible with oxygenation of deoxy HbS, but over time may lead to the formation of irreversibly sickle shaped red blood cells that fail to return to their normal discoid shape with oxygenation because of membrane damage imparted by repeated cycles of sickling and unsickling in the circulation. The rate and extent of polymerization is dependent on several factors, including intracellular Hb concentration, presence of Hbs other than HbS, blood oxygen saturation, pH, temperature, and 2,3-BPG levels.[47] Microvascular occlusion by sickle red blood cells containing polymers is favored by prolonged transit times through the microcirculation as a result of high blood viscosity or adhesion to the endothelium, rapid deoxygenation, and increased numbers of dense sickle red blood cells that contain polymers even at oxygen saturation levels found in the arterial circulation.[47-50] Arguments against HbS polymerization as the sole determinant of sickle cell pathophysiology include lack of clinically significant events despite constant sickling of red blood cells, the association of neutrophilia with vasoocclusive crises (VOCs), and clinical features that imply macrovascular rather than microvascular perturbation, such as large-vessel stroke.[51]

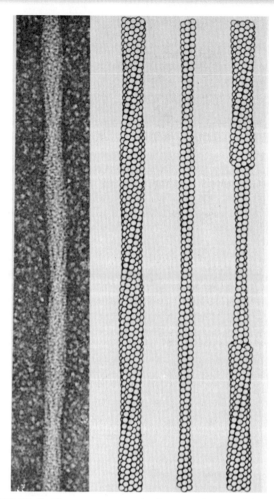

FIGURE 18–6. Electron micrograph of negatively stained fiber of HbS and the structure deduced by three-dimensional image reconstruction. The reconstructed fiber is presented as ball models, with each ball representing a HbS tetramer. The models are presented as the outer sheath *(left)*, the inner core *(center)*, and a combination of both inner and outer filaments *(right). (Used with permission from Dr. Stuart J. Edelstein.)*

Role of Cellular Dehydration in Hemoglobin S Polymerization

Red blood cell membrane injury in sickle cells results in impaired cation homeostasis with decreased ability to maintain intracellular potassium concentrations. The calcium-activated potassium (K^+) channel (Gardos channel), potassium–chloride cotransport channel, and a sickling-induced nonselective cation leak pathway have been implicated in sickle red cell dehydration. The net result is loss of intracellular K^+ and water resulting in cellular dehydration.[52-57] This change effectively increases the red blood cell Hb concentration, favoring sickling.

Hemolysis and Nitric Oxide Scavenging

Nitric oxide (NO), a key signaling molecule of the vascular endothelium, has vasodilatory, antiinflammatory, and anti-platelet properties.[58] NO is a soluble gas synthesized from L-arginine by endothelial NO synthase (NOS).[59] Red cell L-arginase released as a consequence of sickle red blood cell hemolysis converts arginine to ornithine, thereby limiting L-arginine availability for NO synthesis. Decreased NO production resulting from elevated levels of endogenous NOS inhibitors, especially asymmetric dimethylarginine and reduced levels of L-arginine, have been documented in SCD, especially during a VOC.[60-64] Reduced plasma arginine levels and elevated asymmetric dimethylarginine levels also result in NOS uncoupling, causing production of reactive oxygen species rather than NO.[65,66] Chronic hemolysis with release of plasma-free Hb results in scavenging of NO with consequent endothelial dysfunction, which may favor sickle cell adhesion.[67,68]

Abnormal Cell Adhesiveness

Seminal work by several groups showed that sickle red blood cells adhere to stimulated endothelium unlike their normal counterparts.[69,70] Mature sickle red blood cells and reticulocytes recently released from the marrow express high levels of adhesion molecules, integrin $\alpha_4\beta_1$ and CD36, and are more adherent than older circulating dense sickle red blood cells.[71,72] Young, adherent red blood cells may stick to the endothelium first, followed by dense red blood cells, which are trapped in the logjam with white blood cells and platelets, leading to microvascular occlusion.[47] Other molecules involved in sickle red blood cell-endothelium interactions include vascular cell-adhesion molecule 1 (VCAM-1), integrin $\alpha_V\beta_3$, P-selectin, P-selectin glycoprotein ligand-1, E-selectin, Lutheran blood group antigen, and thrombospondin.[73-78] The site of adhesion is purported to be the postcapillary venule at which site sickle red cells appear to interact with white cells adherent to the endothelium rather than engaging the endothelium directly.[49]

Neutrophilia is an adverse prognostic factor in sickle cell anemia. Because of their larger size, adherent leukocytes cause a greater decrease in vessel caliber than red blood cells. Diapedesis, or the passage of blood cells through the intact walls of the capillaries, typically accompanying inflammation, occurs in postcapillary venules, a site of vasoocclusion in sickle cell anemia.[49,79-81] Neutrophil integrin $\alpha_M\beta_2$ microdomains capture sickle red blood cells causing vascular occlusion in sickle cell mouse models. Monocytes are also highly activated in SCD, and they promote increased endothelial activation by increased production of tumor necrosis factor (TNF)-α and interleukin (IL)-1β.[61] Expression of leukocyte adhesion molecules, L-selectin and integrin $\alpha_M\beta_2$, are associated with a severe clinical phenotype.[79,82]

Inflammation and Chronic Vasculopathy

Sickle cell anemia is characterized by chronic leukocytosis, abnormal activation of neutrophils and monocytes, and an increase in several proinflammatory mediators, including TNF-α, IL-6, and IL-1β. Several adhesion molecules are upregulated, including VCAM-1, selectins, integrins, the acute-phase reactants C-reactive protein and secretory phospholipase A_2 (sPLA$_2$), and coagulation factors are activated.[82-93] Placenta growth factor is released from erythrocytes and activates monocytes to produce inflammatory cytokines. In addition, placenta growth factor upregulates endothelin-1 signaling via the endothelin B receptor. Endothelin-1 is a potent vasoconstrictor and upregulation is associated with adverse outcomes in SCD. Placenta growth factor independently correlates with disease severity as well.[94,95] Hemin activates placenta growth factor in mice via the erythroid Krüppel-like factor.[96] It is an open question whether inflammation is caused by abnormally adhesive red blood cells to the vascular endothelium or whether inflammation causes abnormal red blood cell adhesiveness. It is likely that both occur, given that red blood cell adhesiveness incites endothelial activity, and infection-induced inflammation precipitates clinically significant vascular events in patients. Some vascular beds in sickle cell anemia display changes akin to atherosclerotic vascular disease: large vessel intimal hyperplasia and smooth muscle proliferation.[97,98] However, the characteristic lipid-laden plaques of atherosclerotic vascular disease are not present.[82]

Ischemia–Reperfusion Injury

Akin to other disease states, such as myocardial infarction, resolution of vasoocclusion results in reperfusion injury characterized by increased oxygen free radical formation via activation of xanthine oxidase, generation of oxidant stress, lipid peroxidation, upregulation of cellular adhesion molecules, and nuclear factor-κB, a key player in the inflammatory process.[82,99,100] Invariant natural killer T cells propagate the inflammatory cascade in ischemia reperfusion injury and are increased and activated in patients with SCD. Agonists to adenosine 2A receptor on invariant natural killer T cells downregulate their activation and attenuate inflammation in mouse models of SCD.[101] A candidate adenosine 2A receptor agonist, regadenoson, was tested in a randomized phase II trial in individuals with SCD, but no differences between the regadenoson and placebo groups in length of hospital stay, mean total opioid use, or pain scores were found.[102]

Activation of the Coagulation System

The initiator of coagulation, tissue factor (TF), is elevated in the plasma of patients with SCD.[58,91,103-105] Microparticles expressing TF derived from monocytes, macrophages, neutrophils, and endothelial cells have been described in SCD.[106,107] Conflicting results exist in the literature on the presence and contribution of TF and TF-bearing microparticles to procoagulant activity.[108,109] There is a lack of correlation between TF-bearing microparticles and procoagulant activity in SCD.[110] Erythrocyte and platelet microparticles are TF-negative and are the major component of microparticles in SCD. Activation of the intrinsic pathway of coagulation by TF-negative, red blood cell and platelet microparticles through a phosphatidylserine-dependent mechanism appears to be the major contributor of microparticle-dependent coagulation activation in SCD.[111] Perivascular TF interaction with plasma coagulation factors made possible by increased vascular permeability and phosphatidylserine exposure on the surface of red blood cells secondary to repeated cycles of sickling provide an impetus for the coagulation process. Heightened thrombin generation, platelet activation, and decreased protein C and protein S levels favor a procoagulant state.[86,112,113] Increased plasma levels of D-dimers, thrombin–antithrombin complexes, prothrombin fragment 1.2, and plasmin–antiplasmin complexes are indicative of increased thrombin generation and coagulation with subsequent fibrinolysis.[114] Plasma from sickle cell patients contains increased ultralarge von Willebrand factor (vWF) multimers as a result of increased endothelial cell secretion and impaired cleavage by relatively low levels of ADAMTS13 (a disintegrin and metalloprotease with a thrombospondin type 1 motif member 13),[115] and hyperadhesive von Willebrand factor may contribute to VOC in patients with SCD.[116]

Adenosine Signaling

Cellular stress leads to the degradation of adenine nucleotides, resulting in the generation of adenosine. Adenosine homeostasis is maintained by two enzymes: adenosine kinase, which phosphorylates adenosine to adenosine monophosphate and adenosine deaminase, which converts adenosine to inosine. Adenosine signals through 4 different receptors that have differing functions. Signaling via the adenosine A2A receptor expressed on most leukocytes and platelets results in an antiinflammatory effect;[117] however, signaling via the adenosine A2B receptor causes priapism in SCD mice via hypoxia inducible factor-1–mediated decrease of phosphodiesterase.[118] Signaling via the adenosine A2B receptor also leads to increased 2,3-BPG in red cells causing decreased oxygen binding affinity of Hb, which promotes sickling. Pegylated adenosine deaminase treatment of sickle mice resulted in decreased hemolysis and hypoxia reoxygenation injury.[119,120]

SICKLE CELL TRAIT

Inheritance of only one HbS allele along with a normal β-globin gene in trans is termed *sickle cell trait* (HbAS). An estimated 300 million people carry the trait worldwide.[121] The percentage of HbA is always higher (~60%) than HbS (~40%) in sickle cell trait, as the α-globin chain prefers to pair with a normal β-globin chain over HbS, as a consequence of electrostatic interactions governing αβ dimer formation. The amount of HbA in the red blood cells of individuals with sickle cell trait is sufficient to prevent sickling except in the most unusual circumstances. HbAS cells sickle at oxygen (O_2) tension of approximately 15 torr.[122] Plasma myeloperoxidase and red blood cell sickling have been reported to increase during exercise with fluid restriction in HbAS subjects.[123] Plasma levels of VCAM-1 are higher in HbAS subjects and remain elevated following exercise compared to normal controls or HbAS with concomitant α-thalassemia, which is suggestive of subtle microcirculatory dysfunction in this population.[124] Skeletal muscle capillary structures are different in HbAS subjects compared to controls. There is a 30-fold increased risk of sudden death in black army recruits with HbAS.[125] In 2009, the National Collegiate Athletic Association recommended mandatory testing for HbAS for all its student athletes.[126] Sudden exertional death of athletes with sickle cell trait continues to be reported, sometimes associated with heat stroke and rhabdomyolysis.[127,128] The American College of Cardiology recommends preventive strategies for athletes with sickle cell trait, including adequate rest and hydration during exercise, and particular caution for athletes competing or training in high environmental temperatures or at extreme altitude.[129]

HbAS is considered a generally asymptomatic state. Children with sickle cell trait do not have more health encounters than children with normal Hb. However, higher rates of stroke and renal disease have been reported in trait individuals compared to African Americans with normal Hb.[130-132]

Renal abnormalities are among the most common manifestations of HbAS. Anoxia, hyperosmolarity, and low pH of the renal medulla predispose red blood cells to sickling. Microscopic or gross hematuria from renal papillary necrosis is usually painless. Renal neoplasm or stones should be excluded in those with persistent gross hematuria. Isosthenuria may be seen and may contribute to exercise induced rhabdomyolysis and sudden death.[133] Renal medullary carcinoma is a rare but serious complication of HbAS.[134] Risk of urinary tract infection is higher in females with HbAS, especially during pregnancy.[135] End-stage renal disease occurs at an earlier age for HbAS patients with polycystic kidney disease and HbAS may contribute to erythropoietin resistance.[136]

Splenic infarction occurs under extreme environmental conditions in persons with HbAS; most splenic infarctions resolve spontaneously.[137] Caution and immediate intervention is also warranted in those HbAS individuals who develop traumatic hyphema.[138] The risk of venous thromboembolism (VTE) is increased twofold in HbAS subjects compared to those without the trait, and they have a greater risk for pulmonary embolism than for deep vein thrombosis.[126,139] HbAS patients do not have increased perioperative morbidity or mortality.[140] The life span of HbAS individuals is normal.[141]

LABORATORY FEATURES OF SICKLE CELL DISEASE

Individuals with SCD exhibit laboratory evidence of hemolytic anemia, with elevated lactate dehydrogenase (LDH), aspartate aminotransferase, indirect bilirubin, and reticulocyte count, and decreased serum haptoglobin. Unless there is coinheritance of α-thalassemia, the anemia of HbSS individuals is usually normochromic and normocytic with a steady-state Hb level between 50 g/L and 110 g/L.[142] The red cell density is increased with a normal mean cell Hb concentration.[143] Serum erythropoietin level is inappropriately low relative to the degree of anemia.[144] Elevated neutrophil and platelet levels are often observed, even in asymptomatic patients, which is reflective of persistent low-grade inflammation and functional asplenia.[145,146] Platelet levels may be low in individuals with splenic enlargement as a consequence of trapping.[147]

Vitamin E, vitamin D, and zinc levels are often low in individuals with SCD.[148-150] Serum ferritin is often increased at steady-state, especially in patients who have received multiple blood transfusions; this reflects increased iron stores.[151] Elevated brain natriuretic peptide is seen in patients with pulmonary hypertension (PH) and congestive heart failure.[152,153] Morphologically, classic sickle red cells are seen on the blood film examination, and the marrow shows erythroid hyperplasia.

SCD can be accurately diagnosed with high-performance liquid chromatography (HPLC) and isoelectric focusing.[154] No HbA is found in patients with HbSS, HbSC, or HbSβ⁰ diseases. Varying amounts of HbA (depending on the severity of the β-thalassemia mutation) are found in HbSβ⁺ subjects, but HbA is always less than 50% of total hemoglobin in nontransfused HbSβ⁺ patients. Several novel point-of-care tests are under development to diagnose SCD; these will be particularly useful in low-resource countries where incidence is highest, and newborn screening is absent or incomplete. These tests typically exploit some aspect of SCD, such as the tendency to produce dense red blood cells or of HbS to precipitate, or solubility testing and sickling of red cells using sodium metabisulfite. These tests may give a false-negative result for milder SCD genotypes such as HbSβ⁺, or perform poorly in the newborn period when HbF levels are high. A promising point-of-care test that addresses these challenges is the HemoTypeSC, which uses a qualitative lateral flow immunoassay method to detect the presence of HbA, HbS, and HbC with monoclonal antibodies that detect HbA, HbS, and HbC antigens, but are blind to HbF, and so even newborns with elevated HbF and very low levels of HbA or HbS can be diagnosed.[155]

Hemorheologic Abnormalities in Sickle Cell Disease

The clinical complications of SCD can be linked to the abnormal flow properties (blood rheology or hemorheology) of SCD blood.[156] High viscosity (or thickness) of SCD blood contributes to pain crises and organ damage. Dense cells, defined as having more than 111 g/L of Hb, are more likely to sickle. Whole-blood viscosity and percent of dense red blood cells are classical indicators for the severity of SCD.[156,157] Blood viscosity is determined by the hematocrit, red blood cell deformability, red cell aggregation, and plasma viscosity.[156,158] For a given hematocrit, SCD blood is very viscous in deoxygenated conditions as a result of HbS sickling: An individual with SCD with a hematocrit of 21% would have a whole-blood viscosity comparable to that of a normal individual with a hematocrit of 45%.[159,160] Another way of describing viscosity, the hematocrit-to-viscosity ratio, adjusts for differences in hematocrit between individuals, and correlates with oxygen-carrying capacity; a higher hematocrit-to-viscosity ratio indicates improved oxygen-carrying capacity, and it is lower in patients with SCD compared to normal individuals.[161] In patients with SCD, low hematocrit-to-viscosity ratio is associated with recurrent leg ulcers.[156] SCD patients with leg ulcers, renal dysfunction, and priapism also have higher percentage of dense red blood cells and decreased red blood cell deformability compared to SCD patients without these complications.[161,162] Therefore, high viscosity and high percentage of dense red blood cells correlate with SCD complications and disease severity, and suggest a role for measurement of red blood cell rheology in monitoring patients with SCD and their response to therapy.

COURSE AND PROGNOSIS

Mortality from SCD in the United States declined after 1968, coinciding with the introduction of pneumococcal polyvalent conjugate-7 vaccine and the use of penicillin prophylaxis in children with SCD who are younger than 5 years. Comparison of mortality rates between 1979–1998 and 1999–2009 showed a 61% decrease in infants, a 67% decrease in children between ages 1 and 4 years, and a 35% decrease in children and young adults between ages 5 and 19 years. A spike in mortality is observed in the young adult period corresponding to transition from pediatric to adult medical care, although 96% of individuals with SCD living in the United States now reach the age of 18 years.[163,164] In 1994, the average life expectancy of patients with HbSS disease in the United States was estimated to be 42 years for men and 48 years for women.[165] The estimates for median survival range from 48 to 49 years for patients with sickle cell anemia[166,167] and 54 years for HbSC and HbSβ⁺-thalassemia.[167] In Jamaica, the population has a median survival of 53 years for men and 58 years for women, with 44% of individuals born prior to 1943 still living as of 2009.[168]

CLINICAL FEATURES AND MANAGEMENT

The reader is referred to the National Institutes of Health, National Heart, Lung and Blood Institute's guidelines for an extensive review on the topic; revised guidelines were released in the Fall of 2014 at http://www.nhlbi.nih.gov/health-pro/guidelines/sickle-cell-disease-guidelines/.[169] General approaches to SCD management and pain management are described separately (Table 18-1). More guidelines have been issued by the American Society of Hematology.[170-175]

TABLE 18–1. Pathophysiologic Mechanisms and Potential Therapeutic Targets in Sickle Cell Disease

Pathophysiology/ Complication	Therapeutic Interventions
HbS polymerization	HbF induction
Cellular dehydration	Gardos channel inhibition
	Potassium-chloride cotransport channel inhibition
Adhesion to endothelium	
Red blood cells	Antiselectin
	Antiintegrin
White blood cells	Antiselectin
	Intravenous immunoglobulin
	HU
Inflammation	NFκB inhibition
	Immunomodulatory drugs
	HU
	Statins
NO scavenging	Nitric oxide donor (NO, HU, BH4)
	PDE5 inhibition
	Modulation of hemolysis
Coagulation	Tissue factor inhibition
	Antiplatelet therapy
	Anticoagulation
Hyposplenism/infection	Penicillin prophylaxis
Ischemia–reperfusion	Xanthine oxidase inhibition
	Myeloperoxidase inhibition
Iron overload	Chelation

Abbreviations: BH₄, tetrahydrobiopterin; HbF, fetal hemoglobin; HbS, sickle hemoglobin; HU, hydroxyurea; NFκB, nuclear factor κB; NO, nitric oxide; PDE5, phosphodiesterase 5.

Sickle Cell Crises

The typical course for an individual living with SCD is to have periods of relatively normal function despite chronic anemia and ongoing vasoocclusion, punctuated by periods of increased pain and serial changes in various laboratory parameters that are termed *a sickle cell crisis*. Crises have typically been classified as VOC, aplastic crisis, sequestration crisis, and hyperhemolytic crisis.

Vasoocclusive Crisis The clinical hallmark of SCD is the VOC; it occurs with varying frequency in different individuals, and may become more frequent during the transition from teenage years to young adulthood. Pain results from vasoocclusion causing tissue hypoxia and ischemia. Vasoocclusion may affect any tissue, but patients typically report pain in the chest, lower back, and extremities. Patients may also have a VOC of the abdomen, which can mimic acute abdomen from other causes. Alternatively, serious life-threatening pathology may be dismissed in patients with SCD as being a VOC, sometimes with fatal results. Different patients display different patterns of painful sites during a VOC, but patients often report recurrence of VOC in the same site as prior events. Episodes may be precipitated by insomnia, emotional stress, dehydration, infection, and cold weather, although in most cases no precipitating factor is found.[176]

Phases of a typical VOC are shown in Fig. 18-7.[177] Crises requiring readmission within 1 week occur in approximately 20% of patients after hospital discharge.[177] The characterization of crisis phases has implications for clinical research, especially in pain management, wherein interventions early in the course of a crisis could result in better outcomes for patients. The pattern of a VOC may also help distinguish VOC from chronic pain, which may not be the result of ischemic tissue damage, but rather of neuropathic pain, opioid-induced hyperalgesia, or other causes.

Aplastic Crisis Aplastic crisis in SCD results when there is a marked reduction in red blood cell production in the face of ongoing hemolysis, causing an acute, severe drop in Hb level. The characteristic laboratory finding is a reticulocyte count less than 1%. The most common cause is parvovirus B19 infection, which attaches to the P-antigen receptor on erythroid progenitor cells, causing a temporary arrest in red blood cell production (Chaps. 3, 5, and 29). Recurrent aplastic crises induced by parvovirus B19 are rare because of the development of

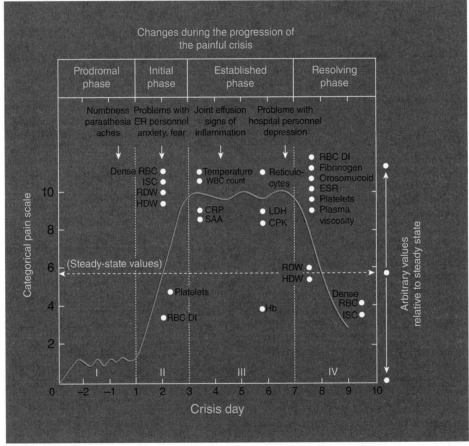

FIGURE 18–7. A typical profile of the events that develop during the evolution of a severe sickle cell painful crisis in an adult in the absence of overt infection or other complications. Such events are usually treated in the hospital with an average stay of 9 to 11 days. Pain becomes severest by day 3 of the crisis and starts decreasing by day 6 or 7. The Roman numerals refer to the phase of the crisis: I indicates prodromal phase; II, initial phase; III, established phase; and IV, resolving phase. *Dots* on the *x*-axis indicate the time when changes became apparent; and *dots* on the *y*-axis indicate the relative value of change compared with the steady state indicated by the horizontal dashed line. *Arrows* indicate the time when certain clinical signs and symptoms may become apparent. Values shown are those reported at least twice by different investigators; values that were anecdotal, unconfirmed, or that were not reported to occur on a specific day of the crisis are not shown. CPK, creatinine phosphokinase; CRP, C-reactive protein; ESR, erythrocyte sedimentation rate; HDW, hemoglobin distribution width; ISC, irreversibly sickled cells; LDH, lactate dehydrogenase; RBC DI, red cell deformability index; RDW, red cell distribution width; SAA, serum amyloid A; WBC, white blood cell. *(Reproduced with permission from Ballas SK, Gupta K, Adams-Graves P. Sickle cell pain: a critical reappraisal.* Blood. *2012 Nov 1;120[18]:3647-3656.)*

protective antibodies, but other viruses may cause transient red blood cell aplasia, particularly in young children with SCD. Other rare complications associated with parvovirus B19 include acute splenic and/or hepatic sequestration, acute chest syndrome, marrow necrosis, and renal dysfunction. Patients usually recover within 2 weeks; those with severe symptomatic anemia need red blood cell transfusion. Concomitant treatment with hydroxyurea seems to attenuate the severity of anemia associated with parvovirus B19 infection.[178] Siblings of SCD patients with parvovirus infections should be monitored closely for aplastic crisis given high secondary attack rates (>50%). Patients need to be isolated from pregnant individuals given increased risk of hydrops fetalis with parvovirus B19 infection.[179]

Sequestration Crisis Sequestration can cause severe, life-threatening anemia due to sudden, massive pooling of red blood cells, typically in the spleen, and less commonly, the liver.[180] Splenic sequestration is typically seen in children younger than 5 years prior to autoinfarction of the spleen, but also can be seen in adolescents or adults with HbSC disease or HbSβ-thalassemia with persisting splenomegaly.[181-183] A minor sequestration episode is usually accompanied by a Hb of more than 70 g/L, and a major episode usually is one in which the Hb is less than 70 g/L or the Hb has decreased by 30 g/L from baseline.[184]

Acute splenic and hepatic sequestration crises can present with rapidly enlarging spleen or liver, pain, hypoxemia, and hypovolemic shock. Treatment consists of small, cautious red blood cell transfusion. Transfusion carries the risk of hyperviscosity when the sequestration crisis resolves and the sequestered red blood cells are returned to the general circulation. Splenic sequestration has a high rate of recurrence, especially in children. Splenectomy, total or partial, to prevent recurrence is debated in very young children. Chronic red blood cell transfusion may be used as a means of delaying splenectomy until the child is 2 years or older, at which time splenectomy may be considered. Splenectomy is recommended after the first episode of life-threatening splenic sequestration crisis or chronic hypersplenism. Emergency splenectomy during a crisis is not recommended. Parents should be instructed on how to palpate the spleen in young children; education is of importance in early recognition of the problem in order to seek medical care promptly.[179]

Hyperhemolytic Crisis The term *hyperhemolytic crisis* is used to describe the occurrence of episodes of accelerated rates of hemolysis characterized by decreased Hb concentration and increased levels of reticulocytes and other markers of hemolysis (hyperbilirubinemia, increased LDH). Hyperhemolysis can occur during resolution of a VOC because irreversibly sickled and dense red blood cells trapped in microcirculation during the crisis are rapidly destroyed, as well as from an acute or delayed hemolytic transfusion reactions.[179,185]

Pain Control

Patients with SCD may have acute pain, chronic pain, or both. As a symptom, pain is often underrated in its intensity and undertreated by caregivers, especially inexperienced physicians. Patients are often perceived as drug-seekers or drug addicts, when in fact fewer than 10% of patients are addicted, a number comparable to other disease states. A study comparing sickle cell anemia patients who use the emergency department frequently or infrequently found significant impairment in quality of life and increased markers of disease severity in those who use the emergency department frequently. This dispels the myth that frequent emergency department use indicates narcotic-addicted individuals when, in fact, they may have more severe disease.[186-191] The landmark Pain in Sickle Cell Epidemiology Study (PiSCES) revealed that adult SCD patients have pain at home approximately 55% of the time, which contrasts sharply to pain studies in children, who report at-home pain approximately 9% of the time.[192,193]

Acute pain is managed with opioids, nonsteroidal anti-inflammatory drugs, acetaminophen, or a combination of these medications. Nonsteroidal anti-inflammatory agents must be used with caution because of the risk of contributing to acute kidney injury or chronic kidney disease.[194] Immediate pain assessment and frequent reassessment with appropriate application of medications until pain relief is obtained is important. For adults and children weighing more than 50 kg, morphine can be started at a dose of 0.1 to 0.15 mg/kg. The hydromorphone dose should be 0.015 to 0.020 mg/kg IV. These are recommended doses for opioid-naive patients and are at the lower end of the dosing range.[169,195,196] The use of meperidine has declined because of neurologic side effects, especially in patients with renal failure, who are at risk for the serotonin syndrome in conjunction with use of other medications.[197-199] However, the use of morphine is not benign and concerns of increased association of acute chest syndrome, dysphoria, and neuroexcitatory side effects have been raised.[177] Prolonged use of opioids can lead to opioid-induced hyperalgesia, contributing to chronic pain. A sign of opioid-induced hyperalgesia is lack of improvement in pain despite dose increase; this can help distinguish it from tolerance, in which a dose increase reduces pain.[200-202]

Prior use of opioid therapy should be taken into consideration when deciding initial opioid doses as patients may be tolerant and require higher doses. Caution should be exercised with nonsteroidal antiinflammatory drugs and acetaminophen if there is renal or hepatic dysfunction. Patients with acute pain are better managed in a setting dedicated to sickle cell patients.[203,204] A multidisciplinary approach is needed for pain management, including screening for neuropathic pain and depression, especially if chronic pain is present.[205,206] Opioid side effects, particularly constipation, should be anticipated and managed. Antidepressants, anticonvulsants, and clonidine can be used for neuropathic pain. Occasionally, severe, unrelenting pain may require red blood cell transfusion to decrease HbS below 30%.[207] Evidence-based guidelines on the management of acute and chronic pain in sickle cell disease have been published by the American Society of Hematology.[208]

Pulmonary Manifestations

Acute Chest Syndrome Acute chest syndrome (ACS) is a constellation of signs and symptoms in patients with SCD that includes a new infiltrate on chest radiograph defined by alveolar consolidation, but not atelectasis, that may be accompanied by chest pain, fever, tachypnea, wheezing, cough and/or hypoxia (Fig. 18-8).[209] Respiratory findings on clinical examination in the absence of radiographic findings should trigger high suspicion for ACS and warrant close monitoring. ACS has been a leading cause of mortality in patients with SCD.[165] Etiology varies depending on age, with viral and bacterial infections dominating in the pediatric age group and unknown causes, infections, infarction, and fat embolization resulting from marrow necrosis during VOC dominating in adults.[210,211] Important pathogens include *Chlamydia pneumoniae*, *Mycoplasma pneumoniae*, *Streptococcus pneumoniae*, *Staphylococcus aureus*, Parvovirus B19, respiratory syncytial virus, and influenza. Regardless of the triggering factor, the pathogenesis of ACS involves increased intrapulmonary sickling, intrapulmonary inflammation with increased microvascular permeability, and alveolar consolidation. ACS can rapidly evolve with bilateral infiltrates and consolidation leading to acute respiratory failure requiring intubation and ventilatory assistance. Independent risk factors for respiratory failure are age older than 20 years, platelet count less than 20×10^9/L, multilobar lung involvement, and a history of cardiac disease.[210] Thrombocytopenia is an independent predictor of neurologic complications during hospitalization for ACS, which were seen in 22% of adult patients in the National Acute Chest Syndrome Study.[212]

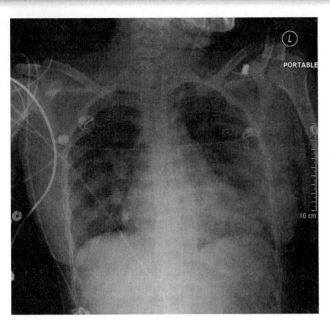

FIGURE 18–8. Anteroposterior view of chest radiograph depicting bilateral, patchy, lung infiltrates in a 30-year-old woman with sickle cell disease and evolving acute chest syndrome.

ACS prevention includes incentive spirometry, adequate pain control to avoid chest splinting, antimicrobial therapy that always covers atypical bacteria and influenza when indicated, avoidance of overhydration, use of bronchodilators, and red blood cell transfusion to decrease intrapulmonary sickling.[210,213-217] Exchange transfusion is ideal, but simple transfusions to a target Hb of 100g/L are most often used for expediency. The use of glucocorticoids may attenuate the course of ACS, but their use is not well established and readmission rates for VOC after ACS resolution are increased.[211,218] Although sPLA$_2$ was reported to be a predictor of ACS,[219] a clinical trial investigating early transfusion based on sPLA$_2$ elevation closed because of poor accrual.[220] Hydroxyurea therapy should be offered to all patients with a history of ACS because it reduces the incidence by 50% in children and 73% in adults.[217,221]

Pulmonary Hypertension PH, defined by a resting mean pulmonary arterial pressure 25 torr or higher on right-heart catheterization, is seen in 6% to 11% of SCD patients. The tricuspid regurgitation velocity measured during echocardiography in combination with estimated right atrial pressure is considered to be a valid estimate of systolic pulmonary artery pressure.[222,223] An elevated tricuspid regurgitation velocity of 2.5 m/s or higher is seen in up to one-third of adults with sickle cell anemia and has a positive predictive value of 25% for PH. An increased risk of mortality is seen with PH documented by right-heart catheterization. Elevated tricuspid regurgitation jet velocity of 2.5 m/s or higher and serum N-terminal pro-brain natriuretic peptide level of 160 pg/mL or higher are observed in considerably greater proportions of patients and are also associated with increased mortality.[224] Abnormalities in NO metabolism, hemolysis, hypoxia, inflammation contribute to the pathophysiology of PH.[224,225] Parenchymal lung disease from repeated episodes of ACS and chronic thromboembolism are other causal factors. Clinical symptoms of PH include fatigue, dizziness, and dyspnea on exertion, chest pain, and syncope. These may be unrecognized as being related to PH, as PH is often undiagnosed in patients with SCD.

Patients with SCD should be screened for PH by echocardiogram at steady-state. A tricuspid regurgitation velocity of 2.5 m/sec should prompt referral to a pulmonary specialist for further evaluation, especially if the brain natriuretic peptide is greater than 160 pg/mL or the tricuspid regurgitation velocity is greater than 2.9 m/s regardless of the brain natriuretic peptide. The optimal treatment of PH in SCD documented by right-heart catheterization has not been defined. PH may be precapillary, postcapillary related to left ventricular dysfunction, or a combination of both. Patients with postcapillary PH should be referred to a cardiologist for optimal management of left ventricular cardiac dysfunction. Whether treatment of precapillary PH in SCD should follow guidelines set for the treatment of primary PH unrelated to SCD is not clear. Two trials looking at bosentan (endothelin receptor antagonist) in SCD patients closed because of sponsor withdrawal. A trial of sildenafil was halted early because of increased incidence of VOC. Patients who have VTE in the setting of PH should be considered for indefinite anticoagulation. Hydroxyurea should be offered to all patients with any of the risk factors for increased mortality described above.[224,225]

Asthma, Abnormal Pulmonary Function Tests, and Airway Hyperreactivity Asthma is a common comorbidity with higher-than-average prevalence in patients with SCD, and is associated with increased risk of ACS, vaso-occlusive episode, stroke, and mortality. Airway hyperreactivity as evidenced by a positive bronchodilator response on pulmonary function testing, irrespective of baseline function, and in response to cold air or methacholine challenge, is seen in approximately two-thirds of SCD patients. Inflammation, hypoxemia, and increased oxidative stress associated with asthma may contribute to the vasculopathy of SCD.[226] Pulmonary function tests collected as part of the Cooperative Study of Sickle Cell Disease revealed abnormalities in 279 (90%) of 310 patients, with the majority having restrictive lung disease. In a prospective study of 146 children, adolescents, and young adults between ages 7 and 20 years with HbSS or HbSβ^0-thalassemia, 28 (19%) had obstructive physiology as defined according to guidelines of the American Thoracic Society, 13 (9%) had restrictive physiology, and 16 (11%) had abnormal but not categorized physiology.[227] Asthma treatment follows general treatment guidelines as in the non-SCD populations.[228,229]

Cardiac Manifestations

Anemia in SCD results in an elevated cardiac output secondary to an increased stroke volume with minimal increase in heart rate.[230,231] Clinical manifestations of a hyperdynamic circulation include a forceful precordial apical impulse, systolic and diastolic flow murmurs, and tachycardia that may increase during periods of increased hemodynamic stress. Diastolic left ventricular dysfunction may begin in early childhood and is an independent risk factor for death, with even greater risk of mortality in those having PH.[232] Left ventricular hypertrophy is common and progressive with age; left ventricular dysfunction is a late event. Myocardial infarction is an underrecognized problem in SCD. Epicardial coronary artery disease is rare; microvascular ischemia is likely causative. Sudden cardiac death was reported in 40% of patients in an autopsy series.[233-235] Previously sudden cardiac death was ascribed to narcotic overdose; currently, it is thought to be secondary to cardiopulmonary causes in the majority of cases. QTc prolongation and nonspecific ST-T wave changes on electrocardiography are common findings in SCD patients, as are atrial and ventricular arrhythmias. Patients presenting with chest pain should have a thorough evaluation to rule out cardiac disease. Cardiac magnetic resonance may be a good modality to image microvascular flow and quantitate cardiac iron overload.[236,237] Blood pressure in patients with SCD is significantly lower than age-matched, sex-matched, and race-matched controls partly secondary to anemia.[238] Relative hypertension is associated with end-organ damage. Diuretics may be used, keeping in mind that SCD patients have obligate hyposthenuria and are prone to dehydration, which can precipitate a VOC.

Central Nervous System

Overt, clinical stroke in SCD is a macrovascular phenomenon with devastating consequences that affects approximately 11% of patients younger than 20 years.[239,240] Risk is highest in the first decade of life followed by a second smaller peak after age 29 years. Ischemic stroke is most common in children and older adults, whereas hemorrhagic stroke predominates in the third decade of life.[240] Recurrent stroke is most common in the first 2 years following the primary event.[241] Silent infarcts, defined as an increased T2 signal abnormality on magnetic resonance imaging (MRI), begins in infancy and has a cumulative incidence of 37% by age 14 years. Silent strokes occur in watershed areas of the brain, are not predicted by abnormal transcranial Doppler (TCD) velocity, and may progress despite chronic transfusion.[242-245] There is evidence of neurocognitive decline in asymptomatic adults despite having normal brain imaging that is attributed to anemia and hypoxemia.[212]

Cerebral blood flow is increased in SCD because of chronic anemia and hypoxemia, but does not increase further in response to increased hypoxic stress, thereby predisposing to ischemia.[246,247] Stenosis of large vessels, especially of the circle of Willis, without the classic atherosclerotic plaque occurs in conjunction with a multitude of other factors, including chronic hemolysis, deranged NO metabolism, and impaired vascular autoregulation, and can lead to stroke.[239] Rare causes of cerebral vascular disease include fat embolization and venous sinus thrombosis. Moyamoya-type fragile collaterals have been reported in more than 20% of patients with prior stroke, possibly leading to hemorrhagic stroke in later life.[248-253]

Risk factors for ischemic stroke include transient ischemic attack, recent or recurrent ACS, nocturnal hypoxemia, silent infarcts, hypertension, elevated LDH, and leukocytosis, whereas anemia, neutrophilia, the use of glucocorticoids, and recent transfusion are independent risk factors for hemorrhagic stroke, especially in children.[240,254-260] Sickle cell genotypes other than HbSS carry a lower risk of stroke, as do patients with coinheritance of α-thalassemia, or Hb levels above 90 g/L.[240,261,262] The best predictor of stroke risk is an increased blood flow velocity in major intracranial arteries on TCD ultrasonography.[262] Blood flow velocities less than 170 cm/s are considered normal. Velocities between 170 and 200 cm/s are termed *conditional*, and velocities faster than 200 cm/s are considered high and are associated with a 10-fold increase in ischemic stroke in children between ages 2 and 16 years.

There is a higher frequency of stroke among siblings of patients with SCD than would be expected by chance alone, raising the possibility of other modifier genes contributing to stroke risk.[248] The *TNF* (−308) G/A promoter polymorphism is associated with increased large-vessel stroke risk.[263,264] Another variant associated with protection against stroke, *ENPP1* K173Q was identified using whole-exome sequencing.[265,266] The clinical features of stroke in SCD encompass the classic findings of stroke in other disorders, including, but not limited to, hemiparesis, seizures, coma, paresthesias, headaches, and cranial nerve palsies. Neurocognitive deficits in IQ, memory, language, and executive function are found.[212,267] Imaging approaches for acute stroke are the same as those for non-SCD patients and include MRI and magnetic resonance angiography.

Based on the results from the Stroke Prevention in Sickle Cell Disease (STOP) Study, it is recommended that asymptomatic children with HbSS disease older than 2 years should be screened for stroke risk using TCD.[262] Those with high TCD velocities should be offered a chronic red blood cell transfusion program for primary stroke prevention. Repeat TCD screenings should be done every 3 to 12 months even in patients who have normal or conditional baseline velocities, because they can evolve into a higher risk category. Despite obstacles to TCD screening, clinical practice changes based on the STOP study translated into

declining stroke rates since 1991, from 5% to 10% of children with SCD experiencing an overt stroke to less than 1%.[268,269]

Prevention of Secondary Stroke Patients with SCD who present with a stroke and are not on chronic transfusion should be placed on a transfusion program to prevent secondary strokes. Exchange transfusion may be preferable to periodic red blood cell transfusion, not only to avoid iron overload, but also to further reduce stroke risk. In a retrospective study, children who received periodic transfusion had a fivefold higher relative risk of a recurrent stroke compared to those on an exchange transfusion regimen.[270] Despite chronic transfusions, patients may have a recurrent stroke, especially in patients with HbS greater than 30%.[271] Hydroxyurea decreased high and conditional TCD velocities in more than 90% of patients studied.[272] A randomized trial that compared transfusions with iron chelation to hydroxyurea with phlebotomy in children with a history of stroke, showed a 10% stroke rate in the hydroxyurea arm, and no strokes in the transfusion arm, thus establishing transfusion as the preferred preventive strategy.[273] A subsequent trial comparing transfusions with iron chelation to hydroxyurea with phlebotomy in children with abnormal TCD velocities, showed that hydroxyurea and phlebotomy was not inferior to transfusion and iron chelation to prevent primary stroke in high-risk children who have received at least 1 year of transfusions.[274]

Treatment guidelines for intracranial hemorrhage are the same as for non–SCD-related intracranial hemorrhage; the role of transfusion in the setting of hemorrhagic stroke in SCD is less clear than for ischemic stroke. Patients with moyamoya disease who have a particularly poor outcome may benefit from revascularization using encephaloduroarteriosynangiosis.[275,276]

Genitourinary Systems

Nephropathy Sickle red blood cells are prone to sickle in the hypoxic, acidic, and hypertonic environment of the renal medulla. Oxidative stress, increase in prostaglandins and endothelin-1, and abnormalities of the renin–angiotensin system contribute to the pathophysiology of kidney disease in SCD.[277] Chronic kidney disease, defined on the basis of abnormal albuminuria and/or low estimated glomerular filtration rate, is observed in up to 68% of SCD adults[278-281] and is a consistent predictor of early mortality.[165,282-285] Once a serum creatinine equal to or greater than 1.5 mg/dL develops, time to death averages 4 years.[285] The incidence of renal failure varies between 4% and 20%.[278,279,282,285] Dehydration is the most common cause of acute renal failure in SCD. Hyposthenuria, or difficulty concentrating urine, is highly prevalent in SCD, may increase the risk of dehydration, and is irreversible.[286] Glomerular hypertrophy, focal and segmental glomerular sclerosis, and hemosiderin deposition in proximal renal tubular epithelium have been described; however, no single lesion is pathognomonic of sickle cell nephropathy. Cystatin C is an accurate marker of glomerular filtration and is preferable to serum creatinine in estimating renal function.[287,288] Glomerular hyperfiltration, microalbuminuria, and macroalbuminuria occur sequentially in SCD patients starting in infancy and increasing in frequency with age.[168,221,289] Incidence of microalbuminuria is greater than 60% in those older than age 35 years.[287] Intravascular hemolysis is associated with chronic kidney disease in SCD.[281,290,291] Hemoglobinuria occurs in up to 42% of patients[281,282,293] and is associated with risk of chronic kidney disease progression.[281,294] End-stage renal disease requiring dialysis carries a poor prognosis and is associated with a median survival of 4 years.[295]

Angiotensin-converting enzyme inhibitors or angiotensin receptor blockers decrease proteinuria in SCD. A study showed that losartan resulted in a decrease in albumin excretion rate and stable glomerular filtration rate in subjects with SCD.[296] Accumulating evidence suggests a role for endothelin-1 in the evolution of glomerulopathy in SCD.

Long-term blockade of endothelin-A receptors produces robust reno-protection as evidenced by decrease in microalbuminuria and preservation of podocyte structure in humanized mouse models of SCD.[297-299]

Treatment of renal disease follows principles used for non-SCD kidney pathology and includes effective blood pressure control, avoidance of nephrotoxic agents, and treatment of urinary tract infection. A relative decrease in serum erythropoietin levels, disproportionate to the degree of anemia is observed; erythropoietin treatment, with its resultant increase in Hb may cause an increase in VOCs because of an increase in blood viscosity.[287] Renal tubular acidosis type IV, secondary to decreased K^+ and hydrogen ion in the distal tubule, can cause disproportionate acidosis and hyperkalemia in patients with declining renal function.[287] SCD patients with evidence of early chronic kidney disease should be offered treatment with hydroxyurea. If kidney disease progresses despite such treatment, some physicians believe that consideration should be given to a chronic exchange transfusion program.

Priapism Priapism affects at least 35% of male patients with SCD, potentially with devastating psychological consequences; true prevalence may be higher as it is often underreported.[299-302] The mean age of onset is 15 years; two-thirds of patients have "stuttering priapism," a term used for episodes that last less than 3 hours.[303] Derangements in NO metabolism and adenosine signaling are thought to be the major contributors to priapism in SCD.[119] More than 95% of priapism is the "low-flow" type resulting from ischemia, is painful, and is a medical emergency.[304]

Aspiration of the corpus cavernosa followed by epinephrine injections, exchange transfusion, and α and β agonists have all been used, but data regarding efficacy are sparse. α-Agonists, etilefrine 50 mg/day and ephedrine 15 to 30 mg/day, have been studied as a strategy to reduce stuttering priapism in a small trial, but no significant difference compared to placebo was found.[305] Hormonal therapies, including antiandrogens and luteinizing hormone–releasing hormone, reduce nocturnal erections but are associated with loss of libido.[304] Transfusion therapy has resulted in neurologic sequelae termed the *ASPEN syndrome* (Association of Sickle Cell Disease, Priapism, Exchange Transfusion) and is thought to be secondary to hyperviscosity; care, therefore, must be taken not to increase the hematocrit above 30%.[306] In recalcitrant cases, a shunt is performed, but this results in permanent impotence.[305] A penile prosthesis is used to ameliorate sexual dysfunction.

Nocturnal Enuresis Nocturnal enuresis is present in 25% to 33% of the pediatric sickle cell population, which is higher than in age-matched controls.[307-309] It tends to decrease with age but is still prevalent in adults. Social and environmental factors, hyposthenuria-decreased functional bladder capacity, and decreased arousal during sleep appear to be contributing factors.

Dactylitis Dactylitis is a painful swelling of digits of the hands and feet ("hand-foot syndrome"). It occurs early in infancy as hematopoietic marrow is still present in these bones at this age. Most episodes resolve within 2 weeks.[310-313] Epiphyseal infarction can result in joint pain and swelling mimicking septic arthritis. Use of hydroxyurea in the BABY HUG trial resulted in significant reduction of the rate of dactylitis.[221]

Osteomyelitis, Septic Arthritis, and Bone Infarction Impaired cellular and humoral immunity together with infarction of bone contribute to osteomyelitis, which has an estimated prevalence of 12% in individuals with SCD. Atypical serotypes of *Salmonella*, *S. aureus*, and Gram-negative bacilli are the principal infectious offenders. No single laboratory or imaging test reliably differentiates osteomyelitis from infarction.[310,313-318] Culture results may be nondiagnostic because patients usually receive antibiotics on presentation with fever; therefore, the presence of leukocytes in bone and joint aspirates should evoke a high suspicion for osteomyelitis.[179] Septic arthritis tends to occur in joints involved with avascular necrosis; it is also seen following hip

arthroplasty. Multiple joints may be involved. An elevated C-reactive protein should raise suspicion for septic arthritis and prompt intervention with appropriate antibiotics as needed to prevent joint deterioration and collapse.[310] Vertebral body infarctions with subsequent collapse causes the classic "fish mouth" appearance of vertebrae on radiographs of the spine.

Osteopenia and Osteoporosis Osteopenia and osteoporosis are prevalent (30%-80%) in patients with SCD, with a predilection for the lumbar spine. Presence of avascular necrosis with local bone remodeling may lead to false-negative results on a bone mineral density test at the femoral neck.[179] Fractures of the long bones are commonly under diagnosed, and self-reported rates of fracture in young adults with SCD are high. Etiology of osteoporosis is multifactorial, with hypogonadism, hypothyroidism, nutritional deficiencies, and iron overload interfering with osteoblast function being the major causes.[179,319-321] More than 50% of patients are vitamin D deficient with the majority (>80%) having less than optimal levels. High doses of vitamin D supplementation have resulted in improvement in chronic pain and higher levels of physical activity, and supplementation may increase HbF levels.[322,323]

Avascular Necrosis Vasoocclusion resulting in infarction of articular surfaces of long bone occurs, most commonly in the femur followed by the humerus, is termed *avascular necrosis* (AVN). It was previously thought to occur with increased frequency in HbSC disease as opposed to patients with HbSS. With increased longevity of HbSS patients, its prevalence is greater in patients with HbSS.[324-326] As per estimates of the Cooperative Study of Sickle Cell Disease (CSSCD), 50% of patients by age 33 years will have AVN of the femoral head (Fig. 18-9). The presence of concurrent deletional α-thalassemia (−α3.7) and a history of frequent VOCs are classic risk factors for AVN. Other risk factors include male gender, higher Hb concentration, low HbF, and vitamin D deficiency.[179,327,328] Polymorphisms in *BMP6*, *ANNEXIN A$_2$*, *KLOTHO*, *IL1B*, and *S100B* genes are associated with AVN.[329-331]

Patients with untreated AVN may progress to femoral head collapse,[332,333] although spontaneous radiographic improvement without intervention may occur, particularly in children.[334] AVN has been

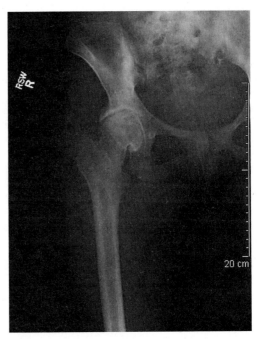

FIGURE 18–9. Avascular necrosis of the right hip in a 31-year-old woman with sickle cell disease depicting a patchy lucency and sclerosis and irregular contour of the femoral head and loss of the joint space.

treated with a number of modalities, including physical therapy, core decompression, osteotomy, bone grafting, surface arthroplasty, and joint replacement. Two randomized trials in individuals with SCD and AVN compared core decompression and physical therapy to physical therapy alone and did not show a difference in outcome; however, follow-up was short, a significant number of stage III hip joints were included in one study, and sample size was limited.[335] Structural bone diseases in SCD make joint replacement challenging.[336-338] It is not clear if hydroxyurea affects the risk of developing AVN.[327,339]

Leg Ulcers

Leg ulcers occur in 2% to 40% of cases with SCD. The incidence varies geographically, with the highest rate reported in Jamaica.[340] In the United States, leg ulcers are seen in 4% to 6% of patients with SCD and are most common in patients older than 10 years.[341] They occur on the lower extremities, especially on the malleoli, and cause chronic pain and disability. Venous stasis is a predisposing factor, while coinheritance of α-thalassemia appears to have a protective effect. The possible relationship between hydroxyurea use and increased occurrence of leg ulcers is controversial.[342] Polymorphisms in *KL* (encoding Klotho), *TEK* (encoding tyrosine kinase endothelial), and several other genes in the transforming growth factor-β and bone morphogenic protein pathways are associated with leg ulcers.[340] Once established, ulcers are recalcitrant and significantly impair quality of life.[343]

Treatment of leg ulcers is largely empiric. Leg elevation, bed rest when practical and feasible, wet-to-dry dressings, gentle debridement, Unna boots, and treatment of infection with topical or systemic antibiotics are commonly used. The peptide encoding integrin-interaction site of many extracellular matrix proteins (RGD peptide) enhanced healing of the ulcers in preliminary studies, but, unfortunately, it never came to clinical practice because of nonmedical reasons.[344] Increase in HbF and transfusions may hasten healing of leg ulcers.[345]

Hepatobiliary Complications

Chronic liver abnormalities in SCD are frequent and of different etiologies that include vasoocclusion, transfusional iron overload, pigmented gallstones with bile duct obstruction, acute or chronic cholecystitis, viral hepatitis, and cholestasis.[346,347] Common clinical manifestations include right upper quadrant pain, fever, hepatomegaly, nausea, and vomiting. Bilirubin levels from chronic hemolysis are usually not above 6 mg/dL, with a majority of it being the indirect fraction.[348] Some degree of aspartate transaminase elevation is seen with hemolysis; therefore, alanine transaminase elevation is a more accurate marker of liver injury.

Vasoocclusion involving the hepatic sinusoids was seen in 39% of patients in one study, while vasoocclusion involving the liver, termed *acute sickle hepatic crisis*, was previously reported in 10% of patients. The differing prevalence is the result of varying criteria used to include biochemical and clinical abnormalities.[349] Acute hepatic sequestration crisis characterized by a rapidly enlarging, tender liver and hypovolemia is akin to splenic sequestration but much rarer. It requires prompt treatment with red cell transfusion. Severe intrahepatic cholestasis with serum bilirubin levels as high as 100 mg/dL is a catastrophic situation needing exchange transfusion for resolution; synthetic liver function is lost as characterized by low serum albumin and coagulation protein abnormalities; renal impairment may occur. A more benign form of cholestasis resolves with conservative measure.[350-355]

Chronic hemolysis results in an increased burden on the heme catabolic pathway leading to increased unconjugated bilirubin and formation of pigmented gallstones. The incidence of gallstones increases with age, with a reported prevalence of 50% at 22 years of age.[356-358] The number of uridine diphosphate glucuronosyltransferase 1 family (UGT1A1) promoter (TA) repeats (the polymorphism associated with Gilbert

syndrome) is strongly associated with increased incidence of gallstones and bilirubin levels, while coinherited α-thalassemia (Chap. 17) decreases bilirubin levels in patients with SCD.[359] Laparoscopic cholecystectomy is recommended in symptomatic patients with cholelithiasis. The treatment of asymptomatic patients with positive findings on abdominal ultrasonography is more controversial. In a Jamaican cohort study, only 7% of patients with positive ultrasounds had symptoms suggestive of biliary tract disease and needed a cholecystectomy. Patients in the United States appear to be more symptomatic, with the majority of gallbladders removed after a positive ultrasound having pathologic evidence of cholecystitis.[356] Asymptomatic patients with negative screening ultrasounds should be observed; however, timing and frequency of screening has not been standardized.

Ophthalmic Complications

The microvasculature of the retina with relative hypoxemia facilitates "sickling" akin to several other vascular beds. Microcirculatory obstruction occurs followed by neovascularization and arteriovenous aneurysms. Hemorrhage, scarring, and retinal detachment leading to blindness are the sequelae. Changes occur at the periphery, thereby sparing central vision at earlier stages. The term *sickle cell retinopathy* encompasses nonproliferative and proliferative changes. Nonproliferative changes include "salmon-patch" hemorrhages, peripheral retinal lesions termed *black sunbursts*, and iridescent spots, whereas neovascularization is characteristic of proliferative changes, giving a pattern of vascular lesions resembling a marine invertebrate that is termed *sea fans*.[360]

Increased levels of plasma and intraocular vascular endothelial growth factor have been documented in proliferative sickle cell retinopathy, as have angiopoietin-1, angiopoietin-2, and vWF. Pigment epithelium-derived factor, an angiogenesis inhibitor, also is increased, especially in nonviable sea fans.[361-363] Proliferative sickle cell retinopathy may differ from other proliferative retinopathies in that spontaneous regression of neovascularization can occur in up to 60% of cases.[364,365] The Jamaican cohort study reported an annual incidence of proliferative retinopathy of 0.5 cases per 100 HbSS patients versus 2.5 cases per 100 HbSC patients. Prevalence was greater in HbSC patients as well, with a 43% rate in the third decade versus 14% for those with HbSS. There was a 32% incidence of spontaneous regression. Irreversible visual loss occurred only in 2% of HbSC patients.[364]

Central retinal artery occlusion is rare in HbSS disease.[366] Conjunctival vascularity is decreased in SCD patients compared to controls with further decreased vascularity and decreased conjunctival red cell velocities during vasoocclusion.[367-370] An orbital compression syndrome characterized by fever, headache, orbital swelling, and visual impairment secondary to optic nerve dysfunction can occur in SCD. Orbital marrow infarction is a common cause.[371]

All patients with sickle hemoglobinopathies should have a yearly ophthalmology examination beginning in childhood. The examination should be carried out by an ophthalmologist and should include slitlamp examination of the anterior chamber and detailed retinal visualization, including fluorescein angiography in addition to visual acuity. The evaluation and treatment of proliferative sickle retinopathy is complicated by the fact that spontaneous regression may occur. Laser photocoagulation is the most commonly performed procedure for this finding. Traumatic hyphema needs urgent ophthalmology referral as sickle red blood cells can cause obstruction of outflow channels, resulting in acute glaucoma. This vascular obstruction may cause a decrease in retinal and optic nerve perfusion, causing further visual problems. Unresolved vitreous hemorrhage and retinal detachment may need surgical intervention. Exchange transfusion to maintain HbA equal to or greater than 50% is recommended. Central retinal artery occlusion needs urgent exchange transfusion and an ophthalmology consultation.[364,372-374] Orbital compression syndrome is treated with glucocorticoids with the addition of antibiotics if concomitant infection cannot be ruled out.[179]

Splenic Complications

Functional asplenia defined as impaired mononuclear phagocyte system functions in the spleen occurs in 86% of infants with SCD.[375] It is defined by the presence of Howell-Jolly bodies and absence of ^{99m}technetium splenic uptake, even in the presence of a palpable spleen. Slow blood flow in the red pulp of the spleen sets the stage for increased red blood cell sickling. Repeated splenic infarctions lead to "autosplenectomy." As a consequence, patients are prone to microbial infections, especially with encapsulated microorganisms such as *S. pneumoniae*, *Haemophilus influenzae*, and *Neisseria meningitidis* and should be vaccinated against these microorganisms (see "Management and prevention of infection"). Chronic transfusion prior to age 7 years may lead to reversal of functional asplenia. Marrow transplantation and hydroxyurea have resulted in reversal of functional asplenia in some older patients. Splenic sequestration typically occurs in children younger than age 5 years.[376-380]

Sickle Cell Disease Management During Pregnancy

Differing morbidity and mortality rates have been reported in pregnant women with SCD, with some of the differences being attributed to geographic location and access to health care. Although the CSSCD data showed low rates of pregnancy loss and mortality, other studies showed an increased mortality 10- to 100-fold greater compared to non-SCD patients. Preterm delivery occurs in 30% to 50% of SCD patients and two-thirds of all deliveries will have infants with birth weights less than the 50th percentile.[381,382] There is an increased frequency of VOC reported during pregnancy. In a study looking at pregnancy outcomes in SCD patients compared to non-SCD patients with comorbidities, patients with SCD displayed a significantly increased incidence of VTE, nonhemorrhagic obstetric shock (defined as pulmonary thromboembolism, amniotic fluid embolism, acute uterine inversion, and sepsis), and infection, despite being significantly younger.[383,384] Other studies have obtained similar findings, especially the fivefold increased risk of VTE in this population.[382,384,385]

Given the increased risk of preeclampsia and eclampsia, patients should have close monitoring of blood pressure and proteinuria after 20 weeks of gestation. Fetal nonstress and umbilical artery Doppler studies should be undertaken after 28 weeks of gestation to identify patients who might benefit from early delivery. Studies examining prophylactic red blood cell transfusions in pregnancy have shown mixed results. A systematic review of the literature and metaanalysis indicated that prophylactic transfusion was associated with reduction in maternal mortality, VOC, pulmonary complications, perinatal mortality, neonatal mortality, and preterm birth, but the studies had a moderate to high risk of bias.[386] Patients should be transfused for a Hb concentration of less than 60 g/L, as abnormal fetal oxygenation and death have been reported below this Hb level in non-SCD populations. They should also be transfused based on guidelines for the nonpregnant patient with SCD.[381] Based on data from animal models and small reports of spontaneous abortion and fetal death, the use of hydroxyurea is not recommended during pregnancy and breastfeeding.[387,388] Because hydroxyurea may decrease spermatogenesis,[389] male patients may need to stop the drug temporarily when their partners are trying to conceive. Narcotics administered for relief of pain have not been shown to cause fetal harm, but babies of mothers exposed to narcotics during pregnancy should be monitored for the neonatal abstinence syndrome.[381]

Given the increased risk of VTE in women with SCD, it is prudent to restrict hormonal contraception advice to progesterone-only preparations.[390,391]

Management and Prevention of Infection

Patients with SCD are predisposed to infections for a variety of reasons, including functional asplenia and defective neutrophil responses.[392-396] The magnitude of this problem was highlighted in a landmark paper by E. Barrett-Connor in 1971.[396] Functional asplenia results in susceptibility to encapsulated microorganisms, particularly to *S. pneumoniae*, especially in children younger than 5 years. The CSSCD data reported an 8 per 100 patient-years rate of invasive bacterial infection in children younger than 3 years.[397]

Given the high incidence of infection, especially in childhood, infection prevention and rapid diagnosis of established infections is of paramount importance.[398-400] The pneumococcal vaccine (7 polyvalent conjugate, PCV7) can be administered in infancy with effective immunologic response prior to 2 years of age; the American Academy of Pediatrics recommends it be administered at age 2, 4, 6, 8, and 12 to 15 months. The PCV7 vaccine decreases invasive pneumococcal disease by as much as 80% to 90%. The pneumococcal polysaccharide vaccine, PPV23, covers more serotypes but is not immunogenic prior to age 24 months and response lasts for 3 years. The first dose is recommended at age 24 months with additional doses 3 to 5 years later.[399,401-404] Non–vaccine-covered strains of *S. pneumoniae* are emerging as important pathogens; therefore, prompt referral of patients with suspected infection to a health care facility is important.[405]

Oral penicillin prophylaxis is recommended at a dose of 125 mg twice a day for children with HbSS or HbSβ⁰ between 0 and 3 years of age and at a dose of 250 mg twice a day between 3 and 5 years of age.[406] Penicillin prophylaxis beyond 5 years is recommended only for patients with recurrent pneumococcal infections or who have had surgical splenectomy. Patients allergic to penicillin are offered erythromycin.

The meningococcal vaccine covers most invasive isolates of *N. meningitidis* and is recommended by the American Academy of Pediatrics.[407] Standard pediatric immunizations protecting against *H. influenzae* and hepatitis B virus should be given. Influenza virus vaccine should be given annually as viral respiratory tract infection favors invasive bacterial infection.

Parents and caregivers of children should be educated to recognize infections and to seek medical attention early. Diagnosis of established infections varies by site and offending agent. For invasive pneumococcal disease, ceftriaxone is the drug of choice despite concerns of immune-mediated hemolysis. *Salmonella* osteomyelitis and atypical bacteria, such as *M. pneumoniae* and *Chlamydia* isolated in ACS,[408,409] should be treated with appropriate antibiotics. Local antibiotic resistance patterns influence decision of empiric antibiotic treatment.

The spectrum of infectious complications in adults may be different.[410] One study reported data on blood infections in adults.[392] Pneumococcal infections were rare. *S. aureus* was the predominant organism. Patients with *S. aureus* had a predilection for bone-joint infection. Those with indwelling venous catheters and a severe disease course appeared to have a high risk for bloodstream infections.

Although SCD confers resistance to malaria, protection is not complete and severe disease and deaths from malaria have been reported in SCD patients. Malaria chemoprophylaxis is recommended for all patients living in or traveling to endemic regions.[411,412]

Management During Anesthesia and Surgery

Patients with SCD should have careful monitoring of Hb concentration, hydration, oxygen, and metabolic studies in the perioperative period. ACS and VOC occur with higher frequency in the perioperative period. Increased age is associated with increased complications.[412-415] Transfusion to keep Hb levels at approximately 100 g/L is recommended. A randomized multicenter trial demonstrated that preoperative transfusion from a median Hb of 80 g/L to 97 g/L was associated with a reduction in perioperative ACS and other complications.[416] A prior randomized trial showed no further benefit in aggressively transfusing patients to a mean HbS of less than 30% preoperatively.[271] Care should be taken to avoid transfusion-induced hyperviscosity.

MODIFIERS OF DISEASE SEVERITY

Some patients have a mild course with few problems related to SCD and survive into the sixth or seventh decade. In contrast, some patients have a difficult course with multiple complications, frequent hospitalizations, severe organ damage, and shortened life expectancy.[417,418] Inheritance of α-thalassemia trait and a high fetal Hb are two factors that ameliorate many complications of SCD. Genome-wide association studies revealed four major loci associated with fetal Hb levels: The β-globin locus on chromosome 11, an intergenic region between *HBSIL* (HBS1-Like Translational GTPase) and *MYB* (MYB Protooncogene, Transcription Factor) genes on chromosome 6, and the *BCL11A* (B-Cell CLL/Lymphoma 11A) gene on chromosome 2.[419] Repression of BCL11A results in increased γ-globin gene expression and, consequently, in increased HbF. The exact mechanism of how BCL11A silences γ-globin expression is unclear; its expression seems to be controlled by an erythroid specific transcription factor, KLF1 (Kruppel-Like Factor 1) with decreased expression of BCL11A upon knockdown of *KLF1* gene transcript.[419,420]

Inheritance of α-thalassemia and higher-than-average HbF levels do not account for all of the clinical diversity of SCD. The completion of the human genome project has provided the impetus to study polymorphisms in candidate genes as potential modifiers of disease severity.

Association of polymorphisms in candidate genes and different features of SCD such as stroke,[421-423] ACS,[424] bilirubin levels and cholelithiasis,[425-428] AVN,[329] priapism,[429] and leg ulcers,[340] as well as HbF levels[430-435] and HbF response to hydroxyurea,[436] have been studied in different groups of patients. Table 18-2 contains some genetic modifiers associated with clinical complications of SCD.

Genome-based approaches to studying phenotypic variability have evolved from linkage-based and candidate gene–based searches to genome-wide detection of rare polymorphisms.[437,438] Using whole-genome sequencing approaches, several reports have identified strong candidate genes that may play a role in complications of SCD; these studies, however, are small and results have been difficult to replicate.[437] Focus has also shifted from global severity as a phenotype, to investigating individual SCD complications.

With the development of whole-exome sequencing and whole-genome sequencing techniques, researchers are now able to identify rare genetic variants. Through older cohorts like CSSCD, and newer collections of genomes from the National Heart, Lung, and Blood Institute's Trans-Omics for Precision Medicine (TOPMed) program and other research initiatives, more than 10,000 SCD genomes with various phenotypes attached are available. Therein lies the problem—phenotypes collected from various institutions, from different decades, and for different purposes will be very difficult to standardize. It is widely acknowledged that one of the most prominent barriers to an effective genomics study is the difficulty in defining and harmonizing phenotypes. For example, frequent, unpredictable pain events are the first complication most clinicians think of when they hear "sickle cell disease," yet it has proven very difficult to study genetically or genomically,

TABLE 18–2. Genetic Modifiers Associated with Clinical Complications of Sickle Cell Disease

Sickle Cell Complication	Gene	Main Function	Genomic Study	References
Pain events (VOCs, ACS)	MBL2	Inflammation	CG	547
	VEGF	Angiogenesis	CG	548
	COMMD7	Copper metabolism	GWAS	549
Nephropathy	APOL1	Resistance to *Trypanosoma brucei*	CG	550
	MYH9	Cell integrity and Bowman capsule		
	BMPR1B	Cartilage formation	GWAS	551
Stroke	VCAM1	Cell adhesion	CG	423
	TNF-α	Inflammation	CG	
	ADYC9	Neuronal signaling	CG	421
	ANXA2	Hypercoagulability		552
	TEK	Cell adhesion		
	TGFRP3	Inflammation		265
	GOLGB1	Golgi apparatus transport	WES	
	ENPP1	Transmembrane glycoprotein		
Pulmonary hypertension	ACVRL1	Inflammation	CG	553
	ADRB1	Signal transduction		554
	eNOS	Nitric oxide synthesis	CG	554
Avascular necrosis	KL	Vitamin D regulation	CG	329
	BMP6	Inflammation and bone formation		
	ANXA2	Signal transduction		

Abbreviations: CG, candidate gene-based studies; GWAS, genome-wide association study; WES, whole-exome sequencing.

because of the subjective nature of pain, difficulties in distinguishing between chronic and acute pain, and variability with age. Before the pain phenotype can be studied effectively, we need a reliable biomarker for an acute pain event.

With these challenges acknowledged, it is still essential to work to apply the power of genomics to major SCD phenotypes that have evidence of heritability and are clinically relevant. Far too many complications of SCD, such as priapism, nephropathy, and leg ulcers, have no evidence-based or targeted therapies. Identifying variants present in the subset of patients who develop these complications, followed by functional studies to verify the association, will be the first steps toward finding effective treatments.

GENERAL MANAGEMENT OF SICKLE CELL DISEASE

Pharmacotherapies to Increase Fetal Hemoglobin Levels

The observation that HbF results in ameliorating the phenotype of SCD[439] led to research focused on HbF modulation as a therapy for SCD. The γ-globin chains of HbF are excluded from the deoxy HbS polymer; thus the presence of HbF in sickle red cells exerts a potent antisickling effect. This effect also has been supported by clinical observations; the manifestations of SCD do not become apparent in the first few months of life, not until the switch from γ-globin chain production to β-globin chain production is almost complete in the postnatal period. Additionally, the phenotypes of some compound heterozygous states with HbS and other inherited globin disorders that lead to increased expression of HbF in the adult life, such as δβ-thalassemias and hereditary persistence of HbF are very mild (Chap. 17). In fact, compound heterozygotes for HbS and deletional hereditary persistence of HbF, in which there is continued high levels of HbF expression (30%-35%) uniformly distributed in all red blood cells (pancellular), are clinically asymptomatic and hematologically normal. In the late 1970s, further evidence in support of the ameliorating effect of high HbF levels came from the observation of Saudi Arabian sickle cell anemia patients who had mild anemia and few, if any, symptoms of SCD, and who were not diagnosed until adult age.[440] These individuals had HbF levels in the 20% to 25% range, as opposed to African patients or American patients of African descent, the majority of whom had HbF levels of approximately 5%. These observations paved the way for intense investigations on the cellular and molecular mechanisms of the fetal-to-adult (γ-to-β) switch during the perinatal period and the search for HbF-inducing agents. The observation that there is a transient increase in HbF production during recovery from marrow aplasia or suppression provided the rationale for the use of myelosuppressive agents as HbF-inducing agents (Table 18-3).

Hydroxyurea Although many myelosuppressive agents have been studied in primates and some have been used in a small number of patients, only hydroxyurea was used in large-scale clinical trials, which started in the early 1980s. This is largely attributable to hydroxyurea's excellent oral bioavailability, relatively short half-life (important from the standpoint of rapid reversibility of toxicity), no evidence that its use would lead to an increase of cancer incidence, and few side effects.

Hydroxyurea is the most widely used oral drug therapy in the treatment of SCD. It is a ribonucleotide reductase inhibitor and is S-phase specific in the cell cycle. The mechanism by which hydroxyurea increases HbF synthesis is not fully understood. It is postulated that the myelosuppressive effect leads to the recruitment of early erythroid progenitors that have retained their fetal (γ) globin synthesis capability, giving rise to the production of red blood cells with a higher HbF content. Some studies have shown that hydroxyurea acts as a NO donor, and increases HbF synthesis via the cyclic guanosine monophosphate pathway.[441,442] Other studies suggest it works by reducing the neutrophil

TABLE 18-3. Hemoglobin F–Inducing Therapies

Drug	Mechanism
Hydroxyurea	Stress erythropoiesis
	Antiinflammatory
	Nitric oxide donor
	Increased cyclic guanosine monophosphate
Decitabine	DNA methyltransferase-1 inhibition, ie, hypomethylation
5'-Azacitidine	DNA methyltransferase-1 inhibition, ie, hypomethylation
Butyrate derivatives	Histone deacetylase inhibition
Histone deacetylase inhibitors	Histone deacetylase inhibition
Immunomodulatory drugs	P38 mitogen-activated protein kinase pathway
Pomalidomide	Reversal of γ-globin silencing
Metformin	Induction of FOXO3

count, thereby reducing the contribution of neutrophils to the abnormal vascular adhesion of sickle red blood cells. It has several other actions that explain its efficacy in SCD other than increasing HbF. These actions include decreasing platelets and reticulocytes, improving red blood cell hydration, and decreasing red blood cell adhesiveness to the vascular endothelium (Fig. 18-10).[443,444]

The landmark Multicenter Study of Hydroxyurea found that hydroxyurea decreased frequency of painful crises, ACS, hospitalizations, and blood transfusions. Follow-up showed a 40% decrease in mortality in patients randomized to the drug.[217,445] Hydroxyurea is recommended in patients with three or more VOCs or a history of ACS. It can be started at a dose of 15 mg/kg given as a single daily dose and escalated by 5 mg/kg per day every 8 weeks until toxicity or a maximum dose of 35 mg/kg is reached. Maximum tolerated dose is defined as the dose that targets an absolute neutrophil count of 2.0 to 4.0×10^9/L and absolute reticulocyte count of 100 to 200×10^9/L.[446,447] Periodic monitoring of blood cell counts and serum chemistries, especially in the first year of treatment, is important. Maximal effect on HbF may not be seen until 6 to 12 months of therapy is completed. The dose should be decreased in renal failure. Although not proven to have teratogenic or leukemogenic potential in SCD patients, it is recommended that it not be used in pregnant or breastfeeding patients. Concerns about detrimental effect on spermatogenesis also have been raised based on studies in mice and humans.[389,448-451]

Several studies have been published on the use of hydroxyurea in infants and children. Therapy started between 6 and 9 months of age and was found to be safe and well-tolerated with improved growth rates and preserved organ function, and with the additional benefits seen in adults.[221,447,452,453] The FDA has approved hydroxyurea for use in children with sickle cell anemia who are 2 years of age or older and have recurrent moderate to severe pain crises.

Other Fetal Hemoglobin–Inducing Agents Although important advances have been made in understanding the basic mechanism(s) of the perinatal switch from γ-globin to β-globin synthesis, this knowledge is far from complete. Certain epigenetic mechanisms (histone deacetylation and DNA methylation) are involved in the silencing of the γ-globin genes postnatally. This has led to the use of agents

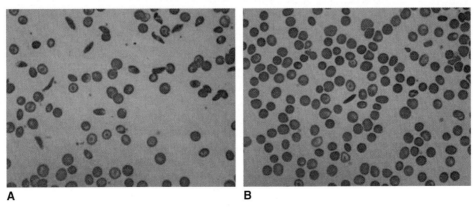

FIGURE 18–10. Blood film from sickle cell disease patients: effect of hydroxyurea therapy. **A.** Blood film before therapy. Note frequent sickled cells. **B.** Marked decrease in sickle cells with therapy. *(Used with permission from Dr. Scott Drury and Dr. Elizabeth Manaloor, Department of Pathology, Medical College of Georgia.)*

that target the two common epigenetic silencing mechanisms: histone deacetylase inhibitors and DNA methyltransferase-1 inhibitors.

The histone deacetylase inhibitors that have been most widely used in early phase, small, clinical trials in SCD, and in some patients with β-thalassemia, are butyrate derivatives (arginine butyrate, sodium phenylbutyrate, isobutyramide). Arginine butyrate has to be administered by intravenous infusion; earlier studies suggested that continuous daily infusions of arginine butyrate were not very effective in leading to a sustained increase in HbF.[345] Later, it was shown that daily continuous infusion induced tachyphylaxis and hence the failure to cause a sustained HbF response. An intermittent schedule of administration (4 days, given every 4 weeks) was efficacious in increasing HbF.[454] Although orally administered sodium phenylbutyrate was effective in increasing HbF, the daily doses needed to maintain a HbF response required the administration of a large number of tablets and was impractical.[455] A phase II trial studying the efficacy of oral 2,2-dimethylbutyrate sodium salt, HQK1001, did not show significant increase in HbF and was associated with a trend for increased VOC.[456]

The 2 DNA methyltransferase inhibitors with HbF inducing activity are 5-azacytidine and decitabine. Both of these agents are myelosuppressive when used in higher doses; however, non-myelosuppressive doses are potent inhibitors of DNA methyltransferase-1 that increase HbF synthesis in baboons and in patients with SCD.[457-464] Unlike 5-azacytidine, which incorporates into both DNA and RNA, decitabine incorporates only into DNA and is believed to have a better genotoxicity profile. It is effective in increasing HbF and ameliorating the disease severity in patients with SCD who are refractory to hydroxyurea.[464] Orally administered decitabine in combination with tetrahydrouridine is effective in increasing HbF percent, HbF-containing red blood cells, and Hb concentration in sickle cell anemia patients,[465] and is a promising combination that is undergoing further study.

Immunomodulatory agents (thalidomide and derivatives) increase HbF synthesis in erythroid colonies from SCD patients.[466] Pomalidomide augments HbF in sickle cell mice.[467] Data from use in sickle cell patients is awaited. The finding that the KLF-1–BCL11A axis is the major factor in the switch from β-globin to γ-globin has made these factors attractive targets for therapy; however, as of this writing, no effective pharmacologic means of targeting these transcription factors has been developed.

Allogeneic Hematopoietic Stem Cell Transplantation

Because SCD is an inherited defect in the hematopoietic stem cell, stem cell transplantation (SCT) is an attractive option to permanently cure the disease rather than manage its sequelae piecemeal. However, the tremendous phenotypic variability that characterizes the disorder combined with lack of an accurate predictive model to foretell which patients are likely to have a catastrophic disease course, make selecting patients for allogeneic hematopoietic stem cell transplantation (AHSCT) challenging. AHSCT should be done in patients who are likely to have a severe disease course, but should be instituted early, prior to end-organ damage. The risk-to-benefit ratio of the morbidity and mortality associated with AHSCT has to be weighed against the disease severity of a nonmalignant hematologic disorder. AHSCT in adults is problematic given the toxicity of the standard myeloablative conditioning regimens.

AHSCT is an underused treatment modality in SCD, even in eligible patients secondary to lack of donor availability and socioeconomic factors.[468] Human leukocyte antigen (HLA)-matched sibling donor transplant with myeloablative conditioning represents the most common transplant type in SCD. Cerebrovascular disease, recurrent ACS, and frequent VOCs despite adequate hydroxyurea therapy are the most common indications for SCT. Data from approximately 1200 patients worldwide show an overall survival of 95%; early or late allograft failure resulting in disease recurrence is seen in 10% to 15% of patients.[468,469] The most common myeloablative regimen used is busulfan, cyclophosphamide, and antithymocyte globulin; the addition of antithymocyte globulin resulted in a significant reduction in allograft rejection. Transplant-related mortality ranges between 2% and 8%.[469] Acute graft-versushost disease occurs in approximately 10% to 15% of patients whereas chronic graft-versus-host disease has been reported in 12% to 20% of patients. Most series have used cyclosporine alone or in combination with methotrexate for graft-versus-host disease prophylaxis.[468,470,471]

Risk of increased incidence of neurologic complications following transplantation may be ameliorated with the use of prophylactic anticonvulsants, strict control of arterial hypertension, correction of hypomagnesemia, and maintenance of Hb at levels greater than 100 g/L and platelets at levels greater than 50×10^9/L. Long-term toxicity remains a concern, especially in relation to growth, reproduction, and secondary malignancies. Follow-up data on AHSCT in children between 1991 and 2000 show significant gonadal toxicity and infertility, especially in females.[472] Cord blood and HLA haploidentical transplantation have been used in a small number of patients with SCD, but graft failure is a significant issue.[468,473,474]

More than 60 adult patients have received hematopoietic stem cells from HLA-matched siblings using a nonmyeloablative conditioning regimen with low-dose total-body irradiation plus alemtuzumab for conditioning followed by sirolimus for graft-versus-host disease prophylaxis and to prevent graft rejection.[470,471] This approach is associated with a greater than 97% overall survival, a greater than 87% event-free survival, and no acute or chronic graft-versus-host disease. These results indicate that future efforts for AHSCT in adults with SCD should focus on nonmyeloablative conditioning regimens.[471]

Gene-Based Therapies

Cellular-based and gene-based therapies are an area of intense investigation; they can provide a means to extend SCT to a larger number of SCD patients, as the patients are their own donors. Hematopoietic stem and progenitor cells are harvested from the patient, modified using lentiviruses or genome editing, and transplanted back into the patient. A particular challenge is the source of autologous CD34$^+$ cells. Patients with SCD cannot be mobilized with granulocyte colony-stimulating factor, limiting the number of available patient CD34$^+$ cells to what can be obtained through marrow harvest. The number of CD34$^+$ cells needed is also greater than for an allogeneic transplant, as ex vivo gene editing is associated with cell death, and edited cells show lower levels of engraftment. Plerixafor mobilization is safe and effective, and has been incorporated into ongoing gene-based therapy trials. Clinical trials studying gene therapy (lentivirus based) and gene editing (CRISPR [clustered regularly interspaced short palindromic repeats]/Cas9 based) approaches are underway.[475-478]

Lentivirus-based gene therapies have been used to treat patients with β-hemoglobinopathies; a number of clinical trials have been performed around the world. For SCD, lentivirus-based therapies have two primary aims: induction of HbF by introducing lentiviruses containing a γ-globin or a hybrid β-promotor/γ-globin gene, or by introducing a mutated β-globin that interferes with HbS and prevents polymerization.[479] The BB305 LentiGlobin (Bluebird Bio, Cambridge, MA) is a self-inactivating lentivirus developed to encode an "antisickling" β-globin. A published report of LentiGlobin gene-based therapy in a 13-year-old with SCD showed approximately 47% HbA^{T87Q} and 2% HbF, and total Hb of 117 g/L.[480]

Other gene-editing therapy strategies include zinc finger nucleases, transcription activator-like effector nucleases, and clustered regulatory interspaced short palindromic repeats and associated Cas9 (CRISPR/Cas9). CRISPR/Cas9 shows a promising editing rate of 85% to 90% after 16 weeks in human marrow cells in preclinical studies.[481]

CRISPR/Cas9 targeting of HbF regulators such as KLF1 can lead to inhibition of the γ-globin-to-β-globin switching process.[482] However, there is concern that these transcription factors have essential roles in native erythropoiesis and/or nonerythroid contexts. For example, BCL11A, a potent HbF silencer, has a significant role in lymphoid and neuronal development, and *BCL11A* knockout mice are perinatal lethal.[483,484] In this regard, instead of complete knockout of the *BCL11A* gene, approaches focusing on the deletion of erythroid-specific BCL11A-binding sequences in the proximity of the γ-globin gene are promising. Another approach is repression of erythroid-specific BCL11A as demonstrated successfully by Canver and colleagues.[485] To interrupt the BCL11A effect on γ-globin silencing, they used CRISPR/Cas9 technology in human umbilical cord blood-derived erythroid progenitor (HUDEP)-2 cells to delete a 12-kb *BCL11A* enhancer located in the first intron of the *BCL11A* gene by introduction of a pair of chimeric single-guide RNAs. This site is targeted by GATA1 and is essential for *BCL11A* expression only in erythroid cells. The result was a significant increase in expression of γ-globin and HbF protein, suggesting that perturbation of defined critical sequences within the *BCL11A* enhancer may result in HbF levels exceeding the clinical threshold required to ameliorate the SCD.[486]

The challenges of these gene-based therapies are significant: potential off-target effects, the need for high levels of correction, and

need for effective engraftment. An additional challenge is that we do not know what level of correction of the sickle mutation or induction of HbF is curative. Therefore, a comprehensive functional analysis of the resulting blood, after a patient has undergone gene-based therapy, is essential for further development of these novel therapies, and verification that a cure has been achieved. To consider a gene-based therapy as curative, the patient should have rheology normalized to at least that of a sickle cell trait individual, who has a relatively benign condition when compared to HbSS.[487,488]

As of this writing, six patients with SCD have been followed for at least half a year (median 18 months) after receiving infusion of autologous CD34+ cells transduced with a lentiviral vector that encodes a short hairpin RNA (shRNA) targeting *BCL11A* mRNA embedded in a microRNA (shmiR), allowing erythroid lineage–specific knockdown. The patients achieved robust and stable HbF induction with HbF broadly distributed in red blood cells, and clinical manifestations of SCD reduced or absent during the follow-up period.[489]

Transfusion

Red cell transfusions are used frequently in SCD on an acute or chronic basis. The rationale for transfusion in SCD is twofold. Besides increasing Hb concentration and thereby increasing oxygen-carrying capacity of the blood, transfusion also decreases the percentage of circulating HbS-containing red blood cells. Hb level alone should not constitute an indication to transfusion as patients adapt to their level. Thus, it is important to know the patient's baseline Hb concentration. It is also important to calculate whether the reticulocyte count, a measure of marrow red blood cell production, is adequate or not. An asymptomatic patient with an Hb level below their typical level with a brisk reticulocytosis can be monitored rather than transfused in many cases.

Indications for red blood cell transfusion include symptomatic anemia, ACS, stroke, aplastic and sequestration crises, other major organ damage secondary to vasoocclusion, and occurrence of unrelenting priapism. Transfusion also may be required prior to major surgery, depending on patient genotype and duration of the procedure.[271,490] Patients with HbSS may benefit from transfusion to 100 g/L, even for low-risk or medium-risk surgery.[416] The best-established indication for chronic transfusion is stroke and an abnormal TCD velocity if obtained while on hydroxyurea, or to prevent stroke while hydroxyurea is being initiated. Patients with other chronic or recurrent events are sometimes placed on chronic transfusion as well. Inappropriate indications for transfusion include chronic steady-state anemia, uncomplicated VOC, minor surgical procedures, infection, and AVN.[491]

Simple or exchange transfusion of red blood cells can be used.[492] Simple transfusion is easier to perform. Exchange transfusion, has the advantage of not raising total Hb, and thereby blood viscosity, while decreasing the percentage of circulating sickle cells as sickle cell patients transport less oxygen to their tissues beyond a hematocrit of 30% as a result of increased blood viscosity.[493-495] Exchange transfusion also has the advantage of reduced iron overload risk.

Alloimmunization occurs in approximately 30% of transfused SCD patients, compared to 2% to 5% of all transfusion recipients.[496-498] In the United States, the majority of blood donors are of European descent, and the majority of SCD patients are of African descent (Chaps. 29 and 30). This results in blood group antigenic disparity, and alloantibodies to E, C, K, Jkb, S, and Fyb are common in transfused individuals with SCD. Age at first transfusion, total number of transfusions, transfusion in the context of inflammation, and influence of immunoregulatory genes may affect the rate and extent of alloimmunization.[498] Whole-exome sequencing identified a novel genetic association between an African-origin haplotype on chromosome 5q33 and the development of multiple alloantibodies in adult transfusion recipients with SCD.[499]

Extended antigen phenotyping (Kell, Duffy, Kidd, Lewis, Lutheran, P, and M&S) in addition to the usual ABO and D antigens (Chaps. 29 and 30) and leukodepletion of blood products is recommended for patients with SCD.[492,496,498,500] Delayed hemolytic transfusion reaction (DHTR) complicates 4% to 11%[501] of transfusions in SCD and may present as a painful crisis a week after transfusion. Hb is typically at pretransfusion levels. DHTR is caused by alloantibodies to non-ABO antigens. Alloantibody-mediated hemolysis will present as a rapid decrease in the percent of HbA compared to HbS. A failure to demonstrate a new alloantibody posttransfusion should not exclude the diagnosis of DHTR (Chaps. 29 and 30).

Even though terminology in the literature is inconsistent, it is important to distinguish DHTR, in which the Hb drops to pretransfusion levels and all HbA is hemolyzed, from hyperhemolysis syndrome, an underrecognized and potentially fatal transfusion reaction seen primarily in patients with SCD. In hyperhemolysis syndrome, Hb falls below pretransfusion levels and can be associated with a depressed reticulocyte count and autoantibodies. HbA may still be present, with the ratio of HbA:HbS expected posttransfusion preserved. Patients should be transfused only if symptomatic under such circumstances as further transfusion can cause further hemolysis and decline in Hb.[491,497] Treatments for hyperhemolysis include steroids, intravenous immunoglobulins, and rituximab.[502] Genetic variants associated with increased risk of hyperhemolysis syndrome in SCD have been identified.[503]

Iron Overload

Iron overload and its attendant complications and infection transmission are major complications of blood transfusion. Iron overload (Chap. 11) in SCD is similar to iron overload in other chronically transfused populations.[234,504,505] The Multicenter Study of Iron Overload research group showed that transfused sickle cell patients had increased morbidity and mortality when compared to transfused β-thalassemia patients and untransfused SCD patients.[506]

Diagnosing significant iron overload accurately and early can be difficult. Serum ferritin is an easy, widely employed method, but is imprecise in SCD as it is an acute-phase reactant. Its measurement can result in overestimation or underestimation of iron stores, and is poorly correlated to liver iron content.[507] As a reflection of iron status, serum ferritin concentration should be measured at steady state, at least 3 weeks after a VOC or infection has resolved. A ferritin value of greater than 1000 ng/L in the steady state has been used as an indication of iron overload. Liver iron concentration of greater than 7.7 mg/g dry weight, as determined by analysis of a liver biopsy specimen, has been used as an indication for treatment. Noninvasive methods of assessment of iron overload, such as MRI T2* (Chap. 11), are becoming standard. Cumulative transfusion of 120 mL of red blood cells/kg of body weight also can be used as a chelation trigger.[496]

Before oral iron chelators were available, iron chelation (Chap. 11) was typically carried out with desferrioxamine at a dose of 25 to 40 mg/kg per day given over 8 hours SQ.[508] Desferrioxamine can reverse cardiac iron overload. The availability of deferasirox, the once-daily oral iron chelator, has made iron-chelation therapy considerably more convenient. Deferasirox is a tridentate ligand that binds iron with a high affinity in a 2:1 ratio. It has a half-life of 8 to 16 hours and is metabolized by glucuronidation and excreted in the feces. Adverse reactions include nausea and vomiting, abdominal pain, and rash, and increases in liver function tests and serum creatinine were reported. Rare cases of anaphylaxis, occurring mostly in the first month of starting treatment, have been reported. Because of the possibility of renal failure, hepatotoxicity, and agranulocytosis, the complete blood count and a chemistry profile must be determined regularly in patients who receive this therapy. Auditory and ophthalmic side effects occur in less than 1% of patients;

however, annual eye and auditory examinations are recommended for patients receiving deferasirox as they are for patients receiving desferrioxamine.[509] Deferiprone, another oral iron chelator, is approved in the United States for the treatment of iron overload in patients with transfusion-dependent thalassemia. It is orally administered and is considered a better chelator of cardiac iron because of its ability to cross cell membranes.[510] Iron chelation in SCD follows the general guidelines of iron chelation in other populations with iron overload, and a number of studies have demonstrated safety and efficacy to reduce iron stores in SCD.[510-513]

Newly FDA Approved Therapies

Novel therapeutic approaches for mitigating the symptoms of SCD and improving clinical outcomes can be categorized based on the SCD pathology they are designed to target. Endari (oral pharmaceutical L-glutamine powder) received FDA approval in 2017 as a treatment for SCD. A pivotal phase 3 clinical study conducted by Emmaus Medical, Inc., showed that L-glutamine resulted in a lower incidence of VOC as well as a lower rate of hospitalizations and shorter hospital stays.[514] No changes in standard clinical laboratory values were noted. The clinical improvements associated with sickle cell complications are believed to be the result of an increase in the proportion of the reduced form of nicotinamide adenine dinucleotides in the red blood cells of patients with SCD, reducing the oxidative stress.

Another therapeutic approach is to modify HbS, so it cannot sickle. Voxelotor (Oxbryta), a small molecule that modifies HbS by binding to the α-globin subunit and stabilizing the R-state of Hb conformation, increasing Hb oxygen affinity and reducing polymerization, was FDA-approved for use in individuals with SCD in 2019.[515] A phase I/II clinical trial for voxelotor showed it was well tolerated and had a dose-dependent increase in oxygen affinity.[516] Patients receiving voxelotor have an increase in Hb level and a reduction of both reticulocytes and indirect bilirubin, indicating a reduction in hemolysis (NCT02285088).[517] A phase III clinical trial investigating both safety and efficacy of voxelotor in adults found voxelotor significantly increased Hb levels and reduced markers of hemolysis compared to placebo (NCT03036813).[517] Patients receiving voxelotor had a sustained decrease of approximately 70% in the number of irreversibly sickled red blood cells after 90 days of treatment.[518] Voxelotor also improved sickle red blood cell deformability as observed using micropipette and filtration techniques and blood viscosity in vitro.[519]

Another SCD therapy, also FDA-approved in 2019, is crizanlizumab (Adakveo; SEG101). Crizanlizumab is a P-selectin monoclonal antibody that blocks interaction of P-selectins with leukocytes. A 12-month-long clinical trial (SUSTAIN Trial; NCT01895361) assessed the safety and efficacy of crizanlizumab for patients both on and off hydroxyurea therapy. Treatment with high-dose crizanlizumab resulted in reduced rates of VOC compared to placebo, and increased the time to the first crisis.[520] No significant changes in Hb, LDH, reticulocyte count, and indirect bilirubin were observed between crizanlizumab and placebo groups.[520] Therefore, it seems that the benefits of crizanlizumab are not related to intrinsic red blood cell changes or inhibition of hemolysis. At least four more clinical studies are investigating dose confirmation and safety with primary end points being frequency of adverse events and organ damage. It would be advantageous to study how crizanlizumab and similar agents affect blood flow through the adhesive microfluidic technologies, considering the main target is the prevention of adhesive events. Adhesion flow devices that run whole blood can investigate the potential efficacy of a drug by directly analyzing leukocyte rolling on devices coated with P-selectins.[521]

Given the complex pathophysiology of SCD, numerous therapies targeting different pathways have been tried to ameliorate disease manifestations. For more than 20 years, hydroxyurea was the only FDA-approved drug for the treatment of SCD. Many drugs failed to show efficacy, especially in phase II/III trials, prior to the three approved drugs described earlier. Table 18-4 is a list of trials and their outcomes.

OTHER ABNORMAL HEMOGLOBINS

The number of Hb variants described at the time of writing is 2028. The vast majority of these variants is benign, without any significant clinical or hematologic problems, but is of interest to geneticists and biochemists (http://globin.cse.psu.edu). Most of the Hb variants are missense mutations in the globin genes (α, β, γ, or δ) resulting from single nucleotide substitutions. Other uncommon mechanisms include (1) deletion or insertion of 1 or more nucleotides altering the reading frame, (2) fusion of globin genes with deletion of intergenic DNA sequences ($\gamma\beta$ fusion in Hb_{Kenya} and $\delta\beta$ fusion in Hb_{Lepore}), and (3) mutations of the termination codon leading to the production of elongated globin chains ($Hb_{Constant\ Spring}$).

Hb variants that significantly alter the structure, stability, synthesis, or function of the molecule have hematologic and/or clinical consequences. These can be classified in certain categories (Table 18-5). HbS and HbC are two examples of mutations on the surface of the Hb molecule that alter both the charge and the physical/chemical properties of

the molecule with polymer formation in the case of deoxyhemoglobin S and crystallization in HbC with profound effects on the function, morphology, rheology, and life span of the red cells. Several mechanisms account for the pathogenesis of unstable Hb variants. The common mechanism involves the precipitation of the unstable Hb molecule within the red cell with attachment to the inner layer of the red cell membrane ("Heinz body" formation); red ells containing membrane-attached Heinz bodies (Chaps. 1 and 2) have impaired deformability and filterability leading to their premature destruction (congenital Heinz body hemolytic anemia). Mutations in certain residues alter the oxygen affinity of the Hb molecule; a stabilization of the R (relaxed, oxy) state will result in high O_2 affinity variants and erythrocytosis. Conversely, a stabilization of the T (tense, deoxy) configuration will result in a variant with low O_2 affinity with enhanced unloading of O_2 to the tissues with resultant cyanosis and anemia in certain cases (because of the suppression of the O_2 sensing pathway) (Chaps. 3 and 19). Mutations of the heme binding site, particularly those affecting the conserved proximal (F8) and distal (E7) histidine residues, lead to the oxidation of the iron atom in heme from ferrous (Fe^{2+}) to ferric (Fe^{3+}) state with resultant methemoglobinemia (M Hbs) and cyanosis (Chap. 19). A group of mutations alter both the structure and the synthetic rate of the globin chain leading to a "β-thalassemia" phenotype (Chap. 17). These include fusion Hbs (eg, Hb_{Lepore}, where the 5' δ-globin sequences are fused to 3' β-globin sequences with deletion of the intergenic DNA; this puts

TABLE 18–4. Novel Therapies for Sickle Cell Disease					
Drug	Mechanism of Action	Pathway Targeted in SCD	Trial Phase/ Type	Outcomes	Ref.
Crizanlizumab	P-selectin inhibitor	Endothelial adhesion	III	Reduction number of VOC per year and in time to next VOC	520
Voxelotor	Antisickling	HbS polymerization	III	Increase in total Hb	517
L-Glutamine	Antioxidant	Red cell oxidative stress	III	Reduction in number of VOC per year	514
Regadenoson	iNKT A_2A receptor agonist	Inflammation	RCT	No change in length of hospital stay, mean total opioid use, or pain scores	102
Rivipansel	E-selectin inhibitor	Red cell adhesion	RCT	No change in length of stay or opioid use	
Omega-3 fatty acid	Reduction in oxidative injury	Red cell adhesion	RCT	Decreased VOE, anemia, and blood transfusion in supplemented group	555
Arginine	Increased NO production	NO signaling	RCT	Decreased parenteral opioids use and pain scores	556, 557
Ticagrelor	P2Y12 ADP receptor antagonist	Platelet activation	IIb	No change in patient reported pain	558
Magnesium sulfate	Increased cellular hydration	Cellular dehydration	RCT	No difference on LOS, pain scores, or analgesia use	559
Prasugrel	P2Y12 ADP receptor antagonist	Platelet activation	RCT	No change in VOC frequency or pain scores	560
Eptifibatide	Platelet $\alpha_{IIb}\beta_3$ inhibitor	Platelet activation	RCT	Safe but no difference in VOE resolution	561
Senicapoc	Gardos channel inhibitor	Cellular dehydration	III	Increased Hb and hematocrit and decreased erythrocytes and reticulocytes	562
Poloxamer-188	Amphipathic copolymer	Tissue oxygenation	III	Safe and well tolerated and demonstrated crisis resolution in a percentage of patients (greater in children than adults)	563

Abbreviations: ADP, adenosine diphosphate; Hb, hemoglobin; HbS, sickle hemoglobin; iNKT, invariant natural killer T cell; LOS, length of stay; NO, nitric oxide; RCT, randomized controlled trial; SCD, sickle cell disease; VOC, vasoocclusive crisis; VOE, vasoocclusive episode.

TABLE 18–5. Clinically Significant Hemoglobin Variants

I. Altered physical/chemical properties:
- a. HbS (deoxyhemoglobin S polymerization): sickle syndromes
- b. HbC (crystallization): hemolytic anemia; microcytosis

II. Unstable Hb variants:
- a. Congenital Heinz body hemolytic anemia (N=135)

III. Variants with altered oxygen affinity
- a. High-affinity variants: erythrocytosis (N=92)
- b. Low-affinity variants: anemia, cyanosis

IV. M-Hbs
- a. Methemoglobinemia, cyanosis (N=9)

V. Variants causing a thalassemic phenotype (N=50)
- a. β-Thalassemia
  - i. Hb_{Lepore} (δβ) fusion (N=3)
  - ii. Aberrant RNA processing (HbE, $Hb_{Knossos}$, Hb_{Malay})
  - iii. Hyperunstable globins (Hb_{Geneva}, $Hb_{Westdale}$, etc)
- b. α-Thalassemia
  - i. Chain-termination mutants ($Hb_{Constant\ Spring}$)
  - ii. Hyperunstable variants ($Hb_{Quong\ Sze}$)

Data from Bunn HF, Forget BG. *Hemoglobin: Molecular, Genetic, and Clinical Aspects.* Philadelphia, PA: WB Saunders; 1986.

the δβ-fusion gene under the transcriptional control of the inefficient δ-globin promoter with low expression of the fusion globin and hence the β-thalassemia phenotype), mutations that cause both a missense mutation and create an aberrant splice site (such as HbE, $Hb_{Knossos}$, and Hb_{Malay}), and "hyperunstable" globins where the nascent globin chains are highly unstable, undergo rapid proteolytic degradation, and result in a reduction in the affected globin.

Except for the commonly occurring variants (HbS, HbC, HbE, and $HbD_{Los\ Angeles}$), very few abnormal Hbs have been observed in the homozygous state. Variant Hbs are usually found in the heterozygous state. Although γ-globin chain variants are expressed in fetal life and their level gradually decreases as the γ-globin–to–β-globin (fetal to adult) switch progresses during the postnatal period, β-globin and α-globin variants are expressed throughout life. δ-Globin variants are expressed at very low levels and can be detected only after the switch to adult globin synthesis is complete. Because α-globin chains are present in all of the Hbs expressed after the embryonic stage (HbF-$α_2γ_2$; HbA-$α_2β_2$, and HbA$_2$-$α_2δ_2$), α-chain variants are associated with the production of variant HbF ($α_2^xγ_2$) and HbA$_2$ ($α_2^xδ_2$) as well. In heterozygous states, β-chain variants constitute 40% to 50% of the Hb in red cells; it should, however, be kept in mind that certain factors affect the amount of variant β-globin in carriers. These include the stability of the variant, the surface charge of the variant β-globin, and the presence of concomitant α-thalassemia or β-thalassemia (Chap. 17). The more unstable the variant, the lower the quantity. Surface charge of the variant also plays a role in determining the quantity in red cells; this is because the formation of the αβ-globin dimers ($α_1β_1$ and $α_2β_2$ contacts) is the critical first step in Hb tetramer formation, and this step is primarily driven by electrostatic interactions between α- and β-globin. The α-globin chains have a relatively positive surface charge; they interact more readily with relatively negatively charged β-globin variants to form αβ dimers. This is reflected in the higher percentage of negatively charged β-globin variants, such as $HbN_{Baltimore}$ (β95Lys→Glu), which are found in approximately 50%

of heterozygotes compared to β-globin variants with a positive surface charge, HbS (β6Glu→Val) or HbC (β6Glu→Lys), whose quantity in the heterozygote is 40% to 45%. In the presence of α-thalassemia, negatively charged β-globin variants compete more favorably for the available α-globin chains; this phenomenon is reflected in even lower percentages of HbS and HbC in heterozygous carriers of these variants in the presence of common deletional forms of α-thalassemia (HbS of 30%-35% in individuals with heterozygous α$^+$-thalassemia, –α/αα; and 25%-30% in homozygous α$^+$-thalassemia, –α/–α).[522,523] Conversely, the amount of a β-globin variant will increase if there is a β-thalassemia allele in *trans*; the percentage of the variant will be inversely proportional to the output of the β-thalassemia allele; thus, the higher the variant the lower the output of the β$^+$-thalassemia allele. In the case of a β^0-thalassemia allele in *trans*, the variant will amount to greater than 90% or more of the Hb in red blood cells, with HbA$_2$ and HbF constituting the remainder. The quantity of α-globin variants is also variable, depending on the α-globin gene involved, and the presence of concomitant α-thalassemia or β-thalassemia. Because there are normally 4 α-globin loci (αα/αα) and the upstream 5′ α-globin gene ($α_2$) is expressed at a higher level, some of the variation in the level of α-globin variants depends on which α-globin gene carries the mutation; $α_2$-globin mutations are usually present at 20% to 25% of the total Hb, whereas 3′ downstream $α_1$-globin variants are expressed at a lower level (15%-20%). Concomitant α-thalassemia results in a higher level of expression of α-globin variants. Observations on the different levels of expression of the common α-globin variant, $HbG_{Philadelphia}$ (α68Asn→Lys), is a case in point.[524] Although this variant has an expression of approximately 25% in Northern Italians, its percentage expression in Americans of African descent can be either 33% or approximately 50%. This is clearly related to the different genotypes found in these two distinct populations; in Northern Italy and Sardinia, the genotype is $α^Gα/αα$, with an expression level of approximately 30%, whereas in Americans of African descent, the $HbG_{Philadelphia}$ mutation is commonly found on a hybrid $α_2α_1$ gene associated with the common 3.7-kb α$^+$-thalassemia deletion ($–α^G/αα$) with approximately 33% expression. When there is an α$^+$-thalassemia deletion in *trans* ($–α^G/–α$ genotype), as expected, the level of $HbG_{Philadelphia}$ will be approximately 50%. Coinheritance of α-chain variants with β-thalassemia results in the increase of the α-chain variant.

HEMOGLOBIN C DISEASE

Definition and History

HbC was the second Hb variant described after HbS.[525] Homozygous HbC was described by Spaet and colleagues[526] and Ranney and colleagues.[527] HbC trait is found in 2% of Americans of African descent, and approximately 1 in 6000 have homozygous HbC.[528] Coinheritance of HbC with HbS results in HbSC disease, which is the second most common form of SCD in the United States, being found in approximately 25% of individuals with SCD. There are also rare cases of HbC-β$^+$-thalassemia and HbC-β^0-thalassemia. HbC is thought to have originated in Central West Africa and in parts of West Africa, where the prevalence of HbC can reach 12.5%. The HbC gene was found on 3 distinct β-globin cluster haplotypes, termed CI, CII, and CIII; the most common is CI, accounting for 70% or more of the HbC studied.[529]

Etiology and Pathogenesis

HbC is the result of a GAG→AAG transition in codon 6 of the β-globin gene, which changes the amino acid residue at this position from glutamic acid to lysine (Glu→Lys). The resultant positively charged Hb variant can easily be distinguished from HbA and HbS by electrophoresis and chromatography, including HPLC. HbC does not differ from HbA in its solubility; however, purified solutions of HbC form tetragonal crystals in high-molarity phosphate buffer. The Hb in red cells from homozygous HbC individuals form crystals when incubated with hypertonic saline; HbC crystals are also observed in vivo, particularly in the red cells of splenectomized HbCC patients (Fig. 18-11D and E). Crystal-containing HbCC red blood cells have impaired deformability and filterability. HbCC red cells have a propensity for K⁺ loss, which is followed by water loss; unlike in sickle red cells, this K⁺ leak does not appear to be mediated through either the K⁺ chloride cotransport or the calcium ion activated K⁺ efflux (Gardos) channel; it is thought to be a volume-stimulated K⁺ efflux.[528] The consequence of this K⁺ loss is dehydrated, often spherocytic, target red cells with increased mean cell Hb concentration, and decreased osmotic fragility. These changes result in impaired rheologic properties of HbCC red cells; their life span is reduced to 40 days.

Clinical Features

Mild to moderate splenomegaly is a common feature of homozygous HbC. Like many other chronic hemolytic states, cholelithiasis may be present. HbCC individuals do not suffer from vasoocclusion or episodic pain. Occasionally, abdominal pain may be present and can be a result of splenomegaly and/or cholelithiasis. Pregnancy does not pose an increased risk to women with HbCC. Life expectancy of HbCC individuals is comparable to non-HbC Americans of African descent. In a single-institution study, splenomegaly and cholelithiasis occurred in approximately 2.5% of patients younger than 8 years, but it was far more common (71%) in individuals older than 8 years.[530]

Laboratory Features

HbCC individuals have a mild to moderate hemolytic anemia. Hb is usually in the 100 to 110 g/L range. There is associated reticulocytosis usually in the 3% to 4% range. There usually is mild microcytosis with mean corpuscular volume of 70 to 75 fL and, often, an elevated mean cell Hb concentration. The blood film from affected individuals shows an abundance of target cells, microspherocytes, and HbC red cell crystals, especially in splenectomized patients (see Fig. 18-11E and F). Indirect bilirubin may be mildly elevated. White cell and platelet counts are normal in the absence of hypersplenism.

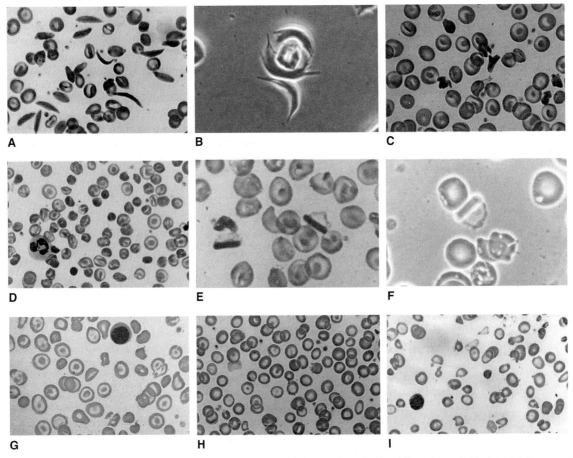

FIGURE 18–11. Blood cell morphology in patients with structural hemoglobinopathies. **A.** Blood film. Hemoglobin (Hb) SS disease with characteristic sickle-shaped cells and extreme elliptocytes with dense central Hb staining. Both shapes are characteristic of sickled cells. Occasional target cells. **B.** Phase-contrast microscopy of wet preparation. Note the three sickled cells with terminal fine-pointed projections as a result of tactoid formation and occasional target cells. **C.** HbSC disease. Blood film. Note the high frequency of target cells characteristic of HbC and the small dense, irregular, contracted cells reflective of their content of HbS. **D.** HbCC disease. Blood film. Characteristic combination of numerous target cells and a population of dense (hyperchromatic) microspherocytes. Of the nonspherocytic cells, virtually all are target cells. **E.** HbCC disease postsplenectomy. Blood film. Note the rod-like inclusions in 2 cells as a result of HbC paracrystallization. These cells are virtually all removed in patients with spleens. **F.** HbCC disease postsplenectomy. Phase-contrast microscopy of wet preparation. Note the HbC crystalline rod in a cell. **G.** HbDD disease. Blood film. Note Frequent target cells admixed with population of small spherocytes, poikilocytes, and tiny red cell fragments. **H.** HbEE disease. Blood film. Hypochromia, anisocytosis, and target cells. **I.** HbE β-thalassemia. Blood film. Marked hypochromia, anisocytosis (primarily microcytes) and poikilocytosis. *(Reproduced with permission from Lichtman MA, Shafer MS, Felgar RE, et al: Lichtman's Atlas of Hematology 2016. New York, NY: McGraw Hill; 2017.)*

Differential Diagnosis

Differential diagnosis is usually achieved by Hb electrophoresis. HbC moves to a cathodic position, comigrating with HbA$_2$, HbE, and HbO$_{Arab}$ on alkaline pH (cellulose acetate) electrophoresis. The distinction from these Hbs can be made by electrophoresis on citrate agar in acid pH where HbE and HbA$_2$ comigrate with HbA; HbO$_{Arab}$ has a HbS-like mobility, and HbC has a unique migration pattern. With isoelectric focusing, HbC can readily be distinguished from other Hbs with similar mobility on cellulose acetate electrophoresis. In cation exchange HPLC and capillary electrophoresis, HbC has a distinct elution pattern and can be distinguished from HbE and HbO$_{Arab}$; HPLC and capillary electrophoresis also have the advantage of separating and quantifying HbA$_2$ in HbC homozygotes and in HbC trait. This confers the advantage of readily differentiating between HbCC and rare cases of HbC-β^0-thalassemia (where HbA$_2$ is significantly higher, ~5%).

Therapy

The vast majority of HbCC individuals do not require any therapeutic intervention. Cholecystectomy may be required in individuals who have symptomatic gallstones. A few patients with HbCC develop hypersplenism with a reduction in white blood cell and platelet counts, and occasionally worsening of anemia. In such instances, splenectomy should be considered. Another indication for splenectomy is pain associated with an enlarged spleen. It is important to apply the usual precautions in patients considered for splenectomy (appropriate vaccinations, prophylactic antibiotic use, and delaying splenectomy in young children). Folic acid supplementation, as usually done in many chronic hemolytic states, is of no proven value.

HEMOGLOBIN E DISEASE

Definition and History

HbE (β26Glu→Lys) was the fourth abnormal Hb described.[531] It is most commonly found in Southeast Asia; in some areas (in the border between Thailand, Laos, and Cambodia, the so-called HbE triangle) the gene frequency may reach as high as 0.50.[532] This high frequency is thought to be the result of a protective effect against malaria. HbE is also found in other malaria-endemic areas, such as Bangladesh, India, and Madagascar. HbE now has a wide distribution as a result of the large population movements from Southeast and South Asia to Western Europe and North America.

Etiology and Pathogenesis

The GAG→AAG mutation in codon 26 of the β-globin gene not only leads to a missense mutation (Glu→Lys) at this position, but also activates a cryptic donor splice site at the boundary of exon 1 and intron 1 by increasing the sequence similarity of this site to a consensus splice sequence. The resultant aberrant splicing through this alternate site leads to a decrease in the correctly spliced mRNA and hence a β$^+$-thalassemic phenotype. This is reflected in the fact that heterozygotes for HbE have 25% to 30% of the variant; in the presence of concomitant α-thalassemia, this quantity decreases even further. The coinheritance of HbE with a host of other globin mutants (α-thalassemia and β-thalassemias, other Hb variants), which are also common in the populations where HbE is prevalent, results in a wide spectrum of hemoglobinopathies with varying degrees of severity (HbE disorders or HbE syndromes). The most significant of these are the HbE-β-thalassemia syndromes. HbE also has been reported in combination with HbS (HbSE disease).

Clinical Features

Individuals with homozygous HbE are asymptomatic. Most patients do not have hepatosplenomegaly or jaundice. They are usually diagnosed during screening programs or family studies of individuals with severe HbE disorders, or on routine evaluation of a blood film with significant microcytosis without anemia. HbE-β-thalassemia is a rather heterogeneous group of disorders varying from a mild thalassemia intermedia–like phenotype to a severe transfusion-dependent thalassemia major phenotype (Chap. 17). Part of this heterogeneity results from the type of coinherited β-thalassemia mutation. Patients who are compound heterozygotes for HbE and one of the mild β$^+$-thalassemia mutations (such as the mild promoter mutation, −28A→G) have a mild to moderate anemia, whereas patients with compound heterozygosity for HbE and one of the more severe β$^+$-thalassemia mutations (such as intervening sequence [IVS] I nucleotide 5 or IVS II nucleotide 654 mutations) have a more severe phenotype with severe anemia and transfusion dependency. There is also a large heterogeneity among patients with HbE-β^0-thalassemia; these patients do not produce any HbA and have only HbE and varying amounts of HbF. Known factors that influence the phenotype include the ability to produce HbF and the presence of concomitant α-thalassemia. Individuals who have the propensity to synthesize significant amounts of HbF (such as those who have the Xmn I C→T mutation in the ^{G}γ-globin promoter, or BCL11A variants) are able to ameliorate the globin chain imbalance and thus have a milder phenotype. Concomitant α-thalassemia also mitigates the course of the disease by decreasing globin chain imbalance. In some cases, there may be nonglobin modifiers that impact the phenotype. Patients with severe forms of HbE-β^0-thalassemia have clinical features very similar to β-thalassemia major; they develop complications such as hypersplenism, iron overload, increased susceptibility to infections, thromboembolic complications, heart failure, and shortened life expectancy.[532] Splenectomized HbE-β-thalassemia patients have more pronounced intravascular hemolysis, markers of endothelial cell activation, and activation of coagulation with increased levels of cell-free Hb, sE-selectin, sP-selectin, high sensitivity C-reactive protein, and thrombin–antithrombin complex compared to nonsplenectomized patients.[533]

Laboratory Features

HbE trait individuals have a borderline microcytosis with mean corpuscular volume in the lower 80-fL range but are not anemic. Homozygotes for HbE are usually only borderline or mildly anemic (Hb 110-130 g/L), but they are microcytic (mean corpuscular volume ~70 fL). Blood films show target cells, hypochromia, and microcytosis (see Fig. 18-11H). Osmotic fragility of the red cells is increased. Hb electrophoresis shows greater than 90% HbE and 5% to 10% HbF. Certain chromatography techniques that can separate HbE from HbA$_2$ reveal elevated levels of HbA$_2$. Patients with mild forms of HbE-β$^+$-thalassemia (Chap. 17) have Hb levels in the 90 to 95 g/L range, whereas those with severe HbE-β$^+$-thalassemia are more severely anemic (Hb 65-80 g/L) and have more severe poikilocytosis and hypochromia (see Fig. 18-11I). Individuals with HbE-β^0-thalassemia have varying degrees of anemia, depending on their ability to produce HbF; these patients have HbE in the 40% to 60% range, with the remainder being HbF. Patients with higher HbF values are less anemic.

Therapy

HbE homozygotes do not require any therapy. Patients with severe HbE-β^0-thalassemia are similar to thalassemia intermedia or thalassemia major; most of the latter patients should be on a chronic transfusion regimen aiming at Hb levels of approximately 100 g/L; iron chelation should be a part of standard therapy. Splenectomy should be considered when hypersplenism develops. Patients with a thalassemia intermedia–like phenotype may require sporadic transfusions. Hydroxyurea can increase HbF levels and decrease ineffective erythropoiesis in HbE-β-thalassemia.[534] AHSCT (including umbilical cord blood-derived stem cells in one patient) also has been used in HbE-β-thalassemia.

Course and Prognosis

The prognosis is dependent upon the clinical phenotype. Patients with milder phenotypes tend to do well. Severe HbE-β-thalassemia patients require chronic red blood cell transfusion and iron-chelation therapy; these place a great burden on the economies of countries where this disease is prevalent. AHSCT, although potentially curative, will not be available for the vast majority of these patients. Prenatal diagnosis and neonatal screening are strategies to decrease the disease burden and improve care. Long-term use of hydroxyurea and other novel HbF-inducing agents as modifiers of disease (histone deacetylase inhibitors and DNA methyltransferase 1 inhibitors) can be an important addition to therapy.

HEMOGLOBIN D DISEASE

HbD is the third variant Hb identified.[535] The substitution in HbD is a glutamic acid to glutamine at the 121st amino acid of the β-globin chain (β121Glu→Gln). HbD has an S-like mobility on alkaline electrophoresis but comigrates with HbA on acid pH. Subsequently, a number of other Hb variants with the same electrophoretic properties were discovered and named HbD (HbD$_{Ibadan}$, HbD$_{Gainesville}$). The most common HbD is HbD$_{Los Angeles}$ (β121Glu→Gln), the originally discovered HbD, which is identical to HbD$_{Punjab}$. It is most commonly found in Punjab, India, where 2% to 3% of the population has the HbD gene. Subsequently, it also has been found in a number of other populations, including Europeans of the Mediterranean region and Americans of African descent.[536]

HbD heterozygotes are asymptomatic, are not anemic, and have normal red cell indices. Homozygotes for HbD$_{Los Angeles}$ are asymptomatic and are hematologically normal with normal red cell indices. Blood films made from affected individuals show target cells (see Fig. 18-11G). Osmotic fragility may be decreased. Compound heterozygotes for HbD$_{Los Angeles}$ and a β^0-thalassemia mutation have mild microcytic anemia and show minimal hemolysis. Coinheritance of HbD$_{Los Angeles}$ with HbS results in a severe SCD phenotype not different from homozygous HbS.

HbD$_{Los Angeles}$ should be distinguished from HbS. This can be done by a combination of routine alkaline and acid Hb electrophoretic methods. Techniques such as isoelectric focusing, HPLC, and capillary electrophoresis readily provide this distinction. Such methods allow accurate diagnosis of SCD because of compound heterozygosity for HbS and HbD$_{Los Angeles}$.

UNSTABLE HEMOGLOBINS

Unstable Hbs form an important group of clinically significant Hb variants. Several different mechanisms lead to the generation of unstable variants, which result in a congenital hemolytic anemia with inclusion bodies in red cells (Heinz bodies), hence the term *congenital Heinz body hemolytic anemia*.[537]

Definition and History

Cathie reported a 10-month-old child with hemolytic anemia, jaundice, and splenomegaly in 1952.[538] Splenectomy did not result in improvement. The patient's red blood cells had large Heinz bodies (Chap. 1). Similar cases were reported from around the world, and the observation that these cases were characterized by the precipitation of their hemolysate upon exposure to heat, suggested an Hb abnormality as the cause. Subsequently, nearly all similar cases were found to have a variant Hb, and Cathie's case was found to have Hb$_{Bristol}$ (β67Val→Asp). As of this writing, 153 unstable variants have been reported; the vast majority is

sporadic cases reported only once. Few have been observed repeatedly in different populations.

Etiology and Pathogenesis

Several different mechanisms lead to the instability of the globin molecule with precipitation in the red blood cell leading to hemolysis. These are summarized below.

Substitutions Near the Heme Pocket Heme is inserted into a hydrophobic pocket in each globin molecule where it is in contact with a number of invariant nonpolar amino acid residues (see Fig. 18-2). Substitution of these invariant nonpolar residues will decrease the stability of heme–globin association and ultimately lead to instability of the globin moiety. Hb$_{Zurich}$[539] (β63His→Arg), Hb$_{Koln}$[540] (β98Val→Met), and Hb$_{Hammersmith}$[541] (β42Phe→Ser) are examples of this group.

Disruption of Secondary Structure (α-Helix) The secondary structure of globin chains is 75% in the conformation of an α helix (see Fig. 18-1). Proline residues cannot participate in an α-helical conformation. Thus, the substitution of a proline residue for any other amino acid except for the first three residues of an α helix will disrupt the secondary structure and lead to the disruption and precipitation of the mutant globin chain.[537]

Mutations in the α$_1$β$_1$ Interface The first step in the assembly of the Hb tetramer is the formation of an αβ dimer. This structure is stabilized by a secondary structure that exposes the charged amino acids (glutamic acid, aspartic acid, lysine, and arginine) on the surface of the molecule in contact with water and stabilizes the interior of the molecule (α$_1$β$_1$ interface) with hydrophobic interactions. Substitution of a charged (polar) residue for a nonpolar amino acid involved in α$_1$β$_1$ contact will disrupt and destabilize this dimer formation and lead to the precipitation of the Hb molecule.

Amino Acid Deletions Deletion of one or more amino acid residues is expected to disrupt the secondary structure of the globin chains and may lead to instability of the mutant chain. Mutant globins with deletion of one or more residues have been reported. Examples of this type include Hb$_{Leiden}$[542] (β6 or β7Glu→0), Hb$_{Gun Hill}$[543] (β91–95→0), and Hb$_{Freiburg}$[544] (β23Val→0).

Elongated Globin Chains Some variants result from either a mutation in the termination codon or a frameshift leading to the synthesis of longer than normal globin chains. These variants tend to be unstable because of the presence of a nonfunctional fragment. Examples include Hb$_{Cranston}$[545] and Hb$_{Tak}$.[546]

Whatever the underlying mechanism may be, unstable Hb variants precipitate within developing red blood cell precursors forming hemichromes (intermediate substances in Hb denaturation) and, ultimately, aggregates that attach to the inner layer of the red blood cell membrane (Heinz bodies). Heinz bodies can be visualized with supravital stains, such as brilliant cresyl blue. Red blood cells with Heinz bodies have impaired rheologic properties (deformability and filterability) and are trapped in the splenic circulation (Chap. 25) with pitting of the membrane attached bodies. Hemolysis ultimately ensues. The degree of hemolysis is proportionate to the quantity and the instability of the variant.

Clinical Features

Patients with unstable Hb variants have varying degrees of hemolytic anemia. This can range from a compensated, asymptomatic hemolytic state to severe, life-threatening hemolysis. Generally, hemolytic anemia is mild to moderate and does not require therapeutic intervention. Typically, hemolysis is exacerbated by increased oxidant stress such as infections and the use of oxidant drugs. Patients may have jaundice and splenomegaly. As is the case with other chronic hemolytic states, gallstones may develop. Hypersplenism can be a problem in some cases.

Many unstable Hb variants that are associated with mild, compensated hemolysis are diagnosed fortuitously or during population screening for hemoglobinopathies. Unstable variants are inherited in a Mendelian pattern; they usually manifest in the heterozygous state. There are instances of de novo mutations without evidence of the variant in parents of an affected individual. Many of the 153 known unstable variants are found in a single individual or in a limited number of instances. However, some unstable variants, like Hb_{Koln} (β98Val→Met) and Hb_{Zurich} (β67His→Arg), are found in many populations around the world.

Laboratory Features

Patients with unstable Hb variants may have varying degrees of anemia. Generally, the anemia is mild and does not require therapeutic intervention. However, exacerbation of anemia during exposure to oxidant stress (such as infections and the use of oxidant drugs) is a common feature. Features of a hemolytic state (reticulocytosis, indirect hyperbilirubinemia, elevated LDH, decreased or undetectable haptoglobin) are present. Red blood cell morphology shows polychromasia, anisocytosis, poikilocytosis, and occasionally basophilic stippling. A typical feature of this disorder is the presence of Heinz bodies. Hb electrophoresis reveals the presence of an additional abnormal Hb band. The quantity of the variant Hb is variable and inversely proportional to the degree of instability of the abnormal Hb (eg, the more unstable the variant, the less the quantity). More accurate quantification can be achieved with cation exchange or reversed-phase HPLC. The presence of an unstable variant in the hemolysate can be demonstrated by simple tests of stability. The most commonly used tests are heat denaturation and isopropanol precipitation. The heat denaturation test is more cumbersome and time-consuming, and is seldom used in practice. The isopropanol precipitation test is a simple screening test for unstable variants and involves the incubation of the hemolysate with a 17% solution of isopropanol; hemolysates containing unstable Hb variants will form a precipitate, whereas a normal hemolysate will remain clear.

HEMOGLOBINS WITH ALTERED OXYGEN AFFINITY

Mutations in certain critical areas of the globin molecule alter the affinity of the globin for oxygen. M Hbs result from mutations around the heme pocket that disrupt the hydrophobic nature of this structure with resultant oxidation of the iron in the heme moiety from ferrous (Fe^{2+}) to ferric (Fe^{3+}) state and cause methemoglobinemia (Chap. 19). In general, mutations that stabilize the molecule in the T (tense, deoxy) state lead to low oxygen affinity variants, which can clinically manifest as cyanosis or mild anemia. Mutations that stabilize the R (relaxed, oxy) state or destabilize the T state result in high O_2 affinity variants. These variants will cause secondary erythrocytosis (Chap. 28).[537] The mutations that affect the ligand binding affinity of the Hb molecule are mostly in the $\alpha_1\beta_2$ interface. Rarely, mutations in the $\alpha_1\beta_1$ interface lead to altered O_2 affinity. Another mechanism in the generation of high O_2 affinity mutants involves mutations that alter the binding of 2,3-BPG.

REFERENCES

1. Ingram VM. Gene mutations in human haemoglobin: the chemical difference between normal and sickle cell haemoglobin. *Nature.* 1957;180:326-328.
2. Travassos MA, Coulibaly D, Laurens MB, et al. Hemoglobin C trait provides protection from clinical falciparum malaria in Malian children. *J Infect Dis.* 2015;212:1778-1786.
3. Ha J, Martinson R, Iwamoto SK, et al. Hemoglobin E, malaria and natural selection. *Evol Med Public Health.* 2019;2019:232-241.
4. Herrick JB. Peculiar elongated and sickle-shaped red corpuscles in a case of severe anemia. *Arch Intern Med.* 1910;6:517-521.
5. Cook JE, Meyer J. Severe anemia with remarkable elongated and sickle-shaped red blood cells and chronic leg ulcers. *Arch Intern Med (Chic).* 1915;XVI:644-651.
6. Emmel VE. A study of the erythrocytes in a case of severe anemia with elongated sickle-shaped red blood corpuscles. *Arch Intern Med (Chic).* 1917;XX:586-598.
7. Mason VR. Sickle cell anemia. *JAMA.* 1922;79:1318-1320.
8. Sydnestricker VP, Mulherin WA, Houseal RW. Sickle cell anemia. Report of two cases in children with necropsy in one case. *Am J Dis Child.* 1923;26:132-154.
9. Huck JG. Sickle-cell anemia. *Bull Johns Hopkins Hosp.* 1923;34:335-344.
10. Huck JG, Bigelow RM. Poikilocytes in otherwise normal blood. *Bull Johns Hopkins Hosp.* 1923;34:390-394.
11. Hahn EV, Gillespie EB. Sickle cell anemia. Report of a case greatly improved by splenectomy. Experimental study of sickle cell formation. *Arch Intern Med (Chic).* 1927;39:233-254.
12. Diggs LW, Ahmann CF, Bibb J. The incidence and significance of the sickle cell trait. *Ann Intern Med.* 1933;7:769-778.
13. Pauling L, Itano HA, et al. Sickle cell anemia a molecular disease. *Science.* 1949;110:543-548.
14. Marotta CA, Wilson JT, Forget BG, et al. Human beta-globin messenger RNA. III. Nucleotide sequences derived from complementary DNA. *J Biol Chem* 1977;252:5040-5053.
15. Kan YW, Dozy AM. Antenatal diagnosis of sickle-cell anaemia by D.N.A. analysis of amniotic-fluid cells. *Lancet.* 1978;2:910-912.
16. Gormley M. The first 'molecular disease': a story of Linus Pauling, the intellectual patron. *Endeavour.* 2007;31:71-77.
17. Haller JO, Berdon WE, Franke H. Sickle cell anemia: the legacy of the patient (Walter Clement Noel), the interne (Ernest Irons), and the attending physician (James Herrick) and the facts of its discovery. *Pediatr Radiol.* 2001;31:889-890.
18. Serjeant GR. The emerging understanding of sickle cell disease. *Br J Haematol.* 2001;112:3-18.
19. Williams VL. Pathways of innovation: a history of the first effective treatment for sickle cell anemia. *Perspect Biol Med.* 2004;47:552-563.
20. Raper AB. The incidence of sicklaemia. *East Afr Med J.* 1949;26:281-282.
21. Mackey JP, Vivarelli F. Sickle-cell anaemia. *Br Med J.* 1954;1:276.
22. Allison AC. Protection afforded by sickle-cell trait against subtertian malareal infection. *Br Med J.* 1954;1:290-294.
23. Goldsmith JC, Bonham VL, Joiner CH, et al. Framing the research agenda for sickle cell trait: building on the current understanding of clinical events and their potential implications. *Am J Hematol.* 2012;87:340-346.
24. Gong L, Parikh S, Rosenthal PJ, et al. Biochemical and immunological mechanisms by which sickle cell trait protects against malaria. *Malar J.* 2013;12:317.
25. De Franceschi L. Pathophisiology of sickle cell disease and new drugs for the treatment. *Mediterr J Hematol Infect Dis.* 2009;1:e2009024.
26. Thein MS, Thein SL. World Sickle Cell Day 2016: a time for appraisal. *Indian J Med Res.* 2016;143:678-681.
27. Serjeant GR, Serjeant BE, Forbes M, et al. Haemoglobin gene frequencies in the Jamaican population: a study in 100,000 newborns. *Br J Haematol.* 1986;64:253-262.
28. Hassell KL. Population estimates of sickle cell disease in the U.S. *Am J Prev Med.* 2010;38:S512-S521.
29. Okumura MJ, Campbell AD, Nasr SZ, et al. Inpatient health care use among adult survivors of chronic childhood illnesses in the United States. *Arch Pediatr Adolesc Med.* 2006;160:1054-1060.
30. Kauf TL, Coates TD, Huazhi L, et al. The cost of health care for children and adults with sickle cell disease. *Am J Hematol.* 2009;84:323-327.
31. Kan YW, Dozy AM. Polymorphism of DNA sequence adjacent to human beta-globin structural gene: relationship to sickle mutation. *Proc Natl Acad Sci U S A.* 1978;75:5631-5635.
32. Nagel RL, Fabry ME, Pagnier J, et al. Hematologically and genetically distinct forms of sickle cell anemia in Africa. The Senegal type and the Benin type. *N Engl J Med.* 1985;312:880-884.
33. Pagnier J, Mears JG, Dunda-Belkhodja O, et al. Evidence for the multicentric origin of the sickle cell hemoglobin gene in Africa. *Proc Natl Acad Sci U S A.* 1984;81:1771-1773.
34. Powars DR. Sickle cell anemia: beta s-gene-cluster haplotypes as prognostic indicators of vital organ failure. *Semin Hematol.* 1991;28:202-208.
35. Shriner D, Rotimi CN. Whole-genome-sequence-based haplotypes reveal single origin of the sickle allele during the Holocene wet phase. *Am J Hum Genet.* 2018;102:547-556.
36. Gordeuk VR, Shah BN, Zhang X, et al. The CYB5R3$^{c.350C>G}$ and G6PD A alleles modify severity of anemia in malaria and sickle cell disease. *Am J Hematol.* 2020;95(11):1269-1279.
37. Dykes GW, Crepeau RH, Edelstein SJ. Three-dimensional reconstruction of the 14-filament fibers of hemoglobin S. *J Mol Biol.* 1979;130:451-472.
38. Fronticelli C, Gold R. Conformational relevance of the beta6Glu replaced by Val mutation in the beta subunits and in the beta(1-55) and beta(1-30) peptides of hemoglobin S. *J Biol Chem.* 1976;251:4968-4972.
39. Wishner BC, Ward KB, Lattman EE, et al. Crystal structure of sickle-cell deoxyhemoglobin at 5 A resolution. *J Mol Biol.* 1975;98:179-194.
40. Ferrone FA, Hofrichter J, Eaton WA. Kinetics of sickle hemoglobin polymerization. I. Studies using temperature-jump and laser photolysis techniques. *J Mol Biol.* 1985;183:591-610.
41. Ferrone FA, Hofrichter J, Eaton WA. Kinetics of sickle hemoglobin polymerization. II. A double nucleation mechanism. *J Mol Biol.* 1985;183:611-631.
42. Huang Z, Hearne L, Irby CE, et al. Kinetics of increased deformability of deoxygenated sickle cells upon oxygenation. *Biophys J.* 2003;85:2374-2383.

43. Carragher B, Bluemke DA, Gabriel B, et al. Structural analysis of polymers of sickle cell hemoglobin. I. Sickle hemoglobin fibers. *J Mol Biol.* 1988;199:315-331.

44. Padlan EA, Love WE. Refined crystal structure of deoxyhemoglobin S. II. Molecular interactions in the crystal. *J Biol Chem.* 1985;260:8280-8291.

45. Vekilov PG. Sickle-cell haemoglobin polymerization: is it the primary pathogenic event of sickle-cell anaemia? *Br J Haematol.* 2007;139:173-184.

46. Ferrone FA. Polymerization and sickle cell disease: a molecular view. *Microcirculation.* 2004;11:115-128.

47. Ballas SK, Mohandas N. Sickle red cell microrheology and sickle blood rheology. *Microcirculation.* 2004;11:209-225.

48. Eaton WA, Hofrichter J. Hemoglobin S gelation and sickle cell disease. *Blood.* 1987;70:1245-1266.

49. Kaul DK, Fabry ME, Nagel RL. Microvascular sites and characteristics of sickle cell adhesion to vascular endothelium in shear flow conditions: pathophysiological implications. *Proc Natl Acad Sci U S A.* 1989;86:3356-3360.

50. Noguchi CT, Schechter AN. The intracellular polymerization of sickle hemoglobin and its relevance to sickle cell disease. *Blood.* 1981;58:1057-1068.

51. Embury SH. The not-so-simple process of sickle cell vasoocclusion. *Microcirculation.* 2004;11:101-113.

52. Steinberg MH. Pathophysiologically based drug treatment of sickle cell disease. *Trends Pharmacol Sci.* 2006;27:204-210.

53. Stuart MJ, Nagel RL. Sickle-cell disease. *Lancet.* 2004;364:1343-1360.

54. Brugnara C. Sickle cell disease: from membrane pathophysiology to novel therapies for prevention of erythrocyte dehydration. *J Pediatr Hematol Oncol.* 2003;25:927-933.

55. Stocker JW, De Franceschi L, McNaughton-Smith GA, et al. ICA-17043, a novel Gardos channel blocker, prevents sickled red blood cell dehydration in vitro and in vivo in SAD mice. *Blood.* 2003;101:2412-2418.

56. Bennekou P, Pedersen O, Moller A, et al. Volume control in sickle cells is facilitated by the novel anion conductance inhibitor NS1652. *Blood.* 2000;95:1842-1848.

57. Joiner CH, Jiang M, Claussen WJ, et al. Dipyridamole inhibits sickling-induced cation fluxes in sickle red blood cells. *Blood.* 2001;97:3976-3983.

58. Aslan M, Freeman BA. Redox-dependent impairment of vascular function in sickle cell disease. *Free Radic Biol Med.* 2007;43:1469-1483.

59. Gladwin MT, Schechter AN. Nitric oxide therapy in sickle cell disease. *Semin Hematol.* 2001;38:333-342.

60. Enwonwu CO, Xu XX, Turner E. Nitrogen metabolism in sickle cell anemia: free amino acids in plasma and urine. *Am J Med Sci.* 1990;300:366-371.

61. Lopez BL, Barnett J, Ballas SK, et al. Nitric oxide metabolite levels in acute vaso-occlusive sickle-cell crisis. *Acad Emerg Med.* 1996;3:1098-1103.

62. Lopez BL, Davis-Moon L, Ballas SK, et al. Sequential nitric oxide measurements during the emergency department treatment of acute vasoocclusive sickle cell crisis. *Am J Hematol.* 2000;64:15-19.

63. Morris CR, Kuypers FA, Larkin S, et al. Arginine therapy: a novel strategy to induce nitric oxide production in sickle cell disease. *Br J Haematol.* 2000;111:498-500.

64. Morris CR, Kuypers FA, Larkin S, et al. Patterns of arginine and nitric oxide in patients with sickle cell disease with vaso-occlusive crisis and acute chest syndrome. *J. Pediatr. Hematol Oncol.* 2000;22:515-520.

65. Kato GJ, Wang Z, Machado RF, et al. Endogenous nitric oxide synthase inhibitors in sickle cell disease: abnormal levels and correlations with pulmonary hypertension, desaturation, haemolysis, organ dysfunction and death. *Br J Haematol.* 2009;145:506-513.

66. Kato GJ, Taylor JGt. Pleiotropic effects of intravascular haemolysis on vascular homeostasis. *Br J Haematol.* 2010;148:690-701.

67. Frenette PS, Atweh GF. Sickle cell disease: old discoveries, new concepts, and future promise. *J Clin Invest.* 2007;117:850-858.

68. Reiter CD, Wang X, Tanus-Santos JE, et al. Cell-free hemoglobin limits nitric oxide bioavailability in sickle-cell disease. *Nat Med.* 2002;8:1383-1389.

69. Hebbel RP, Yamada O, Moldow CF, et al. Abnormal adherence of sickle erythrocytes to cultured vascular endothelium: possible mechanism for microvascular occlusion in sickle cell disease. *J Clin Invest.* 1980;65:154-160.

70. Hoover R, Rubin R, Wise G, et al. Adhesion of normal and sickle erythrocytes to endothelial monolayer cultures. *Blood.* 1979;54:872-876.

71. Barabino GA, McIntire LV, Eskin SG, et al. Rheological studies of erythrocyte-endothelial cell interactions in sickle cell disease. *Prog Clin Biol Res.* 1987;240:113-127.

72. Mohandas N, Evans E. Sickle erythrocyte adherence to vascular endothelium. Morphologic correlates and the requirement for divalent cations and collagen-binding plasma proteins. *J Clin Invest.* 1985;76:1605-1612.

73. Kaul DK, Tsai HM, Liu XD, et al. Monoclonal antibodies to alphaVbeta3 (7E3 and LM609) inhibit sickle red blood cell-endothelium interactions induced by platelet-activating factor. *Blood.* 2000;95:368-374.

74. Frenette PS. Sickle cell vaso-occlusion: multistep and multicellular paradigm. *Curr Opin Hematol.* 2002;9:101-106.

75. Gee BE, Platt OS. Sickle reticulocytes adhere to VCAM-1. *Blood.* 1995;85:268-274.

76. Parsons SF, Lee G, Spring FA, et al. Lutheran blood group glycoprotein and its newly characterized mouse homologue specifically bind alpha5 chain-containing human laminin with high affinity. *Blood.* 2001;97:312-320.

77. Swerlick RA, Eckman JR, Kumar A, et al. Alpha 4 beta 1-integrin expression on sickle reticulocytes: vascular cell adhesion molecule-1-dependent binding to endothelium. *Blood.* 1993;82:1891-1899.

78. Udani M, Zen Q, Cottman M, et al. Basal cell adhesion molecule/lutheran protein. The receptor critical for sickle cell adhesion to laminin. *J Clin Invest.* 1998;101:2550-2558.

79. Okpala I. The intriguing contribution of white blood cells to sickle cell disease-a red cell disorder. *Blood Rev.* 2004;18:65-73.

80. Okpala I. Leukocyte adhesion and the pathophysiology of sickle cell disease. *Curr Opin Hematol.* 2006;13:40-44.

81. Tan P, Luscinskas FW, Homer-Vanniasinkam S. Cellular and molecular mechanisms of inflammation and thrombosis. *Eur J Vasc Endovasc Surg.* 1999;17:373-389.

82. Hebbel RP, Osarogiagbon R, Kaul D. The endothelial biology of sickle cell disease: inflammation and a chronic vasculopathy. *Microcirculation.* 2004;11:129-151.

83. Belcher JD, Marker PH, Weber JP, et al. Activated monocytes in sickle cell disease: potential role in the activation of vascular endothelium and vaso-occlusion. *Blood.* 2000;96:2451-2459.

84. Benkerrou M, Delarche C, Brahimi L, et al. Hydroxyurea corrects the dysregulated L-selectin expression and increased H(2)O(2) production of polymorphonuclear neutrophils from patients with sickle cell anemia. *Blood.* 2002;99:2297-2303.

85. Fadlon E, Vordermeier S, Pearson TC, et al. Blood polymorphonuclear leukocytes from the majority of sickle cell patients in the crisis phase of the disease show enhanced adhesion to vascular endothelium and increased expression of CD64. *Blood.* 1998;91:266-274.

86. Francis R Jr, Hebbel RP, eds. *Hemostasis.* Raven; 1994:299-310.

87. Hofstra TC, Kalra VK, Meiselman HJ, et al. Sickle erythrocytes adhere to polymorphonuclear neutrophils and activate the neutrophil respiratory burst. *Blood.* 1996;87:4440-4447.

88. Inwald DP, Kirkham FJ, Peters MJ, et al. Platelet and leucocyte activation in childhood sickle cell disease: association with nocturnal hypoxaemia. *Br J Haematol.* 2000;111:474-481.

89. Lard LR, Mul FP, de Haas M, et al. Neutrophil activation in sickle cell disease. *J Leukoc Biol.* 1999;66:411-415.

90. Nath KA, Grande JP, Haggard JJ, et al. Oxidative stress and induction of heme oxygenase-1 in the kidney in sickle cell disease. *Am J Pathol.* 2001;158:893-903.

91. Solovey A, Gui L, Key NS, et al. Tissue factor expression by endothelial cells in sickle cell anemia. *J Clin Invest.* 1998;101:1899-1904.

92. Solovey A, Lin Y, Browne P, et al. Circulating activated endothelial cells in sickle cell anemia. *N Engl J Med.* 1997;337:1584-1590.

93. Wun T, Cordoba M, Rangaswami A, et al. Activated monocytes and platelet-monocyte aggregates in patients with sickle cell disease. *Clin Lab Haematol.* 2002;24:81-88.

94. Patel N, Gonsalves CS, Malik P, et al. Placenta growth factor augments endothelin-1 and endothelin-B receptor expression via hypoxia-inducible factor-1 alpha. *Blood.* 2008;112:856-865.

95. Perelman N, Selvaraj SK, Batra S, et al. Placenta growth factor activates monocytes and correlates with sickle cell disease severity. *Blood.* 2003;102:1506-1514.

96. Wang X, Mendelsohn L, Rogers H, et al. Heme-bound iron activates placenta growth factor in erythroid cells via erythroid Kruppel-like factor. *Blood.* 2014;124:946-954.

97. Hillery CA, Panepinto JA. Pathophysiology of stroke in sickle cell disease. *Microcirculation.* 2004;11:195-208.

98. Prengler M, Pavlakis SG, Prohovnik I, et al. Sickle cell disease: the neurological complications. *Ann Neurol.* 2002;51:543-552.

99. Granger DN, Korthuis RJ. Physiologic mechanisms of postischemic tissue injury. *Annu Rev Physiol.* 1995;57:311-332.

100. Grisham MB, Granger DN, Lefer DJ. Modulation of leukocyte-endothelial interactions by reactive metabolites of oxygen and nitrogen: relevance to ischemic heart disease. *Free Radic Biol Med.* 1998;25:404-433.

101. Field JJ, Nathan DG, Linden J. Targeting iNKT cells for the treatment of sickle cell disease. *Clin Immunol.* 2011;140:177-183.

102. Field JJ, Majerus E, Gordeuk VR, et al. Randomized phase 2 trial of regadenoson for treatment of acute vaso-occlusive crises in sickle cell disease. *Blood Adv.* 2017;1:1645-1649.

103. Eilertsen KE, Osterud B. Tissue factor: (patho)physiology and cellular biology. *Blood Coagul Fibrinolysis.* 2004;15:521-538.

104. Key NS, Slungaard A, Dandelet L, et al. Whole blood tissue factor procoagulant activity is elevated in patients with sickle cell disease. *Blood.* 1998;91:4216-4223.

105. Krishnaswamy S. The interaction of human factor VIIa with tissue factor. *J Biol Chem.* 1992;267:23696-23706.

106. Chantrathammachart P, Pawlinski R. Tissue factor and thrombin in sickle cell anemia. *Thromb Res.* 2012;129(suppl 2):S70-S72.

107. Shet AS, Aras O, Gupta K, et al. Sickle blood contains tissue factor-positive microparticles derived from endothelial cells and monocytes. *Blood.* 2003;102:2678-2683.

108. Faes C, Ilich A, Sotiaux A, et al. Red blood cells modulate structure and dynamics of venous clot formation in sickle cell disease. *Blood.* 2019;133:2529-2541.

109. Chantrathammachart P, Mackman N, Sparkenbaugh E, et al. Tissue factor promotes activation of coagulation and inflammation in a mouse model of sickle cell disease. *Blood.* 2012;120:636-646.

110. Brunetta DM, De Santis GC, Silva-Pinto AC, et al. Hydroxyurea increases plasma concentrations of microparticles and reduces coagulation activation and fibrinolysis in patients with sickle cell anemia. *Acta Haematol.* 2015;133:287-294.

111. Camus SM, De Moraes JA, Bonnin P, et al. Circulating cell membrane microparticles transfer heme to endothelial cells and trigger vasoocclusions in sickle cell disease. *Blood.* 2015;125:3805-3814.

112. Kurantsin-Mills J, Ofosu FA, Safa TK, et al. Plasma factor VII and thrombin-antithrombin III levels indicate increased tissue factor activity in sickle cell patients. *Br J Haematol.* 1992;81:539-544.

113. Tomer A, Harker LA, Kasey S, et al. Thrombogenesis in sickle cell disease. *J Lab Clin Med.* 2001;137:398-407.

114. Sparkenbaugh E, Pawlinski R. Interplay between coagulation and vascular inflammation in sickle cell disease. *Br J Haematol.* 2013;162:3-14.

115. Chen J, Hobbs WE, Le J, et al. The rate of hemolysis in sickle cell disease correlates with the quantity of active von Willebrand factor in the plasma. *Blood.* 2011;117:3680-3683.

116. Sins JWR, Schimmel M, Luken BM, et al. Dynamics of von Willebrand factor reactivity in sickle cell disease during vaso-occlusive crisis and steady state. *J Thromb Haemost.* 2017;15:1392-1402.

117. Field JJ, Nathan DG, Linden J. The role of adenosine signaling in sickle cell therapeutics. *Hematol Oncol Clin North Am.* 2014;28:287-299.

118. Ning C, Wen J, Zhang Y, et al. Excess adenosine A2B receptor signaling contributes to priapism through HIF-1alpha mediated reduction of PDE5 gene expression. *FASEB J.* 2014;28:2725-2735.

119. Zhang Y, Dai Y, Wen J, et al. Detrimental effects of adenosine signaling in sickle cell disease. *Nat Med.* 2011;17:79-86.

120. Zhang Y, Xia Y. Adenosine signaling in normal and sickle erythrocytes and beyond. *Microbes Infect.* 2012;14:863-873.

121. Tsaras G, Owusu-Ansah A, Boateng FO, et al. Complications associated with sickle cell trait: a brief narrative review. *Am J Med.* 2009;122:507-512.

122. Harris JW, Brewster HH, Ham TH, et al. Studies on the destruction of red blood cells. X. The biophysics and biology of sickle-cell disease. *AMA Arch Intern Med.* 1956;97:145-168.

123. Bergeron MF, Cannon JG, Hall EL, et al. Erythrocyte sickling during exercise and thermal stress. *Clin J Sport Med.* 2004;14:354-356.

124. Monchanin G, Serpero LD, Connes P, et al. Effects of progressive and maximal exercise on plasma levels of adhesion molecules in athletes with sickle cell trait with or without alpha-thalassemia. *J Appl Physiol.* 2007;102:169-173.

125. Weisman IM, Zeballos RJ, Johnson BD. Cardiopulmonary and gas exchange responses to acute strenuous exercise at 1,270 meters in sickle cell trait. *Am J Med.* 1988;84:377-383.

126. Key NS, Derebail VK. Sickle-cell trait: novel clinical significance. *Hematology Am Soc Hematol Educ Program.* 2010;2010:418-422.

127. Saxena P, Chavarria C, Thurlow J. Rhabdomyolysis in a sickle cell trait positive active duty male soldier. *U S Army Med Dep J.* 2016;20-23.

128. Murugappan KR, Cocchi MN, Bose S, et al. Case study: fatal exertional rhabdomyolysis possibly related to drastic weight cutting. *Int J Sport Nutr Exerc Metab.* 2018;1-4.

129. Maron BJ, Harris KM, Thompson PD, et al. Eligibility and disqualification recommendations for competitive athletes with cardiovascular abnormalities: Task Force 14: sickle cell trait: a scientific statement from the American Heart Association and American College of Cardiology. *Circulation.* 2015;132:e343-e345.

130. Hu J, Nelson DA, Deuster PA, et al. Sickle cell trait and renal disease among African American U.S. Army soldiers. *Br J Haematol.* 2019;185:532-540.

131. Caughey MC, Loehr LR, Key NS, et al. Sickle cell trait and incident ischemic stroke in the Atherosclerosis Risk in Communities study. *Stroke.* 2014;45:2863-2867.

132. Partington MD, Aronyk KE, Byrd SE. Sickle cell trait and stroke in children. *Pediatr Neurosurg.* 1994;20:148-151.

133. Gupta AK, Kirchner KA, Nicholson R, et al. Effects of alpha-thalassemia and sickle polymerization tendency on the urine-concentrating defect of individuals with sickle cell trait. *J Clin Invest.* 1991;88:1963-1968.

134. Alvarez O, Rodriguez MM, Jordan L, et al. Renal medullary carcinoma and sickle cell trait: a systematic review. *Pediatr Blood Cancer.* 2015;62:1694-1699.

135. Pastore LM, Savitz DA, Thorp JM Jr: Predictors of urinary tract infection at the first prenatal visit. *Epidemiology.* 1999;10:282-287.

136. Yium J, Gabow P, Johnson A, et al. Autosomal dominant polycystic kidney disease in blacks: clinical course and effects of sickle-cell hemoglobin. *J Am Soc Nephrol.* 1994;4:1670-1674.

137. Kumar R, Kapoor R, Singh J, et al. Splenic infarct on exposure to extreme high altitude in individuals with sickle trait: a single-center experience. *High Alt Med Biol.* 2019;20:215-220.

138. Hooper CY, Fraser-Bell S, Farinelli A, et al. Complicated hyphaema: think sickle. *Clin Exp Ophthalmol.* 2006;34:377-378.

139. Austin H, Key NS, Benson JM, et al. Sickle cell trait and the risk of venous thromboembolism among blacks. *Blood.* 2007;110:908-912.

140. Heller P, Best WR, Nelson RB, et al. Clinical implications of sickle-cell trait and glucose-6-phosphate dehydrogenase deficiency in hospitalized black male patients. *N Engl J Med.* 1979;300:1001-1005.

141. Castro O, Rana SR, Bang KM, et al. Age and prevalence of sickle-cell trait in a large ambulatory population. *Genet Epidemiol.* 1987;4:307-311.

142. Glader BE, Propper RD, Buchanan GR. Microcytosis associated with sickle cell anemia. *Am J Clin Pathol.* 1979;72:63-64.

143. Mohandas N, Johnson A, Wyatt J, et al. Automated quantitation of cell density distribution and hyperdense cell fraction in RBC disorders. *Blood.* 1989;74:442-447.

144. Sherwood JB, Goldwasser E, Chilcote R, et al. Sickle cell anemia patients have low erythropoietin levels for their degree of anemia. *Blood.* 1986;67:46-49.

145. Boggs DR, Hyde F, Srodes C. An unusual pattern of neutrophil kinetics in sickle cell anemia. *Blood.* 1973;41:59-65.

146. Buchanan GR, Glader BE. Leukocyte counts in children with sickle cell disease. Comparative values in the steady state, vaso-occlusive crisis, and bacterial infection. *Am J Dis Child.* 1978;132:396-398.

147. Zimmerman SA, Ware RE. Palpable splenomegaly in children with haemoglobin SC disease: haematological and clinical manifestations. *Clin Lab Haematol.* 2000;22:145-150.

148. Karayalcin G, Lanzkowsky P, Kazi AB. Zinc deficiency in children with sickle cell disease. *Am J Pediatr Hematol Oncol.* 1979;1:283-284.

149. Natta C, Machlin L. Plasma levels of tocopherol in sickle cell anemia subjects. *Am J Clin Nutr.* 1979;32:1359-1362.

150. Niell HB, Leach BE, Kraus AP. Zinc metabolism in sickle cell anemia. *JAMA.* 1979;242:2686-2687.

151. Drasar E, Vasavda N, Igbineweka N, et al. Serum ferritin and total units transfused for assessing iron overload in adults with sickle cell disease. *Br J Haematol.* 2012;157:645-647.

152. Takatsuki S, Ivy DD, Nuss R. Correlation of N-terminal fragment of B-type natriuretic peptide levels with clinical, laboratory, and echocardiographic abnormalities in children with sickle cell disease. *J Pediatr. Pediatrics.* 2012;160:428-433.e1.

153. Niss O, Fleck R, Makue F, et al. Association between diffuse myocardial fibrosis and diastolic dysfunction in sickle cell anemia. *Blood.* 2017;130:205-213.

154. Mario N, Baudin B, Aussel C, et al. Capillary isoelectric focusing and high-performance cation-exchange chromatography compared for qualitative and quantitative analysis of hemoglobin variants. *Clin Chem.* 1997;43:2137-2142.

155. Mukherjee MB, Colah RB, Mehta PR, et al. Multicenter evaluation of HemoTypeSC as a point-of-care sickle cell disease rapid diagnostic test for newborns and adults across India. *Am J Clin Pathol.* 2020;153:82-87.

156. Connes P, Alexy T, Detterich J, et al. The role of blood rheology in sickle cell disease. *Blood Rev.* 2016;30:111-118.

157. Nader E, Skinner S, Romana M, et al. Blood rheology: key parameters, impact on blood flow, role in sickle cell disease and effects of exercise. *Front Physiol.* 2019;10:e1329.

158. Baskurt OK, Meiselman HJ. Blood rheology and hemodynamics. *Semin Thromb Hemost.* 2003;29:435-450.

159. Li X, Du E, Lei H, et al. Patient-specific blood rheology in sickle-cell anaemia. *Interface Focus.* 2016;6:e20150065.

160. Renoux C, Romana M, Joly P, et al. Effect of age on blood rheology in sickle cell anaemia and sickle cell haemoglobin C disease: a cross-sectional study. *PLoS One.* 2016;11:e0158182.

161. Connes P, Lamarre Y, Hardy-Dessources MD, et al. Decreased hematocrit-to-viscosity ratio and increased lactate dehydrogenase level in patients with sickle cell anemia and recurrent leg ulcers. *PLoS One.* 2013;8:e79680.

162. Bartolucci P, Brugnara C, Teixeira-Pinto A, et al. Erythrocyte density in sickle cell syndromes is associated with specific clinical manifestations and hemolysis. *Blood.* 2012;120:3136-3141.

163. Hamideh D, Alvarez O. Sickle cell disease related mortality in the United States (1999-2009). *Pediatr Blood Cancer.* 2013;60:1482-1486.

164. Quinn CT, Rogers ZR, McCavit TL, et al. Improved survival of children and adolescents with sickle cell disease. *Blood.* 2010;115:3447-3452.

165. Platt OS, Brambilla DJ, Rosse WF, et al. Mortality in sickle cell disease. Life expectancy and risk factors for early death. *N Engl J Med.* 1994;330:1639-1644.

166. Maitra P, Caughey M, Robinson L, et al. Risk factors for mortality in adult patients with sickle cell disease: a meta-analysis of studies in North America and Europe. *Haematologica.* 2017;102:626-636.

167. DeBaun MR, Ghafuri DL, Rodeghier M, et al. Decreased median survival of adults with sickle cell disease after adjusting for left truncation bias: a pooled analysis. *Blood.* 2019;133:615-617.

168. Wierenga KJ, Hambleton R, Lewis NA. Survival estimates for patients with homozygous sickle cell disease in Jamaica: a clinic based population study. *Lancet.* 2001;357:680-683.

169. National Heart, Lung, and Blood Institute. *The Management of Sickle Cell Disease.* 4th ed. NIH Publication No. 02-2117. National Institutes of Health; 2002:59-74.

170. Liem R, Lanzkron S, Coates TD, et al. American Society of Hematology 2019 guidelines for sickle cell disease: cardiopulmonary and kidney disease. *Blood Adv.* 2019;3(23):3867-3897.

171. Murad MH, Liem RI, Lang ES, et al. 2019 sickle cell disease guidelines by the American Society of Hematology: methodology, challenges, and innovations. *Blood Adv.* 2019;3(23):3945-3950.

172. Chou ST, Alsawas M, Fasano RM, et al. American Society of Hematology 2020 guidelines for sickle cell disease: transfusion support. *Blood Adv.* 2020;4(2):327-355.

173. DeBaun MR, Jordan LC, King AA, et al. American Society of Hematology 2020 guidelines for sickle cell disease: prevention, diagnosis, and treatment of cerebrovascular disease in children and adults. *Blood Adv.* 2020;4(8):1554-1588.

174. Izcovich A, Cuker A, Kunkle R, et al. A user guide to the American Society of Hematology clinical practice guidelines. *Blood Adv.* 2020;4(9):2095-2110.

175. O'Neill D, Coakley D, Walsh JB, O'Neill J. HIV seropositivity in a geriatric medical unit. *Postgrad Med J.* 1988;64(756):832.

176. Yale SH, Nagib N, Guthrie T. Approach to the vaso-occlusive crisis in adults with sickle cell disease. *Am Fam Physician.* 2000;61:1349-1356, 1363-1364.

177. Ballas SK, Gupta K, Adams-Graves P. Sickle cell pain: a critical reappraisal. *Blood.* 2012;120:3647-3656.

178. Hankins JS, Penkert RR, Lavoie P, et al. Original research: parvovirus B19 infection in children with sickle cell disease in the hydroxyurea era. *Exp Biol Med (Maywood).* 2016;241:749-754.

179. Ballas SK, Kesen MR, Goldberg MF, et al. Beyond the definitions of the phenotypic complications of sickle cell disease: an update on management. *ScientificWorldJournal.* 2012;2012:949535.

180. Kinney TR, Ware RE, Schultz WH, et al. Long-term management of splenic sequestration in children with sickle cell disease. *J Pediatr.* 1990;117:194-199.

181. Solanki DL, Kletter GG, Castro O. Acute splenic sequestration crises in adults with sickle cell disease. *Am J Med.* 1986;80:985-990.

182. Bowcock SJ, Nwabueze ED, Cook AE, et al. Fatal splenic sequestration in adult sickle cell disease. *Clin Lab Haematol.* 1988;10:95-99.

183. Koduri PR, Agbemadzo B, Nathan S. Hemoglobin S-C disease revisited: clinical study of 106 adults. *Am J Hematol.* 2001;68:298-300.

184. Vichinsky E, Lubin BH. Suggested guidelines for the treatment of children with sickle cell anemia. *Hematol Oncol Clin North Am.* 1987;1:483-501.

185. de Montalembert M, Dumont MD, Heilbronner C, et al. Delayed hemolytic transfusion reaction in children with sickle cell disease. *Haematologica.* 2011;96:801-807.

186. Solomon LR. Treatment and prevention of pain due to vaso-occlusive crises in adults with sickle cell disease: an educational void. *Blood.* 2008;111:997-1003.

187. Grahmann PH, Jackson KC 2nd, Lipman AG. Clinician beliefs about opioid use and barriers in chronic nonmalignant pain. *J Pain Palliat Care Pharmacother.* 2004;18:7-28.

188. Labbe E, Herbert D, Haynes J. Physicians' attitude and practices in sickle cell disease pain management. *J Palliat Care.* 2005;21:246-251.

189. Elander J, Lusher J, Bevan D, et al. Understanding the causes of problematic pain management in sickle cell disease: evidence that pseudoaddiction plays a more important role than genuine analgesic dependence. *J Pain Symptom Manage.* 2004;27:156-169.

190. Ballas SK. Ethical issues in the management of sickle cell pain. *Am J Hematol.* 2001;68:127-132.

191. Aisiku IP, Smith WR, McClish DK, et al. Comparisons of high versus low emergency department utilizers in sickle cell disease. *Ann Emerg Med.* 2009;53:587-593.

192. McClish DK, Smith WR, Dahman BA, et al. Pain site frequency and location in sickle cell disease: the PiSCES project. *Pain.* 2009;145:246-251.

193. Dampier C, Ely E, Brodecki D, et al. Home management of pain in sickle cell disease: a daily diary study in children and adolescents. *J Pediatr Hematol Oncol.* 2002;24:643-647.

194. Han J, Saraf SL, Lash JP, et al. Use of anti-inflammatory analgesics in sickle-cell disease. *J Clin Pharm Ther.* 2017;42:656-660.

195. Rees DC, Olujohungbe AD, Parker NE, et al. Guidelines for the management of the acute painful crisis in sickle cell disease. *Br J Haematol.* 2003;120:744-752.

196. Benjamin L, Dampier CD, Jacox A, et al. *Guideline for the Management of Acute and Chronic Pain in Sickle Cell Disease.* American Pain Society; 1999.

197. Ballas SK. Meperidine for acute sickle cell pain in the emergency department: revisited controversy. *Ann Emerg Med.* 2008;51:217.

198. Howland MA, Goldfrank LR. Why meperidine should not make a comeback in treating patients with sickle cell disease. *Ann Emerg Med.* 2008;51:203-205.

199. Morgan MT. Use of meperidine as the analgesic of choice in treating pain from acute painful sickle cell crisis. *Ann Emerg Med.* 2008;51:202-203.

200. Arout CA, Edens E, Petrakis IL, et al. Targeting opioid-induced hyperalgesia in clinical treatment: neurobiological considerations. *CNS Drugs.* 2015;29:465-486.

201. Bannister K. Opioid-induced hyperalgesia: where are we now? *Curr Opin Support Palliat Care.* 2015;9:116-121.

202. Bantel C, Shah S, Nagy I. Painful to describe, painful to diagnose: opioid-induced hyperalgesia. *Br J Anaesth.* 2015;114:850-851.

203. Benjamin LJ, Swinson GI, Nagel RL. Sickle cell anemia day hospital: an approach for the management of uncomplicated painful crises. *Blood.* 2000;95:1130-1136.

204. Han J, Saraf SL, Kavoliunaite L, et al. Program expansion of a day hospital dedicated to manage sickle cell pain. *Am J Hematol.* 2018;93:E20-E21.

205. Platt OS, Thorington BD, Brambilla DJ, et al. Pain in sickle cell disease. Rates and risk factors. *N Engl J Med.* 1991;325:11-16.

206. Vichinsky EP, Johnson R, Lubin BH. Multidisciplinary approach to pain management in sickle cell disease. *Am J Pediatr Hematol Oncol.* 1982;4:328-333.

207. Styles LA, Vichinsky E. Effects of a long-term transfusion regimen on sickle cell-related illnesses. *J Pediatr.* 1994;125:909-911.

208. Brandow AM, Carroll CP, Creary S, et al. American Society of Hematology 2020 guidelines for sickle cell disease: management of acute and chronic pain. *Blood Adv.* 2020;4(12):2656-2701.

209. Gladwin MT, Vichinsky E. Pulmonary complications of sickle cell disease. *N Engl J Med.* 2008;359:2254-2265.

210. Vichinsky EP, Neumayr LD, Earles AN, et al. Causes and outcomes of the acute chest syndrome in sickle cell disease. National Acute Chest Syndrome Study Group. *N Engl J Med.* 2000;342:1855-1865.

211. Miller ST. How I treat acute chest syndrome in children with sickle cell disease. *Blood.* 2011;117:5297-5305.

212. Vichinsky EP, Neumayr LD, Gold JI, et al. Neuropsychological dysfunction and neuroimaging abnormalities in neurologically intact adults with sickle cell anemia. *JAMA.* 2010;303:1823-1831.

213. Emre U, Miller ST, Gutierez M, et al. Effect of transfusion in acute chest syndrome of sickle cell disease. *J Pediatr.* 1995;127:901-904.

214. Emre U, Miller ST, Rao SP, et al. Alveolar-arterial oxygen gradient in acute chest syndrome of sickle cell disease. *J Pediatr.* 1993;123:272-275.

215. Bellet PS, Kalinyak KA, Shukla R, et al. Incentive spirometry to prevent acute pulmonary complications in sickle cell diseases. *N Engl J Med.* 1995;333:699-703.

216. Uchida K, Rackoff WR, Ohene-Frempong K, et al. Effect of erythrocytapheresis on arterial oxygen saturation and hemoglobin oxygen affinity in patients with sickle cell disease. *Am J Hematol.* 1998;59:5-8.

217. Charache S, Terrin ML, Moore RD, et al. Effect of hydroxyurea on the frequency of painful crises in sickle cell anemia. Investigators of the Multicenter Study of Hydroxyurea in Sickle Cell Anemia. *N Engl J Med.* 1995;332:1317-1322.

218. Bernini JC, Rogers ZR, Sandler ES, et al. Beneficial effect of intravenous dexamethasone in children with mild to moderately severe acute chest syndrome complicating sickle cell disease. *Blood.* 1998;92:3082-3089.

219. Styles LA, Abboud M, Larkin S, et al. Transfusion prevents acute chest syndrome predicted by elevated secretory phospholipase A2. *Br J Haematol.* 2007;136:343-344.

220. Styles L, Wager CG, Labotka RJ, et al. Refining the value of secretory phospholipase A2 as a predictor of acute chest syndrome in sickle cell disease: results of a feasibility study (PROACTIVE). *Br J Haematol.* 2012;157:627-636.

221. Wang WC, Ware RE, Miller ST, et al. Hydroxycarbamide in very young children with sickle-cell anaemia: a multicentre, randomised, controlled trial (BABY HUG). *Lancet.* 2011;377:1663-1672.

222. McQuillan BM, Picard MH, Leavitt M, et al. Clinical correlates and reference intervals for pulmonary artery systolic pressure among echocardiographically normal subjects. *Circulation.* 2001;104:2797-2802.

223. Pyxaras SA, Pinamonti B, Barbati G, et al. Echocardiographic evaluation of systolic and mean pulmonary artery pressure in the follow-up of patients with pulmonary hypertension. *Eur J Echocardiogr.* 2011;12:696-701.

224. Klings ES, Machado RF, Barst RJ, et al. An official American Thoracic Society clinical practice guideline: diagnosis, risk stratification, and management of pulmonary hypertension of sickle cell disease. *Am J Respir Crit Care Med.* 2014;189:727-740.

225. Gordeuk VR, Castro OL, Machado RF. Pathophysiology and treatment of pulmonary hypertension in sickle cell disease. *Blood.* 2016;127:820-828.

226. Morris CR. Asthma management: reinventing the wheel in sickle cell disease. *Am J Hematol.* 2009;84:234-241.

227. Arteta M, Campbell A, Nouraie M, et al. Abnormal pulmonary function and associated risk factors in children and adolescents with sickle cell anemia. *J Pediatr Hematol Oncol.* 2014;36:185-189.

228. Klings ES, Wyszynski DF, Nolan VG, et al. Abnormal pulmonary function in adults with sickle cell anemia. *Am J Respir Crit Care Med.* 2006;173:1264-1269.

229. Newaskar M, Hardy KA, Morris CR. Asthma in sickle cell disease. *Scientific World Journal.* 2011;11:1138-1152.

230. Varat MA, Adolph RJ, Fowler NO. Cardiovascular effects of anemia. *Am Heart J.* 1972;83:415-426.

231. Balfour IC, Covitz W, Davis H, et al. Cardiac size and function in children with sickle cell anemia. *Am Heart J.* 1984;108:345-350.

232. Sachdev V, Machado RF, Shizukuda Y, et al. Diastolic dysfunction is an independent risk factor for death in patients with sickle cell disease. *J Am Coll Cardiol.* 2007;49:472-479.

233. Fitzhugh CD, Lauder N, Jonassaint JC, et al. Cardiopulmonary complications leading to premature deaths in adult patients with sickle cell disease. *Am J Hematol.* 2010;85:36-40.

234. Manci EA, Culberson DE, Yang YM, et al. Causes of death in sickle cell disease: an autopsy study. *Br J Haematol.* 2003;123:359-365.

235. Darbari DS, Kple-Faget P, Kwagyan J, et al. Circumstances of death in adult sickle cell disease patients. *Am J Hematol.* 2006;81:858-863.

236. Chacko P, Kraut EH, Zweier J, et al. Myocardial infarction in sickle cell disease: use of translational imaging to diagnose an under-recognized problem. *J Cardiovasc Transl Res.* 2013;6:752-761.

237. Voskaridou E, Christoulas D, Terpos E. Sickle-cell disease and the heart: review of the current literature. *Br J Haematol.* 2012;157:664-673.

238. Pegelow CH, Colangelo L, Steinberg M, et al. Natural history of blood pressure in sickle cell disease: risks for stroke and death associated with relative hypertension in sickle cell anemia. *Am J Med.J Med.* 1997;102:171-177.

239. Stockman JA, Nigro MA, Mishkin MM, et al. Occlusion of large cerebral vessels in sickle-cell anaemia. *N Engl J Med.* 1972;287:846-849.

240. Ohene-Frempong K, Weiner SJ, Sleeper LA, et al. Cerebrovascular accidents in sickle cell disease: rates and risk factors. *Blood.* 1998;91:288-294.

241. Steen RG, Xiong X, Langston JW, et al. Brain injury in children with sickle cell disease: prevalence and etiology. *Ann Neurol.* 2003;54:564-572.

242. Webb J, Kwiatkowski JL. Stroke in patients with sickle cell disease. *Expert Rev Hematol.* 2013;6:301-316.

243. Bernaudin F, Verlhac S, Arnaud C, et al. Impact of early transcranial Doppler screening and intensive therapy on cerebral vasculopathy outcome in a newborn sickle cell anemia cohort. *Blood.* 2011;117:1130-1140; quiz 1436.

244. DeBaun MR, Sarnaik SA, Rodeghier MJ, et al. Associated risk factors for silent cerebral infarcts in sickle cell anemia: low baseline hemoglobin, sex, and relative high systolic blood pressure. *Blood.* 2012;119:3684-3690.

245. Hulbert ML, McKinstry RC, Lacey JL, et al. Silent cerebral infarcts occur despite regular blood transfusion therapy after first strokes in children with sickle cell disease. *Blood.* 2011;117:772-779.

246. Prohovnik I, Pavlakis SG, Piomelli S, et al. Cerebral hyperemia, stroke, and transfusion in sickle cell disease. *Neurology.* 1989;39:344-348.

247. Wang WC. The pathophysiology, prevention, and treatment of stroke in sickle cell disease. *Curr Opin Hematol.* 2007;14:191-197.

248. Switzer JA, Hess DC, Nichols FT, et al. Pathophysiology and treatment of stroke in sickle-cell disease: present and future. *Lancet Neurol.* 2006;5:501-512.

249. Powars D, Adams RJ, Nichols FT, et al. Delayed intracranial hemorrhage following cerebral infarction in sickle cell anemia. *J Assoc Acad Minor Phys.* 1990;1:79-82.

250. Diggs LW, Brookoff D. Multiple cerebral aneurysms in patients with sickle cell disease. *South Med J.* 1993;86:377-379.

251. Anson JA, Koshy M, Ferguson L, et al. Subarachnoid hemorrhage in sickle-cell disease. *J Neurosurg.* 1991;75:552-558.

252. Oyesiku NM, Barrow DL, Eckman JR, et al. Intracranial aneurysms in sickle-cell anemia: clinical features and pathogenesis. *J Neurosurg.* 1991;75:356-363.

253. Preul MC, Cendes F, Just N, et al. Intracranial aneurysms and sickle cell anemia: multiplicity and propensity for the vertebrobasilar territory. *Neurosurgery.* 1998;42:971-977; discussion 977-978.

254. O'Driscoll S, Height SE, Dick MC, et al. Serum lactate dehydrogenase activity as a biomarker in children with sickle cell disease. *Br J Haematol.* 2008;140:206-209.

255. Miller ST, Macklin EA, Pegelow CH, et al. Silent infarction as a risk factor for overt stroke in children with sickle cell anemia: a report from the Cooperative Study of Sickle Cell Disease. *J Pediatr.* 2001;139:385-390.

256. Pegelow CH, Macklin EA, Moser FG, et al. Longitudinal changes in brain magnetic resonance imaging findings in children with sickle cell disease. *Blood.* 2002;99:3014-3018.

257. Kirkham FJ, Hewes DK, Prengler M, et al. Nocturnal hypoxaemia and central-nervous-system events in sickle-cell disease. *Lancet.* 2001;357:1656-1659.

258. Kinney TR, Sleeper LA, Wang WC, et al. Silent cerebral infarcts in sickle cell anemia: a risk factor analysis. The Cooperative Study of Sickle Cell Disease. *Pediatrics.* 1999;103:640-645.

259. Moser FG, Miller ST, Bello JA, et al. The spectrum of brain MR abnormalities in sickle-cell disease: a report from the Cooperative Study of Sickle Cell Disease. *AJNR Am J Neuroradiol.* 1996;17:965-972.

260. Strouse JJ, Hulbert ML, DeBaun MR, et al. Primary hemorrhagic stroke in children with sickle cell disease is associated with recent transfusion and use of corticosteroids. *Pediatrics.* 2006;118:1916-1924.

261. Adams RJ, Kutlar A, McKie V, et al. Alpha thalassemia and stroke risk in sickle cell anemia. *Am J Hematol.* 1994;45:279-282.

262. Adams R, McKie V, Nichols F, et al. The use of transcranial ultrasonography to predict stroke in sickle cell disease. *N Engl J Med.* 1992;326:605-610.

263. Hoppe C, Klitz W, D'Harlingue K, et al. Confirmation of an association between the TNF(-308) promoter polymorphism and stroke risk in children with sickle cell anemia. *Stroke.* 2007;38:2241-2246.

264. Belisario AR, Nogueira FL, Rodrigues RS, et al. Association of alpha-thalassemia, TNF-alpha (-308G>A) and VCAM-1 (c.1238G>C) gene polymorphisms with cerebrovascular disease in a newborn cohort of 411 children with sickle cell anemia. *Blood Cells Mol Dis.* 2015;54:44-50.

265. Flanagan JM, Sheehan V, Linder H, et al. Genetic mapping and exome sequencing identify 2 mutations associated with stroke protection in pediatric patients with sickle cell anemia. *Blood.* 2013;121:3237-3245.

266. Belisario AR, Sales RR, Toledo NE, et al. Association between ENPP1 K173Q and stroke in a newborn cohort of 395 Brazilian children with sickle cell anemia. *Blood.* 2015;126:1259-1260.

267. Berkelhammer LD, Williamson AL, Sanford SD, et al. Neurocognitive sequelae of pediatric sickle cell disease: a review of the literature. *Child Neuropsychol.* 2007;13:120-131.

268. Fullerton HJ, Gardner M, Adams RJ, et al. Obstacles to primary stroke prevention in children with sickle cell disease. *Neurology.* 2006;67:1098-1099.

269. Fullerton HJ, Adams RJ, Zhao S, et al. Declining stroke rates in Californian children with sickle cell disease. *Blood.* 2004;104:336-339.

270. Hulbert ML, Scothorn DJ, Panepinto JA, et al. Exchange blood transfusion compared with simple transfusion for first overt stroke is associated with a lower risk of subsequent stroke: a retrospective cohort study of 137 children with sickle cell anemia. *J Pediatr.* 2006;149:710-712.

271. Vichinsky EP, Haberkern CM, Neumayr L, et al. A comparison of conservative and aggressive transfusion regimens in the perioperative management of sickle cell disease. The Preoperative Transfusion in Sickle Cell Disease Study Group. *N Engl J Med.* 1995;333:206-213.

272. Zimmerman SA, Schultz WH, Burgett S, et al. Hydroxyurea therapy lowers transcranial Doppler flow velocities in children with sickle cell anemia. *Blood.* 2007;110:1043-1047.

273. Ware RE, Helms RW; SWiTCH Investigators. Stroke with Transfusions Changing to Hydroxyurea (SWiTCH). *Blood.* 2012;119:3925-3932.

274. Ware RE, Davis BR, Schultz WH, et al. Hydroxycarbamide versus chronic transfusion for maintenance of transcranial Doppler flow velocities in children with sickle cell anaemia—TCD With Transfusions Changing to Hydroxyurea (TWiTCH): a multicentre, open-label, phase 3, non-inferiority trial. *Lancet.* 2016;387:661-670.

275. Dobson SR, Holden KR, Nietert PJ, et al. Moyamoya syndrome in childhood sickle cell disease: a predictive factor for recurrent cerebrovascular events. *Blood.* 2002;99:3144-3150.

276. Hankinson TC, Bohman LE, Heyer G, et al. Surgical treatment of moyamoya syndrome in patients with sickle cell anemia: outcome following encephaloduroarteriosynangiosis. *J Neurosurg Pediatr.* 2008;1:211-216.

277. Nur E, Biemond BJ, Otten HM, et al. Oxidative stress in sickle cell disease; pathophysiology and potential implications for disease management. *Am J Hematol.* 2011;86:484-489.

278. Sklar AH, Campbell H, Caruana RJ, et al. A population study of renal function in sickle cell anemia. *Int J Artif Organs.* 1990;13:231-236.

279. Falk RJ, Scheinman J, Phillips G, et al. Prevalence and pathologic features of sickle cell nephropathy and response to inhibition of angiotensin-converting enzyme. *N Engl J Med.* 1992;326:910-915.

280. Guasch A, Navarrete J, Nass K, et al. Glomerular involvement in adults with sickle cell hemoglobinopathies: prevalence and clinical correlates of progressive renal failure. *J Am Soc Nephrol.* 2006;17:2228-2235.

281. Saraf SL, Zhang X, Kanias T, et al. Haemoglobinuria is associated with chronic kidney disease and its progression in patients with sickle cell anaemia. *Br J Haematol.* 2014;164:729-739.

282. Powars DR, Chan LS, Hiti A, et al. Outcome of sickle cell anemia: a 4-decade observational study of 1056 patients. *Medicine (Baltimore).* 2005;84:363-376.

283. Saraf S, Farooqui M, Infusino G, et al. Standard clinical practice underestimates the role and significance of erythropoietin deficiency in sickle cell disease. *Br J Haematol.* 2011;153:386-392.

284. Darbari DS, Wang Z, Kwak M, et al. Severe painful vaso-occlusive crises and mortality in a contemporary adult sickle cell anemia cohort study. *PLoS One.* 2013;8:e79923.

285. Powars DR, Elliott-Mills DD, Chan L, et al. Chronic renal failure in sickle cell disease: risk factors, clinical course, and mortality. *Ann Intern Med.* 1991;115:614-620.

286. Scheinman J. *Sickle Cell Nephropathy.* Williams & Wilkins; 1994:908-919.

287. Sharpe CC, Thein SL. Sickle cell nephropathy—a practical approach. *Br J Haematol.* 2011;155:287-297.

288. Huang SH, Sharma AP, Yasin A, et al. Hyperfiltration affects accuracy of creatinine eGFR measurement. *Clin J Am Soc Nephrol.* 2011;6:274-280.

289. McKie KT, Hanevold CD, Hernandez C, et al. Prevalence, prevention, and treatment of microalbuminuria and proteinuria in children with sickle cell disease. *J Pediatr Hematol Oncol.* 2007;29:140-144.

290. Day TG, Draşar ER, Fulford T, et al. Association between hemolysis and albuminuria in adults with sickle cell disease. *Haematologica.* 2012;97:201-205.

291. Maier-Redelsperger M, Levy P, Lionnet F, et al. Strong association between a new marker of hemolysis and glomerulopathy in sickle cell anemia. *Blood Cells Mol Dis.* 2010;45:289-292.

292. Bolarinwa RA, Akinlade KS, Kuti MA, et al. Renal disease in adult Nigerians with sickle cell anemia: a report of prevalence, clinical features and risk factors. *Saudi J Kidney Dis Transpl.* 2012;23:171-175.

293. Aleem A. Renal abnormalities in patients with sickle cell disease: a single center report from Saudi Arabia. *Saudi J Kidney Dis Transpl.* 2008;19:194-199.

294. Saraf SL, Zhang X, Shah B, et al. Genetic variants and cell-free hemoglobin processing in sickle cell nephropathy. *Haematologica.* 2015;100:1275-1284.

295. Kanso AA, Hassan NMA, Badr KF. Microvascular and macrovascular diseases of the kidney. In: Brenner BM, ed. *Brenner and Rector's The Kidney.* 8th ed. Saunders; 2007:1147-1173.

296. Yee ME, Lane PA, Archer DR, et al. Losartan therapy decreases albuminuria with stable glomerular filtration and permselectivity in sickle cell anemia. *Blood Cells Mol Dis.* 2018;69:65-70.

297. Tharaux PL. Endothelin in renal injury due to sickle cell disease. *Contrib Nephrol.* 2011;172:185-199.

298. Heimlich JB, Speed JS, O'Connor PM, et al. Endothelin-1 contributes to the progression of renal injury in sickle cell disease via reactive oxygen species. *Br J Pharmacol.* 2016;173:386-395.

299. Kasztan M, Fox BM, Speed JS, et al. Long-term endothelin-a receptor antagonism provides robust renal protection in humanized sickle cell disease mice. *J Am Soc Nephrol.* 2017;28:2443-2458.

300. Mantadakis E, Cavender JD, Rogers ZR, et al. Prevalence of priapism in children and adolescents with sickle cell anemia. *J Pediatr Hematol Oncol.* 1999;21:518-522.

301. Fowler JE Jr, Koshy M, Strub M, et al. Priapism associated with the sickle cell hemoglobinopathies: prevalence, natural history and sequelae. *J Urol.* 1991;145:65-68.

302. Emond AM, Holman R, Hayes RJ, et al. Priapism and impotence in homozygous sickle cell disease. *Arch Intern Med.* 1980;140:1434-1437.

303. Adeyoju AB, Olujohungbe AB, Morris J, et al. Priapism in sickle-cell disease; incidence, risk factors and complications-an international multicentre study. *BJU Int.* 2002;90:898-902.

304. Olujohungbe A, Burnett AL. How I manage priapism due to sickle cell disease. *Br J Haematol.* 2013;160:754-765.

305. Olujohungbe AB, Adeyoju A, Yardumian A, et al. A prospective diary study of stuttering priapism in adolescents and young men with sickle cell anemia: report of an international randomized control trial—the priapism in sickle cell study. *J Androl.* 2011;32:375-382.

306. Siegel JF, Rich MA, Brock WA. Association of sickle cell disease, priapism, exchange transfusion and neurological events: ASPEN syndrome. *J Urol.* 1993;150:1480-1482.

307. Field JJ, Austin PF, An P, et al. Enuresis is a common and persistent problem among children and young adults with sickle cell anemia. *Urology.* 2008;72:81-84.

308. Jordan SS, Hilker KA, Stoppelbein L, et al. Nocturnal enuresis and psychosocial problems in pediatric sickle cell disease and sibling controls. *J Dev Behav Pediatr.* 2005;26:404-411.

309. Barakat LP, Smith-Whitley K, Schulman S, et al. Nocturnal enuresis in pediatric sickle cell disease. *J Dev Behav Pediatr.* 2001;22:300-305.

310. Almeida A, Roberts I. Bone involvement in sickle cell disease. *Br J Haematol.* 2005;129:482-490.

311. Kim SK, Miller JH. Natural history and distribution of bone and bone marrow infarction in sickle hemoglobinopathies. *J Nucl Med.* 2002;43:896-900.

312. Smith J. Bone disorders in sickle cell disease. *Hematol Oncol Clin North Am.* 1996;10:1345-1356.

313. Lonergan GJ, Cline DB, Abbondanzo SL. Sickle cell anemia. *Radiographics.* 2001;21:971-994.

314. Atkins BL, Price EH, Tillyer L, et al. Salmonella osteomyelitis in sickle cell disease children in the east end of London. *J Infect.* 1997;34:133-138.

315. Burnett MW, Bass JW, Cook BA. Etiology of osteomyelitis complicating sickle cell disease. *Pediatrics.* 1998;101:296-297.

316. William R, Hussein SS, Jeans WD, et al. A prospective study of soft-tissue ultrasonography in sickle cell disease patients with suspected osteomyelitis. *Clin Radiol.* 2000;55:307-310.

317. Umans H, Haramati, N, Flusser, G. The diagnostic role of gadolinium enhanced MRI in distinguishing between acute medullary bone infarct and osteomyelitis. *Magn Reson Imaging.* 2000;18:255-262.

318. Neonato M, Guilloud-Bataille M, Beauvais P, et al. Acute clinical events in 299 homozygous sickle cell patients living in France. French study group on sickle cell disease. *Eur J Haematol.* 2000;65:155-164.

319. Guggenbuhl P, Fergelot P, Doyard M, et al. Bone status in a mouse model of genetic hemochromatosis. *Osteoporos Int.* 2011;22:2313-2319.

320. Tsay J, Yang Z, Ross FP, et al. Bone loss caused by iron overload in a murine model: importance of oxidative stress. *Blood.* 2010;116:2582-2589.

321. Fung EB, Harmatz PR, Milet M, et al. Fracture prevalence and relationship to endocrinopathy in iron overloaded patients with sickle cell disease and thalassemia. *Bone.* 2008;43:162-168.

322. Osunkwo I, Ziegler TR, Alvarez J, et al. High dose vitamin D therapy for chronic pain in children and adolescents with sickle cell disease: results of a randomized double blind pilot study. *Br J Haematol.* 2012;159:211-215.

323. Dougherty KA, Bertolaso C, Schall JI, et al. Safety and efficacy of high-dose daily vitamin D3 supplementation in children and young adults with sickle cell disease. *J Pediatr Hematol Oncol.* 2015;37:e308-e315.

324. Milner P, Kraus, AP, Sebes, JJ, et al. Sickle cell disease as a cause of osteonecrosis of the femoral head. *N Engl J Med.* 1991;325:1479-1481.

325. Ware H, Brooks AP, Toye R, Berney SI. Sickle cell disease and silent avascular necrosis of the hip. *J Bone Joint Surg Br.* 1991;73:947-949.

326. Adekile AD, Gupta R, Yacoub F, et al. Avascular necrosis of the hip in children with sickle cell disease and high Hb F: magnetic resonance imaging findings and influence of alpha-thalassemia trait. *Acta Haematol.* 2001;105:27-31.

327. Mahadeo KM, Oyeku S, Taragin B, et al. Increased prevalence of osteonecrosis of the femoral head in children and adolescents with sickle-cell disease. *Am J Hematol.* 2011;86:806-808.

328. Akinyoola AL, Adediran IA, Asaleye CM, et al. Risk factors for osteonecrosis of the femoral head in patients with sickle cell disease. *Int Orthop.* 2009;33:923-926.

329. Baldwin C, Nolan VG, Wyszynski DF, et al. Association of klotho, bone morphogenic protein 6, and annexin A2 polymorphisms with sickle cell osteonecrosis. *Blood.* 2005;106:372-375.

330. Zhang X, Shah BN, Zhang W, et al. S100B has pleiotropic effects on vaso-occlusive manifestations in sickle cell disease. *Am J Hematol.* 2020;95:E62-E65.

331. Vicari P, Adegoke SA, Mazzotti DR, et al. Interleukin-1beta and interleukin-6 gene polymorphisms are associated with manifestations of sickle cell anemia. *Blood Cells Mol Dis.* 2015;54:244-249.

332. Hernigou P, Bachir D, Galacteros F. The natural history of symptomatic osteonecrosis in adults with sickle-cell disease. *J Bone Joint Surg Am.* 2003;85:500-504.

333. Hernigou P, Habibi A, Bachir D, et al. The natural history of asymptomatic osteonecrosis of the femoral head in adults with sickle cell disease. *J Bone Joint Surg Am.* 2006;88:2565-2572.

334. Itzep NP, Jadhav SP, Kanne CK, et al. Spontaneous healing of avascular necrosis of the femoral head in sickle cell disease. *Am J Hematol.* 2019;94:E160-E162.

335. Neumayr LD, Aguilar C, Earles AN, et al. Physical therapy alone compared with core decompression and physical therapy for femoral head osteonecrosis in sickle cell disease. Results of a multicenter study at a mean of three years after treatment. *J Bone Joint Surg Am.* 2006;88:2573-2582.

336. Hernigou P, Zilber S, Filippini P, et al. Total THA in adult osteonecrosis related to sickle cell disease. *Clin Orthop Relat Res.* 2008;466:300-308.

337. Moran MC, Huo MH, Garvin KL, et al. Total hip arthroplasty in sickle cell hemoglobinopathy. *Clin Orthop Relat Res.* 1993;140-148.

338. Acurio MT, Friedman RJ. Hip arthroplasty in patients with sickle-cell haemoglobinopathy. *J Bone Joint Surg Br.* 1992;74:367-371.

339. Adesina OO, Neumayr LD. Osteonecrosis in sickle cell disease: an update on risk factors, diagnosis, and management. *Hematology Am Soc Hematol Educ Program.* 2019;2019:351-358.

340. Nolan VG, Adewoye A, Baldwin C, et al. Sickle cell leg ulcers: associations with haemolysis and SNPs in Klotho, TEK and genes of the TGF-beta/BMP pathway. *Br J Haematol.* 2006;133:570-578.

341. Koshy M, Entsuah R, Koranda A, et al. Leg ulcers in patients with sickle cell disease. *Blood.* 1989;74:1403-1408.

342. Best PJ, Daoud MS, Pittelkow MR, et al. Hydroxyurea-induced leg ulceration in 14 patients. *Ann Intern Med.* 1998;128:29-32.

343. Halabi-Tawil M, Lionnet F, Girot R, et al. Sickle cell leg ulcers: a frequently disabling complication and a marker of severity. *Br J Dermatol.* 2008;158:339-344.

344. Wethers DL, Ramirez GM, Koshy M, et al. Accelerated healing of chronic sickle-cell leg ulcers treated with RGD peptide matrix. RGD Study Group. *Blood.* 1994;84:1775-1779.

345. Sher GD, Olivieri NF. Rapid healing of chronic leg ulcers during arginine butyrate therapy in patients with sickle cell disease and thalassemia. *Blood.* 1994;84:2378-2380.

346. Traina F, Jorge SG, Yamanaka A, et al. Chronic liver abnormalities in sickle cell disease: a clinicopathological study in 70 living patients. *Acta Haematol.* 2007;118:129-135.

347. Banerjee S, Owen C, Chopra S. Sickle cell hepatopathy. *Hepatology.* 2001;33:1021-1028.

348. West MS, Wethers D, Smith J, et al. Laboratory profile of sickle cell disease: a cross-sectional analysis. The Cooperative Study of Sickle Cell Disease. *J Clin Epidemiol.* 1992;45:893-909.

349. Koskinas J, Manesis EK, Zacharakis GH, et al. Liver involvement in acute vaso-occlusive crisis of sickle cell disease: prevalence and predisposing factors. *Scand J Gastroenterol.* 2007;42:499-507.

350. Buchanan GR, Glader BE. Benign course of extreme hyperbilirubinemia in sickle cell anemia: analysis of six cases. *J Pediatr.* 1977;91:21-24.

351. Johnson CS, Omata M, Tong MJ, et al. Liver involvement in sickle cell disease. *Medicine (Baltimore).* 1985;64:349-356.

352. Shao SH, Orringer EP. Sickle cell intrahepatic cholestasis: approach to a difficult problem. *Am J Gastroenterol.* 1995;90:2048-2050.

353. Ahn H, Li CS, Wang W. Sickle cell hepatopathy: clinical presentation, treatment, and outcome in pediatric and adult patients. *Pediatr Blood Cancer.* 2005;45:184-190.

354. Sheehy TW. Sickle cell hepatopathy. *South Med J.* 1977;70:533-538.

355. Schubert TT. Hepatobiliary system in sickle cell disease. *Gastroenterology.* 1986;90:2013-2021.

356. Suell MN, Horton TM, Dishop MK, et al. Outcomes for children with gallbladder abnormalities and sickle cell disease. *J Pediatr.* 2004;145:617-621.

357. Rennels MB, Dunne MG, Grossman NJ, et al. Cholelithiasis in patients with major sickle hemoglobinopathies. *Am J Dis Child.* 1984;138:66-67.

358. Bond LR, Hatty SR, Horn ME, et al. Gall stones in sickle cell disease in the United Kingdom. *Br Med J (Clin Res Ed).* 1987;295:234-236.

359. Vasavda N, Menzel S, Kondaveeti S, et al. The linear effects of alpha-thalassaemia, the UGT1A1 and HMOX1 polymorphisms on cholelithiasis in sickle cell disease. *Br J Haematol.* 2007;138:263-270.

360. To KW, Nadel AJ. Ophthalmologic complications in hemoglobinopathies. *Hematol Oncol Clin North Am.* 1991;5:535-548.

361. Mohan JS, Lip PL, Blann AD, et al. The angiopoietin/Tie-2 system in proliferative sickle retinopathy: relation to vascular endothelial growth factor, its soluble receptor Flt-1 and von Willebrand factor, and to the effects of laser treatment. *Br J Ophthalmol.* 2005;89:815-819.

362. Aiello LP, Avery RL, Arrigg PG, et al. Vascular endothelial growth factor in ocular fluid of patients with diabetic retinopathy and other retinal disorders. *N Engl J Med.* 1994;331:1480-1487.

363. Aiello LP, Northrup JM, Keyt BA, et al. Hypoxic regulation of vascular endothelial growth factor in retinal cells. *Arch Ophthal.* 1995;113:1538-1544.

364. Downes SM, Hambleton IR, Chuang EL, et al. Incidence and natural history of proliferative sickle cell retinopathy: observations from a cohort study. *Ophthalmology.* 2005;112:1869-1875.

365. Condon PI, Serjeant GR. Behaviour of untreated proliferative sickle retinopathy. *Br J Ophthalmol.* 1980;64:404-411.

366. Liem RI, Calamaras DM, Chhabra MS, et al. Sudden-onset blindness in sickle cell disease due to retinal artery occlusion. *Pediatr Blood Cancer.* 2008;50:624-627.

367. Paton D. The conjunctival sign of sickle-cell disease. *Arch Ophthal.* 1961;66:90-94.

368. Paton D. The conjunctival sign ox sickle-cell disease. Further observations. *Arch Ophthal.* 1962;68:627-632.

369. Cheung AT, Chen PC, Larkin EC, et al. Microvascular abnormalities in sickle cell disease: a computer-assisted intravital microscopy study. *Blood.* 2002;99:3999-4005.

370. Knisely MH, Bloch EH, Eliot TS, et al. Sludged blood. *Science.* 1947;106:431-440.

371. Curran EL, Fleming JC, Rice K, et al. Orbital compression syndrome in sickle cell disease. *Ophthalmology.* 1997;104:1610-1615.

372. Sayag D, Binaghi M, Souied EH, et al. Retinal photocoagulation for proliferative sickle cell retinopathy: a prospective clinical trial with new sea fan classification. *Eur J Ophthalmol.* 2008;18:248-254.

373. Fox PD, Minninger K, Forshaw ML, et al. Laser photocoagulation for proliferative retinopathy in sickle haemoglobin C disease. *Eye (Lond).* 1993;7(pt 5):703-706.

374. Fox PD, Vessey SJ, Forshaw ML, et al. Influence of genotype on the natural history of untreated proliferative sickle retinopathy—an angiographic study. *Br J Ophthalmol.* 1991;75:229-231.

375. Rogers ZR, Wang WC, Luo Z, et al. Biomarkers of splenic function in infants with sickle cell anemia: baseline data from the BABY HUG Trial. *Blood.* 2011;117:2614-2617.

376. Brousse V, Buffet P, Rees D. The spleen and sickle cell disease: the sick(led) spleen. *Br J Haematol.* 2014;166:165-176.

377. Pearson HA, Spencer RP, Cornelius EA. Functional asplenia in sickle-cell anemia. *N Engl J Med.* 1969;281:923-926.

378. Ferster A, Bujan W, Corazza F, et al. Bone marrow transplantation corrects the splenic reticuloendothelial dysfunction in sickle cell anemia. *Blood.* 1993;81:1102-1105.

379. Buchanan GR, McKie V, Jackson EA, et al. Splenic phagocytic function in children with sickle cell anemia receiving long-term hypertransfusion therapy. *J Pediatr.* 1989;115:568-572.

380. Claster S, Vichinsky E. First report of reversal of organ dysfunction in sickle cell anemia by the use of hydroxyurea: splenic regeneration. *Blood.* 1996;88:1951-1953.

381. Naik RP, Lanzkron S. Baby on board: what you need to know about pregnancy in the hemoglobinopathies. *Hematology Am Soc Hematol Educ Program.* 2012;2012:208-214.

382. Sun PM, Wilburn W, Raynor BD, et al. Sickle cell disease in pregnancy: twenty years of experience at Grady Memorial Hospital, Atlanta, Georgia. *Am J Obstet Gynecol.* 2001;184:1127-1130.

383. Boulet SL, Okoroh EM, Azonobi I, et al. Sickle cell disease in pregnancy: maternal complications in a Medicaid-enrolled population. *Matern Child Health J.* 2013;17:200-207.

384. Villers MS, Jamison MG, De Castro LM, et al. Morbidity associated with sickle cell disease in pregnancy. *Am J Obstet Gynecol.* 2008;199:125.e1-e5.

385. James AH, Jamison MG, Brancazio LR, et al. Venous thromboembolism during pregnancy and the postpartum period: incidence, risk factors, and mortality. *Am J Obstet Gynecol.* 2006;194:1311-1315.

386. Malinowski AK, Shehata N, D'Souza R, et al. Prophylactic transfusion for pregnant women with sickle cell disease: a systematic review and meta-analysis. *Blood.* 2015;126:2424-2435; quiz 2437.

387. Wilson JG, Scott WJ, Ritter EJ, et al. Comparative distribution and embryotoxicity of hydroxyurea in pregnant rats and rhesus monkeys. *Teratology.* 1975;11:169-178.

388. Thauvin-Robinet C, Maingueneau C, Robert E, et al. Exposure to hydroxyurea during pregnancy: a case series. *Leukemia.* 2001;15:1309-1311.

389. Berthaut I, Bachir D, Kotti S, et al. Adverse effect of hydroxyurea on spermatogenesis in patients with sickle cell anemia after 6 months of treatment. *Blood.* 2017;130:2354-2356.

390. Austin H, Lally C, Benson JM, et al. Hormonal contraception, sickle cell trait, and risk for venous thromboembolism among African American women. *Am J Obstet Gynecol.* 2009;200:620.e1-e3.

391. Noubouossie D, Key NS. Sickle cell disease and venous thromboembolism in pregnancy and the puerperium. *Thromb Res.* 2015;135(suppl 1):S46-S48.

392. Zarrouk V, Habibi A, Zahar JR, et al. Bloodstream infection in adults with sickle cell disease: association with venous catheters, *Staphylococcus aureus*, and bone-joint infections. *Medicine (Baltimore).* 2006;85:43-48.

393. Mollapour E, Porter JB, Kaczmarski R, et al. Raised neutrophil phospholipase A2 activity and defective priming of NADPH oxidase and phospholipase A2 in sickle cell disease. *Blood.* 1998;91:3423-3429.

394. Overturf GD. Infections and immunizations of children with sickle cell disease. *Adv Pediatr Infect Dis.* 1999;14:191-218.

395. Sullivan JL, Ochs HD, Schiffman G, et al. Immune response after splenectomy. *Lancet.* 1978;1:178-181.

396. Barrett-Connor E. Bacterial infection and sickle cell anemia. An analysis of 250 infections in 166 patients and a review of the literature. *Medicine (Baltimore).* 1971;50:97-112.

397. Zarkowsky HS, Gallagher D, Gill FM, et al. Bacteremia in sickle hemoglobinopathies. *J Pediatr.* 1986;109:579-585.

398. Leikin SL, Gallagher D, Kinney TR, et al. Mortality in children and adolescents with sickle cell disease. Cooperative Study of Sickle Cell Disease. *Pediatrics.* 1989;84:500-508.

399. Adamkiewicz TV, Sarnaik S, Buchanan GR, et al. Invasive pneumococcal infections in children with sickle cell disease in the era of penicillin prophylaxis, antibiotic resistance, and 23-valent pneumococcal polysaccharide vaccination. *J Pediatr.* 2003;143:438-444.

400. Gaston MH, Verter JI, Woods G, et al. Prophylaxis with oral penicillin in children with sickle cell anemia. A randomized trial. *N Engl J Med.* 1986;314:1593-1599.

401. Halasa NB, Shankar SM, Talbot TR, et al. Incidence of invasive pneumococcal disease among individuals with sickle cell disease before and after the introduction of the pneumococcal conjugate vaccine. *Clin Infect Dis.* 2007;44:1428-1433.

402. Kyaw MH, Lynfield R, Schaffner W, et al. Effect of introduction of the pneumococcal conjugate vaccine on drug-resistant *Streptococcus pneumoniae*. *N Engl J Med.* 2006;354:1455-1463.

403. Health supervision for children with sickle cell disease. *Pediatrics.* 2002;109:526-535.

404. Adamkiewicz TV, Silk BJ, Howgate J, et al. Effectiveness of the 7-valent pneumococcal conjugate vaccine in children with sickle cell disease in the first decade of life. *Pediatrics.* 2008;121:562-569.

405. McCavit TL, Quinn CT, Techasaensiri C, et al. Increase in invasive *Streptococcus pneumoniae* in children with sickle cell disease since pneumococcal conjugate vaccine licensure. *J Pediatr.* 2011;158:505-507.

406. Falletta JM, Woods GM, Verter JI, et al. Discontinuing penicillin prophylaxis in children with sickle cell anemia. Prophylactic Penicillin Study II. *J Pediatr.* 1995;127:685-690.

407. Rice TW, Rubinson L, Uyeki TM, et al. Critical illness from 2009 pandemic influenza A virus and bacterial coinfection in the United States. *Crit Care Med.* 2012;40:1487-1498.

408. Neumayr L, Lennette E, Kelly D, et al. Mycoplasma disease and acute chest syndrome in sickle cell disease. *Pediatrics.* 2003;112:87-95.

409. Dean D, Neumayr L, Kelly DM, et al. *Chlamydia pneumoniae* and acute chest syndrome in patients with sickle cell disease. *J Pediatr Hematol Oncol.* 2003;25:46-55.

410. Claudio AM, Foltanski L, Delay T, et al. Antibiotic use and respiratory pathogens in adults with sickle cell disease and acute chest syndrome. *Ann Pharmacother.* 2019;53:991-996.

411. Makani J, Komba AN, Cox SE, et al. Malaria in patients with sickle cell anemia: burden, risk factors, and outcome at the outpatient clinic and during hospitalization. *Blood.* 2010;115:215-220.

412. McAuley CF, Webb C, Makani J, et al. High mortality from *Plasmodium falciparum* malaria in children living with sickle cell anemia on the coast of Kenya. *Blood.* 2010;116:1663-1668.

413. Koshy M, Weiner SJ, Miller ST, et al. Surgery and anesthesia in sickle cell disease. Cooperative Study of Sickle Cell Diseases. *Blood.* 1995;86:3676-3684.

414. Firth PG, Head CA. Sickle cell disease and anesthesia. *Anesthesiology.* 2004;101:766-785.

415. Griffin TC, Buchanan GR. Elective surgery in children with sickle cell disease without preoperative blood transfusion. *J Pediatr Surg.* 1993;28:681-685.

416. Howard J, Malfroy M, Llewelyn C, et al. The Transfusion Alternatives Preoperatively in Sickle Cell Disease (TAPS) study: a randomised, controlled, multicentre clinical trial. *Lancet.* 2013;381:930-938.

417. Kutlar A. Sickle cell disease: a multigenic perspective of a single gene disorder. *Hemoglobin.* 2007;31:209-224.

418. Steinberg MH. Predicting clinical severity in sickle cell anaemia. *Br J Haematol.* 2005;129:465-481.

419. Sankaran VG. Targeted therapeutic strategies for fetal hemoglobin induction. *Hematology Am Soc Hematol Educ Program.* 2011;2011:459-465.

420. Zhou D, Liu K, Sun CW, et al. KLF1 regulates BCL11A expression and gamma- to beta-globin gene switching. *Nat Genet.* 2010;42:742-744.

421. Hoppe C, Klitz W, Cheng S, et al. Gene interactions and stroke risk in children with sickle cell anemia. *Blood.* 2004;103:2391-2396.

422. Sebastiani P, Ramoni MF, Nolan V, et al. Genetic dissection and prognostic modeling of overt stroke in sickle cell anemia. *Nat Genet.* 2005;37:435-440.

423. Taylor JGt, Tang DC, Savage SA, et al. Variants in the VCAM1 gene and risk for symptomatic stroke in sickle cell disease. *Blood.* 2002;100:4303-4309.

424. Sharan K, Surrey S, Ballas S, et al. Association of T-786C eNOS gene polymorphism with increased susceptibility to acute chest syndrome in females with sickle cell disease. *Br J Haematol.* 2004;124:240-243.

425. Adekile A, Kutlar F, McKie K, et al. The influence of uridine diphosphate glucuronosyl transferase 1A promoter polymorphisms, beta-globin gene haplotype, co-inherited alpha-thalassemia trait and Hb F on steady-state serum bilirubin levels in sickle cell anemia. *Eur J Haematol.* 2005;75:150-155.

426. Fertrin KY, Melo MB, Assis AM, et al. UDP-glucuronosyltransferase 1 gene promoter polymorphism is associated with increased serum bilirubin levels and cholecystectomy in patients with sickle cell anemia. *Clin Genet.* 2003;64:160-162.

427. Haverfield EV, McKenzie CA, Forrester T, et al. UGT1A1 variation and gallstone formation in sickle cell disease. *Blood.* 2005;105:968-972.

428. Passon RG, Howard TA, Zimmerman SA, et al. Influence of bilirubin uridine diphosphate-glucuronosyltransferase 1A promoter polymorphisms on serum bilirubin levels and cholelithiasis in children with sickle cell anemia. *J Pediatr Hematol Oncol.* 2001;23:448-451.

429. Nolan VG, Baldwin C, Ma Q, et al. Association of single nucleotide polymorphisms in klotho with priapism in sickle cell anaemia. *Br J Haematol.* 2005;128:266-272.

430. Close J, Game L, Clark B, et al. Genome annotation of a 1.5 Mb region of human chromosome 6q23 encompassing a quantitative trait locus for fetal hemoglobin expression in adults. *BMC Genomics.* 2004;5:33.

431. Garner CP, Tatu T, Best S, et al. Evidence of genetic interaction between the beta-globin complex and chromosome 8q in the expression of fetal hemoglobin. *Am J Hum Genet.* 2002;70:793-799.

432. Lettre G, Sankaran VG, Bezerra MA, et al. DNA polymorphisms at the BCL11A, HBS1L-MYB, and beta-globin loci associate with fetal hemoglobin levels and pain crises in sickle cell disease. *Proc Natl Acad Sci U S A.* 2008;105:11869-11874.

433. Thein SL, Menzel S. Discovering the genetics underlying foetal haemoglobin production in adults. *Br J Haematol.* 2009;145:455-467.

434. Uda M, Galanello R, Sanna S, et al. Genome-wide association study shows BCL11A associated with persistent fetal hemoglobin and amelioration of the phenotype of beta-thalassemia. *Proc Natl Acad Sci U S A.* 2008;105:1620-1625.

435. Wyszynski DF, Baldwin CT, Cleves MA, et al. Polymorphisms near a chromosome 6q QTL area are associated with modulation of fetal hemoglobin levels in sickle cell anemia. *Cell Mol Biol (Noisy-le-grand).* 2004;50:23-33.

436. Ma Q, Wyszynski DF, Farrell JJ, Kutlar A, et al. Fetal hemoglobin in sickle cell anemia: genetic determinants of response to hydroxyurea. *Pharmacogenomics J.* 2007 Dec;7(6):386-94. doi: 10.1038/sj.tpj.6500433. Epub 2007 Feb 13.

437. Lettre G, Bauer DE. Fetal haemoglobin in sickle-cell disease: from genetic epidemiology to new therapeutic strategies. *Lancet.* 2016;387:2554-2564.

438. Fertrin KY, Costa FF. Genomic polymorphisms in sickle cell disease: implications for clinical diversity and treatment. *Expert Rev Hematol.* 2010;3:443-458.

439. Watson J. The significance of the paucity of sickle cells in newborn Negro infants. *Am J Med Sci.* 1948;215:419-423.

440. Pembrey ME, Wood WG, Weatherall DJ, et al. Fetal haemoglobin production and the sickle gene in the oases of Eastern Saudi Arabia. *Br J Haematol.* 1978;40:415-429.

441. Platt OS. Hydroxyurea for the treatment of sickle cell anemia. *N Engl J Med.* 2008;358:1362-1369.

442. Gladwin MT, Shelhamer JH, Ognibene FP, et al. Nitric oxide donor properties of hydroxyurea in patients with sickle cell disease. *Br J Haematol.* 2002;116:436-444.

443. Hillery CA, Du MC, Wang WC, et al. Hydroxyurea therapy decreases the in vitro adhesion of sickle erythrocytes to thrombospondin and laminin. *Br J Haematol.* 2000;109:322-327.

444. Orringer EP, Blythe DS, Johnson AE, et al. Effects of hydroxyurea on hemoglobin F and water content in the red blood cells of dogs and of patients with sickle cell anemia. *Blood.* 1991;78:212-216.

445. Steinberg MH, Barton F, Castro O, et al. Effect of hydroxyurea on mortality and morbidity in adult sickle cell anemia: risks and benefits up to 9 years of treatment. *JAMA.* 2003;289:1645-1651.

446. Ware RE. How I use hydroxyurea to treat young patients with sickle cell anemia. *Blood.* 2010;115:5300-5311.

447. Ware RE. Hydroxycarbamide: clinical aspects. *C R Biol.* 2013;336:177-182.

448. Brawley OW, Cornelius LJ, Edwards LR, et al. National Institutes of Health Consensus Development Conference statement: hydroxyurea treatment for sickle cell disease. *Ann Intern Med.* 2008;148:932-938.

449. Strouse JJ, Lanzkron S, Beach MC, et al. Hydroxyurea for sickle cell disease: a systematic review for efficacy and toxicity in children. *Pediatrics.* 2008;122:1332-1342.

450. Shelby MD. National Toxicology Program Center for the Evaluation of Risks to Human Reproduction: guidelines for CERHR expert panel members. *Birth Defects Res B Dev Reprod Toxicol.* 2005;74:9-16.

451. Shelby MD. 2007. *Center for the Evaluation of Risks to Human Reproduction.* https://ntp.niehs.nih.gov/ntp/ohat/hydroxyurea/humonograph20090401.pdf

452. Kinney TR, Helms RW, O'Branski EE, et al. Safety of hydroxyurea in children with sickle cell anemia: results of the HUG-KIDS study, a phase I/II trial. Pediatric Hydroxyurea Group. *Blood.* 1999;94:1550-1554.

453. Hankins JS, Ware RE, Rogers ZR, et al. Long-term hydroxyurea therapy for infants with sickle cell anemia: the HUSOFT extension study. *Blood.* 2005;106:2269-2275.

454. Atweh GF, Sutton M, Nassif I, et al. Sustained induction of fetal hemoglobin by pulse butyrate therapy in sickle cell disease. *Blood.* 1999;93:1790-1797.

455. Dover GJ, Brusilow S, Charache S. Induction of fetal hemoglobin production in subjects with sickle cell anemia by oral sodium phenylbutyrate. *Blood.* 1994;84:339-343.

456. Reid ME, El Beshlawy A, Inati A, et al. A double-blind, placebo-controlled phase II study of the efficacy and safety of 2,2-dimethylbutyrate (HQK-1001), an oral fetal globin inducer, in sickle cell disease. *Am J Hematol.* 2014;89:709-713.

457. DeSimone J, Heller P, Hall L, et al. 5-Azacytidine stimulates fetal hemoglobin synthesis in anemic baboons. *Proc Natl Acad Sci U S A.* 1982;79:4428-4431.

458. DeSimone J, Heller P, Schimenti JC, et al. Fetal hemoglobin production in adult baboons by 5-azacytidine or by phenylhydrazine-induced hemolysis is associated with hypomethylation of globin gene DNA. *Prog Clin Biol Res.* 1983;134:489-500.

459. Charache S, Dover G, Smith K, et al. Treatment of sickle cell anemia with 5-azacytidine results in increased fetal hemoglobin production and is associated with nonrandom hypomethylation of DNA around the gamma-delta-beta-globin gene complex. *Proc Natl Acad Sci U S A.* 1983;80:4842-4846.

460. Ley TJ, DeSimone J, Noguchi CT, et al. 5-Azacytidine increases gamma-globin synthesis and reduces the proportion of dense cells in patients with sickle cell anemia. *Blood.* 1983;62:370-380.

461. Mavilio F, Giampaolo A, Care A, et al. Molecular mechanisms of human hemoglobin switching: selective undermethylation and expression of globin genes in embryonic, fetal, and adult erythroblasts. *Proc Natl Acad Sci U S A.* 1983;80:6907-6911.

462. Lowrey CH, Nienhuis AW. Brief report: treatment with azacitidine of patients with end-stage beta-thalassemia. *N Engl J Med.* 1993;329:845-848.

463. Saunthararajah Y, Hillery CA, Lavelle D, et al. Effects of 5-aza-2′-deoxycytidine on fetal hemoglobin levels, red cell adhesion, and hematopoietic differentiation in patients with sickle cell disease. *Blood.* 2003;102:3865-3870.

464. Saunthararajah Y, Molokie R, Saraf S, et al. Clinical effectiveness of decitabine in severe sickle cell disease. *Br J Haematol.* 2008;141:126-129.

465. Molokie R, Lavelle D, Gowhari M, et al. Oral tetrahydrouridine and decitabine for non-cytotoxic epigenetic gene regulation in sickle cell disease: a randomized phase 1 study. *PLoS Med.* 2017;14:e1002382.

466. Moutouh-de Parseval LA, Verhelle D, Glezer E, et al. Pomalidomide and lenalidomide regulate erythropoiesis and fetal hemoglobin production in human CD34+ cells. *J Clin Invest.* 2008;118:248-258.

467. Meiler SE, Wade M, Kutlar F, et al. Pomalidomide augments fetal hemoglobin production without the myelosuppressive effects of hydroxyurea in transgenic sickle cell mice. *Blood.* 2011;118:1109-1112.

468. Gluckman E. Allogeneic transplantation strategies including haploidentical transplantation in sickle cell disease. *Hematology Am Soc Hematol Educ Program.* 2013;2013:370-376.

469. Locatelli F, Pagliara D. Allogeneic hematopoietic stem cell transplantation in children with sickle cell disease. *Pediatr Blood Cancer.* 2012;59:372-376.

470. Hsieh MM, Kang EM, Fitzhugh CD, et al. Allogeneic hematopoietic stem-cell transplantation for sickle cell disease. *N Engl J Med.* 2009;361:2309-2317.

471. Saraf SL, Rondelli D. Allogeneic hematopoietic stem cell transplantation for adults with sickle cell disease. *J Clin Med.* 2019;8:1565.

472. Walters MC, Hardy K, Edwards S, et al. Pulmonary, gonadal, and central nervous system status after bone marrow transplantation for sickle cell disease. *Biol Blood Marrow Transplant.* 2010;16:263-272.

473. Ruggeri A, Eapen M, Scaravadou A, et al. Umbilical cord blood transplantation for children with thalassemia and sickle cell disease. *Biol Blood Marrow Transplant.* 2011;17:1375-1382.

474. Bolanos-Meade J, Fuchs EJ, Luznik L, et al. HLA-haploidentical bone marrow transplantation with posttransplant cyclophosphamide expands the donor pool for patients with sickle cell disease. *Blood.* 2012;120:4285-4291.

475. Boulad F, Shore T, van Besien K, et al. Safety and efficacy of plerixafor dose escalation for the mobilization of CD34(+) hematopoietic progenitor cells in patients with sickle cell disease: interim results. *Haematologica.* 2018;103:770-777.

476. Esrick EB, Manis JP, Daley H, et al. Successful hematopoietic stem cell mobilization and apheresis collection using plerixafor alone in sickle cell patients. *Blood Adv.* 2018;2:2505-2512.

477. Hsieh MM, Tisdale JF. Hematopoietic stem cell mobilization with plerixafor in sickle cell disease. *Haematologica.* 2018;103:749-750.

478. Lagresle-Peyrou C, Lefrere F, Magrin E, et al. Plerixafor enables safe, rapid, efficient mobilization of hematopoietic stem cells in sickle cell disease patients after exchange transfusion. *Haematologica.* 2018;103:778-786.

479. Poletti V, Urbinati F, Charrier S, et al. Pre-clinical development of a lentiviral vector expressing the anti-sickling βAS3 globin for gene therapy for sickle cell disease. *Mol Ther Methods Clin Dev.* 2018;11:167-179.

480. Cavazzana M, Ribeil J-A, Payen E, et al. 279. Clinical outcomes of gene therapy with BB305 lentiviral vector for sickle cell disease and β-thalassemia. *Mol Ther.* 2016;24:S111-S112.

481. Lin MI, Paik E, Mishra B, et al. CRISPR/Cas9 genome editing to treat sickle cell disease and B-Thalassemia: re-creating genetic variants to upregulate fetal hemoglobin appear well-tolerated, effective and durable. *Hematology Am Soc Hematol Educ Program.* 2017;130:10661-10665.

482. Shariati L, Khanahmad H, Salehi M, et al. Genetic disruption of the KLF1 gene to overexpress the gamma-globin gene using the CRISPR/Cas9 system. *J Gene Med.* 2016;18:294-301.

483. John A, Brylka H, Wiegreffe C, et al. Bcl11a is required for neuronal morphogenesis and sensory circuit formation in dorsal spinal cord development. *Development.* 2012;139:1831-1841.

484. Liu P, Keller JR, Ortiz M, et al. Bcl11a is essential for normal lymphoid development. *Nat Immunol.* 2003;4:525-532.

485. Bauer DE, Kamran SC, Lessard S, et al. An erythroid enhancer of BCL11A subject to genetic variation determines fetal hemoglobin level. *Science.* 2013;342:253-257.

486. Canver MC, Smith EC, Sher F, et al. BCL11A enhancer dissection by Cas9-mediated in situ saturating mutagenesis. *Nature.* 2015;527:192-197.

487. Xu M, Papageorgiou DP, Abidi SZ, et al. A deep convolutional neural network for classification of red blood cells in sickle cell anemia. *PLoS Comput Biol.* 2017;13:e1005746.

488. Connes P, Hue O, Tripette J, et al. Blood rheology abnormalities and vascular cell adhesion mechanisms in sickle cell trait carriers during exercise. *Clin Hemorheol Microcirc.* 2008;39:179-184.

489. Erica BE, Lehmann LE, Biffi A, et al. Post-transcriptional genetic silencing of BCL11A to treat sickle cell disease. *N Engl J Med.* 2021;384(3)205-215.

490. Neumayr L, Koshy M, Haberkern C, et al. Surgery in patients with hemoglobin SC disease. Preoperative Transfusion in Sickle Cell Disease Study Group. *Am J Hematol.* 1998;57:101-108.

491. Smith-Whitley K, Thompson AA. Indications and complications of transfusions in sickle cell disease. *Pediatr Blood Cancer.* 2012;59:358-364.

492. Telen MJ. Principles and problems of transfusion in sickle cell disease. *Semin Hematol.* 2001;38:315-323.

493. Chien S, Usami S, Bertles JF. Abnormal rheology of oxygenated blood in sickle cell anemia. *J Clin Invest.* 1970;49:623-634.

494. Morris CL, Gruppo RA, Shukla R, et al. Influence of plasma and red cell factors on the rheologic properties of oxygenated sickle blood during clinical steady state. *J Lab Clin Med.* 1991;118:332-342.

495. Schmalzer EA, Lee JO, Brown AK, et al. Viscosity of mixtures of sickle and normal red cells at varying hematocrit levels. Implications for transfusion. *Transfusion.* 1987;27:228-233.

496. Vichinsky EP. Current issues with blood transfusions in sickle cell disease. *Semin Hematol.* 2001;38:14-22.

497. Rosse WF, Gallagher D, Kinney TR, et al. Transfusion and alloimmunization in sickle cell disease. The Cooperative Study of Sickle Cell Disease. *Blood.* 1990;76:1431-1437.

498. Yazdanbakhsh K, Ware RE, Noizat-Pirenne F. Red blood cell alloimmunization in sickle cell disease: pathophysiology, risk factors, and transfusion management. *Blood.* 2012;120:528-537.

499. Williams LM, Qi Z, Batai K, et al. A locus on chromosome 5 shows African ancestry-limited association with alloimmunization in sickle cell disease. *Blood Adv.* 2018;2:3637-3647.

500. Wahl S, Quirolo KC. Current issues in blood transfusion for sickle cell disease. *Curr Opin Pediatr.* 2009;21:15-21.

501. Talano JA, Hillery CA, Gottschall JL, et al. Delayed hemolytic transfusion reaction/hyperhemolysis syndrome in children with sickle cell disease. *Pediatrics.* 2003;111:e661-e665.

502. Win N. Hyperhemolysis syndrome in sickle cell disease. *Expert Rev Hematol.* 2009;2:111-115.

503. Mwesigwa S, Moulds JM, Chen A, et al. Whole-exome sequencing of sickle cell disease patients with hyperhemolysis syndrome suggests a role for rare variation in disease predisposition. *Transfusion.* 2018;58:726-735.

504. Ballas SK. Iron overload is a determinant of morbidity and mortality in adult patients with sickle cell disease. *Semin Hematol.* 2001;38:30-36.

505. Vichinsky E, Butensky E, Fung E, et al. Comparison of organ dysfunction in transfused patients with SCD or beta thalassemia. *Am J Hematol.* 2005;80:70-74.

506. Fung EB, Harmatz P, Milet M, et al. Morbidity and mortality in chronically transfused subjects with thalassemia and sickle cell disease: a report from the multi-center study of iron overload. *Am J Hematol.* 2007;82:255-265.

507. Brittenham GM, Cohen AR, McLaren CE, et al. Hepatic iron stores and plasma ferritin concentration in patients with sickle cell anemia and thalassemia major. *Am J Hematol.* 1993;42:81-85.

508. Silliman CC, Peterson VM, Mellman DL, et al. Iron chelation by deferoxamine in sickle cell patients with severe transfusion-induced hemosiderosis: a randomized, double-blind study of the dose-response relationship. *J Lab Clin Med.* 1993;122:48-54.

509. Vichinsky E, Onyekwere O, Porter J, et al. A randomised comparison of deferasirox versus deferoxamine for the treatment of transfusional iron overload in sickle cell disease. *Br J Haematol.* 2007;136:501-508.

510. Lucania G, Vitrano A, Filosa A, et al. Chelation treatment in sickle-cell-anaemia: much ado about nothing? *Br J Haematol.* 2011;154:545-555.

511. Brittenham GM. Iron-chelating therapy for transfusional iron overload. *N Engl J Med.* 2011;364:146-156.

512. Antmen B, Karakas Z, Yesilipek MA, et al. Deferasirox in children with transfusion-dependent thalassemia or sickle cell anemia: a large cohort real-life experience from Turkey (REACH-THEM). *Eur J Haematol.* 2019;102:123-130.

513. Coates TD, Wood JC. How we manage iron overload in sickle cell patients. *Br J Haematol.* 2017;177:703-716.

514. Niihara Y, Miller ST, Kanter J, et al. A phase 3 trial of l-glutamine in sickle cell disease. *N Engl J Med.* 2018;379:226-235.

515. Oder E, Safo MK, Abdulmalik O, et al. New developments in anti-sickling agents: can drugs directly prevent the polymerization of sickle haemoglobin in vivo? *Br J Haematol.* 2016;175:24-30.

516. Howard J, Hemmaway CJ, Telfer P, et al. A phase 1/2 ascending dose study and open-label extension study of voxelotor in patients with sickle cell disease. *Blood.* 2019;133:1865-1875.

517. Vichinsky E, Hoppe CC, Ataga KI, et al. A phase 3 randomized trial of voxelotor in sickle cell disease. *N Engl J Med.* 2019;381:509-519.

518. Telfer P, Agodoa I, Fox KM, et al. Impact of voxelotor (GBT440) on unconjugated bilirubin and jaundice in sickle cell disease. *Hematol Rep.* 2018;10:e7643.

519. Dufu K, Patel M, Oksenberg D, et al. GBT440 improves red blood cell deformability and reduces viscosity of sickle cell blood under deoxygenated conditions. *Clin Hemorheol Microcirc.* 2018;70:95-105.

520. Ataga KI, Kutlar A, Kanter J, et al. Crizanlizumab for the prevention of pain crises in sickle cell disease. *N Engl J Med.* 2017;376:429-439.

521. Shimp EA, Alsmadi NZ, Cheng T, et al. Effects of shear on P-selectin deposition in microfluidic channels. *Biomicrofluidics.* 2016;10:024128.

522. Steinberg MH, Adams JG 3rd, Dreiling BJ. Alpha thalassaemia in adults with sickle-cell trait. *Br J Haematol.* 1975;30:31-37.

523. Wong SC, Ali MA, Boyadjian SE. Sickle cell traits in Canada. Trimodal distribution of Hb S as a result of interaction with alpha-thalassaemia gene. *Acta Haematol.* 1981;65:157-163.

524. Sciarratta GV, Sansone G, Ivaldi G, et al. Alternate organization of alpha G-Philadelphia globin genes among U.S. black and Italian Caucasian heterozygotes. *Hemoglobin.* 1984;8:537-547.

525. Itano HA, Neel JV. A new inherited abnormality of human hemoglobin. *Proc Natl Acad Sci U S A.* 1950;36:613-617.

526. Spaet TH, Alway RH, Ward G. Homozygous type c hemoglobin. *Pediatrics.* 1953;12:483-490.

527. Ranney HM, Larson DL, McCormack GH Jr. Some clinical, biochemical and genetic observations on hemoglobin C. *J Clin Invest.* 1953;32:1277-1284.

528. Steinberg MH, Nagel R. Hemoglobin SC Disease and Hb C Disorders. In: Steinberg MH, Forget BG, Higgs DR, Nagel RL, eds. *Disorders of Hemoglobin: Genetics, Pathophysiology, and Clinical Management.* Cambridge University Press; 2001:761-785.

529. Boehm CD, Dowling CE, Antonarakis SE, et al. Evidence supporting a single origin of the beta(C)-globin gene in blacks. *Am J Hum Genet.* 1985;37:771-777.

530. Cook CM, Smeltzer MP, Mortier NA, et al. The clinical and laboratory spectrum of Hb C [beta6(A3)Glu—>Lys, GAG>AAG] disease. *Hemoglobin.* 2013;37:16-25.

531. Itano HA, Bergren WR, Sturgeon P. Identification of fourth abnormal human hemoglobin. *J Am Chem Soc.* 1954;76:2278.

532. Fucharoen S. Hemoglobin E Disorders. In: Steinberg MH, Forget BG, Higgs DR, Nagel RL, eds. *Disorders of Hemoglobin: Genetics, Pathophysiology, and Clinical Management.* Cambridge University Press; 2001:1139-1154.

533. Atichartakarn V, Chuncharunee S, Archararit N, et al. Intravascular hemolysis, vascular endothelial cell activation and thrombophilia in splenectomized patients with hemoglobin E/beta-thalassemia disease. *Acta Haematol.* 2014;132:100-107.

534. Fucharoen S, Siritanaratkul N, Winichagoon P, et al. Hydroxyurea increases hemoglobin F levels and improves the effectiveness of erythropoiesis in beta-thalassemia/hemoglobin E disease. *Blood.* 1996;87:887-892.

535. Itano HA. A third abnormal hemoglobin associated with hereditary hemolytic anemia. *Proc Natl Acad Sci U S A.* 1951;37:775-784.

536. Huisman THJ, Carver MFH, Efremov GD. *A Syllabus of Human Hemoglobin Variants.* The Sickle Cell Anemia Foundation, 1998.

537. Bunn HF, Forget BG. *Hemoglobin: Molecular, Genetic, and Clinical Aspects.* Saunders; 1986.

538. Cathie IAB. Apparent idiopathic Heinz body anaemia. *Great Ormond St J.* 1952;3:343.

539. Huisman TH, Horton B, Bridges MT, et al. A new abnormal human hemoglobin-Hb: Zurich. *Clin Chim Acta.* 1961;6:347-355.

540. Kersten HG, Kleihauer E. Hemoglobin M Cologne, a new hemoglobin variant. Simultaneous report on the differential diagnosis of cyanosis. Article in German. *Med Welt.* 1964;30:1607-1611.

541. White JM, Dacie JV. In vitro synthesis of Hb Hammersmith (CDI phe-ser). *Nature.* 1970;225:860-861.

542. Nagel RL, Rieder RF, Bookchin RM, et al. Some functional properties of hemoglobin Leiden. *Biochem Biophys Res Commun.* 1973;53:1240-1245.

543. Bradley TB Jr, Wohl RC, Rieder RF. Hemoglobin Gun Hill: deletion of five amino acid residues and impaired heme-globin binding. *Science.* 1967;157:1581-1583.

544. Jones RT, Brimhall B, Huisman TH, et al. Hemoglobin Freiburg: abnormal hemoglobin due to deletion of a single amino acid residue. *Science.* 1966;154:1024-1027.

545. Bunn HF, Schmidt GJ, Haney DN, et al. Hemoglobin Cranston, an unstable variant having an elongated beta chain due to nonhomologous crossover between two normal beta chain genes. *Proc Natl Acad Sci U S A.* 1975;72:3609-3613.

546. Flatz G, Kinderlerer JL, Kilmartin JV, et al. Haemoglobin Tak: a variant with additional residues at the end of the beta-chains. *Lancet.* 1971;1:732-733.

547. Mendonca TF, Oliveira MC, Vasconcelos LR, et al. Association of variant alleles of MBL2 gene with vasoocclusive crisis in children with sickle cell anemia. *Blood Cells Mol Dis.* 2010;44:224-228.

548. Redha NA, Mahdi N, Al-Habboubi HH, et al. Impact of VEGFA -583C > T polymorphism on serum VEGF levels and the susceptibility to acute chest syndrome in pediatric patients with sickle cell disease. *Pediatr Blood Cancer.* 2014;61:2310-2312.

549. Galarneau G, Coady S, Garrett ME, et al. Gene-centric association study of acute chest syndrome and painful crisis in sickle cell disease patients. *Blood.* 2013;122:434-442.

550. Ashley-Koch AE, Okocha EC, Garrett ME, et al. MYH9 and APOL1 are both associated with sickle cell disease nephropathy. *Br J Haematol.* 2011;155:386-394.

551. Nolan VG, Ma Q, Cohen HT, et al. Estimated glomerular filtration rate in sickle cell anemia is associated with polymorphisms of bone morphogenetic protein receptor 1B. *Am J Hematol.* 2007;82:179-184.

552. Ware RE, Despotovic JM, Mortier NA, et al. Pharmacokinetics, pharmacodynamics, and pharmacogenetics of hydroxyurea treatment for children with sickle cell anemia. *Blood.* 2011;118:4985-4991.

553. Ashley-Koch AE, Elliott L, Kail ME, et al. Identification of genetic polymorphisms associated with risk for pulmonary hypertension in sickle cell disease. *Blood.* 2008;111:5721-5726.

554. Yousry SM, Ellithy HN, Shahin GH. Endothelial nitric oxide synthase gene polymorphisms and the risk of vasculopathy in sickle cell disease. *Hematology.* 2016;21:359-367.

555. Daak AA, Dampier CD, Fuh B, et al. Double-blind, randomized, multicenter phase 2 study of SC411 in children with sickle cell disease (SCOT trial). *Blood Adv.* 2018;2:1969-1979.

556. Morris CR, Kuypers FA, Lavrisha L, et al. A randomized, placebo-controlled trial of arginine therapy for the treatment of children with sickle cell disease hospitalized with vaso-occlusive pain episodes. *Haematologica.* 2013;98:1375-1382.

557. Eleuterio RMN, Nascimento FO, Araujo TG, et al. Double-blind clinical trial of arginine supplementation in the treatment of adult patients with sickle cell anaemia. *Adv Hematol.* 2019;2019:4397150.

558. Kanter J, Abboud MR, Kaya B, et al. Ticagrelor does not impact patient-reported pain in young adults with sickle cell disease: a multicentre, randomised phase IIb study. *Br J Haematol.* 2019;184:269-278.

559. Goldman RD, Mounstephen W, Kirby-Allen M, et al. Intravenous magnesium sulfate for vaso-occlusive episodes in sickle cell disease. *Pediatrics.* 2013;132:e1634-e1641.

560. Heeney MM, Hoppe CC, Abboud MR, et al. A multinational trial of prasugrel for sickle cell vaso-occlusive events. *N Engl J Med.* 2016;374:625-635.

561. Desai PC, Brittain JE, Jones SK, et al. A pilot study of eptifibatide for treatment of acute pain episodes in sickle cell disease. *Thromb Res.* 2013;132:341-345.

562. Ataga KI, Reid M, Ballas SK, et al. Improvements in haemolysis and indicators of erythrocyte survival do not correlate with acute vaso-occlusive crises in patients with sickle cell disease: a phase III randomized, placebo-controlled, double-blind study of the Gardos channel blocker senicapoc (ICA-17043). *Br J Haematol.* 2011;153:92-104.

563. Orringer EP, Casella JF, Ataga KI, et al. Purified poloxamer 188 for treatment of acute vaso-occlusive crisis of sickle cell disease: a randomized controlled trial. *JAMA.* 2001;286:2099-2106.

CHAPTER 19
METHEMOGLOBINEMIA AND OTHER DYSHEMOGLOBINEMIAS

Josef T. Prchal

SUMMARY

Methemoglobin is a metalloprotein, in which the iron in the heme group is in the Fe^{3+}(ferric), not the Fe^{2+}(ferrous), state of normal hemoglobin (Hb). Methemoglobinemia occurs because of either increased production of oxidized Hb due to exposure to environmental agents or diminished reduction of oxidized Hb because of underlying germline mutations. Cyanosis occurs when methemoglobin exceeds 15g/L; in comparison, cyanosis is discernible with deoxyhemoglobin at 40 g/L and sulfhemoglobin at 5g/L. Hb can also bind carbon monoxide (CO) and nitric oxide, resulting in the formation of carboxyhemoglobin (COHb) and nitrosohemoglobin. Sulfhemoglobinemia occurs because of occupational exposure to sulfa compounds or exposure to oxidants. These modified Hbs are known as dyshemoglobins. Depending on the severity, the presence of dyshemoglobins can result in varying degree of clinical manifestations. Prompt diagnosis is the key to the specific treatment.

● METHEMOGLOBINEMIA

CYANOSIS: DEFINITION AND HISTORY

A bluish discoloration of the skin and mucous membrane, designated *cyanosis*, has been recognized since antiquity as a manifestation of lung or heart disease; however, in methemoglobinemia and sulfhemoglobinemia, it has a different molecular basis than hemoglobin (Hb) oxygen desaturation. Cyanosis resulting from drug administration has also been recognized since before 1890. Toxic methemoglobinemia occurs when various drugs or toxic substances either oxidize Hb directly in the circulation, or facilitate its oxidation by molecular oxygen.[1]

Acronyms and Abbreviations: AOP2, antioxidant protein 2; 2,3-BPG, 2,3-bisphosphoglycerate; cytochrome b5R, cytochrome b_5 reductase; CO, carbon monoxide; COHb, carboxyhemoglobin; cGMP, cyclic guanosine monophosphate; ETCO, end-tidal CO; GSH, reduced glutathione; iNO, inhaled nitric oxide; M, hemoglobins; those hemoglobin mutants associated with methemoglobinemia; NADH, nicotinamide adenine dinucleotide (reduced form); N_2O_3, dinitrogen trioxide; NADPH, reduced nicotinamide adenine dinucleotide phosphate; NO, nitric oxide; NOS, nitric oxide synthase; p50, the oxygen tension at which hemoglobin is 50% saturated; pO_2, partial pressure of oxygen; RBC, red blood cells; SNO-Hb, S-nitroso hemoglobin; SpO2, arterial oxygen saturation; SpCO, arterial COHb concentration; SpMet, arterial methemoglobin concentration.

In 1912, Sloss and Wybauw[2] reported a case of a patient with idiopathic methemoglobinemia. Later, Hitzenberger[3] suggested that a hereditary form of methemoglobinemia might exist, and subsequently, numerous such cases were reported.[4] In 1948, Hörlein and Weber[5] described a family in which eight members over four generations had cyanosis. The absorption spectrum of methemoglobin was abnormal, and the authors demonstrated that the defect must reside in the globin portion of the molecule. Subsequently, Singer[6] proposed the abnormal Hbs associated with methemoglobinemia be given the designation Hb M. The cause of another form of methemoglobinemia that occurs independently of drug administration and without the existence of any abnormality of the globin portion of Hb was first explained by Gibson,[7] who clearly pointed to the nature of the enzyme defect, the reduced form of nicotinamide adenine dinucleotide (NADH) diaphorase also designated as methemoglobin reductase and now known as cytochrome b_5 reductase (cytochrome b5R) (Chap. 16). More than 40 years after Gibson's insightful studies, the genetic disorder that he had predicted was verified at the DNA level.[8]

The most potent initiator of cyanosis is *sulfhemoglobin*. When hydrogen sulfide combine with ferric iron of Hb, a greenish pigment is formed, that is, sulfhemoglobin; it does not transport oxygen. It is the most potent cause of cyanosis; the clinical cyanosis is noted when the level of sulfhemoglobin exceeds 5 g/L.[9]

The existence of abnormal Hbs that cause cyanosis through quite another mechanism was first recognized in 1968 with the description of Hb_{Kansas}.[10] Here the cyanosis resulted not from methemoglobin, as occurs in Hb M, but rather from an abnormally low oxygen affinity of the mutant Hb. Thus, at normal oxygen tensions, a large amount of deoxygenated Hb is present in the blood.

EPIDEMIOLOGY

Methemoglobinemia occurring as a result of cytochrome b5R deficiency is more common than those associated with M Hbs. It is endemic among Native Americans both in Alaska (Athabascans) and in the continental United States (Navajo) and among the Evenk People of Yakutia of Russian Siberia.[11-13] Methemoglobinemia resulting from Hbs M is sporadic, as is the occurrence of toxic methemoglobinemia. Toxic methemoglobinemia is related to chemical industrial exposure and certain medications and is therefore most common among patients receiving methemoglobinemia-inducing medications, workers in the chemical industry, and drug abusers.

ETIOLOGY AND PATHOGENESIS

Methemoglobinemia decreases the oxygen-carrying capacity of blood because the oxidized ferric iron cannot reversibly bind oxygen. Moreover, when one or more iron atoms have been oxidized, the conformation of Hb is changed so as to increase the oxygen affinity of the remaining ferrous heme groups. In this way, methemoglobinemia exerts a dual effect in impairing the supply of oxygen to tissues.[14]

Toxic Methemoglobinemia

Hb is continuously oxidized in vivo from the ferrous to the ferric state. The rate of such oxidation is accelerated by many drugs and toxic chemicals, including sulfonamides, especially dapsone, lidocaine, and other aniline derivatives, and nitrites. A vast number of chemical substances may cause methemoglobinemia.[9,15-17] Table 19-1 lists some of the agents that are responsible for clinically significant methemoglobinemia in clinical practice.

The most common offenders include benzocaine and lidocaine[18-20] and increasingly dapsone.[21,22] In some cases, the patients have been

TABLE 19–1. Some Drugs That Cause Methemoglobinemia

Phenazopyridine (Pyridium)[70]

Sulfamethoxazole[180]

Dapsone[23,24]

Aniline[93,94]

Paraquat/monolinuron[181,182]

Nitrate[25,26,32]

Nitroglycerin[183]

Amyl nitrite[184]

Isobutyl nitrite[30]

Sodium nitrite[27]

Benzocaine[185-187]

Prilocaine[188,189]

Methylene blue[92] (Although it is also the principal treatment of methemoglobinemia, this paradoxical effect is dose dependent.)

Chloramine[189,190]

unaware that they have been ingesting one of the drugs known to produce methemoglobinemia; dapsone is apparently used in some "street drugs."[23,24] Nitrates and the nitrites contaminating water supplies or used as preservatives in foods are also common offending agents.[25-33]

Cytochrome b5R Reductase Deficiency

Cytochrome b5R, also known as NADH diaphorase and methemoglobin reductase,[9] catalyzes a step in the major pathway for methemoglobin reduction. This enzyme reduces cytochrome b_5 using NADH as a hydrogen donor. The reduced cytochrome b_5 reduces, in turn, methemoglobin to Hb. A steady-state methemoglobin level is achieved when the rate of methemoglobin formation equals the rate of methemoglobin reduction either through the cytochrome b5R or through a relatively minor auxiliary mechanism such as direct chemical reduction by ascorbate and reduced glutathione (GSH). A reduced nicotinamide adenine dinucleotide phosphate (NADPH)–linked enzyme, NADPH diaphorase, does not play a role in methemoglobin reduction except when an electron acceptor, such as methylene blue, is supplied (see "Therapy, Course, and Prognosis" further). A marked diminution in the activity of cytochrome b5R results in the accumulation of methemoglobin.

A balance to methemoglobin formation is antioxidant protein 2 (AOP2), which is present in high concentrations in human and mouse red cells (Chap. 1). This member of the peroxiredoxin protein family binds to Hb and prevents spontaneous as well as oxidant-induced methemoglobin formation.[34] Mutations of this gene or its acquired deficiency are theoretical candidates responsible for congenital and acquired methemoglobinemia but have not yet been described. Cyanosis resulting from abnormal HbM and low-oxygen affinity Hbs is inherited as an autosomal dominant disorder. In contrast, hereditary methemoglobinemia resulting from cytochrome b5R deficiency is inherited in an autosomal recessive fashion.

Accordingly, hereditary deficiency of the enzyme that reduces cytochrome b_5, cytochrome b5R, is one of the causes of methemoglobinemia. Many mutations of cytochrome b5R have been identified at the nucleotide level,[8,9] and the functional effects of some of these have been deduced from the structure of the enzyme.[35,36] Although most of the mutants have been found in persons of European descent, unique mutations were found in Chinese,[37] Thais,[38] Americans of African descent,[39,40] and Asian Indians.[41,42] In addition, a common polymorphism (allele

frequency = 0.023) has been identified in Americans of African descent; it does not appear to impair the activity of the enzyme.[43] Most of the patients with cytochrome b5R deficiency merely have methemoglobinemia, and the enzyme deficiency is limited to the red cells; these have been classified as having type I disease. Although most patients with methemoglobinemia are cyanotic, those with modest elevations of methemoglobin below 15 g/L are seen in some affected Puerto Rican patients.[44]

In contrast, type II cytochrome b5R deficiency, which represents 10% to 15% of cases of enzyme deficient congenital methemoglobinemia, cytochrome b5R is decreased in all cells. Type II cytochrome b5R deficiency is a grave disease. In addition to cyanosis, severe developmental abnormalities, a progressive encephalopathy, and mental retardation generally occur, and most affected infants die in the first year of life.[45,46] The finding that fatty acid elongation is defective in the platelets and leukocytes of such patients[47] provides a clue to the type of defect that could occur in the central nervous system, where fatty acid elongation plays an important role in myelination. Rare patients with deficiency of cytochrome b5R in nonerythroid cells do not have any neurologic disorder, and it has been suggested that they be designated as having type III disease.[48] However, existence of type III disease is not firmly established.[49]

Heterozygosity for Cytochrome b5R Deficiency

Heterozygotes for cytochrome b5R deficiency are not usually methemoglobinemic. However, under the stress of administration of drugs that normally induce only slight, clinically unimportant, methemoglobinemia, such persons have been reported to become severely cyanotic because of methemoglobinemia.[50] Although in this report, the affected patients were Ashkenazi Jews, the prevalence of cytochrome b5R deficiency in 500 unselected Jewish subjects was found to be low.[51] In addition, predisposition to acute toxic methemoglobinemia in heterozygous subjects for cytochrome b5R deficiency seems to be quite uncommon.[49]

Animal models of cytochrome b5R deficiency have been described in dogs, cats, and horses.[52,53]

Infant Susceptibility

A combination of both increased Hb oxidation and decreased methemoglobin reduction also may occur. Because the activity of cytochrome b5R is normally low in newborn infants,[54] they are particularly susceptible to the development of methemoglobinemia. Thus, serious degrees of methemoglobinemia have been observed in infants as a result of toxic materials, such as aniline dyes used on diapers,[55] and the ingestion of nitrate-contaminated water[27,33] and even of beets.[56] Bacterial action in the intestinal tract may reduce nitrates to nitrites, which, in turn, cause methemoglobinemia. In rural areas, fatal methemoglobinemia in infants caused by drinking water from wells contaminated with nitrates still occurs.[57]

Inhaled nitric oxide (iNO) is approved for treatment of infants with pulmonary hypertension because of its vasodilatory effect on pulmonary vessels. During the binding and release of nitric oxide (NO) from Hb, methemoglobin is formed at a higher rate. In one study of 81 premature and 82 term infants, methemoglobin was greater than 5% in preterm infants and between 2.5% and 5% in 16 infants.[58]

Methemoglobinemia occurring in acidotic infants with diarrhea is a syndrome that may have a fatal outcome.[59] Such infants were reported to have normal red cell cytochrome b5R activity, and the mechanism by which methemoglobinemia occurs is unknown. However, the syndrome seems most common when soy formula is being fed,[60] and breastfeeding appears to be protective.[57]

Cytochrome b5 Deficiency

Rarely, the defect leading to methemoglobinemia may not be in the cytochrome b5R that transfers hydrogen to the cytochrome b_5 but rather to a deficiency in the cytochrome b_5 itself.[61]

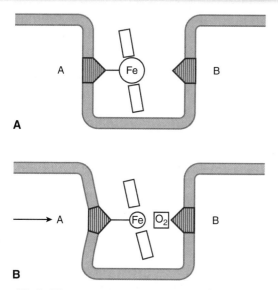

Figure 19–1. Diagrammatic representation of the heme group inserted into the heme pocket. **A.** proximal histidine. In the deoxygenated form, the larger ferrous atom lies out of the place of the porphyrin ring. **B.** Distal histidine. In the oxygenated form, the now smaller "ferric-like" atom can slip into the plane of the porphyrin ring. As a result, the proximal histidine and helix F into which it is incorporated are displaced. *(Reproduced with permission from Lehmann H, Huntsman RG. Man's Haemoglobins. Philadelphia PA: Lippincott Williams & Wilkins; 1974.)*

Hemoglobin M

The molecular mechanisms by which Hb binds oxygen and releases it are discussed in Chap. 18. Heme is held in a hydrophobic "heme pocket" between the E and F α-helices of each of the four globin chains. The iron atom in the heme forms four bonds with the pyrrole nitrogen atoms of the porphyrin ring and a fifth covalent bond with the imidazole nitrogen of a histidine residue in the nearby F α-helix (Fig. 19-1).[62] This histidine, residue 87 in the α chain and 92 in the β chain, is designated as the proximal histidine. On the opposite side of the porphyrin ring, the iron atom lies adjacent to another histidine residue to which, however, it is not covalently bonded. This distal histidine occupies position 58 in the α chain and position 63 in the β chain. Under normal circumstances, oxygen is occasionally discharged from the heme pocket as a superoxide anion, removing an electron from the iron and leaving it in the ferric state. The enzymatic machinery of the red cell efficiently reduces the iron to the divalent form, converting the methemoglobin to Hb (Chap. 16).

In most of the HbMs, tyrosine has been substituted for either the proximal or the distal histidine. Tyrosine can form an iron-phenolate complex that resists reduction to the divalent state by the normal metabolic systems of the erythrocyte. Four Hb Ms are a consequence of substitution of tyrosine for histidine in the proximal and distal sites of the α and β chains. As Table 19-2 shows, these four Hb Ms have been designated by the geographic names Boston, Saskatoon, Iwate, and Hyde Park.

Analogous His→Tyr substitutions in the γ chain of fetal Hb have also been documented and have been designated Hb FM-Osaka[63] and FM-Fort Ripley.[64]

TABLE 19–2.	Properties of Hemoglobin Ms			
Hemoglobin[96]	Amino Acid Substitution	Oxygen Dissociation and Other Properties	Clinical Effect	References
Hb M$_{Boston}$	α58 (E7)His→Tyr	Very low O_2 affinity; almost nonexistent heme-heme interaction; no Bohr effect	Cyanosis resulting from formation of methemoglobin	179
Hb M$_{Saskatoon}$	β63 (E7)His→Tyr	Increased O_2 affinity; reduced heme-heme interaction; normal Bohr effect; slightly unstable	Cyanosis resulting from methemoglobin formation; mild hemolytic anemia exacerbated by ingestion of sulfonamides	179
Hb M$_{Iwate}$	α87 (F8)His→Tyr	Low O_2 affinity; negligible heme-heme interaction; no Bohr effect	Cyanosis resulting from formation of methemoglobin	179
Hb M$_{Kankakee}$				
Hb M$_{Oldenburg}$				
HB MS$_{endai}$				
Hb M$_{Hyde park}$	β92 (F8)His→Tyr	Increased O_2 affinity; reduced heme-heme interaction; normal Bohr effect; slightly unstable	Cyanosis resulting from formation of methemoglobin; mild hemolytic anemia	84
Hb M$_{Milwaukee 2}$				
Hb M$_{Akita}$				
Hb M$_{Milwaukee}$	β67 (E11)Val →Glu	Low O_2 affinity; reduced heme-heme interaction; normal Bohr effect; slightly unstable	Cyanosis resulting from methemoglobin formation	193
Hb FM$_{Osaka}$	^{G}γ63His→Tyr	Low O_2 affinity; increased Bohr effect; methemoglobinemia	Cyanosis at birth	63
Hb FM$_{Fort Ripley}$	^{G}γ92His→Tyr	Slightly increased O_2 affinity	Cyanosis at birth	194

Hb, hemoglobin.

Another Hb M, Hb M$_{Milwaukee}$, is formed by substitution of glutamic acid for valine in the 67th residue of the β chain rather than substitution of tyrosine for histidine. The glutamic acid side chain points toward the heme group, and its γ-carboxyl group interacts with the iron atom, stabilizing it in the ferric state.

It is rare for methemoglobinemia to occur as a result of hemoglobinopathies other than Hb Ms, but hemoglobin$_{Chile}$ (β28 Leu→Met) is such a Hb. Producing hemolysis only with drug administration, this unstable Hb is characterized clinically by chronic methemoglobinemia.[65]

CLINICAL FEATURES

Drug Ingestion

Methemoglobinemia may be chronic or acute and acquired or congenital. Acquired severe acute methemoglobinemia, usually the consequence of drug ingestion or toxic exposure, can produce symptoms of hypoxia and anemia because methemoglobin lacks the capacity to transport oxygen. Symptoms may include shortness of breath, palpitations, and vascular collapse, and arterial blood gases reveal a large discrepancy between PaO$_2$ and O$_2$ saturation. Chemicals that induce methemoglobinemia may also be capable of causing hemolysis, and a combination of hemolytic anemia and methemoglobinemia may occur. Chronic methemoglobinemia, typically from hereditary causes, is usually asymptomatic. Cyanosis, even if present, may not be discernable in persons with very dark skin coloration.[39,40] In instances when the methemoglobin levels are very high (>20% of the total pigment), mild erythrocytosis is occasionally noted (Chap. 28).

Hemoglobin M

Patients with Hb M also manifest cyanosis. In the case of α-globin M variants, the methemoglobinemia persists from birth. In contrast, the clinical manifestations of β-globin M variants become apparent only after β chains have largely replaced the fetal γ chains at 6 to 9 months of age, but those inheriting γ globin M variants have methemoglobinemia at birth that subsides after about 6 months of age. Despite the impaired Hb function, no cardiopulmonary symptoms are observed, and there is no digital clubbing. In the case of Hb M$_{Saskatoon}$ and Hb M$_{Hyde Park}$, hemolytic anemia with jaundice may be present. The hemolytic state may be exacerbated by administration of oxidant medications or chemicals.[66]

Cytochrome b5R Deficiency

Hereditary methemoglobinemia resulting from cytochrome b5R deficiency may, in addition to cyanosis, as noted earlier, be also associated with mental retardation, failure to thrive, and early death. In one case, skeletal anomalies were documented as well.[67]

LABORATORY FEATURES

Toxic Methemoglobinemia

In toxic methemoglobinemia, an elevated level of methemoglobin is found, but the activity of cytochrome b5R is normal. Methemoglobin levels are best measured using the change of absorbance of methemoglobin at 630 nm that occurs when cyanide is added, converting the methemoglobin to cyanmethemoglobin, a principle used in the Evelyn-Malloy method.[68,69] Errors in diagnosis can be made when automated instruments designed to estimate levels of reduced Hb, oxygenated Hb, methemoglobin, and carboxyhemoglobin (COHb) are used. Most automated instruments do not properly make this distinction.[70,71] Clinical incidence of methemoglobinemia can be overestimated by cooximetry measurements compared with the more specific Evelyn-Malloy method.[72] This method involves direct spectrophotometric analysis and should be optimally used when methemoglobinemia is suspected. This is achieved by lysing the blood in a slightly acid buffer and measuring the optical density at 630 nm before and after adding a small amount of neutralized cyanide. The absorption of methemoglobin at this wavelength disappears when it is converted to cyanmethemoglobin. Although this method was described in 1938,[68] it remains the most accurate technique for the estimation of methemoglobin in the blood. Details of its performance can be found in an earlier edition of this text[73] and elsewhere.[66]

Routine pulse oximetry is generally inaccurate for monitoring oxygen saturation in the presence of methemoglobinemia because pulse oximetry only measures the relative absorbance of two wavelengths (ie, 660 nm and 940 nm), and the methemoglobin absorbs light at these pulse oximeter's two wavelengths. This leads to error in estimating the percentages of reduced and oxyhemoglobins. An eight-wavelength pulse oximeter, Masimo Rad-57 (the Rainbow-SET Rad-57 Pulse CO-Oximeter, Masimo Inc.), has been approved by the U.S. Food and Drug Administration (FDA) for the measurement of both COHb and methemoglobin. The Rad-57 uses eight wavelengths of light instead of the usual two and is thereby able to measure more than two species of human Hb.[74] In addition to the usual SpO$_2$ value, the Rad-57 displays SpCO and SpMet, which are the pulse oximeter's estimates of COHb and methemoglobin concentrations, respectively. In a study on healthy human volunteers in whom controlled levels of methemoglobin and COHb were induced, the Rad-57 measured COHb with an uncertainty of ± 2% within a range of 0% to 15% and measured methemoglobin with an uncertainty of 0.5% within a range of 0% to 12%.[74] The usefulness of this instrument was also verified also by other studies.[75,76]

Cytochrome b5R Deficiency

In hereditary methemoglobinemia resulting from cytochrome b5R deficiency, between 8% and 40% of the Hb is in the form of methemoglobin. The blood may have a chocolate-brown color, and cyanosis may be present. Cytochrome b5R activity is best measured using ferricyanide as a receptor, measuring the rate of oxidation of NADH.[77,78] The residual level of enzyme activity is usually less than 20% of normal in patients with methemoglobinemia, resulting from deficiency of this enzyme. An immunoassay has been described,[79] but such an assay would not detect mutants in which enzyme molecules with impaired catalytic activity are present. For unknown reasons, GSH reductase activity (Chap. 16) is usually also diminished.[80]

Cytochrome b5 Deficiency

Cytochrome b$_5$ assays may be useful if cytochrome b5R activity is normal and the presence of Hb M is ruled out.[81]

M Hemoglobin

Optical Spectrum The spectrum of normal methemoglobin A at a pH of 7.0 is illustrated in Figure 19-2.[82] Hb Ms may be differentiated from methemoglobin formed from HbA by its absorption spectrum in the range of 450 to 750 nm. Because only some 20% to 35% of the total Hb will ordinarily be the Hb M, the mixed spectra of methemoglobin A and the Hb M may be difficult to interpret. Therefore, it is preferable to perform these spectral studies on purified Hb M isolated by electrophoretic or chromatographic means.[62]

Electrophoresis All Hb M samples should be converted to methemoglobin so that any difference found in electrophoresis will be the result of the amino acid substitution and not the different charge of the iron atom. Electrophoresis at a pH of 7.1 is most useful for separation of Hb Ms because the imidazole groups of histidine have a net positive charge at this pH, but at higher pH levels, the histidines and the substituting tyrosines are both neutral.

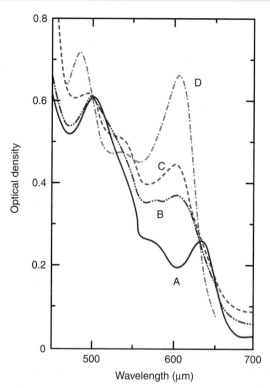

Figure 19–2. Absorption spectra at a pH of 7.0. **A.** Methemoglobin A. **B.** Methemoglobin M$_{Boston}$; C, methemoglobin M$_{Saskatoon}$; D, methemoglobin A fluoride complex. For purposes of comparison, all the optical densities have been made equal to 0.61 at 500 nm. *(Data from Gerald PS, Efron ML. Chemical studies of several varieties of Hb M. Proc Natl Acad Sci USA. 1961 Nov 15;47(11):1758-1767.)*

Other Biochemical Methods The Hb Ms differ in their reactivity to cyanide and to azide ions.[83] This property may help to identify the subunit affected because the iron-phenolate bonds are stronger in the α-chain variants than in the β-chain variants. However, definitive identification of the variant requires DNA analysis. Hbs that cause cyanosis because of a diminished oxygen affinity may be detected by determining the oxygen dissociation curve of blood (see later), being certain that the 2,3-bisphosphoglycerate (2,3-BPG) level is normal, or by estimating the oxygen dissociation curve of Hb, which has been stripped of 2,3-BPG by extensive dialysis against an appropriate buffer. Many of the Hbs with decreased oxygen affinity are unstable (Chap. 18) and precipitate in the isopropanol or heat stability test.[83] Over the past several years, it has become easier to analyze the coding sequence of the globin chains at the DNA level than to attempt to determine the properties of the Hb.[84]

TREATMENT AND COURSE

Toxic Methemoglobinemia

Acute toxic methemoglobinemia may represent a serious medical emergency. Because of the loss of oxygen-carrying capacity of the blood and because of the left shift in the oxygen dissociation curve that occurs when methemoglobin is present in high concentration,[85] acute methemoglobinemia may be life threatening when the level of the pigment exceeds third of the total circulating Hb. Levels of methemoglobin exceeding 50% of the total pigment may be associated with vascular collapse, coma, and death,[86,87] but recovery was documented in one patient with a level as high as 81.5% of the total pigment.[88]

Methylene blue[89] is an effective treatment for patients with methemoglobinemia because NADPH formed in the hexose monophosphate pathway can rapidly reduce this dye to leukomethylene blue in a reaction catalyzed by NADPH diaphorase (Chap. 16). Leukomethylene blue, in turn, nonenzymatically reduces methemoglobin to Hb.[90] An exception to the efficacy of this treatment exists in patients who are glucose-6-phosphate dehydrogenase (G6PD) deficient (Chap. 16). In these patients, methylene blue would not only fail to give the desired effect on methemoglobin levels but might compound the patient's difficulty by inducing an acute hemolytic episode[91] or by increasing the level of methemoglobin.[92]

Methylene blue, if given to patients taking serotonergic psychiatric medications, may cause toxicity referred to as *serotonin syndrome* (https://www.fda.gov/drugs/drug-safety-and-availability/fda-drug-safety-communication-serious-cns-reactions-possible-when-methylene-blue-given-patients). While it would be prudent to ascertain that patients with acute methemoglobinemia do not take serotonergic psychiatric medications; however, to our knowledge, that has not yet been reported in subjects receiving methylene blue for treatment of methemoglobinemia.

In patients with acute toxic methemoglobinemia who are symptomatic or whose methemoglobin level is rising rapidly, the IV administration of 1 or 2 mg methylene blue per kilogram body weight over a period of 5 minutes is the preferred treatment because of its very rapid action.[93] Use of excessive amounts of methylene blue should be avoided: the administration of repeated doses of 2 mg methylene blue per kilogram body weight has produced acute hemolysis even in patients with normal G6PD levels.[94] If methylene blue is unavailable, or in case of G6PD deficiency, the administration of ascorbic acid, 300 to 600 mg orally is beneficial.

The response to treatment is so rapid, with marked lowering or normalization of methemoglobin levels within an hour or two, that no other treatment is usually needed, but the patient should be observed carefully because continued absorption of a toxic substance from the gastrointestinal tract may cause recurrence of the methemoglobinemia. In patients who are in shock, blood transfusion may be helpful. Cimetidine, used as a selective inhibitor of N-hydroxylation, may decrease the methemoglobinemia produced by dapsone in patients with dermatitis herpetiformis.[95]

Hereditary Methemoglobinemia

The course of hereditary methemoglobinemia is generally benign (but not in type II cytochrome b5R deficiency), but patients with this disorder should be shielded from exposure to aniline derivatives, nitrites, and other agents that may, even in normal persons, induce methemoglobinemia.

Hereditary methemoglobinemia resulting from cytochrome b5R deficiency is readily treated by the administration of ascorbic acid, 300 to 600 mg orally daily divided into three or four doses. Although intravenously administered methylene blue is very effective in correcting this type of methemoglobinemia, it is not suitable for the long-term therapy that needs to be given if the state is to be treated at all. Riboflavin administration seems to benefit some patients[96] but not others.[97]

The iron-phenolate complex that exists in the Hb Ms prevents the reduction of ferric to ferrous iron. For this reason, the methemoglobinemia does not respond to administration of ascorbic acid or of methylene blue. No effective treatment exists for the cyanosis that is present in patients with abnormal Hbs with reduced oxygen affinity.

⬤ SULFHEMOGLOBIN

DEFINITION AND HISTORY

Sulfhemoglobinemia refers to the presence in the blood of Hb derivative that is defined by their characteristic absorption of light at 620 nm and, unlike in methemoglobinemia, even in the presence of cyanide. Sulfhemoglobin derives its name from the fact that it can be produced in vitro from the action of hydrogen sulfide on Hb[98] and that the feeding of dogs with elemental sulfur has been associated with sulfhemoglobinemia.[99]

ETIOLOGY AND PATHOGENESIS

Sulfhemoglobin may contain one excess sulfur atom. The sulfur atom is bound to a β-pyrrole carbon atom at the periphery of the porphyrin ring.[100-102] Sulfhemoglobinemia has been associated with the ingestion of various drugs, particularly sulfonamides, phenacetin, acetanilide, and phenazopyridine.[70,103] It also occurs independently of drug use and has been thought to be related to chronic constipation or to purging.[104] The non–drug-induced sulfhemoglobinemia was reported in a 7-day-old preterm infant associated with intestinal *Morganella morganii* infection. These bacteria are capable of producing hydrogen sulfide, and the sulfhemoglobinemia resolved after eradication of *M. morganii* with the third-generation cephalosporins.[105] A similar case was reported in a 7-year-old girl with urinary infection; however, her suspected *M. morganii* infection was not definitely proven.[106]

Fatal sulfhemoglobinemia after inhalation of volcanic gases was reported in three family members upon their fall in a volcanic pothole while they were visiting the Solfatara Park near Naples.[107]

Some patients with sulfhemoglobinemia or a past history of this disorder appear to have increased levels of red blood cell reduced GSH.[108] The reason for this and its relationship to sulfhemoglobinemia is not clearly understood, but it may be of significance that some of the types of drugs that have been associated with sulfhemoglobinemia cause an elevation of red cell GSH levels, probably by activating the enzyme GSH synthase[109] or by increasing intracellular glutamate levels.[110]

Evidence for the occurrence of hereditary sulfhemoglobinemia is not convincing,[111] and it is likely that the single family reported represents an Hb M hemoglobinopathy.

CLINICAL FEATURES

Sulfhemoglobinemia is characterized by cyanosis. Drugs that cause sulfhemoglobinemia often have the capacity to produce accelerated red cell destruction as well. Thus, mild hemolysis is sometimes observed in patients with sulfhemoglobinemia.

LABORATORY FEATURES

Sulfhemoglobin is detected in the lysate of blood treated with ferricyanide, cyanide, and ammonia by comparing the optical density at 620 nm with that at 540 nm.[68,69]

TREATMENT AND COURSE

Sulfhemoglobinemia is usually a benign disorder; however, fatalities have been reported. Unlike methemoglobin, sulfhemoglobin does not produce a left shift in the oxygen dissociation curve but rather decreases the affinity of Hb for oxygen.[103] The disorder tends to recur in the same persons after exposure to drugs but does not generally appear to affect their overall health. Unlike methemoglobin, sulfhemoglobin cannot be converted to Hb. Thus, when sulfhemoglobinemia occurs, it will persist until the erythrocytes carrying the abnormal pigment reach the end of their life span.

● LOW-OXYGEN AFFINITY HEMOGLOBINS: A CAUSE OF CYANOSIS

ETIOLOGY AND PATHOGENESIS

In some Hb variants, the deoxy conformation of the Hb molecule is favored because the angle of the heme is altered from that found normally in deoxyhemoglobin. Such changes occur in $Hb_{Hammersmith}$, $Hb_{Bucuresti}$, Hb_{Torino}, and $Hb_{Peterborough}$. In other instances, the quaternary conformation is changed by mutations involving the $\alpha_1\beta_2$ contact (Hb_{Kansas}, $Hb_{Titusville}$, and $Hb_{Yoshizuka}$). Properties of abnormal Hbs associated with low-oxygen affinity are summarized in Table 19-3.

CLINICAL FEATURES

In response to the improved tissue oxygen supply brought about by a right-shifted oxygen dissociation curve, the "oxygen sensor" of the body decreases the output of erythropoietin.[112] As a result, the steady-state level of Hb is diminished; mild anemia is characteristic of patients with Hbs with a decreased oxygen affinity.

LABORATORY FEATURES

Affinity of Hb with oxygen is expressed as the P50, which is the partial pressure of oxygen at which 50% of the blood Hb is saturated with oxygen. The Hb P50 can be measured directly using a cooximeter, which is no longer easily available in routine and even reference laboratories. Lichtman and colleagues have reported a mathematical formula that can be used to calculate P50 reliably from a venous blood sample.[113] Calculating P50 using this formula requires the following *venous* gas parameters—partial pressure of oxygen (venous pO2), venous pH, and venous oxygen saturation—and uses anti-log mathematical function that many clinicians find difficult to use for calculation. An electronic version (in Microsoft Excel) of this mathematical formula is available for rapid calculation of P50 from venous blood gases.[114] The P50 of a healthy person with normal Hb is 26 ± 1.3 mm Hg. An abnormally low P50 reflects an increased affinity of Hb for oxygen and vice versa and is especially useful for detecting high-affinity Hb mutants and congenital enzyme disorder associated with low 2,3-BPG levels associated with erythrocytosis (Chaps. 16 and 28).

TABLE 19–3. Some Abnormal Hemoglobins Associated with Low-Oxygen Affinity

Hemoglobin	Amino Acid Substitution	Oxygen Dissociation and Other Properties	Clinical Effect	References
$Hb_{Seattle}$	β70 (E14)Ala→Asp	Decreased O_2 affinity; normal heme-heme interaction	Mild chronic anemia associated with reduced urinary erythropoietin; physiologic adaptation to more efficient O_2 release to tissues	112
Hb_{Kansas}	β102 (G4)Asn→Thr	Very low O_2 affinity; low heme-heme interaction; dissociates into dimers in ligand form	Cyanosis resulting from deoxyhemoglobin,[195] mild anemia	

Hb, hemoglobin.

DIFFERENTIAL DIAGNOSIS

Cyanosis resulting from low-oxygen affinity Hbs, methemoglobinemia, or sulfhemoglobinemia should be differentiated from cyanosis resulting from cardiac or pulmonary disease, particularly when right-to-left shunting is present. Whereas in the latter instances, the arterial oxygen tension will be low, in methemoglobinemia and sulfhemoglobinemia, it should be normal. One should be certain, however, that the oxygen tension was measured directly and not deduced from the percent saturation of Hb. Blood from a patient with cyanosis because of arterial oxygen desaturation promptly becomes bright red upon being shaken with air. In addition, these causes of cyanosis are readily differentiated by carrying out quantitative blood methemoglobin and sulfhemoglobin levels. Because of the potential lethal nature of high levels of methemoglobin and because prompt treatment may be lifesaving, a high index of suspicion is important. A patient with cyanosis whose arterial blood is brown with a SpO_2 that is found to be normal on blood gas examination is likely to have methemoglobinemia. One should not rely on the readings of a standard pulse oximeter because false readings may be obtained in the presence of methemoglobin. Rapid examination of a blood sample using an automatic analyzer such as a cooximeter is the first step in confirming the diagnosis. Treatment should not be delayed, but as pointed out earlier in "Laboratory Features," direct spectrophotometric analysis should be carried out on the pretreatment sample as soon as possible to distinguish between methemoglobinemia and sulfhemoglobinemia.

A family history, as well as any information whether acquired or congenital, is helpful in differentiating hereditary methemoglobinemia as a result of cytochrome b5R deficiency from Hb M disease or cytochrome b_5 deficiency. The former has a recessive mode of inheritance and the latter two a dominant mode. Thus, cyanosis in successive generations suggests the presence of Hb M or cytochrome b_5 deficiency; having normal parents but possibly affected siblings implies the presence of cytochrome b5R. Consanguinity is more common in cytochrome b5R deficiency. In cytochrome b5R deficiency, incubation of the blood with small amounts of methylene blue results in rapid reduction of the methemoglobin; in Hb M disease, such reduction does not take place. The absorption spectra of methemoglobin and its derivatives are normal in cytochrome b5R deficiency; they are abnormal in Hb M disease. In the case of toxic methemoglobinemia, cyanosis is generally of relatively recent origin, and a history of exposure to drug or toxin may usually be obtained; in hereditary methemoglobinemia, a history of lifelong cyanosis may usually be elicited.

● OTHER DYSHEMOGLOBINS

CARBON MONOXIDE AND CARBOXYHEMOGLOBIN

Carbon monoxide (CO) is a toxic, odorless, colorless, and tasteless gas that binds with high affinity to Hb, generating COHb. It can be unknowingly inhaled to dangerous levels when present in the high concentration in the atmosphere with serious clinical implications.[115]

Epidemiology

Acute CO intoxication is one of the most common causes of morbidity from poisoning in the United States. In the United States, CO poisoning results in approximately 50,000 emergency department visits per year,[116,117] and approximately 500 accidental deaths caused by CO poisoning occur annually with the number of intentional CO-related deaths being 5 to 10 times higher.[118,119] Primary sources of CO are home appliances, and the majority of exposures occur during the fall

and winter months and during weather-related disasters.[120,121] During warmer months, boating activities are another source of exposure.[122] The death rate is highest among older adults and can be attributed to delayed diagnosis because symptoms often resemble those of associated comorbidities.[123,124] The exhaust produced by the typical home-use 5.5-kW generator contains as much CO as that of six idling automobiles.[125]

Chronic CO intoxication is commonly caused by cigarette smoking, leading to an average percent COHb of 4%, with a usual range of 3 to 8.[126] Heavy smokers may have COHb levels of 10% to 15%.[118] The elevated COHb was also reported in barbecue workers with the average COHb of 6.5%.[127] In this profession, "warehouse workers' headache" was described.[118] Houses with defective heating exhaust systems and vehicles that leak CO into the passenger compartment, either because of mechanical failure or driving with the rear hatch-door open, are the second most common cause of chronic CO exposure. Occupations that involve a high risk for CO intoxication include garage work with improper ventilation, toll booth attendants, tunnel workers, firefighters, and workers exposed to paint remover, aerosol propellant, or organic solvents containing dichloromethane.[128]

Etiology and Pathogenesis

CO binds with high affinity with the heme and with lesser affinities to myoglobin and cytochromes at the iron core, a site that it shares with O_2.[129]

At equilibrium in physiological conditions, CO affinity for Hb is approximately 240 times greater than that of O_2. This very high equilibrium constant is the result of reaction kinetics. Contrary to popular belief, CO reacts more slowly than O_2 with the heme of Hb. When CO is bound to heme, its "off" rate is only 0.015 mol/L/s in contrast to 35 mol/L/s for O_2.[129] This extraordinarily slow-release process produces a very high affinity constant of CO for heme and a life-threatening danger for individuals exposed to high levels of CO. When two molecules of CO are bound to Hb, the Hb switches to the relaxed state, which increases the affinity of Hb for oxygen. As a consequence of this phenomenon, called the Darling-Roughton effect,[85] the Hb O_2 affinity increases in parallel with increasing CO levels, further impairing tissue oxygen delivery.

In the absence of environmental CO, the blood of adults contains approximately 1% COHb. This represents approximately 80% of the total body CO, the remainder probably sequestered in myoglobin and other heme binding proteins. This CO is endogenously produced,[130] originating from the degradation of heme by the rate-limiting heme oxygenase-cytochrome P450 complex, which produces CO and biliverdin. Caloric restriction, dehydration, infancy, and the genetic variations reported in Japanese and Native Americans generate higher endogenous levels of CO. Hemolytic anemia (Chap. 2), hematomas, and infection tend to increase CO production several-fold. Fetuses and newborns have double the normal adult levels of COHb. Drugs such as diphenylhydantoin and phenobarbital, by inducing the cytochrome P450 complex, increase CO production. Normal adult level of COHb is less than 1.5%. In the absence of severe hemolysis, levels more than 3% have an exogenous origin, except for rare conditions as occur in carriers of abnormal Hbs such as Hb_{Zurich}. The affinity of Hb_{Zurich} for CO is approximately 65 times that of normal Hb.[131]

Pregnant women and fetuses are particularly at risk. CO readily crosses the placenta, and the half-life of CO in a fetus is as much as five times longer than it is in the mother.[132] The O_2 affinity of HbF is shifted to the left[133,134] owing to its lack of 2,3-BPG binding (Chaps. 2 and 18), making the Darling-Roughton effect particularly pernicious. This is one of the reasons why cigarette smoking during pregnancy is hazardous to fetuses.

Clinical and Laboratory Features

CO poisoning is a clinical diagnosis that is confirmed by laboratory testing. Signs and symptoms consistent with CO poisoning in certain circumstances should raise the suspicion of CO intoxication. A higher index of suspicion should attend the simultaneous presentation of multiple patients from the same family or housing complex. The eight-wavelength pulse oximeter, Masimo Rad-57, has been reported to be accurate in measuring COHb concentration in normal healthy volunteers[74] as well as in emergency department patients.[135]

Acute intoxication with CO rapidly affects the central and peripheral nervous systems and cardiopulmonary functions. Cerebral edema is common, as is an impaired peripheral nervous system. CO induces increased capillary permeability in the lung, resulting in acute pulmonary edema. Cardiac arrhythmias, generalized hypoxemia, and respiratory failure are the common causes of CO-related death. In survivors, considerable neuropsychological deficits might remain. In a prospective longitudinal study, approximately 45% of patients with CO poisoning had cognitive sequelae after 6 weeks of poisoning.[136,137] Acute CO intoxication in children[138] sometimes has unique symptomatology resembling gastroenteritis. Surviving children are more likely to have severe sequelae such as leukoencephalopathy and severe myocardial ischemia.[139]

Chronic intoxication in adults might result in irritability, nausea, lethargy, headaches, and sometimes a flulike condition. Higher COHb levels produce somnolence, palpitations, cardiomegaly, and hypertension and could contribute to atherosclerosis. Chronic CO poisoning can produce erythrocytosis, the magnitude of which varies with the level of COHb. By increasing red cell production, chronic CO poisoning can mask the mild anemia of acquired or congenital hemolytic disorders.

Therapy, Course, and Prognosis

The most important step in the treatment for CO poisoning is prompt removal of patients from the source of CO followed by administering 100% supplemental O_2 via a tight-fitting mask. The serum elimination half-lives of CO are 5 hours when breathing room air and 30 minutes with O_2 therapy (100% O_2 at 3 atm).[132]

For mild to moderate cases of CO poisoning, which more often happens with chronic intoxication, removing the patient from the source of environmental CO is usually curative. If the COHb level is high, breathing 100% O_2 will increase the rate of CO removal.

In severe cases of CO poisoning, which more often occur with acute intoxication, after identification and removal of the source of CO, 100% O_2 should be administered with cardiac monitoring. Management should primarily be guided by clinical signs and symptoms because COHb levels correlate imprecisely with the degree of poisoning and are not predictive of neurologic sequelae. Endotracheal intubation should be done in all patients with impaired mental status.

Because of conflicting evidence, there is no absolute indication for the use of hyperbaric O_2 treatment for patients with CO poisoning. Hyperbaric O_2 might be indicated in patients who have obvious neurologic abnormalities, have cardiac dysfunction, have persistent symptoms despite normobaric O_2, or have metabolic acidosis.[140] Hyperbaric oxygen treatment has no added value when the patient is intubated and receives 100% oxygen via an endotracheal tube, and it has complications of its own such as bronchial irritation and pulmonary edema. Locations of hyperbaric chambers throughout the world and in the United States can be found at the Undersea and Hyperbaric Medical Society's website at www.uhms.org under "Chamber Directory."

Pregnant women exposed to CO are at particularly high risk. CO poisoning is especially dangerous to fetuses because CO readily crosses the placenta, and the half-life of CO in fetuses is as much as five times longer than it is in pregnant women. For these reasons, treatment with hyperbaric O_2 should be carried during pregnancy when the COHb levels exceed 15%. In limited number of studies done on pregnant patients, hyperbaric O_2 does not seem to adversely affect fetuses.[141,142]

Use of Carboxyhemoglobin and Exhaled Carbon Monoxide in Clinical Hematology

The value of determination of COHb in differential diagnosis of elevated Hb and hematocrit is discussed in Chap. 28.

Carboxyhemoglobin for Blood Volume Measurements Furthermore, to differentiate true from relative or spurious erythrocytosis (Chap. 28), CO inhalation with rebreathing has been used as a simple method to determine directly Hb content and indirectly red cell and plasma volumes. This approach was developed more than 100 years ago; previously standard methods of measuring red cell and plasma volume using radioactive chromium-labeled red cells and radioiodine-labeled albumin are no longer available in the United States because of concern of radiation risk.[143] With CO rebreathing, COHb levels increases, and using the *dilution principle*, Hb content and indirectly red cell and plasma volumes can be calculated.[144] The commercial equipment (Detalo Instruments ApS) has been developed and approved and used in Europe. This procedure takes 10 minutes, and exposure time to CO is hence short.

Exhaled Carbon Monoxide for Estimation of the Presence of Hemolysis Previously standard methods of measuring red cell survival used in vitro labeling of red cells with radioactive chromium, injecting these to the studied subject, and following radioactivity of peripheral blood over 14 days. That method is no longer available in the United States because of concern of radiation risk. To rapidly measure red cell survival by noninvasive technique, one can use exhaled CO (end-tidal CO [ETCO]). ETCO can be measured by a nonradioactive method using FDA-approved equipment, the CoSense ETCO Monitor made by Capnia, Inc. The measured exhaled CO (the product of Hb catabolism, hence hemolysis) uses single-use disposable cannulas with reading available in 5 minutes, making this method fast safe, simple, noninvasive, and nonradioactive.[145] However, the current version of the equipment is relatively nonsensitive, with the background of the difference of ETCO from ambient CO measurement set up too high by the manufacturer, and is thus only useful for detection of moderate to severe hemolysis (Chap. 2).

NITRIC OXIDE AND NITRIC OXIDE HEMOGLOBINS

PHYSIOLOGY AND CHEMISTRY

NO, a soluble gas, is continuously synthesized in endothelial cells by isoforms of the NOS enzyme, eNOS. A functional NOS transfers electrons from NADPH to its heme center, where L-arginine is oxidized to L-citrulline and NO.[146] Vasodilation is caused by diffusion of NO into the smooth muscle cells wherein NO binds avidly to the heme of soluble guanylyl cyclase, producing cyclic guanosine monophosphate (cGMP), which activates cGMP-dependent protein kinases and ultimately produces smooth muscle relaxation.[146]

Blood NO levels are set by the balance between the production of NO by NOS and the binding or scavenging of NO by the heme groups of erythrocyte Hb. The half-life of NO in whole blood is extremely short and is estimated to be 1.8 ms.[147] The short half-life of NO greatly limits its diffusional distance in blood and only maintain NO as a paracrine vasoregulator.[148,149] This does not explain how Hb is capable of transducing NO bioactivity far from their location of formation.

Interaction of the red blood cells (RBCs) with NO is a complex phenomenon (Fig. 19-3). Two models have been proposed. The S-nitrosohemoglobin (SNO-Hb)–dependent mechanism proposes that NO binds to heme when the Hb is in T-state (deoxygenated). In the oxygenated state, NO gets transferred from heme to a cysteine residue

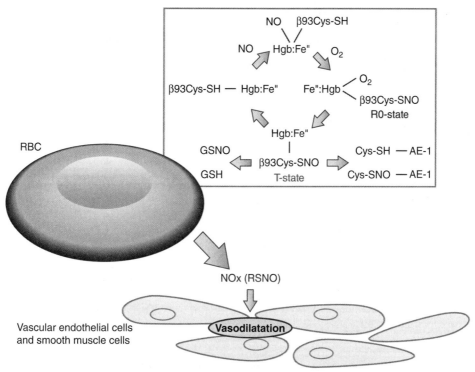

Figure 19–3. S-nitrosylated hemoglobin (SNO-Hb) and hypoxic vasodilation. GSH, reduced glutathione; GSNO, S-nitrosoglutathione; RSNO, S-nitrosothiol; RBC, red blood cell. *(Reproduced with permission from Parker C. Is SNO-Hgb a Snow Job? I Still Can't Decide,* The Hematologist. *2009 Jan 1;6(1):12.)*

on the globin portion of Hb, forming S-nitrosohemoglobin.[150,151] NO is transported by RBCs from the lungs to the hypoxic tissues in protected form as SNO-Hb and is delivered in the hypoxic microvasculature at the same time as oxygen, coupling Hb deoxygenation to vasodilatation. The other model is of deoxyhemoglobin-mediated nitrite reduction to NO.[152] In the blood, deoxygenated Hb functions as the predominant nitrite reductase.[153] Deoxygenated Hb reacts with nitrite to form NO and methemoglobin and causes vasodilation along the physiological oxygen gradient. Although this reaction is experimentally associated with NO generation, kinetic analysis suggests that NO should not be able to escape inactivation in the erythrocyte.[154] This inactivation or scavenging of NO is avoided by the formation of an intermediate species, dinitrogen trioxide (N_2O_3). Products of the nitrite-Hb reaction generate N_2O_3 via a novel reaction of NO and nitrite-bound methemoglobin.[155] N_2O_3 diffuses out of the red cell and later forms NO and effects vasodilation and/or forms nitrosothiols (SNO) (Fig. 19-4). According to this paradigm, nitrite, previously thought to be an inert end products of endogenous NO metabolism, is the main stable NO reservoir in blood and tissues.[156-158] Nitrite is formed during normoxic condition and then reduced to NO and N_2O_3 along the physiological oxygen and pH gradient by the heme globins.[155] However, erythrocytes have the ability to export NO bioactivity by a mechanism that is not yet fully understood, and this occurs independently of SNO formation.[159]

Cell-free Hb and red cell microparticles formed during hemolytic conditions and long storage of RBCs lead to NO scavenging 1000 times faster than regular RBCs, leading to insufficient NO bioavailability.[160] Stored RBCs are also stored in acidic solution that also leads to decrease in SNO-Hb levels.[161] This has been further substantiated by the fact that renitrosylated RBCs lead to improved oxygen delivery in animal models.[162] This could explain the mortality and morbidity associated with stored RBCs.[161] Moreover, underlying recipient endothelial dysfunction (eg, obesity or hypertension) can also induce increased RBC membrane

damage in the transfused blood, leading to increased microparticle formation and increased NO scavenging.[163,164]

PATHOPHYSIOLOGY AND POTENTIAL THERAPEUTIC APPLICATIONS

NO was long considered highly toxic. Exogenous administration of NO by inhalation activates cytosolic guanylate cyclase increases intracellular levels of cGMP, resulting in relaxation of the smooth muscles in the pulmonary arteries.

Based on this observation, iNO has been used to manage the acute pulmonary hypertension seen in adult respiratory distress syndrome, sickle cell disease, and primary or secondary pulmonary hypertension. Even though NO lowers the pulmonary artery pressure and improves oxygenation in acute respiratory distress syndrome, in both adults and children, it has not consistently resulted in an improvement in mortality and leads to methemoglobinemia (see "Infant Susceptibility" to methemoglobinemia in the earlier section).

At present, prolonged administration of iNO is not considered as first-line therapy for pulmonary artery hypertension and instead is used only for vasoreactivity testing in these patients.[165] iNO has been shown to have beneficial effects in animal models and in preliminary human trials of acute vasoocclusive crisis and acute chest syndrome associated with sickle cell disease.[166-168] Some animal data suggest beneficial effects of iNO therapy in the setting of ischemia-reperfusion injury (lung, heart, and intestine).[169] However, iNO has also been associated with multiple side effects such as methemoglobinemia,[58,170] left heart failure,[171] renal insufficiency,[172] and a "rebound" increase in pulmonary artery pressure upon discontinuation of iNO that may result in cardiovascular collapse.[173]

Direct repletion of S-nitrosothiol in the lung and blood has the potential to avoid toxicities related to iNO. In an animal model of acute lung injury, inhaled ethyl nitrite but not iNO efficiently repleted lung

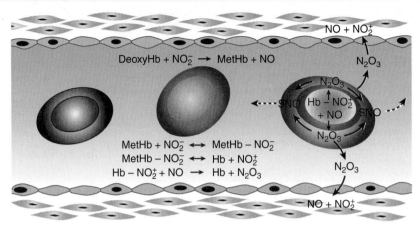

Figure 19–4. Hemoglobin deoxygenation (*purple*) occurs in capillaries. Nitrite reacts with deoxyHb that is oxidized to methemoglobin (MetHb) and nitric oxide (NO). The NO binds to hemes of deoxyHb and undergoes dioxygenation to form nitrate and MetHb from oxyHb. MetHb binds nitrite to form an adduct with some Fe(II)-NO$_2$, ie, Hb-NO. This species reacts quickly with NO to form N$_2$O$_3$, which can diffuse out of the red cell, forming NO and effecting vasodilation and/or forming nitrosothiols (SNOs).

SNOs, lowered pulmonary vascular resistance, improved oxygenation dose dependently,[174] and had a protective effect against a decline in cardiac output.[175]

In humans, newborns with persistent pulmonary hypertension improved oxygenation and hemodynamics after ethyl nitrite inhalation.[176] Use of cell-free Hb has been associated with vasoconstriction and subsequent development of hypertension. Increased vascular resistance and vasoconstriction has been shown to be mediated mainly by the scavenging of NO because of high affinity of free Hb for NO.[177,178]

Several patients with SARS-CoV-2 infection have developed methemoglobinemia following treatment with hydroxychloroquine. In two of these patients, methemoglobinemia improved after methylene blue therapy; in a third it did not. The latter patient had hemolysis and died. He was later found to be G6PD deficient.[196] In a retrospective review, 14 patients were described who developed acute methemoglobinemia as a result of acetaminophen poisoning. Most patients had used the drug therapeutically; a few had used it in a suicide attempt.[197]

REFERENCES

1. Hsieh HS, Jaffe ER. The metabolism of methemoglobin in human erythrocytes. In: Surgenor DM, ed. *The Red Blood Cell*. Academic Press; 1975:799.
2. Sloss A, Wybauw R. Un Cas de methemoglobinemie idiopathique. *Ann Soc R Sci Med Nat Bruxelles*. 1912;70:206.
3. Hitzenberger K. Autotoxic cyanosis due to intraglobular methemoglobinemia. *Wien Arch Med*. 1932;23:85.
4. Jaffe E. Hereditary methemoglobinemias associated with abnormalities in the metabolism of erythrocytes. *Am J Med*. 1966;41:786.
5. Horlein H, Weber G. Über Chronische familiare Methämoglobinamie und eine neue Modification des Methämoglobins. *Dtsch Med Wochenschr*. 1948;73:476.
6. Singer K. Hereditary hemolytic disorders associated with abnormal hemoglobins. *Am J Med*. 1955;18:633.
7. Gibson QH. The reduction of methaemoglobin in red blood cells and studies on the cause of idiopathic methaemoglobinaemia. *Biochem J*. 1948;42:13.
8. Percy M, Gillespie M, Savage G, et al. Familial idiopathic mutations in NADH-cytochrome b5 reductase. *Blood*. 2002;100:3447.
9. Cortazzo JA, Lichtman AD. Methemoglobinemia: a review and recommendations for management. *J Cardiothorac Vasc Anesth*. 2014;28(4):1043.
10. Bonaventura J, Riggs A. Hemoglobin Kansas, a human hemoglobin with a neutral amino acid substitution and an abnormal oxygen equilibrium. *J Biol Chem*. 1968;243:980.
11. Scott E, Hoskins D. Hereditary methemoglobinemia in Alaskan Eskimos and Indians. *Blood*. 1958;13:795.
12. Balsamo P, Hardy W, Scott E. Hereditary methemoglobinemia due to diaphorase deficiency in Navajo Indians. *J Pediatr*. 1964;65:928.
13. Burtseva T, Prchal JT, Chasnyk V, et al. Type I methemoglobinemia caused by the cytochrome b5 reductase 806C>T mutation is present in the indigenous Evenk people of Yakutia. ASH Annual Meeting; 2009.
14. Sorensen PR. The influence of pH, pCO2 and concentrations of dyshemoglobins on the oxygen dissociation curve (ODC) of human blood determined by non-linear least squares regression analysis. *Scand J Clin Lab Invest Suppl*. 1990;203:163.
15. Bodansky O. Methemoglobinemia and methemoglobin-producing compounds. *Pharmacol Rev*. 1951;3:144.
16. Kiese M. The biochemical production of ferrihemoglobin-forming derivatives from aromatic amines and mechanisms of ferrihemoglobin formation. *Pharmacol Rev*. 1966;18:1091.
17. Dean BS, Lopez G, Krenzelok EP. Environmentally-induced methemoglobinemia in an infant. *J Toxicol Clin Toxicol*. 1992;30:127.
18. McGuigan MA. Benzocaine-induced methemoglobinemia. *Can Med Assoc J*. 1981;125:816.
19. O'Donohue WJ Jr, Moss LM, Angelillo VA. Acute methemoglobinemia induced by topical benzocaine and lidocaine. *Arch Intern Med*. 1980;140:1508.
20. Kane GC, Hoehn SM, Behrenbeck TR, et al. Benzocaine-induced methemoglobinemia based on the Mayo Clinic experience from 28,478 transesophageal echocardiograms: incidence, outcomes, and predisposing factors. *Arch Intern Med*. 2007;167:1977.
21. Ash-Bernal R, Wise R, Wright SM. Acquired methemoglobinemia: a retrospective series of 138 cases at 2 teaching hospitals. *Medicine (Baltimore)*. 2004;83:265.
22. Swartzentruber GS, Yanta JH, Pizon AF. Methemoglobinemia as a complication of topical dapsone. *N Engl J Med*. 2015;372:491.
23. Lee SW, Lee JY, Lee KJ, et al. A case of methemoglobinemia after ingestion of an aphrodisiac, later proven as dapsone. *Yonsei Med J*. 1999;40:388.
24. Esbenshade AJ, Ho RH, Shintani A, et al. Dapsone-induced methemoglobinemia: a dose-related occurrence? *Cancer*. 2011;117:3485.
25. Johnson CJ, Kross BC. Continuing importance of nitrate contamination of groundwater and wells in rural areas. *Am J Ind Med*. 1990;18:449.
26. Chan TY. Food-borne nitrates and nitrites as a cause of methemoglobinemia. *Southeast Asian J Trop Med Public Health*. 1996;27:189.
27. Knobeloch L, Proctor M. Eight blue babies. *WMJ*. 2001;100:43.
28. Askew GL, Finelli L, Genese CA, et al. Boilerbaisse: an outbreak of methemoglobinemia in New Jersey in 1992. *Pediatrics*. 1994;94:381.
29. Bakshi SP, Fahey JL, Pierce LE. Brief recording: sausage cyanosis—acquired methemoglobinemic nitrite poisoning. *N Engl J Med*. 1967;277:1072.
30. Bradberry SM, Whittington RM, Parry DA, et al. Fatal methemoglobinemia due to inhalation of isobutyl nitrite. *J Toxicol Clin Toxicol*. 1994;32:179.
31. Bradberry SM, Gazzard B, Vale JA. Methemoglobinemia caused by the accidental contamination of drinking water with sodium nitrite. *J Toxicol Clin Toxicol*. 1994;32:173.
32. Harris JC, Rumack BH, Peterson RG, et al. Methemoglobinemia resulting from absorption of nitrates. *JAMA*. 1979;242:2869.
33. Lukens JN. Landmark perspective: the legacy of well-water methemoglobinemia. *JAMA*. 1987;257:2793.
34. Stuhlmeier KM, Kao JJ, Wallbrandt P, et al. Antioxidant protein 2 prevents methemoglobin formation in erythrocyte hemolysates. *Eur J Biochem*. 2003;270:334.
35. Bewley M, Marohnic C, Barber M. The structure and biochemistry of NADH-dependent cytochrome b5 reductase are now consistent. *Biochemistry*. 2001;40:13574.
36. Yamada M, Tamada T, Takeda K, et al. Elucidations of the catalytic cycle of NADH-cytochrome b5 reductase by X-ray crystallography: new insights into regulation of efficient electron transfer. *J Mol Biol*. 2013;425:4295.
37. Wang Y, Wu Y, Zheng P, et al. A novel mutation in the NADH-cytochrome b5 reductase gene of a Chinese patient with recessive congenital methemoglobinemia. *Blood*. 2000;95:3250.
38. Shotelersuk V, Tosukhowong P, Chotivitayatarakorn P, et al. A Thai boy with hereditary enzymopenic methemoglobinemia type II. *J Med Assoc Thai*. 2000;83:1380.

39. Jenkins MM, Prchal JT. A novel mutation found in the 3′ domain of NADH-cytochrome b5 reductase in an African-American family with type I congenital methemoglobinemia. *Blood.* 1996;87:2993.

40. Prchal JT, Borgese N, Moore M, et al. Congenital methemoglobinemia due to methemoglobin reductase deficiency in two unrelated American black families. *Am J Med.* 1990;89:516.

41. Nussenzveig RH, Lingam HB, Gaikwad A, et al. A novel mutation of the cytochrome-b5 reductase gene in an Indian patient: the molecular basis of type I methemoglobinemia. *Haematologica.* 2006;91:1542.

42. Kedar PS, Gupta V, Warang P, et al. Novel mutation (R192C) in CYB5R3 gene causing NADH-cytochrome b5 reductase deficiency in eight Indian patients associated with autosomal recessive congenital methemoglobinemia type-I. *Hematology.* 2018;23:567.

43. Jenkins MM, Prchal JT. A high frequency polymorphism of NADH-cytochrome b5 reductase in African-Americans. *Hum Genet.* 1997;99:248.

44. Reading NS, Ruiz-Bonilla JA, Christensen RD, et al. A patient with both methemoglobinemia and G6PD deficiency: a therapeutic conundrum. *Am J Hematol.* 2017;92:474.

45. Leroux A, Junien C, Kaplan JC, et al. Generalised deficiency of cytochrome b5 reductase in congenital methaemoglobinaemia with mental retardation. *Nature.* 1975;258:619.

46. Ewenczyk C, Leroux A, Roubergue A, et al. Recessive hereditary methaemoglobinaemia, type II: delineation of the clinical spectrum. *Brain.* 2008;131:760.

47. Takeshita M, Tamura M, Kugi M, et al. Decrease of palmitoyl-CoA elongation in platelets and leukocytes in the patient of hereditary methemoglobinemia associated with mental retardation. *Biochem Biophys Res Commun.* 1987;148:384.

48. Tanishima K, Tanimoto K, Tomoda A, et al. Hereditary methemoglobinemia due to cytochrome b5 reductase deficiency in blood cells without associated neurologic and mental disorders. *Blood.* 1985;66:1288.

49. Maran J, Guan Y, Ou CN, et al. Heterogeneity of the molecular biology of methemoglobinemia: a study of eight consecutive patients. *Haematologica.* 2005;90:687.

50. Cohen R, Sachs J, Wicker D, et al. Methemoglobinemia provoked by malarial chemoprophylaxis in Vietnam. *N Engl J Med.* 1968;279:1127.

51. Moore MR, Conrad ME, Bradley EL Jr, et al. Studies of nicotinamide adenine dinucleotide methemoglobin reductase activity in a Jewish population. *Am J Hematol.* 1982;12:13.

52. Fine DM, Eyster GE, Anderson LK, et al. Cyanosis and congenital methemoglobinemia in a puppy. *J Am Anim Hosp Assoc.* 1999;35:33.

53. Harvey JW, Ling GV, Kaneko JJ. Methemoglobin reductase deficiency in a dog. *J Am Vet Med Assoc.* 1974;164:1030.

54. Lo SC, Agar NS. NADH-methemoglobin reductase activity in the erythrocytes of newborn and adult mammals. *Experientia.* 1986;42:1264.

55. Graubarth J, Bloom CJ, Coleman FC, et al. Dye poisoning in the nursery: a review of seventeen cases. *JAMA.* 1945;128:1155.

56. Sanchez-Echaniz J, Benito-Fernandez J, Mintegui-Raso S. Methemoglobinemia and consumption of vegetables in infants. *Pediatrics.* 2001;107:1024.

57. Hanakoglu A, Danon PN. Endogenous methemoglobinemia associated with diarrheal disease in infancy. *J Pediatr Gastroenterol Nutr.* 1996;23:1.

58. Hamon I, Gauthier-Moulinier H, Grelet-Dessioux E, et al. Methaemoglobinaemia risk factors with inhaled nitric oxide therapy in newborn infants. *Acta Paediatr.* 2010;99:1467.

59. Bricker T, Jefferson LS, Mintz AA. Methemoglobinemia in infants with enteritis. *J Pediatr.* 1983;102:161.

60. Murray KF, Christie DL. Dietary protein intolerance in infants with transient methemoglobinemia and diarrhea. *J Pediatr.* 1993;122:90.

61. Hegesh E, Hegesh J, Kaftory A. Congenital methemoglobinemia with a deficiency of cytochrome b5. *N Engl J Med.* 1986;314:757.

62. Lehmann H, Huntsman RG. *Man's Haemoglobins.* Lippincott; 1974:213.

63. Hayashi A, Fujita T, Fujimura M, et al. A new abnormal fetal hemoglobin, Hb FM-Osaka (alpha 2 gamma 2 63His replaced by Tyr). *Hemoglobin.* 1980;4:447.

64. Priest JR, Watterson J, Jones RT, et al. Mutant fetal hemoglobin causing cyanosis in a newborn. *Pediatrics.* 1989;83:734.

65. Hojas-Bernal R, McNab-Martin P, Fairbanks VF, et al. Hb Chile [beta28(B10) Leu-->Met]: an unstable hemoglobin associated with chronic methemoglobinemia and sulfonamide or methylene blue-induced hemolytic anemia. *Hemoglobin.* 1999;23:125.

66. Dacie JV, Lewis SM. Chemical and physico-chemical methods of haematological importance. *Practical Hematology.* Grune & Stratton; 1998:476.

67. Yawata Y, Ding L, Tanishima K, et al. New variant of cytochrome b5 reductase deficiency (b5RKurashiki) in red cells, platelets, lymphocytes, and cultured fibroblasts with congenital methemoglobinemia, mental and neurological retardation, and skeletal anomalies. *Am J Hematol.* 1992;40:299.

68. Evelyn K, Malloy H. Microdetermination of oxyhemoglobin, methemoglobin, and sulfhemoglobin in a single sample of blood. *J Biol Chem.* 1938;126:655.

69. Beutler E. Carboxyhemoglobin, methemoglobin, and sulfhemoglobin determinations. In: Beutler E, Lichtman MA, Coller BS, et al, eds. *Hematology.* McGraw Hill; 1995:L50.

70. Halvorsen SM, Dull WL. Phenazopyridine-induced sulfhemoglobinemia: inadvertent rechallenge. *Am J Med.* 1991;91:315.

71. Watcha MF, Connor MT, Hing AV. Pulse oximetry in methemoglobinemia. *Am J Dis Child.* 1989;143:845.

72. Molthrop DJ, Wheeler R, Hall K, et al. Evaluation of the methemoglobinemia associated with sulofenur. *Invest New Drugs.* 1994;12:99.

73. Beutler E, Gelbart T. Carboxyhemoglobin, methemoglobin, and sulf-hemoglobin determinations. In: Williams WJ, Beutler E, Erslev AJ, et al, eds. *Hematology.* McGraw-Hill; 1990:1732.

74. Barker SJ, Curry J, Redford D, et al. Measurement of carboxyhemoglobin and methemoglobin by pulse oximetry: a human volunteer study. *Anesthesiology.* 2006;105:892.

75. Annabi EH, Barker SJ. Severe methemoglobinemia detected by pulse oximetry. *Anesth Analg.* 2009;108:898.

76. Hampson NB. Noninvasive pulse CO-oximetry expedites evaluation and management of patients with carbon monoxide poisoning. *Am J Emerg Med.* 2012;30:2021.

77. Beutler E. *Red Cell Metabolism: A Manual of Biochemical Methods.* Grune & Stratton; 1984.

78. Board P. NADH-ferricyanide reductase, a convenient approach to the evaluation of NADH-methemoglobin reductase in human erythrocytes. *Clin Chim Acta.* 1981;109:233.

79. Lan FH, Tang YC, Huang CH, et al. Antibody-based spot test for NADH-cytochrome b5 reductase activity for the laboratory diagnosis of congenital methemoglobinemia. *Clin Chim Acta.* 1998;273:13.

80. Das Gupta A, Vaidya MS, Bapat JP, et al. Associated red cell enzyme deficiencies and their significance in a case of congenital enzymopenic methemoglobinemia. *Acta Haematol.* 1980;64:285.

81. Kaftory A, Hegesh E. Improved determination of cytochrome b5 in human erythrocytes. *Clin Chem.* 1984;30:1344.

82. Gerald PS, George P. Second spectroscopically abnormal methemoglobin associated with hereditary cyanosis. *Science.* 1959;129:393.

83. Carrell RW, Kay R. A simple method for the detection of unstable haemoglobins. *Br J Haematol.* 1972;23:615.

84. Hutt PJ, Pisciotta AV, Fairbanks VF, et al. DNA sequence analysis proves Hb M-Milwaukee-2 is due to beta-globin gene codon 92 (CAC->TAC), the presumed mutation of Hb M-Hyde Park and Hb M-Akita. *Hemoglobin.* 1998;22:1.

85. Darling RC, Roughton F. The effect of methemoglobin on the equilibrium between oxygen and hemoglobin. *Am J Physiol.* 1942;137:56.

86. Johnson CJ, Bonrud PA, Dosch TL, et al. Fatal outcome of methemoglobinemia in an infant. *JAMA.* 1987;257:2796.

87. Ellis M, Hiss Y, Shenkman L. Fatal methemoglobinemia caused by inadvertent contamination of a laxative solution with sodium nitrite. *Isr J Med Sci.* 1992;28:289.

88. Caudill L, Walbridge J, Kuhn G. Methemoglobinemia as a cause of coma. *Ann Emerg Med.* 1990;19:677.

89. Clifton J 2nd, Leikin JB. Methylene blue. *Am J Ther.* 2003;10:289.

90. Beutler E, Baluda MC. Methemoglobin reduction. Studies of the interaction between cell populations and of the role of methylene blue. *Blood.* 1963;22:323.

91. Rosen PJ, Johnson C, McGehee WG, et al. Failure of methylene blue treatment in toxic methemoglobinemia: associations with glucose-6-phosphate dehydrogenase deficiency. *Ann Intern Med.* 1971;75:83.

92. Bilgin H, Ozcan B, Bilgin T. Methemoglobinemia induced by methylene blue perturbation during laparoscopy. *Acta Anaesthesiol Scand.* 1998;42:594.

93. Kearney TE, Manoguerra AS, Dunford JV Jr. Chemically induced methemoglobinemia from aniline poisoning. *West J Med.* 1984;140:282.

94. Harvey J, Keitt A. Studies of the efficacy and potential hazards of methylene blue therapy in aniline-induced methemoglobinemia. *Br J Haematol.* 1983;54:29.

95. Coleman MD, Rhodes LE, Scott AK, et al. The use of cimetidine to reduce dapsone-dependent methaemoglobinaemia in dermatitis herpetiformis patients. *Br J Clin Pharmacol.* 1992;34:244.

96. Kaplan JC, Chirouze M. Therapy of recessive congenital methaemoglobinaemia by oral riboflavine. *Lancet.* 1978;2:1043.

97. Beutler E. Important recent advances in the field of red cell metabolism: practical implications. In: Gerlach E, Moser K, Deutsch E, et al, eds. *Erythrocytes, Thrombocytes, Leukocytes.* George Thieme Verlag; 1973:123.

98. Lemberg R, Legge JW. *Hematin Compounds and Bile Pigments.* Inter-Science Publishers; 1949.

99. Harrop GA Jr, Waterfield RL. Sulphemoglobinemia. *JAMA.* 1930;95:647.

100. Nichol AW, Hendry I, Movell DB, et al. Mechanism of formation of sulfhemoglobin. *Biochim Biophys Acta.* 1986;156:97.

101. Berzofsky JA, Peisach J, Horecker BL. Sulfheme proteins. IV. The stoichiometry of sulfur incorporation and the isolation of sulfhemin, the prosthetic group of sulfmyoglobin. *J Biol Chem.* 1972;247:3783.

102. Berzofsky JA, Peisach J, Blumberg WE. Sulfheme proteins. II. The reversible oxygenation of ferrous sulfmyoglobin. *J Biol Chem.* 1971;246:7366.

103. Park CM, Nagel RL. Sulfhemoglobinemia. Clinical and molecular aspects. *N Engl J Med.* 1984;310:1579.

104. Discombe G. Sulphaemoglobinaemia and glutathione. *Lancet.* 1960;2:371.

105. Murphy K, Ryan C, Dempsey EM, et al. Neonatal sulfhemoglobinemia and hemolytic anemia associated with intestinal Morganella morganii. *Pediatrics.* 2015;136:e1641.

106. George A, Goetz D. A case of sulfhemoglobinemia in a child with chronic constipation. *Respir Med Case Rep.* 2017;21:21.

107. Carfora A, Campobasso CP, Cassandro P, et al. Fatal inhalation of volcanic gases in three tourists of a geothermal area. *Forensic Sci Int.* 2019;297:e1.

108. McCutcheon A. Sulphaemoglobinaemia and glutathione. *Lancet.* 1960;2:290.

109. Paniker NV, Beutler E. The effect of methylene blue and diaminodiphenylsulfone on red cell reduced glutathione synthesis. *J Lab Clin Med.* 1972;80:481.

110. Smith JE, Mahaffey E, Lee M. Effect of methylene blue on glutamate and reduced glutathione of rabbit erythrocytes. *Biochem J.* 1977;168:587.

111. Pandey J, Chellani H, Garg M, et al. Congenital sulfhemoglobin and transient methemoglobinemia secondary to diarrhoea. *Indian J Pathol Microbiol.* 1996;39:217.

112. Stamatoyannopoulos G, Parer JT, Finch CA. Physiologic implications of a hemoglobin with decreased oxygen affinity (hemoglobin Seattle). *N Engl J Med.* 1996;281:916.

113. Lichtman MA, Murphy MS, Adamson JW. Detection of mutant hemoglobins with altered affinity for oxygen. A simplified technique. *Ann Intern Med.* 1976;84:517.

114. Agarwal N, Mojica-Henshaw MP, Simmons ED, et al. Familial polycythemia caused by a novel mutation in the beta globin gene: essential role of P50 in evaluation of familial polycythemia. *Int J Med Sci.* 2007;4:232.

115. Vreman HJ, Mahoney JJ, Stevenson DK. Carbon monoxide and carboxyhemoglobin. *Adv Pediatr.* 1995;42:303.

116. Hampson NB, Weaver LK. Carbon monoxide poisoning: a new incidence for an old disease. *Undersea Hyperb Med.* 2007;34:163.

117. Weaver LK. Carbon monoxide poisoning. *Crit Care Clin.* 1999;15:297.

118. Ernst A, Zibrak JD. Carbon monoxide poisoning. *N Engl J Med.* 1998;339:1603.

119. Centers for Disease Control and Prevention (CDC). Epidemiologic assessment of the impact of four hurricanes: Florida 2004. *MMWR Morb Mortal Wkly Rep.* 2005;54:693.

120. Chen BC, Shawn LK, Connors NJ, et al. Carbon monoxide exposures in New York City following Hurricane Sandy in 2012. *Clin Toxicol (Phila).* 2013;51:879.

121. Centers for Disease Control and Prevention (CDC). Carbon monoxide exposures after hurricane Ike—Texas, September 2008. *MMWR Morbid Mortal Wkly Rep.* 2009;58:845.

122. Centers for Disease Control and Prevention (CDC). Unintentional non-fire-related carbon monoxide exposures—United States, 2001-2003. *MMWR Morb Mortal Wkly Rep.* 2005;54:36.

123. Mott JA, Wolfe MI, Alverson CJ, et al. National vehicle emissions policies and practices and declining US carbon monoxide-related mortality. *JAMA.* 2002;288:988.

124. Harper A, Croft-Baker J. Carbon monoxide poisoning: undetected by both patients and their doctors. *Age Ageing.* 2004;33:105.

125. US Environmental Protection Agency (EPA). *Emission Facts: Idling Vehicle Emissions.* US Environmental Protection Agency, Publication EPA420-F-98-014; 1998.

126. Radford EP, Drizd TA. Blood carbon monoxide levels in persons 3-74 years of age: United States, 1976-80. *Adv Data.* 1982;1.

127. Sari I, Zengin S, Ozer O, et al. Chronic carbon monoxide exposure increases electrocardiographic P-wave and QT dispersion. *Inhal Toxicol.* 2008;20:879.

128. Stewart RD, Fisher TN, Hosko MJ, et al. Carboxyhemoglobin elevation after exposure to dichloromethane. *Science.* 1972;176:295.

129. Antonini E, Brunori M. Hemoglobin and myoglobin in their reactions with ligands. In: Neuberger A, Taum EL, eds. *Frontiers of Biology.* Elsevier. 1971:19.

130. Sjostrand T. Endogenous formation of carbon monoxide in man. *Nature.* 1949;164:580.

131. Giacometti GM, Brunori M, Antonini E, et al. The reaction of hemoglobin Zurich with oxygen and carbon monoxide. *J Biol Chem.* 1980;255:6160.

132. Hampson NB, Dunford RG, Kramer CC, et al. Selection criteria utilized for hyperbaric oxygen treatment of carbon monoxide poisoning. *J Emerg Med.* 1995;13:227.

133. Benesch RE, Maeda N, Benesch R. 2,3-Diphosphoglycerate and the relative affinity of adult and fetal hemoglobin for oxygen and carbon dioxide. *Biochim Biophys Acta.* 1972;257:178.

134. Engel RR, Rodkey FL, O'Neal JD, et al. Relative affinity of human fetal hemoglobin for CO and O_2. *Blood.* 1969;33:37.

135. Suner S, Partridge R, Sucov A, et al. Non-invasive screening for carbon monoxide toxicity in the emergency department is valuable. *Ann Emerg Med.* 2007;49:718.

136. Weaver LK. Clinical practice. Carbon monoxide poisoning. *N Engl J Med.* 2009;360:1217.

137. Jasper BW, Hopkins RO, Duker HV, et al. Affective outcome following carbon monoxide poisoning: a prospective longitudinal study. *Cogn Behav Neurol.* 2005;18:127.

138. Gemelli F, Cattani R. Carbon monoxide poisoning in childhood. *Br Med J.* 1985;291:1197.

139. Lacey D. Neurologic sequelae of acute carbon monoxide intoxication. *Am J Dis Child.* 1981;135:145.

140. Buckley NA, Juurlink DN, Isbister G, et al. Hyperbaric oxygen for carbon monoxide poisoning. *Cochrane Database Syst Rev.* 2011;CD002041.

141. Elkharrat D, Raphael, JC, Korach, JM, et al. Acute carbon monoxide intoxication and hyperbaric oxygen in pregnancy. *Intensive Care Med.* 1991;17:289.

142. Koren G, Sharav T, Pastuszak A, et al. A multicenter, prospective study of fetal outcome following accidental carbon monoxide poisoning in pregnancy. *Reprod Toxicol.* 1991;5:397.

143. Haldane J, Smith JL. The mass and oxygen capacity of the blood in man. *J Physiol.* 1900;25:331.

144. Ahlgrim C, Birkner P, Seiler F, et al. Applying the optimized CO rebreathing method for measuring blood volumes and hemoglobin mass in heart failure patients. *Front Physiol.* 2018;9:1603.

145. Christensen RD, Malleske DT, Lambert DK, et al. Measuring end-tidal carbon monoxide of jaundiced neonates in the birth hospital to identify those with hemolysis. *Neonatology.* 2016;109:1.

146. Ignarro LJ. Nitric oxide: a novel signal transduction mechanism for transcellular communication. *Hypertension.* 1990;16:477.

147. Liu X, Miller MJ, Joshi MS, et al. Diffusion-limited reaction of free nitric oxide with erythrocytes. *J Biol Chem.* 1998;273:18709.

148. Azarov I, Huang KT, Basu S, et al. Nitric oxide scavenging by red blood cells as a function of hematocrit and oxygenation. *J Biol Chem.* 2005;280:39024.

149. Kim-Shapiro DB, Schechter AN, Gladwin MT. Unraveling the reactions of nitric oxide, nitrite, and hemoglobin in physiology and therapeutics. *Arterioscler Thromb Vasc Biol.* 2006;26:697.

150. Stamler JS, Jia L, Eu JP, et al. Blood flow regulation by S-nitrosohemoglobin in the physiological oxygen gradient. *Science.* 1997;276:2034.

151. Stamler JS, Singel DJ, Piantadosi CA. SNO-hemoglobin and hypoxic vasodilation. *Nat Med.* 2008;14:1008.

152. Vitturi DA, Teng X, Toledo JC, et al. Regulation of nitrite transport in red blood cells by hemoglobin oxygen fractional saturation. *Am J Physiol Heart Circ Physiol.* 2009;296:H1398.

153. Gladwin MT, Kim-Shapiro DB. The functional nitrite reductase activity of the heme-globins. *Blood.* 2008;112:2636.

154. Gladwin MT, Schechter AN, Kim-Shapiro DB, et al. The emerging biology of the nitrite anion. *Nat Chem Biol.* 2005;1:308.

155. Basu S, Grubina R, Huang J, et al. Catalytic generation of N2O3 by the concerted nitrite reductase and anhydrase activity of hemoglobin. *Nat Chem Biol.* 2007;3:785.

156. Lauer T, Preik M, Rassaf T, et al. Plasma nitrite rather than nitrate reflects regional endothelial nitric oxide synthase activity but lacks intrinsic vasodilator action. *Proc Natl Acad Sci U S A.* 2001;98:12814.

157. Shiva S, Wang X, Ringwood LA, et al. Ceruloplasmin is a NO oxidase and nitrite synthase that determines endocrine NO homeostasis. *Nat Chem Biol.* 2006;2:486.

158. Bailey DM, Rasmussen P, Overgaard M, et al. Nitrite and S-nitrosohemoglobin exchange across the human cerebral and femoral circulation: relationship to basal and exercise blood flow responses to hypoxia. *Circulation.* 2017;135:166.

159. Sun CW, Yang J, Kleschyov AL, et al. Hemoglobin beta93 cysteine is not required for export of nitric oxide bioactivity from the red blood cell. *Circulation.* 2019;139:2654.

160. Liu C, Zhao W, Christ GJ, et al. Nitric oxide scavenging by red cell microparticles. *Free Radic Biol Med.* 2013;65:1164.

161. Matto F, Kouretas PC, Smith R, et al. S-nitrosohemoglobin levels and patient outcome after transfusion during pediatric bypass surgery. *Clin Transl Sci.* 2018;11:237.

162. Reynolds JD, Bennett KM, Cina AJ, et al. S-nitrosylation therapy to improve oxygen delivery of banked blood. *Proc Natl Acad Sci U S A.* 2013;110:11529.

163. Kanias T, Gladwin MT. Nitric oxide, hemolysis, and the red blood cell storage lesion: interactions between transfusion, donor, and recipient. *Transfusion.* 2012;52:1388.

164. Kahn MJ, Maley JH, Lasker GF, et al. Updated role of nitric oxide in disorders of erythrocyte function. *Cardiovasc Hematol Disord Drug Targets.* 2013;13:83.

165. Badesch DB, Abman SH, Ahearn GS, et al. Medical therapy for pulmonary arterial hypertension: ACCP evidence-based clinical practice guidelines. *Chest.* 2004;126 (1 suppl):35S.

166. Martinez-Ruiz R, Montero-Huerta P, Hromi J, et al. Inhaled nitric oxide improves survival rates during hypoxia in a sickle cell (SAD) mouse model. *Anesthesiology.* 2001;94:1113.

167. Weiner DL, Hibberd PL, Betit P, et al. Preliminary assessment of inhaled nitric oxide for acute vaso-occlusive crisis in pediatric patients with sickle cell disease. *JAMA.* 2003;289:1136.

168. Sullivan KJ, Goodwin SR, Evangelist J, et al. Nitric oxide successfully used to treat acute chest syndrome of sickle cell disease in a young adolescent. *Crit Care Med.* 1999;27:2563.

169. McMahon TJ, Doctor A. Extrapulmonary effects of inhaled nitric oxide: role of reversible S-nitrosylation of erythrocytic hemoglobin. *Proc Am Thorac Soc.* 2006;3:153.

170. Young JD, Dyar O, Xiong L, et al. Methaemoglobin production in normal adults inhaling low concentrations of nitric oxide. *Intensive Care Med.* 1994;20: 581.

171. Loh E, Stamler JS, Hare JM, et al. Cardiovascular effects of inhaled nitric oxide in patients with left ventricular dysfunction. *Circulation.* 1994;90:2780.

172. Lundin S, Mang H, Smithies M, et al. Inhalation of nitric oxide in acute lung injury: results of a European multicentre study. The European Study Group of Inhaled Nitric Oxide. *Intensive Care Med.* 1999;25:911.

173. Christenson J, Lavoie A, O'Connor M, et al. The incidence and pathogenesis of cardiopulmonary deterioration after abrupt withdrawal of inhaled nitric oxide. *Am J Respir Crit Care Med.* 2000;161:1443.

174. Reynolds JD, Jenkins T, Matto F, et al. Pharmacologic targeting of red blood cells to improve tissue oxygenation. *Clin Pharmacol Ther.* 2018;104:553.

175. Moya MP, Gow AJ, McMahon TJ, et al. S-nitrosothiol repletion by an inhaled gas regulates pulmonary function. *Proc Natl Acad Sci U S A.* 2001;98:5792.

176. Moya MP, Gow AJ, Califf RM, et al. Inhaled ethyl nitrite gas for persistent pulmonary hypertension of the newborn. *Lancet.* 2002;360:141.

177. Gulati A, Sen AP, Sharma AC, et al. Role of ET and NO in resuscitative effect of diaspirin cross-linked hemoglobin after hemorrhage in rat. *Am J Physiol.* 1997;273:H827.

178. Gibson JB, Maxwell RA, Schweitzer JB, et al. Resuscitation from severe hemorrhagic shock after traumatic brain injury using saline, shed blood, or a blood substitute. *Shock.* 2002;17:234.

179. Gerald PS, Efron ML. Chemical studies of several varieties of Hb M. *Proc Natl Acad Sci U S A.* 1961;47:1758.

180. Lloyd CJ. Chemically induced methaemoglobinaemia in a neonate. *Br J Oral Maxillofac Surg.* 1992;30:63.

181. Ng LL, Nai KR, Polak A. Paraquat ingestion with methaemoglobinaemia treated with methylene blue. *Br Med J (Clin Res Ed).* 1982;284:1445.

182. Proudfoot AT. Methaemoglobinaemia due to monolinuron-not paraquat. *Br Med J (Clin Res Ed).* 1982;285:812.

183. Paris PM, Kaplan RM, Stewart RD, et al. Methemoglobin levels following sublingual nitroglycerin in human volunteers. *Ann Emerg Med.* 1986;15:171.

184. Forsyth RJ, Moulden A. Methaemoglobinaemia after ingestion of amyl nitrite. *Arch Dis Child.* 1991;66:152.

185. Kuschner WG, Chitkara RK, Canfield J Jr, et al. Benzocaine-associated methemoglobinemia following bronchoscopy in a healthy research participant. *Respir Care.* 2000;45:953.

186. Abdallah HY, Shah SA. Methemoglobinemia induced by topical benzocaine: a warning for the endoscopist. *Endoscopy.* 2002;34:730.

187. Novaro G, Aronow, H, Militello, M, et al. Benzocaine-induced methemoglobinemia: experience from a high-volume transesophageal echocardiography laboratory. *J Am Soc Echocardiogr.* 2003;16:170.

188. Nilsson A, Engberg G, Henneberg S, et al. Inverse relationship between age-dependent erythrocyte activity of methaemoglobin reductase and prilocaine-induced methaemoglobinaemia during infancy. *Br J Anaesth.* 1990;64:72.

189. Davidovits M, Barak A, Cleper R, et al. Methaemoglobinaemia and haemolysis associated with hydrogen peroxide in a paediatric haemodialysis centre: a warning note. *Nephrol Dial Transplant.* 2003;18:2354.

190. de Torres JP, Strom JA, Jaber BL, et al. Hemodialysis-associated methemoglobinemia in acute renal failure. *Am J Kidney Dis.* 2002;39:1307.

191. Stavem P, Stromme J, Lorkin PA, et al. Haemoglobin M Saskatoon with slight constant haemolysis, markedly increased by sulphonamides. *Scand J Haematol.* 1972;9:566.

192. Hayashi N, Motokawa Y, Kikuchi G. Studies on relationships between structure and function of hemoglobin M-Iwate. *J Biol Chem.* 1966;241:79.

193. Horst J, Schafer R, Kleihauer, et al. Analysis of the Hb M Milwaukee mutation at the DNA level. *Br J Haematol.* 1983;54:643.

194. Hain RD, Chitayat D, Cooper R, et al. Hb FM-Fort Ripley: confirmation of autosomal dominant inheritance and diagnosis by PCR and direct nucleotide sequencing. *Hum Mutat.* 1994;3:239.

195. Reissmann KR, Ruth WE, Nomura T. A human hemoglobin with lowered oxygen affinity and impaired heme-heme interactions. *J Clin Invest.* 1961;40:1826.

196. Naymagon L, Berwick S, Kessler A, et al. The emergence of methemoglobinemia amidst the COVID-19 pandemic. *Am J Hematol.* 2020;95(8):E196-E197.

197. Sahu KK, George SV, Siddiqui AD. Systematic review of methemoglobinemia in acetaminophen poisoning. *QJM.* May 19 2020; hcaa174.

CHAPTER 20
POLYCLONAL AND HEREDITARY SIDEROBLASTIC ANEMIAS

Amel Hamdi and Josef T. Prchal

SUMMARY

Sideroblastic anemias are characterized by the presence of ring sideroblasts in the marrow. These cells are erythroid precursors that have accumulated abnormal amounts of mitochondrial iron. A variety of abnormalities of porphyrin metabolism in affected erythroid cells have been documented. Hereditary sideroblastic anemias are usually X-linked, as the result of mutations in the erythroid form of 5-aminolevulinic acid synthase. Inherited autosomal and mitochondrial forms are seen occasionally. Acquired sideroblastic anemias can occur as a result of copper deficiency or the ingestion of drugs, alcohol, or toxins such as lead or zinc. Patients with acquired sideroblastic macrocytic anemia and variable degrees of thrombocytopenia and leukopenia caused by copper deficiency have been recognized more frequently; the hematologic abnormalities typically resolve after copper replacement. Ring sideroblasts are also a feature of myelodysplastic neoplasms. Some patients with sideroblastic anemia may respond to pharmacologic doses of pyridoxine. Iron loading is common in the sideroblastic anemias and can be treated by phlebotomy when the anemia is mild or with iron chelators (Chap. 11) when it is more severe.

DEFINITION AND HISTORY

Sideroblastic anemias are a heterogeneous group of disorders that have as a common feature the presence of (1) large numbers of pathological sideroblasts in the marrow, which characteristically display abnormal mitochondrial iron accumulation in a circumnuclear position, the location of mitochondria in erythroblasts; these are referred to as ring sideroblasts; (2) ineffective erythropoiesis; (3) increased levels of tissue iron;

Acronyms and Abbreviations: ABCB7, ATP-binding cassette; ALA; 5-aminolevulinic acid; ALAS; 5-aminolevulinic acid synthase; ALAS2, gene encoding erythroid-specific ALA synthase 2; ATP, adenosine triphosphate; CoA, coenzyme A; FC, ferrochelatase; GLRX5, glutaredoxin 5; Fe-S, iron sulfur cluster; Hb, hemoglobin; IRE, the iron-responsive element; HSP70, heat shock protein 70; IRP1, iron regulatory protein 1; MDS, myelodysplastic syndrome; MLASA, mitochondrial myopathy and sideroblastic anemia; mRNA, messenger RNA; NDUFB11, NADH:ubiquinone oxidoreductase subunit B11; PUS1, pseudouridine synthase 1 gene; SLC25A38, mitochondrial carrier family gene; Steap3, ferric reductase; TfR, transferrin receptor; tRNA, mitochondrial transfer RNA; XLSA/A, X-linked sideroblastic anemia, associated with ataxia.

and (4) varying proportions of hypochromic erythrocytes in the blood. They may be acquired or hereditary (Table 20-1).

Acquired monoclonal sideroblastic anemia is a neoplastic disease, that is, it is a clonal cytopenia or oligoblastic myelogenous leukemia that can progress to acute leukemia. Acquired polyclonal sideroblastic anemia may also develop as a result of the administration of certain drugs, exposure to toxins, or coincident to neoplastic or inflammatory disease. Hereditary sideroblastic anemias include X-linked, autosomal, and mutations of mitochondrial genome. Occasionally, a patient with familial disease develops a myelodysplastic syndrome (MDS) later,[1,2] but with these rare exceptions, the disorders are distinct and do not coexist or evolve one from the other.

Although the perinuclear distribution of siderotic granules in the erythroblasts of patients with various types of anemia was described in 1947,[3,4] the concept of sideroblastic anemia as a generic designation was not generally accepted until the publications of Björkman,[5] Dacie and coworkers,[6] Heilmeyer and coworkers,[7,8] Bernard and coworkers,[9] and Mollin.[10] After these descriptions of the acquired, "primary adult form of refractory sideroblastic anemia,"[5,6] similar to the morphological changes in hereditary (sex-linked) hypochromic anemia was recognized. Cooley[11] described a patient with anemia and ovalocytosis who was shortly thereafter shown to have a hereditary sex-linked disorder[12] that we now know resulted from an aminolevulinic acid (ALA) synthase mutation.[13] Autosomally inherited cases were also described,[14] and prominent sideroblastic changes of the marrow were found in Pearson marrow–pancreas syndrome, a disorder that is caused by mutations of mitochondrial DNA.[15-19] Sideroblastic anemia can also be associated with a wide variety of diseases,[20] therapy with antituberculosis drugs,[21,22] lead intoxication,[23-26] and copper deficiency.[27,28] In some patients, the anemia responded to large doses of pyridoxine and was designated "pyridoxine-responsive anemia."[10,29-31] These "secondary" acquired disorders were then incorporated into the classification.

EPIDEMIOLOGY

All of the hereditary forms are rare, and no particular ethnic predilection is known. Drug-induced forms occur sporadically among subjects taking the drugs listed in Table 20-1.

ETIOLOGY AND PATHOGENESIS
MORPHOLOGICAL ASPECTS: THE SIDEROBLASTS

Sideroblasts are erythroblasts containing aggregates of nonheme iron appearing as one or more Prussian blue–positive granules on light microscopy.[32] The morphology of these cells in normal and abnormal states is discussed in detail in Chap. 1. In normal marrow, virtually every erythroblast has siderosomes, iron-containing organelles that are demonstrable by transmission electron microscopy. Light microscopy of Prussian blue–stained marrow aspirates or biopsy sections is a relatively insensitive method to identify these structures. One can usually identify about 25% to 35% of erythroblasts with one to three very fine Prussian blue–stained granules in the cytoplasm of a well-prepared marrow sample. Pathological sideroblasts may be of two types: erythroblasts with a marked increase in the number and size of siderotic granules in the cytoplasm (seen in individuals with iron saturated transferrin[33]), compared with normal erythroblasts, or ring sideroblasts. Ring sideroblasts are the hallmark of the sideroblastic anemias. They are defined as erythroblasts characterized by at least five siderotic granules surrounding at least one-third of the nuclear circumference.[34] In contrast to the normal

TABLE 20–1. Classification of Sideroblastic Anemias

I. Acquired
  A. Primary sideroblastic anemia (myelodysplastic syndromes)
    1. Subunit 1 of the mitochondrial cytochrome oxidase[59,60]
  B. Sideroblastic anemia secondary to:
    1. Isoniazid[21,22]
    2. Pyrazinamide[21,22]
    3. Copper deficiency[27,28]
    4. Cycloserine[158]
    5. Chloramphenicol[158]
    6. Ethanol[129]
    7. Lead[24]
    8. Chronic neoplastic disease
    9. Zinc-induced copper deficiency[133,134]
II. Hereditary
  A. X chromosome-linked
    1. Defects in the erythroid specific ALAS
    2. Defects in ABCB7[53,57,101]
    3. Defects in NDUFB11[105]
    4. Defects in HSPA9[106] (an autosomal recessive trait)
  B. Autosomal
    1. Defects in the erythroid specific mitochondrial carrier family protein SLC25A38[51]
    2. Mitochondrial myopathy and sideroblastic anemia (*PSU1* mutations)[62,118,119]
  C. Mitochondrial
    1. Pearson marrow–pancreas syndrome[15-19]
    2. Heteroplasmic point mutations in subunit 1 of the *mitochondrial cytochrome oxidase* gene
    3. Mutation of *ABCB7*
    4. *NDUFB11*, encoding NADH:ubiquinone oxidoreductase subunit B11, a mitochondrial respiratory complex I
    5. Mutations of *HSPA9*

ALAS, 5-aminolevulinic acid synthase.

cytoplasmic location of siderotic granules, the pathologic sideroblasts in the sideroblastic anemias have large amounts of iron deposited as dust- or plaque-like ferruginous micelles between the cristae of mitochondria (Fig. 20-1).[35] The iron-loaded mitochondria are distorted and swollen, their cristae are indistinct, and identification of mitochondria may itself be difficult. In humans, the mitochondria of the erythroblast are distributed perinuclearly,[23] which accounts for the distinctive "ring" sideroblast identified by Prussian blue staining or electron microscopy when mitochondrial iron overload is present (see Fig. 20-1). The morphological features that characterize pathologic sideroblasts in various disorders have been summarized elsewhere.[36]

PATHOGENESIS

The pathogenesis of most of the sideroblastic anemias is not well understood.[37,38] It is not clear whether the basic mechanism by which abnormal accumulations of intramitochondrial iron occurs is the same in inherited and acquired forms of the disease. However, it seems appropriate, given the present state of knowledge, to discuss both forms together. The pathogenesis of the disorder may be viewed from two standpoints: the underlying biochemical lesions and the mechanism(s) of the anemia itself.

Biochemical Lesions and Genetics

In the search for the biochemical lesions responsible for the development of sideroblastic anemia, attention has been focused on an intramitochondrial defect in heme synthesis and on possible disturbances in pyridoxine metabolism.

Defects in Heme Synthesis

The role of defects in heme biosynthesis has occupied a central stage since the early studies of Garby and colleagues,[39] who postulated that such a defect might exist; they demonstrated that the level of free erythrocyte protoporphyrin was decreased. Subsequently, a variety of abnormalities of the levels of protoporphyrin IX precursors and of their rate of incorporation into heme was documented (Chap. 21).[40-45] However, the findings have not all been consistent because levels of free erythrocyte protoporphyrin have often been increased,[46,47] not diminished. The role of mitochondria in the etiology of sideroblastic anemia gained further credence when mutations of the mitochondrial genome were found in patients with Pearson syndrome.[15-19]

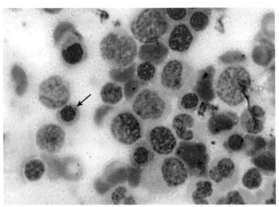

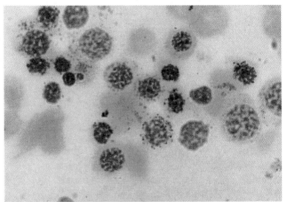

A **B**

FIGURE 20–1. Bone marrow films. **A.** Normal marrow stained with Prussian blue. Note several erythroblasts without apparent siderotic (blue-stained) granules. The *arrow* indicates erythroblast with several very small cytoplasmic blue–stained granules. It is very difficult to see siderosomes in most erythroblasts in normal marrow because they are often below the resolution of the light microscope. **B.** Sideroblastic anemia. Note the florid increase in Prussian blue–staining granules in the erythroblasts, most with circumnuclear locations. In some cases, cytoplasmic iron granules are also increased in size and number, also a pathologic change. *(Reproduced with permission from Lichtman MA, Shafer MS, Felgar RE, et al: Lichtman's Atlas of Hematology 2016. New York, NY: McGraw Hill; 2017.)*

Hereditary Sideroblastic Anemias

Shortly after the identification of erythroid-specific 5-aminolevulinic acid synthase (ALAS2, the first enzyme in heme synthesis; Fig. 20-2), it became apparent that most patients with hereditary X-linked sideroblastic anemias (XLSA) had mutations in the *ALAS2* gene.[48-50] However, a proportion of patients with congenital sideroblastic anemia has autosomal recessive inheritance. At least some such patients have a defect in the gene encoding the erythroid specific mitochondrial carrier protein, *SLC25A38*.[51] This transporter imports glycine into mitochondria,[51,52] where it serves as one of the substrates for ALAS2, the first enzyme in heme biosynthesis. Hence, *SLC25A38* defects would be expected to generate a phenotype identical to that seen in patients with defects in ALAS2. One can speculate that, in erythroid cells, a common control mechanism exists that regulates acquisition of the two substrates for heme synthesis (iron and glycine).

Hereditary sideroblastic anemia with spinocerebellar degeneration with ataxia is a rare X-linked syndrome that appears to be distinct from the other forms of sideroblastic anemia.[53-56] It is caused by mutation of adenosine triphosphate (ATP)-binding cassette (*ABCB7* gene).[53,57,58]

Heteroplasmic point mutations in subunit 1 of the *mitochondrial cytochrome oxidase* gene have been documented in some patients with sideroblastic anemia.[59-61]

Rare autosomal forms of inherited sideroblastic anemia have also been reported,[62,63] including those with a deficiency of uroporphyrinogen decarboxylase[64,65] and ferrochelatase (FC)[40,45,66-68] enzymes, both necessary for the synthesis of heme (Chap. 21). The other reported defects, such as that of heme synthetase (currently FC), could result from the inhibitory effect of mitochondrial iron overload on enzyme activity.[45] A defect in coproporphyrinogen oxidase could not be confirmed by direct measurement.[69]

An unusual phenotype of inherited sideroblastic anemia, developmental delay with variable neurologic defects and B-cell lymphopenia with hypogammaglobulinemia is caused by mutations of (tRNA nucleotidyltransferase 1).[70,71]

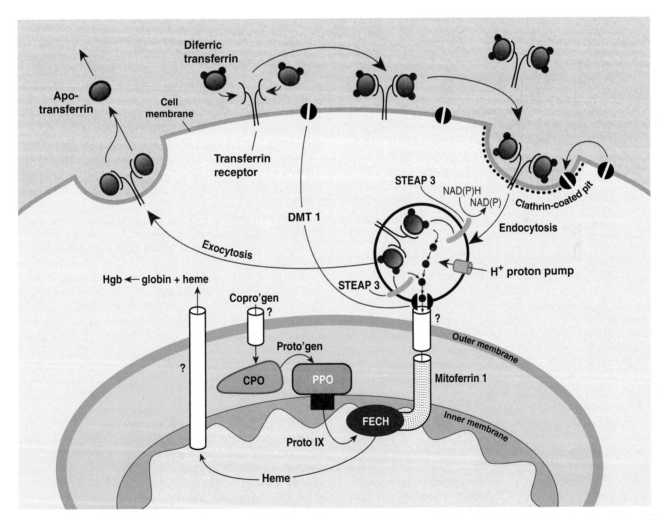

FIGURE 20–2. Schematic representation of iron uptake from transferrin and its delivery to the hemoglobin (Hb) molecule. Extracellular diferric transferrin is bound by the membrane-bound transferrin receptor (TfR) and internalized via receptor-mediated endocytosis into an endosome. Iron is released from transferrin by a decrease in pH (~pH 5.5), reduced by Steap 3, after which the metal is transported through the endosomal membrane by DMT1. In erythroid cells, more than 90% of iron must enter mitochondria via the "kiss-and-run" mechanism. Mitochondrial ferrochelatase (FC, the enzyme that inserts Fe^{2+} into protoporphyrin IX) resides on the inner leaflet of the inner mitochondrial membrane. The transport of coproporphyrinogen (Copro'gen) into mitochondria is not fully understood. Neither mechanisms nor the regulation of the transport of heme from mitochondria to globin polypeptides are known; however, it has been proposed that a carrier protein, heme binding protein 1 (gene: *HEBP1*), is involved in this process. CPO, coproporphyrinogen oxidase; PPO, protoporphyrinogen oxidase.

Pyridoxine Metabolism

A role for pyridoxine has been supported by the demonstration that pyridoxine deficiency in animals is a prototype of sideroblastic anemia.[35] Sideroblastic anemia can be induced by drugs that reduce the level of pyridoxal phosphate in blood, which decreases the ALAS2 activity in normoblasts.[22,40,44] Moreover, certain sideroblastic disorders, although not caused by pyridoxine deficiency, are nonetheless responsive to pharmacologic doses of pyridoxine.[48,72-74] The pyridoxal phosphate is a necessary coenzyme for the first enzyme of heme synthesis, the condensation of glycine and succinyl coenzyme A (CoA) to form ALA, a reaction mediated by ALAS (Chap. 21). Furthermore, pyridoxal phosphate is a factor in the enzymatic conversion of serine to glycine (Chap. 9). This reaction generates a form of folate coenzyme necessary for the formation of thymidylate, an important step in DNA synthesis. Pyridoxal 5′-phosphate, the active form of the coenzyme, must itself be enzymatically synthesized from pyridoxine. Deficiencies in its biosynthesis have also been invoked as the possible cause of certain sideroblastic anemias,[29,75] but direct measurements of pyridoxal kinase failed to confirm that the postulated lesion was present.[76]

Other Metabolic Defects and Acquired Associations with Sideroblastic Anemia

Increased levels of uroporphyrinogen 1 synthase are commonly encountered in patients with sideroblastic anemias.[43] Alcoholism, a common cause of secondary sideroblastic anemia, inhibits heme synthesis at several steps.[42] Dramatically altered activity ratios of a wide diversity of enzymes have been described[77,78] (eg, elevated arginase activity).

Sideroblastic anemia has been found in a patient with apparent antibody-mediated red cell aplasia.[79] There are alterations in red cell antigen patterns frequently with an increase of i and a loss of A$_1$ antigens (Chap. 29).[80] Similar findings occur in certain hereditary and acquired refractory anemias with cellular marrows but without ring sideroblasts.[78] Such dyscrasias are also characterized by ineffective erythropoiesis and, except for the lack of ring sideroblasts, may in some instances be virtually indistinguishable from their sideroblastic counterparts.[81]

Pathogenesis of Ring Sideroblast Formation

Iron accumulation within mitochondria is an unusual pathological phenomenon occurring only in erythroblasts of patients with sideroblastic anemias and, to a much lesser degree, in cardiomyocytes of patients with Friedreich ataxia.[82,83] Mitochondrial iron accumulation has not been demonstrated in patients with either primary or secondary iron overload. The pathophysiology of ring sideroblast formation in patients with ALAS2 defects and those caused by inhibitors of porphyrin biosynthesis (see Table 20-1) is likely because of the unique aspects of the regulation of iron metabolism and heme synthesis in erythroid cells.[84] These differences can account for the accumulation of nonheme iron in erythroid mitochondria of sideroblastic anemia patients. In hemoglobin (Hb)-synthesizing cells, iron is specifically targeted toward mitochondria that avidly take up iron even when the synthesis of protoporphyrin IX is suppressed.[85-88] In contrast, nonerythroid cells store iron in excess of metabolic needs within ferritin.[89] Hence, erythroid-specific mechanisms and controls are involved in the transport of iron into mitochondria in erythroid cells, but the nature of these processes, including the role of mitoferrin 1 (Chap. 10), an inner mitochondrial membrane protein that presumably provides Fe^{2+} to FC,[90] is poorly understood. The transferrin-bound iron is used for Hb synthesis[84,88] with a high degree of efficiency and is targeted into erythroid mitochondria, and because no intermediate for cytoplasmic iron transport has ever been identified in erythroid cells, the following hypothesis of intracellular iron trafficking in developing red cells has been proposed[84] and then experimentally

confirmed.[91-93] These reports have demonstrated that iron released from transferrin in the endosome is passed directly from protein to protein until it reaches FC, which incorporates Fe^{2+} into protoporphyrin IX[94] in the mitochondrion. Such a transfer bypasses the cytosol as the movement of iron between proteins could be mediated by a direct interaction of the endosome with the mitochondrion.[84,91-93,95] It has been shown that (1) endosome mobility is essential for the efficient incorporation of Fe from diferric transferrin into heme[92,93]; (2) confocal microscopy showed that in reticulocytes, endosomes continuously traverse the cytosol[91,92]; and (3) the highly efficient transport of Fe toward erythroid cell mitochondria requires a direct interaction between endosomes and mitochondria in a "kiss-and-run" mechanism[91-93] (see Fig. 20-2). These studies also revealed that cytoplasmic iron not bound to transferrin is inefficiently used for heme biosynthesis and that the endosome–mitochondrion interaction increases chelatable mitochondrial iron.

An important distinction between erythroid and nonerythroid cells is the presence of a feedback mechanism in which "uncommitted" heme inhibits iron acquisition from transferrin.[96-99] Although it is still unresolved whether heme inhibits transferrin endocytosis[96,97] or iron release from transferrin,[99] the lack of heme plays an important role in mitochondrial iron accumulation. Additionally, nonheme iron, which accumulates in erythroid mitochondria, cannot be released from the organelle unless it is inserted into heme.[88] This suggests that mitochondria can release iron only when the metal is in a proper chemical form, in this case, inserted into protoporphyrin IX. These considerations provide a framework to the pathogenesis of mitochondrial iron accumulation in erythroblasts of patients with sideroblastic anemia caused by ALAS2 defects as well as those caused by agents inhibiting porphyrin biosynthesis (see Table 20-1).

It was also demonstrated that mutations in an enhancer element in ALAS2 intron 1,[100] which contains a GATA-binding site, cause a clinical phenotype similar to patients with XLSA caused by mutations in the ALAS2 coding sequence itself.

A distinct form of X-linked sideroblastic anemia associated with ataxia (XLSA/A) was described in several families with putative mutations mapped to chromosome region Xq13.[55] In contrast to ALAS2-linked disease, the XLSA/A syndrome is associated with elevated erythrocyte protoporphyrin IX levels. It was demonstrated that mutations of ABCB7 gene is responsible for XLSA/A.[53,57,101] The ABCB7 protein is thought to transfer iron sulfur [Fe-S] clusters from mitochondria to the cytosol.[82,102,103] How the disruption of [Fe-S] cluster export might impede heme biosynthesis is, however, not clear, but the accumulation of erythrocyte zinc–protoporphyrin IX is found in XLSA/A.[53,55,57] Additionally, mouse erythrocytes with mutated ABCB7 (E433K) have an increase in zinc-protoporphyrin IX/heme ratios.[104] Because the formation of zinc–protoporphyrin IX requires FC, ABCB7 mutations cannot interfere with the activity of this enzyme. Instead, the loss of function of ABCB7 may, by a yet-to-be-defined mechanism, diminish the availability of reduced iron (the only substrate of iron for FC) required for the assembly of heme from protoporphyrin IX. In this ABCB7 mutated X-linked sideroblastic anemia, as in ALAS2-associated sideroblastic anemia, decreased levels of heme likely contribute to the pathogenesis of ring sideroblast formation.

A new mutation in NDUFB11, encoding NADH:ubiquinone oxidoreductase subunit B11, a mitochondrial respiratory complex I–associated protein located on the X chromosome, was described in five men with a variably syndromic, normocytic congenital sideroblastic anemia. The NDUFB11's p.F93del mutation results in respiratory insufficiency and loss of complex I stability and activity in patient-derived fibroblasts.[105] The pathogenesis of the sideroblast formation is likely caused by a defect in the electron transport chain.

A mutation in *HSPA9*, a mitochondrial *HSP70* homolog involved in mitochondrial [Fe-S] biogenesis was described to cause congenital sideroblastic anemia. *HSPA9* is one of the genes in the 5′ region in the acquired 5q deletion of MDS coined *5q minus syndrome*. The 5q minus syndrome is characterized by a defect in erythroid maturation, but ring sideroblasts are uncommon.[106]

Another type of hereditary hypochromic anemia was described in *shiraz* zebrafish mutants.[107] These mutants have a deficiency of glutaredoxin 5 encoded by (*GLRX5*) whose product is required for [Fe-S] cluster assembly. This study demonstrated that the loss of the [Fe-S] cluster in the iron regulatory protein 1 (IRP1) blocked *ALAS2* translation by binding to the iron-responsive element (IRE) located in the 5′-untranslated region of *ALAS2* messenger RNA (mRNA). Subsequently, a case of GLRX5 deficiency in an anemic male with iron overload and a low number of ring sideroblasts was reported.[108] As in zebrafish with *shiraz* mutants, ferritin levels were low, and transferrin receptor levels were high in the patient's cells; this can be explained by increased IRP1 binding to IREs in mRNAs of these two proteins. However, erythroblasts from zebrafish *shiraz* mutants were not found to contain iron-loaded mitochondria.

Sideroblasts were reported in some β-thalassemia patients.[109] The mechanism of ring sideroblast formation in β-thalassemia is obscure.

Primary Acquired Sideroblastic Anemia (Refractory Anemia with Ring Sideroblasts or Myelodysplastic Syndrome with Ring Sideroblasts)

The pathophysiology of acquired idiopathic sideroblastic anemia as a manifestation of MDS is distinct from the already discussed X-linked congenital sideroblastic anemias. In these patients, there is no evidence for a decrease in the formation protoporphyrin IX levels; instead, the amount of protoporphyrin IX is moderately increased.[47] Impaired iron reduction could cause intramitochondrial iron accumulation in patients with MDSs. The ferric reductase, Steap3, is involved in the reduction of Fe^{3+} to Fe^{2+} in endosomes.[110] Based on the model of the direct inter-organellar transfer of iron (see Fig. 20-2), it can be assumed that there is only one reduction step during the path of iron from endosomes to FC. However, the efficient insertion of ferrous ions into protoporphyrin IX may still require a reducing environment in mitochondria that would be provided by an uninterrupted respiratory chain. This proposal is compatible with the fact that sideroblastic anemia accompanying Pearson marrow–pancreas syndrome[111] is caused by deletions of mitochondrial DNA genes; products of these are involved in electron transport.[112] Indeed, there are at least some myelodysplasia-associated sideroblastic anemia patients described caused by acquired mutations in cytochrome oxidase, encoded by mitochondrial DNA.[59,60,113-115] However, a rigorous study failed to find cytochrome oxidase mutations in 10 patients with myelodysplasia-associated sideroblastic anemia.[116] Alternatively, there is some evidence that *ABCB7* (see the earlier discussion of XLSA/A) could be a possible candidate gene for the formation of ring sideroblasts in refractory anemia with ring sideroblasts.[117]

Mitochondrial Myopathy and Sideroblastic Anemia

There are some similarities and some dissimilarities between Pearson marrow–pancreas syndrome and patients with mitochondrial myopathy and sideroblastic anemia (MLASA).[62,118,119] In both cases, there are defects in mitochondrial electron transport chain, likely creating an environment that retards iron access to FC in the reduced form. Both disorders are hereditary, but Pearson syndrome is caused by large deletions of mitochondrial DNA, whereas MLASA results from a homozygous missense mutation in the genomic DNA of pseudouridine synthase 1 gene (*PUS1*) encoding pseudouridine synthase 1.[118]

It has been proposed that deficient pseudouridylation of mitochondrial tRNAs explains the pathogenesis of MLASA type of sideroblastic anemia.[118]

Mitochondrial Ferritin

Mitochondrial ferritin is a ferritin isoform with ferroxidase activity that is expressed only in mitochondria. This protein is encoded by an intronless nuclear gene and can store iron within a shell of homopolymers.[120-122] Although the function and regulation of expression of this protein is not fully understood, the induction of mitochondrial ferritin causes the transfer of iron from cytosolic ferritin to mitochondrial ferritin.[123] The mitochondrial ferritin has a very low expression in all tissues except testes.[120,122] Mitochondrial ferritin is not expressed in normal erythroblasts, but it is expressed in ring sideroblasts of patients with sideroblastic anemias,[124] caused by ALAS2 defects as well as those associated with MDS. In both, iron is sequestered within mitochondrial ferritin.[124] Because mitochondrial ferritin has ferroxidase activity, it likely protects mitochondria by converting the toxic ferrous iron to ferric iron that is stored. Further research is needed to explain the mechanism of mitochondrial ferritin induction in erythroblasts of patients with sideroblastic anemias, both hereditary and acquired. Whether the mitochondrial ferritin also accumulates iron in ring sideroblasts of patients with XLSA/A has not yet been studied.

Mechanism of Anemia

The dominant factor that determines anemia is ineffective erythropoiesis (intramedullary apoptosis of late erythroid precursors); the rate of red cell destruction is usually near normal or only moderately accelerated to levels for which a normally functioning marrow can compensate.[125] The half-time of disappearance of intravenously injected tracer doses of radioactive iron is usually is rapid (25-50 minutes; normal mean, 90-100 minutes) but in some patients may be normal. The plasma iron turnover tends to be increased (0.15-0.59 mg/L of blood per day; normal, ~0.030-0.070 mg/L per day), but incorporation of radioactive iron into heme and its delivery to the blood as newly synthesized Hb are depressed (15%-30% of tracer dose; normal, 70%-90%). Red cell survival ranges between 40 and 120 days, indicating some cases have moderate or only very slightly shortened red cell life span, but in other cases, red cell survival is normal. As in other kinds of anemia characterized by ineffective erythropoiesis, the fecal stercobilin excreted per day may be greater than can be accounted for by the daily catabolism of circulating Hb.

● CLINICAL AND LABORATORY FEATURES

PRIMARY ACQUIRED (CLONAL) SIDEROBLASTIC ANEMIA

The acquired monoclonal sideroblastic anemia is a subtype of MDS. Anemia is present in more than 90% of patients. Patients may be asymptomatic or, if anemia is more severe, have the nonspecific symptoms of anemia, including pallor, weakness, loss of a sense of well-being, and exertional dyspnea that may require red cell transfusions and other interventions. A small proportion of patients have infections related to severe granulocytopenia or hemorrhage related to severe thrombocytopenia at the time of diagnosis; however, this variant of MDS has the lowest probability of symptomatic neutropenia, thrombocytopenia, and acute leukemic transformation. Hepatomegaly or splenomegaly also occurs rarely in this type of MDS. Iron overloading regularly accompanies this disorder, usually in those who have a large requirement for transfusion, and may be the cause of death (Chap. 11).

Mutations of *SF3B1*, a splicing factor gene, are closely associated with ring sideroblasts. Approximately 85% of patients with MDS and ring sideroblasts have an *SF3B1* mutation. *SF3B1* mutant patients with MDS are less likely to have cytogenetic abnormalities or other mutations in genes associated with a poor prognosis. Thus, *SF3B1*-mutant MDS represents a nosologic entity.[126]

SECONDARY ACQUIRED (POLYCLONAL) SIDEROBLASTIC ANEMIA

Drugs and Alcohol

Administration of certain drugs and the ingestion of alcohol may cause sideroblastic anemia (see Table 20-1). The drugs that are most commonly associated with this type of anemia are isonicotinic acid hydrazide,[127] pyrazinamide,[21,22,128] and cycloserine,[21,22,128] all pyridoxine antagonists. Although plasma pyridoxal phosphate levels are often low in patients with alcoholism, there is no correlation between these levels and the appearance of ring sideroblasts in the marrow.[129]

Anemia secondary to drugs may be quite severe, even necessitating transfusion,[22] but characteristically, the anemia improves rapidly when the patient is given pyridoxine and/or when administration of the offending drug is discontinued. The red cells are hypochromic, and a dimorphic appearance of the erythrocytes in the blood film may be notable, that is, two populations of red cells can be distinguished (hypochromic and anisocytic along with normochromic and normocytic). The reticulocyte count is low or normal.[130] In rare instances, a sideroblastic anemia first observed during the course of drug administration has progressed in the face of discontinuing the putative offending drug. In such cases, the patient presumably had an unmasked underlying myelodysplastic neoplasm.

Copper Deficiency

In 1974, two patients with sideroblastic anemia, one also with neutropenia, after extensive bowel surgery and long-term parenteral nutrition were described.[27] In 2002, another patient was described who developed progressive macrocytic anemia, thrombocytopenia, and leukopenia with ring sideroblasts after gastroduodenal bypass (Billroth II procedure); she was considered to have MDS and scheduled to have marrow transplant until her copper deficiency was discovered. This patient also had optic neuritis and other neurologic abnormalities.[28] The hematologic abnormalities, but not neurologic defects, resolved fully with copper therapy. Since that time, numerous similar cases, with and without neurologic abnormalities, have been reported.[131,132] A similar hematologic picture can be seen with zinc-induced copper deficiency.[133,134]

HEREDITARY SIDEROBLASTIC ANEMIA

Hereditary sideroblastic anemia is very uncommon. More instances of the X chromosome–linked varieties than of apparently autosomally inherited cases have been documented.[135] The disorder is heterogeneous. The variant with ataxia is characterized by neurologic impairment and typically mild anemia in males. The neurologic symptoms include ataxia, dysmetria, dysdiadochokinesis, dysarthria, and intention tremor that are referred as spinocerebellar syndrome. A mild intellectual impairment may also be seen.

In some of the cases, either the presence of the sideroblasts in the marrow or the hereditary nature of the disorder is documented in others presumed but not clearly documented in each case. Anemia is usually apparent during the first few months[136] or years[39,41] of life; it may even occur prenatally.[113] However, there are patients in whom microcytic anemia first became evident in the eighth and ninth decade of life and were found to have a microcytic, pyridoxine response anemia

apparently related to inherited mutations of the *ALAS2* gene.[137,138] Splenomegaly may be present[139] but not universally so.[39,136] The anemia is characteristically microcytic and hypochromic, and prominent dimorphism of the red cell population has been noted in carrier females of the sex-linked form of the anemia.[12,136,140] This has been regarded as evidence of X-inactivation affecting the locus responsible for this disorder,[41,136,140,141] but it is notable that marked dimorphism is sometimes seen in the red cells of affected males as well[12,39] and in autosomal forms of the disease.[142] The degree of anisocytosis and poikilocytosis is usually striking. Sometimes the anemia can be macrocytic,[2,143] especially in mitochondrial forms of the disease. The red cells show marked heterogeneity with respect to resistance to osmotic lysis: A flattened curve indicates that cells with both increased and decreased resistance to lysis are present.[39,144] The white cell count is usually normal or slightly decreased unless splenectomy has been performed. Then it may be greatly elevated.[145] In one family, a platelet function abnormality resembling a storage pool defect was noted,[146] but this could have been an independently inherited disorder.

Pearson marrow–pancreas syndrome is a refractory sideroblastic anemia with vacuolization of marrow precursors and exocrine pancreatic dysfunction.[61,147] It may be fatal in infancy or early childhood and is characterized by marrow failure with macrocytic sideroblastic anemia, which is typically transfusion dependent. Neutropenia and thrombocytopenia may also be present. However, the invariable dysfunction of the exocrine pancreas caused by fibrosis and acinar atrophy resulting in chronic malabsorption and diarrhea may in some affected patients be dominant features of its morbidity and mortality. Lactic acidosis caused by a defect in oxidative phosphorylation and other organ dysfunction including liver impairment is also common. The usual causes of death are bacterial sepsis caused by neutropenia, metabolic crisis, and hepatic failure. However, there is considerable phenotypic variation, presumably depending on the number of mitochondria affected and their tissue distribution.

●TREATMENT

Many patients with hereditary sideroblastic anemia have some response to treatment with pyridoxine in doses of 0.05–0.20 g/day,[12,136,140,145,148-150] but failures have also been observed.[8,39,46] Some patients have responded to doses as low as 0.0025 g/day.[145] An additional effect may be achieved by the administration of folic acid.[136] *pyridoxine is given orally but it has been reported that, rarely,* adding parenteral crude liver extract anemias can improve the likelihood of a response.[151,152] Responses to pyridoxine may result in an increase in the steady-state Hb level of the blood or a decrease in the transfusion requirement, but normalization of the Hb level does not usually occur and the anemia relapses when pyridoxine administration is discontinued.

Iron overloading regularly accompanies this disorder and may be the cause of death[45] (Chap. 11). Iron storage may be enhanced when any of the mutations of hereditary hemochromatosis are co-inherited.[153] If the anemia is not too severe or if it can be partially corrected by the administration of pyridoxine, phlebotomy may be used to diminish the iron burden.[154,155] Otherwise, it may be advisable to attempt to decrease the amount of body iron by iron chelation (Chap. 11).

Marrow transplantation, both ablative[156] and nonmyeloablative,[157] has been used on rare occasions to treat patients with severe hereditary sideroblastic anemia.

REFERENCES

1. Kardos G, Veerman AJ, de Waal FC, et al. Familial sideroblastic anemia with emergence of monosomy 5 and myelodysplastic syndrome. *Med Pediatr Oncol.* 1996;26(1):54-56.
2. Tuckfield A, Ratnaike S, Hussein S, et al. A novel form of hereditary sideroblastic anaemia with macrocytosis. *Br J Haematol.* 1997;97(2):279-285.

3. Dacie JV, Doniach I. The basophilic property of the iron-containing granules in sidero-cytes. *J Pathol Bacteriol.* 1947;59(4):684-686.

4. McFadzean AJ, Davis LJ. Iron-staining erythrocyte inclusions with special reference to acquired haemolytic anaemia. *Glasg Med J.* 1947;28.

5. Bjorkman SE. Chronic refractory anemia with sideroblastic bone marrow; a study of four cases. *Blood.* 1956;11(3):250-259.

6. Dacie JV, Smith MD, White JC, et al. Refractory normoblastic anaemia: a clinical and haematological study of seven cases. *Br J Haematol.* 1959;5(1):56-82.

7. Heilmeyer L, Emmrich J, Hennemann HH, et al. [Chronic hypochromic anemia in two siblings based on iron metabolism disorders (anemia hypochromica sideroachrestica hereditaria).]. *Folia Haematol (Frankf).* 1958;2(1):61-75.

8. Heilmeyer L, Keiderling W, Bilger R, et al. [Chronic refractory anemia with sideroblastic bone marrow (Anemia refractoria sideroblastica).]. *Folia Haematol (Frankf).* 1958;2(1):49-60.

9. Bernard J, Lortholary P, Levy JP, et al. [Primary sideroblastic normochromic anemia.]. *Nouv Rev Fr Hematol.* 1963;71:723-748.

10. Mollin DL. Sideroblasts and sideroblastic anaemia. *Br J Haematol.* 1965;11:41-48.

11. Cooley TB. A severe type of hereditary anemia with elliptocytosis. Interesting sequence of splenectomy. *Am J Med. Sci.* 1945;209.

12. Rundles R. Hereditary (sex-linked) anemia. *Am J Med Sci.* 1946;211.

13. Cotter PD, Rucknagel DL, Bishop DF. X-linked sideroblastic anemia: identification of the mutation in the erythroid-specific delta-aminolevulinate synthase gene (ALAS2) in the original family described by Cooley. *Blood.* 1994;84(11):3915-3924.

14. Kasturi J, Basha HM, Smeda SH, et al. Hereditary sideroblastic anaemia in 4 siblings of a Libyan family—autosomal inheritance. *Acta Haematol.* 1983;68(4):321-324.

15. Cormier V, Rotig A, Quartino AR, et al. Widespread multi-tissue deletions of the mitochondrial genome in the Pearson marrow-pancreas syndrome. *J Pediatr.* 1990;117(4):599-602.

16. Danse PW, Jakobs C, Rotig A, et al. [Pearson's syndrome: a multi-system disorder based on a mt-DNA deletion]. *Tijdschr Kindergeneeskd.* 1991;59(6):196-202.

17. Gurgey A, Rotig A, Gumruk F, et al. Pearson's marrow-pancreas syndrome in 2 Turkish children. *Acta Haematol.* 1992;87(4):206-209.

18. McShane MA, Hammans SR, Sweeney M, et al. Pearson syndrome and mitochon-drial encephalomyopathy in a patient with a deletion of mtDNA. *Am J Hum Genet.* 1991;48(1):39-42.

19. Rotig A, Cormier V, Blanche S, et al. Pearson's marrow-pancreas syndrome. A multisys-tem mitochondrial disorder in infancy. *J Clin Invest.* 1990;86(5):1601-1608.

20. Macgibbon BH, Mollin DL. Sideroblastic anaemia in man: observations on seventy cases. *Br J Haematol.* 1965;11:59-69.

21. Hines JD, Grasso JA. The sideroblastic anemias. *Semin Hematol.* 1970;7(1):86-106.

22. Verwilghen R, Reybrouck G, Callens L, et al. Antituberculous drugs and sideroblastic anaemia. *Br J Haematol.* 1965;11:92-98.

23. Bessis MC, Jensen WN. Sideroblastic anaemia, mitochondria and erythroblastic Iron. *Br J Haematol.* 1965;11:49-51.

24. Griggs RC. Lead poisoning: hematologic aspects. *Prog Hematol.* 1964;4:117-137.

25. Jensen WN, Moreno G. [The ribosomes and basophilic granulations of erythrocytes in lead poisoning.] *C R Hebd Seances Acad Sci.* 1964;258:3596-3597.

26. Jensen WN, Moreno GD, Bessis MC. An electron microscopic description of basophilic stippling in red cells. *Blood.* 1965;25:933-943.

27. Dunlap WM, James GW 3rd, Hume DM. Anemia and neutropenia caused by copper deficiency. *Ann Intern Med.* 1974;80(4):470-476.

28. Gregg XT, Reddy V, Prchal JT. Copper deficiency masquerading as myelodysplastic syndrome. *Blood.* 2002;100(4):1493-1495.

29. Gehrmann G. Pyridoxine-responsive anaemias. *Br J Haematol.* 1965;11:86-91.

30. Harris JW, Whittington RM, Weisman R Jr, et al. Pyridoxine responsive anemia in the human adult. *Proc Soc Exp Biol Med.* 1956;91(2):427-432.

31. Horrigan DL, Harris JW. Pyridoxine-responsive anemias in man. *Vitam Horm.* 1968;26:549-571.

32. Cartwright GE, Deiss A. Sideroblasts, siderocytes, and sideroblastic anemia. *N Engl J Med.* 1975;292(4):185-193.

33. Bainton DF, Finch CA. The diagnosis of iron deficiency anemia. *Am J Med.* 1964;37:62-70.

34. Mufti GJ, Bennett JM, Goasguen J, et al. Diagnosis and classification of myelodysplastic syndrome: International Working Group on Morphology of myelodysplastic syndrome (IWGM-MDS) consensus proposals for the definition and enumeration of myeloblasts and ring sideroblasts. *Haematologica.* 2008;93(11):1712-1717.

35. Hammond E, Deiss A, Carnes WH, et al. Ultrastructural characteristics of siderocytes in swine. *Lab Invest.* 1969;21(4):292-297.

36. Koc S, Harris JW. Sideroblastic anemias: variations on imprecision in diagnostic cri-teria, proposal for an extended classification of sideroblastic anemias. *Am J Hematol.* 1998;57(1):1-6.

37. Fleming MD. The genetics of inherited sideroblastic anemias. *Semin Hematol.* 2002;39(4):270-281.

38. Furuyama K, Sassa S. Multiple mechanisms for hereditary sideroblastic anemia. *Cell Mol Biol (Noisy-le-grand).* 2002;48(1):5-10.

39. Garby L, Sjolin S, Vahlquist B. Chronic refractory hypochromic anaemia with dis-turbed haem-metabolism. *Br J Haematol.* 1957;3(1):55-67.

40. Konopka L, Hoffbrand AV. Haem synthesis in sideroblastic anaemia. *Br J Haematol.* 1979;42(1):73-83.

41. Lee GR, MacDiarmid WD, Cartwright GE, et al. Hereditary, X-linked, sideroachrestic anemia. The isolation of two erythrocyte populations differing in Xga blood type and porphyrin content. *Blood.* 1968;32(1):59-70.

42. McColl KE, Thompson GG, Moore MR, et al. Acute ethanol ingestion and haem bio-synthesis in healthy subjects. *Eur J Clin Invest.* 1980;10(2 Pt 1):107-112.

43. Pasanen AV, Vuopio P, Borgstrom GH, et al. Haem biosynthesis in refractory side-roblastic anaemia associated with the preleukaemic syndrome. *Scand J Haematol.* 1981;27(1):35-44.

44. Tanaka M, Bottomley SS. Bone marrow delta-aminolevulinic acid synthetase activity in experimental sideroblastic anemia. *J Lab Clin Med.* 1974;84(1):92-98.

45. Vogler WR, Mingioli ES. Porphyrin synthesis and heme synthetase activity in pyridoxine-responsive anemia. *Blood.* 1968;32(6):979-988.

46. Heilmeyer L. *Disturbances in Heme Synthesis.* Charles C. Thomas; 1966.

47. Kushner JP, Lee GR, Wintrobe MM, et al. Idiopathic refractory sideroblastic anemia: clinical and laboratory investigation of 17 patients and review of the literature. *Medicine (Baltimore).* 1971;50(3):139-159.

48. Cotter PD, Baumann M, Bishop DF. Enzymatic defect in "X-linked" sideroblastic ane-mia: molecular evidence for erythroid delta-aminolevulinate synthase deficiency. *Proc Natl Acad Sci U S A.* 1992;89(9):4028-4032.

49. Bottomley SS. Congenital sideroblastic anemias. *Curr Hematol Rep.* 2006;5(1):41-49.

50. Fleming MD. Congenital sideroblastic anemias: iron and heme lost in mitochondrial translation. *Hematology Am Soc Hematol Educ Program.* 2011;2011:525-531.

51. Guernsey DL, Jiang H, Campagna DR, et al. Mutations in mitochondrial carrier family gene SLC25A38 cause nonsyndromic autosomal recessive congenital sideroblastic ane-mia. *Nat Genet.* 2009;41(6):651-653.

52. Lunetti P, Damiano F, De Benedetto G, et al. Characterization of human and yeast mito-chondrial glycine carriers with implications for heme biosynthesis and anemia. *J Biol Chem.* 2016;291(38):19746-19759.

53. Allikmets R, Raskind WH, Hutchinson A, et al. Mutation of a putative mitochondrial iron transporter gene (ABC7) in X-linked sideroblastic anemia and ataxia (XLSA/A). *Hum Mol Genet.* 1999;8(5):743-749.

54. Hellier KD, Hatchwell E, Duncombe AS, et al. X-linked sideroblastic anaemia with ataxia: another mitochondrial disease? *J Neurol Neurosurg Psychiatry.* 2001;70(1):65-69.

55. Pagon RA, Bird TD, Detter JC, et al. Hereditary sideroblastic anaemia and ataxia: an X linked recessive disorder. *J Med Genet.* 1985;22(4):267-273.

56. Raskind WH, Wijsman E, Pagon RA, et al. X-linked sideroblastic anemia and ataxia: linkage to phosphoglycerate kinase at Xq13. *Am J Hum Genet.* 1991;48(2):335-341.

57. Maguire A, Hellier K, Hammans S, et al. X-linked cerebellar ataxia and sideroblastic anaemia associated with a missense mutation in the ABC7 gene predicting V411L. *Br J Haematol.* 2001;115(4):910-917.

58. Shimada Y, Okuno S, Kawai A, et al. Cloning and chromosomal mapping of a novel ABC transporter gene (hABC7), a candidate for X-linked sideroblastic anemia with spinocerebellar ataxia. *J Hum Genet.* 1998;43(2):115-122.

59. Broker S, Meunier B, Rich P, et al. MtDNA mutations associated with sideroblas-tic anaemia cause a defect of mitochondrial cytochrome c oxidase. *Eur J Biochem.* 1998;258(1):132-138.

60. Gattermann N, Retzlaff S, Wang YL, et al. Heteroplasmic point mutations of mitochon-drial DNA affecting subunit I of cytochrome c oxidase in two patients with acquired idiopathic sideroblastic anemia. *Blood.* 1997;90(12):4961-4972.

61. Seneca S, De Meirleir L, De Schepper J, et al. Pearson marrow pancreas syndrome: a molecular study and clinical management. *Clin Genet.* 1997;51(5):338-342.

62. Casas K, Bykhovskaya Y, Mengesha E, et al. Gene responsible for mitochondrial myop-athy and sideroblastic anemia (MSA) maps to chromosome 12q24.33. *Am J Med Genet A.* 2004;127A(1):44-49.

63. Jardine PE, Cotter PD, Johnson SA, et al. Pyridoxine-refractory congenital sideroblastic anaemia with evidence for autosomal inheritance: exclusion of linkage to ALAS2 at Xp11.21 by polymorphism analysis. *J Med Genet.* 1994;31(3):213-218.

64. Goodman JR, Hall SG. Accumulation of iron in mitochondria of erythroblasts. *Br J Haematol.* 1967;13(3):335-340.

65. Kushner JP, Barbuto AJ. Decreased activity of hepatic uroporphyrinogen decarboxylase (Urodecarb) in porphyria cutanea tarda (PCT). *Clin Res.* 1974;22.

66. Chauhan MS, Dakshinamurti K. Fluorometric assay of B6 vitamers in biological material. *Clin Chim Acta.* 1981;109(2):159-167.

67. Lee GR, Cartwright GE, Wintrobe MM. The response of free erythrocyte protopor-phyrin to pyridoxine therapy in a patient with sideroachrestic (sideroblastic) anemia. *Blood.* 1966;27(4):557-567.

68. Pasanen AV, Salmi A, Vuopio P, et al. Heme biosynthesis in sideroblastic anemia. *Int J Biochem.* 1980;12(5-6):969-974.

69. Pasanen AV, Eklof M, Tenhunen R. Coproporphyrinogen oxidase activity and porphy-rin concentrations in peripheral red blood cells in hereditary sideroblastic anaemia. *Scand J Haematol.* 1985;34(3):235-237.

70. Wiseman DH, May A, Jolles S, et al. A novel syndrome of congenital sideroblastic ane-mia, B-cell immunodeficiency, periodic fevers, and developmental delay (SIFD). *Blood.* 2013;122(1):112-123.

71. Chakraborty PK, Schmitz-Abe K, Kennedy EK, et al. Mutations in TRNT1 cause con-genital sideroblastic anemia with immunodeficiency, fevers, and developmental delay (SIFD). *Blood.* 2014;124(18):2867-2871.

72. Barton JR, Shaver DC, Sibai BM. Successive pregnancies complicated by idiopathic sideroblastic anemia. *Am J Obstet Gynecol.* 1992;166(2):576-577.

73. Breton-Gorius J BD, Rochant H. Congenital sideroblastic anemia without clinical iron overload. A case report. *Am J Hematol.* 1989;32.

74. Murakami R, Takumi T, Gouji J, et al. Sideroblastic anemia showing unique response to pyridoxine. *Am J Pediatr Hematol Oncol.* 1991;13(3):345-350.

75. Mason DY, Emerson PM. Primary acquired sideroblastic anaemia: response to treatment with pyridoxal-5-phosphate. *Br Med J.* 1973;1(5850):389-390.

76. Chillar RK, Johnson CS, Beutler E. Erythrocyte pyridoxine kinase levels in patients with sideroblastic anemia. *N Engl J Med.* 1976;295(16):881-883.

77. Nishibe H, Yamagata K, Goto H. A case of sideroblastic anaemia associated with marked elevation of erythrocytic arginase activity. *Scand J Haematol.* 1975;15(1):17-21.

78. Valentine WN, Konrad PN, Paglia DE. Dyserythropoiesis, refractory anemia, and "preleukemia:" metabolic features of the erythrocytes. *Blood.* 1973;41(6):857-875.

79. Ritchey AK, Hoffman R, Dainiak N, et al. Antibody-mediated acquired sideroblastic anemia: response to cytotoxic therapy. *Blood.* 1979;54(3):734-741.

80. Rochant H DB, Bouguerra M, Hoi T-H. Hypothesis: refractory anemias, preleukemic conditions, and fetal erythropoiesis. *Blood.* 1972;39.

81. Geschke W, Beutler E. Refractory sideroblastic and nonsideroblastic anemia: a review of 27 cases. *West J Med.* 1977;127(2):85-92.

82. Napier I, Ponka P, Richardson DR. Iron trafficking in the mitochondrion: novel pathways revealed by disease. *Blood.* 2005;105(5):1867-1874.

83. Pandolfo M. Frataxin deficiency and mitochondrial dysfunction. *Mitochondrion.* 2002;2(1-2):87-93.

84. Ponka P. Tissue-specific regulation of iron metabolism and heme synthesis: distinct control mechanisms in erythroid cells. *Blood.* 1997;89(1):1-25.

85. Adams ML, Ostapiuk I, Grasso JA. The effects of inhibition of heme synthesis on the intracellular localization of iron in rat reticulocytes. *Biochim Biophys Acta.* 1989;1012(3):243-253.

86. Borova J, Ponka P, Neuwirt J. Study of intracellular iron distribution in rabbit reticulocytes with normal and inhibited heme synthesis. *Biochim Biophys Acta.* 1973;320(1):143-156.

87. Ponka P, Wilczynska A, Schulman HM. Iron utilization in rabbit reticulocytes. A study using succinylacetone as an inhibitor or heme synthesis. *Biochim Biophys Acta.* 1982;720(1):96-105.

88. Richardson DR, Ponka P, Vyoral D. Distribution of iron in reticulocytes after inhibition of heme synthesis with succinylacetone: examination of the intermediates involved in iron metabolism. *Blood.* 1996;87(8):3477-3488.

89. Harrison PM, Arosio P. The ferritins: molecular properties, iron storage function and cellular regulation. *Biochim Biophys Acta.* 1996;1275(3):161-203.

90. Shaw GC, Cope JJ, Li L, et al. Mitoferrin is essential for erythroid iron assimilation. *Nature.* 2006;440(7080):96-100.

91. Hamdi A, Roshan TM, Kahawita TM, et al. Erythroid cell mitochondria receive endosomal iron by a "kiss-and-run" mechanism. *Biochim Biophys Acta.* 2016;1863(12):2859-2867.

92. Sheftel AD, Zhang AS, Brown C, et al. Direct interorganellar transfer of iron from endosome to mitochondrion. *Blood.* 2007;110(1):125-132.

93. Zhang AS, Sheftel AD, Ponka P. Intracellular kinetics of iron in reticulocytes: evidence for endosome involvement in iron targeting to mitochondria. *Blood.* 2005;105(1):368-375.

94. Ajioka RS, Phillips JD, Kushner JP. Biosynthesis of heme in mammals. *Biochim Biophys Acta.* 2006;1763(7):723-736.

95. Ponka P, Sheftel AD, Zhang AS. Iron targeting to mitochondria in erythroid cells. *Biochem Soc Trans.* 2002;30(4):735-738.

96. Cox TM, O'Donnell MW, Aisen P, et al. Hemin inhibits internalization of transferrin by reticulocytes and promotes phosphorylation of the membrane transferrin receptor. *Proc Natl Acad Sci U S A.* 1985;82(15):5170-5174.

97. Iacopetta B, Morgan E. Heme inhibits transferrin endocytosis in immature erythroid cells. *Biochim Biophys Acta.* 1984;805(2):211-216.

98. Ponka P, Neuwirt J. Regulation of iron entry into reticulocytes. I. Feedback inhibitory effect of heme on iron entry into reticulocytes and on heme synthesis. *Blood.* 1969;33(5):690-707.

99. Ponka P, Schulman HM, Martinez-Medellin J. Haem inhibits iron uptake subsequent to endocytosis of transferrin in reticulocytes. *Biochem J.* 1988;251(1):105-109.

100. Campagna DR, de Bie CI, Schmitz-Abe K, et al. X-linked sideroblastic anemia due to ALAS2 intron 1 enhancer element GATA-binding site mutations. *Am J Hematol.* 2014;89(3):315-319.

101. Bekri S, Kispal G, Lange H, et al. Human ABC7 transporter: gene structure and mutation causing X-linked sideroblastic anemia with ataxia with disruption of cytosolic iron-sulfur protein maturation. *Blood.* 2000;96(9):3256-3264.

102. Csere P, Lill R, Kispal G. Identification of a human mitochondrial ABC transporter, the functional orthologue of yeast Atm1p. *FEBS Lett.* 1998;441(2):266-270.

103. Lill R, Muhlenhoff U. Iron-sulfur protein biogenesis in eukaryotes: components and mechanisms. *Annu Rev Cell Dev Biol.* 2006;22:457-486.

104. Pondarre C, Campagna DR, Antiochos B, et al. Abcb7, the gene responsible for X-linked sideroblastic anemia with ataxia, is essential for hematopoiesis. *Blood.* 2007;109(8):3567-3569.

105. Lichtenstein DA, Crispin AW, Sendamarai AK, et al. A recurring mutation in the respiratory complex 1 protein NDUFB11 is responsible for a novel form of X-linked sideroblastic anemia. *Blood.* 2016;128(15):1913-1917.

106. Schmitz-Abe K, Ciesielski SJ, Schmidt PJ, et al. Congenital sideroblastic anemia due to mutations in the mitochondrial HSP70 homologue HSPA9. *Blood.* 2015;126(25):2734-2738.

107. Wingert RA, Galloway JL, Barut B, et al. Deficiency of glutaredoxin 5 reveals Fe-S clusters are required for vertebrate haem synthesis. *Nature.* 2005;436(7053):1035-1039.

108. Camaschella C, Campanella A, De Falco L, et al. The human counterpart of zebrafish shiraz shows sideroblastic-like microcytic anemia and iron overload. *Blood.* 2007;110(4):1353-1358.

109. Cattivelli K, Campagna DR, Schmitz-Abe K, et al. Ringed sideroblasts in beta-thalassemia. *Pediatr Blood Cancer.* 2017;64(5).

110. Ohgami RS, Campagna DR, Greer EL, et al. Identification of a ferrireductase required for efficient transferrin-dependent iron uptake in erythroid cells. *Nat Genet.* 2005;37(11):1264-1269.

111. Pearson HA, Lobel JS, Kocoshis SA, et al. A new syndrome of refractory sideroblastic anemia with vacuolization of marrow precursors and exocrine pancreatic dysfunction. *J Pediatr.* 1979;95(6):976-984.

112. Fontenay M, Cathelin S, Amiot M, et al. Mitochondria in hematopoiesis and hematological diseases. *Oncogene.* 2006;25(34):4757-4767.

113. Andersen K, Kaad PH. Congenital sideroblastic anaemia with intrauterine symptoms and early lethal outcome. *Acta Paediatr.* 1992;81(8):652-653.

114. Gattermann N. From sideroblastic anemia to the role of mitochondrial DNA mutations in myelodysplastic syndromes. *Leuk Res.* 2000;24(2):141-151.

115. Inoue S, Yokota M, Nakada K, et al. Pathogenic mitochondrial DNA-induced respiration defects in hematopoietic cells result in anemia by suppressing erythroid differentiation. *FEBS Lett.* 2007;581(9):1910-1916.

116. Shin MG, Kajigaya S, Levin BC, et al. Mitochondrial DNA mutations in patients with myelodysplastic syndromes. *Blood.* 2003;101(8):3118-3125.

117. Boultwood J, Pellagatti A, Nikpour M, et al. The role of the iron transporter ABCB7 in refractory anemia with ring sideroblasts. *PLoS One.* 2008;3(4):e1970.

118. Bykhovskaya Y, Casas K, Mengesha E, et al. Missense mutation in pseudouridine synthase 1 (PUS1) causes mitochondrial myopathy and sideroblastic anemia (MLASA). *Am J Hum Genet.* 2004;74(6):1303-1308.

119. Casas KA, Fischel-Ghodsian N. Mitochondrial myopathy and sideroblastic anemia. *Am J Med Genet A.* 2004;125A(2):201-204.

120. Drysdale J, Arosio P, Invernizzi R, et al. Mitochondrial ferritin: a new player in iron metabolism. *Blood Cells Mol Dis.* 2002;29(3):376-383.

121. Levi S, Arosio P. Mitochondrial ferritin. *Int J Biochem Cell Biol.* 2004;36(10):1887-1889.

122. Levi S, Corsi B, Bosisio M, et al. A human mitochondrial ferritin encoded by an intronless gene. *J Biol Chem.* 2001;276(27):24437-24440.

123. Nie G, Sheftel AD, Kim SF, et al. Overexpression of mitochondrial ferritin causes cytosolic iron depletion and changes cellular iron homeostasis. *Blood.* 2005;105(5):2161-2167.

124. Cazzola M, Invernizzi R, Bergamaschi G, et al. Mitochondrial ferritin expression in erythroid cells from patients with sideroblastic anemia. *Blood.* 2003;101(5):1996-2000.

125. Singh AK, Shinton NK, Williams JD. Ferrokinetic abnormalities and their significance in patients with sideroblastic anaemia. *Br J Haematol.* 1970;18(1):67-77.

126. Mallcovati L, Karimi M, Papaemmanuil E, et al. SF3B1 mutation identifies a distinct subset of myelodysplastic syndrome with ring sideroblasts. Blood. 2015; 126:233-241.

127. Sharp RA, Lowe JG, Johnston RN. Anti-tuberculous drugs and sideroblastic anaemia. *Br J Clin Pract.* 1990;44(12):706-707.

128. Harriss EB, Macgibbon BH, Mollin DL. Experimental sideroblastic anaemia. *Br J Haematol.* 1965;11:99-106.

129. Pierce HI, McGuffin RG, Hillman RS. Clinical studies in alcoholic sideroblastosis. *Arch Intern Med.* 1976;136(3):283-289.

130. McCurdy PR, Donohoe RF. Pyridoxine-responsive anemia conditioned by isonicotinic acid hydrazide. *Blood.* 1966;27(3):352-362.

131. Fong T, Vij R, Vijayan A, et al. Copper deficiency: an important consideration in the differential diagnosis of myelodysplastic syndrome. *Haematologica.* 2007;92(10):1429-1430.

132. Kumar N, Elliott MA, Hoyer JD, et al. "Myelodysplasia," myeloneuropathy, and copper deficiency. *Mayo Clin Proc.* 2005;80(7):943-946.

133. Broun ER, Greist A, Tricot G, et al. Excessive zinc ingestion. A reversible cause of sideroblastic anemia and bone marrow depression. *JAMA.* 1990;264(11):1441-1443.

134. Patterson WP, Winkelmann M, Perry MC. Zinc-induced copper deficiency: megamineral sideroblastic anemia. *Ann Intern Med.* 1985;103(3):385-386.

135. Nusbaum NJ. Concise review: genetic bases for sideroblastic anemia. *Am J Hematol.* 1991;37(1):41-44.

136. Weatherall DJ, Pembrey ME, Hall EG, et al. Familial sideroblastic anaemia: problem of Xg and X chromosome inactivation. *Lancet.* 1970;2(7676):744-748.

137. Cotter PD, May A, Fitzsimons EJ, et al. Late-onset X-linked sideroblastic anemia. Missense mutations in the erythroid delta-aminolevulinate synthase (ALAS2) gene in two pyridoxine-responsive patients initially diagnosed with acquired refractory anemia and ringed sideroblasts. *J Clin Invest.* 1995;96(4):2090-2096.

138. Furuyama K, Harigae H, Kinoshita C, et al. Late-onset X-linked sideroblastic anemia following hemodialysis. *Blood.* 2003;101(11):4623-4624.

139. Buchanan GR, Bottomley SS, Nitschke R. Bone marrow delta-aminolaevulinate synthase deficiency in a female with congenital sideroblastic anemia. *Blood.* 1980;55(1):109-115.

140. Prasad AS, Tranchida L, Konno ET, et al. Hereditary sideroblastic anemia and glucose-6-phosphate dehydrogenase deficiency in a Negro family. *J Clin Invest.* 1968;47(6):1415-1424.

141. Beutler E. The distribution of gene products among populations of cells in heterozygous humans. *Cold Spring Harb Symp Quant Biol.* 1964;29.

142. van Waveren Hogervorst GD, van Roermund HP, Snijders PJ. Hereditary sideroblastic anaemia and autosomal inheritance of erythrocyte dimorphism in a Dutch family. *Eur J Haematol.* 1987;38(5):405-409.

143. Fitzsimons EJ, May A. The molecular basis of the sideroblastic anemias. *Curr Opin Hematol.* 1996;3(2):167-172.

144. Seip M, Gjessing LR, Lie SO. Congenital sideroblastic anaemia in a girl. *Scand J Haematol.* 1971;8(6):505-512.

145. Horrigan DL, Harris JW. Pyridoxine-responsive anemia: analysis of 62 cases. *Adv Intern Med.* 1964;12:103-174.

146. Soslau G, Brodsky I. Hereditary sideroblastic anemia with associated platelet abnormalities. *Am J Hematol.* 1989;32(4):298-304.

147. Smith OP, Hann IM, Woodward CE, et al. Pearson's marrow/pancreas syndrome: haematological features associated with deletion and duplication of mitochondrial DNA. *Br J Haematol.* 1995;90(2):469-472.

148. Bishop RC, Bethell FH. Hereditary hypochromic anemia with transfusion hemosiderosis treated with pyridoxine: report of a case. *N Engl J Med.* 1959;261:486-489.

149. Harris JW, Horrigan DL. Pyridoxine-responsive anemia—prototype and variations on the theme. *Vitam Horm.* 1964;22:721-753.

150. Vogler WR, Mingioli ES. Heme synthesis in pyridoxine responsive anemia. *N Engl J Med.* 1965;273:347-353.

151. Albahary C, Boiron M. [Primary refractory anemia with medullary and hepatic hypersiderosis of blood in a woman.] *Acta Med Scand.* 1959;163(5):429-438.

152. Horrigan DL. Pyridoxine-responsive anemia: influence of tryptophan on pyridoxine responsiveness. *Blood.* 1973;42(2):187-193.

153. Yaouanq J, Grosbois B, Jouanolle AM, et al. Haemochromatosis Cys282Tyr mutation in pyridoxine-responsive sideroblastic anaemia. *Lancet.* 1997;349(9063):1475-1476.

154. French TJ, Jacobs P. Sideroblastic anaemia associated with iron overload treated by repeated phlebotomy. *S Afr Med J.* 1976;50(15):594-596.

155. Weintraub LR, Conrad ME, Crosby WH. Iron-loading anemia. Treatment with repeated phlebotomies and pyridoxine. *N Engl J Med.* 1966;275(4):169-176.

156. Urban C, Binder B, Hauer C, et al. Congenital sideroblastic anemia successfully treated by allogeneic bone marrow transplantation. *Bone Marrow Transplant.* 1992;10(4):373-375.

157. Medeiros BC, Kolhouse JF, Cagnoni PJ, et al. Nonmyeloablative allogeneic hematopoietic stem cell transplantation for congenital sideroblastic anemia. *Bone Marrow Transplant.* 2003;31(11):1053-1055.

158. Yunis AA, Salem Z. Drug-induced mitochondrial damage and sideroblastic change. *Clin Haematol.* 1980;9(3):607-619.

CHAPTER 21
THE PORPHYRIAS

John D. Phillips and Karl E. Anderson

SUMMARY

Porphyrias are diseases that result from derangements of specific enzymes in the heme biosynthetic pathway that lead to overproduction and accumulation of pathway intermediates that cause neurologic symptoms, photocutaneous symptoms, or both. Inherited mutations within the genes encoding the eight committed steps in heme synthesis have been identified in each of the porphyrias. An acquired form of porphyria cutanea tarda (PCT) is caused by an inhibitor of the fifth enzyme in the heme biosynthetic pathway, specifically in the liver, and is usually not associated with a mutation of this enzyme.

Porphyrias can be classified as either hepatic or erythropoietic, depending on the principal site of initial accumulation of excess pathway intermediates. Erythropoietic porphyrias are characterized by childhood onset and a generally stable clinical course. Hepatic porphyrias almost always develop during adult life, and are more variable because of multiple influences of drugs, hormones, and nutritional factors on the heme biosynthetic pathway in the liver.

Porphyrias are also classified as acute or cutaneous. The four acute porphyrias are associated with neurologic manifestations that usually occur as acute attacks. δ-Aminolevulinate dehydratase porphyria (ADP) is an autosomal recessive disorder caused by a deficiency of the second enzyme in the pathway

Acronyms and Abbreviations: ADP, δ-aminolevulinate dehydratase deficiency; AIP, acute intermittent porphyria; ALA, δ-aminolevulinic acid; ALAD, δ-aminolevulinic acid dehydratase; AUG, codon for initial methionine; ALAS, δ-aminolevulinic acid synthase; ALAS1, δ-aminolevulinic acid synthase, housekeeping form; ALAS2, δ-aminolevulinic acid synthase, erythroid-specific form; CAAT, CAAT-enhancer binding protein (C/EBP); cDNA, complementary DNA; CEP, congenital erythropoietic porphyria; CoA, coenzyme A; CLPX, member of the family of the AAA protease (AAA+ ATPase); CPO, coproporphyrinogen oxidase; CPRE, coproporphyrinogen oxidase gene promoter regulatory element; CRIM, cross-reactive immunologic material; CYP, cytochrome P450; Da, Dalton; DNA, deoxyribonucleic acid; EC, enzyme commission; EPP, erythropoietic protoporphyria; FECH, ferrochelatase; FOXO-1, forkhead transcription factor; GATA-1, transcription factor 1 binding to the DNA sequence GATA; HCP, hereditary coproporphyria; HemY, bacterial homolog of PPO; HEP, hepatoerythropoietic porphyria; HFE, hemochromatosis gene; HIV, human immunodeficiency virus; HMB, hydroxymethylbilane; Mr, relative molecular weight; mRNA, messenger RNA; NF-E2, transcription factor that binds in complex to promoters, for example, in β-globin; NRF-1, nuclear regulatory factor 1 transcription factor; PBG, porphobilinogen; PBGD, porphobilinogen deaminase; PCT, porphyria cutanea tarda; PGC-1α, peroxisomal proliferator-activated cofactor 1α; PPO, protoporphyrinogen oxidase; PXR, pregnane X receptor; RNA, ribonucleic acid; SCS-βA, β subunit of ATP-specific succinyl coenzyme A synthetase; Sp1, transcription factor; TATA, DNA sequence binding TBP (TATA Binding Protein); TCDD, 2,3,7,8-Tetrachlorodibenzodioxin; UROD, uroporphyrinogen decarboxylase; UROS, uroporphyrinogen III synthase; VP, variegate porphyria; XLP, X-linked protoporphyria; XLSA, X-linked sideroblastic anemia.

and is the rarest type of porphyria. ADP is classified as hepatic, but also has erythropoietic features. The three other acute porphyrias, namely acute intermittent porphyria (AIP), hereditary coproporphyria (HCP), and variegate porphyria (VP), are autosomal dominant hepatic porphyrias, and result from deficiencies of the third (porphobilinogen deaminase [PBGD]), sixth (coproporphyrinogen oxidase [CPO]), and seventh (protoporphyrinogen oxidase [PPO]) enzymes in the pathway, respectively. HCP and VP are also classified as cutaneous, because photocutaneous lesions may develop, especially in VP. AIP is the most common acute porphyria and the second most common porphyria. Disease expression is highly variable in the acute hepatic porphyrias, and the great majority of individuals who inherit mutations of these enzymes remain latent through all or most of their lives. Attacks are precipitated by factors that increase hepatic heme synthesis, including certain drugs, sex steroid hormones and their metabolites, and restriction of dietary calories and carbohydrate. Treatment of acute porphyrias includes glucose loading, hemin infusions, and RNA interference, all of which target δ-aminolevulinic acid synthase-1 (ALAS1), the rate-limiting enzyme of the heme biosynthetic pathway in the liver.

Cutaneous porphyrias are associated with either blistering skin lesions or, in the protoporphyrias, with acute nonblistering photosensitivity. Blistering skin manifestations are nearly identical in PCT, HCP, and VP. In congenital erythropoietic porphyria (CEP), the cutaneous manifestations are much more severe and are often associated with loss of digits and facial mutilation. CEP results from a severe deficiency of the fourth enzyme in the pathway, uroporphyrinogen III synthase (UROS), and is inherited in an autosomal recessive fashion. Hemolytic anemia is common, and severe cases may be transfusion dependent, and may even present in utero with fetal hydrops. Hematopoietic stem cell transplantation in early childhood is the most effective treatment.

Erythropoietic protoporphyria (EPP) is the third most common porphyria and the most common in children, and is caused by a deficiency of the final enzyme in the pathway. Inheritance of EPP is best described as autosomal recessive, with a severe ferrochelatase (FECH) mutation inherited from one parent and a low-expression variant allele from the other. X-linked protoporphyria (XLP) has the same phenotype as EPP, but is the result of gain-of-function mutations of δ-aminolevulinic acid synthase-2, which is expressed only in erythroblasts and reticulocytes. Protoporphyrin-containing gallstones may develop in EPP and XLP. An uncommon but potentially life-threatening complication is protoporphyric liver failure, which is a result of the cholestatic effects of protoporphyrin, and may require liver transplantation. Sequential or combined hematopoietic stem cell transplantation can reduce the continued contribution of porphyrins from the red cell compartment and prevent recurrent liver failure in the transplanted liver.

PCT is an iron-related hepatic porphyria that usually begins in middle or late adult life. Activity of hepatic uroporphyrinogen decarboxylase (UROD) is reduced in the presence of iron to approximately 20% of normal in PCT by an uroporphomethene inhibitor probably derived from uroporphyrinogen. Multiple susceptibility factors, including use of alcohol, smoking, estrogens, hepatitis C, and HIV, contribute HFE (hemochromatosis gene) mutations that cause excess iron absorption are common in PCT. A minority of patients are heterozygous for UROD mutations and are said to have familial PCT. Polyhalogenated aromatic hydrocarbons cause PCT in laboratory animals and occasionally in humans. PCT responds well to treatment by repeated phlebotomy, which reduces hepatic iron, or low-dose hydroxychloroquine or chloroquine, which mobilizes accumulated hepatic porphyrins. Hepatoerythropoietic porphyria (HEP) is the homozygous form of familial PCT, and is usually a severe disorder that starts in childhood and resembles CEP clinically.

●DEFINITION AND HISTORY

The porphyrias are a group of metabolic diseases resulting from derangements, usually of a genetic nature, in the activity of specific enzymes in the heme biosynthetic pathway, leading to overproduction and accumulation of pathway intermediates. Symptoms of these diseases can be neurologic, photocutaneous, or both. The intermediates that accumulate include porphyrins and the porphyrin precursors δ-aminolevulinic acid (ALA) and porphobilinogen (PBG) and their derivatives. Characteristic patterns of these metabolic intermediates in plasma, erythrocytes, urine, and feces are the basis for diagnostic screening tests and more comprehensive biochemical characterization.

Porphyrias are classified as either *erythropoietic* or *hepatic*, depending on the principal site of accumulation of pathway intermediates. The erythropoietic porphyrias include congenital erythropoietic porphyria (CEP), which is very rare, erythropoietic protoporphyria (EPP), the third most common porphyria and the most common in children, and X-linked protoporphyria (XLP), which has the same phenotype as EPP but is less common. Hepatic porphyrias include the acute porphyrias, which cause neurologic symptoms usually in the form of acute attacks, and porphyria cutanea tarda (PCT), which causes chronic blistering lesions on sun-exposed areas of the skin. Porphyrias that are classified as acute include ALA dehydratase porphyria (ADP), acute intermittent porphyria (AIP), hereditary coproporphyria (HCP), and variegate porphyria (VP). VP, and less commonly HCP, can also cause skin manifestations identical to those caused by PCT.

A porphyria type is associated with *loss-of-function mutations* of seven of the eight enzymes in the heme biosynthetic pathway (Table 21-1 and Fig. 21-1). PCT is primarily caused by an acquired deficiency of uroporphyrinogen decarboxylase (UROD), the fifth pathway enzyme in the liver, with heterozygous mutations of that enzyme contributing in some cases. *Gain-of-function mutations* of ALAS2, the erythroid form of the first pathway enzyme, cause XLP, whereas loss-of-function mutations of this enzyme cause X-linked sideroblastic anemia (Chap. 20). Tables 21-1 and 21-2 summarize the genetic defects and laboratory features of the porphyrias.

A case of CEP reported by Schultz in 1874 was the first description of porphyria in the literature. This case was a 33-year-old man with photosensitivity since age 3 months, anemia, splenomegaly, red-wine-colored urine as a result of a pigment resembling hematoporphyrin, and brown-colored bones at autopsy.[1,2] In 1898, T. McCall Anderson described two brothers (ages 23 and 26 years) who most likely had CEP[3] and suffered from *hydroa aestivale*, including a recurrent erythema, with red urine, pruritus, and blistering of sun-exposed skin, especially in summer, leading to extensive scarring and mutilation of the ears and nose (see Fig. 21-1). Using available methods, their urine was also shown to contain a substance related to hematoporphyrin.[4] In 1889, Stokvis first described a case of acute porphyria in an elderly woman who developed dark-red urine and later died after taking sulfonal, a drug related to the barbiturates.[5]

Hans Günther[6] published a monograph on porphyrins in 1911 and classified porphyrias into four groups: (1) those that have an acute onset without association with drug ingestion, (2) those that are caused by sulfonal or trional, (3) hematoporphyria congenita, and (4) chronic hematoporphyria. The first two groups correspond to the acute porphyrias, which may present with attacks sometimes related to ingestion of certain drugs; the second group corresponds to CEP and hepatoerythropoietic porphyria (HEP); and the fourth group corresponds to PCT. In 1923, Archibald Garrod proposed the term *inborn errors of metabolism* for a number of inherited metabolic disorders, including the porphyrias.[7]

Sachs noted an Ehrlich-positive chromogen that was not urobilinogen in urine of patients with acute porphyria in 1931. In the late 1930s, Waldenström noted that excretion of this chromogen, which

TABLE 21-1. Human Porphyrias: Specific Enzymes Affected by Mutations, Modes of Inheritance, Classification, and Major Types of Clinical Features of Each of the Human Porphyrias

Porphyria[a]	Affected Enzyme	Known Mutations	Inheritance	Classification	Principal Clinical Features
X-linked protoporphyria	ALA synthase-erythroid-specific form (ALAS2)	4 (gain of function)	Sex-linked	Erythropoietic	Nonblistering photosensitivity
ADP	ALAD	15	Autosomal recessive	Hepatic[b]	Neurovisceral
AIP	PBGD	>300	Autosomal dominant	Hepatic	Neurovisceral
CEP	UROS	36	Autosomal recessive	Erythropoietic	Blistering photosensitivity
PCT	UROD	70 (includes HEP)	Autosomal dominant[c]	Hepatic	Blistering photosensitivity
HEP	UROD	–	Autosomal recessive	Hepatic[b]	Blistering photosensitivity
HCP	CPO	42	Autosomal dominant	Hepatic	Neurovisceral; blistering photosensitivity (uncommon)
VP	PPO	130	Autosomal dominant	Hepatic	Neurovisceral; blistering photosensitivity (common)
EPP	FECH	90	Autosomal recessive	Erythropoietic	Nonblistering photosensitivity

ADP, δ-aminolevulinic acid dehydratase porphyria; AIP, acute intermittent porphyria; ALA, δ-aminolevulinic acid; ALAD, ALA dehydratase; CEP, congenital erythropoietic porphyria; CPO, coproporphyrinogen oxidase; EPP, erythropoietic protoporphyria; FECH, ferrochelatase; HCP, hereditary coproporphyria; HEP, hepatoerythropoietic porphyria; PBGD, porphobilinogen deaminase; PCT, porphyria cutanea tarda; PPO, protoporphyrinogen oxidase; UROD, uroporphyrinogen decarboxylase; UROS, uroporphyrinogen III synthase; VP, variegate porphyria.

[a]Porphyrias are listed in the order of the affected enzyme in the heme biosynthetic pathway.

[b]These autosomal recessive porphyrias also have erythropoietic features, including increases in erythrocyte zinc protoporphyrin.

[c]UROD inhibition in PCT is mostly acquired, but an inherited deficiency of the enzyme predisposes in familial (type 2) disease.

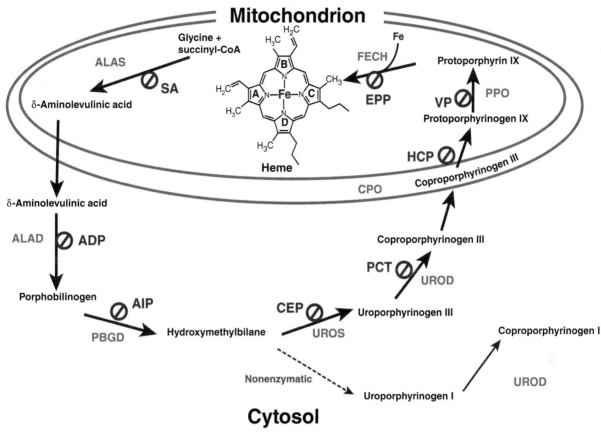

Figure 21–1. Enzymes and intermediates in the heme biosynthetic pathway and the type of porphyria associated with a deficiency of each enzyme (indicated by Ø). Gain-of-function mutation of the erythroid form of ALA synthase is not shown. ADP, ALA dehydratase porphyria; AIP, acute intermittent porphyria; ALA, δ-aminolevulinic acid; ALAD, δ-aminolevulinic acid dehydratase; ALAS, δ-aminolevulinic acid synthase; CEP, congenital erythropoietic porphyria; CPO, coproporphyrinogen oxidase; EPP, erythropoietic protoporphyria; FECH, ferrochelatase; HCP, hereditary coproporphyria; PBG, porphobilinogen; PBGD, porphobilinogen deaminase; PCT, porphyria cutanea tarda; PPO, protoporphyrinogen oxidase; SA, sideroblastic anemia (X-linked); UROD, uroporphyrinogen decarboxylase; UROS, uroporphyrinogen III synthase; VP, variegate porphyria.

he identified as PBG in 1939, was an autosomal dominant trait in AIP families.[8] The classification of porphyrias as erythropoietic and hepatic was proposed in 1954 by Schmid, Schwartz, and Watson.[9] An epidemic of hexachlorobenzene-induced PCT in eastern Turkey in 1957[10,11] provided the foundation for the development of animal models of this disorder using halogenated polyaromatic hydrocarbons.[12,13] Strand and coworkers described the enzyme deficiency in AIP for the first time in 1970,[14] and Bonkovsky and coworkers first reported treatment of an AIP patient with hemin in 1971.[15] The enzymes of the heme biosynthetic pathway have been defined in terms of their amino acid composition, genomic and complementary DNA (cDNA) sequences, and crystal structures. Erythroid-specific and housekeeping transcripts have been described for at least four enzymes in the pathway, and progress has been made in understanding the regulation of heme synthesis in specific tissues, especially the marrow and liver. Multiple mutations have been described in each of the human porphyrias, and some specific treatments introduced.

● ETIOLOGY AND PATHOGENESIS

HEME

Heme (iron protoporphyrin IX; Fig. 21-2) is essential for all cells and functions as the prosthetic group of numerous hemoproteins such as hemoglobin, myoglobin, respiratory cytochromes, cytochromes P450

(CYPs), catalase, peroxidase, tryptophan pyrrolase, and nitric oxide synthase. Approximately 85% of heme is synthesized in the marrow to meet the requirement for hemoglobin formation; the remainder is synthesized largely in the liver.[16] Most heme synthesized in the liver is required for CYPs, which are located primarily in the endoplasmic reticulum, where they turn over rapidly and oxidize a variety of chemicals, including drugs, environmental carcinogens, endogenous steroids, vitamins, fatty acids, and prostaglandins.[17]

The term *heme* may refer more specifically to ferrous protoporphyrin IX, and is readily oxidized in vitro to hemin, that is, ferric protoporphyrin IX. Hemin has one residual positive charge and is isolated as a halide, most commonly as the chloride. In alkaline solution, the halide is replaced by a hydroxyl ion to form hematin (Fig. 21-3). Heme can form further hexacoordinated complexes with nitrogenous bases to form a *hemochrome* or *hemochromogen*; for example, pyridine hemochromogen is useful for identification and quantification of heme and hemoproteins. In medicine, hemin is also a generic term for heme preparations used as IV therapies for acute porphyrias, such as lyophilized hematin and heme arginate.

The ferrous iron atom (Fe^{2+}) in heme has six electron pairs, of which four are bound to the pyrrolic nitrogens of the porphyrin macrocycle, leaving two unoccupied electron pairs, one above and the other below the plane of the porphyrin ring. In hemoglobin, one of these pairs is coordinated with a histidine residue of the globin chain. The other coordination site in deoxyhemoglobin is protected from oxidation by

TABLE 21–2. Biochemical Findings Including Major Increases in Porphyrins and Porphyrin Precursors in the Human Porphyrias

Porphyria	Erythrocytes	Plasma	Urine	Stool
XLP[a]	Metal-free and zinc protoporphyrin	Protoporphyrin[d] (~634 nm)[b]	[e]	Protoporphyrin[a]
ADP	Zinc protoporphyrin	ALA[a]	ALA, coproporphyrin III	[a]
AIP	Decreased PBGD activity (most cases)[a]	ALA, PBG[a] (~620 nm, some cases)[b]	ALA, PBG, uroporphyrin	[a]
CEP	Uroporphyrin I; coproporphyrin I	Uroporphyrin I, coproporphyrin I (~620 nm)[b]	Uroporphyrin I; coproporphyrin I	Coproporphyrin I
PCT and HEP	Zinc protoporphyrin (in HEP)	Uroporphyrin, heptacarboxyl porphyrin (~620 nm)[b]	Uroporphyrin, heptacarboxyl porphyrin	Heptacarboxyl porphyrin, isocoproporphyrins
HCP	[a]	[c] (~620 nm, some cases)[b]	ALA, PBG, coproporphyrin III	Coproporphyrin III
VP	[a]	Protoporphyrin (~628 nm)[b]	ALA, PBG, coproporphyrin III	Coproporphyrin III, protoporphyrin
EPP	Metal-free protoporphyrin	Protoporphyrin[d] (~634 nm)[b]	[e]	Protoporphyrin[a]

ADP, δ-aminolevulinate dehydratase porphyria; AIP, acute intermittent porphyria; ALA, δ-aminolevulinic acid; CEP, congenital erythropoietic porphyria; EPP, erythropoietic protoporphyria; HCP, hereditary coproporphyria; HEP, hepatoerythropoietic porphyria; PBG, porphobilinogen; PCT, porphyria cutanea tarda; VP, variegate porphyria; XLP, X-linked protoporphyria.

[a]Porphyrin levels normal or slightly increased.

[b]Fluorescence emission peak of diluted plasma at neutral pH.

[c]Plasma porphyrins usually normal, but increased when blistering skin lesions develop.

[d]Zinc protoporphyrin ≤15% of total in EPP, but 15%-50% in XLP.

[e]Increase in urine porphyrins (especially coproporphyrin) only with liver failure.

the nonpolar environment of surrounding amino acid residues, and is available to bind molecular oxygen for transport from the lung to other tissues. To reversibly bind oxygen, the iron in hemoglobin must be in the ferrous state. Methemoglobin (oxidized hemoglobin) that is generated in erythrocytes is continuously reduced to ferrous hemoglobin by the reduced form of nicotinamide adenine dinucleotide-cytochrome b_5 reductase-cytochrome b_5 system (Chaps. 16 and 19).

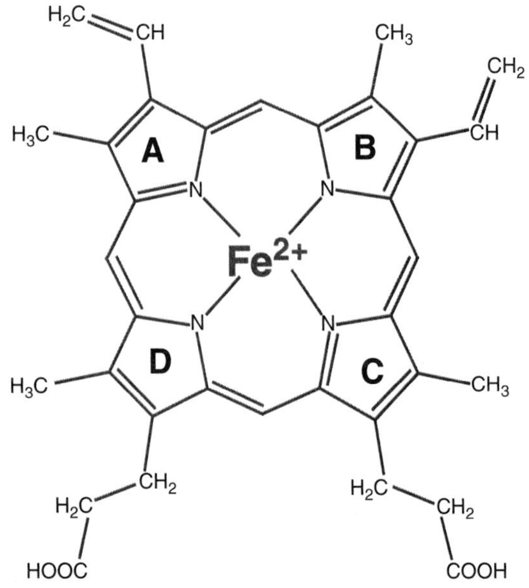

Heme Biosynthesis

Figure 21-4 shows the enzymatic steps involved in heme biosynthesis in eukaryotic cells. The first, ALAS and last three enzymes (CPO, PPO, FECH) are mitochondrial and the intermediate four (ALAD, PBGD, UROS, UROD) are cytosolic. Erythroid heme synthesis occurs in marrow erythroblasts and reticulocytes, which contain mitochondria. Circulating erythrocytes lack mitochondria and no longer synthesize heme. They contain residual cytosolic enzymes of the heme biosynthetic pathway, zinc protoporphyrin, and a smaller amount of metal-free protoporphyrin. These enzyme activities and protoporphyrin decline during the life span of erythrocytes in the circulation.

δ-Aminolevulinate Synthase (Succinyl-Coenzyme A: Glycine C-Succinyl Transferase, Decarboxylating; Enzyme Commission [EC] 2.3.1.37) The first enzyme in the heme biosynthetic pathway catalyzes

HEME

Figure 21–2. Structure of heme. The pyrrole rings are labeled A through D, according to the nomenclature of Hans Fischer.

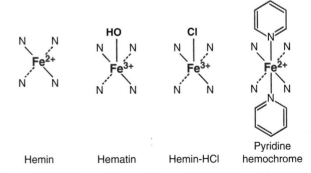

Figure 21–3. Forms of iron protoporphyrin IX. The porphyrin macrocycle is represented only by its pyrrole nitrogen atoms.

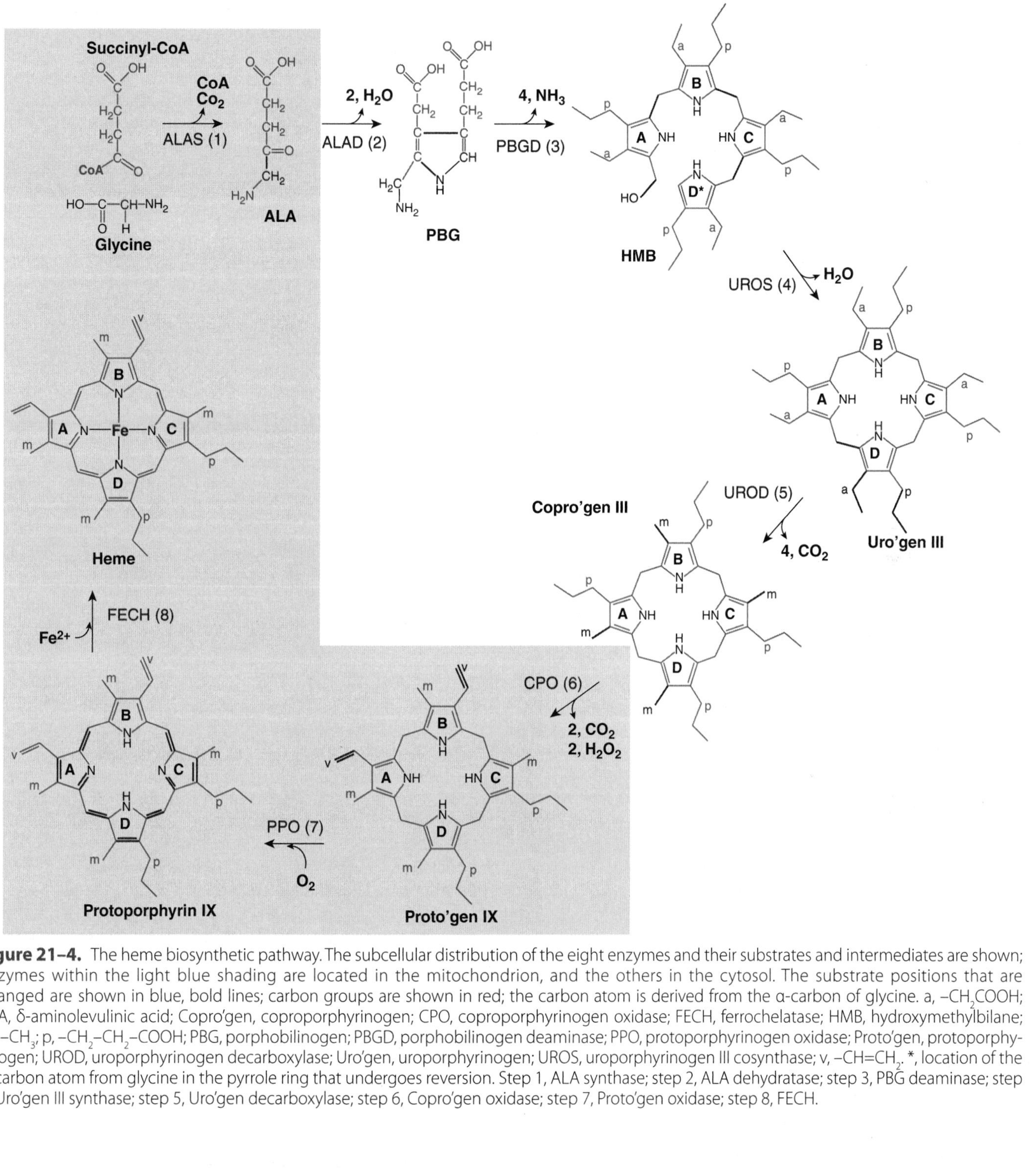

Figure 21–4. The heme biosynthetic pathway. The subcellular distribution of the eight enzymes and their substrates and intermediates are shown; enzymes within the light blue shading are located in the mitochondrion, and the others in the cytosol. The substrate positions that are changed are shown in blue, bold lines; carbon groups are shown in red; the carbon atom is derived from the α-carbon of glycine. a, –CH₂COOH; ALA, δ-aminolevulinic acid; Copro'gen, coproporphyrinogen; CPO, coproporphyrinogen oxidase; FECH, ferrochelatase; HMB, hydroxymethylbilane; m, –CH₃; p, –CH₂–CH₂–COOH; PBG, porphobilinogen; PBGD, porphobilinogen deaminase; PPO, protoporphyrinogen oxidase; Proto'gen, protoporphyrinogen; UROD, uroporphyrinogen decarboxylase; Uro'gen, uroporphyrinogen; UROS, uroporphyrinogen III cosynthase; v, –CH=CH₂. *, location of the α-carbon atom from glycine in the pyrrole ring that undergoes reversion. Step 1, ALA synthase; step 2, ALA dehydratase; step 3, PBG deaminase; step 4, Uro'gen III synthase; step 5, Uro'gen decarboxylase; step 6, Copro'gen oxidase; step 7, Proto'gen oxidase; step 8, FECH.

the condensation of glycine and succinyl-coenzyme A to form ALA (see Fig. 21-4, *step 1*), and requires pyridoxal 5′-phosphate as a cofactor. δ-Aminolevulinic acid synthase (ALAS) in mammalian cells is localized to the mitochondrial matrix.[18] The enzyme is synthesized as a precursor protein in the cytosol and transported into mitochondria. Two separate ALAS genes encode housekeeping (tissue nonspecific) and erythroid specific forms of the enzyme (ALAS1 and ALAS2, respectively).[19,20] The gene locus for human ALAS1 is at 3p.21, and for ALAS2 it is at Xp11.2. The human ALAS2 gene encodes a precursor of 587 amino acids, with an Mr of 64,600 Da. Nucleotide sequences for the ALAS2 and the ALAS1

isoforms are approximately 60% similar. No homology is observed between the aminoterminal regions, whereas high homology (approximately 73%) is seen after residue 197 of the housekeeping form.[21] The two human ALAS genes appear to have evolved by duplication of a common ancestral gene that encoded a primitive catalytic site. Subsequently the DNA sequences were modified to encode gene-specific regulatory regions, functioning mostly at the amino termini.[22] The promoter in the human ALAS2 gene contains several putative erythroid-specific *cis*-acting elements including both a GATA-1 and an NF-E2 binding site.[22,23] Both GATA-1 and NF-E2 are erythroid transcription factors that also bind other DNA sites, such as the promoters of the human β-globin, porphobilinogen deaminase (PBGD), and uroporphyrinogen synthase (UROS) genes.[24] Thus, expression of ALAS2 is under the regulatory influence of erythroid transcription factors such as GATA-1 and is coordinated with expression of other genes involved in hemoglobin synthesis. Additionally, ALAS2 mRNA contains an iron-responsive element in its 5′-untranslated region,[23] similar to mRNAs encoding ferritin and the transferrin receptor (Chap. 10).[25] Gel retardation analysis showed that the iron-responsive element in ALAS2 mRNA is functional and suggests that translation of the erythroid-specific mRNA is directly linked to the availability of iron, or heme, in erythroid cells.[26] In the liver, synthesis of ALAS1 is induced by a variety of chemicals including drugs and steroids that increase the demand for hepatic CYPs. Upstream enhancer elements in the ALAS1 gene and certain hepatic CYP genes respond to inducing chemicals and interact with the pregnane X receptor.[27] Hemin represses synthesis of ALAS1 in liver,[28] accounting for the beneficial effects of intravenous treatment of the acute porphyrias with hemin. At higher concentrations, heme induces heme oxygenase, resulting in its enhanced catabolism.[29] Thus, hepatic heme availability is balanced between the rate of synthesis controlled primarily by ALAS1 and the rate of degradation controlled by heme oxygenase, both of which are regulated by heme at different intracellular concentrations. ALAS1 is also upregulated by the peroxisomal proliferator-activated cofactor 1α (PGC-1α),[30] a coactivator of nuclear receptors and transcription factors. Transcriptional regulation of ALAS1 by PGC-1α is mediated by interaction of NRF-1 (nuclear regulatory factor 1) and FOXO-1 (a forkhead family member) with the ALAS1 promoter.[31] When glucose levels are low, transcription of PGC-1α is upregulated,[32] in turn, increasing ALAS1, which might precipitate an attack of acute porphyria in an individual with the appropriate inherited enzyme deficiency. Thus, upregulation of PGC-1α provides an explanation for the induction of acute attacks of porphyria with fasting, as well as the therapeutic value of glucose loading. Regulation of heme synthesis in erythroid cells is distinct from the liver. ALAS2 expression in erythroid cells is increased during erythroid differentiation when heme synthesis is increased.[33,34] Experimentally, ALAS2 is often upregulated by heme, whereas in liver, ALAS1 is downregulated by heme. The β subunit of human ATP-specific succinyl coenzyme A synthetase (SCS-βA) associates with human ALAS2 but not with ALAS1, and thereby contributes to heme synthesis in the marrow.[35] Multiple ALAS2 mutations have been associated with X-linked sideroblastic anemia (Chap. 20); many are in exon 9, which contains the binding site for pyridoxal 5′-phosphate (K391), and these cases typically respond favorably to high doses of pyridoxine. At least one mutant enzyme (D190V) in a patient with pyridoxine-refractory X-linked sideroblastic anemia,[36] failed to associate with SCS-βA, whereas other ALAS2 mutants did not have this property. The mature D190V mutant protein, but not its precursor protein, underwent abnormal processing, indicating that appropriate association of SCS-βA and ALAS2 is necessary for functioning of ALAS2 in mitochondria.[36] Gain-of-function mutations of ALAS2 have been identified in patients with XLP.[37] The crystal structure of ALAS2 has been solved to 1.5 A resolution.[38] In the models of ALAS2 the C-terminal end of the protein loops back across the active site inhibiting access of succinyl-CoA to the active site, acting as an auto-regulatory domain, and provides the basis for the increased activity seen in individuals with XLP.[38,39]

δ-Aminolevulinate Dehydratase (PBG Synthase; δ-Aminolevulinate Hydrolase; EC 4.2.1.24) ALA dehydratase (ALAD) is a cytosolic enzyme that catalyzes the condensation of two molecules of ALA to form the monopyrrole PBG, with removal of two molecules of water (see Fig. 21-4, *step 2*). The enzyme functions as a homooctamer, and requires intact sulfhydryl groups and zinc for activity, and was recognized to contain an iron-sulfur (^{2}Fe-^{2}S) cluster.[40] ALAD activity is inhibited by

sulfhydryl reagents[41] and by lead, which displaces zinc.[42] In lead poisoning (Chap. 23), erythrocyte ALAD activity is markedly inhibited, urinary ALA and coproporphyrin excretion increased, erythrocyte zinc protoporphyrin elevated, and neurologic symptoms resemble those seen in acute porphyrias.[43] 4,6-Dioxoheptanoic acid (succinylacetone) is a substrate analogue and potent inhibitor of ALAD,[44,45] and a byproduct of the enzyme deficiency in hereditary tyrosinemia type I. This substance is found in urine and blood of patients with this disease, who may also have increased ALA and symptoms resembling acute porphyrias.[46] Human ALAD mRNA has an open-reading frame of 990 bp, encoding a protein with an Mr of 36,274 Da (Chap. 10).[47] Sequences known to be essential for enzymatic activity are those with active site lysine residues and for the cysteine-rich and histidine-rich zinc-binding sites. The gene for human ALAD is localized to chromosome 9p34.[48] Studies using [^{14}C]-ALA have shown that of the two ALA molecules used as substrate, the ALA molecule contributing the propionic acid side is initially bound to the enzyme.[49] The tertiary structure of the yeast ALAD has been solved to 2.3-Å resolution, revealing that each subunit adopts a triosephosphate isomerase barrel fold with a 39-residue N-terminal arm. Pairs of monomers then wrap their arms around each other to form compact dimers, and these dimers associate to form a 422 symmetric octamer.[50] All eight active sites are on the surface of the octamer and possess two lysine residues (210 and 263). The Lys263 residue forms a Schiff base link to the substrate. The two lysine side chains are close to two zinc-binding sites. One binding site is formed by three cysteine residues; the other involves Cys234 and His142. Although there are no tissue-specific ALAD isozymes, the ALAD mRNA has two splice variants, a housekeeping (1A) and an erythroid-specific (1B) form.[48] In both humans and mice, the promoter region upstream of exon 1B contains GATA-1 sites, providing for significant tissue-specific control of these transcripts.[51] The human enzyme is polymorphic with two common alleles that occur in three combinations (1–1, 1–2, and 2–2).[52] The allele 2 sequence differs from allele 1 only by a G to C transversion of nucleotide 177 in the coding region, resulting in replacement of lysine by asparagine, a more electronegative amino acid. ALAD exists primarily as a homooctamer. Mutations associated with δ-aminolevulinate dehydratase deficiency (ADP) favor formation of the less-active hexamer.[53,54]

Porphobilinogen Deaminase (Hydroxymethylbilane Synthase; PBG Ammonia-Lyase [Polymerizing]; EC 4.3.1.8) The fourth enzyme in the heme biosynthetic pathway catalyzes the deamination and condensation of four molecules of PBG to yield the linear tetrapyrrole hydroxymethylbilane (HMB) (see Fig. 21-4, *step 3*).[49] PBG deaminase (PBGD) was previously known as *uroporphyrinogen I synthase*, and the enzyme activity is commonly measured in the laboratory after converting HMB to uroporphyrin I. This enzyme has a unique cofactor, which is a dipyrromethane that binds the pyrrole intermediates at the catalytic site until six pyrroles (including the dipyrrole cofactor) are assembled in a linear fashion, after which the tetrapyrrole HMB is released.[55] The apo-deaminase generates the dipyrrole cofactor to form the holo-deaminase, and this occurs more readily from HMB than from PBG.[56] High concentrations of PBG may inhibit formation of the holo-deaminase. The gene encoding human PBGD maps to chromosome 11q23-11qter,[57] and consists of 15 exons spread over 10 kb of DNA.[58] Distinct erythroid-specific and housekeeping isoforms are produced through alternative splicing of two distinct primary mRNA transcripts arising from two promoters.[59] The housekeeping promoter is upstream of exon 1 and is active in all tissues, while the erythroid-specific promoter, which is upstream of exon 2, is active only in erythroid cells. The human housekeeping and erythroid-specific enzymes isoforms contain 361 and 344 amino acid residues, respectively.[60] Of the additional 17 residues at the N-terminal end of the housekeeping form, 11 are encoded by exon 1, and 6 by a short segment of exon 3 that immediately precedes a methionine codon that initiates translation of the erythroid isoform. Erythroid-specific *trans*-acting factors, such as GATA-1 and NF-E2, recognize sequences in the erythroid promoter.[61] A 1320-bp stretch of perfect identity is present between the erythroid and the nonerythroid PBGD, but with a mismatch in the first exon at their 5′ extremities. An additional in-frame AUG codon that is present 51 bp upstream from the initiating codon of the erythroid cDNA, accounts for the additional 17 amino acid residues at the N-terminus of the housekeeping isoform. Accordingly, a splice-site mutation at the last position of exon 1, or a base transition in intron 1, in certain patients with AIP, results in decreased PBGD expression in nonerythroid tissues including the liver, but not in erythroid cells, because transcription of the gene in erythroid cells starts downstream of the site of the genetic lesion.[62]

Uroporphyrinogen III Synthase (Uroporphyrinogen III Cosynthase; EC 4.2.1.75) UROS, a cytosolic enzyme, catalyzes the formation of uroporphyrinogen III from HMB. The process involves an intramolecular rearrangement that affects only ring D of the porphyrin macrocycle (see Fig. 21-4, *step 4*).[49] In the absence of this enzyme, HMB *spontaneously* forms the ring structure uroporphyrinogen I, which, like the III isomer, is a substrate for UROD. However, because coproporphyrinogen I is not a substrate for coproporphyrinogen oxidase (CPO), the type I porphyrinogen isomers are not further metabolized, and only the type III isomers are precursors of heme. The UROS cDNA has an open-reading frame of 798 bp, and the predicted protein product consists of 263 amino acid residues, with an Mr of 28,607 Da.[20] The amino acid compositions of the hepatic and the purified erythrocyte enzyme are identical, and no tissue-specific isoforms have been described. The interspecies homology for the UROS proteins is below 10%, depending on the number and divergence of the species being compared. However, the crystal structures of uroporphyrinogen III cosynthase from humans and *Thermus thermophilus* have been solved and are very similar.[63,64] The structure supports a mechanism that includes the formation of a spirolactam intermediate by positioning the A and D rings such that the noncatalytic closure, to form uroporphyrinogen I, is not possible.[63]

Uroporphyrinogen Decarboxylase (EC 4.1.1.37) UROD is a cytosolic enzyme that catalyzes the sequential removal of the four carboxylic groups of the carboxymethyl side chains in uroporphyrinogen to yield coproporphyrinogen (see Fig. 21-4, *step 5*). The four successive decarboxylation reactions yield 7-, 6-, 5-, and 4-carboxylated porphyrinogens. Increased amounts of these intermediates can be identified as the corresponding oxidized porphyrins in liver, plasma, urine, and stool in human PCT and in laboratory animal models in which hepatic UROD is inhibited. An inhibitor of UROD activity, a partially oxidized substrate molecule,[65] is produced in liver of mice with inherited partial UROD deficiency and hemochromatosis, as well as in experimental animals in response to halogenated polycyclic aromatic hydrocarbons such as hexachlorobenzene, dioxin, polychlorinated biphenyls, or other compounds able to activate the Ah receptor.[66] This porphomethene compound is believed to explain UROD inhibition in human PCT.[65] Humans UROD is a 42,000-kDa polypeptide encoded by a single gene containing 10 exons spread over 3 kb and functions as a homodimer.[67] The gene has been mapped to chromosome 1p34.[68] Although the UROD gene contains two initiation sites, both sites are used with the same frequencies in all tissues, and the gene is transcribed into a single mRNA.[69] Recombinant human UROD purified to homogeneity has been crystallized, and its crystal structure was determined at 1.60-Å resolution.[70] The purified protein is a dimer with a dissociation constant of 0.1 μM.[70] The 40.8-kDa polypeptide forms a single domain with a distorted $(\beta/\alpha)_8$-barrel fold, and a distinctive deep cleft for the enzyme's active site is formed by loops at the C-terminal ends of the barrel strands. The protein forms a homodimer with one active-site cleft per monomer located adjacent to

its neighbor in the dimer. The structure creates a single extended cleft that is large enough to accommodate two substrate molecules in close proximity. Although both uroporphyrinogen I and uroporphyrinogen III are metabolized by UROD, only the coproporphyrinogen III isomer is further metabolized to heme.[71]

Coproporphyrinogen Oxidase (EC 4.1.1.37) CPO is located on the outer surface of the inner mitochondrial membrane in mammalian cells, with a C-terminal tail that anchors it to the membrane.[72] The enzyme catalyzes the removal of the carboxyl group and two hydrogens from the propionic groups of pyrrole rings A and B, forming vinyl groups at these positions (see Fig. 21-4, *step 6*). The enzyme is isomer-specific for coproporphyrinogen III, yielding protoporphyrinogen IX (see Fig. 21-4, *step 6*). The gene for human CPO has been assigned to chromosome 3q12, spans approximately 14 kb, and consists of 7 exons and 6 introns.[73] cDNA cloning for this enzyme was first reported in mouse erythroleukemia cells.[74] The predicted protein comprises 354 amino acid residues (Mr = 40,647 Da), with a putative leader sequence of 31 amino acid residues. The result is a mature protein consisting of 323 amino acid residues (Mr = 37,225 Da).[74] Potential regulatory elements exist in the GC-rich promoter region of the gene, such as 6 Sp1, 4 GATA-1, 1 CACCC site, and the *CPO* gene promoter regulatory element (CPRE).[75] CPRE binds specifically to a CPRE-binding protein, which has a leucine-zipper-like structure and serves as a DNA sequence-specific transcription factor that regulates gene expression.[75] Tissue-specific expression of CPO is significant. For example, binding proteins to the Spl-like element, CPRE, and GATA-1, cooperatively function in *CPO* gene expression in erythroid cells. The CPRE-binding protein by itself plays a principal role in basal expression of CPO in nonerythroid cells. *CPO* mRNA increases during erythroid cell differentiation.[76] Newly synthesized human CPO contains a 110-amino-acid N-terminal signal peptide,[76] which is removed during transport into the intermembrane space of mitochondria, yielding a mature protein of 354 amino acid residues (Mr = 36,842 Da). A 5-base insertional mutation in the middle of this presequence has been described in one patient with HCP.[77]

Protoporphyrinogen Oxidase (EC 1.3.3.4) The penultimate step in heme biosynthesis is the oxidation of protoporphyrinogen IX to protoporphyrin IX, with removal of six hydrogen atoms. This reaction is mediated by the mitochondrial enzyme protoporphyrinogen oxidase (PPO) (see Fig. 21-4, *step 7*). Human PPO cDNA has been cloned.[78] The gene is present as a single copy per haploid genome, at chromosome 1q22.[79] PPO consists of 477 amino acids with an Mr of 50,800 Da. The deduced protein exhibits a high degree of homology over its entire length to the amino acid sequence of PPO encoded by the *HemY* gene of *Bacillus subtilis*. PPO has been crystallized and the structure shows that the enzyme is a homodimer.[80,81] Sequences required for import into the mitochondria have been identified.[82] Expression of PPO is upregulated, approximately fourfold, in the developing erythron from two GATA-1 binding sites located in exon 1.[83]

Ferrochelatase (Protoheme-Ferrolyase; EC 4.99.1.1) The final step of heme biosynthesis is the insertion of iron into protoporphyrin IX. This reaction is catalyzed by mitochondrial ferrochelatase (FECH) (see Fig. 21-4, *step 8*). The enzyme uses protoporphyrin IX, rather than its reduced form, as substrate, but requires the reduced ferrous form of iron.[84] The gene encoding *FECH* has been assigned to chromosome 18q.[85] Two *FECH* mRNA species, one being approximately 2.5 kb and the other being approximately 1.6 kb in size, are derived from the use of two alternative polyadenylation sites in the mRNA. The human *FECH* gene contains a total of 11 exons and has a minimum size of approximately 45 kb. A major site of transcription initiation is at an adenine 89 bp upstream from the translation-initiating ATG. The promoter region contains a potential binding site for several transcription factors, Sp1,

NF-E2, and GATA-1, but not a typical TATA or CAAT sequence. The transcripts are identical in all tissues examined. The crystal structure of *B. subtilis* FECH has been determined at 1.9-Å resolution.[86] Subsequently, the structure of human FECH was solved and the location of the substrate binding site determined. The enzyme functions as a homodimer and associates with the inside of the inner mitochondrial membrane.[87] The mechanism of catalysis has not been identified nor has a function been assigned to the ^{2}Fe-^{2}S cluster that is present in human FECH. Lead inhibits FECH, and a structure of the protein-lead complex has been solved, indicating a critical role for the pi helix in catalysis.[88] FECH seems to have a structurally conserved core region that is common to the enzyme from bacteria, plants, and mammals.

Control of Heme Synthesis in the Liver and Erythroid Cells

Tissue-specific aspects of heme synthesis have been studied mostly in erythroid cells and hepatocytes, as the marrow and liver have the greatest requirements for heme. The rate of heme synthesis in the liver is largely regulated by ALAS1 activity. The synthesis of ALAS1, in turn, is under feedback control by heme, which regulates ALAS1 at the levels of transcription, translation, and transfer into mitochondria. Many chemicals, hormones, and drugs increase the synthesis of hepatic CYPs, which increases the demand for heme and lead to induction of ALAS1. In addition, the ALAS1 gene contains upstream enhancer elements that are responsive to inducing chemicals and interact with the pregnane X receptor. Therefore, ALAS1 and CYPs are subject to direct induction by xenobiotics and certain steroids.[27] Chemical exposures that induce hepatic heme oxygenase and accelerate the destruction of hepatic heme, or inhibit heme formation, can also induce hepatic ALAS1.

ALAS2 is not inducible in erythroid cells by drugs that induce ALAS1 in hepatocytes. The synthesis of ALAS2 is uninfluenced, or often upregulated, by hemin, at both the transcriptional and the translational levels.[26,34,89] Hemin treatment of marrow cultures increases erythroid colony-forming units,[90] whereas hemin treatment of hepatocytes inhibits synthesis of ALAS1 and CYPs. An additional distinct difference in these ALAS isoforms is that SCS-βA associates with ALAS2[35] but not with ALAS1, suggesting a tissue-specific difference in mitochondrial transport of these isoforms.

●ERYTHROPOIETIC PORPHYRIAS

There are two major erythropoietic porphyrias in humans. CEP is caused by mutations of the *UROS* gene. It is one of the least-common porphyrias, but is well known as a result of its long history and the severe photomutilation of exposed areas such as the face and fingers that is a dramatic feature in many cases (Fig. 21-5). EPP, which is caused by *FECH* mutations, is the third most common porphyria, and the most common in children, but was not well described until 1965. XLP is much less common, has the same phenotype as EPP, but normal FECH activity. In 2008, the discovery of gain-of-function mutations in the last exon of ALAS2 provided an explanation for the increased level of erythrocyte protoporphyrin seen in this type of protoporphyria.[37] Characteristics in most patients with erythropoietic porphyrias that are distinct from the hepatic porphyrias include childhood onset, stable symptoms and levels of porphyrins over time, and severity largely determined by genotype rather than factors that affect the heme pathway primarily in the liver. Substantial increases in erythrocyte zinc protoporphyrin in ADP and homozygous forms of other hepatic porphyrias, such as HEP (the homozygous form of familial PCT), AIP, HCP, and VP, suggest that an erythropoietic component may be important in these conditions.[91]

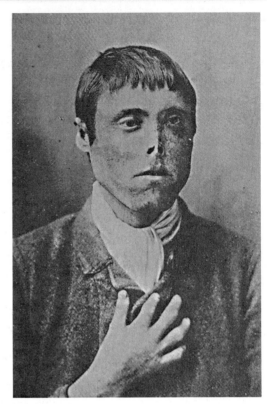

Figure 21–5. A 23-year-old Scottish fisherman with congenital erythropoietic porphyria and scarring and mutilation of the face, ears, and digits as a consequence of repeated sun exposure. He was described in 1898 as having red urine containing excess porphyrins and "hydroa aestivale," because the symptoms, which began at age 3 years, worsened in early summer. A 26-year-old brother was similarly affected. *(Reproduced with permission from Anderson TM. Hydroa aestivale in two brothers, complicated with the presence of haematoporphyrin in the urine.* Br J Dermatol. *1898;10:1)*

CONGENITAL ERYTHROPOIETIC PORPHYRIA

Definition and History

CEP is caused by a deficiency of UROS (see Fig. 21-4, *step 4*), is an autosomal recessive condition, and is also known as Günther disease. It results in accumulation and excretion of isomer I porphyrins, especially uroporphyrin I and coproporphyrin I (see Table 21-2 and Fig. 21-1). Characteristic manifestations of CEP include chronic, severe photosensitivity and hemolytic anemia evident in early childhood. Atypical presentations include milder disease that resembles PCT, and onset during adult life, often in association with a myeloproliferative disorder.[92] Early case descriptions of CEP appeared in 1874 and 1898,[3] and approximately 140 cases were reported up to 1997.[93] However, some of these patients may have had HEP, which has very similar clinical features. Perhaps the most well-known patient was Mathias Petry, who survived until age 34, and, beginning in 1915, worked with the porphyrin chemist Hans Fisher, providing samples for early studies of porphyrin chemistry.[94]

Pathophysiology

The uroporphyrinogen III synthase defects in CEP are remarkably heterogeneous at the molecular level, with at least 46 different mutations of the *UROS* gene, and one *GATA-1* mutation reported as of this writing.[93] The UROS mutations include deletions, insertions, rearrangements, splicing abnormalities, and both missense and nonsense mutations. The missense mutations are well distributed throughout the gene. Of the 12 single-base substitutions, 4 (T228M, G225S, A66V, A104V) were hotspot mutations, occurring at CpG (cytosine-phosphate-guanine) dinucleotides.[95] A mutation that altered the penultimate nucleotide in exon 4, resulting in an E81D mutation, also produced exon skipping on approximately 85% of the transcripts from that allele. With the exception of V82F, all CEP missense mutations occurred in amino acid residues that are conserved in both the mouse and the human enzyme. Genotype-phenotype correlation in CEP was studied by prokaryotic expression of mutant *UROS* cDNAs. Mean activities of the mutant enzymes expressed in *Escherichia coli* ranged from 0% to 36% of the activity expressed by the normal cDNA. The majority of the mutant cDNAs expressed polypeptides with no enzymatic activity. However, V82F, E81D, A66V, A104V, and V99A showed 36%, 30%, 15%, 8%, and 6% enzyme activity, respectively, compared with the normal control. A66V and V82F were thermodynamically unstable mutants.[95] Homoallelism for C73R, the most common mutation, found in five patients, was associated clinically with the most severe phenotypes, such as hydrops fetalis and transfusion dependency from birth.

Pathogenesis of the Clinical Findings

Porphyrins in their oxidized state are reddish, fluorescent, and photosensitizing, whereas porphyrin precursors and the reduced porphyrinogens are colorless and nonfluorescent. Most marrow normoblasts in CEP display marked fluorescence as a result of porphyrin accumulation (located principally in the nuclei, probably the result of fixation artifact).[96] Anemia and the excess production and excretion of porphyrins is largely accounted for by ineffective erythropoiesis in the marrow. Porphyrin concentrations are also increased in circulating erythrocytes, and intravascular hemolysis may result from exposure to light in the dermal capillaries, causing erythrocyte damage and lysis or uptake by the spleen. Splenomegaly is very common in CEP and is presumed to be secondary to the hemolytic process. The excess porphyrins that are produced by the marrow or released by hemolysis are transported in plasma to the skin, leading to photosensitivity.

Clinical Features

Severe cutaneous photosensitivity is noted soon after birth in most cases. The disease may be recognized even earlier as a cause of hydrops fetalis. Phototherapy for hyperbilirubinemia may cause severe cutaneous burns and scarring in newborns with unrecognized CEP. Brown staining of the teeth by porphyrins (erythrodontia) is evident when the teeth erupt. Blistering and scarring resemble those found in PCT, but are usually much more severe, reflecting the much higher plasma porphyrin levels observed in CEP. Some cases are relatively mild, and can closely mimic PCT. Late-onset cases are often associated with myeloproliferative disorders, with expansion of a clone of erythroid cells bearing a mutation and displaying UROS deficiency.[92] Subepidermal bullous lesions are characteristic, and progress to crusted erosions that heal with scarring and areas of hyperpigmentation and hypopigmentation. Also common is hypertrichosis, which is sometimes severe, and alopecia. Loss of facial features and digits are common and result from recurrent blisters, infection, and scarring. Fingers may be shortened and tapered as a consequence of scarring and contraction of the skin during childhood growth. *Erythrodontia*, with brown staining and red fluorescence of the teeth under long-wave ultraviolet light is characteristic, and results from deposition of porphyrins in the developing deciduous and permanent teeth in utero. Porphyrins are also deposited in bone. The skeleton is also affected by expansion of the marrow, leading to pathologic fractures, vertebral compression, short stature, and osteolytic and sclerotic lesions. Vitamin D deficiency resulting from avoiding sunlight might also contribute.

Anemia may be severe and lead to transfusion dependence in the more severe cases. Uncorrected anemia can increase erythropoiesis,

TABLE 21–3. Common Clinical Features of Erythropoietic Protoporphyria from a Series of 32 Cases[135]

Symptoms and Signs	Incidence (% of Total)
Burning	97
Edema	94
Itching	88
Erythema	69
Scarring	19
Vesicles	3
Anemia	27
Cholelithiasis	12
Abnormal liver function results	4

which, in turn, is a stimulus to porphyrin production by the abnormal erythropoietic cells in the marrow. Erythrocytes exhibit polychromasia, poikilocytosis, anisocytosis, and basophilic stippling, and reticulocytes and nucleated red blood cells are increased.[97] Table 21-3 summarizes the clinical features of the porphyrias.

Diagnosis

CEP may be suspected even before birth if a sibling is known to have CEP. However, the family history is often negative. CEP should be suspected as a cause of hydrops fetalis, as the disease can be diagnosed and treated in utero. Aspirated amniotic fluid is dark brown and contains large amounts of porphyrins. The diagnosis of CEP is often made after birth when pink to dark-brown staining of the diapers, with red fluorescence under long-wave ultraviolet light, is noted. Cutaneous vesicles and bullae on sun-exposed areas may be severe, with scarring.

Urinary porphyrin excretion is markedly increased, and often in the range of 50 to 100 mg/day (normal: up to ~0.3 mg/day). Uroporphyrin I and coproporphyrin I account for most of the increase, although the III isomers and heptacarboxyl, hexacarboxyl, and pentacarboxyl porphyrins are also increased. Fecal porphyrins are increased, and are predominantly coproporphyrin I. Plasma total porphyrins are markedly increased as well, with a pattern of individual porphyrins similar to that in urine. Markedly increased erythrocyte porphyrins are predominantly uroporphyrin I and coproporphyrin I, although protoporphyrin IX may predominate especially in milder cases.

CEP must be distinguished by biochemical testing from other causes of blistering skin lesions. HEP can present with photosensitivity in early childhood. Mild cases of CEP may be misdiagnosed as PCT.

The diagnosis should be confirmed in all cases by DNA studies, which can identify causative mutations in almost all cases. This is especially important for genetic counseling and for prenatal diagnosis in subsequent pregnancies. Demonstration of a GATA-1 mutation in one case illustrates that on occasion a genetic defect outside the heme biosynthetic pathway can cause CEP.[97]

Therapy

To avoid severe scarring and loss of facial features and digits, it is essential to avoid sunlight, trauma to the skin, and infections. Topical sunscreens that block long-wave ultraviolet light (ultraviolet A light) and oral treatment with β-carotene[98] are marginally beneficial in most cases. Erythrocyte transfusions are essential in patients with severe anemia.[99] Transfusions to maintain the hematocrit above 35%, with an iron chelator to avoid iron overload, has been beneficial in some cases.[100]

Hydroxyurea to reduce erythropoiesis and porphyrin production also may be considered.[101] Splenectomy has provided short-term benefit. Oral charcoal reportedly was quite effective in one patient,[102] and ascorbic acid and α-tocopherol improved anemia in another.[103] Unaffected infants born to mothers with CEP may have erythrodontia as a result of exposure to maternal porphyrins before birth.[104] Hematopoietic stem cell transplantation is the treatment of choice when a suitable donor is available, especially for young patients.[105] When transplantation is successful, there is marked clinical improvement and reduction in porphyrin levels, even if these are not completely normalized. Because iron upregulates ALAS2, the initial enzyme in the heme biosynthetic pathway in the marrow, it was considered that iron deficiency or removal might be beneficial in CEP. One patient experienced spontaneous improvement in photosensitivity and hemolysis after developing iron deficiency from gastrointestinal bleeding, worsened when the bleeding stopped, and improved when treated with an iron chelating agent.[106] In another patient with CEP, iron depletion by phlebotomy improved hemolysis and photosensitivity and reduced plasma and urine porphyrins.[107] But iron deficiency might also have adverse effects, so the effects of altered iron status in CEP requires further study. Gene therapy is being explored using retroviral and lentiviral vectors and hematopoietic stem cells from patients with CEP.[108,109]

ERYTHROPOIETIC PROTOPORPHYRIA

Definition and History

EPP is caused by a partial deficiency of FECH (see Fig. 21-4, *step 8*) activity, which results in the accumulation of the substrate protoporphyrin in the marrow. XLP has the same phenotype but is much less common, and is a result of ALAS2 gain-of-function mutations (ALAS; see Fig. 21-1).[37] EPP and XLP are characterized by onset of nonblistering cutaneous photosensitivity in early childhood. EPP is the most common porphyria in children and the third most common in adults. Reported prevalence varies between 5 and 15 cases per 1 million individuals.[110-112] A recent study of the UK Biobank suggests that EPP is substantially underrecognized.[113] Protoporphyric liver failure is a potentially fatal complication estimated to occur in less than 5% of patients.

Pathophysiology

EPP is an autosomal recessive disease. In most families, a severe *FECH* mutation is inherited from one parent and a low-expression (hypomorphic) *FECH* allele from the other. More than 75 different severe mutations, including nonsense, missense, and splice-site mutations, and deletions, insertions, and rearrangements, have been described. Splicing mutations are most common. Recombinant human FECH, when engineered to have individual exon skipping for exons 3 through 11, lacks significant enzyme activity when expressed in *E. coli* and almost all such variants lacked the [2Fe-2S] cluster.[114] EPP was usually described in the past as an autosomal dominant disorder, with variable penetrance. However, it was noted that EPP patients have only 30% or less of normal FECH activity, rather than 50%, which would be expected in an autosomal dominant condition. It was then shown that, in addition to a severe *FECH* mutation, a low-expression (hypomorphic) intronic polymorphism (a −23C to T transition) is found in the other *FECH* allele of most patients with EPP, which is inherited from the other parent.[115-117] This transition favors the use of a cryptic acceptor splice site 63 bases upstream of the normal splice site. The aberrantly spliced mRNA contains a premature stop codon and is degraded by a nonsense-mediated decay mechanism.[117] The result is a lower steady-state level of wild-type *FECH* mRNA. Coinheritance of the hypomorphic allele in *trans* to a loss-of-function mutant allele was found in 98% of French cases with EPP,[118] and with a similar frequency in South African patients.[112] The

intervening sequence (IVS) 3–48C hypomorphic allele is common in the European (white) population. By itself it has no major phenotype, but may slightly decrease MCV and hemoglobin.[113] Its frequency varies widely in different populations and relates to the observed differences in the prevalence of EPP.[110-112]

Other underlying genetic mechanisms must be considered in newly identified EPP families. In a few families, a severe *FECH* mutation, at least one of which must produce some FECH enzyme, is inherited from each parent and the hypomorphic allele is not present. Interestingly, EPP in such families is sometimes associated with seasonal palmar keratoderma, unusual neurologic symptoms, less-than-expected increases in erythrocyte protoporphyrin, and absence of liver dysfunction.[110]

XLP was first perceived as a variant form of EPP in which *FECH* mutations were absent. After family studies suggested sex-linked inheritance, gain-of-function mutations of *ALAS2* (the only heme pathway enzyme found on the X chromosome) were discovered.[37] This is the only porphyria to result from mutations of ALAS, the first enzyme in the pathway. Additionally, in 2017 a single family was described with autosomal dominant protoporphyria associated with a point mutation in the *CLPX* gene.[119] CLPX is involved in synthesis and inactivation of ALAS2, and this mutation impaired ALAS2 inactivation, leading to accumulation of ALA and protoporphyrin.

EPP can develop late in life in patients with clonal hematologic disorders and expansion of a clone of hematopoietic cells with mutations of a *FECH* allele.[120,121] For example, a patient with a myeloproliferative disorder later developed severe EPP because of clonal expansion of a cell of erythropoietic lineage with a *FECH* deletion and the IVS3–48C/T polymorphism, and died of EPP-induced liver disease.[122]

Pathogenesis of the Clinical Findings

Marrow reticulocytes are thought to be the primary source of the excess protoporphyrin in EPP.[123,124] Most of the excess erythrocyte protoporphyrin in circulating erythrocytes is found in younger cells as metal-free protoporphyrin (ie, not complexed with zinc), in contrast to other conditions associated with increased erythrocyte protoporphyrin content. Metal-free protoporphyrin declines much more rapidly with red cell age than does zinc protoporphyrin.[123,124] Metal-free protoporphyrin, but not zinc protoporphyrin, is released from erythrocytes following solar irradiation, which may explain why lead intoxication and iron deficiency, which are associated with elevated erythrocyte zinc protoporphyrin levels, are not associated with photosensitivity.[125] Excess metal-free protoporphyrin enters plasma from reticulocytes as well as circulating erythrocytes and is taken up by hepatocytes, excreted in bile and feces, and may undergo enterohepatic recirculation. Hepatocytes may also provide a limited additional source of excess protoporphyrin in this disease. Light-excited protoporphyrin in EPP generates free radicals and singlet oxygen,[126] which in EPP can lead to peroxidation of lipids[127] and crosslinking of membrane proteins. Skin irradiation in EPP patients leads to complement activation and polymorphonuclear chemotaxis, which contributes to the development of skin pathology.[128] Skin histopathology is not specific, but may include thickened capillary walls in the papillary dermis surrounded by amorphous hyaline-like deposits, immunoglobulin, complement, and periodic acid-Schiff–positive mucopolysaccharides.[129] Basement membrane abnormalities are less marked than in other forms of porphyria.[130,131] Protoporphyric liver failure is a feared complication that develops in approximately 5% of patients, and is attributed to the cholestatic effects of excess protoporphyrin presented to the liver. This complication may begin with chronic abnormalities in liver function tests and then progress rapidly as a vicious cycle of increasing protoporphyrin levels in plasma and erythrocytes and worsening liver function and photosensitivity. Liver failure is sometimes precipitated by another cause of liver dysfunction, such as viral or alcoholic hepatitis. Protoporphyrin is cholestatic, and can form crystalline structures in hepatocytes and impair mitochondrial function, leading to decreased hepatic bile formation and flow.[132,133] Accumulated protoporphyrin may appear as brown pigment in hepatocytes, Kupffer cells, and biliary canaliculi and these deposits are doubly refractive with a Maltese cross appearance under polarizing microscopy.[134] DNA microarray studies in explanted livers of patients with liver failure revealed significant changes in expression of several genes involved in wound-healing, organic anion transport, and oxidative stress.[135]

Clinical Features

Photosensitivity is present from early childhood in almost all cases. Parents may observe that an affected infant cries and develops skin swelling and erythema when exposed to sunlight. Although EPP is the most common porphyria in children, there is often considerable delay in diagnosis.[136] Cutaneous photosensitivity in EPP is acute and nonblistering, which is distinctly different from the more chronic, blistering skin manifestations of the other cutaneous porphyrias. Table 21-3 tabulates the symptoms in a series of 32 patients with EPP. Skin symptoms are usually worse during spring and summer and affect light-exposed areas, especially the face and hands. Characteristically, stinging or burning pain develops within 1 hour of sunlight exposure, and if exposure continues is followed by erythema and edema—resembling solar urticaria, sometimes with petechiae, and less commonly purpura. Blistering and crusted lesions are uncommon. Artificial lights may contribute to photosensitivity.[137,138] Patients typically avoid sunlight and may display no objective cutaneous signs. Repeated light exposure can lead to chronic changes including leathery hyperkeratotic skin especially on the dorsa of the hands and finger joints, mild scarring, and separation of the nail plate (onycholysis). Mild anemia with microcytosis, hypochromia, and reduced iron stores, but usually normal serum iron and serum transferrin receptor-1, is a common feature of EPP and XLP,[123,139–141] but there is little evidence for impaired erythropoiesis or abnormal iron metabolism, and hemolysis is absent or very mild.[142] Iron accumulation in erythroblasts and ring sideroblasts have been noted in marrow in some patients.[143] Cytokine and erythropoietin levels are normal, and hepcidin is not inappropriately increased and responds as expected to orally administered iron.[144] Because this unexplained iron deficiency may be detrimental and further limit heme synthesis and increase protoporphyrin accumulation, iron status should be carefully evaluated in EPP patients, keeping in mind that serum ferritin in the lower part of the reference range, especially in women, may be indicative of depleted iron stores. Also, iron is proposed to have a role in splicing of the *FECH* mRNA, where decreased iron leads to an increase in incorrect splicing of the mRNA.[145] Although there are reports that giving iron can increase photosensitivity in EPP, recent findings suggest that iron repletion can correct microcytic anemia and even decrease protoporphyrin levels.[145] However, further studies of iron supplementation in EPP and XLP are needed.[145,146] Precipitating factors that are important in the hepatic porphyrias do not appear to play an important role in EPP. Although more long-term followup studies are needed, porphyrin levels and symptoms typically do not change over time, unless liver dysfunction develops. Concurrent iron deficiency or other marrow problems might also lead to further increases in porphyrin levels and photosensitivity. Pregnancy is reported to lower erythrocyte protoporphyrin levels somewhat and increase tolerance to sunlight.[131] Neurovisceral manifestations are absent in uncomplicated EPP. Patients with severe protoporphyric liver failure may develop a severe motor neuropathy similar to that seen in the acute porphyrias.[147] Autosomal recessive EPP associated with palmar keratoderma also has been associated with unexplained neurologic symptoms.[148] Gallstones containing large amounts of protoporphyrin are common, and may require cholecystectomy at an unusually

early age.[149] Liver function and liver protoporphyrin content are usually normal in EPP. Protoporphyric liver failure, which is the most life-threatening complication of EPP, results from the cholestatic effects of protoporphyrin presented in excess amounts to the liver. It can be the major presenting feature of EPP,[150] and may be chronic or progress rapidly to death from liver failure. Unnecessary surgery for suspected biliary obstruction can be detrimental and should be avoided.[133] Operating room lights during liver transplantation or other surgery, especially in patients with liver failure, can cause marked photosensitivity with extensive burns of the skin, and peritoneum and photodamage of circulating erythrocytes.[151] Table 21-3 summarizes the clinical features of the porphyrias.

Diagnosis

Painful, nonblistering photosensitivity suggests the diagnosis. A substantial elevation of erythrocyte protoporphyrin is expected, but is not specific, because erythrocyte zinc protoporphyrin is increased in conditions such as homozygous porphyrias (other than most cases of CEP), iron deficiency, lead poisoning, anemia of chronic disease,[152] hemolytic conditions,[153] and many other erythrocyte disorders. A unique finding in EPP is increased erythrocyte protoporphyrin with a predominance of metal-free protoporphyrin rather than zinc protoporphyrin. This occurs because FECH, which can use metals in addition to iron, catalyzes the formation of zinc protoporphyrin, and this activity is deficient in EPP. Because FECH is not deficient in XLP, erythrocytes contain increased amounts of both zinc protoporphyrin and metal-free protoporphyrin, although the metal-free protoporphyrin still predominates in most cases. Consequently, the diagnosis of EPP requires demonstration of an increase in metal-free protoporphyrin in red cells. Amounts of metal-free protoporphyrin and zinc protoporphyrin in erythrocytes can be measured by ethanol or acetone extraction, or by HPLC. Confusion arises because laboratories do not use the same terminology when reporting. For example, the term *free erythrocyte protoporphyrin*, when reporting results measured with a hematofluorometer as an indicator of lead exposure, actually refers to zinc protoporphyrin rather than metal-free or total protoporphyrin. At this writing, we are aware of only two laboratories in the United States, the Mayo Clinic Laboratories and the Porphyria Laboratory at the University of Texas Medical Branch, that reliably report the amounts of total, metal-free, and zinc protoporphyrin, as is needed for confirmation of a diagnosis of EPP. The proportions of metal-free and zinc protoporphyrin can also usually distinguish XLP (50% to ~85% metal-free protoporphyrin) from EPP (>85% metal-free protoporphyrin).[154] The plasma porphyrin concentration is almost always at least mildly increased in EPP, but often less than in other cutaneous porphyrias, and may be normal in mild cases. Plasma porphyrins in EPP are particularly subject to photodegradation during sample processing unless great care is taken to shield the sample from natural or fluorescent light.[155] For these reasons, measurement of erythrocyte rather than plasma porphyrin should be relied upon for diagnosis of EPP and XLP. Fecal porphyrins are increased in most cases, and consist mostly of protoporphyrin. Urine porphyrins are normal, except after liver failure develops, which causes increases in urinary coproporphyrin as is typical for other forms of liver diseases.

Therapy

Avoidance of sunlight exposure is important, and often requires changes in lifestyle and working environment. Topical sunscreens are not effective, and sunblocks containing zinc oxide or titanium dioxide may be helpful. Orally administered β-carotene, which probably quenches activated oxygen radicals,[138,156] may afford some protection after 1 to 3 months of therapy, but results are variable. A daily dose of 120 to 180 mg is recommended to achieve a serum β-carotene level of 600 to 800 mcg/dL.[137]

Oral cysteine may also quench excited oxygen species and increase tolerance to sunlight in EPP.[157] Other treatments that aim to either increase skin pigmentation or scavenge activated oxygen species have been reviewed[156] and include dihydroxyacetone and lawsone, vitamin C, and narrow-wave ultraviolet B phototherapy to increase melanin.[158] Afamelanotide, an α-melanocyte–stimulating hormone analogue that increases skin melanin, has shown benefit in clinical trials, and is now approved by the FDA for use.[159,160] It is advisable to monitor protoporphyrin levels and liver function tests at least yearly, avoid iron deficiency as assessed by serum ferritin, and avoid severe caloric restriction and drugs or hormone preparations that impair hepatic excretory function.[161,162] Because patients avoid sunlight exposure, vitamin D supplementation is recommended. Little longitudinal data is available, but variation of erythrocyte total protoporphyrin up to 25% is expected over time, and greater increases might raise early concern for protoporphyric liver failure.[163] Management of protoporphyric liver disease is difficult. The condition may resolve spontaneously especially if another reversible cause of liver dysfunction, such as viral hepatitis or alcohol, is contributing.[164,165] Cholestyramine,[133,166,167] ursodeoxycholic acid,[168] vitamin E, red blood cell transfusions,[169] plasma exchange, and intravenous hemin may be given in combination to bridge patients to liver transplantation or spontaneous improvement.[170] Success of liver transplantation is comparable to that in other liver diseases, even though protoporphyric liver failure may recur in the new liver, a result of the continued erythrocyte protoporphyrin release by the marrow.[151,171] Acute motor neuropathy has developed in some patients with protoporphyric liver disease after transfusion[172] or liver transplantation,[173,174] and is sometimes reversible.[173] Marrow transplantation can achieve remission in human EPP,[175] as well in murine models of protoporphyria.[176] Sequential liver and marrow transplantation can correct the overproduction of protoporphyrin by the marrow and prevent recurrence of liver disease.[177] Promising studies in murine models suggest a future role for gene therapy in human EPP.[178]

● ACUTE PORPHYRIAS

The acute porphyrias are comprised of four disorders caused by different enzyme deficiencies, and are distinctive for neurologic symptoms that usually occur as acute exacerbations during adult life. Similar neurologic symptoms occur in lead poisoning and hereditary tyrosinemia type I.

δ-AMINOLEVULINIC ACID DEHYDRATASE PORPHYRIA

Definition and History
ADP is an autosomal recessive disorder resulting from severe deficiency of ALAD activity (see Table 21-1 and Fig. 21-1). This is the rarest of the porphyrias, with only eight cases documented at the molecular level.[50,178-183]

Pathophysiology
In all reported cases, the patients have been male. Compound heterozygosity for two distinct ALAD mutations was responsible for the disease in all but one case (see Fig. 21-4, *step 2*).[182,184] Four (three in Germany and one in the United States) patients experienced onset of symptoms in their teens, whereas one Swedish patient developed severe symptoms in infancy.[181] The sixth patient was a Belgian male who developed ADP at age 63 years and was found to have two inherited base transitions in one allele, and was therefore heterozygous for ALAD deficiency.[179,185] He also developed polycythemia vera and his erythrocyte ALAD activity was less than 1% of normal, while his lymphocyte ALAD activity was

greater than 20% of normal. Heterozygous ALAD deficiency was apparently clinically silent in this patient until there was expansion of a clone of erythroid cells that carried the mutant ALAD allele.[186] Thus ADP is highly heterogeneous at the molecular level, with a total of 15 mutant alleles identified in these eight patients.[184] An additional mutation was found in a healthy Swedish girl with markedly decreased ALAD activity (12% of normal), which was detected by ALAD measurement during neonatal screening for hereditary tyrosinemia.[187] The same mutation was found in a U.S. male patient with acute porphyria who also had a *CPO* mutation and an unusual pattern of porphyrin precursors and porphyrins reflecting dual enzyme deficiencies.[188] Thus, heterozygous ALAD deficiency may rarely be combined with another enzyme deficiency, or may itself cause porphyria if a marrow disorder leads to clonal expansion of the mutant *ALAD* allele. Human ALAD consists of eight identical oligomers, each with two zinc-binding sites. Lead can bind at least one of these sites and impair enzyme activity. Some mutations found in ADP may affect zinc binding or the site of the iron-sulfur cluster [189], or favor assembly of a hexameric enzyme with decreased activity. Thus, ADP has been described as a conformational disease.[54] ADP is classified as one of the hepatic porphyrias because it closely resembles the other acute porphyrias. In one patient, ALAS1 mRNA, presumably of hepatic origin, was elevated in exosomes to a degree comparable to that seen in AIP. [190] However, a substantial increase in erythrocyte zinc protoporphyrin also suggests an erythroid component. The Swedish infant with severe, early onset disease did not benefit from liver transplantation,[191] and another patient was reported to benefit from suppression of erythropoiesis by treatment with blood transfusions and hydroxyurea.[183] The excess urinary coproporphyrin III in ADP may originate from metabolism of ALA to porphyrinogens in a tissue other than the site of ALA overproduction. Indeed, ALA loading in normal patients has been shown to cause substantial coproporphyrinuria.[192] As in other acute porphyrias, the pathogenesis of the neurologic symptoms is poorly understood.

Clinical Features
Four adolescent males had intermittent symptoms resembling other acute porphyrias, including abdominal pain, vomiting, extremity pain, and motor neuropathy, although exacerbating factors were less evident.[184,193] Of these, two German patients had initial acute attacks and then remained well during 20 years of followup.[194] A third German patient[195] and a U.S. patient[184] had further attacks and were maintained on prophylactic hemin infusions. The Swedish infant had more severe neurologic disease, including failure to thrive, and died after liver transplantation.[196] The 63-year-old man in Belgium developed an acute motor polyneuropathy concurrently with a myeloproliferative disorder.[92,179,197]

Diagnosis
A biochemical diagnosis of ADP includes demonstration of markedly deficient erythrocyte ALAD activity, marked elevation in urinary ALA and coproporphyrin III and erythrocyte zinc protoporphyrin, with little or no increase in urinary PBG. Erythrocyte ALAD activity is approximately half-normal in both parents. Lead poisoning is differentiated by increased blood lead and restoration of ALAD activity in vitro by reduced glutathione or dithiothreitol.[182,198] Although biochemical measurements can strongly suggest ADP, the diagnosis must be confirmed by DNA studies.

Patients with hereditary tyrosinemia type I may also have ALAD inhibition and increased excretion of ALA.[46] Dioxoheptanoic acid (succinylacetone), a structural analogue of ALA and a potent ALAD inhibitor, accumulates as a result of the inherited deficiency of fumarylacetoacetate hydrolase in these patients. The presence of this inhibitor can be demonstrated in urine by measuring ALAD activity in normal blood after addition of a patient's urine. ALAD protein is not reduced in this disease.[199]

Therapy

Because few cases have been documented, treatment recommendations are based on limited experience. Hemin was beneficial in the four male patients with onset near puberty, but there was little or no response to glucose. A long-term preventive hemin regimen was effective in two of these patients. The Swedish infant did not respond to glucose or hemin, and did not improve greatly after liver transplantation.[191] Whether transplantation would benefit less-severe cases is unknown. Hemin produced a biochemical response but no clinical improvement in the late-onset case in Belgium, where the patient had a peripheral neuropathy but no acute attacks.[197] Suppression of erythropoiesis was beneficial in one patient.[183] Elevation of ALAS mRNA was found in one patient,[200] which suggests that RNA interference using givosiran might be effective.

ACUTE INTERMITTENT PORPHYRIA

Definition and History

AIP is an autosomal dominant disorder caused by a partial deficiency of PBGD (see Table 21-1 and Fig. 21-1). Symptoms usually occur as acute attacks, are neurologic in origin and may become chronic. This is the most common acute porphyria and the second most common porphyria worldwide. Most individuals who inherit the enzyme deficiency never develop symptoms. Indeed, penetrance may be as low as 1%.[209] However, some heterozygotes are at risk to develop symptoms after puberty. The first case of acute porphyria was described in 1889 by Stokvis[5] who noted a relationship of the symptoms to the drug sulfonal, which is related to the barbiturates. The prevalence of AIP was estimated to be 1 to 2 per 100,000 in Europe,[201] and 2.4 per 100,000 in Finland.[202] But heterozygous mutations are much more prevalent in genomic databases.[209] More than 300 *PBGD* mutations have been described in AIP, with many found in only one or a few families.[203-205] The disease occurs in all races, but clusters as a result of founder effects occur in some countries. A founder mutation in northern Sweden is associated with a disease prevalence of 1 per 1500.[206] The prevalence of low erythrocyte PBGD activity, which includes latent gene carriers of AIP, is as high as 1 per 500 in the general population of Finland.[207] The minimal prevalence of the AIP-associated genes was calculated to be 1 per 1675 by DNA studies in France[208] and 1 per 1786 in genomic multinational database,[209] suggesting that the penetrance of acute attacks is only approximately 1% and that both modifying genes and environmental modifiers play an important role in causing or preventing attacks.

Pathophysiology

PBGD is also known as HMB synthase (HMBS), and formerly as uroporphyrinogen I synthase. *PBGD* mutations have been classified based in part on the presence or absence of cross-reactive immunologic material (CRIM), which indicates the presence of inactive enzyme protein. *Type I* mutations are CRIM-negative, with reduction of both enzyme activity and protein to approximately 50% of normal in heterozygotes. *Type II* mutations are associated with reduced PBGD activity only in nonerythroid tissue. These patients with "variant AIP" comprise less than 5% of AIP patients, and have normal erythrocyte PBGD activity and decreased hepatic activity because, as explained earlier, transcription of the gene to form the erythroid-specific enzyme starts downstream of the site of the mutation. *Type III* are CRIM-positive mutations that result in decreased activity with structurally abnormal enzyme protein.[210]

Pathogenesis of the Clinical Findings

A partial deficiency of PBGD rarely causes clinical expression of AIP, and most individuals who inherit this enzyme deficiency remain healthy with normal porphyrin precursor excretion throughout life. Unidentified modifying genes almost certainly contribute to disease activation. Certain drugs and hormones exacerbate AIP by directly inducing hepatic ALAS1[27] and also inducing CYP enzymes, thereby increasing the demand for heme. CYP enzymes are abundant, turn over rapidly, and use most of the heme synthesized in the liver.[211] When heme synthesis is stimulated, the partial enzyme deficiency in AIP apparently impairs heme synthesis sufficiently to deplete the regulatory heme pool, which controls synthesis of the rate-limiting enzyme ALAS1. This compromises negative feedback by heme, and leads to marked induction of ALAS1 and overproduction of ALA, PBG, and porphyrins in the liver.

It is generally accepted, although not proven, that hepatic PBGD remains constant at approximately 50% of normal activity during exacerbations and remissions of AIP, as in erythrocytes. An early report suggested that the enzyme activity is considerably less than half-normal in liver during an acute attack,[14] but additional data are lacking. It has been suggested that once the disease becomes activated, excess PBG may interfere with assembly of the dipyrromethane cofactor for this enzyme. Clinical improvement and normalization of porphyrin precursor excretion after liver transplantation in patients with severe AIP is a clear indication that the liver plays an essential role in neuropathic processes in this disease.[212] Proposed explanations for neurologic dysfunction in the acute porphyrias include the following: (a) Heme pathway intermediates or products derived from them may be neurotoxic. This hypothesis is the most favored hypothesis, although the evidence is not conclusive. (b) PBGD deficiency in the nervous system tissues may limit heme synthesis and formation of important hemoproteins. For example, decreased activity of the hemoprotein nitric oxide synthase might decrease production of nitric oxide and cause vasospasm, which might account for some cerebral manifestations of AIP[213,214] and possibly compromise intestinal blood flow.[215] Because regulation of heme and hemoprotein synthesis in nervous tissue and blood vessels is difficult to study, convincing evidence for this hypothesis is lacking. (c) Impaired hepatic heme synthesis during an attack may lead to decreased activity of hepatic tryptophan pyrrolase, which might increase levels of tryptophan in plasma and brain, leading to increased synthesis of the neurotransmitter 5-hydroxytryptamine. ALA is increased in a number of disorders with similar neurologic manifestations, including all four of the acute porphyrias, lead poisoning, and hereditary tyrosinemia type I, which favors a neuropathic role for this porphyrin precursor or perhaps a derivative. ALA can enter cells readily and be converted to porphyrins, which, in turn, may have toxic potential.[216] ALA is also structurally similar to γ-aminobutyric acid and can interact with γ-aminobutyric acid receptors.[217,218] However, studies of ALA loading have not shown adverse effects. Impaired motor function with ataxia develops in mice with PBGD deficiency as a result of compound heterozygous or homozygous mutations induced by gene targeting.[219] Induction of hepatic CYPs is impaired in these animals and corrected by heme.[220] But motor neuropathy can develop even with normal or only slightly increased ALA in plasma and urine, suggesting a primary role for heme deficiency in porphyric neuropathy in this murine model.[221]

Precipitating Factors Acute attacks are precipitated in some heterozygotes by various endogenous or exogenous factors that are additive. Some individuals remain susceptible to repeated attacks even after avoidance of known precipitants, suggesting that additional unknown genetic factors contribute. Many precipitating factors cause *induction* *of hepatic ALAS1*, which is closely associated with induction of CYPs and leads to overproduction of ALA and other pathway intermediates.

Drugs and Other Exogenous Chemicals Most drugs that are harmful in acute porphyrias are known inducers of hepatic CYPs. These drugs increase de novo heme synthesis, thereby derepressing hepatic ALAS1, and also directly induce this rate-limiting enzyme.[27] Table 21-4 lists some drugs known to be harmful or safe. Information regarding safety of many drugs in clinical practice is uncertain or lacking. More extensive drug safety databases are available at the websites of the American Porphyria Foundation (www.porphyriafoundation. com/) and the European Porphyria Network (EPNET: www.porphyria-europe.com/). These drug classifications are often based on limited evidence and may be controversial. Ethanol and other alcohols are inducers of hepatic ALAS1 and some CYPs.[222] Smoking is known to increase CYPs in humans, probably from effects of polycyclic aromatic hydrocarbons, and has been associated with more frequent symptoms of acute porphyria.[223]

Endocrine Factors Rarity of symptoms before puberty and more common clinical expression in women point to hormonal factors as important contributors in AIP. Although estrogens are considered harmful, it is likely that progesterone is mostly responsible for cyclic premenstrual attacks that occur in some women. Progesterone, certain metabolites of testosterone, and synthetic progestins are potent inducers of ALAS1. Thus, administration of progestational agents should be avoided. Diabetes mellitus is not known to precipitate attacks of porphyria, and has been observed to decrease the frequency of attacks and lower porphyrin precursor levels, possibly in relation to high circulating glucose levels.[224]

Pregnancy Pregnancy is usually well tolerated.[225] Attacks during pregnancy are sometimes a result of harmful drugs or reduced caloric intake. Metoclopramide, considered at least by some a contraindicated drug, is associated with exacerbation of the disease when used to treat hyperemesis gravidarum.[226,227] But for reasons that are not clear, some women experience attacks during pregnancy even when harmful factors are avoided.

Nutrition Reduced intake of calories and carbohydrate can exacerbate acute porphyrias. This may occur from efforts to lose weight, bariatric surgery or from metabolic stress from an illness or surgery. Under these conditions, upregulation of PGC-1α can lead to induction of ALAS1, increases in ALA and PBG, and symptoms of acute porphyria, and these effects are reversed by administration of carbohydrate.[30,228] Starvation, may also induce hepatic heme oxygenase,[229] which may deplete hepatic heme and contribute to ALAS1 induction.

Stress Various forms of physical or psychological stress may exacerbate acute porphyrias, although the mechanisms are not well defined. Medical illnesses, fever, infections, alcoholic excess, and surgery may decrease food intake and contribute to induction of hepatic ALAS1 and heme oxygenase. Psychological stress may also lead to decreased food intake and have other metabolic effects.

Clinical Features

Symptoms are almost never seen before puberty, but may develop especially in women in the third or fourth decade of life. Acute attacks are life-threatening but rarely fatal if promptly recognized and treated. Attacks that recur frequently and chronic symptoms can be disabling. Although the most prominent symptoms are a result of effects on the nervous system, liver and kidney damage may be important in the long-term. In very rare homozygous patients, severe neurologic manifestations are seen early in childhood, and acute attacks are not prominent.[230,231] Symptoms and signs are nonspecific and highly variable. Abdominal pain is the most common symptom, occurring in 85% to 95% of patients.[232,233] It is usually severe, steady, and poorly localized, but may be cramping, and is often accompanied by nausea, vomiting, constipation, and abdominal distention because of ileus. Pain in the chest and extremities are also common. Tachycardia is the most common physical sign, occurring in up to 80% of acute attacks,[233,234] and often accompanied by hypertension, sweating, tremors, and other effects of sympathetic overactivity and excess catecholamine production. There is little or no abdominal tenderness, fever, or leukocytosis because inflammation is not prominent. Bowel sounds are usually decreased, but are sometimes increased with diarrhea. The urine is often dark (because of porphobilin, a degradation product of PBG) or reddish (because of porphyrins, including uroporphyrin formed enzymatically and nonenzymatically from PBG). Bladder dysfunction may cause hesitancy and dysuria. Acute mental symptoms may include insomnia, anxiety, restlessness, disorientation, paranoia, and hallucinations. Paresis from peripheral motor neuropathy is a feature of prolonged, severe attacks, but is sometimes an early or even initial manifestation.[235,236] Porphyric neuropathy is primarily motor and results from axonal degeneration, which may be followed by demyelinization.[237] Muscle weakness may not be detected until it is quite advanced because it usually begins in the proximal muscles of the upper extremities. Paresis is usually symmetrical, but may be asymmetrical or focal. Course tremors, clonus and increased reflexes are sometimes prominent. Magnetic resonance

---

TABLE 21–4. A Partial List of Drugs Known to Be Unsafe or Safe in the Acute Porphyrias

Unsafe		Safe
Alcohol	Meprobamate[a] (also mebutamate,[a] tybamate[a])	Acetaminophen
Barbiturates[a]		Aspirin
Carbamazepine[a]	Methyprylon	Atropine
Carisoprodol[a]	Metoclopramide[a]	Bromides
Clonazepam (high doses)	Phenytoin[a]	Cimetidine
	Primidone[a]	Erythropoietin[a,b]
Danazol[a]	Progesterone and synthetic progestins[a]	Gabapentin
Diclofenac[a] and possibly other NSAIDs		Glucocorticoids
Ergots	Pyrazinamide[a]	Insulin
Estrogens[a,c]	Pyrazolones (aminopyrine, antipyrine)	Narcotic analgesics
Ethchlorvynol[a]		Penicillin and derivatives
Glutethimide[a]	Rifampin[a]	Phenothiazines
Griseofulvin[a]	Succinimides (ethosuximide, methsuximide)	Ranitidine[a,b]
Mephenytoin		Streptomycin
	Sulfonamide antibiotics[a]	Vigabatrin
	Valproic acid[a]	

NSAIDs, nonsteroidal anti-inflammatory drugs.

[a]Porphyria is listed as a contraindication, warning, precaution, or adverse effect in U.S. labeling for these drugs.

[b]Although porphyria is listed as a precaution in U.S. labeling, these drugs are regarded as safe by other sources.

[c]Estrogens are unsafe for porphyria cutanea tarda, but can be used with caution in the acute porphyrias.

Note: More complete sources, such as the websites of the American Porphyria Foundation (www.porphyriafoundation.com/) and the European Porphyria Network (www.porphyria-europe.com/) should be consulted before using drugs not listed here, keeping in mind that classifications may not be supported by high-quality evidence.

imaging may demonstrate cortical densities resembling the posterior reversible encephalopathy syndrome.[214] Sensory loss may develop, especially in the distal extremities. Cranial nerve involvement and cortical blindness have been described. Motor neuropathy may progress to respiratory and bulbar paralysis and death especially if diagnosis and treatment are delayed and harmful drugs continued. Death also may result from respiratory arrest or cardiac arrhythmia.[238,239] Most attacks that are treated promptly resolve within days or even hours. Advanced neuropathy from a severe attack is potentially completely reversible, with improvement continuing for as long as 2 years.[240] Hyponatremia is common during severe attacks and is sometimes a result of hypothalamic involvement and the syndrome of inappropriate antidiuretic hormone secretion. However, hyponatremia may be accompanied by reductions in blood volume,[241] indicating that increased antidiuretic hormone secretion in this setting is an appropriate physiologic response.[239] Hyponatremia may sometimes result from gastrointestinal loss, poor intake, and excess renal sodium loss.[239,242] A possible nephrotoxic effect of ALA may explain renal tubular sodium loss and impaired renal function in some patients.[242] Other electrolyte abnormalities may include hypomagnesemia and hypercalcemia.[243] Seizures may result from hyponatremia or represent a neurologic effect of acute porphyria.[244] Chronic mental symptoms, such as depression, are difficult to attribute to AIP. But chronic pain accompanied by depression develops in some patients after frequent exacerbations, and risk for suicide is increased. The disease also predisposes to chronic arterial hypertension and impaired renal function.[224,245,246] A common variant of peptide transporter 2 (PEPT2), which encodes a transporter for ALA in the kidney, predisposes to development of renal disease in AIP.[247] [Impaired renal function may progress and require renal transplantation.[248,249] Mild abnormalities in serum transaminases are common in AIP.[250] More advanced liver disease may develop and the risk of primary liver cancer is greatly increased (60–70-fold) in AIP, and is not related to specific *PBGD* mutations. They develop without an increase in serum α-fetoprotein and usually in the absence of cirrhosis.[251] Increased serum thyroxin levels because of increased thyroxin-binding globulin occurs in some patients with AIP, and occasionally hyperthyroidism and porphyria occur together.[252] Elevated low-density lipoprotein cholesterol is apparently less often observed in this disorder than it was in the past.[253]

Diagnosis

Suspecting AIP even when the index of suspicion is not high contributes to making an *initial diagnosis*. Because the disease so often remains latent, there is often no family history of porphyria. Acute porphyria should be considered in patients with unexplained abdominal pain or other characteristic symptoms when initial evaluation does not suggest another more common explanation. This diagnosis is readily ruled in or out by measuring urinary PBG, which is both sensitive and specific.[232] A substantial increase in PBG establishes that a patient has either AIP, HCP, or VP. Unfortunately, a commercial kit for rapid, semiquantitative PBG determination[254] is no longer available, making it difficult to follow consensus recommendations that all major medical centers should retain the capacity for rapid urinary PBG testing. If the sample is sent out, the referral laboratory may be contacted and asked to expedite the PBG measurement. A single-void urine specimen is recommended, with normalization of the result by creatinine, because collection of a 24-hour urine can greatly delay diagnosis and treatment. The urine specimen should be saved for later measurement of total porphyrin levels, which may be more persistently elevated, especially in HCP and VP, and is substantially elevated in ADP. If PBG is substantially increased, samples of plasma, erythrocytes, and feces should also be obtained prior to treatment with hemin. In patients with renal failure, PBG can be measured in serum by a specialized laboratory. Figure 21-6 presents

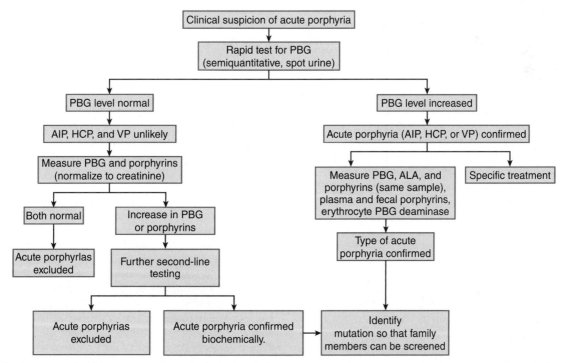

Figure 21–6. Recommended laboratory evaluation of patients with concurrent symptoms suggesting an acute porphyria, indicating how the diagnosis is established or excluded by biochemical testing and when specific therapy should be initiated. This schema is not applicable to patients who were treated with hemin or who have recovered from past symptoms suggestive of porphyria. Levels of δ-aminolevulinic acid (*ALA*) and porphobilinogen may be less increased in hereditary coproporphyria (*HCP*) and variegate porphyria (*VP*) and decrease more quickly with recovery than in acute intermittent porphyria (*AIP*). Mutation detection provides confirmation and greatly facilitates detection of relatives with latent porphyria. CPO, coproporphyrinogen oxidase; PBG, porphobilinogen; PPO, protoporphyrinogen oxidase.

a diagnostic flowchart for use when acute porphyria is suspected. PBG excretion is generally 50 to 200 mg/day (reference range: 0 to ~4 mg/day) during acute attacks of AIP. Similar elevations occur with spot urine samples when results are expressed per gram or millimoles creatinine. Excretion of ALA is usually about half that of PBG (expressed in milligrams). Increases in ALA and PBG can persist for prolonged periods between attacks, especially in AIP. Increases in ALA and PBG are less striking during acute attacks of HCP and VP and often decrease more rapidly.

The *diagnosis of an acute attack* is largely clinical, and is not based on a specific level of PBG. Levels of ALA and PBG during an acute attack may be increased compared to baseline levels, which fluctuate considerably. However, baseline levels between attacks are difficult to establish. Intravenous hemin causes dramatic, rapid but often transient decreases in these levels. Urinary porphyrins are increased in AIP, are predominantly uroporphyrin and account for reddish urine (ALA and PBG are colorless). Uroporphyrin can form nonenzymatically from PBG in urine even prior to excretion. However, there is evidence that porphyrins in this condition are predominantly isomer III, and formed enzymatically,[255] perhaps from ALA transported to tissues other than the liver.[216] Total fecal porphyrins and plasma porphyrins are normal or slightly increased in AIP, and erythrocyte zinc protoporphyrin concentrations may be modestly and nonspecifically increased. Erythrocyte PBGD activity is approximately half-normal in most (70%-80%) patients with AIP. However, this measurement is not definitive for confirming or excluding the diagnosis. As described earlier, some PBGD mutations cause the enzyme to be deficient only in nonerythroid tissues. Moreover, the ranges of activity are wide for both normal and AIP subjects and overlap, and the erythrocyte enzyme is highly age-dependent, such that an increase in the proportion of younger cells in the circulation can raise the activity into the reference range in AIP patients with a concurrent condition such as hemolytic anemia or hepatic disease.[256,257] A decrease in this enzyme also does not distinguish between latent and active disease. For these reasons, and because it does not detect other acute porphyrias, erythrocyte PBGD measurement in not useful for initial diagnosis of ill patients.

Once the diagnosis of AIP is established by biochemical methods, the underlying *PBGD* mutation should be identified. This confirms the diagnosis and, most importantly, enables reliable and definitive identification of other gene carriers by DNA testing. Erythrocyte PBGD measurement is useful for screening of asymptomatic family members if a known case in the family has low erythrocyte enzyme activity, but is less dependable than DNA testing. Prenatal diagnosis is possible by identifying the familial mutation in amniotic fluid cells, but is usually not indicated because the great majority of heterozygous carriers of PBGD mutations have a good prognosis.

Therapy

Hospitalization is usually required for treatment of attacks. Well-characterized patients with frequently recurring mild attacks that respond rapidly to treatment are sometimes managed as outpatients. Hospitalization facilitates treatment of severe symptoms, intravenous therapies, and monitoring of respiration, electrolytes, and nutritional status. Admission to intensive care is warranted if the vital capacity is impaired. Harmful drugs should be discontinued whenever possible. Pain, nausea, and vomiting are generally severe and require narcotic analgesics, chlorpromazine or another phenothiazine, or ondansetron. Low doses of short-acting benzodiazepines are considered safe for anxiety and insomnia. β-Adrenergic blocking agents may be useful to control tachycardia and hypertension, but may be hazardous in patients with hypovolemia or incipient cardiac failure.[258] Seizures are treated by correcting hyponatremia, if present. Almost all anticonvulsant drugs have

at least some potential for exacerbating acute porphyrias. Clonazepam may be less harmful than phenytoin, barbiturates, or valproic acid.[259,260] Bromides, gabapentin, levetiracetam, and vigabatrin are safe.

Carbohydrate Loading Glucose and other carbohydrates repress hepatic ALAS1 and reduce porphyrin precursor excretion, but the effects are weak compared to those of hemin. Attacks with mild pain (not requiring narcotics) and without severe manifestations such as paresis, seizures, severe central nervous system symptoms or hyponatremia may be treated with carbohydrate loading. Oral glucose polymer solutions may be given if tolerated. Intravenous treatment with 300 to 500 g of intravenous glucose, usually administered as a 10% solution, is recommended. However, the dilutional effects of a large volume of free water may increase risk of hyponatremia. A more complete parenteral nutrition regimen may be needed if oral or enteral feeding is not possible.

Intravenous Hemin Hemin is much more potent in reducing levels of ALA and PBG compared to glucose. Although controlled clinical trials are lacking for all current therapies for acute attacks of porphyria, consensus recommendations are that the clinical benefits of hemin are superior to other available therapies.[261,262] Hemin is available in the United States as a lyophilized hematin preparation (Panhematin), and was the first drug approved under the Orphan Drug Act. Heme arginate (Normosang), which is a stable preparation of heme and arginine, is available in Europe and South Africa.[262,263] Hemin, when infused intravenously as hematin or heme arginate, becomes bound to circulating hemopexin and albumin and is then taken up primarily by hepatocytes. It then enters and reconstitutes the regulatory heme pool and represses the synthesis of hepatic ALAS1. This results in a dramatic reduction in porphyrin precursor excretion within a few days. The standard regimen for treatment of acute attacks is 3 to 4 mg/kg daily for 4 days. Treatment may be extended if a response is not observed within this time. Hemin has been administered safely during pregnancy.[262,263] Product labeling recommends reconstitution of hematin with sterile water. But it was subsequently discovered that degradation of hematin begins immediately upon reconstitution with water, and degradation products are responsible for phlebitis at the site of infusion and a transient anticoagulant effect.[264] Infusion site phlebitis is frequent and can lead to loss of venous access with repeated dosing. Stabilization of hematin with 25% human albumin can prevent these adverse effects,[265] and is currently recommended.[266] Uncommon side effects include fever, aching, malaise, hemolysis, anaphylaxis, and circulatory collapse.[267,268] Excessive dosing caused reversible acute renal tubular damage in one case.[269]

Controlled trials comparing initial treatment with either glucose or hemin are lacking, except for 1 randomized, double-blind, placebo-controlled trial of heme arginate for acute attacks of porphyria, which was underpowered (only 12 patients) and treatment was delayed for 2 days; nonetheless striking decreases in urinary PBG and trends in clinical benefit were noted.[270] In contrast, a larger uncontrolled study enrolled 22 patients who had 51 acute attacks, and heme arginate was initiated within 24 hours of admission in 37 attacks (73%); all patients responded and hospitalization was less than 7 days in 90% of cases.[262] Based on this and numerous other uncontrolled clinical studies, it is now recommended that most acute attacks of porphyria be treated promptly with intravenous hemin, without an initial trial of intravenous glucose. Response to hemin may be delayed or incomplete when there is advanced neurologic damage. Subacute or chronic symptoms are unlikely to respond.

Prevention of Acute Attacks Multiple inciting factors must be avoided especially in patients who continue to have repeated attacks. Consultation with a dietitian may be useful to identify dietary indiscretions, and to help maintain a well-balanced diet somewhat high in carbohydrate (60%-70% of total calories). There is little evidence that additional dietary carbohydrate helps further in preventing attacks. Iron deficiency, if present, should be corrected. Patients who wish to lose excess weight should do so gradually and when they are clinically stable.

Givosiran An RNA interference agent that inhibits hepatic ALAS1 synthesis by reducing the levels of mRNA for ALAS1 was approved for treatment of acute hepatic porphyrias. Givosiran given monthly as a subcutaneous injection leads to sustained reduction in ALAS1 mRNA, ALA, PBG, and recurrent attack rates in acute hepatic porphyria patients. The recommended dose is 2.5 mg/kg body weight. Abnormalities in liver and kidney function were seen more frequently with givosiran than placebo treatment.[244] This new approach is a major advance for preventing attacks, but experience in treating acute attacks, in pregnancy or in patients with significant liver or renal impairment in lacking.

Gonadotropin-Releasing Hormone Analogues These agents can interrupt ovulation and prevent repeated attacks that are confined to the luteal phase of the menstrual cycle,[271-273] but are less effective in patients with attacks partially associated with the cycle. If treatment is effective after several months, low-dose estradiol, preferably by the transdermal route, or a bisphosphonate may be added to prevent bone loss and other side effects, or treatment changed to a low-dose oral contraceptive.

Hemin Prophylaxis Hemin administered once or twice weekly can prevent frequent, noncyclic attacks of porphyria in some patients. This treatment is difficult long-term because hemin is a short-acting agent and intravenous access is required.

Liver Transplantation Liver transplantation has been highly effective in patients who were disabled by recurrent attacks of AIP.[212] This may be an option for severely affected patients.

Other Therapies

Cimetidine has been recommended for human acute porphyrias based on uncontrolled observations in small numbers of patients.[274,275] This drug inhibits hepatic CYPs, and can prevent experimental forms of porphyria induced by agents such as allylisopropylacetamide that undergo activation by these enzymes.[276] However, these mechanisms are not immediately relevant to inherited porphyrias in humans. Therefore, cimetidine cannot be recommended as an alternative treatment.

Long-Term Monitoring Patients with acute porphyrias are at risk for renal damage and hepatocellular carcinoma. Renal function should be monitored, hypertension controlled, and nephrotoxic drugs avoided. Current recommendations are that patients with acute porphyrias who are older than 50 years, and especially those with continued elevations of ALA and PBG, be screened at least annually by ultrasonogram or an alternative imaging method to detect hepatocellular carcinoma at an early stage.[233]

HEREDITARY COPROPORPHYRIA AND VARIEGATE PORPHYRIA

Definition

Hereditary coproporphyria (HCP) and variegate porphyria (VP), are closely related hepatic porphyrias that are caused by deficiencies of CPO and PPO, the sixth and seventh enzymes of the heme biosynthetic pathway. They present with neurovisceral symptoms, as in AIP, or with blistering skin lesions identical to those seen in PCT. Cutaneous manifestations are much more common in VP than in HCP. The enzyme deficiency in each is inherited as an autosomal dominant trait with variable penetrance (see Table 21-1 and Fig. 21-1). As in AIP, most individuals who inherit the trait remain asymptomatic. Both disorders are less common in most countries, and generally less severe, than AIP.

The incidence of HCP was estimated to be 2 per 1,000,000 population in Denmark,[277] and the incidence of VP in Finland is reported to be 1.3 per 100,000 population.[278] Because of a founder effect, VP is especially common among Europeans of Dutch descent in South Africa, where almost all cases share the same *PPO* mutation (R59W). The incidence of VP in South Africa was estimated at 3 per 1000 in the white population.[279] Very rare cases of homozygous HCP and VP are manifested by severe neurologic impairment early in life, but not acute attacks, and severe photosensitivity.[280]

Pathophysiology

Like other porphyrias, HCP and VP are heterogeneous at the molecular level. At least 43 *CPO* mutations, mostly missense mutations, have been identified in HCP,[281] and 187 *PPO* mutations in VP (see Table 21-1).[282] Clinical expression is variable and onset of neurologic manifestations is influenced by the same factors that are important in AIP. CPO catalyzes the two-step decarboxylation of coproporphyrinogen III to yield protoporphyrinogen IX, with intermediate formation of harderoporphyrinogen, a tricarboxyl porphyrinogen. A single active site carries out both decarboxylations, and most of the harderoporphyrinogen formed is not released before being further decarboxylated to protoporphyrinogen IX. However, a variant form of HCP termed *harderoporphyria* is a result of *CPO* mutations that favor premature release of harderoporphyrinogen from the enzyme.[283,284]

Clinical Features

Neurovisceral manifestations are identical to those in other acute porphyrias. Although both HCP and VP are generally less severe than AIP, attacks may be life-threatening. Blistering skin lesions may be seen, and are much more common in VP than in HCP. Factors that contribute to attacks, including drugs, hormones, and dietary factors, are also the same as in AIP. Oral contraceptives may precipitate cutaneous manifestations of VP. Risk of chronic hypertension, renal disease, and hepatocellular carcinoma are increased, as in AIP.

Diagnosis

Urinary PBG is elevated during acute attacks, and usually is the basis for diagnosis of these acute porphyrias. However, increases in PBG may be less than in AIP, and more transient. Levels of coproporphyrin III are markedly increased in urine and feces, whereas in AIP fecal porphyrins are normal or only slightly increased. Fecal porphyrins in HCP are almost entirely coproporphyrin III, whereas in VP both coproporphyrin III and protoporphyrin are approximately equally increased. The fecal coproporphyrin III:I ratio is sensitive for diagnosis of HCP, even in asymptomatic stages of the disease.[285] Plasma porphyrin concentration is commonly increased in VP, seldom increased in HCP unless there are cutaneous manifestations, and are normal or only slightly increased in AIP. A characteristic plasma porphyrin fluorescence maximum observed at neutral pH is a very specific marker for VP, and is believed to represent protoporphyrin bound covalently to plasma proteins.[286] The fluorescence maximum is at approximately 626 nm in VP, approximately 634 in EPP, and approximately 620 in other porphyrias. This fluorometric method is more effective than examination of fecal porphyrins for detecting asymptomatic VP,[286] and is useful for rapidly differentiating VP and PCT. Erythrocyte PBGD activity is normal in HCP and VP, and usually deficient in AIP. Assays for CPO and PPO are not widely available. DNA studies are most reliable for identifying asymptomatic carriers, once the mutation affecting the family is identified. In homozygous HCP and VP, increases in porphyrin precursors and porphyrins may be more severe with substantial increases in erythrocyte zinc protoporphyrin. Harderoporphyria is a variant form of HCP that results from a homozygous defect of a structurally altered CPO, such that harderoporphyrinogen is released prematurely from the enzyme. This variant is identified by finding large amounts of harderoporphyrin in feces and erythrocytes. Neonatal hemolytic anemia is a distinctive feature of this condition.[287]

Therapy

The identification and avoidance of precipitating factors is essential. Treatment of acute attacks is the same as in AIP. Treatment of the phototoxic manifestations is not satisfactory. Although the lesions are identical to the blistering skin lesions seen in PCT, there is no response in HCP and VP to phlebotomies or low-dose chloroquine or hydroxychloroquine. Therefore, avoidance of sunlight and use of protective clothing is most important. Yearly screening for hepatocellular carcinoma by imaging is recommended after age 50 years, especially in individuals with persistent increases in porphyrin precursors or porphyrins.[233]

PORPHYRIA CUTANEA TARDA AND HEPATOERYTHROPOIETIC PORPHYRIA

Definition

PCT is caused by a deficiency of hepatic UROD activity and is manifested by the development of chronic, blistering skin lesions on the dorsal aspects of the hands and other sun-exposed areas of skin in middle or late life. This iron-related disorder is the most common and readily treated form of porphyria (see Table 21-1 and Fig. 21-1). The enzyme deficiency develops specifically in the liver as a result of generation of a UROD inhibitor in the presence of iron and multiple susceptibility factors. The disease has been classified as types 1 to 3, based on the presence or absence of heterozygous *UROD* mutations. Patients with familial (type 2) PCT are heterozygous for *UROD* mutations, which are inherited as an autosomal dominant trait with low penetrance. HEP is the homozygous (or compound heterozygous) form of familial (type 2) PCT, which usually presents in childhood and resembles CEP clinically. Rarely, hepatocellular carcinomas may generate excess porphyrins and simulate PCT; however, the enzyme defect was not established in such cases.[288] PCT must be differentiated from other porphyrias that cause identical blistering skin lesions and from pseudoporphyria (also known as pseudo-PCT). Pseudoporphyria is a poorly understood condition that presents with lesions that closely resemble PCT, but with plasma porphyrins that are not significantly increased. Potentially photosensitizing drugs, such as nonsteroidal antiinflammatory agents, are sometimes implicated.

Pathophysiology

UROD sequentially decarboxylates uroporphyrinogen (which has 8 carboxyl side chains) to yield coproporphyrinogen (with 4 carboxyl groups). When hepatic UROD is profoundly inhibited, the substrate and the intermediate and final products of the reaction accumulate as the oxidized porphyrins in the liver (mostly uroporphyrin and heptacarboxylporphyrin), and then appear in plasma and urine. Photosensitivity results from activation of porphyrins in the skin by light and generation of reactive oxygen species. Hepatic UROD activity is inhibited to less than approximately 20% of normal in all patients with PCT. Types 1, 2, and 3 are not fundamentally different or clinically distinguishable from each other. Patients with type 1 or "sporadic" PCT have no *UROD* mutations and no family history of PCT. In most geographic areas, approximately 80% of patients fall into this category. Type 2 or "familial" PCT comprises approximately 20% of patients who are heterozygous for *UROD* mutations, but because the penetrance of this trait is low there are usually no other documented cases in the family. In families with type 3, which is rare, more than one member has PCT, but there is no *UROD* mutation; these familial cases may share other inherited or environmental susceptibility factors.

Although hepatic UROD activity must be reduced to approximately 20% of normal for PCT to be manifest, the amount of enzyme protein, when measured immunochemically in liver, remains at its genetically determined level, which in type 2 cases is approximately 50% of normal.[289] Mice heterozygous for mutant *UROD* alleles are much more sensitive to porphyrinogenic stimuli than wild-type animals.[290] In heterozygous mice that display porphyric phenotypes, hepatic UROD protein is half normal, but the catalytic activity of the enzyme is reduced to approximately 20%, suggesting the existence of an inhibitor of hepatic UROD.[290] Although iron does not directly inhibit UROD, there is considerable evidence that PCT is an iron-related disease, with hepatic siderosis seen in many cases. This explains why *HFE* (hemochromatosis gene) mutations that lead to increased intestinal iron absorption predispose to development of PCT (Chaps. 10 and 11). Individuals who inherit a *UROD* mutation have approximately 50% of normal enzyme activity from birth, such that a UROD inhibitor can more readily reduce enzyme activity to less than approximately 20% of normal. How iron and other known or suspected susceptibility factors, such as alcohol, smoking, estrogens, hepatitis C, HIV, hepatic steatosis, and other suspected factors, contribute to the development of PCT is less-well understood, but these may act in part by increasing oxidative stress in hepatocytes. A deficiency of ascorbic acid[291] and perhaps other antioxidants[292] may play a role in some patients. Smoking may also act by inducing hepatic CYPs, including CYP1A2, which is essential for causing uroporphyria in rodent models,[293,294] and may produce a UROD inhibitor, which has been characterized as a uroporphomethene—a product of partial oxidation of uroporphyrinogen. This inhibitor was found in the liver of mice heterozygous for a *UROD* mutation and homozygous for an *HFE* mutation (C282Y) who spontaneously developed uroporphyria.[65] Other potential mechanisms for lowering of hepatic UROD activity in PCT, such as oxidative damage to UROD active site residues, are less favored but have not been excluded.[295]

At least 70 different *UROD* mutations have been identified in type 2 PCT and HEP (see Table 21-1). These reduce UROD activity and immunoreactivity to approximately 50% of normal in all tissues from birth in heterozygous individuals. Most are missense mutations, with each occurring in one or a few families. Homozygosity for a null *UROD* mutation is lethal in early neonatal life. Therefore, in HEP at least one of the mutant *UROD* alleles must preserve at least some catalytic activity. Knowledge of the crystal structure of UROD allows mapping of specific mutations and prediction of their impact on enzyme structure and function. Expression studies in eukaryotic cells suggest that some mutations may destabilize the enzyme protein in a tissue-specific manner.[296]

Pathogenesis of the Clinical Findings

A distinctive feature of PCT is massive accumulation of porphyrins in the liver. As a result, fresh hepatic tissue shows strong red fluorescence on exposure to long-wave ultraviolet light. Microscopic, birefringent, needle-like inclusions are found in lysosomes, and paracrystalline inclusions in mitochondria. Increased stainable iron is very common. Other nonspecific hepatic findings are probably partly a result of the disease itself, although the effects of associated factors such as alcohol and hepatitis C are difficult to differentiate. Liver histopathology includes hepatocyte necrosis, inflammation, increased iron, and increased fat. Mild abnormalities in liver function tests, especially serum transaminases and γ-glutamyltranspeptidase, are present in almost all cases, but cirrhosis is unusual. The risk of hepatocellular carcinoma is increased, especially in those with more prolonged disease, cirrhosis, or other risk factors such as hepatitis C or alcoholic liver disease.[297-299] Excess porphyrins are transported in plasma from the liver. Skin histopathology includes subepidermal blistering and deposition of periodic acid-Schiff–positive material around blood vessels and fine fibrillar material in the upper dermis and at the dermoepithelial junction. Immunoglobulin G, other immunoglobulins, and complement are deposited around dermal blood vessels and at the dermoepithelial junction. Splits in the lamina lucida of the basement membrane lead to formation of fluid-containing bullae.[300] These histologic changes are found in other cutaneous porphyrias as well as pseudoporphyria, a dermal condition that resembles PCT but has no significant increase in plasma or urinary porphyrins. Activation of the complement system after irradiation has been demonstrated in PCT patients both in vivo and in vitro in sera,[301] and is thought to result from generation of reactive oxygen species.

Susceptibility Factors PCT is a highly heterogeneous disease, with multiple susceptibility factors expected in the individual patient.[302] Multiple factors are important in familial as well as sporadic PCT, because heterozygosity for a *UROD* mutation is a susceptibility factor that does not of itself reduce hepatic enzyme activity sufficiently to cause the disease. The environmental, infectious, and inherited factors discussed below, none of which is invariably present, are known or suspected to play an important role. Their prevalence may show considerable geographic variation in PCT patients as well as healthy subjects.

Alcohol PCT has long been associated with excess alcohol use. Alcohol and its metabolites may induce ALAS1 and CYP2E1, generate active oxygen species that contribute to oxidative damage, cause mitochondrial injury, deplete reduced glutathione and other antioxidant defenses, increase production of endotoxin, activate Kupffer cells, decrease the iron regulatory hormone hepcidin,[303] and increase iron retention within hepatocytes.

Smoking and Cytochrome P450 Enzymes Smoking is less-extensively studied as a risk factor but is commonly associated with alcohol use in PCT.[302] Smoking may increase oxidative stress in hepatocytes, and induces CYP1A2, which is essential to the development of uroporphyria in rodent models. CYP levels are increased in liver in human PCT, but it is not clear which CYP might be important in pathogenesis of the human disease. A study of caffeine metabolism did not find evidence for increased CYP1A2 activity in vivo in PCT, even when smokers and nonsmokers were analyzed separately.[304] However, a more inducible polymorphism of CYP1A2 is more common in PCT than in normal subjects.[305]

Estrogens Estrogen use is very common in women with PCT.[302,306,307] In the past, some men developed the disease after treatment of prostate cancer with estrogens.[306] Female rats or male rats treated with estrogens are more susceptible to development of chemically induced uroporphyria than untreated male rats.[308] The mechanism is not established, although estrogens can generate reactive oxygen species in some experimental systems.[295] The porphyrinogenic risk from estrogen is minimized by selecting a transdermal form of estrogen rather than use of an oral form.[304]

Hepatitis C Reported prevalence of hepatitis C in PCT has ranged from 21% to 92% in various countries, and greatly exceeds the prevalence of this viral infection in healthy subjects, which shows considerable geographic variation. Hepatitis C is associated with excess fat, some iron accumulation, mitochondrial dysfunction, and oxidative stress in hepatocytes, which may contribute to the development of PCT. Dysregulation of hepcidin may contribute to iron accumulation in hepatitis C.[309]

Human Immunodeficiency Virus PCT is less commonly associated with HIV infection than with hepatitis C.[310] Occasionally PCT is the initial manifestation of this infection. The mechanism is unknown.

Iron and *HFE* Mutations Mild to moderate iron overload is found in most patients with PCT, and iron deficiency is protective. The importance of iron has been confirmed in animal models, such as rodents treated with hexachlorobenzene and other halogenated polyaromatic hydrocarbons.[295] Mice with disruption of 1 *UroD* allele (*UroD[+/−]*)

and 2 disrupted *Hfe* alleles (*Hfe[−/−]*) develop uroporphyria without administration of exogenous chemicals.[290] Prevalence of the *C282Y* mutation of the *HFE* gene, which is the major cause of hemochromatosis in whites, is increased in both sporadic and familial PCT, and 10% to 20% of patients may be *C282Y* homozygotes (Chap. 11).[311] In southern Europe, where the *C282Y* is less prevalent, the *H63D* mutation is more commonly associated with PCT.[312] Excess iron may contribute to UROD inhibition by providing an oxidative environment that is apparently needed for generation of a UROD inhibitor. Hepatic hepcidin expression is reduced in hemochromatosis, and is also reduced in PCT patients without hemochromatosis genotypes when compared to patients without PCT and comparable iron overload, suggesting that reduced expression of this peptide is important in causing hepatic siderosis in PCT.[313]

Antioxidants Substantial reductions in plasma levels of ascorbate and carotenoids have been noted in some patients with PCT.[292] Ascorbate deficiency in rodents enhances susceptibility to development of uroporphyria, and ascorbate decreases uroporphyrin accumulation except in animals treated with large amounts of iron.[291]

Halogenated Chemicals A large outbreak of PCT occurred during a period of food shortage in a population in eastern Turkey in the 1950s from consumption of seed wheat treated with the fungicide hexachlorobenzene.[11] Smaller outbreaks and individual cases have occurred after exposures to other chemicals such as 2,3,7,8-tetrachlorodibenzo-*p*-dioxin (TCDD, dioxin).[314] These chemicals were subsequently shown to cause hepatic UROD deficiency and biochemical features resembling PCT in laboratory animals, and many studies that followed have greatly increased our understanding of this acquired enzyme deficiency.[295,315] But such exposures are rarely identified in PCT patients in current clinical practice.

Clinical Features

Disease onset is usually in the fourth or fifth decade of life, and is more common in men. Onset may occur earlier in familial (type 2) disease or in cases with the C282Y/C282Y *HFE* genotype.[316] Fluid-filled vesicles develop most commonly on the backs of the hands (Fig. 21-7A). Skin friability is increased and blisters often follow minor trauma. These also occur on the forearms, face, ears, neck, legs, and feet. The blisters often rupture, crust over, and are prone to infection before healing slowly. Milia may precede or follow vesicle formation. Facial hypertrichosis and hyperpigmentation are particularly noticed by female patients (Fig. 21-7B). Severe thickening of affected areas of skin sometimes occurs, is termed *pseudoscleroderma*, and resembles systemic scleroderma. Blistering skin lesions in VP and HCP are identical to those in PCT. Those in CEP and HEP resemble PCT but are usually much more severe and mutilating. Mild or moderate erythrocytosis is common in PCT; chronic lung disease from smoking may contribute.

Drugs that exacerbate the acute porphyrias are only occasionally reported to play a role in PCT.[317] PCT may occur with other conditions predisposing to iron overload, such as myelofibrosis[318,319] and end-stage renal disease,[316] and with diabetes mellitus[299] and cutaneous and systemic lupus erythematosus. PCT associated with end-stage renal disease is usually more severe, sometimes with severe mutilation. Lack of urinary porphyrin excretion in these patients often leads to much higher concentrations of porphyrins in plasma, and the excess porphyrins are poorly dialyzable.[320] The disease occasionally develops during pregnancy, perhaps related to effects of estrogen.

The clinical manifestations of HEP usually resemble CEP, with onset of blistering skin lesions, hypertrichosis, scarring, and red urine in infancy or childhood. Sclerodermoid skin changes are sometimes prominent. Excess porphyrins originate mostly from the liver in this condition. Unusually mild cases have been described.[321]

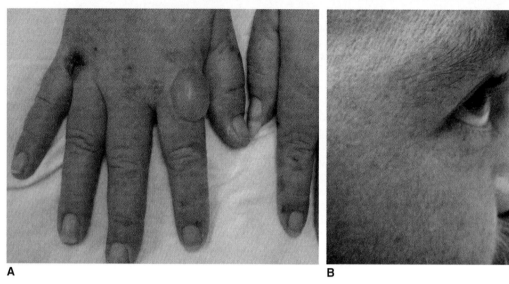

Figure 21–7. Cutaneous findings in porphyria cutanea tarda include (**A**) bullous lesions most commonly on the dorsal aspects of the hands and fingers, which rupture and crust over, and (**B**) facial hirsutism most noticeable on the upper cheeks.

Diagnosis

A diagnosis of PCT is established by finding a substantial elevation of porphyrins in urine or plasma, with a predominance of highly carboxylated porphyrins (uroporphyrin and heptacarboxylporphyrin, hexacarboxylporphyrin, and pentacarboxylporphyrin); coproporphyrin is also increased. Levels of PBG are normal, and urinary ALA is normal or slightly increased. The pattern of porphyrins in feces is complex, and includes heptacarboxylporphyrin and isocoproporphyrins. Isocoproporphyrins are overproduced in the presence of UROD deficiency because pentacarboxylporphyrinogen is a substrate for CPO, leading to formation of dehydroisocoproporphyrinogen, which is excreted in bile and undergoes oxidation by intestinal bacteria to isocoproporphyrins.[322] Measurement of plasma porphyrins and determination of the fluorescence emission peak at neutral pH is especially useful for screening patients with blistering skin lesions. A substantial increase with a peak at approximately 620 nm is most commonly caused by PCT, although not specific, excludes VP and pseudoporphyria, which are the most common conditions that mimic PCT clinically.[323] Plasma porphyrin measurements are essential for diagnosis of PCT in patients with advanced renal disease; the reference range is higher in patients with renal failure than in normal patients.[323] Erythrocyte porphyrins are substantially increased in CEP, HEP, and other homozygous porphyrias, but are normal or only modestly increased in PCT. Rare cases of HCP with blistering lesions are identified by a predominance of coproporphyrin III in urine and especially feces. Familial (type 2) cases of PCT are identified by half-normal erythrocyte UROD activity or, preferably, by DNA studies to identify a *UROD* mutation. Erythrocyte UROD activity is 5% to 30% of normal in HEP, and DNA studies reveal that a *UROD* mutation is inherited from each parent. Biochemical findings in HEP resemble PCT, with predominant accumulation and excretion of highly carboxylated porphyrins and isocoproporphyrins. However, in contrast to PCT, erythrocyte zinc protoporphyrin is substantially increased. At least one genotype may be associated with predominant excretion of pentacarboxylporphyrin.[321]

Therapy

Treatment is highly effective but specific in both sporadic and familial PCT, and therefore should be initiated only after the diagnosis is well established. It is sometimes reasonable to start treatment after PCT is

validated with a plasma porphyrin screen that excludes VP and pseudoporphyria (see "Diagnosis" above). Patients should be questioned and tested for all known susceptibility factors, including use of alcohol, tobacco, and estrogens, hepatitis C, HIV, *HFE* mutations, and inherited UROD deficiency (erythrocyte UROD activity or preferably *UROD* mutations), because their presence influences management. Serum ferritin should be measured before starting treatment. Patients should be advised to stop drinking and smoking and to discontinue oral estrogens. A nutritionally adequate intake of ascorbic acid and other nutrients should be assured, but treatment with this vitamin should not be used as primary therapy. Initial treatment of hepatitis C is an option (see further), but recovery is slow after removing other susceptibility factors without phlebotomy or low-dose hydroxychloroquine recovery.[324] Repeated phlebotomy is the preferred treatment at most centers. The original rationale proposed by Ippen in 1961 was to decrease the commonly associated mild or moderately increased hemoglobin, stimulate erythropoiesis, and perhaps channel excess heme pathway intermediates to hemoglobin synthesis.[325] However the oxidized porphyrins that accumulate in PCT cannot reenter the heme biosynthetic pathway and be converted to heme, and it is now understood that phlebotomy is effective by reducing body iron stores and liver iron content. Treatment with an iron chelator, such as desferrioxamine, is less efficient, but may be tried when preferred treatment (phlebotomy or low-dose hydroxychloroquine) are contraindicated.[326] Approximately 450 mL of blood is removed, usually at 2-week intervals. In one series, an average of 5.4 phlebotomies was required for remission, but many more are needed in some patients with coexisting hemochromatosis and marked increases in serum ferritin levels. Hemoglobin or hematocrit levels are followed as safety (not therapeutic) targets, to prevent symptomatic anemia. Usually, the hemoglobin should not fall below 100 to 110 g/L, but the baseline value and the age and clinical condition of the patient also need to be considered. The therapeutic target is a serum ferritin near 15 mcg/L, which is during treatment close to the lower limit of normal and associated with tissue iron depletion, but usually not anemia. Additional iron depletion is not beneficial, and causes anemia. Treatment is also guided by plasma (or serum) porphyrin levels, which are more convenient to measure repeatedly than urine porphyrins, and fall more slowly than the serum ferritin. Plasma porphyrins usually decline during treatment from initial levels of 10 to 25 mcg/dL during treatment, to below the upper limit of normal (~1 mcg/dL) within weeks after phlebotomies are completed.[327] New skin lesions are generally decreased at the end of treatment, but some may occur for a few weeks after plasma porphyrin levels become normal. Severe sclerodermatous changes and liver function abnormalities can also improve.

After a remission, continued phlebotomies are generally not needed. However, relapses may occur, especially in patients who resume use of alcohol, and are treated by another course of phlebotomies. For patients with the *C282Y/C282Y* or *C282Y/H63D HFE* genotypes, management guidelines for hemochromatosis should be followed. Continuing phlebotomies on an as needed basis to maintain a serum ferritin below approximately 100 mcg/L also may be beneficial in patients who experience recurrences of PCT, although published experience is limited. It is also advisable to follow porphyrin levels and reinstitute phlebotomies promptly if porphyrin levels begin to rise. Liver imaging and a serum α-fetoprotein determination should be repeated as surveillance for primary liver cancer in patients with increased fibrosis or cirrhosis. After remission, transdermal estrogen can be resumed in women, if needed, with little risk for recurrence of PCT.[304]

A low-dose regimen of hydroxychloroquine or chloroquine is also effective,[295,328-333] and most appropriate when phlebotomy is contraindicated or poorly tolerated, if iron overload is not severe. This treatment is preferred at some centers because it is more convenient and much less expensive. Hydroxychloroquine is felt to have a better safety profile than chloroquine. These 4-aminoquinoline antimalarials do not appear to deplete hepatic iron, and the mechanism for their effect in PCT is not fully understood. Full therapeutic doses of these drugs exacerbate photosensitivity in PCT, induce fever, malaise, and nausea, markedly increase urinary and plasma porphyrins, and increase serum transaminases, other liver function tests, and ferritin. This reaction can even unmask previously unrecognized PCT.[334] Although these adverse effects, which are unique to PCT, are followed by complete remission,[335] they should be avoided by a low-dose treatment regimen (hydroxychloroquine 100 mg—one-half of a standard tablet—twice weekly) at least until plasma or urine porphyrins are normalized.[328,331,332] However, some patients may respond poorly and require later treatment with larger doses or phlebotomy.[335] There is a small risk of retinopathy,[336] which may be lower with hydroxychloroquine. A prospective comparative study found that time to biochemical remission with low-dose hydroxychloroquine was comparable to that with phlebotomy.[337] In a retrospective study, low-dose chloroquine was ineffective in patients homozygous for the *C282Y* mutation of the *HFE* gene,[338] which suggests that the degree of excess hepatic iron may influence response to this treatment. These 4-aminoquinolines are not effective in other porphyrias, and do not mobilize all types of porphyrins from liver and other tissues.[339] These drugs may form complexes with a variety of porphyrins, which might promote their mobilization from liver,[340,341] but this does not appear to explain their effects in PCT. It was suggested that mobilization of hepatic iron may be important,[332,342,343] but serum ferritin concentrations do not change significantly during treatment. Most likely, these drugs colocalize with excess porphyrins in lysosomes and other intracellular organelles and promote their release by a process that involves transient cell damage.

There is increasing evidence that PCT improves after treatment of coexisting hepatitis C.[344,345] This is being examined prospectively in a study by the Porphyrias Consortium. Treatment of PCT associated with end-stage renal disease is more difficult, as phlebotomy is often contraindicated because of anemia. Erythropoietin administration can correct anemia, mobilize iron, and support phlebotomy in many cases.[320,346,347] High-flux hemodialysis may remove porphyrins from plasma and provide some benefit.[348] PCT is not a contraindication to renal transplantation, which is likely to lead to remission[349] partly because of resumption of endogenous erythropoietin production. Levels of plasma porphyrins are often especially high in these patients, and should be assessed prior to surgery, because there may be some risk of skin and peritoneal burns from exposure to operating room lights.

Management of HEP emphasizes avoiding sunlight, as in CEP. Oral charcoal was helpful in a severe case associated with dyserythropoiesis.[102] Phlebotomy has shown little or no benefit. Retrovirus-mediated gene transfer can correct porphyria in cell lines from patients with this disease, which suggests that gene therapy may be applicable in the future.[350]

REFERENCES

1. Moore MR, McColl KE. *Disorders of Porphyrin Metabolism.* Plenum; 1987.
2. Schultz JH. *Ein Fall von Pemphigus Leprosus kompliziert durch Lepra visceralis.* PhD thesis. Greifswald, Germany; 1874.
3. Anderson TM. Hydroa aestivale in two brothers, complicated with the presence of hematoporphyrin in the urine. *Br J Dermatol.* 1898;10:1.
4. Harris DF. Haematoporphyrinuria and its relations to the source of urobilin. *J Anat Physiol.* 1897;31:383.
5. Stokvis BJ. Over Twee Zeldsame Kleuerstoffen in Urine van Zieken. *Ned Tijdschr Geneeskd.* 1889;13:409.
6. Günther H. Die haematoporphyrie. *Deutsche Archiv für Klinische Medizin.* 1911;105:89.
7. Garrod AE. *Inborn Errors of Metabolism.* Hodder & Stoughton; 1923.
8. Waldenström J, Vahlquist BC. Studien uber die entstehung der roten harnpigmente (uroporphyrin und porphobilin) bein der akuten porphyrie aus iher farblosen vorstufe (porphobilinogen). *Hoppe Seylers Z Physiol Chem.* 1939;260:189.
9. Schmid R, Schwartz S, Watson CJ. Porphyrin content of bone marrow and liver in the various forms of porphyria. *Arch Intern Med.* 1954;93:167.
10. Cam C, Nigogosyan G. Acquired toxic porphyria cutanea tarda due to hexachlorobenzene. *JAMA.* 1963;183:90.
11. Schmid R. Cutaneous porphyria in Turkey. *N Engl J Med.* 1960;263:397.
12. Ockner RK, Schmid R. Acquired porphyria in man and rat due to hexachlorobenzene intoxication. *Nature.* 1961;189:499.
13. Schmid R. Hepatoxic drugs causing porphyria in man and animals. *S Afr J Lab Clin Med.* 1963;14:212.
14. Strand LJ, Felsher BF, Redeker AG, et al. Heme biosynthesis in intermittent acute porphyria: decreased hepatic conversion of porphobilinogen to porphyrins and increased delta-aminolevulinic acid synthetase activity. *Proc Natl Acad Sci U S A.* 1970;67:1315.
15. Bonkowsky HL, Tschudy DP, Collins A, et al. Repression of the overproduction of porphyrin precursors in acute intermittent porphyria by intravenous infusions of hematin. *Proc Natl Acad Sci U S A.* 1971;68:2725.
16. Granick S, Sassa S. δ-Aminolevulinic acid synthase and the control of heme and chlorophyll synthesis. In: Vogel HJ, ed. *Metabolic Regulation.* Academic Press; 1971:77.
17. Sassa S, Kappas A. Genetic, metabolic and biochemical aspects of the porphyrias. In: Harris H, Hirschhorn K, eds. *Advances in Human Genetics.* Plenum Publications; 1981:121.
18. McKay R, Druyan R, Getz GS, et al. Intramitochondrial localization of delta-aminolaevulate synthetase and ferrochelatase in rat liver. *Biochem J.* 1969;114:455.
19. Riddle RD, Yamamoto M, Engel JD. Expression of delta-aminolevulinate synthase in avian cells: separate genes encode erythroid-specific and nonspecific isozymes. *Proc Natl Acad Sci U S A.* 1989;86:792.
20. Tsai SF, Bishop DF, Desnick RJ. Human uroporphyrinogen III synthase: molecular cloning, nucleotide sequence, and expression of a full-length cDNA. *Proc Natl Acad Sci U S A.* 1988;85:7049.
21. Bishop DF. Two different genes encode delta-aminolevulinate synthase in humans: nucleotide sequences of cDNAs for the housekeeping and erythroid genes. *Nucleic Acids Res.* 1990;18:7187.
22. Cox TC, Bawden MJ, Martin A, et al. Human erythroid 5-aminolevulinate synthase: promoter analysis and identification of an iron-responsive element in the mRNA. *EMBO J.* 1991;10:1891.
23. Aziz N, Munro HN. Iron regulates ferritin mRNA translation through a segment of its 5′ untranslated region. *Proc Natl Acad Sci U S A.* 1987;84:8478.
24. Lowry JA, Mackay JP. GATA-1: one protein, many partners. *Int J Biochem Cell Biol.* 2006;38:6.
25. Casey JL, Di Jeso B, Rao K, et al. The promoter region of the human transferrin receptor gene. *Ann N Y Acad Sci.* 1988;526:54.
26. Melefors O, Goossen B, Johansson HE, et al. Translational control of 5-aminolevulinate synthase mRNA by iron-responsive elements in erythroid cells. *J Biol Chem.* 1993;268:5974.
27. Podvinec M, Handschin C, Looser R, et al. Identification of the xenosensors regulating human 5-aminolevulinate synthase. *Proc Natl Acad Sci U S A.* 2004;101:9127.
28. Elferink CJ, Srivastava G, Maguire DJ, et al. A unique gene for 5-aminolevulinate synthase in chickens. Evidence for expression of an identical messenger RNA in hepatic and erythroid tissues. *J Biol Chem.* 1987;262:3988.
29. Kitchin KT. Regulation of rat hepatic delta-aminolevulinic acid synthetase and heme oxygenase activities: evidence for control by heme and against mediation by prosthetic iron. *Int J Biochem.* 1983;15:479.

30. Handschin C, Lin J, Rhee J, et al. Nutritional regulation of hepatic heme biosynthesis and porphyria through PGC-1alpha. *Cell.* 2005;122:505.

31. Virbasius JV, Scarpulla RC. Activation of the human mitochondrial transcription factor A gene by nuclear respiratory factors: a potential regulatory link between nuclear and mitochondrial gene expression in organelle biogenesis. *Proc Natl Acad Sci U S A.* 1994;91:1309.

32. Scassa ME, Guberman AS, Ceruti JM, et al. Hepatic nuclear factor 3 and nuclear factor 1 regulate 5-aminolevulinate synthase gene expression and are involved in insulin repression. *J Biol Chem.* 2004;279:28082.

33. Dandekar T, Stripecke R, Gray NK, et al. Identification of a novel iron-responsive element in murine and human erythroid delta-aminolevulinic acid synthase mRNA. *EMBO J.* 1991;10:1903.

34. Fujita H, Yamamoto M, Yamagami T, et al. Erythroleukemia differentiation. Distinctive responses of the erythroid-specific and the nonspecific delta-aminolevulinate synthase mRNA. *J Biol Chem.* 1991;266:17494.

35. Furuyama K, Sassa S. Interaction between succinyl CoA synthetase and the heme-biosynthetic enzyme ALAS-E is disrupted in sideroblastic anemia. *J Clin Invest.* 2000;105:757.

36. Furuyama K, Fujita H, Nagai T, et al. Pyridoxine refractory X-linked sideroblastic anemia caused by a point mutation in the erythroid 5-aminolevulinate synthase gene. *Blood.* 1997;90:822.

37. Whatley SD, Ducamp S, Gouya L, et al. C-terminal deletions in the ALAS2 gene lead to gain of function and cause X-linked dominant protoporphyria without anemia or iron overload. *Am J Hum Genet.* 2008;83:408.

38. Bailey H, Bezerra G, Marcero J, et al. Human aminolevulinate synthase structure reveals a eukaryotic-specific autoinhibitory loop regulating substrate binding and product release. *Nat Commun.* 2020 Jun 4;11(1):2813. doi: 10.1038/s41467-020-16586.

39. Liu J, Li Y, Tong J, Gao J, et al. Long non-coding RNA-dependent mechanism to regulate heme biosynthesis and erythrocyte development. *Nat Commun.* 2018 Oct 22; 9(1):4386.

40. Liu G, Sil D, Maio N, et al. Heme biosynthesis depends on previously unrecognized acquisition of iron-sulfur cofactors in human amino-levulinic acid dehydratase. *Nat Commun.* 2020 Dec 9;11(1):6310. doi: 10.1038/s41467-020-20145-9.

41. Sassa S. Delta-aminolevulinic acid dehydratase assay. *Enzyme.* 1982;28:133.

42. Tsukamoto I, Yoshinaga T, Sano S. The role of zinc with special reference to the essential thiol groups in delta-aminolevulinic acid dehydratase of bovine liver. *Biochim Biophys Acta.* 1979;570:167.

43. Granick JL, Sassa S, Kappas A. Some biochemical and clinical aspects of lead intoxication. In: Bodansky O, Latner AL, eds. *Advances in Clinical Chemistry.* Academic Press; 1978:287.

44. Sassa S, Kappas A. Hereditary tyrosinemia and the heme biosynthetic pathway. Profound inhibition of delta-aminolevulinic acid dehydratase activity by succinylacetone. *J Clin Invest.* 1983;71:625.

45. Tschudy DP, Hess RA, Frykholm BC. Inhibition of delta-aminolevulinic acid dehydrase by 4,6-dioxoheptanoic acid. *J Biol Chem.* 1981;256:9915.

46. Lindblad B, Lindstedt S, Steen G. On the enzymic defects in hereditary tyrosinemia. *Proc Natl Acad Sci U S A.* 1977;74:4641.

47. Wetmur JG, Bishop DF, Cantelmo C, et al. Human delta-aminolevulinate dehydratase: nucleotide sequence of a full-length cDNA clone. *Proc Natl Acad Sci U S A.* 1986;83:7703.

48. Potluri VR, Astrin KH, Wetmur JG, et al. Human delta-aminolevulinate dehydratase: chromosomal localization to 9q34 by in situ hybridization. *Hum Genet.* 1987; 76:236.

49. Battersby AR, Fookes CJ, Matcham GW, et al. Biosynthesis of the pigments of life: formation of the macrocycle. *Nature.* 1980;285:17.

50. Erskine PT, Senior N, Awan S, et al. X-ray structure of 5-aminolaevulinate dehydratase, a hybrid aldolase. *Nat Struct Biol.* 1997;4:1025.

51. Bishop TR, Miller MW, Beall J, et al. Genetic regulation of delta-aminolevulinate dehydratase during erythropoiesis. *Nucleic Acids Res.* 1996;24:2511.

52. Wetmur JG, Bishop DF, Ostasiewicz L, et al. Molecular cloning of a cDNA for human delta-aminolevulinate dehydratase. *Gene.* 1986;43:123.

53. Inoue R, Akagi R. Co-synthesis of human delta-aminolevulinate dehydratase (ALAD) mutants with the wild-type enzyme in cell-free system-critical importance of conformation on enzyme activity. *J Clin Biochem Nutr.* 2008;43:143.

54. Jaffe EK, Stith L. ALAD porphyria is a conformational disease. *Am J Hum Genet.* 2007;80:329.

55. Jordan PM. The biosynthesis of 5-aminolevulinic acid and its transformation into coproporphyrinogen in animals and bacteria. In: Dailey HA, ed. *Biosynthesis of Heme and Chlorophylls.* McGraw-Hill; 1990:55.

56. Awan SJ, Siligardi G, Shoolingin-Jordan PM, et al. Reconstitution of the holoenzyme form of *Escherichia coli* porphobilinogen deaminase from apoenzyme with porphobilinogen and preuroporphyrinogen: a study using circular dichroism spectroscopy. *Biochemistry.* 1997;36:9273.

57. Wang AL, Arredondo-Vega FX, Giampietro PF, et al. Regional gene assignment of human porphobilinogen deaminase and esterase A4 to chromosome 11q23 leads to 11qter. *Proc Natl Acad Sci U S A.* 1981;78:5734.

58. Chretien S, Dubart A, Beaupain D, et al. Alternative transcription and splicing of the human porphobilinogen deaminase gene result either in tissue-specific or in housekeeping expression. *Proc Natl Acad Sci U S A.* 1988;85:6.

59. Grandchamp B, De Verneuil H, Beaumont C, et al. Tissue specific expression of porphobilinogen deaminase. Two isoenzymes from a single gene. *Eur J Biochem.* 1987;162:105.

60. Raich N, Romeo PH, Dubart A, et al. Molecular cloning and complete primary sequence of human erythrocyte porphobilinogen deaminase. *Nucleic Acids Res.* 1986;14:5955.

61. Mignotte V, Eleouet JF, Raich N, et al. *Cis-* and *trans*-acting elements involved in the regulation of the erythroid promoter of the human porphobilinogen deaminase gene. *Proc Natl Acad Sci U S A.* 1989;86:6548.

62. Grandchamp B, Picat C, de Rooij F, et al. A point mutation G—A in exon 12 of the porphobilinogen deaminase gene results in exon skipping and is responsible for acute intermittent porphyria. *Nucleic Acids Res.* 1989;17:6637.

63. Mathews MA, Schubert HL, Whitby FG, et al. Crystal structure of human uroporphyrinogen III synthase. *EMBO J.* 2001;20:5832.

64. Schubert HL, Phillips JD, Heroux A, et al. Structure and mechanistic implications of a uroporphyrinogen III synthase-product complex. *Biochemistry.* 2008;47:8648.

65. Phillips JD, Bergonia HA, Reilly CA, et al. A porphomethene inhibitor of uroporphyrinogen decarboxylase causes porphyria cutanea tarda. *Proc Natl Acad Sci U S A.* 2007;104:5079.

66. Smith AG, Clothier B, Robinson S, et al. Interaction between iron metabolism and 2,3,7,8-tetrachlorodibenzo-p-dioxin in mice with variants of the Ahr gene: a hepatic oxidative mechanism. *Mol Pharmacol.* 1998;53:52.

67. Romana M, Dubart A, Beaupain D, et al. Structure of the gene for human uroporphyrinogen decarboxylase. *Nucleic Acids Res.* 1987;15:7343.

68. de Verneuil H, Grandchamp B, Foubert C, et al. Assignment of the gene for uroporphyrinogen decarboxylase to human chromosome 1 by somatic cell hybridization and specific enzyme immunoassay. *Hum Genet.* 1984;66:202.

69. Romeo P-H, Raich N, Dubart A, et al. Molecular cloning and nucleotide sequence of a complete human uroporphyrinogen decarboxylase cDNA. *J Biol Chem.* 1986; 261:9825.

70. Whitby FG, Phillips JD, Kushner JP, et al. Crystal structure of human uroporphyrinogen decarboxylase. *EMBO J.* 1998;17:2463.

71. Phillips JD, Whitby FG, Kushner JP, et al. Structural basis for tetrapyrrole coordination by uroporphyrinogen decarboxylase. *EMBO J.* 2003;22:6225.

72. Rhee HW, Zou P, Udeshi ND, et al. Proteomic mapping of mitochondria in living cells via spatially restricted enzymatic tagging. *Science.* 2013;339:1328.

73. Cacheux V, Martasek P, Fougerousse F, et al. Localization of the human coproporphyrinogen oxidase gene to chromosome band 3q12. *Hum Genet.* 1994;94:557.

74. Kohno H, Furukawa T, Tokunaga R, et al. Mouse coproporphyrinogen oxidase is a copper-containing enzyme: expression in Escherichia coli and site-directed mutagenesis. *Biochim Biophys Acta.* 1996;1292:156.

75. Takahashi S, Furuyama K, Kobayashi A, et al. Cloning of a coproporphyrinogen oxidase promoter regulatory element binding protein. *Biochem Biophys Res Commun.* 2000;273:596.

76. Conder LH, Woodard SI, Dailey HA. Multiple mechanisms for the regulation of haem synthesis during erythroid cell differentiation. Possible role for coproporphyrinogen oxidase. *Biochem J.* 1991;275:321.

77. Lamoril J, Deybach JC, Puy H, et al. Three novel mutations in the coproporphyrinogen oxidase gene. *Hum Mutat.* 1997;9:78.

78. Nishimura K, Taketani S, Inokuchi H. Cloning of a human cDNA for protoporphyrinogen oxidase by complementation in vivo of a hemG mutant of *Escherichia coli. J Biol Chem.* 1995;270:8076.

79. Taketani S, Inazawa J, Abe T, et al. The human protoporphyrinogen oxidase gene (PPOX): organization and location to chromosome 1. *Genomics.* 1995;29:698.

80. Koch M, Breithaupt C, Kiefersauer R, et al. Crystal structure of protoporphyrinogen IX oxidase: a key enzyme in haem and chlorophyll biosynthesis. *EMBO J.* 2004;23:1720.

81. Wang B, Wen X, Qin X, et al. Quantitative structural insight into human variegate porphyria disease. *J Biol Chem.* 2013;288:11731.

82. Morgan RR, Errington R, Elder GH. Identification of sequences required for the import of human protoporphyrinogen oxidase to mitochondria. *Biochem J.* 2004;377:281.

83. de Vooght KM, van Wijk R, van Solinge WW. GATA-1 binding sites in exon 1 direct erythroid-specific transcription of PPOX. *Gene.* 2008;409:83.

84. Porra RJ, Jones OT. Studies on ferrochelatase. 1. Assay and properties of ferrochelatase from a pig-liver mitochondrial extract. *Biochem J.* 1963;87:181.

85. Whitcombe DM, Carter NP, Albertson DG, et al. Assignment of the human ferrochelatase gene (FECH) and a locus for protoporphyria to chromosome 18q22. *Genomics.* 1991;11:1152.

86. Al-Karadaghi S, Hansson M, Nikonov S, et al. Crystal structure of ferrochelatase: the terminal enzyme in heme biosynthesis. *Structure.* 1997;5:1501.

87. Medlock A, Swartz L, Dailey TA, et al. Substrate interactions with human ferrochelatase. *Proc Natl Acad Sci U S A.* 2007;104:1789.

88. Medlock AE, Dailey TA, Ross TA, et al. A pi-helix switch selective for porphyrin deprotonation and product release in human ferrochelatase. *J Mol Biol.* 2007;373:1006.

89. Ross J, Sautner D. Induction of globin mRNA accumulation by hemin in cultured erythroleukemic cells. *Cell.* 1976;8:513.

90. Sassa S, Nagai T. The role of heme in gene expression. *Int J Hematol.* 1996;63:167.

91. Erwin A, Balwani M, Desnick RJ; Porphyrias Consortium of the NIH-Sponsored Rare Diseases Clinical Research Network. Congenital erythropoietic porphyria. In: Adam MP, Ardinger HH, Pagon RA, et al, eds. *GeneReviews.* University of Washington, Seattle; 1993.

92. Sassa S, Akagi R, Nishitani C, et al. Late-onset porphyrias: what are they? *Cell Mol Biol (Noisy-le-grand France).* 2002;48:97.

93. Erwin AL, Desnick RJ. Congenital erythropoietic porphyria: recent advances. *Mol Genet Metab.* 2019;128:288.

94. Günther H. Hämatoporphyrie. In: Aschoff L, Bürger M, Frank E, et al, eds. *Handbuch der Krankheiten des Blutes und der Blutbildenden Organe.* Springer-Verlag, Berlin, 1925:622.

95. Desnick RJ, Glass IA, Xu W, et al. Molecular genetics of congenital erythropoietic porphyria. *Semin Liver Dis.* 1998;18:77.

96. Watson CJ, Perman V, Spurrell FA, et al. Some studies of the comparative biology of human and bovine porphyria erythropoietica. *Trans Assoc Am Physicians.* 1958;71:196.

97. Phillips JD, Steensma DP, Pulsipher MA, et al. Congenital erythropoietic porphyria due to a mutation in GATA1: the first trans-acting mutation causative for a human porphyria. *Blood.* 2007;109:2618.

98. Seip M, Thune PO, Eriksen L. Treatment of photosensitivity in congenital erythropoietic porphyria (CEP) with beta-carotene. *Acta Derm Venereol.* 1974;54:239.

99. Haining RG, Cowger ML, Labbe RF, et al. Congenital erythropoietic porphyria. II. The effects of induced polycythemia. *Blood.* 1970;36:297.

100. Piomelli S, Poh-Fitzpatrick MB, Seaman C, et al. Complete suppression of the symptoms of congenital erythropoietic porphyria by long-term treatment with high-level transfusions. *N Engl J Med.* 1986;314:1029.

101. Guarini L, Piomelli S, Poh-Fitzpatrick MB. Hydroxyurea in congenital erythropoietic porphyria (letter). *N Engl J Med.* 1994;330:1091.

102. Pimstone NR, Gandhi SN, Mukerji SK. Therapeutic efficacy of oral charcoal in congenital erythropoietic porphyria. *N Engl J Med.* 1987;316:390.

103. Fritsch C, Bolsen K, Ruzicka T, et al. Congenital erythropoietic porphyria. *J Am Acad Dermatol.* 1997;36:594.

104. Hallai N, Anstey A, Mendelsohn S, et al. Pregnancy in a patient with congenital erythropoietic porphyria. *N Engl J Med.* 2007;357:622.

105. Dupuis-Girod S, Akkari V, Ged C, et al. Successful match-unrelated donor bone marrow transplantation for congenital erythropoietic porphyria (Gunther disease). *Eur J Pediatr.* 2005;164:104.

106. Egan DN, Yang Z, Phillips J, et al. Inducing iron deficiency improves erythropoiesis and photosensitivity in congenital erythropoietic porphyria. *Blood.* 2015;126:257.

107. Mirmiran A, Poli A, Ged C, et al. Phlebotomy as an efficient long-term treatment of congenital erythropoietic porphyria. *Haematologica.* 2021;106(3):913-917.

108. Geronimi F, Richard E, Lamrissi-Garcia I, et al. Lentivirus-mediated gene transfer of uroporphyrinogen III synthase fully corrects the porphyric phenotype in human cells. *J Mol Med (Berl).* 2003;81:310.

109. Kauppinen R, Glass IA, Aizencang G, et al. Congenital erythropoietic porphyria: prolonged high-level expression and correction of the heme biosynthetic defect by retroviral-mediated gene transfer into porphyric and erythroid cells. *Mol Genet Metab.* 1998;65:10.

110. Holme SA, Anstey AV, Finlay AY, et al. Erythropoietic protoporphyria in the U.K.: clinical features and effect on quality of life. *Br J Dermatol.* 2006;155:574.

111. Marko PB, Miljkovic J, Gorenjak M, et al. Erythropoietic protoporphyria patients in Slovenia. *Acta Dermatovenerol Alp Pannonica Adriat.* 2007;16:99.

112. Parker M, Corrigall AV, Hift RJ, et al. Molecular characterization of erythropoietic protoporphyria in South Africa. *Br J Dermatol.* 2008;159:182.

113. Dickey AK, Quick C, Ducamp S, et al. Evidence in the UK Biobank for the underdiagnosis of erythropoietic protoporphyria. *Genet. Med.* 2021;23:140-148.

114. Nakahashi Y, Fujita H, Taketani S, et al. The molecular defect of ferrochelatase in a patient with erythropoietic protoporphyria. *Proc Natl Acad Sci U S A.* 1992;89:281.

115. Gouya L, Deybach JC, Lamoril J, et al. Modulation of the phenotype in dominant erythropoietic protoporphyria by a low expression of the normal ferrochelatase allele. *Am J Hum Genet.* 1996;58:292.

116. Gouya L, Puy H, Lamoril J, et al. Inheritance in erythropoietic protoporphyria: a common wild-type ferrochelatase allelic variant with low expression accounts for clinical manifestation. *Blood.* 1999;93:2105.

117. Gouya L, Puy H, Robreau AM, et al. The penetrance of dominant erythropoietic protoporphyria is modulated by expression of wildtype FECH. *Nat Genet.* 2002;30:27.

118. Gouya L, Martin-Schmitt C, Robreau AM, et al. Contribution of a common single-nucleotide polymorphism to the genetic predisposition for erythropoietic protoporphyria. *Am J Hum Genet.* 2006;78:2.

119. Yien YY, Ducamp S, van der Vorm LN, et al. Mutation in human CLPX elevates levels of delta-aminolevulinate synthase and protoporphyrin IX to promote erythropoietic protoporphyria. *Proc Natl Acad Sci U S A.* 2017;114:E8045.

120. Aplin C, Whatley SD, Thompson P, et al. Late-onset erythropoietic porphyria caused by a chromosome 18q deletion in erythroid cells. *J Invest Dermatol.* 2001;117:1647.

121. Shirota T, Yamamoto H, Hayashi S, et al. Myelodysplastic syndrome terminating in erythropoietic protoporphyria after 15 years of aplastic anemia. *Int J Hematol.* 2000;72:44.

122. Goodwin RG, Kell WJ, Laidler P, et al. Photosensitivity and acute liver injury in myeloproliferative disorder secondary to late-onset protoporphyria caused by deletion of a ferrochelatase gene in hematopoietic cells. *Blood.* 2006;107:60.

123. Bottomley SS, Tanaka M, Everett MA. Diminished erythroid ferrochelatase activity in protoporphyria. *J Lab Clin Med.* 1975;86:126.

124. Piomelli S, Lamola AA, Poh-Fitzpatrick MB, et al. Erythropoietic protoporphyria and Pb intoxication: The molecular basis for difference in cutaneous photosensitivity. I. Different rates of disappearance of protoporphyrin from the erythrocytes, both in vivo and in vitro. *J Clin Invest.* 1975;56:1519.

125. Sandberg S, Brun A, Hovding G, et al. Effect of zinc on protoporphyrin induced photohaemolysis. *Scand J Clin Lab Invest.* 1980;40:185.

126. Spikes JD. Porphyrins and related compounds as photodynamic sensitizers. *Ann N Y Acad Sci.* 1975;244:496.

127. Goldstein BD, Harber LC. Erythropoietic protoporphyria: lipid peroxidation and red cell membrane damage associated with photohemolysis. *J Clin Invest.* 1972;51:892.

128. Lim HW, Poh-Fitzpatrick MB, Gigli I. Activation of the complement system in patients with porphyrias after irradiation in vivo. *J Clin Invest.* 1984;74:1961.

129. Ryan EA. Histochemistry of the skin in erythropoietic protoporphyria. *Br J Dermatol.* 1966;78:501.

130. Poh-Fitzpatrick MB. Molecular and cellular mechanisms of porphyrin photosensitization. *Photodermatol.* 1986;3:148.

131. Poh-Fitzpatrick MB. Human protoporphyria: reduced cutaneous photosensitivity and lower erythrocyte porphyrin levels during pregnancy. *J Am Acad Dermatol.* 1997;36:40.

132. Berenson MM, Kimura R, Samowitz W, et al. Protoporphyrin overload in unrestrained rats: biochemical and histopathologic characterization of a new model of protoporphyric hepatopathy. *Int J Exp Pathol.* 1992;73:665.

133. Bloomer JR. The liver in protoporphyria. *Hepatology.* 1988;8:402.

134. Bloomer JR, Enriquez R. Evidence that hepatic crystalline deposits in a patient with protoporphyria are composed of protoporphyrin. *Gastroenterology.* 1982;82:569.

135. Bloomer J, Wang Y, Singhal A, et al. Molecular studies of liver disease in erythropoietic protoporphyria. *J Clin Gastroenterol.* 39:S167, 2005.

136. Lala SM, Naik H, Balwani M. Diagnostic delay in erythropoietic protoporphyria. *J Pediatr.* 2018;202:320.

137. Mathews-Roth MM. Systemic photoprotection. *Dermatol Clin.* 1986;4:335.

138. Mathews-Roth MM, Pathak MA, Fitzpatrick TB, et al. Beta carotene therapy for erythropoietic protoporphyria and other photosensitivity diseases. *Arch Dermatol.* 1977;113:1229.

139. DeLeo VA, Poh-Fitzpatrick M, Mathews-Roth M, et al. Erythropoietic protoporphyria: 10 years experience. *Am J Med.* 1976;60:8.

140. Delaby C, Lyoumi S, Ducamp S, et al. Excessive erythrocyte ppix influences the hematologic status and iron metabolism in patients with dominant erythropoietic protoporphyria. *Cell Mol Biol (Noisy-le-grand).* 2009;55:45.

141. Turnbull A, Baker H, Vernon-Roberts B, et al. Iron metabolism in porphyria cutanea tarda and in erythropoietic protoporphyria. *Q J Med.* 1973;42:341.

142. Holme SA, Worwood M, Anstey AV, et al. Erythropoiesis and iron metabolism in dominant erythropoietic protoporphyria. *Blood.* 2007;110:4108.

143. Rademakers LH, Koningsberger JC, Sorber CW, et al. Accumulation of iron in erythroblasts of patients with erythropoietic protoporphyria. *Eur J Clin Invest.* 1993;23:130.

144. Bossi K, Lee J, Schmeltzer P, et al. Homeostasis of iron and hepcidin in erythropoietic protoporphyria. *Eur J Clin Invest.* 2015;45:1032.

145. Barman-Aksozen J, Beguin C, Dogar AM, et al. Iron availability modulates aberrant splicing of ferrochelatase through the iron- and 2-oxoglutarate dependent dioxygenase Jmjd6 and U2AF(65.). *Blood Cells Mol Dis.* 2013;51:151.

146. Balwani M. Erythropoietic protoporphyria and X-linked protoporphyria: pathophysiology, genetics, clinical manifestations, and management. *Mol Genet Metab.* 2019;128:298.

147. Rank JM, Carithers R, Bloomer J. Evidence for neurological dysfunction in end-stage protoporphyric liver disease. *Hepatology.* 1993;18:1404.

148. Holme SA, Whatley SD, Roberts AG, et al. Seasonal palmar keratoderma in erythropoietic protoporphyria indicates autosomal recessive inheritance. *J Invest Dermatol.* 2009;129:599.

149. Doss MO, Frank M. Hepatobiliary implications and complications in protoporphyria, a 20-year study. *Clin Biochem.* 1989;22:223.

150. Singer JA, Plaut AG, Kaplan MM. Hepatic failure and death from erythropoietic protoporphyria. *Gastroenterology.* 1978;74:588.

151. Singal AK, Parker C, Bowden C, et al. Liver transplantation in the management of porphyria. *Hepatology.* 2014;60:1082.

152. Hastka J, Lasserre JJ, Schwarzbeck A, et al. Zinc protoporphyrin in anemia of chronic disorders. *Blood.* 1993;81:1200.

153. Anderson KE, Sassa S, Peterson CM, et al. Increased erythrocyte uroporphyrinogen-L-synthetase, delta-aminolevulinic acid dehydratase and protoporphyrin in hemolytic anemias. *Am J Med.* 1977;63:359.

154. Gou EW, Balwani M, Bissell DM, et al. Pitfalls in erythrocyte protoporphyrin measurement for diagnosis and monitoring of protoporphyrias. *Clin Chem.* 2015;61:1453.

155. Poh-Fitzpatrick MB, DeLeo VA. Rates of plasma porphyrin disappearance in fluorescent vs. red incandescent light exposure. *J Invest Dermatol.* 1977;69:510.

156. Minder EI, Schneider-Yin X, Steurer J, et al. A systematic review of treatment options for dermal photosensitivity in erythropoietic protoporphyria. *Cell Mol Biol (Noisy-le-grand).* 2009;55:84.

157. Mathews-Roth MM, Rosner B. Long-term treatment of erythropoietic protoporphyria with cysteine. *Photodermatol Photoimmunol Photomed.* 2002;18:307.

158. Warren LJ, George S. Erythropoietic protoporphyria treated with narrow-band (TL-01) UVB phototherapy. *Australas J Dermatol.* 1998;39:179.

159. Harms J, Lautenschlager S, Minder CE, et al. An alpha-melanocyte-stimulating hormone analogue in erythropoietic protoporphyria. *N Engl J Med.* 2009;360:306.

160. Langendonk JG, Balwani M, Anderson KE, et al. Afamelanotide for erythropoietic protoporphyria. *N Engl J Med.* 2015;373:48.

161. Gordeuk VR, Brittenham GM, Hawkins CW, et al. Iron therapy for hepatic dysfunction in erythropoietic protoporphyria. *Ann Intern Med.* 1986;105:27.

162. Mercurio MG, Prince G, Weber FL, et al. Terminal hepatic failure in erythropoietic protoporphyria. *J Am Acad Dermatol.* 1993;29:829.

163. Gou E, Weng C, Greene T, et al. A longitudinal analysis of erythrocyte and plasma protoporphyrin levels in patients with protoporphyria. *J Appl Lab Med.* 2018;3:213.

164. Bonkovsky HL, Schned AR. Fatal liver failure in protoporphyria. Synergism between ethanol excess and the genetic defect. *Gastroenterology.* 1986;90:191.

165. Poh-Fitzpatrick MB. The erythropoietic porphyrias. *Dermatol Clin.* 1986;4:291.

166. Bloomer JR. Pathogenesis and therapy of liver disease in protoporphyria. *Yale J Biol Med.* 1979;52:39.

167. Kniffen JC. Protoporphyrin removal in intrahepatic porphyrastasis. *Gastroenterology.* 1970;58:1027.

168. Gross U, Frank M, Doss MO. Hepatic complications of erythropoietic protoporphyria. *Photodermatol Photoimmunol Photomed.* 1998;14:52.

169. Bechtel MA, Bertolone SJ, Hodge SJ. Transfusion therapy in a patient with erythropoietic protoporphyria. *Arch Dermatol.* 1981;117:99.

170. Van Wijk HJ, Van Hattum J, Delafaille HB, et al. Blood exchange and transfusion therapy for acute cholestasis in protoporphyria. *Dig Dis Sci.* 1988;33:1621.

171. McGuire BM, Bonkovsky HL, Carithers RL Jr, et al. Liver transplantation for erythropoietic protoporphyria liver disease. *Liver Transpl.* 2005;11:1590.

172. Todd DJ, Callender ME, Mayne EE, et al. Erythropoietic protoporphyria, transfusion therapy and liver disease. *Br J Dermatol.* 1992;127:534.

173. Muley SA, Midani HA, Rank JM, et al. Neuropathy in erythropoietic protoporphyrias. *Neurology.* 1998;51:262.

174. Nordmann Y. Erythropoietic protoporphyria and hepatic complications. *J Hepatol.* 1992;16:4.

175. Poh-Fitzpatrick MB, Wang X, Anderson KE, et al. Erythropoietic protoporphyria: altered phenotype after bone marrow transplantation for myelogenous leukemia in a patient heteroallelic for ferrochelatase gene mutations. *J Am Acad Dermatol.* 2002;46:861.

176. Fontanellas A, Mazurier F, Landry M, et al. Reversion of hepatobiliary alterations by bone marrow transplantation in a murine model of erythropoietic protoporphyria. *Hepatology.* 2000;32:73.

177. Rand EB, Bunin N, Cochran W, et al. Sequential liver and bone marrow transplantation for treatment of erythropoietic protoporphyria. *Pediatrics.* 2006;118:e1896.

178. Richard E, Robert E, Cario-Andre M, et al. Hematopoietic stem cell gene therapy of murine protoporphyria by methylguanine-DNA-methyltransferase-mediated in vivo drug selection. *Gene Ther.* 2004;11:1638.

179. Hassoun A, Verstraeten L, Mercelis R, et al. Biochemical diagnosis of an hereditary aminolaevulinate dehydratase deficiency in a 63-year-old man. *J Clin Chem Clin Biochem.* 1989;27:781.

180. Pawliuk R, Tighe R, Wise RJ, et al. Prevention of murine erythropoietic protoporphyria-associated skin photosensitivity and liver disease by dermal and hepatic ferrochelatase. *J Invest Dermatol.* 2005;124:256.

181. Plewinska M, Thunell S, Holmberg L, et al. delta-Aminolevulinate dehydratase deficient porphyria: identification of the molecular lesions in a severely affected homozygote. *Am J Hum Genet.* 1991;49:167.

182. Sassa S. ALAD porphyria. *Semin Liver Dis.* 1998;18:95.

183. Neeleman RA, van Beers EJ, Friesema EC, et al. Clinical remission of delta-aminovulinic acid dehydratase deficiency through suppression of erythroid heme synthesis. *Hepatology.* 2019;70:434.

184. Akagi R, Kato N, Inoue R, et al. delta-Aminolevulinate dehydratase (ALAD) porphyria: The first case in North America with two novel ALAD mutations. *Mol Genet Metab.* 2006;87:329.

185. Akagi R, Shimizu R, Furuyama K, et al. Novel molecular defects of the delta-aminovulinate dehydratase gene in a patient with inherited acute hepatic porphyria. *Hepatology.* 2000;31:704.

186. Akagi R, Nishitani C, Harigae H, et al. Molecular analysis of delta-aminolevulinate dehydratase deficiency in a patient with an unusual late-onset porphyria. *Blood.* 2000;96:3618.

187. Akagi R, Yasui Y, Harper P, et al. A novel mutation of delta-aminolevulinate dehydratase in a healthy child with 12% erythrocyte enzyme activity. *Br J Haematol.* 1999;106:931.

188. Akagi R, Inoue R, Muranaka S, et al. Dual gene defects involving delta-aminolaevulinate dehydratase and coproporphyrinogen oxidase in a porphyria patient. *Br J Haematol.* 2006;132:237.

189. Liu G, Sil D, Tong WH, et al. Dependence of heme biosynthesis on iron-sulfur cluster biogenesis: human ALAD is an unrecognized iron-sulfur protein. *Nat Commun.* 2020 Dec 9;11(1):6310. doi: 10.1038/s41467-020-20145-9.

190. Lahiji AP, Anderson KE, Chan A, et al. 5-Aminolevulinate dehydratase porphyria: update on hepatic 5-aminolevulinic acid synthase induction and long-term response to hemin. *Mol Genet Metab.* 2020;131(4):418-423.

191. Thunell S, Henrichson A, Floderus Y, et al. Liver transplantation in a boy with acute porphyria due to aminolaevulinate dehydratase deficiency. *Eur J Clin Chem Clin Biochem.* 1992;30:599.

192. Shimizu Y, Ida S, Naruto H, et al. Excretion of porphyrins in urine and bile after the administration of delta-aminolevulinic acid. *J Lab Clin Med.* 1978;92:795.

193. Doss M, von Tiepermann R, Schneider J, et al. New type of hepatic porphyria with porphobilinogen synthase defect and intermittent acute clinical manifestation. *Klin Wochenschr.* 1979;57:1123.

194. Gross U, Sassa S, Jacob K, et al. 5-Aminolevulinic acid dehydratase deficiency porphyria: a twenty-year clinical and biochemical follow-up. *Clin Chem.* 1998;44:1892.

195. Doss MO, Stauch T, Gross U, et al. The third case of Doss porphyria (delta-aminolevulinic acid dehydratase deficiency) in Germany. *J Inherit Metab Dis.* 2004;27:529.

196. Thunell S, Holmberg L, Lundgren J. Aminolaevulinate dehydratase porphyria in infancy. A clinical and biochemical study. *J Clin Chem Clin Biochem.* 1987;25:5.

197. Mercelis R, Hassoun A, Verstraeten L, et al. Porphyric neuropathy and hereditary d-aminolevulinic acid dehydratase deficiency in an adult. *J Neurol Sci.* 1990;95:39.

198. Fujita H, Sato K, Sano S. Increase in the amount of erythrocyte delta-aminolevulinic acid dehydratase in workers with moderate lead exposure. *Int Arch Occup Environ Health.* 1982;50:287.

199. Sassa S, Fujita H, Kappas A. Succinylacetone and delta-aminolevulinic acid dehydratase in hereditary tyrosinemia: immunochemical study of the enzyme. *Pediatrics.* 1990;86:84.

200. Gou E, Chan A, Penz C, et al. 5-Aminolevulinate dehydratase porphyria (ADP): evidence for hepatic ALAS1 induction. Oral presentation. *International Conference on Porphyrins and Porphyrias.* Bordeaux, France; June 27, 2017.

201. Goldberg A, Moore MR, McColl KEL, et al. Porphyrin metabolism and the porphyrias. In: Ledingham, DA, Warrell, DA, Wetherall, DJ, eds. *Oxford Textbook of Medicine.* Oxford University Press; 1987:9136.

202. Mustajoki P, Koskelo P. Hereditary hepatic porphyrias in Finland. *Acta Med Scand.* 1976;200:171.

203. Chen B, Solis-Villa C, Erwin AL, et al. Identification and characterization of 40 novel hydroxymethylbilane synthase mutations that cause acute intermittent porphyria. *J Inherit Metab Dis.* 2019;42:186.

204. Grandchamp B. Acute intermittent porphyria. *Semin Liver Dis.* 1998;18:17.

205. Kauppinen R, von und zu Fraunberg M. Molecular and biochemical studies of acute intermittent porphyria in 196 patients and their families. *Clin Chem.* 2002;48:1891.

206. Wetterberg L. *A Neuropsychiatric and Genetical Investigation of Acute Intermittent Porphyria.* Scandinavian University Books; 1967.

207. Mustajoki P, Kauppinen R, Lannfelt L, et al. Frequency of low erythrocyte porphobilinogen deaminase activity in Finland. *J Intern Med.* 1992;231:389.

208. Nordmann Y, Puy H, Da Silva V, et al. Acute intermittent porphyria: prevalence of mutations in the porphobilinogen deaminase gene in blood donors in France. *J Intern Med.* 1997;242:213.

209. Chen B, Solis-Villa C, Hakenberg J, et al. Acute intermittent porphyria: predicted pathogenicity of HMBS variants indicates extremely low penetrance of the autosomal dominant disease. *Hum Mutat.* 2016;37(11):1215–1222.

210. Grandchamp B, Picat C, De Rooij FWM, et al. Molecular analysis of acute intermittent porphyria in a Finnish family with normal erythrocyte porphobilinogen deaminase. *Eur J Clin Invest.* 1989;19:415.

211. Anderson KE, Freddara U, Kappas A. Induction of hepatic cytochrome P-450 by natural steroids: relationships to the induction of delta-aminolevulinate synthase and porphyrin accumulation in the avian embryo. *Arch Biochem Biophys.* 1982;217:597.

212. Lissing M, Nowak G, Adam R, et al. Liver transplantation for acute intermittent porphyria. *Liver transpl.* 2020;27(4):491-501.

213. Kauppinen R, Mustajoki P. Prognosis of acute porphyria: occurrence of acute attacks, precipitating factors, and associated diseases. *Medicine (Baltimore).* 1992;71:1.

214. Kuo HC, Huang CC, Chu CC, et al. Neurological complications of acute intermittent porphyria. *Eur Neurol.* 2011;66:247.

215. Lithner F. Could attacks of abdominal pain in cases of acute intermittent porphyria be due to intestinal angina? *J Intern Med.* 2000;247:407.

216. Anderson KE, Drummond GS, Freddara U, et al. Porphyrogenic effects and induction of heme oxygenase in vivo by D-aminolevulinic acid. *Biochim Biophys Acta.* 1981;676:289.

217. Brennan MJW, Cantrill RC. delta-Aminolaevulinic acid is a potent agonist for GABA autoreceptors. *Nature.* 1979;280:514.

218. Müller WE, Snyder SH. delta-Aminolevulinic acid: influences on synaptic GABA receptor binding may explain CNS symptoms of porphyria. *Ann Neurol.* 1977;2:340.

219. Meyer UA, Schuurmans MM, Lindberg RLP. Acute porphyrias: pathogenesis of neurological manifestations. *Semin Liver Dis.* 1998;18:43.

220. Jover R, Hoffmann F, Scheffler-Koch V, et al. Limited heme synthesis in porphobilinogen deaminase-deficient mice impairs transcriptional activation of specific cytochrome P450 genes by phenobarbital. *Eur J Biochem.* 2000;267:7128.

221. Lindberg RL, Martini R, Baumgartner M, et al. Motor neuropathy in porphobilinogen deaminase-deficient mice imitates the peripheral neuropathy of human acute porphyria. *J Clin Invest.* 1999;103:1127.

222. Louis CA, Sinclair JF, Wood SG, et al. Synergistic induction of cytochrome-P450 by ethanol and isopentanol in cultures of chick embryo and rat hepatocytes. *Toxicol Appl Pharmacol.* 1993;118:169.

223. Lip GY, McColl KE, Goldberg A, Moore MR. Smoking and recurrent attacks of acute intermittent porphyria. *Br Med J.* 1991;302:507.

224. Andersson C, Bylesjo I, Lithner F. Effects of diabetes mellitus on patients with acute intermittent porphyria. *J Intern Med.* 1999;245:193.

225. Kauppinen R. *Prognosis of Acute Porphyrias and Molecular Genetics of Acute Intermittent Porphyria in Finland.* Thesis. University of Helskinki; 1992.

226. Milo R, Neuman M, Klein C, et al. Acute intermittent porphyria in pregnancy. *Obstet Gynecol.* 1989;73:450.

227. Shenhav S, Gemer O, Sassoon E, et al. Acute intermittent porphyria precipitated by hyperemesis and metoclopramide treatment in pregnancy. *Acta Obstet Gynecol Scand.* 1997;76:484.

228. Welland FH, Hellman ES, Gaddis EM, et al. Factors affecting the excretion of porphyrin precursors by patients with acute intermittent porphyria. I. The effect of diet. *Metabolism.* 1964;13:232.

229. Thaler MM, Dawber NH. Stimulation of bilirubin formation in liver of newborn rats by fasting and glucagon. *Gastroenterology.* 1977;72:312.

230. Bernstein HD, Rapport TA, Walter P. Cytosolic protein translocatioin factors. Is SRP still unique? *Cell.* 1989;58:1017.

231. Picat C, Delfau MH, De Rooij FWM, et al. Identification of the mutations in the parents of a patient with a putative compound heterozygosity for acute intermittent porphyria. *J Inherit Metab Dis.* 1990;13:684.

232. Bonkovsky HL, Maddukuri VC, Yazici C, et al. Acute porphyrias in the USA. Features of 108 subjects from Porphyria Consortium. *Am J Med.* 2014;127:1233.

233. Balwani M, Wang B, Anderson KE, et al. Acute hepatic porphyrias: recommendations for evaluation and long-term management. *Hepatology.* 2017;66:1314.

234. Stein JA, Tschudy DP. Acute intermittent porphyria. A clinical and biochemical study of 46 patients. *Medicine (Baltimore).* 1970;49:1.

235. Barohn RJ, Sanchez JE, Anderson KE. Acute peripheral neuropathy due to hereditary coproporphyria. *Muscle Nerve.* 1994;17:793.

236. Greenspan GH, Block AJ. Respiratory insufficiency associated with acute intermittent porphyria. *South Med J.* 1981;74:954.

237. Kazamel M, Desnick RJ, Quigley JG. Porphyric neuropathy: pathophysiology, diagnosis, and updated management. *Curr Neurol Neurosci Rep.* 2020;20:56. https://doi.org/10.1007/s11910-020-01089-5.

238. Ridley A. Porphyric neuropathy. In: Dyck PJ, Thomas PK, Lambert EH, Bunge R, eds. *Peripheral Neuropathy.* WB Saunders; 1984:1704.

239. Stein JA, Curl FD, Valsamis M, et al. Abnormal iron and water metabolism in acute intermittent porphyria with new morphologic findings. *Am J Med.* 1972;53:784.

240. Goldberg A. Acute intermittent porphyria. A study of 50 cases. *Q J Med.* 1959;28:183.

241. Bloomer JR, Berk PD, Bonkowsky HL, et al. Blood volume and bilirubin production in acute intermittent porphyria. *N Engl J Med.* 1971;284:17.

242. Eales L, Dowdle EB, Sweeney GD. The acute porphyric attack. I. The electrolyte disorder of the acute porphyric attack and the possible role of delta-aminolaevulic acid. *S Afr Med J.* September 1971:89.

243. Tschudy DP, Valsamis M, Magnussen CR. Acute intermittent porphyria: clinical and selected research aspects. *Ann Intern Med.* 1975;83:851.

244. Balwani M, Sardh E, Ventura P, et al. Phase 3 Trial of RNAi Therapeutic Givosiran for Acute Intermittent Porphyria. *New England Journal of Medicine.* 2020;382:(24):2289-2301.

245. Andersson C, Wikberg A, Stegmayr B, et al. Renal symptomatology in patients with acute intermittent porphyria. A population-based study. *J Intern Med.* 2000;248:319.

246. Church SE, McColl KE, Moore MR, et al. Hypertension and renal impairment as complications of acute porphyria. *Nephrol Dial Transplant.* 1992;7:986.

247. Tchernitchko D, Tavernier Q, Lamoril J, et al. A variant of peptide transporter 2 predicts the severity of porphyria-associated kidney disease. *J Am Soc Nephrol.* 2017;28:1924.

248. Barone GW, Gurley BJ, Anderson KE, et al. The tolerability of newer immunosuppressive medications in a patient with acute intermittent porphyria. *J Clin Pharmacol.* 2001;41:113.

249. Nunez DJ, Williams PF, Herrick AL, et al. Renal transplantation for chronic renal failure in acute porphyria. *Nephrol Dial Transplant.* 1987;2:271.

250. Ostrowski J, Kostrzewska E, Michalak T, et al. Abnormalities in liver function and morphology and impaired aminopyrine metabolism in hereditary hepatic porphyrias. *Gastroenterology.* 1983;85:1131.

251. Saberi B, Naik H, Overbey JR, et al. Hepatocellular carcinoma in acute hepatic porphyrias: results from the longitudinal study of the US Porphyrias Consortium. *Hepatology.* 2020 Jul 18.

252. Hollander CS, Scott RL, Tschudy DP, et al. Increased protein bound iodine and thyroxine binding globulin in acute intermittent porphyria. *N Engl J Med.* 1967;277:995.

253. Mustajoki P, Nikkila EA. Serum lipoproteins in asymptomatic acute porphyria: no evidence for hyperbetalipoproteinemia. *Metabolism.* 1984;33:266.

254. Deacon AC, Peters TJ. Identification of acute porphyria: evaluation of a commercial screening test for urinary porphobilinogen. *Ann Clin Biochem.* 1998;35(pt 6):726.

255. Minder EI. Coproporphyrin isomers in acute-intermittent porphyria. *Scand J Clin Lab Invest.* 1993;53:87.

256. Blum M, Koehl C, Abecassis J. Variations in erythrocyte uroporphyrinogen I synthetase activity in non porphyrias. *Clin Chim Acta.* 1978;87:119.

257. Kostrzewska E, Gregor A. Increased activity of porphobilinogen deaminase in erythrocytes during attacks of acute intermittent porphyria. *Ann Clin Res.* 1986;18:195.

258. Bonkowsky HL, Tschudy DP. Hazard of propranolol in treatment of acute porphyria (letter). *Br Med J.* 1974;4:47.

259. Bonkowsky HL, Sinclair PR, Emery S, et al. Seizure management in acute hepatic porphyria: risks of valproate and clonazepam. *Neurology.* 1980;30:588.

260. Larson AW, Wasserstrom WR, Felsher BF, et al. Posttraumatic epilepsy and acute intermittent porphyria: effects of phenytoin, carbamazepine, and clonazepam. *Neurology.* 1978;28:824.

261. Harper P, Wahlin S. Treatment options in acute porphyria, porphyria cutanea tarda, and erythropoietic protoporphyria. *Curr Treat Options Gastroenterol.* 2007;10:444.

262. Mustajoki P, Nordmann Y. Early administration of heme arginate for acute porphyric attacks. *Arch Intern Med.* 1993;153:2004.

263. Tenhunen R, Mustajoki P. Acute porphyria: treatment with heme. *Semin Liver Dis.* 1998;18:53.

264. Jones RL. Hematin-derived anticoagulant. Generation in vitro and in vivo. *J Exp Med.* 1986;163:724.

265. Bonkovsky HL, Healey JF, Lourie AN, et al. Intravenous heme-albumin in acute intermittent porphyria: evidence for repletion of hepatic hemoproteins and regulatory heme pools. *Am J Gastroenterol.* 1991;86:1050.

266. Anderson KE, Bonkovsky HL, Bloomer JR, et al. Reconstitution of hematin for intravenous infusion. *Ann Intern Med.* 2006;144:537.

267. Daimon M, Susa S, Igarashi M, et al. Administration of heme arginate, but not hematin, caused anaphylactic shock. *Am J Med.* 2001;110:240.

268. Khanderia U. Circulatory collapse associated with hemin therapy for acute intermittent porphyria. *Clin Pharm.* 1986;5:690.

269. Jeelani Dhar G, Bossenmaier I, Cardinal R, et al. Transitory renal failure following rapid administration of a relatively large amount of hematin in a patient with acute intermittent porphyria in clinical remission. *Acta Med Scand.* 1978;203:437.

270. Herrick AL, McColl KE, Moore MR, et al. Controlled trial of haem arginate in acute hepatic porphyria. *Lancet.* 1989;1:1295.

271. Anderson KE, Spitz IM, Bardin CW, et al. A gonadotropin releasing hormone analogue prevents cyclical attacks of porphyria. *Arch Intern Med.* 1990;150:1469.

272. Yamamori I, Asai M, Tanaka F, et al. Prevention of premenstrual exacerbation of hereditary coproporphyria by gonadotropin-releasing hormone analogue. *Intern Med.* 1999;38:365.

273. Schulenburg-Brand D, Gardiner T, Guppy S, et al. An audit of the use of gonadorelin analogues to prevent recurrent acute symptoms in patients with acute porphyria in the United Kingdom. *JIMD Rep.* 2017;36:99.

274. Cherem JH, Malagon J, Nellen H. Cimetidine and acute intermittent porphyria. *Ann Intern Med.* 2005;143:694.

275. Horie Y, Tanaka K, Okano J, et al. Cimetidine in the treatment of porphyria cutanea tarda. *Intern Med.* 1996;35:717.

276. Marcus DL, Nadel H, Lew G, et al. Cimetidine suppresses chemically induced experimental hepatic porphyria. *Am J Med Sci.* 1990;300:214.

277. With TK. Hereditary coproporphyria and variegate porphyria in Denmark. *Dan Med Bull.* 1983;30:106.

278. Mustajoki P. Variegate porphyria. Twelve years' experience in Finland. *Q J Med.* 1980;49:191.

279. Eales L, Day RS, Blekkenhorst GH. The clinical and biochemical features of variegate porphyria: an analysis of 300 cases studied at Groote Schuur Hospital, Cape Town. *Int J Biochem.* 1980;12:837.

280. Grandchamp B, Phung N, Nordmann Y. Homozygous case of hereditary coproporphyria. *Lancet.* 1977;2:1348.

281. To-Figueras J, Badenas C, Enriquez MT, et al. Biochemical and genetic characterization of four cases of hereditary coproporphyria in Spain. *Mol Genet Metab.* 2005;85:160.

282. Stenson PD, Mort M, Ball EV, et al. The Human Gene Mutation Database: towards a comprehensive repository of inherited mutation data for medical research, genetic diagnosis and next-generation sequencing studies. *Hum Genet.* 2017;136:665.

283. Nordmann Y, Grandchamp B, de Verneuil H, et al. Harderoporphyria: a variant hereditary coproporphyria. *J Clin Invest.* 1983;72:1139.

284. Moghe A, Ramanujam VMS, Phillips JD, et al. Harderoporphyria: case of lifelong photosensitivity associated with compound heterozygous coproporphyrinogen oxidase (CPOX) mutations. *Mol Genet Metab Rep.* 2019;19:100457.

285. Blake D, McManus J, Cronin V, et al. Fecal coproporphyrin isomers in hereditary coproporphyria. *Clin Chem.* 1992;38:96.

286. Hift RJ, Davidson BP, van der Hooft C, et al. Plasma fluorescence scanning and fecal porphyrin analysis for the diagnosis of variegate porphyria: precise determination of sensitivity and specificity with detection of protoporphyrinogen oxidase mutations as a reference standard. *Clin Chem.* 2004;50:915.

287. Lamoril J, Puy H, Gouya L, et al. Neonatal hemolytic anemia due to inherited harderoporphyria: clinical characteristics and molecular basis. *Blood.* 1998;91:1453.

288. Tio TH, Leijnse B, Jarrett A, et al. Acquired porphyria from a liver tumor. *Clin Sci Mol Med.* 1959;16:517.

289. Elder GH, Urquhart AJ, de Salamanca RE, et al. Immunoreactive uroporphyrinogen decarboxylase in the liver in porphyria cutanea tarda. *Lancet.* 1985;2:229.

290. Phillips JD, Jackson LK, Bunting M, et al. A mouse model of familial porphyria cutanea tarda. *Proc Natl Acad Sci U S A.* 2001;98:259.

291. Gorman N, Zaharia A, Trask HS, et al. Effect of iron and ascorbate on uroporphyria in ascorbate-requiring mice as a model for porphyria cutanea tarda. *Hepatology.* 2007;45:187.

292. Rocchi E, Casalgrandi G, Masini A, et al. Circulating pro- and antioxidant factors in iron and porphyrin metabolism disorders. *Ital J Gastroenterol Hepatol.* 1999;31:861.

293. Sinclair PR, Gorman N, Walton HS, et al. CYP1A2 is essential in murine uroporphyria caused by hexachlorobenzene and iron. *Toxicol Appl Pharmacol.* 2000;162:60.

294. Smith AG, Francis JE, Walters DG, et al. Protection against iron-induced uroporphyria in C57BL/10ScSn mice by the peroxisome proliferator nafenopin. *Biochem Pharmacol.* 1990;40:2564.

295. Elder GH. Porphyria cutanea tarda and related disorders. In: Kadish KM, Smith K, Guilard R, eds. *Porphyrin Handbook, Part II.* Vol 14. Academic Press; 2003:67.

296. Phillips JD, Parker TL, Schubert HL, et al. Functional consequences of naturally occurring mutations in human uroporphyrinogen decarboxylase. *Blood.* 2001;98:3179.

297. Cassiman D, Vannoote J, Roelandts R, et al. Porphyria cutanea tarda and liver disease. A retrospective analysis of 17 cases from a single centre and review of the literature. *Acta Gastroenterol Belg.* 2008;71:237.

298. Gisbert JP, Garcia-Buey L, Alonso A, et al. Hepatocellular carcinoma risk in patients with porphyria cutanea tarda. *Eur J Gastroenterol Hepatol.* 2004;16:689.

299. Rossmann-Ringdahl I, Olsson R. Porphyria cutanea tarda in a Swedish population: risk factors and complications. *Acta Derm Venereol.* 2005;85:337.

300. Dabski C, Beutner EH. Studies of laminin and type IV collagen in blisters of porphyria cutanea tarda and drug-induced pseudoporphyria. *J Am Acad Dermatol.* 1991;25:28.

301. Pigatto PD, Polenghi MM, Altomare GF, et al. Complement cleavage products in the phototoxic reaction of porphyria cutanea tarda. *Br J Dermatol.* 1986;114:567.

302. Egger NG, Goeger DE, Payne DA, et al. Porphyria cutanea tarda: multiplicity of risk factors including HFE mutations, hepatitis C, and inherited uroporphyrinogen decarboxylase deficiency. *Dig Dis Sci.* 2002;47:419.

303. Darwich E, To-Figueras J, Molina-Lopez RA, et al. Increased serum hepcidin levels in patients with porphyria cutanea tarda. *J Eur Acad Dermatol Venereol.* 2013;27:e68.

304. Bulaj ZJ, Franklin MR, Phillips JD, et al. Transdermal estrogen replacement therapy in postmenopausal women previously treated for porphyria cutanea tarda. *J Lab Clin Med.* 2000;136:482.

305. Wickliffe JK, Abdel-Rahman SZ, Lee C, et al. *CYP1A2*1F* and *GSTM1* alleles are associated with susceptibility to porphyria cutanea tarda. *Mol Med.* 2011;17:241-247

306. Grossman ME, Bickers DR, Poh-Fitzpatrick MB, et al. Porphyria cutanea tarda. Clinical features and laboratory findings in 40 patients. *Am J Med.* 1979;67:277.

307. Sixel-Dietrich F, Doss M. Hereditary uroporphyrinogen-decarboxylase deficiency predisposing porphyria cutanea tarda (chronic hepatic porphyria) in females after oral contraceptive medication. *Arch Dermatol Res.* 1985;278:13.

308. Legault N, Sabik H, Cooper SF, et al. Effect of estradiol on the induction of porphyria by hexachlorobenzene in the rat. *Biochem Pharmacol.* 1997;54:19.

309. Fujita N, Sugimoto R, Motonishi S, et al. Patients with chronic hepatitis C achieving a sustained virological response to peginterferon and ribavirin therapy recover from impaired hepcidin secretion. *J Hepatol.* 2008;49:702.

310. Wissel PS, Sordillo P, Anderson KE, et al. Porphyria cutanea tarda associated with the acquired immune deficiency syndrome. *Am J Hematol.* 1987;25:107.

311. Roberts AG, Whatley SD, Nicklin S, et al. The frequency of hemochromatosis-associated alleles is increased in British patients with sporadic porphyria cutanea tarda. *Hepatology.* 1997;25:159.

312. Dereure O, Aguilar-Martinez P, Bessis D, et al. HFE mutations and transferrin receptor polymorphism analysis in porphyria cutanea tarda: a prospective study of 36 cases from southern France. *Br J Dermatol.* 2001;144:533.

313. Ajioka RS, Phillips JD, Weiss RB, et al. Down-regulation of hepcidin in porphyria cutanea tarda. *Blood.* 2008;112:4723.

314. Calvert GM, Sweeney MH, Fingerhut MA, et al. Evaluation of porphyria cutanea tarda in U.S. workers exposed to 2,3,7,8-tetrachlorodibenzo-p-dioxin. *Am J Ind Med.* 1995;25:559.

315. Smith A. Porphyria caused by chlorinated AH receptor ligands and associated mechanisms of liver injury and cancer. In: Kadish KM, Smith K, Guilard R, eds. *Porphyrin Handbook, Part II.* Vol 14. Academic Press; 2003:169.

316. Brady JJ, Jackson HA, Roberts AG, et al. Co-inheritance of mutations in the uroporphyrinogen decarboxylase and hemochromatosis genes accelerates the onset of porphyria cutanea tarda. *J Invest Dermatol.* 2000;115:868.

317. Barzilay D, Orion E, Brenner S. Porphyria cutanea tarda triggered by a combination of three predisposing factors. *Dermatology.* 2001;203:195.

318. Au WY, Tam SC, Ho KM, et al. Hypertrichosis due to porphyria cutanea tarda associated with blastic transformation of myelofibrosis. *Br J Dermatol.* 1999;141:932.

319. Lee SC, Yun SJ, Lee JB, et al. A case of porphyria cutanea tarda in association with idiopathic myelofibrosis and CREST syndrome. *Br J Dermatol.* 2001;144:182.

320. Anderson KE, Goeger DE, Carson RW, et al. Erythropoietin for the treatment of porphyria cutanea tarda in a patient on long-term hemodialysis. *N Engl J Med.* 1990;322:315.

321. Armstrong DK, Sharpe PC, Chambers CR, et al. Hepatoerythropoietic porphyria: a missense mutation in the UROD gene is associated with mild disease and an unusual porphyrin excretion pattern. *Br J Dermatol.* 2004;151:920.

322. Elder GH. The metabolism of porphyrins of the isocoproporphyrin series. *Enzyme.* 1974;17:61.

323. Poh-Fitzpatrick MB, Sosin AE, Bemis J. Porphyrin levels in plasma and erythrocytes of chronic hemodialysis patients. *J Am Acad Dermatol.* 1982;7:100.

324. Topi GC, Amantea A, Griso D. Recovery from porphyria cutanea tarda with no specific therapy other than avoidance of hepatic toxins. *Br J Dermatol.* 1984;111:75.

325. Ippen H. Treatment of porphyria cutanea tarda by phlebotomy. *Semin Hematol.* 1977;14:253.

326. Rocchi E, Cassanelli M, Ventura E. High weekly intravenous doses of desferrioxamine in porphyria cutanea tarda. *Br J Dermatol.* 1987;117:393.

327. Ratnaike S, Blake D, Campbell D, et al. Plasma ferritin levels as a guide to the treatment of porphyria cutanea tarda by venesection. *Australas J Dermatol.* 1988;29:3.

328. Ashton RE, Hawk JLM, Magnus IA. Low-dose oral chloroquine in the treatment of porphyria cutanea tarda. *Br J Dermatol.* 1984;3:609.

329. Bruce AJ, Ahmed I. Childhood-onset porphyria cutanea tarda: successful therapy with low-dose hydroxychloroquine (Plaquenil). *J Am Acad Dermatol.* 1998;38:810.

330. Freesemann A, Frank M, Sieg I, et al. Treatment of porphyria cutanea tarda by the effect of chloroquine on the liver. *Skin Pharmacol.* 1995;8:156.

331. Kordac V, Semradova M. Treatment of porphyria cutanea tarda with chloroquine. *Br J Dermatol.* 1974;90:95.

332. Taljaard JJF, Shanley BC, Stewart-Wynne EG, et al. Studies on low dose chloroquine therapy and the action of chloroquine in symptomatic porphyria. *Br J Dermatol.* 1972;87:261.

333. Timonen K, Niemi KM, Mustajoki P. Skin morphology in porphyria cutanea tarda does not improve despite clinical remission. *Clin Exp Dermatol.* 1991;16:355.

334. Thornsvard CT, Guider BA, Kimball DB. An unusual reaction to chloroquine-primaquine. *JAMA.* 1976;235:1719.

335. Sweeney GD, Jones KG. Porphyria cutanea tarda: clinical and laboratory features. *Can Med Assoc J.* 1979;120:803.

336. Malkinson FD, Levitt L. Hydroxychloroquine treatment of porphyria cutanea tarda. *Arch Dermatol.* 1980;116:1147.

337. Singal AK, Kormos-Hallberg C, Lee C, et al. Low-dose hydroxychloroquine is as effective as phlebotomy in treatment of patients with porphyria cutanea tarda. *Clin Gastroenterol Hepatol.* 2012;10:1402.

338. Stolzel U, Kostler E, Schuppan D, et al. Hemochromatosis (HFE) gene mutations and response to chloroquine in porphyria cutanea tarda. *Arch Dermatol.* 2003;139:309.

339. Egger NG, Goeger DE, Anderson KE. Effects of chloroquine in hematoporphyrin-treated animals. *Chem Biol Interact.* 1996;102:69.

340. Cohen SN, Phifer KO, Yielding KL. Complex formation between chloroquine and ferrihaemic acid in vitro, and its effect on the antimalarial action of chloroquine. *Nature.* 1964;202:805.

341. Scholnick PL, Epstein J, Marver HS. The molecular basis of the action of chloroquine in porphyria cutanea tarda. *J Invest Dermatol.* 1973;61:226.

342. Chlumska A, Chlumsky J, Malina L. Liver changes in porphyria cutanea tarda patients treated with chloroquine. *Br J Dermatol.* 1980;102:261.

343. Vizethum W, Dahlmann D, Bolsen K, et al. Influence of chloroquine (Resochin) on hexachlorobenzene (HCB) induced porphyria of the rat. *Arch Dermatol Res.* 1979;264:125.

344. Singal AK, Venkata KVR, Jampana S, et al. Hepatitis C treatment in patients with porphyria cutanea tarda. *Am J Med Sci.* 2017;353:523.

345. To-Figueras J. Association between hepatitis C virus and porphyria cutanea tarda. *Mol Genet Metab.* 2019;128:282.

346. Shieh S, Cohen JL, Lim HW. Management of porphyria cutanea tarda in the setting of chronic renal failure: a case report and review. *J Am Acad Dermatol.* 2000;42:645.

347. Yaqoob M, Smyth J, Ahmad R, et al. Haemodialysis-related porphyria cutanea tarda and treatment by recombinant human erythropoietin. *Nephron.* 1992;60:428.

348. Carson RW, Dunnigan EJ, DuBose TDJ, et al. Removal of plasma porphyrins with high-flux hemodialysis in porphyria cutanea tarda associated with end-stage renal disease. *J Am Soc Nephrol.* 1992;2:1445.

349. Stevens BR, Fleischer AB, Piering F, et al. Porphyria cutanea tarda in the setting of renal failure: response to renal transplantation. *Arch Dermatol.* 1993;129:337.

350. Fontanellas A, Mazurier F, Moreau-Gaudry F, et al. Correction of uroporphyrinogen decarboxylase deficiency (hepatoerythropoietic porphyria) in Epstein-Barr virus-transformed B- cell lines by retrovirus-mediated gene transfer: fluorescence-based selection of transduced cells. *Blood.* 1999;94:465.

Part V Anemia as a Result of Exogenous Factors

CHAPTER 22
FRAGMENTATION HEMOLYTIC ANEMIA

Kelty R. Baker and Joel Moake

SUMMARY

Erythrocyte fragmentation and hemolysis occur when red cells are forced through partial vascular occlusions or over abnormal vascular surfaces at high shear stress. "Split" red cells, or schistocytes, are prominent on blood films under these conditions, and considerable quantities of lactate dehydrogenase (LDH) are released into the blood from traumatized red cells. In the high-flow (high-shear) microvascular (arteriolar or capillary) or arterial circulation, partial vascular obstructions are caused by platelet aggregates in the systemic microvasculature during episodes of thrombotic thrombocytopenic purpura (TTP), by platelet-fibrin thrombi in the renal microvasculature in the hemolytic uremic syndrome, and by malfunction of a cardiac prosthetic valve in valve-related hemolysis. Less-extensive red cell fragmentation, hemolysis, and schistocytosis occur under conditions of more moderate vascular occlusion or endothelial surface abnormalities, sometimes under conditions of lower shear stress. These latter entities include (i) excessive platelet aggregation, fibrin polymer formation, and secondary fibrinolysis in the arterial or venous microcirculation (eg, disseminated intravascular coagulation [DIC]); (ii) in the placental vasculature in preeclampsia or eclampsia and the syndrome of hemolysis, elevated liver enzymes and low platelets (HELLP); (iii) in march hemoglobinuria; and (iv) in giant cavernous hemangiomas (the Kasabach-Merritt phenomenon).

● PREECLAMPSIA OR ECLAMPSIA AND HELLP SYNDROME

DEFINITION AND HISTORY

A life-threatening condition of pregnancy denoted by eclampsia, hemolysis, and thrombocytopenia was first noted in the German literature

Acronyms and Abbreviations: ADAMTS13, a disintegrin and metalloproteinase with thrombospondin domain 13; ALT, alanine transaminase; aPTT, activated partial thromboplastin time; AST, aspartic acid transaminase; AT, antithrombin; DIC, disseminated intravascular coagulation; HELLP, hemolysis, elevated liver enzymes, and low platelet count; LDH, lactate dehydrogenase; MAHA, microangiopathic hemolytic anemia; NO, nitrous oxide; PGF, placental growth factor; PGI_2, prostaglandin I_2; PT, prothrombin time; PTT, partial thromboplastin time; sEng, soluble endoglin; sFlt-1, soluble form of fms-like tyrosine kinase 1; sVEGFR-1, soluble vascular endothelial growth factor receptor-1; TGF-β, transforming growth factor-β; TTP, thrombotic thrombocytopenic purpura; VEGF, vascular endothelial growth factor; VWF, von Willebrand factor.

by Stahnke in 1922.[1] Subsequently, Pritchard and coworkers described three cases in English and suggested that an immunologic process might account for both the preeclampsia or eclampsia and the hematologic abnormalities.[2] Although initially known as edema-proteinuria-hypertension gestosis type B,[3] a catchier phrase, HELLP syndrome (H for hemolysis, EL for elevated liver function tests, and LP for low platelet counts), was later applied by Louis Weinstein in 1982.[4]

EPIDEMIOLOGY

HELLP syndrome occurs in approximately 0.5% of pregnancies,[5] in 4% to 12% of those complicated by preeclampsia (hypertension + proteinuria), and in 30% to 50% of those complicated by eclampsia (hypertension + proteinuria + seizures); however, approximately 15% of patients ultimately diagnosed with HELLP syndrome present with neither hypertension nor proteinuria.[6] Two-thirds of HELLP patients are diagnosed antepartum, usually between 27 and 37 weeks. The remaining third are diagnosed in the postpartum period, from a few to 48 hours after delivery (occasionally as long as 6 days).[7,8]

Risk factors for HELLP syndrome include European ancestry, multiparity, maternal age (older than age 34 years), and a personal or familial history of the disorder.[5] Although the presence of homozygosity for the 677 (C→T) polymorphism of the methylenetetrahydrofolate reductase gene may be a modest risk factor for the development of preeclampsia, this weak association does not exist for HELLP syndrome.[9] More promising are studies indicating that heterozygosity for the factor V Leiden mutation, missense mutations of the Toll-like receptor-4 gene, decreased expression of the syncytin envelope gene (essential for mediating cytotrophoblasts cell-cell fusion and differentiation), and polymorphisms of the genes coding for mannose-binding lectin, vascular endothelial growth factor, angiotensin converting enzyme, the glucocorticoid receptor, and Fas receptor may increase the risk of the HELLP syndrome. The aforementioned abnormalities could predispose to aberrant placental growth and ischemia as a result of arterial thrombosis, impaired syncytiotrophoblast formation, complement- and lymphocyte-mediated destruction of invading extravillous trophoblasts, and abnormal remodeling of the spiral arteries.[10] There is evidence that activation of the alternative complement pathway (ACP) and mutations in ACP genes may be associated with HELLP.[11]

ETIOLOGY AND PATHOGENESIS

A developing embryo must acquire a supply of maternal blood to survive. During a normal pregnancy, the first wave of trophoblastic invasion into the decidua occurs at 10 to 12 days. This is followed by a second wave at 16 to 22 weeks, when these specialized placental epithelial cells replace the endothelium of the uterine spiral arteries and intercalate within the muscular tunica, increasing the vessels' diameters and decreasing their resistance. As a result, the spiral arteries are remodeled into unique hybrid vessels composed of fetal and maternal cells, and the vasculature is converted into a high-flow–low-resistance system resistant to vasoconstrictors circulating in the maternal blood.[12] In a preeclamptic pregnancy, the second wave fails to penetrate adequately the spiral arteries of the uterus, perhaps as a result of reduced placental expression of syncytin and subsequent altered cell fusion processes during placentogenesis.[13] The resultant poorly perfused, hypoxic placenta then releases the extracellular domain (soluble) form of fms-like tyrosine kinase 1 (sFLT-1), also known as soluble vascular endothelial growth factor receptor-1 (sVEGF receptor-1, or sVEGFR-1). sVEGFR-1 functions as an antiangiogenic protein because it binds to vascular endothelial growth factor (VEGF) and placental growth factor (PGF) and prevents their interaction with endothelial cell receptors.

The ratio of sVEGFR-1 to PGF levels is increased in the maternal circulation.[14] The result is maternal glomerular endothelial cell and placental dysfunction.[15-17]

Direct and indirect sequelae of this dysfunction include increased vascular tone, hypertension, proteinuria, enhanced platelet activation and aggregation, and decreased levels of the vasodilators prostaglandin I_2 (PGI_2) and nitrous oxide (NO).[5,17] Concurrent activation of the coagulation cascade results in platelet-fibrin deposition in the capillaries, multiorgan microvascular injury, microangiopathic hemolytic anemia (MAHA), elevated liver enzymes because of hepatic necrosis, and thrombocytopenia because of peripheral consumption of platelets.[5]

Another antiangiogenic molecule, a soluble form of endoglin (sEng), also increases in patient serum during early and severe preeclampsia.[18] Endoglin is part of the transforming growth factor-β (TGF-β) complex and is expressed on vascular endothelial cells and syncytiotrophoblasts. The shed extracellular domain of endoglin, sEng, is capable of binding to and inactivating the proangiogenic growth factors, TGF-β_1 and TGF-β_3. The presence of elevated serum levels of both sFLT-1 (sVEGFR-1) and sEng may be associated with the progression of preeclampsia to HELLP.[17,18]

CLINICAL FEATURES

Ninety percent of patients with HELLP syndrome present with malaise and right upper quadrant or epigastric pain. Approximately two-thirds have nausea or vomiting, somewhat over half have edema, and nearly half of patients have headache. A smaller percentage complains of visual changes. Fever is not typically seen. Although hypertension is found in approximately 85% of affected patients, 15% of those with HELLP syndrome do not develop either hypertension or proteinuria.[6]

LABORATORY FEATURES

There is no consensus regarding the laboratory criteria necessary to diagnose HELLP syndrome, so clinical judgment in conjunction with judicious interpretation of a variety of laboratory tests constitute the diagnostic standard. In two-thirds of the patients, the blood film has schistocytes, helmet cells, and burr cells consistent with MAHA. Reticulocytosis can be present. Low haptoglobin levels are both sensitive (~85%) and specific (~95%) for confirming the presence of hemolysis and return to normal within 24 to 30 hours postpartum.[6]

Lactate dehydrogenase (LDH) levels are usually above normal. The ratio of LDH-5 (an isoenzyme found specifically in the liver) to total LDH is elevated in proportion to the severity of HELLP. The high LDH seen in HELLP is most likely the result, principally, of liver damage rather than hemolysis. Serum levels of aspartic acid transaminase (AST) and alanine transaminase (ALT) can be more than 100 times normal, whereas alkaline phosphatase values are typically only about twice normal, and total bilirubin ranges between 1.2 and 5.0 mg/dL. Liver enzymes usually return to normal within 3 to 5 days postpartum.[6]

The degree of thrombocytopenia has been used in a classification system to predict maternal morbidity and mortality: the rapidity of postpartum recovery, the risk of disease recurrence, and perinatal outcome. This *Mississippi triple-class system* places those patients with platelet counts less than 50×10^9/L in class 1 (~13% incidence of bleeding), those with platelet counts between 50 and 100×10^9/L in class 2 (~8% incidence of bleeding), and those with a platelet count greater than 100×10^9/L in class 3 (no increased bleeding risk). Patients with class 1 HELLP syndrome have the highest incidence of perinatal morbidity and mortality and have the most protracted recovery periods postpartum.[19] There is a direct correlation between the extent of thrombocytopenia and measurements of liver function,[20] but the same cannot

be said for the severity of associated hepatic histopathologic changes.[21] If a marrow aspiration and biopsy are performed, abundant megakaryocytes are found consistent with a consumptive thrombocytopenia causing reduction of the normal platelet lifespan of approximately 10 days to 3-5 days.[19] The platelet count nadir occurs 23 to 29 hours postpartum, with subsequent normalization within 6 days.[7]

The prothrombin time (PT) and activated partial thromboplastin time (aPTT) are usually within normal limits, although one report cited a prolonged aPTT in 50% of patients.[22] Although low fibrinogen levels are inconsistently found, other measures of increased coagulation and secondary fibrinolysis may be present. These include decreased protein C and antithrombin (AT) levels and increased D-dimer and thrombin-AT values. von Willebrand factor (VWF) antigen levels increase in proportion to the severity of the disease, reflecting the extent of endothelial damage; however, no unusually large VWF multimers are present in plasma,[23] and ADAMTS13 (a disintegrin and metalloproteinase with thrombospondin domains-13) levels are within a broad normal range. ADAMTS13 normally declines moderately during pregnancy.[24,25] This finding is in contrast to the severe deficiency of ADAMTS13 in familial and autoantibody-mediated types of thrombotic thrombocytopenic purpura (TTP).[26] Unlike TTP, the thrombi found in organs involved in the HELLP syndrome contain increased amounts of fibrin and low levels of VWF.[23]

In patients with severe liver involvement, hepatic ultrasonography shows large, irregular, well-demarcated (or "geographical") areas of increased echogenicity.[27] Liver biopsy shows periportal or focal necrosis, platelet-fibrin deposits in the sinusoids, and vascular microthrombi. As the disease progresses, large areas of necrosis can coalesce and dissect into the liver capsule. This produces a subcapsular hematoma and the risk of hepatic rupture.[5]

DIFFERENTIAL DIAGNOSIS

Other complications of pregnancy that can be confused with HELLP include TTP[28] and the hemolytic uremic syndrome, sepsis, disseminated intravascular coagulation (DIC), connective tissue disease, antiphospholipid antibody syndrome, and acute fatty liver of pregnancy. The latter entity is also seen in the last trimester or postpartum and presents with thrombocytopenia and right upper quadrant pain, but the levels of AST and ALT only rise to one to five times normal, and the PT and aPTT are both prolonged. Oil-red-O staining of liver biopsies demonstrates fat in the cytoplasm of centrilobular hepatocytes, and stains show inflammation and patchy hepatocellular necrosis as a result of the HELLP syndrome. Because it causes right upper quadrant pain and nausea, HELLP has also been misdiagnosed as viral hepatitis, biliary colic, esophageal reflux, cholecystitis, and gastric cancer. Conversely, other conditions misdiagnosed as HELLP syndrome include cardiomyopathy, dissecting aortic aneurysm, acute cocaine intoxication, essential hypertension and renal disease, and alcoholic liver disease.[19]

THERAPY

Supportive care of HELLP includes IV administration of magnesium sulfate to control hypertension and prevent eclamptic seizures, treatment of severe hypertension with agents such as labetalol, management of fluids and electrolytes, judicious transfusion of blood products, stimulation of fetal lung maturation with beclomethasone, and delivery of the fetus as soon as possible.[19] Indications for delivery include a severe disease presentation, maternal DIC, fetal distress, and a gestational age greater than 32 weeks with evidence of lung maturity.[6] Cesarean section under general anesthesia is used most frequently, but vaginal delivery after induction can be attempted if the fetus is older than 32 weeks of age and the mother's cervical anatomy is favorable. Postpartum curettage is helpful in lowering the mean arterial pressure and increasing the urine output and platelet count. Transfusion therapy with packed red cells, platelets, or fresh-frozen plasma is indicated in cases complicated by severe anemia or bleeding because of coagulopathy.

Although previously thought to be beneficial based on the results of observational studies and small randomized trials, the use of dexamethasone has fallen out of favor after large randomized trials found that it did not reduce the duration of hospitalization, amount of blood products transfused, maternal complications, or time to normalization of laboratory abnormalities.[29]

Plasma exchange cannot arrest or reverse HELLP syndrome when used antepartum but may minimize hemorrhage and morbidity when used peripartum. It can also be tried postpartum in the 5% of patients who fail to improve within 72 to 96 hours of delivery. These women are more likely to be younger than 20 years of age or nulliparous.[7] Whether or not plasma exchange can effectively lower circulating levels of sVEGF, or sEng is not known. Liver transplantation may be necessary in occasional patients with HELLP complicated by large hematomas or total hepatic necrosis. It is not yet known if replacement with some (possibly modified) form of VEGF or TGF-β may have future therapeutic use in preeclampsia or HELLP. A single case report describes the successful use of eculizumab to prolong by 17 days a pregnancy affected by severe HELLP, without associated maternal or fetal morbidity or mortality.[30]

COURSE AND PROGNOSIS

Most patients stabilize within 24 to 48 hours after delivery; however, maternal death still occurs in 3% to 5% even with best supportive care. Mortality rates as high as 25% were reported before 1980. Events leading to maternal death include cerebral hemorrhage, cardiopulmonary arrest, DIC, acute respiratory distress syndrome (ARDS), and hypoxic ischemic encephalopathy.[5] Other complications include infection, placenta abruptio, postpartum hemorrhage, intraabdominal bleeding, and subcapsular liver hematomas with resultant rupture (a fatal event in 50% of those in whom it occurs).[6] The latter patients complain of right-sided shoulder pain and are found to be in shock with ascites or pleural effusions. The hematoma is usually present in the anterior superior portion of the right lobe of the liver.[5] If the liver remains intact when discovered, abdominal palpation, seizures, and emesis should be avoided or prevented. Emergency surgery is required for hepatic artery embolization or ligation, hepatic lobectomy, or even liver transplantation in patients with total hepatic necrosis.[5,19]

Renal complications of HELLP include acute renal failure, hyponatremia, and nephrogenic diabetes insipidus as a result of impaired hepatic metabolism of vasopressinase and resultant "resistance to vasopressin" (antidiuretic hormone). Pulmonary complications of HELLP include pleural effusions, pulmonary edema, and ARDS. Neurologic sequelae of HELLP not mentioned earlier include retinal detachment, postictal cortical blindness, and hypoglycemic coma.[31]

Fetal morbidity and mortality rates are each approximately 15%.[6] Complications arise as a result of prematurity, placental abruption, and intrauterine asphyxia. Intrauterine growth retardation is seen in approximately one-third of infants. One-third of all babies born to mothers with HELLP have thrombocytopenia, but intraventricular hemorrhage is seen very infrequently in thrombocytopenic infants.[32]

HELLP syndrome complicates approximately 3% of all pregnancies[5] and can recur in as many as 25% of those affected during subsequent pregnancies.[33] Other hypertensive disorders of pregnancy (preeclampsia or pregnancy-induced hypertension) are also relatively common in future pregnancies (~25% of second and subsequent pregnancies).[34] Women who recover from preeclampsia or HELLP may also be more likely to develop subsequent hypertension and cardiovascular disorders, possibly because of some persistent abnormal balance between proangiogenic and antiangiogenic factors.[17]

● DISSEMINATED MALIGNANCY

DEFINITION AND HISTORY

The association between widespread malignancy and hemolytic anemia associated with pathologic changes in small blood vessels was first noted by Brain and colleagues in 1962.[35]

EPIDEMIOLOGY

Cancer-associated MAHA has been described in a wide variety of malignancies (Table 22-1). MAHA is more likely to be associated with metastatic malignant disease than with localized cancers or benign tumors.[36] Approximately 80% of the tumors are mucinous adenocarcinomas of either the stomach (55%), breast (13%), or lung (10%). The median age at diagnosis is 50 years, with a slight male predominance.[37]

ETIOLOGY AND PATHOGENESIS

MAHA as a result of malignancy can be caused by either of two distinct mechanisms: (i) DIC with intravascular occlusions (often partial) of small vessels by platelet-fibrin thrombi or (ii) intravascular tumor emboli.[35,38] In the first mechanism,[1] intravascular activation of coagulation may occur from excessive exposure of tissue factor on phagocytes, activated endothelial cells, or tumor cells. Alternatively, a protease in the mucin secreted by adenocarcinomas may directly activate factor X.[39] Subsequent activation of coagulation factors, thrombin generation, fibrin polymer deposition, and platelet aggregation result in the formation of intravascular platelet-fibrin thrombi and the shearing of red cells attempting to maneuver past the partial platelet-fibrin occlusions in the high-flow microvasculature. Also, circulating carcinoma mucins

TABLE 22–1. Cancers Associated with Microangiopathic Hemolytic Anemia

Gastric (55%)[37,40]

Breast (13%)[127]

Lung (10%)[35]

Other adenocarcinomas

    Unknown primary[38]

    Prostate[35]

    Colon[38]

    Gallbladder

    Pancreas

    Ovary

Other malignancies

    Hemangiopericytoma[36]

    Hepatoma

    Melanoma

    Small cell cancer of the lung[128]

    Testicular cancer

    Squamous cell cancer of the oropharynx

    Thymoma

    Erythroleukemia[129]

may interact with leukocyte L-selectin and platelet P-selectin, causing the rapid generation of platelet-rich microthrombi.[40] In the second mechanism,[2] intravascular tumor emboli partially occlude small vessels, mechanically or chemically disrupt the endothelium, and promote platelet adherence to exposed subendothelium, coagulation activation and fibrin polymer formation, intimal hyperplasia, and vascular hypertrophy.[35,37,38]

LABORATORY FEATURES

Patients with cancer-associated DIC or MAHA present with moderate to severe anemia. The blood film reveals schistocytes (accounting for approximately 5%-21% of the red cells), burr cells, microspherocytes, polychromasia (reticulocytes), and nucleated red cells.[38] Although the reticulocyte count can be high, it is an unreliable measure of hemolysis because extensive replacement of the marrow by metastatic tumor (Chap. 13) may prevent the reticulocytosis expected with MAHA. Other indicators of hemolysis that could be more reliable include increased levels of serum unconjugated bilirubin and LDH, the presence of plasma hemoglobin, and elevated urine urobilinogen and hemoglobinuria (as αβ dimers).[37] Absent or low levels of haptoglobin may also be found; however, haptoglobin is an acute-phase reactant that may be increased in malignancy.[38] The direct antiglobulin test result is negative.[37,41]

Additional findings in MAHA include thrombocytopenia, with mean platelet counts of approximately 50×10^9/L (range, 3-225 × 10^9/L),[37] caused by a shortened platelet lifespan without demonstrable sequestration of platelets in the liver or spleen. Some patients with malignant tumors, however, may have preexisting thrombocytosis, so superimposed MAHA may reduce the platelet count only toward "normal" values.[38] A normal to high white cell count with immature myeloid precursors may also be seen.[37,38,41] Leukoerythroblastosis caused by marrow invasion (Chap. 13), along with MAHA, is highly suggestive of metastatic malignancy.[38] Marrow aspiration and biopsy demonstrate erythroid hyperplasia, normal to high numbers of megakaryocytes, and (in 55% of patients) cancer cells.[41]

Additional laboratory evidence of DIC has been reported in approximately 50% of patients with MAHA secondary to malignancy. Findings include reduced levels of fibrinogen (mean, 177 g/dL; range, 8-490 mg/dL), increased levels of D-dimers (or fibrin degradation products), and prolonged prothrombin and thrombin times.[37] In the early phase of DIC, aPTTs may be shortened (eg, to <23 seconds).[42-45] It is not known if shortened aPTT values reflect the presence of activated coagulation factors in the plasma, consumption of coagulation inhibitor proteins faster than their production by hepatic cells (eg, protein C, protein S, AT, tissue factor pathway inhibitor), or the presence in plasma of a cysteine protease capable of directly activating factor X.[39] Cancer-related DIC has been reported to be associated with a deficiency of the VWF-cleaving protease, ADAMTS13.[46] Although this has been disputed by some investigators,[47] ADAMTS13 levels gradually decrease in DIC patients with poor survival rates,[48] perhaps as a result of ADAMTS13 consumption onto the long VWF multimeric strings released from cytokine-stimulated endothelial cells.[49]

DIFFERENTIAL DIAGNOSIS

The most common cause of anemia in malignancy is anemia of inflammation (Chap. 6). Other diagnostic considerations include blood loss, myelophthisis as a result of disease metastatic to the marrow (Chap. 13), MAHA associated with DIC, and autoimmune hemolytic anemia (Chap. 26). The latter is more often found with lymphoproliferative disease but is occasionally seen with carcinoma of the stomach, colon, breast, and cervix.[50] The treatment of cancer can also induce anemia by causing myelosuppression, oxidative hemolysis (doxorubicin, pentostatin), autoimmune hemolysis (cisplatin, chlorambucil, cyclophosphamide, melphalan, teniposide, methotrexate), or thrombotic microangiopathic anemia (mitomycin C, cisplatin, gemcitabine, and targeted cancer agents[51]).

THERAPY

Heparin, glucocorticoids, dipyridamole, indomethacin, and ε-aminocaproic acid have all been tested without success for malignancy-associated DIC/MAHA. Plasma infusion and platelet transfusions, sometimes with additional cryoprecipitate containing fibrinogen, may be useful during bleeding episodes associated with prolonged PT and aPTT, low fibrinogen levels, and thrombocytopenia, but available evidence does not support the use of antithrombin concentrate, recombinant activated protein C, or recombinant thrombomodulin.[52] Control of the underlying metastatic malignancy, if achievable, is known to be beneficial.[53]

COURSE AND PROGNOSIS

MAHA caused by cancer is usually a preterminal event. Life expectancy after diagnosis is 2 to 150 days, with a mean of 21 days.[37,38]

● HEART VALVE HEMOLYSIS

DEFINITION AND HISTORY

Anemia arising after cardiac valve replacement was first described in 1954,[54] soon after corrective valvular surgery was initiated. This anemia was subsequently shown to be caused by erythrocyte shearing and fragmentation as the red cells traversed the turbulent flow through or around the prosthetic valve.[55] Since then, prevention of irreversible red cell injury has been a goal when designing new prostheses; as a result, the incidence of significant valve-associated hemolysis has declined from 5% to 15% in the 1960s and 1970s[56,57] to less than 1% with newer-generation prostheses.[58] However, compensated hemolysis can occur with any type of valve prosthesis and can be detected in almost every patient when assayed using appropriate methods.[59,60] However, artificial valves are not the only cause. Intravascular hemolysis can be seen after mitral valve repair[61] and wrap aortoplasty,[62] in unoperated patients with native valvular disease[56] and hypertrophic obstructive cardiomyopathy,[63] and with mechanical circulatory assist devices.[64] In fact, much engineering work using hemolysis prediction models in computational fluid dynamics is being done to predict a given assist device's potential hemolytic risk.[65]

EPIDEMIOLOGY

A variety of factors can increase the chance of valvular hemolysis: the presence of central or paravalvular regurgitation,[57,66] placement of small valve prostheses with resultant high transvalvular pressure gradients,[57] and regurgitation because of bioprosthetic valve failure, seen especially when the valve is more than 10 to 15 years old.[66] Patients with ball-and-cage valves,[59] bileaflet valves versus tilting disk valves,[67] mechanical valve prostheses versus xenograft tissue prostheses,[68] and double-valve as compared with single-valve replacement[67] are more likely to experience clinically significant hemolysis. Some studies have found no difference in the degree of hemolysis when comparing aortic and mitral valve prostheses,[60,67] whereas others have found that the aortic location is associated with slightly greater hemolysis than the mitral location.[69-71]

ETIOLOGY AND PATHOGENESIS

Valve-related hemolysis occurs when red cells are exposed to the shearing stresses created by turbulent blood flow through and around a valve prosthesis, impaction against foreign surfaces or cardiac structures such as the wall of the atrial appendage,[66] or large pressure fluctuations between cardiac chambers. A transvalvular pressure gradient of more than 50 torr can generate shearing forces exceeding 4000 dynes/cm², more than the 3000 dynes/cm² usually needed to cause red cell fragmentation.[72] In a study looking at malfunctioning mitral valve prostheses, sophisticated computer modeling using transesophageal echocardiography demonstrated a maximal shear value of 6000 dynes/cm² when the regurgitant jet was divided by a solid structure such as a loose suture or dehisced annuloplasty ring. A maximal shear rate of 4500 dynes/cm² was found when the regurgitant jet was suddenly decelerated by a solid structure like the left atrial appendage or when the blood was regurgitated through a small orifice (<2 mm in diameter) such as a leaflet perforation or a paravalvular leak.[66] Lack of endothelialization of the prosthetic ring may contribute to the severity of hemolysis after valve repair or replacement, but it is unclear if this is primary or secondary to the high-velocity jet of blood preventing fibrous incorporation of the prosthetic materials.[66,73] Similarly, lack of endothelialization of the Teflon patch can result in clinically significant hemolysis necessitating reoperation after repair of a ventricular septal defect.[74] These sorts of surface interactions depends more directly on the area of the contact surface and the time of exposure.[75]

CLINICAL FEATURES

Patients with valve-induced hemolysis can present with symptoms caused by anemia or congestive heart failure, pallor, icterus, and dark urine (described variously as red, brown, or black). Urine excreted during periods of physical activity may be darker than that excreted at rest.[76] Similarly, hemolysis can be exacerbated by supraventricular tachycardia or other tachyarrhythmias and regress once normal sinus rhythm is restored.[77] Anecdotally, some patients with severe valve hemolysis complain of chest pain subsequently proven to be caused by esophageal spasm, and one can speculate that the cause is nitric oxide depletion such as that reported in paroxysmal nocturnal hemoglobinuria.[78]

LABORATORY FEATURES

Helpful laboratory studies include review of the blood film, which will reveal moderate poikilocytosis, schistocytosis, and polychromasia (Fig. 22-1). The red cells are usually normochromic and normocytic

TABLE 22–2. Severity of Prosthetic Valve Hemolysis

	Mild	Moderate	Severe
Hemosiderinuria	Present	Present	Marked
Hemoglobinuria	Absent	Absent	Absent
Schistocytosis (%)	<1	>1	>>1
Reticulocytosis (%)	<5	>5	>>5
Haptoglobin	Decreased	Absent	Absent
LDH (U/L)	<500	>500	>>500

LDH, lactate dehydrogenase.

Data from Eyster E, Rothchild J, Mychajliw O. Chronic intravascular hemolysis after aortic valve replacement. *Circulation.* 1971 Oct;44(4):657-665.

but can occasionally be hypochromic and microcytic as a result of longstanding urinary iron loss[61] and increased erythropoiesis caused by ongoing hemolysis.[62] The reticulocyte count, urine hemosiderin, plasma hemoglobin, and serum levels of total and indirect bilirubin and LDH can be elevated, whereas the serum haptoglobin will be depressed. Both the number of schistocytes in the blood[61,64] and the elevation of LDH[64,65,79,80] correlate with the severity of hemolysis. Hemoglobinuria is usually seen only in those with particularly severe hemolysis and high LDH levels. There is no correlation between the severity of hemolysis and bilirubin levels, however, and whether the reticulocyte count is helpful in assessing the severity of hemolysis is controversial.[64,65] The aforementioned laboratory tests can be used as a means to determine the degree of hemolysis and to help guide management (Table 22-2).[64]

Red cell labeling studies demonstrate that erythrocyte lifespan is markedly shortened to between 6 and 9 days.[74,76] Measurement of erythrocyte creatine, a relatively simple but not yet widely available assay, can be performed in lieu of red cell labeling studies. Young erythrocytes contain much higher levels of creatine than older cells. Thus, an increase in erythrocyte creatine represents shortened red cell survival and is significantly correlated with total peak flow velocity across the valve and the severity of any associated hemolysis.[81] When performed, marrow aspiration will show erythroid hyperplasia.[75,76] As a result of hemosiderin deposition, magnetic resonance imaging of the kidneys reveal reduced signal intensity of the renal cortex compared with the medulla on T1- and T2-weighted images, both with and without gadolinium enhancement.[82]

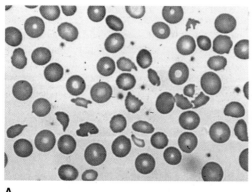
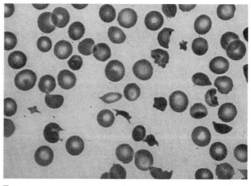

A   B

Figure 22–1. A and **B.** Two cases of fragmentation hemolytic anemia as a result of heart valve hemolysis. The red cell shape abnormalities are varied and characteristic of fragmentation hemolysis, although they are not specific for the cause. *(Reproduced with permission from Lichtman MA, Shafer MS, Felgar RE, et al: Lichtman's Atlas of Hematology 2016. New York, NY: McGraw Hill; 2017.)*

DIFFERENTIAL DIAGNOSIS

Factors that can promote valve-associated hemolysis or worsen the resultant anemia include iron deficiency (Chap. 11), because anemia increases cardiac output and shear stress and iron-poor red cells are more fragile than normal; folate deficiency (Chap. 9) arising from increased erythropoiesis; anemia of chronic disease because of endocarditis; anticoagulant-induced gastrointestinal hemorrhage; and increased cardiac output as a consequence of strenuous physical exertion.[78]

THERAPY

Appropriate therapy for hemolytic anemia arising from valvular dysfunction consists of iron and folate replacement (if deficient) and surgical repair or replacement of the malfunctioning prosthesis (if indicated).[83] Poor surgical candidates with perivalvular leaks may benefit from percutaneous closure with an Amplatzer occluder device.[84] Adjunctive measures to be tried include β-blockade to slow the velocity of the circulation,[85] erythropoietin therapy to stimulate erythropoiesis further,[86] and pentoxifylline therapy to increase the deformability of red cells.[87]

Although some authors have not found the use of pentoxifylline to be beneficial,[88] several case reports have described amelioration of valve-related hemolysis and resultant decreased need for red cell transfusion in patients receiving pentoxifylline.[89-91] A prospective study of 40 individuals with double (mitral and aortic) valve replacements randomized patients to receive either no treatment or pentoxifylline 400 mg orally three times daily for 120 days. The group that received pentoxifylline had significantly higher hemoglobin and haptoglobin levels and significantly lower LDH, total and indirect bilirubin, and corrected reticulocyte levels after 4 months of treatment. Of the nine patients with severe hemolysis (LDH >1500 U/L), six individuals had amelioration or complete resolution of their disease, but three patients' hemolysis persisted unchecked, suggesting that pentoxifylline therapy is beneficial in more than 60% of those with valve-related hemolysis.[92]

Between 15% and 30% of patients develop black pigment gallstones after valve surgery, the majority occurring within 6 months of the procedure. Whether this is a result of acute hemolysis associated with use of the heart-lung machine[93] or chronic hemolysis because of the valve replacement itself[94,95] is uncertain; however, therapy with ursodeoxycholic acid 600 mg daily beginning 1 week before surgery significantly decreases the incidence of gallstone formation from approximately 29% in those who were left untreated to approximately 8% (P < .01).[96]

COURSE AND PROGNOSIS

Evidence of hemolysis can be seen within days[60] or weeks[64,74,76] after valve surgery. If reoperation is required, reported mortality rates range between 0% and 6%,[75,97] and hemolytic anemia can occasionally recur.[60,97]

● OTHER CAUSES OF NONIMMUNE HEMOLYSIS

MARCH HEMOGLOBINURIA

In 1881, Fleischer described a German soldier in whom hemoglobinuria was brought on by marching.[98] Although usually reported in young men, no doubt explained by their more frequent participation in severe and prolonged exertion, it can also be seen in women.[99,100] The presenting complaint is passage of dark urine immediately after physical exertion in the upright position, occasionally accompanied by nausea,

abdominal cramps, aching in the back or legs, a "stitch in the side," or a burning feeling in the soles of the feet. Physical examination is usually unrevealing, although hepatosplenomegaly and transient jaundice have been rarely reported.[101]

Davidson proved definitively in 1969 that march hemoglobinuria is caused by red cell trauma within the vessels of the soles of the feet, and its severity is influenced by the hardness of the running surface, the distance run, the heaviness of the athlete's stride, and the protective adequacy of the footwear.[101] In addition, the condition could be prevented by using padded insoles, a finding later substantiated by other authors.[102,103] Hemoglobinuria has also been seen after other types of trauma in activities as diverse as repetitive slapping of the forehead,[104] karate exercises,[105] basketball followed by congo drum playing,[106] and kendo (a Japanese martial art in which heavily padded combatants strike each other repeatedly with bamboo swords).[99]

Because the estimated quantity of blood hemolyzed in an average paroxysm is only 6 to 40 mL, anemia is uncommon and if present is usually mild[101]; however, repeated episodes can cause iron deficiency, which may lead to or accentuate anemia (Chap. 11). Morphologic evidence of red cell damage is not seen, although one patient was found to have poikilocytes and occasional "four-leaf clover" cells after exercise.[107] Renal damage is also not commonly seen, but cases of acute tubular necrosis and resultant acute renal insufficiency have been described.[108-111]

KASABACH-MERRITT PHENOMENON

First described in 1940,[112] the Kasabach-Merritt phenomenon is a syndrome that usually develops in early childhood and is characterized by thrombocytopenia, MAHA, consumptive coagulopathy, and hypofibrinogenemia caused by an enlarging kaposiform hemangioendothelioma or tufted angioma.[113] Kaposiform hemangioendotheliomas are highly aggressive, vascular tumors that occur equally in males and females and show little tendency to resolve spontaneously. They can be locally invasive but have never been reported to metastasize.[114] Complications can include hemothorax or pericardial effusion.[114,115] It is postulated that endothelial cell abnormalities and vascular stasis lead to activation of platelets and the coagulation cascade within the tumor's vessels, with subsequent depletion of both platelets and clotting factors. MAHA results from mechanical trauma sustained by the erythrocytes traversing the tumor's abnormal, partially thrombosed vascular channels.[116]

Although numerous therapies are used, the mortality rate of Kasabach-Merritt phenomenon can be as high as 30%.[117] Even though surgical resection is always followed by normalization of hematologic parameters, many lesions are too large to be resected without severe disfigurement. Other treatments include glucocorticoids, interferon-α, antifibrinolytic agents, and the antiplatelet agents ticlopidine and aspirin, low-molecular-weight heparin, embolization, radiation, laser therapy, and chemotherapy using vincristine, cyclophosphamide, actinomycin D, or methotrexate.[113,114,116,118,119] Intralesion injections of absolute ethanol were reported in 2014 to be effective in eight pediatric patients.[120]

MISCELLANEOUS

MAHA has also been seen in malignant systemic hypertension, pulmonary hypertension, giant cavernous hemangiomas of the liver,[121] and various vasculitides, including Wegener granulomatosis[122,123] and giant cell arteritis.[124] Osmotically induced hemolysis has occurred when distilled water was used as an irrigant during transurethral resection of the prostate[125] or inadvertently used as a dialysate.[126]

REFERENCES

1. Stahnke E. Über das Verhalten der Blutplättchen bei Eklampsie. *Zentralbl Gynakol.* 1922;46:391.

2. Pritchard JA, Weisman R Jr, Ratnoff OD, et al. Intravascular hemolysis, thrombocytopenia and other hematologic abnormalities associated with severe toxemia of pregnancy. *N Engl J Med.* 1954;250:89.

3. Goodlin RC, Cotton DB, Haesslein HC. Severe edema-proteinuria-hypertension gestosis. *Am J Obstet Gynecol.* 1978;132:595.

4. Weinstein L. Syndrome of hemolysis, elevated liver enzymes, and low platelet count: a severe consequence of hypertension in pregnancy. *Am J Obstet Gynecol.* 1982;142:159.

5. Rahman TM, Wendon J. Severe hepatic dysfunction in pregnancy. *Q J Med.* 2002; 95:343.

6. Rath W, Faridi A, Dudenhausen JW. HELLP syndrome. *J Perinat Med.* 2000;28:249.

7. Martin JN Jr, Magann EF, Blake PG, et al. Analysis of 454 pregnancies with severe preeclampsia/eclampsia HELLP syndrome using the 3-class system of classification. *Am J Obstet Gynecol.* 1993;68:386.

8. Sibai BM, Ramadan MK, Usta I, et al. Maternal morbidity and mortality in 442 pregnancies with hemolysis, elevated liver enzymes, and low platelets (HELLP syndrome). *Am J Obstet Gynecol.* 19;93169:1000.

9. Zusterzeel PLM, Visser W, Blom HJ, et al. Methylenetetrahydrofolate reductase polymorphisms in preeclampsia and the HELLP syndrome. *Hypertens Pregnancy.* 2000;19:299.

10. Haram K, Mortensen JH, Nagy B. Genetic aspects of preeclampsia and the HELLP syndrome. *J Pregnancy.* 2014;2014:910751.

11. Vaught AJ, Braunstein EM, Jasem J, et al. Germline mutations in the alternative pathway of complement predispose to HELLP syndrome. *JCI Insight.* 2018;3:1.

12. Zhou Y, McMaster M, Woo K, et al. Vascular endothelial growth factor ligands and receptors that regulate human cytotrophoblast survival are dysregulated in severe preeclampsia and hemolysis, elevated liver enzymes, and low platelets syndrome. *Am J Pathol.* 2002;160:1405.

13. Knerr I, Beinder E, Rascher W. Syncytin, a novel human endogenous retroviral gene in human placenta: evidence for its dysregulation in preeclampsia and HELLP syndrome. *Am J Obstet Gynecol.* 2002;186:210.

14. Sovio U, Gaccioli F, Cook E, et al. Prediction of preeclampsia using the soluble fms-like tyrosine kinase 1 to placental growth factor ratio: a prospective cohort study of unselected nulliparous women. *Hypertension.* 2017;69:731.

15. Levine RJ, Maynard SE, Qian C, et al. Circulating angiogenic factors and the risk of preeclampsia. *N Engl J Med.* 2004;350:672.

16. Widmer M, Villar J, Benigni A, et al. Mapping the theories of preeclampsia and the role of angiogenic factors: a systematic review. *Obstet Gynecol.* 2007;109:168.

17. Mutter WP, Karumanchi SA. Molecular mechanisms of preeclampsia. *Microvasc Res.* 2008;75:1.

18. Kim YN, Lee DS, Jeong DH, et al. The relationship of the level of circulating antiangiogenic factors to the clinical manifestations of preeclampsia. *Prenat Diagn.* 2009;29:464.

19. Magann EF, Martin JN Jr. Twelve steps to optimal management of HELLP syndrome. *Clin Obstet Gynecol.* 1999;42:532.

20. Thiagarajah S, Bourgeois FJ, Harbert GM, et al. Thrombocytopenia in preeclampsia: associated abnormalities and management principles. *Am J Obstet Gynecol.* 1984;150:1.

21. Barton JR, Riely CA, Adamed TA, et al. Hepatic histopathologic condition does not correlate with laboratory abnormalities in HELLP syndrome (hemolysis, elevated liver enzymes, and low platelet count). *Am J Obstet Gynecol.* 1992;167:1538.

22. De Boer K, Büller HR, Ten Cate JW, et al. Coagulation studies in the syndrome of haemolysis, elevated liver enzymes and low platelets. *Br J Obstet Gynaecol.* 1991;98:42.

23. Thorp JM Jr, Gilbert GC II, Moake JL, et al. von Willebrand factor multimeric levels and patterns in patients with severe preeclampsia. *Obstet Gynecol.* 1990;75:163.

24. Lattuada A, Rossi E, Calzarossa C, et al. Mild to moderate reduction of a von Willebrand factor cleaving protease (ADAMTS13) in pregnant women with HELLP microangiopathic syndrome. *Haematologica.* 2003;88:1029.

25. Molvarec A, Rigo J, Boze T, et al. Increased plasma von Willebrand factor antigen levels but normal von Willebrand factor cleaving protease (ADAMTS13) activity in preeclampsia. *Thromb Haemost.* 2009;101:305.

26. Lopez JA, Chen J, Ozpolot T, et al. Thrombotic thrombocytopenic purpura and related thrombotic microangiopathies. In: C.S. Kitchens, C.M. Kessler, B.A. Konkle, et al, eds. *Consultative Hemostasis and Thrombosis.* 4th ed. Elsevier; 2019:448-472.

27. Thomas EA, Copplestone JA, Dubbins PA, et al. The radiologist cries "HELLP"! *Br J Radiol.* 1991;64:964.

28. Rehberg JF, Briery CM, Hudson WT, et al. Thrombotic thrombocytopenic purpura masquerading as hemolysis, elevated liver enzymes, low platelets (HELLP) syndrome in late pregnancy. *Obstet Gynecol.* 2006;108:817.

29. Fonseca JE, Mendez F, Catano C. Dexamethasone treatment does not improve the outcome of women with HELLP syndrome: a double-blind, placebo-controlled, randomized clinical trial. *Am J Obstet Gynecol.* 2005;193:1591.

30. Burwick RM, Feinberg BB. Eculizumab for the treatment of preeclampsia/HELLP syndrome. *Placenta.* 2012;34:201.

31. Reubinoff BE, Schenker JG. HELLP syndrome—a syndrome of hemolysis, elevated liver enzymes and low platelet count—complicating preeclampsia-eclampsia. *Int J Gynaecol Obstet.* 1991;36:95.

32. Harms K, Rath W, Herting E, et al. Maternal hemolysis, elevated liver enzymes, low platelet count, and neonatal outcome. *Am J Perinatol.* 1995;12:1.

33. Sullivan CA, Magann EF, Perry KG Jr, et al. The recurrence risk of the syndrome of hemolysis, elevated liver enzymes, and low platelets: subsequent pregnancy outcome and long term prognosis. *Am J Obstet Gynecol.* 1995;172:125.

34. van Pampus MG, Wolf H, Mayruhu G, et al. Long-term follow-up in patients with a history of (H)ELLP syndrome. *Hypertens Pregnancy.* 2001;20:15.

35. Brain MC, Dacie JV, Hourihane DO. Microangiopathic haemolytic anemia: the possible role of vascular lesions in pathogenesis. *Br J Haematol.* 1962;8:358.

36. Kupers EC, Friedman NB, Lee S, et al. Metastatic hemangiopericytoma associated with microangiopathic hemolytic anemia: review and report of a case. *J Am Geriatr Soc.* 1975;23:411.

37. Antman KH, Skarin AT, Mayer RJ, et al. Microangiopathic hemolytic anemia and cancer: a review. *Medicine (Baltimore).* 1979;58:377.

38. Lohrmann H-P, Adam W, Heymer B, et al. Microangiopathic hemolytic anemia in metastatic carcinoma. Report of eight cases. *Ann Intern Med.* 1973;79:368.

39. Gordon SG, Cross BA. A factor X-activating cysteine protease from malignant tissue. *J Clin Invest.* 1981;67:1665.

40. Wahrenbrock M, Borsig L, Le D, et al. Selectin-mucin interactions as a probable molecular explanation for the association of Trousseau syndrome with mucinous adenocarcinomas. *J Clin Invest.* 2003;112:853.

41. Lynch EC, Bakken CL, Casey TH, et al. Microangiopathic hemolytic anemia in carcinoma of the stomach. *Gastroenterology.* 1967;52:88.

42. Mandernach MW, Kitchens CS. Disseminated intravascular coagulation. In: Kitchens CS, Kessler CM, Konkle BA, et al, eds. *Consultative Hemostasis and Thrombosis.* 4th ed. Elsevier; 2019:207-225.

43. Reddy NM, Hall SW, MacKintosh R. Partial thromboplastin time: prediction of adverse events and poor prognosis by low abnormal values. *Arch Intern Med.* 1999;159:2706.

44. Tripodi A, Chantarangkul V, Martinelli I, et al. A shortened activated partial thromboplastin time is associated with the risk of venous thromboembolism. *Blood.* 2004;104:3631.

45. Lippi G, Favaloro EJ. Activated partial thromboplastin time: new tricks for an old dogma. *Semin Thromb Hemost.* 2008;34:604.

46. Oleksowicz L, Bhagwati N, DeLeon-Fernandez M. Deficient activity of von Willebrand's factor-cleaving protease in patients with disseminated malignancies. *Cancer Res.* 1999;59:2244.

47. Fontana S, Gerritsen HE, Hovinga JK, et al. Microangiopathic haemolytic anaemia in metastasizing malignant tumours is not associated with a severe deficiency of the von Willebrand factor-cleaving protease. *Br J Haematol.* 2001;113:100.

48. Hyun J, Kim HK, Kim JE, et al. Correlation between plasma activity of ADAMTS13 and coagulopathy, and prognosis in disseminated intravascular coagulation. *Thromb Res.* 2009;124:75.

49. Bernardo A, Ball C, Nolasco L, et al. Effects of inflammatory cytokines on the release and cleavage of the endothelial cell-derived ultra-large von Willebrand factor multimers under flow. *Blood.* 2004;104:100.

50. Ellis LD, Westerman MP. Autoimmune hemolytic anemia and cancer. *JAMA.* 1965;193:962.

51. Blake-Haskins JA, Lechleider RJ, Kreitman RJ. Thrombotic microangiopathy with targeted cancer agents. *Clin Cancer Res.* 2011;17:5858.

52. Murao S, Yamakawa K. A systematic summary of systemic reviews on anticoagulant therapy in sepsis. *J Clin Med.* 2019;8:E1869.

53. Kayatani H, Matsuo K, Ueda Y, et al. Pulmonary tumor thrombotic microangiopathy diagnosed antemortem and treated with combination chemotherapy. *Intern Med.* 2012;51:2767.

54. Rose JC, Hufnagel CA, Fries ED, et al. The hemodynamic alterations produced by plastic valvular prosthesis for severe aortic insufficiency in man. *J Clin Invest.* 1954;33:891.

55. Rodgers BM, Sabiston DC Jr. Hemolytic anemia following prosthetic valve replacement. *Circulation.* 1969;39:155.

56. Marsh GW, Lewis SM. Cardiac haemolytic anaemia. *Semin Hematol.* 1969;6:133.

57. Kloster FE. Diagnosis and management of complications of prosthetic heart valves. *Am J Cardiol.* 1975;35:872.

58. Iguro Y, Moriyama Y, Yamaoka A, et al. Clinical experience of 473 patients with the Omnicarbon prosthetic heart valve. *J Heart Valve Dis.* 1999;8:674.

59. Eyster E, Rothchild J, Mychajliw O. Chronic intravascular hemolysis after aortic valve replacement. *Circulation.* 1971;44:657.

60. Crexells C, Aerichide N, Bonny Y, et al. Factors influencing hemolysis in valve prosthesis. *Am Heart J.* 1972;84:161.

61. Demirsoy E, Yilmaz O, Sirin G, et al. Hemolysis after mitral valve repair; a report of five cases and literature review. *J Heart Valve Dis.* 2008;17:24.

62. Davison MA, Morton DM, Popoff AM, et al. Hemolysis following wrap aortoplasty for type A aortic dissection repair: case report and review of the literature. *Vasc Med.* 2018;23:400.

63. Kubo T, Kitaoka H, Terauchi Y, et al. Hemolytic anemia in a patient with hypertrophic obstructive cardiomyopathy. *J Cardiol.* 2010;55:125.

64. Olia SE, Maul TM, Antaki JF, et al. Mechanical blood trauma in assisted circulation: sublethal RBC damage preceding hemolysis. *Int J Artif Organs.* 2016;39:150.

65. Yu H, Engel S, Janiga G, et al. A review of hemolysis prediction models for computational fluid dynamics. *Artif Organs.* 2017;41:603.

66. Garcia MJ, Vandervoort P, Stewart WJ, et al. Mechanisms of hemolysis with mitral prosthetic regurgitation. *J Am Coll Cardiol.* 1996;27:399.

67. Skoularigis J, Essop MR, Skudicky D, et al. Frequency and severity of intravascular hemolysis after left-sided cardiac valve replacement with Medtronic Hall and St. Jude

Medical prostheses, and influence of prosthetic type, position, size and number. *Am J Cardiol.* 1993;71:587.

68. Chang H, Lin FY, Hung CR, et al. Chronic intravascular hemolysis after valvular surgery. *J Formos Med Assoc.* 1990;89:880.

69. Yacoub MH, Keeling DH. Chronic haemolysis following insertion of ball valve prostheses. *Br Heart J.* 1968;30:676.

70. Falk RH, Mackinnon J, Wainscoat J, et al. Intravascular haemolysis after valve replacement: comparative study between Starr-Edwards (ball valve) and Bjork-Shiley (disc valve) prosthesis. *Thorax.* 1979;34:746.

71. Febres-Roman PR, Bourg WC, Crone RA, et al. Chronic intravascular hemolysis after aortic valve replacement with Ionescu-Shiley xenograft: comparative study with Bjork-Shiley prosthesis. *Am J Cardiol.* 1980;46:735.

72. Nevaril CG, Lynch EC, Alfrey CP, et al. Erythrocyte damage and destruction induced by shearing stress. *J Lab Clin Med.* 1968;71:784.

73. Cerfolio RJ, Orszulak TA, Daly RC, et al. Reoperation for hemolytic anaemia complicating mitral valve repair. *Eur J Cardiothorac Surg.* 1997;11:479.

74. Sayed HM, Dacie JV, Handley DA, et al. Haemolytic anaemia of mechanical origin after open heart surgery. *Thorax.* 1961;16:356.

75. Leverett LB, Hellums JD, Alfrey CP, et al. Red blood cell damage by shear stress. *Biophys J.* 1972;12:257.

76. Sears DA, Crosby WH. Intravascular hemolysis due to intracardiac prosthetic devices. *Am J Med.* 1965;39:341.

77. Papadogiannakis A, Xydakis D, Sfakianaki M, et al. An unusual cause of severe hyperkalemia in a dialysis patient. *J Cardiovasc Med (Hagerstown).* 2007;8:541.

78. Pu JJ, Brodsky RA. Paroxysmal nocturnal hemoglobinuria from bench to bedside. *Clin Transl Sci.* 2011;4:219.

79. Myhre E, Rasmussen K, Andersen A. Serum lactic dehydrogenase activity in patients with prosthetic heart valves: a parameter of intravascular hemolysis. *Am Heart J.* 1970;80:463.

80. Thompson ME, Lewis JH, Prokolab FL, et al. Indexes of intravascular hemolysis quantification of coagulation factors, and platelet survival in patients with porcine heterograft valves. *Am J Cardiol.* 1983;51:489.

81. Okumiya T, Ishikawa-Nishi M, Doi T, et al. Evaluation of intravascular hemolysis with erythrocyte creatine in patients with cardiac valve prostheses. *Chest.* 2004;125:2115.

82. Lee JW, Kim SH, Yoon CJ. Hemosiderin deposition on the renal cortex by mechanical hemolysis due to malfunctioning prosthetic cardiac valve: report of MR findings in two cases. *J Comput Assist Tomogr.* 1999;23:445.

83. Amidon TM, Chou TM, Rankin JS, et al. Mitral and aortic paravalvular leaks with hemolytic anemia. *Am Heart J.* 1993;125:122.

84. Shapira Y, Hirsch R, Kornowski R, et al. Percutaneous closure of perivalvular leaks with Amplatzer occluders: feasibility, safety, and short-term results. *J Heart Valve Dis.* 2007;16:305.

85. Okita Y, Miki S, Kusuhara K, et al. Propranolol for intractable hemolysis after open heart operation. *Ann Thorac Surg.* 1991;52:1158.

86. Shapira Y, Bairey O, Vatury M, et al. Erythropoietin can obviate the need for repeated heart valve replacement in high-risk patients with severe mechanical hemolytic anemia: case reports and literature review. *J Heart Valve Dis.* 2001;10:431.

87. Ward A, Clissold SP. Pentoxifylline. A review of its pharmacodynamic and pharmacokinetic properties, and its therapeutic efficacy. *Drugs.* 1987;34:50.

88. Okita Y, Miki S. Reply to the editor. *Ann Thorac Surg.* 1992;54:7.

89. Jim RT. New therapy for cardiac valve prosthesis caused by microangiopathic hemolytic anemia: a case report. *Hawaii Med J.* 1988;47:285.

90. Golino A, Stassano P, Spampinato N. Hemolysis after open heart operations [letter]. *Ann Thorac Surg.* 1992;54:1246.

91. Geller S, Gelber R. Pentoxifylline treatment for microangiopathic hemolytic anemia caused by mechanical heart valves. *Md Med J.* 1999;48:173.

92. Golbasi I, Turkay C, Timuragaoglu A, et al. The effect of pentoxifylline on haemolysis in patients with double cardiac prosthetic valves. *Acta Cardiol.* 2003;58:379.

93. Azemoto R, Tsuchiya Y, Ai T, et al. Does gallstone formation after open cardiac surgery result only from latent hemolysis by replaced valves? *Am J Gastroenterol.* 1996;91:2185.

94. Merendino KA, Manhas DR. Man-made gallstones: a new entity following cardiac valve replacement. *Ann Surg.* 1973;177:694.

95. Harrison EC, Roschke EJ, Meyers HI, et al. Cholelithiasis: a frequent complication of artificial heart valve replacement. *Am Heart J.* 1978;95:483.

96. Ai T, Azemoto R, Saisho H. Prevention of gallstones by ursodeoxycholic acid after cardiac surgery. *J Gastroenterol.* 2003;38:1071.

97. Lam BK, Cosgrove DM, Bhudia SK, et al. Hemolysis after mitral valve repair: mechanisms and treatment. *Ann Thorac Surg.* 2004;77:191.

98. Fleischer R. Ueber eine neue Form von Haemoglobinurie beim Menschen. *Berl Klin Wschr.* 1881;18:691.

99. Urabe M, Hara Y, Hokama A, et al. A female case of march hemoglobinuria induced by kendo (Japanese fencing) exercise. *Nippon Naika Gakkai Zasshi.* 1986;75:1657.

100. Gilligan A. March hemoglobinuria in a woman. *N Engl J Med.* 1950;243:944.

101. Davidson RJL. March or exertional haemoglobinuria. *Semin Hematol.* 1969;6:150.

102. Buckle RM. Exertional (march) haemoglobinuria: reduction of haemolytic episodes by use of Sorbo-rubber insoles in shoes. *Lancet.* 1965;68:1136.

103. Sagov SE. March hemoglobinuria treated with rubber insoles: two case reports. *J Am Coll Health Assoc.* 1970;19:146.

104. Ensor CW, Barrett JO. Paroxysmal haemoglobinuria of traumatic origin. *Med Chir Trans.* 1903;86:165.

105. Streeton JA. Traumatic haemoglobinuria caused by karate exercises. *Lancet.* 1967;2:191.

106. Schwartz KA, Flessa HC. March hemoglobinuria. Report of a case after basketball and congo drum playing. *Ohio State Med J.* 1973;69:448.

107. Watson EM, Fischer LC. Paroxysmal "march" haemoglobinuria with a report of a case. *Am J Clin Pathol.* 1935;5:151.

108. Pollard TD, Weiss IW. Acute tubular necrosis in a patient with march hemoglobinuria. *N Engl J Med.* 1970;283:803.

109. Susa S, Dumovic B, Pantovic R. March hemoglobinuria associated with acute renal failure. *Vojnosanit Pregl.* 1972;29:407.

110. Ciko Z, Radojicic B, Lazic D. Pathogenesis of acute renal insufficiency in march hemoglobinuria. *Vojnosanit Pregl.* 1973;30:198.

111. Yashpal M, Abdulkader TA, Chatterji JC. Acute tubular necrosis in march haemoglobinuria. *J Assoc Physicians India.* 1970;28:145.

112. Kasabach HH, Merritt KK. Capillary hemangioma with extensive purpura: report of a case. *Am J Dis Child.* 1940;59:1063.

113. Haisley-Royster C, Enjolras O, Frieden IJ, et al. Kasabach-Merritt phenomenon: a retrospective study of treatment with vincristine. *J Pediatr Hematol Oncol.* 2002;24:459.

114. San Miguel FL, Spurbeck W, Budding C, et al. Kaposiform hemangioendothelioma: a rare cause of spontaneous hemothorax in infancy. Review of the literature. *J Pediatr Surg.* 2008;43:E37.

115. Walsh MA, Carcao M, Pope E, et al. Kaposiform hemangioendothelioma presenting antenatally with a pericardial effusion. *J Pediatr Hematol Oncol.* 2008;30:761.

116. Ortel TL, Onorato JJ, Bedrosian CL, et al. Antifibrinolytic therapy in the management of the Kasabach Merritt syndrome. *Am J Hematol.* 1988;29:44.

117. Esterly NB. Kasabach-Merritt syndrome in infants. *J Am Acad Dermatol.* 1983;8:504.

118. Hall GW. Kasabach-Merritt syndrome: pathogenesis and management. *Br J Haematol.* 2001;112:851.

119. Hauer J, Graubner U, Konstantopoulos N, et al. Effective treatment of kaposiform hemangioendotheliomas associated with Kasabach-Merritt phenomenon using four-drug regimen. *Pediatr Blood Cancer.* 2006;49:852.

120. Shen W, Cui J, Chen J, et al. Treating kaposiform hemangioendothelioma with Kasabach-Merritt phenomenon by intralesional injection of absolute ethanol. *J Carniofac Surg.* 2014;25:2188.

121. Shimizu M, Miura J, Itoh H, et al. Hepatic giant cavernous hemangioma with microangiopathic hemolytic anemia and consumption coagulopathy. *Am J Gastroenterol.* 1990;85:1411.

122. Crummy CS, Perlin E, Moquin RB. Microangiopathic hemolytic anemia in Wegener's granulomatosis. *Am J Med.* 1971;51:544.

123. Jordan JM, Manning M, Allen NB. Multiple unusual manifestations of Wegener's granulomatosis: breast mass, microangiopathic hemolytic anemia, consumptive coagulopathy, and low erythrocyte sedimentation rate. *Arthritis Rheum.* 1986;29:1527.

124. Zauber NP, Echikson AB. Giant cell arteritis and microangiopathic hemolytic anemia. *Am J Med.* 1982;73:928.

125. Chen SS, Lin AT, Chen KK, et al. Hemolysis in transurethral resection of the prostate using distilled water as the irrigant. *J Chin Med Assoc.* 2006;69:270.

126. Pendergrast JM, Hiadunewich MA, Richardson RM. Hemolysis due to inadvertent hemodialysis against distilled water: perils of bedside dialysate preparation. *Crit Care Med.* 2006;34:2866.

127. Stratford EC, Tanaka KR. Microangiopathic hemolytic anemia in metastatic carcinoma. Report of a case and biochemical studies. *Arch Intern Med.* 1965;116:346.

128. Davis S, Rambotti P, Grignani F, et al. Microangiopathic hemolytic anemia and pulmonary small-cell carcinoma [letter]. *Ann Intern Med.* 1985;103:638.

129. Atkins JN, Muss HB. Case report: schistocytes in erythroleukemia. *Am J Med Sci.* 1985;289:110.

CHAPTER 23
ERYTHROCYTE DISORDERS AS A RESULT OF TOXIC AGENTS

Paul C. Herrmann

SUMMARY

Erythrocyte disorders can be caused by a wide variety of toxic agents. Whereas some erythrocyte toxins damage red blood cells through well-defined mechanisms, others have mechanisms that are incompletely defined or for which there is complexity involving multiple simultaneous pathways. The well-defined mechanisms include neocytolysis, damage from oxidation, damage to structural proteins, damage to erythrocyte membranes, and direct damage to metabolic pathways. Incompletely defined mechanisms are responsible for toxicity from nanoparticles and metals with broad biological activity spectra such as lead. A table of other toxins not specifically described in the text is included.

● ERYTHROCYTE TOXINS ACTING THROUGH WELL-DEFINED MECHANISMS

Certain toxins cause erythrocyte damage through clearly defined mechanisms, in some cases affecting the processes or functions of single subcellular systems. Other mechanisms causing erythrocyte damage within the context of enzyme deficiency, unstable hemoglobins, or immune dysfunction are discussed in Chaps. 16, 18, and 26. The present chapter deals with cell destruction from toxic agents that are not discussed elsewhere within this textbook.

DAMAGE FROM OXIDATION

The earth's oxidizing atmosphere, although necessary for metabolic processes, also provides a ubiquitous source of potential oxidizing toxins. Oxidative damage affects a number of the erythrocyte structural and functional elements that tend to lead to red cell destruction through the final common pathway of eryptosis.[1]

Neocytolysis

Astronauts experience significant anemia after space flight in the presence of normal or elevated ambient oxygen concentration.[2] Neocytolysis

describes this phenomenon of rapid hemolysis observed after transition from acclimated hypoxic or hypobaric environments to normoxic atmospheric conditions. Observations of altered erythropoietin levels and research with radiolabeled erythrocytes from astronauts suggest there is selective hemolysis of young erythrocytes less than 12 days old.[3] In addition to space flight, neocytolysis has been invoked to explain the anemia resulting when high-altitude dwellers relocate to sea level and has also been demonstrated within the first neonatal week of life.[4,5] Although long a mechanistic mystery, neocytolysis has recently been convincingly demonstrated to be induced by intrinsically generated toxic agents within the cell. Reticulocytes generated within hypoxic or hypobaric environments contain expanded mitochondria and low levels of catalase. In the presence of suddenly increased oxygen levels, oxidant radicals are rapidly generated by the expanded mitochondria at levels, which overwhelm the decreased catalase enzyme activity, resulting in cell lysis.[5]

Oxygen Gas

Oxygen is a powerful oxidizing agent. Fortunately, quantum mechanical properties of the oxygen molecule prevent spontaneous oxidation of biological membranes under normal atmospheric conditions.[6] However, when bound to hemoglobin, oxygen has significantly different quantum mechanical properties and occasionally, an exceptionally reactive superoxide molecule escapes.[7] It is estimated that 2% to 3% of total hemoglobin would be oxidized daily in the absence of enzyme systems to protect against escaped superoxide.[8,9] Hemolytic anemia can occur when ambient oxygen concentration is increased markedly, presumably overwhelming these protective mechanisms.[1] Hyperbaric oxygenation has been associated with acute hemolysis.[10]

Chlorates and Chloramines

Sodium and potassium chlorate are oxidative drugs that produce methemoglobinemia, Heinz bodies, and hemolytic anemia.[11,12] Although it has been presumed that the mechanism of hemolysis is similar to that resulting from other oxidative drugs, enigmatically, no cases have been observed in patients deficient in glucose-6-phosphate dehydrogenase (G6PD). Hemolytic anemia with Heinz body formation has also occurred in patients undergoing dialysis when the water contained a substantial amount of chloramines. Oxidative damage to the red cells of these patients was demonstrated by the presence of Heinz bodies, a positive ascorbate-cyanide test result, and methemoglobinemia.[13,14]

Arsenic Hydride

Arsenic exposure is a major cause of anemia in regions with high environmental arsenic concentrations. Examples include Bangladesh's tainted water supply and areas of China where arsenic laden coal is used.[15] Arsine gas (arsenic hydride, AsH$_3$) is the most erythrotoxic form of arsenic, and inhalation of arsine gas is a well-recognized cause of hemolytic anemia.[16-18] Arsine is formed during many industrial processes, including the reaction of hydrogen with available arsenic compounds in metallurgical processes. The arsenic is usually a contaminant, so contact with arsenic compounds may not be apparent from the patient's history. The mechanism of erythrocyte damage by arsenic involves oxidation of sulfhydryl groups in the erythrocyte membrane and associated cytoskeleton. As expected, decreased levels of reduced glutathione in erythrocytes exposed to AsH$_3$ are observed.[19-21]

DAMAGE TO SKELETAL OR STRUCTURAL PROTEINS

A normal erythrocyte in liquid behaves physically as a drop of fluid because the flexible membrane allows the surface of the cell to rotate around the intracellular contents.[22] These fluidlike properties couple collisional energy between the erythrocyte membrane and the viscous hemoglobin solution within the cell, allowing dissipation of collisional energy through the entire cell and ultimately protecting the cell membrane.

Heat

Heat decreases erythrocyte resilience. When heated, the spectrin comprising the erythrocyte cytoskeleton denatures and, upon cooling, renatures into a rigid conformation. This rigidity prevents collisional energy dissipation as described earlier, making such cells particularly susceptible to membrane damage.[23,24] The ensuing damage to the erythrocyte membrane structure results in splenic sequestration and cell removal.[25] Gross hemoglobinemia was observed in 11 of 40 patients with second- and third-degree burns involving 15% to 65% of body surface area.[26] Within the first 24 hours after a burn, hemolytic anemia resulted. Blood heated to temperatures above 47°C demonstrated morphologically similar damage (Fig. 23-1A), consistent with increased osmotic and mechanical fragility caused by reduced erythrocyte resilance.[27,28]

Venom

Band 3 of the red cell membrane protein has dual functions related to ion exchange in addition to serving as an anchor of the cell membrane to the underlying cellular skeleton.[29] It appears disruption of the structural role of band 3 leads to cell lysis. Spider and scorpion bites occasionally are followed by hemolytic anemia and hemoglobinuria.[30-35] The spiders usually responsible are *Loxosceles laeta* and *Loxosceles recluse* with sphingomyelinase D as one of the causative toxins. This venom preferentially hydrolyzes band 3 of the red cell membrane protein.[36] In addition, bee[37,38] and wasp[39-41] stings as well as contact with caterpillar bristle from *Lonomia obliqua*[42] are associated with severe hemolysis.

DAMAGE TO THE ERYTHROCYTE MEMBRANE

The erythrocyte membrane serves as an important barrier holding hemoglobin intracellularly as well as protecting vascular and contiguous structures such as renal tubules from exposure to free hemoglobin. Hence, damage to the erythrocyte membrane is particularly problematic because it often leads to hemolysis.

Cytotoxins

One of the most intriguing mechanisms of membrane damage is that induced by a class of pore-forming cytotoxins found in marine invertebrate organisms including jelly fish (*Chironex fleckeri*),[43] sea anemones (*Stichodactyla helianthus*),[44] and echinoderms such as sea cucumbers (*Cucumaria echinata*).[45] X-ray crystallography reveals these toxins to be composed of proteins that associate together to span the erythrocyte membrane, forming an ion permeable pore.[46]

Hypotonic Lysis

When large amounts of distilled water gain access to the systemic circulation, either by IV injection or when used as an irrigating solution during surgery, hemolysis will occur.[47] Severe hemolysis may also result from water inhalation in near-drowing.[48] Occasionally, self-induced hypotonic lysis secondary to water intoxication from polydipsia in the setting of psychiatric illness or hazing rituals occurs.[49] In all cases, hemolysis follows expansion of the erythrocyte volume, transition to a spherical shape, and ultimately cell rupture when the erythrocyte volume exceeds that which can be encompassed by the cell membrane.[50]

DAMAGE TO METABOLIC PATHWAYS

As metabolic pathways are responsible for cell homeostasis, toxic agents that alter these pathways also alter erythrocyte homeostasis. Hence, although the metabolic mechanisms disrupted by a particular toxin may be rather simple, the effects of the toxin may be observed as damage to a number of the cell's structural and functional elements.

Copper

Erythrocyte damage has resulted from ingestion of copper sulfate in suicide attempts and from copper accumulation when hemodialysis fluid is contaminated by copper pipes.[51,52] Hemolysis in Wilson disease has been attributed to the elevated plasma copper levels characteristic of that disorder.[53-55] Spherocytic anemia with a hematocrit below 25% may be the presenting symptom (see Fig. 23-1A-C).[56] The pathogenesis may be related to oxidation of intracellular glutathione, hemoglobin, and NADPH (reduced form of nicotinamide adenine dinucleotide), along with inhibition of G6PD by copper.[57] However, the amount of copper required to inhibit G6PD is large. Copper, in much

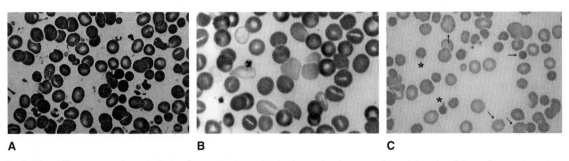

A   B   C

Figure 23–1. A. Blood film prepared at admission from a patient who had sustained a severe burn injury involving a large percentage of the body surface. Note the presence of normal erythrocytes (apparently from vessels not exposed to heat damage) along with populations of normocytic and microcytic spherocytes. In addition, there are numerous red cell fragments, some smaller than platelets. **B.** Blood film prepared from a patient exposed to arsenic hydride. Note the very pale red cells resulting from partial hemoglobin loss secondary to membrane damage. An extreme example, represented by the virtual ghost thinly rimmed with scant residual hemoglobin, can be found in the upper left-hand corner. **C.** Wilson disease. In this image from a patient with Wilson disease, there are numerous visible sequelae of oxidative damage caused by excess copper. The striking microspherocytosis indicates damage to the membrane. Damage to hemoglobin is demonstrated by the Heinz bodies projecting from red cells (*asterisks* show two examples). The *horizontal arrow* points to one of several spherocytes. The *vertical arrow* points to a macrocyte (reticulocyte). An occasional cell shows damage to both membrane and hemoglobin. The presence of echinocytes (*oblique arrows* show two examples) suggests that the liver is also affected. *(Part A & B, Reproduced with permission from Lichtman MA, Shafer MS, Felgar RE, et al: Lichtman's Atlas of Hematology 2016. New York, NY: McGraw Hill; 2017. Part C, Kindly provided by Barbara J. Bain, Imperial College, London, UK.)*

lower concentrations, inhibits pyruvate kinase, hexokinase, phosphogluconate dehydrogenase, phosphofructokinase, and phosphoglycerate kinase, suggesting the potential for a global metabolic insult.[58,59] Plasma exchange successfully prevents hemolytic anemia in Wilson disease.[60]

Formaldehyde

Leaching of formaldehyde from plastic used in water filters used for hemodialysis is also a cause of hemolytic anemia. The effect of the low levels of formaldehyde found in the water has not been mediated through a fixative effect but rather by inducing metabolic changes within the erythrocytes.[61]

● ERYTHROCYTE TOXINS ACTING THROUGH INCOMPLETELY DEFINED MECHANISMS

A variety of toxic agents cause erythrocyte disorder through poorly defined or multiple complex mechanisms. What follows is the description of a couple of erythrocyte-damaging agents and processes that, although not clearly defined, have mechanisms that are beginning to be elucidated. Ongoing research will likely clarify the complex processes involved in these described toxicities. Table 23-1 lists additional toxins described in isolated reports to cause hemolytic anemia, which are not further described within the chapter.

NANOPARTICLES

Nanoparticles are defined as inorganic particles with diameters between 1 and 100 nanometers.[62] Nanoparticles have been used in the glass and pottery trades for at least a millennium. Mesopotamian lustrous pottery glazes from the ninth century were based on dispersed nanoparticles.[63] Within the past few decades, there has been an explosion of interest in nanoparticles and related technology. There are a plethora of applications within diverse industries ranging from agriculture to cosmetics and pharmaceutical agents. Although nanoparticles are in common use, their toxicity is still in the early stages of investigation.[64] The major mechanisms of nanoparticle toxicity appear to result from the high surface area to volume ratio of the particles that become very active when composed of a compound with high catalytic potential along with the nanoparticles' propensity for adherence to, and crossing of, biological membranes.[65] One important sequela of nanoparticle exposure to blood is hemolysis. Research has demonstrated some unique features of this red cell toxicity, which varies based on composition, as well as size of the nanoparticles involved. Unexpectedly, the nanoparticle size dependence of the potential for hemolysis differs among various materials, with some materials demonstrating increasing toxicity with decreasing particle diameter, but other materials showing the highest toxicity from intermediate-sized particles.[66,67] In addition to the effects of size described earlier, there is toxicity seemingly caused by dissolution of the particles within the blood. This toxicity is clearly related to the chemical properties of elements and compounds present that are indistinguishable from those demonstrated by the same elements and compounds fully dissolved in solution.[68]

LEAD

Lead poisoning (plumbism) has been recognized since antiquity. The ingestion of beverages containing lead leached from highly soluble lead-based glazes or earthenware containers has been blamed for the decline and fall of the Roman aristocracy and is still an occasional cause of lead intoxication.[69] The distillation of alcohol in leaded flasks is another rare case of plumbism, although the practice was prohibited in 1723 by the Massachusetts Bay Colony after it was noticed that consumption of rum so distilled resulted in abdominal pain known as the "dry gripes." Among the earliest published descriptions of lead poisoning is a letter written in 1786 by Benjamin Franklin.[70]

Lead intoxication in children generally results from ingestion of flaking lead paint or chewing lead-painted articles. Lead poisoning tends to be more severe in iron-deficient children, a relatively close relationship existing between blood lead levels and hematocrit.[71] In certain parts of the world, including several countries in Africa, control of lead additives to petrol and paint lag behind that of European and North American countries, and creates serious risks of the effects of lead in children exposed to lead paint in homes, schools, toys, and playground equipment as well as other locales. In adults, lead poisoning primarily occurs as the result of inhalation of lead compounds from industrial processes such as battery manufacture,[72,73] or ingestion of food having leached lead from pottery or dishes.[74,75] Lead poisoning from restoring tapestries and producing ceramics also has been noted.[76,77]

Generally, the erythrocyte disorder associated with lead intoxication in vivo is thought to be caused by interference with normal production of erythrocytes. There is direct evidence that lead inhibits red blood cell 5′-nucleotidase and results in basophilic stippling and hemolysis indistinguishable from the morphologic changes observed with inherited deficiency of this enzyme. The other lead poisoning–associated morphologic changes are observed when chronic lead exposure is associated with sideroblastic anemia but are not observed in acute lead poisoning.[78,79] The literature describes a number of tantalizing observations and proposed mechanisms. For instance, in vitro treatment of red cells with lead produces membrane damage and inhibition of the hexose monophosphate shunt.[80] Lead also interferes with the erythrocyte cation pump,[81,82] possibly by inhibiting membrane adenosine triphosphatase.[83,84] Free radical and Fenton-type chemistry around the iron atoms of hemoglobin have also been described.[85]

Microscopic examination of the blood provides the key diagnostic clue to lead poisoning. Complete observations of the acute hematologic changes, including erythrocyte distortion, occurring after the IV injection of lead in an attempt to treat malignant disease were first published in 1928.[86] Lead induces normocytic and slightly hypochromic erythrocytes, with the hypochromia possibly resulting from coexisting iron deficiency.[87] Basophilic stippling of the erythrocytes may be fine or coarse, and the number of granules seen in each cell may be quite variable. Blood collected in heparin may most reliably demonstrate basophilic stippling because storage of red blood cells in ethylenediaminetetraacetic acid (EDTA) is associated with the disappearance of

TABLE 23–1. Drugs and Chemicals That Have Been Reported to Cause Hemolytic Anemia Secondary to Erythrocyte Damage

Chemicals	Drugs
Aniline[90]	Amyl nitrite[98]
Apiol[91]	Meyanesin[99]
Dichlorprop (herbicide)[92]	Methylene blue[100]
Hydroxylamines[93]	Omeprazole[101]
Lysol[94]	Pentachlorophenol[102]
Mineral spirits[95]	Salicylazosulfapyridine (Azulfidine)[103]
Nitrobenzene[96]	Sulfonamide[104]
Resorcin[97]	Tacrolimus[105]

stippling.[88] Young polychromatophilic cells are most likely to be stippled. Electron microscopic studies have demonstrated that the basophilic granules represent abnormally aggregated ribosomes. Iron-laden mitochondria are present but do not appear to contribute to the basophilic stippling that is observed on light microscopy.[89] Ringed sideroblasts are frequently found within the marrow (Chap. 20).

REFERENCES

1. Lang F, Lang E, Foller M. Physiology and pathophysiology of eryptosis. *Transfus Med Hemother.* 2012;39:308.
2. Tavassoli M. Anemia of spaceflight. *Blood.* 1982;60:1059.
3. Rice L, Alfrey CP. The negative regulation of red cell mass by neocytolysis: physiologic and pathophysiologic manifestations. *Cell Physiol Biochem.* 2005;15:245.
4. Risso A, Turello M, Biffoni F, et al. Red blood cell senescence and neocytolysis in humans after high altitude acclimatization. *Blood Cells Mol Dis.* 2007;38:83.
5. Song J, Yoon D, Christensen RD, et al. HIF-mediated increased ROS from reduced mitophagy and decreased catalase causes neocytolysis. *J Mol Med.* 2015;93:857.
6. Taube H. Mechanisms of oxidation with oxygen. *J Gen Physiol.* 1965;49:29.
7. Collman JP, Hermann PC, Fu L, et al. Aza-crown capped porphyrin models of myoglobin: studies of the steric interactions of gas binding. *J Am Chem Soc.* 1997;119:3481.
8. Harris JW, Kellermeyer RW. *The Red Cell: Production, Metabolism, Destruction: Normal and Abnormal.* Rev. ed. Harvard University Press; 1970.
9. Bunn HF, Forget BG. *Hemoglobin—Molecular, Genetic, and Clinical Aspects.* WB Saunders; 1986.
10. Mengel CE, Kann HE Jr, Heyman A, et al. Effects of in vivo hyperoxia on erythrocytes. II. Hemolysis in a human after exposure to oxygen under high pressure. *Blood.* 1965;25:822.
11. Eysseric H, Vincent F, Peoc'h M, et al. A fatal case of chlorate poisoning: confirmation by ion chromatography of body fluids. *J Forensic Sci.* 2000;45:474.
12. Romanovsky A, Djogovic D, Chin D. A case of sodium chlorite toxicity managed with concurrent renal replacement therapy and red cell exchange. *J Med Toxicol.* 2013;9:67.
13. Caterson RJ, Savdie E, Raik E, et al. Heinz-body hemolysis in hemodialyzed patients caused by chloramines in Sydney tap water. *Med J Aust.* 1982;2:367.
14. Eaton JW, Kolpin CF, Swofford HS, et al. Chlorinated urban water—cause of dialysis-induced hemolytic-anemia. *Science.* 1973;181:463.
15. Biswas D, Banerjee M, Sen G, et al. Mechanism of erythrocyte death in human population exposed to arsenic through drinking water. *Toxicol Appl Pharmacol.* 2008;230:57.
16. Mahmud H, Foller M, Lang F. Arsenic-induced suicidal erythrocyte death. *Arch Toxicol.* 2009;83:107.
17. Phoon WH, Chan MO, Goh CH, et al. Five cases of arsine poisoning. *Ann Acad Med Singapore.* 1984;13:394.
18. Romeo L, Apostoli P, Kovacic M, et al. Acute arsine intoxication as a consequence of metal burnishing operations. *Am J Ind Med.* 1997;32:211.
19. Rael LT, Ayala-Fierro F, Carter DE. The effects of sulfur, thiol, and thiol inhibitor compounds on arsine-induced toxicity in the human erythrocyte membrane. *Toxicol Sci.* 2000;55:468.
20. Winski SL, Barber DS, Rael LT, et al. Sequence of toxic events in arsine-induced hemolysis in vitro: implications for the mechanism of toxicity in human erythrocytes. *Fundam Appl Toxicol.* 1997;38:123.
21. Blair PC, Thompson MB, Bechtold M, et al. Evidence for oxidative damage to red blood cells in mice induced by arsine gas. *Toxicology.* 1990;63:25.
22. Schmid-Schonbein H, Wells R. Fluid drop-like transition of erythrocytes under shear. *Science.* 1969;165:288.
23. Bull B. Red-cell biconcavity and deformability—macromodel based on flow chamber observations. *Nouv Rev Fr Hematol.* 1972;12:835.
24. Bull BS, Brailsford JD. Red-cell membrane deformability—new data. *Blood.* 1976;48:663.
25. Ham TH, Shen SC, et al. Studies on the destruction of red blood cells; thermal injury; action of heat in causing increased spheroidicity, osmotic and mechanical fragilities and hemolysis of erythrocytes; observations on the mechanisms of destruction of such erythrocytes in dogs and in a patient with a fatal thermal burn. *Blood.* 1948;3:373.
26. Shen SC, Ham TH, Fleming EM. Studies on the destruction of red blood cells. III. Mechanism and complications of hemoglobinuria in patients with thermal burns: spherocytosis and increased osmotic fragility of red blood cells. *N Engl J Med.* 1943;229:701.
27. Zarkowsky HS, Mohandas N, Speaker CB, et al. A congenital hemolytic-anemia with thermal sensitivity of the erythrocyte membrane. *Br J Haematol.* 1975;29:537.
28. Prchal JT, Castleberry RP, Parmley RT, et al. Hereditary pyropoikilocytosis and elliptocytosis: clinical, laboratory and ultrastructural features in infants and children. *Pediatr Res.* 1982;16:484.
29. Tanner MJ. The structure and function of band 3 (AE1): Recent developments (review). *Mol Membr Biol.* 1997;14:155.
30. Barretto OC, Cardoso JL, Decillo D. Viscerocutaneous form of loxoscelism and erythrocyte glucose-6-phosphate deficiency. *Rev Inst Med Trop Sao Paulo.* 1985;27:264.
31. Chadha JS, Leviav A. Hemolysis, renal-failure, and local necrosis following scorpion sting. *JAMA.* 1979;241:1038.
32. Madrigal GC, Wenzl JE, Ercolani RL. Toxicity from a bite of brown spider (*Loxosceles reclusus*)—skin necrosis, hemolytic anemia, and hemoglobinuria in a 9-year-old child. *Clin Pediatr (Phila).* 1972;11:641.
33. Nance WE. Hemolytic anemia of necrotic arachnidism. *Am J Med.* 1961;31:801.
34. Wasserman GS, Siegel C. Loxoscelism (brown recluse spider bites)—review of the literature. *Clin Toxicol.* 1979;14:353.
35. McDade J, Aygun B, Ware RE. Brown recluse spider (*Loxosceles reclusa*) envenomation leading to acute hemolytic anemia in six adolescents. *J Pediatr.* 2010;156:155.
36. Barretto OC, Satake M, Nonoyama K, et al. The calcium-dependent protease of *Loxosceles gaucho* venom acts preferentially upon red cell band 3 transmembrane protein. *Braz J Med Biol Res.* 2003;36:309.
37. Bresolin NL, Carvalho FLC, Goes JEC, et al. Acute renal failure following massive attack by Africanized bee stings. *Pediatr Nephrol.* 2002;17:625.
38. Dacie JV. *The Hæmolytic Anæmias: Congenital and Acquired.* 2nd ed. Grune & Stratton; 1960.
39. Monzon C, Miles J. Hemolytic-anemia following a wasp sting. *J Pediatr.* 1980;96:1039.
40. Schulte KL, Kochen MM. Hemolytic-anemia in an adult after a wasp sting. *Lancet.* 1981;2:478.
41. Vachvanichsanong P, Dissaneewate P, Mitarnun W. Non-fatal acute renal failure due to wasp stings in children. *Pediatr Nephrol.* 1997;11:734.
42. Seibert CS, Santoro ML, Tambourgi DV, et al. *Lonomia obliqua* (Lepidoptera, Saturniidae) caterpillar bristle extract induces direct lysis by cleaving erythrocyte membrane glycoproteins. *Toxicon.* 2010;55:1323.
43. Brinkman DL, Konstantakopoulos N, McInerney BV, et al. *Chironex fleckeri* (box jellyfish) venom proteins: expansion of a cnidarian toxin family that elicits variable cytolytic and cardiovascular effects. *J Biol Chem.* 2014;289:4798.
44. Celedon G, Gonzalez G, Barrientos D, et al. Stycholysin II, a cytolysin from the sea anemone *Stichodactyla helianthus* promotes higher hemolysis in aged red blood cells. *Toxicon.* 2008;51:1383.
45. Uchida T, Yamasaki T, Eto S, et al. Crystal structure of the hemolytic lectin CEL-III isolated from the marine invertebrate *Cucumaria echinata*: implications of domain structure for its membrane pore-formation mechanism. *J Biol Chem.* 2004;279:37133.
46. Fagerlund A, Lindback T, Storset AK, et al. *Bacillus cereus* Nhe is a pore-forming toxin with structural and functional properties similar to the ClyA (HlyE, SheA) family of haemolysins, able to induce osmotic lysis in epithelia. *Microbiology.* 2008;154:693.
47. Landsteiner EK, Finch CA. Hemoglobinemia accompanying transurethral resection of the prostate. *N Engl J Med.* 1947;237:310.
48. Rath CE. Drowning hemoglobinuria. *Blood.* 1953;8:1099.
49. Farrell DJ, Bower L. Fatal water intoxication. *J Clin Pathol.* 2003;56:803.
50. Delano MD. Simple physical constraints in hemolysis. *J Theoret Biol.* 1995;175:517.
51. Klein WJ Jr, Metz EN, Price AR. Acute copper intoxication. A hazard of hemodialysis. *Arch Intern Med.* 1972;129:578.
52. Manzler AD, Schreiner AW. Copper-induced acute hemolytic anemia. A new complication of hemodialysis. *Ann Intern Med.* 1970;73:409.
53. Deiss A, Lee GR, Cartwright GE. Hemolytic anemia in Wilson's disease. *Ann Intern Med.* 1970;73:413.
54. Hansen PB. Wilson's disease presenting with severe hemolytic anemia. *Ugeskr Laeger.* 1988;150:1229.
55. McIntyre N, Clink HM, Levi AJ, et al. Hemolytic anemia in Wilson's disease. *N Engl J Med.* 1967;276:439.
56. Grudeva-Popova JG, Spasova MI, Chepileva KG, et al. Acute hemolytic anemia as an initial clinical manifestation of Wilson's disease. *Folia Med (Plovdiv).* 2000;42:42.
57. Fairbanks VF. Copper sulfate-induced hemolytic anemia. Inhibition of glucose-6-phosphate dehydrogenase and other possible etiologic mechanisms. *Arch Intern Med.* 1967;120:428.
58. Blume KG, Hoffbauer RW, Lohr GW, et al. Genetische und biochemische Aspekte der Pyruvatkinase menschlicher Erythrozyten. *Verh Dtsch Ges Inn Med.* 1969;75:450.
59. Boulard M, Beutler E, Blume KG. Effect of copper on red-cell enzyme-activities. *J Clin Invest.* 1972;51:459.
60. Kiss JE, Berman D, Van Thiel D. Effective removal of copper by plasma exchange in fulminant Wilson's disease. *Transfusion.* 1998;38:327.
61. Orringer EP, Mattern WD. Formaldehyde-induced hemolysis during chronic-hemodialysis. *N Engl J Med.* 1976;294:1416.
62. Batista CAS, Larson RG, Kotov NA. Nonadditivity of nanoparticle interactions. *Science.* 2015;350(6257):1242477.
63. Reiss G, Hutten A. Magnetic nanoparticles. In: Sattler KD, ed. *Handbook of Nanophysics: Nanoparticles and Quantum Dots.* CRC Press. 2010;20-21.
64. Zoroddu, MA, Medici S, Ledda A, et al. Toxicity of nanoparticles. *Curr Med Chem.* 2014;21(33):3837.
65. Thake THF, Webb JR, Nash A, et al. Permeation of polystyrene nanoparticles across model lipid bilayer membranes. *Soft Matter.* 2013;9:10265.
66. Zook JM, Maccuspie RI, Locascio LE, et al. Stable nanoparticle aggregates/agglomerates of different sizes and the effect of their size on hemolytic cytotoxicity. *Nanotoxicology.* 2011;5(4):517.
67. Yu T, Malugin A, Ghandehari H. The impact of silica nanoparticle design on cellular toxicity and hemolytic activity. *ACS Nano.* 2011;5(7):5717.
68. Chen LQ, Fang L, Ling J, et al. Nanotoxicity of silver nanoparticles to red blood cells: size dependent adsorption, uptake and hemolytic activity. *Chem Res Toxicol.* 2015;28:501.
69. Klein M, Namer R, Harpur E, Corbin R. Earthenware containers as a source of fatal lead poisoning—case study and public-health considerations. *N Engl J Med.* 1970;283:669.

70. Andreasen NJ. Benjamin Franklin: physicus et medicus. *JAMA*. 1976;236:57.

71. Bradman A, Eskenazi B, Sutton P, et al. Iron deficiency associated with higher blood lead in children living in contaminated environments. *Environ Health Perspect*. 2001;109:1079.

72. Staudinger KC, Roth VS. Occupational lead poisoning. *Am Fam Physician*. 1998;57:719.

73. Froom P, Kristal-Boneh E, Benbassat J, et al. Predictive value of determinations of zinc protoporphyrin for increased blood lead concentrations. *Clin Chem*. 1998;44:1283.

74. Autenrieth T, Schmidt T, Habscheid W. Lead poisoning caused by a Greek ceramic cup. *Dtsch Med Wochenschr*. 1998;123:353.

75. Kakosy T, Hudak A, Naray M. Lead intoxication epidemic caused by ingestion of contaminated ground paprika. *J Toxicol Clin Toxicol*. 1996;34:507.

76. Fischbein A, Wallace J, Sassa S, et al. Lead poisoning from art restoration and pottery work: unusual exposure source and household risk. *J Environ Pathol Toxicol Oncol*. 1992;11:7.

77. Vahter M, Counter SA, Laurell G, et al. Extensive lead exposure in children living in an area with production of lead-glazed tiles in the Ecuadorian Andes. *Int Arch Occup Environ Health*. 1997;70:282.

78. Valentine WN, Paglia DE, Fink K, et al. Lead-poisoning: association with hemolytic-anemia, basophilic stippling, erythrocyte pyrimidin 5′-nucleotidase deficiency, and intraery-throcytic accumulation of pyrimidines. *J Clin Invest*. 1976;58:926.

79. Paglia DE, Valentine WN, Dahlgren JG. Effects of low-level lead-exposure on pyrimidine 5′-nucleotidase and other erythrocyte enzymes: possible role of pyrimidine 5′-nucleotidase in pathogenesis of lead-induced anemia. *J Clin Invest*. 1975;56:1164.

80. Lachant NA, Tomoda A, Tanaka KR. Inhibition of the pentose-phosphate shunt by lead—a potential mechanism for hemolysis in lead-poisoning. *Blood*. 1984;63:518.

81. Khalil-Manesh F, Tartaglia-Erler J, Gonick HC. Experimental model of lead nephropathy. IV. Correlation between renal functional changes and hematological indices of lead toxicity. *J Trace Elem Electrolytes Health Dis*. 1994;8:13.

82. Vincent PC, Blackburn CRB. The effects of heavy metal ions on the human erythrocyte. I Comparisons of the action of several heavy metals. *Aust J Exp Biol Med Sci*. 1958;36:471.

83. Hasan J, Vihko V, Hernberg S. Deficient red cell membrane/Na⁺ + K⁺/-ATPase in lead poisoning. *Arch Environ Health*. 1967;14:313.

84. Hernberg S, Nikkanen J. Enzyme inhibition by lead under normal urban conditions. *Lancet*. 1970;1:63.

85. Casado MF, Cecchini AL, Simao AN, et al. Free radical-mediated pre-hemolytic injury in human red blood cells subjected to lead acetate as evaluated by chemiluminescence. *Food Chem Toxicol*. 2007;45:945.

86. Brookfield RW. Blood changes occurring during the course of treatment of malignant disease by lead, with special reference to punctate basophilia and the platelets. *J Pathol*. 1928;31:277.

87. Clark M, Royal J, Seeler R. Interaction of iron deficiency and lead and the hematologic findings in children with severe lead poisoning. *Pediatrics*. 1988;81:247.

88. White JM, Selhi HS. Lead and Red-Cell. *Br J Haematol*. 1975;30:133.

89. Jensen WN, Moreno GD, Bessis MC. An electron microscopic description of basophilic stippling in red cells. *Blood*. 1965;25:933.

90. Lubash GD, Phillips RE, Bonsnes RW, et al. Acute aniline poisoning treated by hemodialysis—report of case. *Arch Intern Med*. 1964;114:530.

91. Lowenstein L, Ballew DH. Fatal acute haemolytic anaemia, thrombocytopenic purpura, nephrosis and hepatitis resulting from ingestion of a compound containing apiol. *Can Med Assoc J*. 1958;78:195.

92. Schroder C, Kruger E, Abel J. Acute poisoning caused by the herbicide dichlorprop (preparation SYS 67 PROP). *Kinderarztl Prax*. 1991;59:81.

93. Martin H, Woerner W, Rittmeister B. Hemolytic anemia by inhalation of hydroxy-lamines, with a contribution to the problem of Heinz body formation. *Klin Wochenschr*. 1964;42:725.

94. Fisher B. The significance of Heinz bodies in anemias of obscure etiology. *Am J Med Sci*. 1955;230:143.

95. Nierenberg DW, Horowitz MB, Harris KM, et al. Mineral spirits inhalation associated with hemolysis, pulmonary edema, and ventricular fibrillation. *Arch Intern Med*. 1991;151:1437.

96. Hunter D. Industrial toxicology. *QJM*. 1943;12:185.

97. Gasser C. Perakute hämolytische Innenkörperanämie mit Methämoglobinämie nach Behandlung eines Säuglingsekzems mit Resorcin. *Helv Paediatr Acta*. 1954;9:285.

98. Graves TD, Mitchell S. Acute haemolytic anaemia after inhalation of amyl nitrite. *J R Soc Med*. 2003;96:594.

99. Pugh JI, Enderby GEH. Haemoglobinuria after intravenous myanesin. *Lancet*. 1947;2:387.

100. Sills MR, Zinkham WH. Methylene blue-induced Heinz body hemolytic anemia. *Arch Pediatr Adolesc Med*. 1994;148:306.

101. Davidson S, Seldon M, Jones B. Omeprazole and Heinz-body haemolytic anaemia. *Aust N Z J Med*. 1997;27:441.

102. Hassan AB, Seligmann H, Bassan HM. Intravascular haemolysis induced by pentachlo-rophenol. *Br Med J (Clin Res Ed)*. 1985;291:21.

103. Kaplinsky N, Frankl O. Salicylazosulphapyridine-induced Heinz body anemia. *Acta Haematol*. 1978;59:310.

104. Adams JG, Heller P, Abramson RK, Vaithianathan T. Sulfonamide-induced hemolytic anemia and hemoglobin Hasharon. *Arch Intern Med*. 1977;137:1449.

105. Lin CC, King KL, Chao YW, et al. Tacrolimus-associated hemolytic uremic syndrome: a case analysis. *J Nephrol*. 2003;16:580.

CHAPTER 24
HEMOLYTIC ANEMIA RESULTING FROM INFECTIONS WITH MICROORGANISMS

Marshall A. Lichtman

SUMMARY

Hemolytic anemia is a prominent part of the clinical presentation of patients infected with certain organisms such as *Plasmodium*, *Babesia*, and *Bartonella* spp., which directly invade the erythrocyte. Malaria is the most common cause of hemolytic anemia worldwide, and much has been learned about how the parasite enters the erythrocyte and the mechanism of the development of anemia. Falciparum malaria, in particular, can cause severe and sometimes fatal hemolysis (blackwater fever). The zoonotic malaria parasite *Falciparum knowlesi*, prevalent in Southeast Asia, is also associated with severe hemolytic anemia. Other organisms cause hemolytic anemia by producing a hemolysin (eg, *Clostridium perfringens*), by stimulating an immune response (eg, *Mycoplasma pneumoniae*), by enhancing macrophage recognition and hemophagocytosis, or by as yet unknown mechanisms. The many different infections that have been associated with hemolytic anemia are tabulated and references to the relevant studies provided.

Shortening of erythrocyte life span occurs commonly in the course of inflammatory and infectious diseases. This effect may occur particularly in patients with glucose-6-phosphate dehydrogenase (G6PD) deficiency (Chap. 16), splenomegaly (Chap. 25), and in the microvascular red cell fragmentation syndrome (Chap. 22). In some infections, however, rapid destruction of erythrocytes represents a prominent part of the overall clinical picture (Table 24-1).[1-49] This chapter deals only with the latter states.

Several distinct mechanisms may lead to hemolysis during infections.[49] These include direct invasion of or injury to the erythrocytes by the infecting organism, as in malaria, babesiosis, and bartonellosis; elaboration of hemolytic toxins, as by *Clostridium perfringens*;

Acronyms and Abbreviations: ADAMTS-13, a disintegrin and metalloprotease with a thrombospondin type 1 motif member 13; CDC, Centers for Disease Control and Prevention; CR1, complement receptor-1; EBA, erythrocyte-binding antigen; G6PD, glucose-6-phosphate dehydrogenase; ICAM, intercellular adhesion molecule; PCR, polymerase chain reaction; PfEMP, *Plasmodium falciparum* erythrocyte membrane protein; RH, reticulocyte homology; RSP-2, ring surface protein 2; VCAM, vascular cell adhesion molecule; VWF, von Willebrand factor.

and development of antibodies, either autoantibodies against red cell antigens or deposition of microbial antigens or immune complexes on erythrocytes, which result in hemolytic anemia.[50]

● MALARIA

EPIDEMIOLOGY

A disease known since antiquity, malaria is the world's most common cause of hemolytic anemia.[36] Human malaria is caused by one of five species of the protozoan *Plasmodium*. In 2018, an estimated 228 million episodes of malaria occurred worldwide, resulting in approximately 500,000 deaths, mainly among inhabitants of sub-Saharan Africa, where the disease is endemic.[51] The incidence rate of malaria has decreased by approximately 25% from 2010, indicating progress in disease prevention. The decrease in morbidity and mortality has been ascribed to (1) vector control through the use of indoor spraying of insecticide and insecticide impregnated mosquito netting, (2) use of rapid diagnosis kits, (3) improved access to antimalarial drugs, and (4) the effect of preventive treatment in pregnant women.[52] Unfortunately, these techniques have decreased in effectiveness as a result of acquired resistance of mosquitoes to pesticides and the change in mosquito habits, biting earlier in the evening before bedtime and later in the morning after leaving net covered beds, which had heretofore been very effective at decreasing incidence of bites and disease. In addition, drug resistance of plasmodia, has decreased drug effectiveness. Experimentation using gene editing to alter the ability of the mosquito vector to transmit the disease to humans has been accomplished but has been limited to the laboratory because of potential issues regarding broader risks to biodiversity. Severe malarial anemia is most commonly seen in young children and pregnant women.[51,52] The disease has a particular propensity to affect children younger than 5 years and as many as 200,000 deaths in this age group occur in Africa per year.

Malaria transmission depends on geography, rainfall patterns, and the breeding sites of the *Anopheles* mosquito, the specific vector. Some regions have conditions that make malaria common throughout the year, so-called endemic areas; in other places, there are seasonal peaks, usually the rainy season when mosquito breeding is enhanced. Persons in Africa, Asia, the Middle East, and southern parts of Europe may be at risk. Travelers to such places are at high risk because of lack of immunity and because when they return home, the diagnosis might not be considered promptly.

Malaria may also be transmitted by blood transfusion[53] or organ transplantation[54] from an infected donor. Treatment of blood with extracorporeal ultraviolet light and riboflavin may reduce the risk of transmission by transfusion.[53]

LIFE CYCLE

Sporozoites enter the circulation while the female *Anopheles* mosquito takes a blood meal. They invade and multiply in hepatocytes. The latter cells rupture when engorged and release merozoites that invade the red cell. In the red cell, the merozoites also cycle through these stages: trophozoites (ring-forms), which then can convert to schizonts. Schizonts are spherical structures that contain numerous merozoites. Mature schizonts burst the red cells and release their merozoites that invade other red cells. The bursting and release coincides with the abrupt rises in temperature and related signs and symptoms seen in malaria. A small fraction of merozoites in red cells convert to male and female gametocytes that are ingested when the mosquito bites. In the mosquito, they fuse and form an oocyst that divides asexually into numerous sporozoites. The sporozoites migrate to the mosquito's salivary glands from

TABLE 24–1. Organisms That Cause Hemolytic Anemia

Aspergillus spp.[1]

Bacillus anthracis[2]

Babesia microti and *Babesia divergens*[3]

Bartonella bacilliformis[4,5]

Campylobacter jejuni[6,7]

Clostridium perfringens (Welchii)[8,9]

Coxsackievirus[10]

Cytomegalovirus[11]

Diplococcus pneumoniae[12]

Epstein-Barr virus[13,14]

Escherichia coli[15,16,137]

Fusobacterium necrophorum[17]

Haemophilus influenzae[12,23]

Hepatitis A[18-20]

Hepatitis B[19,21]

Hepatitis C[22]

Herpes simplex virus[10]

Human immunodeficiency virus[24-26] (Chap. 80)

Influenza A virus[27,28]

Leishmania donovani[30]

Leptospira interrogans serovar *ballum* and *Leptospira kirschneri* serovar *butembo*[29]

Mumps virus[31]

Mycobacterium tuberculosis[12,32]

Mycoplasma pneumoniae[33]

Neisseria intracellularis[12]

Parvovirus B19[34]

Plasmodium falciparum[35]

Plasmodium malariae[35]

Plasmodium vivax[36]

Rubella virus[37,38]

Rubeola virus[10]

Salmonella spp.[12,39]

Shigella spp.[40,41,137]

Streptococcus spp.[12,42-45]

Toxoplasma spp.[12]

Trypanosoma brucei[46]

Varicella virus[10,47]

Vibrio cholerae[12]

Yersinia enterocolitica[48]

where they reenter a victim's blood upon the next bite, initiating a malarial infection. *P. vivax* and *P.m ovale* can persist in the liver in a dormant stage (hypnozoites) and produce relapses months or years later.

ALTERATIONS IN THE INFECTED RED CELL

After the host is bitten by an infected female *Anopheles* mosquito, the sporozoites invade the liver and possibly other internal organs in the asymptomatic tissue stage of malaria. Merozoites, emerging at first from the tissues and later from previously parasitized red cells, use specialized invasion proteins such as the erythrocyte-binding antigen (EBA)

and reticulocyte homology (RH) protein families, which bind to receptors on the erythrocyte surface, including glycophorins A/B/C, CR1 (CD35), and basigin (CD147).[55-57] A complex series of events eventuates in invasion of the interior of the red cell by the parasite.[35,55] Having entered the erythrocyte, the parasite grows intracellularly, nourished by the cell's contents, and modifies the host cell by exporting hundreds of proteins into the cytoplasm, some of which are inserted into the red cell membrane.[57]

Erythrocytes infected with *P. falciparum* develop surface knobs[58] that contain receptors, especially the *P. falciparum* erythrocyte membrane protein-1 (PfEMP-1), for endothelial proteins. All parasites bind to CD36 antigen (platelet glycoprotein IV) and thrombospondin found on endothelial surfaces, whereas some bind to the intercellular adhesion molecule-1 (ICAM-1), and a few bind to the vascular cell adhesion molecule (VCAM)[59-64] and mediate the adherence of parasitized cells to endothelium. Activated endothelium secretes strands of ultralarge von Willebrand factor (VWF), which bind platelets, allowing PfEMP-1 to interact with platelet CD36 and this effect provides an additional means of cytoadherence.[65] Rosetting of parasitized cells with unparasitized cells also occurs through a mechanism mediated by complement receptor-1 (CR1) on uninfected erythrocytes.[66] One of the membrane proteins of *P. falciparum* binds specifically to the protein spectrin on the inner surface of the red cell membrane.[67]

The anemia of falciparum malaria is characteristically a normocytic-normochromic anemia with a paucity of reticulocytes (see "Pathogenesis of the Anemia" later). If microcytosis is present, the concomitant presence of α- or β-thalassemia or iron deficiency should be considered.[68] A large number of genetic polymorphisms that interfere with invasion of erythrocytes by parasites and their proliferation have developed in areas where malaria has been a leading cause of death for many generations.[66,69-71] These include G6PD deficiency (Chap. 16), Southeast Asian ovalocytosis (Chap. 15), CR1 deficiency, the thalassemias (Chap. 17), sickle cell anemia (Chap. 18), and other hemoglobinopathies (Chaps. 17 and 18).

PLASMODIUM SPECIES AND SEVERITY OF ANEMIA

The five plasmodial species that cause human malaria are *P. falciparum*, *P. vivax*, *P. malariae*, *P. ovale*, and the zoonotic malarial parasite *P. knowlesi*. The first two cause the most cases worldwide and are notably associated with hemolytic anemia. *P. vivax* invades only young red cells, whereas *P. falciparum* attacks both young and old cells. Thus, anemia tends to be more severe in the latter form of malaria and is the most deadly type.[35,51] *P. knowlesi* is the only plasmodium that infects humans that is zoonotic, notably in Southeast Asia, and is transmitted from an animal reservoir, macaques, to humans by mosquito. It is not transmitted from human to human by a mosquito vector as are the other four species of *Plasmodia*.[51] *P. knowlesi* causes severe malaria with a frequency similar to *P. falciparum*, and this includes a high frequency of intravascular hemolysis.

PATHOGENESIS OF THE ANEMIA

Hemolytic Mechanisms

Destruction of parasitized red cells appears to occur largely in the spleen, and splenomegaly typically is present in chronic malarial infection. The "pitting" of parasites from infected erythrocytes may also occur in the spleen.[72] The degree of parasitemia, in part, determines the destruction of infected erythrocytes. Low rates of red cell parasitemia may have little effect on the development of anemia, whereas high rates (eg, ≥10% of red cells infected) may have very significant effects.[73]

The degree to which anemia develops often seems to be disproportionate to the number of cells infected with the parasite. It is estimated that 10 times the number of uninfected red cells are removed for each infected red cell, dramatically magnifying the hemolytic rate. Osmotic fragility is increased in nonparasitized cells, as well as in cells containing plasmodia.[74] The erythrocyte cation permeability is altered in monkeys with malaria.[75] Hemin accumulation facilitates hemolytic cell loss via a process of programmed cell death, referred to as eryptosis. This suicidal death pathway is mediated by increased cell calcium, increased annexin-V binding, and ceramide formation.[76] Oxidative damage to red cell lipids occurs,[77,78] and there is an abnormality in the phosphorylation of membranes of parasitized red cells.[79] P. falciparum–infected red cells have a highly irregular surface produced by the intracellular growth of the plasmodium, but nonparasitized cells often have similar surface defects.[80] Activation of hepatosplenic macrophages enhance red cell clearance supported by red cell surface changes in both parasitized and nonparasitized cells that foster recognition and erythrophagocytosis by macrophages. Both marked loss of red cell deformability and deposition of immunoglobulin G and complement (C3d), sometimes resulting in a positive direct antiglobulin reaction, may enhance red cell removal by macrophages.[81,82] Parasite products are part of the immune complexes on the red cell surface. The P. falciparum ring surface protein 2 (RSP-2) mediates adhesion of infected red cells to endothelial cells and is deposited on uninfected cells, undoubtedly providing a mechanism for removal of these cells by mediating complement-dependent phagocytosis.[68] Splenomegaly further enhances red cell removal from the circulation.

An additional explanation of malaria-associated anemia is the occurrence of thrombotic microangiopathy, with high levels of (ultralarge) VWF multimers and low levels of ADAMTS-13 (a disintegrin and metalloprotease with a thrombospondin type 1 motif member 13). The proposed mechanism behind the drop in ADAMTS-13 activity in malaria is endothelial activation caused by parasitized erythrocytes. Subsequent release of ultralarge VWF multimers could lead to a decrease in ADAMTS-13 levels through consumption. The extent of ADAMTS-13 deficiency is related to malaria severity and parasitemia.[83,84]

Decrease in Erythropoiesis

P. falciparum also decreases the erythropoietin response, resulting in less erythropoiesis than expected for the degree of anemia, reticulocytopenia, and, coincidentally, striking dyserythropoiesis with red cell stippling, cytoplasmic vacuolization, nuclear fragmentation, and multinuclearity.[68] The inhibition of the erythroid response (anemia of inflammation) is secondary to release of the cytokines interferon-γ and tumor necrosis factor-α, and the interleukin-10–to–tumor-necrosis-factor ratio, which when low correlates with severe malarial anemia in children (Chap. 6).[68]

TISSUE EFFECTS OF HEMOLYSIS IN MALARIA

In P. knowlesi malaria, intravascular hemolysis, which is associated with malarial parasite mass, results in increased circulating free hemoglobin with its iron, in the absence of intact cell-reducing systems, oxidized to the ferric state. Intravascular hemolysis in P. knowlesi malaria may be more frequent than in any other type of malaria. This event facilitates the release of heme, which results in oxidant damage of endothelial cells, upregulation of endothelial cell adhesion molecules, and the release of reactive oxygen molecules and of proinflammatory cytokines. Evidence of endothelial activation is also evident by the release of the contents of Weibel-Palade bodies (eg, VWF, angiopoietin-2). In P. falciparum malaria, intravascular hemolysis is accompanied by nitrous-oxide-dependent endothelial dysfunction. These alterations subsequent to hemolysis are very likely to contribute to microvascular damage and end-organ damage (eg, kidney) that occurs in these malarial types.[85]

BLACKWATER FEVER

The fever associated with malaria, accompanied by rigors, headache, abdominal pain, nausea and vomiting, and extreme fatigue, is characteristically cyclic, varying in frequency according to the malaria type. Although classic periodicity is often absent, febrile paroxysms of P. vivax malaria tend to occur every 48 hours; those of P. malariae infection occur each 72 hours; and those of P. falciparum malaria occur daily. In the latter cases, the periodicity is the result the synchronization of schizogony with schizont rupture occurring at regular intervals. Schizont rupture accounts for the fever and associated symptoms. Falciparum malaria is occasionally associated with particularly severe hemolysis, hemoglobinemia, hemoglobinuria, and the passage of dark, almost black, urine. This degree of severity, also called blackwater fever, is no longer common. At one time it was seen frequently among Europeans in Africa and in India, usually after quinine was given to treat malaria. The event seems to be related to the intermittent use of antimalarials.[86]

DIAGNOSTIC METHODS

Diagnosis of malaria depends on demonstration of the parasites on the blood film, or the presence of antigenic parasite proteins using rapid detection tests in circumstances in which microscopic examination is unavailable.[87] Identification of the malarial parasite on the blood film is considered the standard of diagnosis and involves examination of a thick and thin blood film preparation. In some rural areas of Africa, electricity is limited and, thus, light microscopy can be difficult. If financing permits, rapid diagnostic tests are being instituted to supplant microscopy. Alternative and supplementary techniques involve polymerase chain reaction (PCR) to demonstrate the appropriate DNA sequences in the blood[88,89] or the use of automated hematology analyzers to identify parasites as part of a routine complete blood count investigation.[90,91]

The morphologic differentiation of P. falciparum from other forms of malaria, principally P. vivax, is clinically important because P. falciparum infection may constitute a clinical emergency. If more than 5% of the red cells infected contain parasites, the infection is almost certainly with P. falciparum. In an infection with this organism, rings are practically the only form of parasite evident on the blood film. The finding of two or more rings within the same red cells is regarded as pathognomonic of P. falciparum (Fig. 24-1). In nonimmune patients, examination of the blood film for malarial parasites should be made for at least 3 days after onset of symptoms because parasitemia may not reach detectable levels for several days. (Access the United States Centers for Disease Control and Prevention [CDC] at www.cdc.gov/malaria/diagnosis_treatment/diagnosis.html) for detailed information on diagnostic approaches and techniques and Plasmodium spp. identification.)

TREATMENT

Early treatment is important. The spread of antimalarial therapy has resulted in major problems with drug resistance. Eradication of blood forms can be achieved with individual agents or combinations of antimalarials.[92]

The treatment of patients with malaria is complex and continually evolving as a result of new agents and development of drug resistance. As many as 12 antimalarial drugs are currently available. Their use may vary with the species of Plasmodium involved, the geographic area of

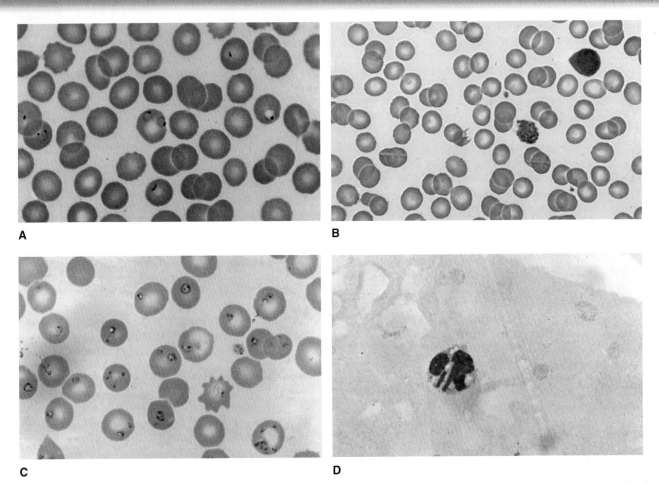

FIGURE 24–1. **A.** Blood film from a patient with malaria caused by *Plasmodium falciparum*. Several red cells contain ring forms. Note red cell with double ring form in center of the field, characteristic of *P. falciparum* infection. Note the ring form with double dots at the left edge of figure, suggestive of *P. falciparum* infection. Note also high rate of parasitemia (~10% of red cells in this field) characteristic of *P. falciparum* infection. **B.** Blood film from a patient with malaria caused by *Plasmodium vivax*. Note mature schizont. **C.** Blood film from a patient with *Babesia microti* infection. The heavy parasitemia is characteristic of babesiosis (approximately two-thirds of red cells infected). **D.** Blood film from a patient with *Clostridium perfringens* septicemia. Few red cells evident as a result of intense erythrolysis. Neutrophil with two bacilli *(C. perfringens)*. *(Reproduced with permission from Lichtman MA, Shafer MS, Felgar RE, et al: Lichtman's Atlas of Hematology 2016. New York, NY: McGraw Hill; 2017.)*

the infection, the clinical status of the patient (eg, pregnancy), and drug allergies or interactions with other drugs in use by the patient. In 2015, there were 1517 cases of malaria in the United States. Approximately 15% of the cases were severe as indicated by one or more of the following: hemoglobin less than 70 g/L, parasitemia of greater than 5% of red cells, acute renal injury, acute respiratory distress syndrome, or jaundice and requiring rapid treatment and intensive care. Treatment of severe malaria in the United States is threatened by the unavailability of timely and effective treatment.[93] The United States CDC provides 24-hour guidance to therapists seeking advice as to the approach to a specific case. (Malaria Hotline, 770-488-7788, Monday-Friday, 9 am to 5 pm; outside these hours: 770-488-7100 and ask to speak to CDC malaria expert. These access numbers were last confirmed on August 2020.) Some antimalarials are capable of producing severe hemolysis in patients with G6PD deficiency, which is relevant in areas with endemic malaria (Chap. 16).[94]

PREVENTION

An initial test of a *P. falciparum* sporozoite vaccine, administered intravenously in five doses, has shown efficacy in a small number of experimental subjects. The immunologic responses were closely correlated with vaccine dose. Although a very important step forward, the practical limitations of five IV doses will have to be circumvented for extensive application to susceptible populations.[95] In 2015, another vaccine, RTS, S (Mosquirix) was the first to be approved for use. It acts to protect against *P. falciparum* and requires four sequential injections. Protection against clinical malaria in infants ranged between 30% and 50% and the effect waned after several months, but it has been deemed of significant benefit to a significant minority of inoculated infants.[96,97]

COURSE AND PROGNOSIS

When acute unusually severe hemolysis occurs in the course of falciparum malaria (blackwater fever), the physician should be certain that a hemolytic drug is not being administered to a G6PD-deficient individual. Transfusions may be needed with severe hemolysis, and if renal failure occurs, extracorporeal dialysis may be required. With early institution of therapy, the prognosis of patients with malaria is excellent. However, when treatment is delayed or there is resistant to the administered agent, *P. falciparum* malaria may follow a rapid, fatal course.

BARTONELLOSIS (OROYA FEVER)

EPIDEMIOLOGY

In 1885, Daniel A. Carrión, a medical student, inoculated himself with blood obtained from a verrucous nodule from the skin of a patient with verruca peruviana. He developed a fatal hemolytic anemia with the characteristics of Oroya fever, a disease that had first been observed some years earlier among workers in a railroad construction project near the city of Oroya in the Peruvian Andes. This fatal self-experiment established the identity of the verrucosa form and the hemolytic phase of human bartonellosis, an infection that now bears the eponymic designation Carrión disease.[5,98,99] Human bartonellosis is transmitted by the sand fly (*Lutzomyia* spp). The only reservoir for this organism is human beings. The disease is found in the countries of the South American Andes Mountains, notably Peru, Columbia, and Ecuador, principally at altitudes above 600 m. The reservoir for the organism is asymptomatic human carriers who represent as many as one-third of persons in regions after an outbreak or in endemic areas.

PATHOGENESIS

After a sand fly bite, the red blood cells become infected with *Bartonella bacilliformis*. It is believed that the organism does not grow within the red cell but rather adheres to its exterior surface. When infected red cells are washed with citrated plasma, numerous free organisms are found, but the red cells are not hemolyzed. In hanging-drop cultures, masses of organisms are seen outside the erythrocytes, but the cells themselves are intact. The osmotic fragility of the red cells is normal. Red cells are rapidly removed from the circulation, apparently both by liver and spleen. Normal red cells transfused into patients with bartonellosis also have a short survival. A 130-kDa *Bartonella* protein that causes erythrocytes to acquire trenches, indentations, and invaginations has been purified from culture broths and has been called *deformin*.[100] Confirmation of the pathogenetic role of this protein has not been established. Two *B. bacilliformis* genes that encode for invasion-associated locus proteins A and B, designated *ialA* and *ialB*, predicted to encode polypeptides of 170 amino acids (20.1 kDa) and of 186 amino acids (19.9 kDa), respectively, greatly enhance the ability of *Escherichia coli* to invade erythrocytes.[101]

CLINICAL FINDINGS

As demonstrated by Carrión's experiment, bartonellosis has two clinical stages. The acute hemolytic anemia, *Oroya fever*, represents the early, invasive stage of a chronic granulomatous disorder, the late stage of which is designated *verruca peruviana* (also called *verruca peruana*). The latter phase is manifest by soft conic or pedunculated papules or nodules on the skin or mucous membranes ranging up to several centimeters in diameter. These two phases usually occur sequentially but may occur independently of one another. Patients may manifest fever, sweating, myalgia, headache, and anorexia during the Oroya fever phase. The spleen and liver may be enlarged. Lymphadenopathy may be prominent. Asymptomatic infection may also occur.

The onset of anemia is usually dramatic. Red counts as low as 0.750×10^{12}/L have been documented.[102] Large numbers of nucleated red cells appear in the blood film, and reticulocytosis is often striking. The white cell count is variable. Diagnosis is established by demonstrating the presence of the organism on the erythrocytes. Giemsa-stained blood films reveal red-violet rods varying in length from 1 to 3 μm and in width from 0.25 to 0.2 μm. Although molecular methods for diagnosis of *Bartonella* spp. are available,[103] in a person with the clinical picture, the examination of the blood film can be accomplished and therapy initiated rapidly.

Immunosuppression is an accompaniment of *B. bacilliformis* infection, leading to secondary infections, exemplified by staphylococcal and *Salmonella* bacteremia or *Toxoplasma* bacteremia and myocarditis.

In those who survive the first phase of the disease, the second stage of *B. bacilliformis* infection, verruca peruviana, can occur. It is characterized by a skin eruption of cutaneous vascular nodular tumors (hemangioma-like) often on the face and extremities. The lesions may last for months. They are thought to be the result of organisms entering the vascular endothelium.

TREATMENT AND COURSE

Patients with Oroya fever respond to treatment with appropriate antibiotics. Sensitivity has been shown in vitro to a wide range of antibiotic classes, including aminoglycosides, cephalosporins, macrolides, quinolones, penicillins, tetracyclines, and others (eg, rifampin).[104,105] The mortality rate among untreated patients is very high, but those who do survive undergo a sudden transitional period in which the *Bartonellae* change from an elongated to a coccoid form, the number of parasitized cells decreases, and the red cell count increases. Lymphocytosis and improved neutrophil count are observed with disappearance of the fever and abatement of other symptoms.

Other species of *Bartonella* cause human febrile infections such as "cat-scratch fever" or "trench fever" or can infect individuals with acquired immunodeficiency disease, but these disorders are not ordinarily associated with severe hemolytic anemia.

BABESIOSIS

EPIDEMIOLOGY

Babesiae are intraerythrocytic protozoa known as piroplasms. They are transmitted by the bite of the tick, *Ixodes scapularis*, which may infect many species of wild and domestic animals. More than 100 species of *Babesia* infect animals. Humans can become infected with *B. microti, B. divergens, B. duncani,* and *B. venatorum.* These species can parasitize rodents, deer, elk, and cattle.[106-110] Once thought to be rare, babesiosis has been recognized with increasing frequency.[109] For example, in New York State the incidence increased threefold from 2006 to 2015, and in Pennsylvania, the incidence increased 10-fold over the same period of time.[109] The disease is usually tickborne in humans but has also been transmitted by transfusion.[111] Cases of babesiosis, mostly caused by *B. microti* but also by *B. duncani,* have been transmitted by transfusion of blood from asymptomatic infected blood donors.[112] The risk of transfusion-transmitted babesiosis is higher than generally appreciated and represents a threat to the blood supply in endemic areas.[113] Presumably because of the distribution of the vector in the United States, the disease is most common in the northeastern coastal and Great Lakes regions, where it became known as "Nantucket fever," but it is more broadly distributed in the East and Midwest United States and has now been identified in 22 states.[109,114,115]

CLINICAL FINDINGS

The symptoms are prompted by reproduction of the organisms in the red cell and subsequent cell lysis. The clinical expression is broad, reflecting the degree of parasitemia.[107,116] The incubation period ranges from 1 week to 3 months but usually is about 3 weeks. The disease generally has a gradual onset with malaise, anorexia, and fatigue followed by fever (sometimes as high as 40°C), chills, sweats, and muscle and joint pains. Hepatic and splenic enlargement may be evident.

The onset, occasionally, may be fulminant and can include acute respiratory distress syndrome, renal failure, and disseminated intravascular coagulation.

A moderate degree of hemolytic anemia is usually present; on occasion it has been sufficiently severe to cause hypotension,[117] and transfusion has occasionally been required. The hemolysis may last a few days, but in asplenic, older, or otherwise immunocompromised patients, it can go on for months. Elevations in serum transaminases, lactic dehydrogenase, unconjugated bilirubin, and alkaline phosphatase correlate with the severity of the parasitemia. Thrombocytopenia and leukopenia may occur, which may be the result of inflammatory cytokine release.[116] The disease has simulated thrombotic thrombocytopenic purpura[118] and the HELLP syndrome in pregnant women.[119]

DIAGNOSIS

The history may indicate exposure to a tick-infested area, recent blood transfusion, or asplenia. Parasites can be seen in the red cells in Giemsa-stained thin blood films. They appear as darkly stained ring forms with light blue cytoplasm. Merozoites may also be visible. Infrequently, the classical Maltese cross tetrad can be found. This intraerythrocytic structure consists of four daughter cells of *Babesia* connected by cytoplasmic bridges, resembling a Maltese cross. The parasitemia can be very high, affecting more than 75% of red cells (see Fig. 24-1C).[116] Immunofluorescent tests for antibodies to *Babesia* are available, and PCR-based diagnostic tests are the test of choice for confirmation of an active infection in an individual bearing antibodies to *Babesia* and for following the response to therapy.[120]

The onset of fever and hemolytic anemia after transfusion should lead to the consideration of babesiosis.

TREATMENT AND COURSE

Most mild *B. microti* infections respond without treatment. The infection has responded to drug therapy with clindamycin and quinine,[120,121] but failure to respond to antibiotics has also been encountered. The two-drug combination can increase rate of clearance of parasites, but they have consequential side effects. A combination of atovaquone and azithromycin has also been proposed as treatment.[108,115,120,121] Tafenoquine, an antimalarial, is being explored as a possible therapy for babesiosis.[122] Whole-blood or red cell exchange can result in marked improvement in recalcitrant cases[114,120].

COINFECTION

In endemic areas, two or more parasites may coinfect an individual by a tick bite. *B. microti* and *Borrelia burgdorferi* (Lyme disease) may both enter the human circulation as a result of the *Ixodes* tick bite, as can several other parasites (eg, human granulocytic ehrlichiosis caused by the rickettsia, *Ehrlichia chaffeensis*). Initial signs and symptoms may be similar. Successful early treatment for Lyme disease may leave a residual *B. microti* infection because antibiotic therapy for the former will not eradicate the latter.[116]

●*CLOSTRIDIUM PERFRINGENS* SEPTICEMIA

EPIDEMIOLOGY

Clostridium perfringens (formerly *Clostridium welchii*) sepsis is most likely to occur in patients who have undergone septic abortion. It has also been observed after acute cholecystitis,[123] as a result of an intrahepatic abscess,[9] and, rarely, after amniocentesis (amnionitis).[124]

PATHOGENESIS

C. perfringens are gram-positive, encapsulated, spore-forming, anaerobic bacilli. The organism causes gas gangrene in soft tissues. The α-toxin of *C. perfringens* is a lecithinase C that reacts with lipoprotein complexes at cell surfaces, liberating potent hemolytic substances, lysolecithins. This toxin is the agent that causes intravascular hemolysis and its subsequent effects. It has also been suggested that erythrocyte membrane proteolysis plays an important role in hemolysis.[125] Fortunately, the frequency of profound intravascular hemolysis is uncommon in patients with *C. perfringens* infections.[126]

CLINICAL FEATURES

Severe, often fatal hemolysis occurs in patients with *C. perfringens* septicemia. Striking hemoglobinemia and hemoglobinuria occur. The serum may become a brilliant red, and the urine is a dark-brown mahogany color. The lysis of red cells (decreasing packed red cell volume) and the high plasma hemoglobin can produce a marked dissociation between the blood hemoglobin and hematocrit level. For example, hematocrits approaching zero with blood hemoglobins as high as 8 g/dL can occur. Dehemoglobinized red cells ("ghosts") may be evident on the blood film (see Fig. 24-1D). Microspherocytes are prominent, and both leukocytosis with occasional myelocytes and band neutrophils (left shift) and thrombocytopenia are often present. Acute renal and hepatic failure often develops, and the prognosis is grave; more than half of the patients die, even with appropriate treatment.[8,126-128]

THERAPY AND COURSE

Therapy consists of antibiotic therapy, fluid support, red cell transfusion, and when appropriate surgical debridement.[126] The infection is often of abrupt onset and overwhelming, and the profundity of the hemolysis and secondary organ damage (eg, renal) results in a high mortality rate.

●OTHER INFECTIONS

A variety of other infections occasionally have been associated with hemolytic anemia. The mechanisms involved vary. Some organisms, among them such common pathogens as *Haemophilus influenzae*, *E. coli*, and *Salmonella* spp., can produce red cell agglutination in vitro, but it is not known whether this phenomenon is important in initiating in vivo hemolysis.[129] Bacteria may also produce destruction of red cells indirectly when bacterial polysaccharides are adsorbed onto erythrocytes. Action of an antibody directed against the antigen-coated cells results in their agglutination[130] or in complement-mediated lysis.[23] The unmasking of T-type antigens by bacteria renders the cell polyagglutinable. This may be a rare cause of hemolysis occurring in the course of bacterial infections.[131-133]

Many different types of microorganisms may play a role in precipitating autoimmune hemolytic disease, such as *Mycoplasma pneumoniae* (Chap. 26). In one study of 234 patients, 55 were found to have an antecedent bacterial infection, 18 of these exhibiting an "unequivocal etiologic relationship" of infection to anemia.[10] However, the principal evidence for such a relationship was a temporal one. A number of viral agents, including measles, cytomegalovirus, varicella, herpes simplex, influenzas A and B, Epstein-Barr, human immunodeficiency virus,[24-26,134] and coxsackievirus have also been associated with immune hemolytic disease.[10,133] Various mechanisms have been postulated, including absorption of immune complexes and complement, cross-reacting antigen, and a true autoimmune state with possible loss of tolerance secondary to the infectious organism.[10,133,135] Histopathologic and sometimes virologic evidence of infection with cytomegalovirus has been reported in a high percentage of children with lymphadenopathy and hemolytic anemia.[135] A positive antiglobulin reaction was demonstrated in some of these patients.

The high cold agglutinin titer that sometimes develops in the course of *M. pneumoniae* (Chap. 26) may occasionally result in hemolytic anemia[1,33,136] or compensated hemolysis, although most patients with high cold agglutinin titers do not become anemic. The red cells of a number of patients with kala azar were found to be agglutinated with anticomplement and anti–non-γ-globulin serum.[30] Both splenic and hepatic sequestration of red cells appears to occur in this disease.[13]

Microangiopathic hemolytic anemia, a form of fragmentation hemolytic anemia is discussed in Chap. 22. This form of hemolytic anemia may be triggered by a variety of infections, some of which are caused by well-characterized organisms such as Shiga toxin-producing *E. coli*, *Shigella dysenteriae* type 1,[137,138] *Campylobacter* spp.,[139] and *Aspergillus* spp.[1]

CO-INFECTION BY GRAM-NEGATIVE BACTERIA AS A RESULT OF HEMOLYSIS

An increased risk of acquiring a gram-negative bacterial infection, notably a nontyphoidal *Salmonella* spp., has been observed in patients with malaria and bartonellosis. There is both epidemiologic and experimental mouse and human evidence to indicate this is an etiologic relationship and not coincidence. Study indicates that one mechanism involves the induction of heme oxygenase in marrow, impairing the ability of maturing neutrophils to develop a potent oxidative response mechanism. Macrophage and neutrophil dysfunction impairs innate immunity, and impotent phagocytes provide a site for proliferation of intracellular bacteria.[140]

REFERENCES

1. Robboy SJ, Salisbury K, Ragsdale B, et al. Mechanism of *Aspergillus*-induced microangiopathic hemolytic anemia. *Arch Intern Med.* 1971;128:790.
2. Freedman A, Afonja O, Chang MW, et al. Cutaneous anthrax associated with microangiopathic hemolytic anemia and coagulopathy in a 7-month-old infant. *JAMA.* 2002;287:869.
3. Pruthi RK, Marshall WF, Wiltsie JC, Persing DH. Human babesiosis. *Mayo Clin Proc.* 1995;70:853.
4. Reynafarje C, Ramos J. The hemolytic anemia of human bartonellosis. *Blood.* 1961;17:562.
5. Schultz MG. A history of Bartonellosis (Carrión's disease). *Am J Trop Med Hygiene.* 1968;17:503.
6. Smith MA, Shah NR, Lobel JS, Hamilton W. Methemoglobinemia and hemolytic anemia associated with *Campylobacter jejuni* enteritis. *Am J Pediatr Hematol Oncol.* 1988;10:3588.
7. Damani NN, Humphrey CA, Bell B. Haemolytic anaemia in *Campylobacter* enteritis. *J Infect.* 1993;26:109.
8. Rogstad B, Ritland S, Lunde S, Hagen AG. *Clostridium perfringens* septicemia with massive hemolysis. *Infection.* 1993;21:54.
9. Kreidl KO, Green GR, Wren SM. Intravascular hemolysis from a *Clostridium perfringens* liver abscess. *J Am Coll Surg.* 2002;194:387.
10. Pirofsky B. Infectious disease and autoimmune hemolytic anemia. In: *Autoimmunization and the Autoimmune Hemolytic Anemias.* Waverly Press; 1969:147.
11. van Spronsen DJ, Breed WP. Cytomegalovirus-induced thrombocytopenia and haemolysis in an immunocompetent adult. *Br J Haematol.* 1996;92:218.
12. Dacie JV. Secondary or symptomatic hemolytic anemias. In: Dacie JV, ed. *The Haemolytic Anaemias, Part III.* Grune & Stratton; 1967:908.
13. Tonkin AM, Mond HG, Alford FP, Hurley TH. Severe acute haemolytic anaemia complicating infectious mononucleosis. *Med J Aust.* 1973;2:1048.
14. Whitelaw F, Brook MG, Kennedy N, Weir WR. Haemolytic anaemia complicating Epstein-Barr virus infection. *Br J Clin Pract.* 1995;49:212.
15. Ludwig K, Ruder H, Bitzan M, et al. Outbreak of *Escherichia coli* O157: H7 infection in a large family. *Eur J Clin Microbiol Infect Dis.* 1997;16:238.
16. Pennings CM, Seitz RC, Karch H, Lenard HG. Haemolytic anaemia in association with *Escherichia coli* O157 infection in two sisters. *Eur J Pediatr.* 1994;153:656.
17. Chand DH, Brady RC, Bissler JJ. Hemolytic uremic syndrome in an adolescent with *Fusobacterium necrophorum* bacteremia. *Am J Kidney Dis.* 2001;37:E22.
18. Gundersen SG, Bjoerneklett A, Bruun JN. Severe erythroblastopenia and hemolytic anemia during a hepatitis A infection. *Scand J Infect Dis.* 1989;21:225.
19. Kanematsu T, Nomura T, Higashi K, Ito M. Hemolytic anemia in association with viral hepatitis. *Nippon Rinsho.* 1996;54:2539.
20. Urganci N, Akyildiz B, Yildirmak Y, Ozbay G. A case of autoimmune hepatitis and autoimmune hemolytic anemia following hepatitis A infection. *Turk J Gastroenterol.* 2003;14:204.
21. Gurgey A, Yuce A, Ozbek N, Kocak N. Acute hemolysis in association with hepatitis B infection in a child with beta-thalassemia trait. *Turk J Pediatr.* 1994;36:259.
22. Etienne A, Gayet S, Vidal F, et al. Severe hemolytic anemia due to cold agglutinin complicating untreated chronic hepatitis C: efficacy and safety of anti-CD20 (rituximab) treatment. *Am J Hematol.* 2004;75:243.
23. Shurin SB, Anderson P, Zollinger J, Rathbun RK. Pathophysiology of hemolysis in infections with *Haemophilus influenzae* type B. *J Clin Invest.* 1986;77:1340.
24. Rheingold SR, Burnham JM, Rutstein R, Manno CS. HIV infection presenting as severe autoimmune hemolytic anemia with disseminated intravascular coagulation in an infant. *J Pediatr Hematol Oncol.* 2004;26:9.
25. Koduri PR, Singa P, Nikolinakos P. Autoimmune hemolytic anemia in patients infected with human immunodeficiency virus-1. *Am J Hematol.* 2002;70:174.
26. Saif MW. HIV-associated autoimmune hemolytic anemia: an update. *AIDS Patient Care STDS.* 2001;15:217.
27. Watanabe T. Hemolytic uremic syndrome associated with influenza A virus infection. *Nephron.* 20001;89:359.
28. Asaka M, Ishikawa I, Nakazawa T, et al. Hemolytic uremic syndrome associated with influenza A virus infection in an adult renal allograft recipient: case report and review of the literature. *Nephron.* 2000;84:258.
29. Trowbridge AA, Green JB III, Bonnett JD, et al. Hemolytic anemia associated with leptospirosis. Morphologic and lipid studies. *Am J Clin Pathol.* 1981;76:493.
30. Woodruff AW, Topley E, Knight R, Downie CGB. The anaemia of kala azar. *Br J Haematol.* 1972;22:319.
31. Ozen S, Damarguc I, Besbas N, et al. A case of mumps associated with acute hemolytic crisis resulting in hemoglobinuria and acute renal failure. *J Med.* 1994;25:255.
32. Kuo PH, Yang PC, Kuo SS, Luh KT. Severe immune hemolytic anemia in disseminated tuberculosis with response to antituberculosis therapy. *Chest.* 2001;119:1961.
33. Fiala M, Myhre BA, Chinh LT, et al. Pathogenesis of anemia associated with *Mycoplasma pneumoniae. Acta Haematol.* 1974;51:297.
34. Chambers LA, Rauck AM. Acute transient hemolytic anemia with a positive Donath-Landsteiner test following parvovirus B19 infection. *J Pediatr Hematol Oncol.* 1996;18:178.
35. Weatherall DJ, Miller LH, Baruch DI, et al. Malaria and the red cell. *Hematology Am Soc Hematol Educ Program.* 2002;35.
36. White NJ. The treatment of malaria. *N Engl J Med.* 1996;335:800.
37. Moriuchi H, Yamasaki S, Mori K, et al. A rubella epidemic in Sasebo, Japan in 1987, with various complications. *Acta Paediatr Jpn.* 1990;32:67.
38. Yoneda S, Yoshikawa M, Yamane Y, et al. A case of rubella complicated by hemolytic anemia. *Kansenshogaku Zasshi.* 2000;74:724.
39. Albaqali A, Ghuloom A, Al Arrayed A, et al. Hemolytic uremic syndrome in association with typhoid fever. *Am J Kidney Dis.* 2003;41:709.
40. Houdouin V, Doit C, Mariani P, et al. A pediatric cluster of Shigella dysenteriae serotype 1 diarrhea with hemolytic uremic syndrome in 2 families from France. *Clin Infect Dis.* 2004;38:e96.
41. Kavaliotis J, Karyda S, Konstantoula T, et al. Shigellosis of childhood in northern Greece: epidemiological, clinical and laboratory data of hospitalized patients during the period 1971–1996. *Scand J Infect Dis.* 1994;26:207.
42. Shepherd AB, Palmer AL, Bigler SA, Baliga R. Hemolytic uremic syndrome associated with group A beta-hemolytic streptococcus. *Pediatr Nephrol.* 2003;18:949.
43. Apilanez UM, Areses TR, Ruiz Benito MA, et al. Hemolytic uremic syndrome secondary to Streptococcus pneumoniae pulmonary infection. *An Esp Pediatr.* 2002; 57:378.
44. Reynolds E, Espinoza M, Monckeberg G, Graf J. Hemolytic-uremic syndrome and *Streptococcus pneumoniae. Rev Med Chil.* 2002;130:677.
45. Brandt J, Wong C, Mihm S, et al. Invasive pneumococcal disease and hemolytic uremic syndrome. *Pediatrics.* 2002;110:371.
46. Wéry M, Mulumba PM, Lambert PH, Kazyumba L. Hematologic manifestations, diagnosis, and immunopathology of African trypanosomiasis. *Semin Hematol.* 1982;19:83.
47. Papalia MA, Schwarer AP. Paroxysmal cold haemoglobinuria in an adult with chicken pox. *Br J Haematol.* 2000;109:328.
48. Von Knorring J, Pettersson T. Haemolytic anaemia complicating *Yersinia enterocolitica* infection. Report of a case. *Scand J Haematol.* 1972;9:149.
49. Berkowitz FE. Hemolysis and infection: categories and mechanisms of their interrelationship. *Rev Infect Dis.* 1991;13:1151.
50. Seitz RC, Buschermohle G, Dubberke G, et al. The acute infection-associated hemolytic anemia of childhood: immunofluorescent detection of microbial antigens altering the erythrocyte membrane. *Ann Hematol.* 1993;67:191.
51. World Health Organization. Fact Sheet. Malaria. https://www.who.int/news-room/fact-sheets/detail/malaria.
52. Thellier M, Simard F, Musset L, et al. Changes in malaria epidemiology in France and worldwide, 2000-2015. *Med Mal Infect.* 2019;pii:S0399-077X(18)30592-4.
53. Allain JP, Owusu-Ofori AK, Assennato SM, et al. Effect of Plasmodium inactivation in whole blood on the incidence of blood transfusion-transmitted malaria in endemic

regions: the African Investigation of the Mirasol System (AIMS) randomised controlled trial. *Lancet.* 2016;387:1753-1761.

54. Martín-Dávila P, Norman F, Fortún-Abete J, et al. Donor-derived multiorgan transmission of mixed P. malariae and P. ovale infection: impact of globalization on post-transplant infections. *Transpl Infect Dis.* 2018;20:e12938.

55. Miller LH, Ackerman HC, Su X, Wellems TE. Malaria biology and disease pathogenesis: insights for new treatments. *Nature.* 2013;19:156.

56. Tham WH, Healer, J Cowman A. Erythrocyte and reticulocyte binding-like proteins of *Plasmodium falciparum*. *Trends Parasitol.* 2012;28:23.

57. Matthews KM, Pitman EL, de Koning-Ward TF. Illuminating how malaria parasites export proteins into host erythrocytes. *Cell Microbiol.* 2019;21:e13009.

58. Wong W, Huang R, Menant S, et al. Structure of Plasmodium falciparum Rh5-CyRPA-Ripr invasion complex. *Nature.* 2019;565:118-121.

59. Salinas ND, Tolia NH. Red cell receptors as access points for malaria infection. *Curr Opin Hematol.* 2016;23(3):215-223.

60. Newbold C, Warn P, Black G, et al. Receptor-specific adhesion and clinical disease in *Plasmodium falciparum*. *Am J Trop Med Hyg.* 1997;57:389.

61. Baruch DI, Ma XC, Singh HB, et al. Identification of a region of PfEMP1 that mediates adherence of *Plasmodium falciparum* infected erythrocytes to CD36: conserved function with variant sequence. *Blood.* 1997;90:3766.

62. Sherman IW, Eda S, Winograd E. Cytoadherence and sequestration in *Plasmodium falciparum*: defining the ties that bind. *Microbes Infect.* 2003;5:897.

63. Udomsangpetch R, Taylor BJ, Looareesuwan S, et al. Receptor specificity of clinical *Plasmodium falciparum* isolates: nonadherence to cell-bound E-selectin and vascular cell adhesion molecule-1. *Blood.* 1996;88:2754.

64. McCormick CJ, Craig A, Roberts D, et al. Intercellular adhesion molecule-1 and CD36 synergize to mediate adherence of *Plasmodium falciparum*-infected erythrocytes to cultured human microvascular endothelial cells. *J Clin Invest.* 1997;100:2521.

65. Bridges DJ, Bunn J, van Mourik JA, et al. Rapid activation of endothelial cells enables *Plasmodium falciparum* adhesion to platelet-decorated von Willebrand factor strings. *Blood.* 2010;115:1472.

66. Cockburn IA, MacKinnon MJ, O'Donnell A, et al. A human complement receptor 1 polymorphism that reduces *Plasmodium falciparum* rosetting confers protection against severe malaria. *Proc Natl Acad Sci U S A.* 2004;101:272.

67. Herrera S, Rudin W, Herrera M, et al. A conserved region of the MSP-1 surface protein of *Plasmodium falciparum* contains a recognition sequence for erythrocyte spectrin. *EMBO J.* 1993;12:1607.

68. Lamikanra AA, Brown D, Potocnik A, et al. Malarial anemia: of mice and men. *Blood.* 2007;110:18.

69. Mombo LE, Ntoumi F, Bisseye C, et al. Human genetic polymorphisms and asymptomatic *Plasmodium falciparum* malaria in Gabonese school-children. *Am J Trop Med. Hyg.* 2003;68:186.

70. Clegg JB, Weatherall DJ. Thalassemia and malaria: new insights into an old problem. *Proc Assoc Am Physician.* 1999;111:278.

71. Zimmerman PA, Patel SS, Maier AG, et al. Erythrocyte polymorphisms and malaria parasite invasion in Papua New Guinea. *Trends Parasitol.* 2003;19:250.

72. Angus BJ, Chotivanich K, Udomsangpetch R, White NJ. In vivo removal of malaria parasites from red blood cells without their destruction in acute falciparum malaria. *Blood.* 1997;90:2037.

73. Jakeman GN, Saul A, Hogarth WL, Collins WE. Anaemia of acute malaria infections in non-immune patients primarily results from destruction of uninfected erythrocytes. *Parasitology.* 1999;119(pt 2):127.

74. George JN, Wicker DJ, Fogel BJ, et al. Erythrocytic abnormalities in experimental malaria. *Proc Soc Exp Biol Med.* 1967;124:1086.

75. Overman RR. Reversible cellular permeability alterations in disease. In vivo studies on sodium, potassium and chloride concentrations in erythrocytes of the malarious monkey. *Am J Physiol.* 1948;152:113.

76. Gatidis S, Föller M, Lang F. Hemin-induced suicidal erythrocyte death. *Ann Hematol.* 2009;88:721.

77. Clark IA, Hunt NH. Evidence for reactive oxygen intermediates causing hemolysis and parasite death in malaria. *Infect Immun.* 1983;39:1.

78. Stocker R, Cowden WB, Tellan RL, et al. Lipids from *Plasmodium vinckei*-infected erythrocytes and their susceptibility to oxidative damage. *Lipids.* 1987;22:51.

79. Yuthavong Y, Limpaiboon T. The relationship of phosphorylation of membrane proteins with the osmotic fragility and filterability of *Plasmodium berghei*-infected mouse erythrocytes. *Biochim Biophys Acta.* 1987;929:278.

80. Balcerzak SP, Arnold JD, Martin DC. Anatomy of red cell damage by *Plasmodium falciparum* in man. *Blood.* 1972;40:98.

81. Jenkins NE, Chakravorty SJ, Urban BC, et al. The effect of *Plasmodium falciparum* infection on expression of monocyte surface molecules. *Trans R Soc Trop Med Hyg.* 2006;100:1007.

82. Helegbe GK, Goka BQ, Kurtzhals JA, et al. Complement activation in Ghanaian children with severe *Plasmodium falciparum* malaria. *Malar J.* 2007;6:165.

83. De Mast Q, Groot E, Asih PB. ADAMTS13 deficiency with elevated levels of ultra-large and active von Willebrand factor in P. falciparum and P. vivax malaria. *Am J Trop Med Hyg.* 20009;80:492-8.

84. Löwenberg EC, Charunwatthana P, Cohen S, et al. Severe malaria is associated with a deficiency of von Willebrand factor cleaving protease, ADAMTS13. *Thromb Haemost.* 2010;103:181-187.

85. Barber BE, Grigg MJ, Piera KA, et al. Intravascular haemolysis in severe *Plasmodium Kownlesi* malaria: association with endothelial activation, microvascular dysfunction, and acute kidney injury. *Emerg Microbes Infect.* 2018;7:106-116.

86. Price R, van Vugt M, Phaipun L, et al. Adverse effects in patients with acute falciparum malaria treated with artemisinin derivatives. *Am J Trop Med Hyg.* 1999;60:547.

87. Mouatcho JC, Goldring JP. Malaria rapid diagnostic tests: challenges and prospects. *J Med Microbiol.* 2013;62(pt 10):1491.

88. Weiss JB. DNA probes and PCR for diagnosis of parasitic infections. *Clin Microbiol Rev.* 1995;8:113.

89. Mangold KA, Manson RU, Koay ES, et al. Real time PCR for detection and identification of *Plasmodium* spp. *J Clin Microbiol.* 2005;43:2435.

90. Tedla M. A focus on improving molecular diagnostic approaches to malaria control and elimination in low transmission settings: review. *Parasite Epidemiol Control.* 2019;6:e00107.

91. Campuzano-Zuluaga G, Hanscheid T, Grobusch MP. Automated haematology analysis to diagnose malaria. *Malar J.* 2010;9:346.

92. Flannery EL, Chatterjee AK, Winzeler EA. Antimalarial drug discovery—approaches and progress towards new medicines. *Nat Rev Microbiol.* 2013;11:849.

93. Krey RA, Travassos MA. Severe malaria treatment in the United States at the precipice. *Ann Intern Med.* 2019;171:362-363.

94. Beutler E, Duparc S; G6PD Deficiency Working Group. Glucose-6-phosphate dehydrogenase deficiency and antimalarial drug development. *Am J Trop Med Hyg.* 2007;77:779.

95. Seder RA, Chang LJ, Enama ME, et al. Protection against malaria by intravenous immunization with a nonreplicating sporozoite vaccine. *Science.* 2013;341:1359.

96. Riley EM, Stewart VA. Immune mechanisms in malaria: new insights in vaccine development. *Nat Med.* 2013;19:168.

97. Ashley EA, Poespoprodjo JR. Treatment and prevention of malaria in children. *Lancet Child Adolescent Hlth* 2020;4:775.

98. Aldana L. Bacteriologia de la enfermedad de carrion. *Cron Med.* 1929;46:235.

99. Garcia-Quintanilla M, Dichter AA, Guerra H, Kempf VA. Carrion's disease: more than a neglected disease. *Parasit Vectors.* 2019;12:141.

100. Xu YH, Lu ZY, Ihler GM. Purification of deformin, an extracellular protein synthesized by *Bartonella bacilliformis* which causes deformation of erythrocyte membranes. *Biochim Biophys Acta.* 1995;1234:173.

101. Mitchell SJ, Minnick MF. Characterization of a two-gene locus from *Bartonella bacilliformis* associated with the ability to invade human erythrocytes. *Infect Immun.* 1995;63:1552.

102. Weinman D. Human *Bartonella* infection and African sleeping sickness. *Bull N Y Acad Med.* 1946;22:647.

103. García-Esteban C, Gil H, Rodríguez-Vargas M, et al. Molecular method for *Bartonella* species identification in clinical and environmental samples. *J Clin Microbiol.* 2008;46:776.

104. Rolain JM, Brouqui P, Koehler JE, et al. Recommendations for treatment of human infections caused by Bartonella species. *Antimicrob Agents Chemother.* 2004;48(6):1921-33.

105. Biswas S, Rolain JM. Bartonella infection: treatment and drug resistance. *Future Microbiol.* 2010;5:1719-31.

106. Gray EB, Herwaldt BL. Babesiosis surveillance—United States, 2011-2015. *MMWR Surveill Summ.* 2019;68:1-11.

107. Vannier E, Krause PJ. Human babesiosis. *N Engl J Med.* 2012;366:239712.

108. Vannier EG, Diuk-Wasser MA, Ben Mamoun C, Krause PJ. Babesiosis. *Infect Dis Clin North Am.* 2015;29:357-370.

109. Westblade LF, Simon MS, Mathison BA, Kirkman LA. Babesia microti: from mice to ticks to an increasing number of highly susceptible humans. *J Clin Microbiol.* 2017;55:2903-2912.

110. Steketee RW, Eckman MR, Burgess EC, et al. Babesiosis in Wisconsin. A new focus of disease transmission. *JAMA.* 1985;253:2675.

111. Herwaldt BL, McGovern PC, Gerwel MP, et al. Endemic babesiosis in another eastern state: New Jersey. *Emerg Infect Dis.* 2003;9:184.

112. Tonnetti L, Townsend RL, Dodd RY, Stramer SL. Characteristics of transfusion-transmitted Babesia microti, American Red Cross 2010-2017. *Transfusion.* 2019;59(9):2908-2912.

113. Levin AE, Krause PJ. Transfusion-transmitted babesiosis: is it time to screen the blood supply? *Curr Opin Hematol.* 2016;23:573-580.

114. Reubush TK II, Cassaday PB, Marsh HJ, et al. Human babesiosis on Nantucket Island. *Ann Intern Med.* 1977;86:6.

115. Kletsova EA, Spitzer ED, Fries BC, Marcos LA. Babesiosis in Long Island: review of 62 cases focusing on treatment with azithromycin and atovaquone. *Ann Clin Microbiol Antimicrob.* 2017;16:26.

116. Homer MJ, Aguilar-Delfin I, Telford SR 3rd, et al. Babesiosis. *Clin Microbiol Rev.* 2000;13:451.

117. Cheng D, Yakobi-Shvilli R, Fernandez J. Life-threatening hypotension from babesiosis hemolysis. *Am J Emerg Med.* 2002;20:367.

118. Chang D, Hossain M, Hossain MA. Severe babesiosis masquerading as thrombotic thrombocytopenic purpura: a case report. *Cureus.* 2019;11:e4459.

119. Khangura RK, Williams N, Cooper S, Prabulos AM. Babesiosis in pregnancy: an imitator of HELLP syndrome. *AJP Rep.* 2019;9:e147-e152.

120. Wittner M, Rowin KS, Tanowitz HB, et al. Successful chemotherapy of transfusion babesiosis. *Ann Intern Med.* 1982;96:601.

121. Weiss LM, Babesiosis in humans: a treatment review. *Expert Opin Pharmacother.* 2002;3:1109.

122. Mordue DG, Wormser GP. Could the drug tafenoquine revolutionize treatment of Babesia microti infection? *J Infect Dis.* 2019;220(3):442-447.

123. van Bunderen CC, Bomers MK, Wesdorp E, et al. Clostridium perfringens septicaemia with massive intravascular haemolysis: a case report and review of the literature. *Neth J Med.* 2010;68:343-346.

124. Hamoda H, Chamberlain PF. *Clostridium welchii* infection following amniocentesis: a case report and review of the literature. *Prenat Diagn.* 2002;22:783.

125. Simpkins H, Kahlenberg A, Rosenberg A, et al. Structural and compositional changes in the red cell membrane during *Clostridium welchii* infection. *Br J Haematol.* 1971;21:173.

126. Shindo Y, Dobashi Y, Sakai T, et al. Epidemiological and pathobiological profiles of Clostridium perfringens infections: review of consecutive series of 33 cases over a 13-year period. *Int J Clin Exp Pathol.* 2015;8:569-577.

127. Mahn HE, Dantuono LM. Postabortal septicotoxemia due to *Clostridium welchii. Am J Obstet Gynecol.* 1955;70:604.

128. Moustoukas NM, Nichols RL, Voros D, Clostridial sepsis: unusual clinical presentations. *South Med J.* 1985;78:440.

129. Neter E. Bacterial hemagglutination and hemolysis. *Bacteriol Rev.* 1956;20:166.

130. Ceppellini R, De Gregorio M. Crisi emolitica in animali batterio-immuni transfusi con sangue omologo sensibilizzato in vitro mediante l'antigene batterico specifico. *Boll Ist Sieroter Milan.* 1953;32:445.

131. Dausset J, Moullec J, Bernard J. Acquired hemolytic anemia with polyagglutinability of red blood cells due to a new factor. *Blood.* 1959;14:1079.

132. Klein PJ, Vierbuchen M, Roth B, et al. Hemolytic anemia in infections caused by neuraminidase-producing bacteria. *Verh Dtsch Ges Pathol.* 1983;67:415.

133. McCullough J. RBCs as targets of infection. *Hematol Am Soc Hematol Educ Prog.* 2014;2014:404-9.

134. McGinniss MH, Macher AM, Rook AH, Alter HJ. Red cell autoantibodies in patients with acquired immune deficiency syndrome. *Transfusion.* 1986;26:405.

135. Zuelzer WW, Stulberg CS, Page RH, et al. The Emily Cooley lecture. Etiology and pathogenesis of acquired hemolytic anemia. *Transfusion.* 1966;6:438.

136. He J, Liu M, Ye Z, et al. Insights into the pathogenesis of Mycoplasma pneumoniae [review]. *Mol Med Rep.* 2016;14:4030-4036.

137. Walker CL, Applegate JA, Black RE. Haemolytic-uraemic syndrome as a sequela of diarrhoeal disease. *J Health Popul Nutr.* 2012;30:257.

138. Binks S, Regan K, Richenberg J, Chevassut T. Microbes without frontiers: severe haemolytic-uraemic syndrome due to E coli O104:H4. *BMJ Case Rep.* 2012;2012:21.

139. Dickgiesser A. Campylobacter infection and the hemolytic-uremic syndrome. *Immun Infekt.* 1983;11:71.

140. Orf K, Cunnington AJ. Infection-related hemolysis and susceptibility to Gram-negative bacterial co-infection. *Front Microbiol.* 2015;6:666.

CHAPTER 25
HYPERSPLENISM AND HYPOSPLENISM

Srikanth Nagalla and Jaime Caro

SUMMARY

The spleen culls aged and abnormal cells from the blood; removes intraery-throcytic inclusions through a process called *pitting*; sequesters approximately one-third of the normal intravascular platelet pool; removes bacteria, foreign particles, and tumor cells from the blood; and by virtue of the T and B lymphocytes and macrophages in the white pulp, plays a role in immune surveillance and antibody formation. Splenomegaly can occur as a result of vascular engorgement or cellular infiltration, and it is frequently associated with a combination of neutropenia, thrombocytopenia, and anemia. Hypersplenism is defined as one or more blood cytopenias in the setting of splenomegaly. Hypersplenism can occur with moderate or minimal splenic enlargement as a result of exaggerated removal of physically abnormal (eg, as in hereditary spherocytosis) or antibody-coated blood cells (eg, as in autoimmune hemolytic anemia). The presence of splenomegaly in a patient with blood cytopenias is useful to narrow the cause of the cytopenias, although the cause of the blood cytopenias may not be solely or principally as a result of hypersplenism (eg, as in hairy cell leukemia). Thrombocytopenia in the setting of cirrhosis and splenomegaly is the result of pooling in the enlarged spleen and a relative decrease in thrombopoietin. The role of the spleen in the anemia and neutropenia associated with cirrhosis with splenomegaly is poorly understood, but a relative reduction in erythropoietin levels and decreased marrow myeloid progenitor cells have been proposed. Splenectomy has been used in cases of severe thrombocytopenia requiring chronic platelet transfusions or leading to bleeding, especially for immune thrombocytopenia. Thrombopoietin receptor agonists are another option in the management of thrombocytopenia, and nonpeptide thrombopoietin receptor agonists have been shown to increase platelet counts in patients with thrombocytopenia associated with hepatitis C virus–related cirrhosis and splenomegaly. Splenectomy may be justified in the case of massive splenomegaly, infarction, or disabling symptoms of pain and compression of neighboring structures. In some circumstances, benefit can be achieved by partial destruction of splenic tissue by embolization using intraarterial infusion of gel microparticles. Hyposplenism can result from agenesis, atrophy, surgical removal of the spleen, or reduction of splenic function by disease. In the latter case, disturbance in splenic circulation disrupts the specific architecture required for the spleen's culling, phagocytic, and pitting functions. Hyposplenism may be suspected by alterations in red cell morphology, such as target cells or acanthocytes; red cell inclusions, specifically Howell-Jolly

and Pappenheimer bodies (siderotic granules highlighted with polychrome stains); pitted red cells; or an elevated platelet count. The presence of pitted red cells identified by interference-contrast microscopy is perhaps the most specific blood finding of hyposplenism followed by Howell-Jolly bodies. The most devastating consequence of hyposplenism is sudden overwhelming sepsis by encapsulated bacteria. Immunizations and prophylactic antibiotics can decrease the risk of sepsis. A high awareness and prompt antibiotic treatment of febrile episodes are warranted.

● HYPERSPLENISM

HISTORY

The spleen has intrigued physicians and philosophers since ancient times[1] and has been assigned mysterious powers, but its association with destruction of blood cells was not elucidated until the turn of the 20th century. The exaggerated and unfounded worry about somatic complaints often reflected by the sense of pain in the spleen (left hypochondrium) led to the term *hypochondriac*. In 1899, Chauffard proposed that increased splenic activity causes hemolysis.[2] This proposal provided the impetus for therapeutic splenectomy, which was performed first in 1910 by Sutherland and Burghard[3] in a patient with splenic anemia (hereditary spherocytosis) and subsequently by Kaznelson[4] in a patient with essential thrombocytopenia (immune thrombocytopenia) in 1916.

DEFINITION

Hypersplenism is defined as blood cytopenias in the setting of splenomegaly. This is usually accompanied by hyperplasia of the affected cell precursors in the marrow. There can be a disproportional decrease in the blood platelets, white cells, and red cells, with thrombocytopenia and leukopenia being disproportionate to the anemia as a result of hypersplenism. Splenomegaly can occur as a result of elevated splenic venous pressures and vascular congestion, histiophagocytic hyperplasia, or other cellular infiltration or because of the inability of physically abnormal red cells, such as sickle cells in infants and children (before infarction atrophy), or antibody-coated cells, such as in autoimmune hemolytic anemia, to navigate the circulation or avoid engulfment by the mononuclear phagocyte population of the normal spleen.[5] The blood cytopenias are not generally corrected by relief of portal hypertension.[6,7]

ONTOGENY

The embryonic spleen appears in the first trimester of gestation as a multiply lobulated condensation of highly vascular mesenchymal cell aggregates interposed in the arterial circulation in the dorsal mesogastrium. The full scope of the molecular basis of splenic organogenesis is not known. The *HOX11 and WT1* genes are essential for its formation, and defects in their expression result in hyposplenia or asplenia.[8-10]

The lymphoid compartment, the white pulp, begins its development early in the second trimester of gestation, when mature T cells, principally CD4+ lymphocytes, form a continuous layer along the length of the vessels (periarteriolar sheaths). CD8+ cells reside in splenic cords and a specialized subset of γδT cells home to the pulp. Immunoglobulin (Ig) D+ and IgG+ B lymphocytes form localized deposits, the primary lymph follicles. Secondary follicles arise later in life, after exposure to immunologic stimuli, and have a distinctive structure that includes a germinal center, a mantle zone, and a marginal zone containing IgM+ and IgG+ B lymphocytes.[11,12]

Acronyms and Abbreviations: G-CSF, granulocyte colony-stimulating factor; Ig, immunoglobulin; TRA, thrombopoietin-receptor agonist.

STRUCTURE AND FUNCTIONAL ORGANIZATION

The normal adult spleen weighs 135 ± 30 g and has a blood flow that is approximately 5% of the cardiac output. In addition to serving as a filter, the spleen plays a role in innate and adaptive immunity and protection against microbes. The spleen is composed of white pulp, a marginal zone, and red pulp. The spleen's principal structure is organized around an arborizing array of arterioles that branch and narrow until they terminate in either (a) the stroma of cords, forming the open circulation, or (b) the sinusoids, forming the closed circulation of the spleen. The cordal elements include histiocytes, antigen-presenting cells, pericytes, fibroblasts, and other cells necessary to maintain the discontinuous basal lamina that separates cords from sinusoid lumen.[13] Lymphatic tissue is inconspicuous and found in T cell–rich zones in the periarteriolar lymphoid sheaths.

The arterial vascular tree, which is lined by conventional CD31+ and CD34+ endothelial cells, branches into arterioles that terminate abruptly in caps of cordal macrophages. Blood cells must pass clusters of macrophages to enter the sinusoids.[13] The sinusoids, the origin of the venous circulation, are lined by specialized cells having combined phagocytic and endothelial activities and a distinctive CD31+, CD34–, CD68+, CD8+ phenotype. A principal function of the spleen is to serve as a filter, removing aged or defective red cells and foreign particles by macrophages. This function is facilitated by diverting part of the splenic blood supply into the red pulp, where the blood slowly percolates through the nonendothelialized mesh studded with macrophages. Abnormal or senescent red cells and pathogens undergo phagocytosis by the macrophages. The blood then reenters the circulation through narrow slits, measuring 1 to 3 μm, in the endothelium of the venous sinuses. The bulk of the blood is rapidly channeled through vessels that link the arterioles with the venous sinuses. This blood is not filtered or modified.[14]

Approximately one-third of platelets are normally sequestered in the spleen.[15] In many animals, such as dogs and horses, the red pulp is a reservoir for red cells, and splenic contraction provides the red cell volume with a functionally important boost.[16] In humans, however, the splenic capsule is poorly contractile, and the spleen does not store red cells to any significant degree.[17] Although margination of neutrophils occurs in the spleen, it is unclear to what degree it occurs in that site.[18] Granulocyte colony-stimulating factor (G-CSF) administered to cirrhotic patients caused a rise in the blood neutrophil count; thereafter, indium scans of the spleen were performed, which did not show significant uptake by white cells.[19]

The slow transit of blood through the red pulp permits macrophages to recognize and destroy antibody- or complement-coated red cells and microorganisms and to ingest poorly deformable red cells or particles retained mechanically by the narrow exit slits in the venous sinuses. The white pulp plays a major role in adaptive immunity. The spleen is involved in the phagocytosis of encapsulated bacteria, including *Streptococcus pneumoniae*, *Haemophilus influenzae*, and *Neisseria meningitidis*.

PATHOPHYSIOLOGY

Filtration and elimination of defective cells occur notably in hereditary abnormalities of the red cell membranes, such as spherocytosis, elliptocytosis, or stomatocytosis, or with antibody-coated red cells, neutrophils, or platelets. In these circumstances, cytopenias of varying severity may ensue. The spleen not only removes antibody-coated cells but also produces antibodies, especially antiplatelet antibodies.[20] Thus, the benefits of splenectomy in immune thrombocytopenia is a result of both the decreased production of antiplatelet antibodies as well as decreased clearance by macrophages of antibody-coated platelets through the Fc recognition function of its large macrophage population.

Splenomegaly increases the proportion of blood channeled through the red pulp.[13,21] Spleen enlargement may result from expansion of the red pulp compartment with increased blood flow; extramedullary hematopoiesis, notable in primary myelofibrosis; hyperplasia or neoplasia involving the white pulp, such as in infectious mononucleosis or lymphoma; or histiophagocytic hyperplasia.

The increased size of the filtering bed is more pronounced when the splenomegaly is caused by congestion as in portal hypertension than when it is caused by cellular infiltration as in leukemias, extramedullary hematopoiesis, or amyloidosis. Even in space-occupying disorders such as Gaucher disease and primary myelofibrosis, splenomegaly may be associated with hypersplenic sequestration of normal cells.

Splenomegaly increases the vascular surface area and thereby the marginated neutrophil pool.[18,19] Platelets are especially likely to be sequestered in an enlarged spleen. However, sequestered white cells and platelets survive in the spleen and may be available when increased demand requires neutrophils or platelets, although their release may be slow.[22]

Some patients with anemia and splenomegaly have a relative erythropoietin deficiency.[23] In one study of cirrhotic patients, 30% had a blunted erythropoietin response to anemia.[24] Dilution of red cells in an expanded plasma volume is another commonly cited cause of a decreased blood hemoglobin concentration,[25] although some studies do not demonstrate hemodilution.[26] Iron deficiency associated with chronic blood loss, folic acid and vitamin B_{12} deficiency, and increased red cell destruction are frequently investigated, although rarely found in patients with liver disease.[27] Red cells are destroyed prematurely in the red pulp in the setting of splenomegaly but only rarely does this explain the anemia.[28]

Varying amounts of erythrophagocytosis are present, reflecting the normal culling of senescent red cells. Erythrophagocytosis increases as a result of hemolytic anemia and viral infections and in alloimmunized transfusion recipients. Macrophages within the sinusoids contain red cell fragments. When the process is pronounced, the littoral cells become cuboidal and stand out on the basement membrane ("hobnails"). Sickle cell disease and red cell membrane disorders such as hereditary spherocytosis lead to sequestration of the poorly deformed red cells in the cords, but little extrasinusoidal erythrophagocytosis is seen, in contrast to immune hemolytic anemia, in which macrophage erythrophagocytosis is prominent.[13]

The increased blood flow from an enlarged spleen expands the splenic and portal veins. A significant increase in portal venous pressure may occur when hepatic vessel compliance is decreased, as in cirrhosis or myelofibrosis. This process initiates a vicious cycle in which portal hypertension contributes to splenomegaly and organ enlargement leads to increased arterial blood flow, which in turn increases portal pressure.

Table 25-1 lists causes of splenomegaly, and Table 25-2 lists causes of massive splenic enlargement.

CLINICAL FEATURES

Slight to moderate enlargement of the spleen usually does not produce local symptoms. Even massive splenomegaly can be well tolerated if it develops gradually. However, frequently, the patient complains of a sagging feeling or other types of abdominal discomfort, early satiety from gastric encroachment, and trouble sleeping on one side. Pleuritic pain in the left upper quadrant or referred to the left shoulder may accompany splenic infarcts, which may be recurrent.

TABLE 25–1. Classification and Most Common Causes of Splenomegaly

1. Congestive
   a. Right-sided congestive heart failure
   b. Budd-Chiari syndrome (inferior vena cava and hepatic vein thrombosis)
   c. Cirrhosis with portal hypertension
   d. Portal or splenic vein thrombosis
2. Immunologic
   a. Viral infection
      i. Acute HIV infection or chronic infection
      ii. Acute mononucleosis
      iii. Dengue fever
      iv. Rubella (rare except in newborns)
      v. Cytomegalovirus (rare except in newborns)
      vi. Herpes simplex (rare except in newborns)
   b. Bacterial infection
      i. Subacute bacterial endocarditis
      ii. Brucellosis
      iii. Tularemia
      iv. Melioidosis
      v. Listeriosis
      vi. Plague
      vii. Secondary syphilis
      viii. Relapsing fever
      ix. Psittacosis
      x. Ehrlichiosis
      xi. Rickettsial diseases (scrub typhus, Rocky Mountain spotted fever, Q fever)
      xii. Tuberculosis
      xiii. Splenic abscess (most common organisms are *Enterobacteriaceae*, *Staphylococcus aureus*, *Streptococcus* group D, and anaerobic organisms as part of mixed flora infections)
   c. Fungal infection
      i. Blastomycosis
      ii. Histoplasmosis
      iii. Systemic candidiasis; hepatosplenic candidiasis

   d. Parasitic infection
      i. Malaria
      ii. Kala-Azar
      iii. Leishmaniasis
      iv. Schistosomiasis
      v. Babesiosis
      vi. Coccidioidomycosis
      vii. Paracoccidioidomycosis
      viii. Trypanosomiasis (cruzi, brucei)
      ix. Toxoplasmosis (rare except newborns)
      x. Echinococcosis
      xi. Cysticercosis
      xii. Visceral larva migrans (*Toxocara* infection)
   e. Inflammatory or autoimmune
      i. Systemic lupus erythematosus
      ii. Felty syndrome
      iii. Juvenile rheumatoid arthritis
      iv. Autoimmune lymphoproliferative syndrome
      v. Hemophagocytic syndrome
      vi. Common variable immunodeficiency
      vii. Splenomegaly caused by granulocyte colony-stimulating factor administration
      viii. Anti-D immunoglobulin administration (RhoGAM)
3. Secondary to hemolysis
   a. Thalassemia major
   b. Pyruvate kinase deficiency
   c. Hereditary spherocytosis
   d. Autoimmune hemolytic anemia (uncommon)
   e. Sickle cell disease in early childhood (splenic sequestration)
4. Infiltrative
   a. Nonmalignant
      i. Splenic hematoma (splenic cysts are usually a late complication of a hematoma)
      ii. Littoral cell angioma

      iii. Disorders of sphingolipid metabolism
         1. Gaucher disease
         2. Niemann-Pick disease
      iv. Cystinosis
      v. Amyloidosis (light chain amyloid and amyloid A protein)
      vi. Multicentric Castleman disease
      vii. Mastocytosis
      viii. Hypereosinophilic syndrome
      ix. Sarcoidosis
   b. Extramedullary hematopoiesis
      i. Primary myelofibrosis
      ii. Osteopetrosis (childhood)
      iii. Thalassemia major
   c. Malignant
      i. Hematologic
         1. Chronic lymphocytic leukemia (especially prolymphocytic variant)
         2. Chronic myeloid leukemia
         3. Polycythemia vera
         4. Hairy cell leukemia
         5. Heavy chain disease
         6. Hepatosplenic lymphoma
         7. Acute leukemia (acute lymphoblastic leukemia/acute myeloid leukemia)
         8. Hodgkin lymphoma
      ii. Nonhematologic
         1. Metastatic carcinoma (rare)
         2. Neuroblastoma
         3. Wilms tumor
         4. Leiomyosarcoma
         5. Fibrosarcoma
         6. Malignant fibrous histiocytoma
         7. Kaposi sarcoma
         8. Hemangiosarcoma
         9. Lymphangiosarcoma
         10. Hemangioendothelial sarcoma

In children with sickle cell anemia or patients with malaria, the spleen may become acutely enlarged and painful as a result of a sudden increase in red cell pooling and sequestration. These sequestration crises are characterized by sudden aggravation of the anemia. Splenic rupture is uncommon but can occur spontaneously with most causes of splenic enlargement or after blunt trauma. Rupture related to the splenic enlargement in infectious mononucleosis is a classic example.

The volume of an enlarged spleen is difficult to assess by palpation and percussion. Children and thin patients with low diaphragms may have a palpable spleen tip without splenomegaly.[29] Generally, a palpable spleen signifies splenomegaly and is measured by the number of centimeters the spleen extends below the left costal margin. Splenic size is most accurately measured with abdominal ultrasound (Fig. 25-1) or computed tomographic scans (Fig. 25-2). Magnetic resonance imaging is used primarily to identify cysts, abscesses, and infarcts.[30]

SPLENOPTOSIS

A wandering spleen (splenoptosis) is an uncommon phenomenon in which the spleen hangs by a long pedicle of mesentery. The spleen could

TABLE 25–2. Causes of Massive Splenomegaly

1. Myeloproliferative disorders
   a. Primary myelofibrosis
   b. Chronic myeloid leukemia
2. Lymphomas
   a. Hairy cell leukemia
   b. Chronic lymphocytic leukemia (especially prolymphocytic variant)
3. Infectious
   a. Malaria
   b. Leishmaniasis (kala azar)
4. Extramedullary hematopoiesis
   a. Thalassemia major
5. Infiltrative
   a. Gaucher disease

shift into the lower part of the abdomen or pelvis because of defects in the ligaments that fix the spleen.[31] The condition may present in three ways: (1) an asymptomatic mass in the pelvis; (2) intermittent abdominal pain with or without gastrointestinal symptoms; or less often, (3) an acute abdomen resulting from torsion. The diagnosis of splenoptosis may be made coincidentally on an imaging study.[32] The condition may be accompanied by signs of hypersplenism or hyposplenism and often, when developing slowly, is initially mistaken for a pelvic or lower abdominal tumor.

LABORATORY FEATURES

The characteristic features of hypersplenism are splenomegaly, blood cytopenias, and absence of other causes of cytopenias (eg, anemia caused by bleeding). The blood cell morphology usually is normal, although a few spherocytes may result from metabolic conditioning of red cells during repeated slow transits through the expanded red pulp. Tests, such as epinephrine mobilization, were used in the past to try to distinguish sequestration from ineffective cellular production, but results are difficult to interpret because epinephrine also releases platelets and neutrophils from marginal pools.[33]

Thrombocytopenia is a common finding in patients with hepatic cirrhosis, portal hypertension, and splenomegaly. In a retrospective study, 64% of patients with nonalcoholic cirrhosis had thrombocytopenia.[34] Other studies have found that approximately one-third of patients with cirrhosis develop severe thrombocytopenia or neutropenia.[35,36] Decompensated liver disease and history of alcohol consumption are independent risk factors for hypersplenism,[37] but why some patients develop marked blood cytopenias is not clear, although folate deficiency is a factor in some instances. The presence of thrombocytopenia or leukopenia in patients with chronic liver disease is associated with increased mortality.[38]

Ultrasound-guided fine-needle biopsy of the spleen can be useful in circumstances in which the spleen holds the tissue required for diagnosis, such as splenic lymphoma. However, fine-needle aspiration is rarely a definitive diagnostic tool but can indicate monoclonality of splenic lymphocytes, which is helpful and forces further diagnostic evaluation. Aspiration cytology and core biopsy can be obtained with relative safety in experienced hands using image-guided fine needles.[39]

The response to transfusion of blood products, especially platelets, may be significantly impaired in patients with massive splenomegaly.[40]

THERAPY, COURSE, AND PROGNOSIS

Total Splenectomy

Splenectomy is indicated as an emergency procedure after abdominal trauma and partial rupture of the spleen. It also may be indicated when splenic size or infarcts causes sustained left upper abdominal pain or discomfort. Splenectomy has been used for the treatment of functionally significant blood cytopenias.[40] In such circumstances, case reports have described dramatic restoration of blood counts to normal levels within days to weeks after splenectomy; however, the only controlled trial evaluating relief of cytopenias showed no improvement.[7] Orthotopic liver transplant corrects the cytopenias in the majority of patients with cirrhosis.[41]

Hereditary spherocytosis, immune thrombocytopenia, and immune hemolytic anemia are the most common indications for splenectomy. Splenectomy exerts its effect in autoimmune cytopenias by improving cell survival and also by decreasing autoantibody production. In thalassemia major, an improvement in the anemia is well described after splenectomy. In such cases, splenectomy may improve the response to transfusion. Some children with sickle cell anemia may benefit from splenectomy if repeated sequestration crises with abdominal pain occur before autosplenectomy renders the spleen atrophic.[42]

Splenectomy in patients with a massive spleen size (>1500 g), especially in primary myelofibrosis, is accompanied by higher morbidity and mortality than is removal of the spleen for immune blood cytopenia.[43]

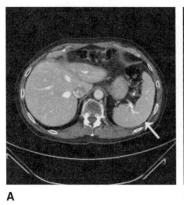   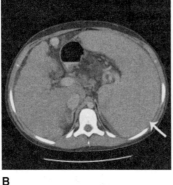   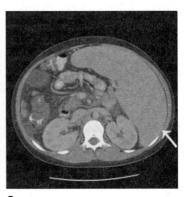

A   **B**   **C**

FIGURE 25–1. A three-way composite of abdominal computerized tomography. **A.** Normal spleen size. **B.** Enlarged spleen. **C.** Massively enlarged spleen at the level of the midkidney. Normally, the spleen would either not be visualized, or only a small lower pole would be evident at the level of the mid-kidney. The *white arrow* in each of the three images marks the edge of the splenic silhouette. *(Kindly provided by Deborah Rubens, MD, The University of Rochester Medical Center.)*

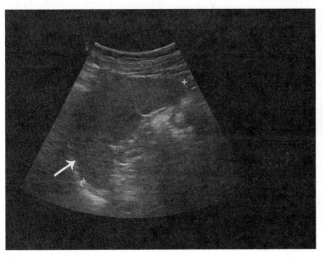

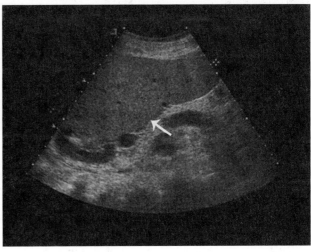

A

B

FIGURE 25–2. A two-way composite of ultrasonography examination for spleen size. **A.** Image of echo indicating the normal spleen size with cranial to caudal longitudinal dimension of 10.3 cm. **B.** Image of echo indicating an enlarged spleen with a cranial-to-caudal longitudinal dimension of 16.2 cm. The *white arrow* in each image marks the edge of the splenic silhouette. The normal spleen is usually less than 13 cm in length, but the examiner has to consider other dimensions in assessing spleen size (volume). *(Kindly provided by Deborah Rubens, MD, The University of Rochester Medical Center.)*

Possible postoperative complications include extensive adhesions with collateral blood vessels, hepatic or portal vein thrombosis, injury to the tail of the pancreas, operative site infections, and subdiaphragmatic abscesses.

Laparoscopic splenectomy performed by experienced surgeons for suitable hematologic conditions can result in less abdominal trauma and pain, shorter hospital stays, and smaller abdominal scars.[44] Laparoscopic splenectomy has lower mortality and complication rates than open splenectomy in immune thrombocytopenia.[45] It could be safely performed in patients with very low platelet counts.[46] An advantage of open splenectomy in hematologic conditions such as the treatment of immune thrombocytopenia is the increased ease of searching assiduously for accessory spleens.

Infections from encapsulated organisms and venous and arterial thromboembolic events are some of the systemic complications after splenectomy.[47-49]

Partial Splenectomy

Partial splenectomy has been explored because it may minimize the risks of immediate postsplenectomy thrombocytosis and overwhelming sepsis that may result from a complete absence of splenic function.[50] However, the degree of thrombocytosis after splenectomy wanes to some degree with time since splenectomy. Reduction of the splenic volume has been performed with ligation of some of the splenic arteries or the intraarterial infusion of Gelfoam particles causing embolization.[51-54] These procedures induce large splenic infarcts and reduce the functional splenic mass. Arterial embolization can be performed percutaneously or intravascularly, but the patients must be observed closely for a number of days to weeks to detect signs of intraabdominal rupture of the splenic infarcts. The long-term results of embolization have been encouraging.[52-56] Treatment with partial arterial embolization for recurrent thrombocytopenia in children temporarily improved the platelet count in approximately 70% of patients.[57]

Splenic Radiation

Splenic radiation for treatment of an enlarged spleen is used sparingly. The procedure may be associated with severe cytopenias and especially thrombocytopenia (abscopal effect). It can be used in patients with an absolute contraindication to splenectomy who might benefit symptomatically from reduction of a massively enlarged spleen.[58]

Liver Transplantation

Thrombopoietin synthesis and secretion are impaired in liver failure and this is corrected after liver transplantation.[59,60] However, thrombocytopenia may not be corrected after liver transplant if the splenomegaly persists.

Thrombopoietin Receptor Agonists

After thrombopoietin was cloned,[61,62] several thrombopoietin mimetic drugs have been developed and tested. A phase II study reported that the oral thrombopoietin-receptor agonist (TRA) eltrombopag increases platelet counts in patients with thrombocytopenia as a result of hepatitis C virus–related cirrhosis.[63] A phase III study done in cirrhotic patients who received eltrombopag for 2 weeks before elective procedures had to be terminated prematurely because of the increased incidence of portal vein thrombosis in the treatment group compared to the placebo group. Although 72% of the eltrombopag patients avoided platelet transfusions compared with 19% of the placebo group patients, there was no significant difference in the incidence of major bleeding.[64] A small study using the TRA romiplostim administered subcutaneously in cirrhotic patients demonstrated the usefulness of the drug in reducing platelet transfusions in preparation for an elective surgical procedure.[65] Patients with chronic liver disease undergoing radiofrequency ablation were able to achieve a sustained increase in platelet counts with lusutrombopag, an oral TRA.[66] Another oral TRA, avatrombopag, was effective in increasing the platelet counts ($\geq 50 \times 10^9$/L) in patients with chronic liver disease undergoing procedures compared with a placebo. There was no increase in the incidence of thrombosis between avatrombopag and placebo groups.[67]

Erythropoietin and Granulocyte Colony-Stimulating Factor

There are minimal data to support the use of erythropoietic or myeloid growth factors in patients with splenomegaly and blood cytopenias.

Patients with cirrhosis who have inappropriately low serum erythropoietin levels may benefit from treatment with exogenous erythropoietin; however, it may increase spleen size. Two reports documented the use of erythropoietin before and after liver transplantation to amplify marrow erythropoiesis in patients who refused blood transfusions for religious reasons.[68,69] These reports demonstrated that liver transplantation in the setting of advanced cirrhosis can be successfully undertaken without the use of blood products.

A rise in the neutrophil count after G-CSF administration was described in patients with cirrhosis and leukopenia. The mean absolute neutrophil count increased from $1300 \pm 200/\mu L$ to $4100 \pm 200/\mu L$ after subcutaneous administration of G-CSF for 7 days.[19] However, the clinical benefit of such treatment is not clear.

⬤ HYPOSPLENISM

DEFINITION

Hyposplenism is the designation for decreased splenic function resulting from diseases that impair function or from the absence of splenic tissue because of agenesis, atrophy (eg, autoinfarction of sickle cell disease), or splenectomy. Splenic hypofunction may be associated with a normal spleen size. In some cases, engorgement of ingested materials impairs the macrophage-dependent functions of the spleen. Impaired filtering function may cause a mild thrombocytosis. Functional or anatomical asplenia, especially after surgical removal in infants and children, increases the risk of an overwhelming bacterial infection. Table 25-3 lists conditions associated with hyposplenism.

CLINICAL FEATURES

Normal neonates and older adults may have findings suggestive of impaired splenic function.[70] These include the presence of Howell-Jolly bodies and erythrocyte pits (see "Laboratory Features" later). However, the clinical significance of functional hyposplenism is uncertain.[71-73]

Sickle cell anemia and surgical splenectomy are the most common causes of hyposplenism. In sickle cell anemia, hyposplenism may be functional in young children with enlarged spleens and disordered circulation and may be the result of atrophy after repeated infarcts have destroyed splenic tissue in older children and adults. Although the presence of an enlarged spleen usually suggests hypersplenism, spleen size is not a reliable index of splenic function. Complete splenic replacement by cysts, neoplastic tissue, or amyloid is an example of hyposplenic splenomegaly.[74] Acute sequestration crises in children with sickle hemoglobinopathies, and occasionally in patients with malaria, may clog the red cell pulp with cellular debris and lead to hyposplenism.[75,76]

Congenital asplenia may be found in infants with situs inversus and other developmental abnormalities.[39] Autoimmune disorders, such as glomerulonephritis,[77] systemic lupus erythematosus,[78,79] and rheumatoid arthritis,[80] are occasionally associated with laboratory evidence and clinical manifestations (overwhelming sepsis with encapsulated bacteria) of functional hyposplenism. Hyposplenism also occurs in chronic graft-versus-host disease,[81,82] sarcoidosis,[83] alcoholic liver cirrhosis,[84,85] hepatic amyloidosis,[86,87] celiac disease,[88,89] and inflammatory bowel disease.[90,91] The mechanisms for these associations are unknown.

Splenic replacement by neoplastic cells, as in lymphomas and leukemias, usually does not cause hyper- or hyposplenism. Splenic irradiation[92] and vascular obstruction[93] may also lead to functional hyposplenism.

TABLE 25-3. Conditions Associated with Hyposplenism
MISCELLANEOUS
Surgical splenectomy
Splenic irradiation
Sickle hemoglobinopathies
Congenital agenesis
Thrombosis of splenic artery or vein
Normal infants
GASTROINTESTINAL AND HEPATIC DISEASES
Celiac disease
Dermatitis herpetiformis
Inflammatory bowel disease
Cirrhosis
AUTOIMMUNE DISORDERS
Systemic lupus erythematosus
Rheumatoid arthritis
Vasculitis
Glomerulonephritis
Hashimoto thyroiditis
Sarcoidosis
HEMATOLOGIC AND NEOPLASTIC DISORDERS
Graft-versus-host disease
Essential thrombocytosis
Chronic lymphocytic leukemia
Non-Hodgkin lymphoma
Hodgkin lymphoma
Amyloidosis
Advanced breast cancer
Hemangiosarcoma
SEPSIS AND INFECTIOUS DISEASES
Malaria
Disseminated meningococcemia

Overwhelming Sepsis

Absence of a functional spleen may lead to life-threatening infections by removal of an efficient filtering bed in which opsonized organisms are engulfed and destroyed by splenic macrophages. The responsible organism is typically an encapsulated bacterium, such as *S. pneumoniae*, *N. meningitidis*, or *H. influenzae*. Unrestrained in vivo proliferation of such microorganisms may cause fatal septicemia.[94-96] The risk is greatest among infants whose general immunologic system has not matured enough to counteract bacterial infections, although the risk is present regardless of the patient's age. For this reason, splenectomy in children should be deferred until 5 years of age, if possible. The risk of sepsis varies depending on the reason for the splenectomy. In a child with an underlying immune disorder, such as Wiskott-Aldrich syndrome, the risk is very high. The infectious risk is higher in children with thalassemia than in those with hereditary spherocytosis and lowest in those with splenectomy for splenic trauma. The risk is reduced by the use of pneumococcal and *H. influenzae* vaccines before splenectomy and prophylactic penicillin therapy.[97]

Because the spleen is a major component of the mononuclear phagocyte system and has substantial lymphatic tissue in the white pulp, hyposplenism or splenectomy can also reduce antibody synthesis that may be beneficial in the management of autoimmune disorders.

LABORATORY FEATURES

The reduction or absence of normal splenic function is accompanied by a slight to moderate increase in white cell and platelet counts. Howell-Jolly bodies, target cells, Pappenheimer (siderotic) bodies, and occasional acanthocytes often are present in the blood film, but the finding of pitted erythrocytes in wet preparations is the most specific of all the blood findings.[98] Target cells reflecting an increased red cell surface[99] are almost always present in the asplenic state, but only 1 in 100 to 1 in 1000 red cells is affected. A sensitive indication of hyposplenism is the appearance of pits or pocks on the cell surface.[100] These pits consist of submembranous vacuoles and can be seen only in wet preparations of red cells using direct interference-contrast microscopy. Intracellular vesiculation containing hemoglobin is a normal occurrence during aging of the red cell in the circulation. This process is intensified in the last half of the erythrocyte lifespan and leads to a decreased mean cell hemoglobin level as the vesicles are removed (pitted) by the spleen. In asplenic individuals, the vesicles are more numerous and enlarge, forming vacuoles that are evident by interference-phase microscopy.[98] This finding is the most specific evidence of hyposplenism followed by the presence of DNA inclusions in circulating red cells (Howell-Jolly bodies; Fig. 25-3).

Oxidative drugs may produce Heinz bodies even in normal individuals, but the spleen effectively removes these red cell inclusions, as well as Pappenheimer bodies. Heinz bodies may be observed in supravitally stained blood films after splenectomy. Nucleated red cells rarely are seen on blood films after splenectomy, except in patients with hemolytic disorders in whom the number of nucleated red cells may increase dramatically. The reticulocyte count remains within normal values, and the lifespan of red cells is unchanged as other organs take up the function of removing senescent erythrocytes.

Technetium-99m sulfur-colloid particles are used for spleen scanning, a reliable measure of the capacity of the spleen to clear particulate matter from the bloodstream.[101]

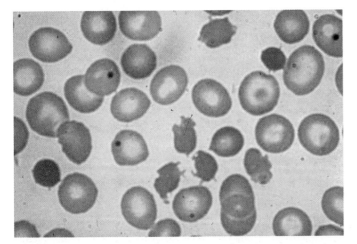

FIGURE 25–3. Blood film of splenectomized patient showing three red cells with Howell-Jolly bodies (nuclear remnants). Note also the cluster of acanthocytes and scattered spheroacanthocytes and the target cell. These changes are also indicative of postsplenectomy red cell changes. (*Reproduced with permission from Lichtman MA, Shafer MS, Felgar RE, et al: Lichtman's Atlas of Hematology 2016. New York, NY: McGraw Hill; 2017.*)

THERAPY, COURSE, AND PROGNOSIS

Vaccination against *H. influenzae*, *N. meningitidis*, and *S. pneumoniae* is recommended in previously unvaccinated individuals prior to splenectomy.[102] Prophylactic immunization has significantly reduced, but not eliminated, the risk of overwhelming infection.[97,103-105] Oral penicillin or a macrolide antibiotic as prophylaxis for asplenic patients is recommended based on publicized guidelines despite problems with compliance and resistance.[106,107] Physicians should advise all asplenic patients that any febrile episode (>38°C) should be considered an emergency requiring immediate medical attention. A febrile asplenic patient must have blood and urine cultures drawn followed by antibiotic treatment. Patients should be given written information about asplenia and carry a card or medical alert bracelet to alert health professionals of the risk of overwhelming infection.[106,107] Dental work, especially tooth extraction, should be preceded by broad-spectrum antibiotics, such as amoxicillin, if the patient is not taking prophylactic antibiotics. Patients should be educated about risks of travel, including risk of malaria infection or animal bites, which could be deadly unless promptly treated.[106,107]

REFERENCES

1. Crosby WH. The spleen. In: Wintrobe MM, ed. *Blood, Pure and Eloquent: A Story of Discovery, of People, and of Ideas.* McGraw Hill; 1980:96.
2. Chauffard AME. Des hepatites d'origine splenique. *Semin Med.* 1899;19.
3. Sutherland GA BF. The treatment of splenic anaemia by splenectomy. *Lancet.* 1910;2.
4. Kaznelson P. Verschwinden der hamorrhagischen Diathesis bei einen falle von "Essentieller Thrombopenia." *Wien Klin Wochenschr.* 1916;29:1451.
5. Crosby WH. Hypersplenism. *Annu Rev Med.* 1962;13:127-146.
6. Jabbour N, Zajko A, Orons P, et al. Does transjugular intrahepatic portosystemic shunt (TIPS) resolve thrombocytopenia associated with cirrhosis? *Dig Dis Sci.* 1998;43(11):2459-2462.
7. Mutchnick MG, Lerner E, Conn HO. Effect of portacaval anastomosis on hypersplenism. *Dig Dis Sci.* 1980;25(12):929-938.
8. Dear TN, Colledge WH, Carlton MB, et al. The Hox11 gene is essential for cell survival during spleen development. *Development.* 1995;121(9):2909-2915.
9. Roberts CW, Shutter JR, Korsmeyer SJ. Hox11 controls the genesis of the spleen. *Nature.* 1994;368(6473):747-749.
10. Roberts CW, Sonder AM, Lumsden A, Korsmeyer SJ. Development expression of Hox11 and specification of splenic cell fate. *Am J Pathol.* 1995;146(5):1089-1101.
11. Bordessoule D, Gaulard P, Mason DY. Preferential localisation of human lymphocytes bearing gamma delta T cell receptors to the red pulp of the spleen. *J Clin Pathol.* 1990;43(6):461-464.
12. Steiniger B, Barth P, Herbst B, et al. The species-specific structure of microanatomical compartments in the human spleen: strongly sialoadhesin-positive macrophages occur in the perifollicular zone, but not in the marginal zone. *Immunology.* 1997;92(2):307-316.
13. Kraus MD. Splenic histology and histopathology: an update. *Semin Diagn Pathol.* 2003;20(2):84-93.
14. Rosse WF. The spleen as a filter. *N Engl J Med.* 1987;317(11):704-706.
15. Bowdler AJ. Splenomegaly and hypersplenism. *Clin Haematol.* 1983;12(2):467-488.
16. Elenes NA, Ewald RA, Crosby WH. The reservoir function of the spleen and its relation to postsplenectomy anemia in the dog. *Blood.* 1964;24:299-304.
17. Wadenvik H, Kutti J. The spleen and pooling of blood cells. *Eur J Haematol.* 1988;41(1):1-5.
18. Aster RH. Pooling of platelets in the spleen: role in the pathogenesis of "hypersplenic" thrombocytopenia. *J Clin Invest.* 1966;45(5):645-657.
19. Gurakar A, Fagiuoli S, Gavaler JS, et al. The use of granulocyte-macrophage colony-stimulating factor to enhance hematologic parameters of patients with cirrhosis and hypersplenism. *J Hepatol.* 1994;21(4):582-586.
20. Karpatkin S. The spleen and thrombocytopenia. *Clin Haematol.* 1983;12(2):591-604.
21. Zwiebel WJ, Mountford RA, Halliwell MJ, Wells PN. Splanchnic blood flow in patients with cirrhosis and portal hypertension: investigation with duplex Doppler US. *Radiology.* 1995;194(3):807-812.
22. Brubaker LH, Johnson CA. Correlation of splenomegaly and abnormal neutrophil pooling (margination). *J Lab Clin Med.* 1978;92(4):508-515.
23. Siciliano M, Tomasello D, Milani A, et al. Reduced serum levels of immunoreactive erythropoietin in patients with cirrhosis and chronic anemia. *Hepatology.* 1995;22(4 pt 1):1132-1135.
24. Vasilopoulos S, Hally R, Caro J, et al. Erythropoietin response to post-liver transplantation anemia. *Liver Transpl.* 2000;6(3):349-355.
25. Hess CE, Ayers CR, Sandusky WR, et al. Mechanism of dilutional anemia in massive splenomegaly. *Blood.* 1976;47(4):629-644.
26. Zhang B, Lewis SM. Splenic haematocrit and the splenic plasma pool. *Br J Haematol.* 1987;66(1):97-102.

27. Jandl JH. The anemia of liver disease: observations on its mechanism. *J Clin Invest.* 1955;34(3):390-404.

28. Christensen BE. Quantitative determination of splenic red blood cell destruction in patients with splenomegaly. *Scand J Haematol.* 1975;14(4):295-302.

29. McIntyre OR, Ebaugh FG Jr. Palpable spleens in college freshmen. *Ann Intern Med.* 1967;66(2):301-306.

30. Sty JR, Wells RG. Imaging the spleen, in *Disorders of the Spleen: Pathophysiology and Management*, edited by Pochedly C, Sills RH, Schwartz AD. Marcel Dekker, 1989,355.

31. Varga I, Babala J, Kachlik D. Anatomic variations of the spleen: current state of terminology, classification, and embryological background. *Surg Radiol Anat.* 2018;40(1):21-29.

32. Buehner M, Baker MS. The wandering spleen. *Surg Gynecol Obstet.* 1992;175(4):373-387.

33. Joyce RA, Boggs DR, Hasiba U, Srodes CH. Marginal neutrophil pool size in normal subjects and neutropenic patients as measured by epinephrine infusion. *J Lab Clin Med.* 1976;88(4):614-620.

34. Alvarez OA, Lopera GA, Patel V, et al. Improvement of thrombocytopenia due to hypersplenism after transjugular intrahepatic portosystemic shunt placement in cirrhotic patients. *Am J Gastroenterol.* 1996;91(1):134-137.

35. Bashour FN, Teran JC, Mullen KD. Prevalence of peripheral blood cytopenias (hypersplenism) in patients with nonalcoholic chronic liver disease. *Am J Gastroenterol.* 2000;95(10):2936-2939.

36. Peck-Radosavljevic M. Hypersplenism. *Eur J Gastroenterol Hepatol.* 2001;13(4):317-323.

37. Liangpunsakul S, Ulmer BJ, Chalasani N. Predictors and implications of severe hypersplenism in patients with cirrhosis. *Am J Med Sci.* 2003;326(3):111-116.

38. Qamar AA, Grace ND, Groszmann RJ, et al. Incidence, prevalence, and clinical significance of abnormal hematologic indices in compensated cirrhosis. *Clin Gastroenterol Hepatol.* 2009;7(6):689-695.

39. Civardi G, Vallisa D, Berte R, et al. Ultrasound-guided fine needle biopsy of the spleen: high clinical efficacy and low risk in a multicenter Italian study. *Am J Hematol.* 2001;67(2):93-99.

40. Pouchedly C. Sills RH, Schwartz AD eds. *Disorders of the Spleen: Pathophysiology and Management.* New York: Marcel Dekker, Inc.; 1989:1-472.

41. Yanaga K, Tzakis AG, Shimada M, et al. Reversal of hypersplenism following orthotopic liver transplantation. *Ann Surg.* 1989;210(2):180-183.

42. al-Salem AH, Qaisaruddin S, Nasserallah Z, et al. Splenectomy in patients with sickle-cell disease. *Am J Surg.* 1996;172(3):254-258.

43. Mohren M, Markmann I, Dworschak U, et al. Thromboembolic complications after splenectomy for hematologic diseases. *Am J Hematol.* 2004;76(2):143-147.

44. Caprotti R, Porta G, Franciosi C, et al. Laparoscopic splenectomy for hematological disorders. Our experience in adult and pediatric patients. *Int Surg.* 1998;83(4):303-307.

45. Kojouri K, Vesely SK, Terrell DR, George JN. Splenectomy for adult patients with idiopathic thrombocytopenic purpura: a systematic review to assess long-term platelet count responses, prediction of response, and surgical complications. *Blood.* 2004;104(9):2623-2634.

46. Agcaoglu O, Aksakal N, Tukenmez M, et al. Is laparoscopic splenectomy safe in patients with immune thrombocytopenic purpura and very low platelet count? A single-institution experience. *Ann Ital Chir.* 2019;90:417-420.

47. Rorholt M, Ghanima W, Farkas DK, Norgaard M. Risk of cardiovascular events and pulmonary hypertension following splenectomy—a Danish population-based cohort study from 1996-2012. *Haematologica.* 2017;102(8):1333-1341.

48. Thomsen RW, Schoonen WM, Farkas DK, et al. Risk of venous thromboembolism in splenectomized patients compared with the general population and appendectomized patients: a 10-year nationwide cohort study. *J Thromb Haemost.* 2010;8(6):1413-1416.

49. Yong M, Thomsen RW, Schoonen WM, et al. Mortality risk in splenectomised patients: a Danish population-based cohort study. *Eur J Intern Med.* 2010;21(1):12-16.

50. Bar-Maor JA. Partial splenectomy in Gaucher's disease: follow-up report. *J Pediatr Surg.* 1993;28(5):686-688.

51. Banani SA. Partial dearterialization of the spleen in thalassemia major. *J Pediatr Surg.* 1998;33(3):449-453.

52. Palsson B, Hallen M, Forsberg AM, Alwmark A. Partial splenic embolization: long-term outcome. *Langenbecks Arch Surg.* 2003;387(11-12):421-426.

53. Petersons A, Volrats O, Bernsteins A. The first experience with non-operative treatment of hypersplenism in children with portal hypertension. *Eur J Pediatr Surg.* 2002;12(5):299-303.

54. Stanley P, Shen TC. Partial embolization of the spleen in patients with thalassemia. *J Vasc Interv Radiol.* 1995;6(1):137-142.

55. Kis B, Mills M, Smith J, et al. Partial splenic artery embolization in 35 cancer patients: results of a single institution retrospective study. *J Vasc Interv Radiol.* 2020;31(4):584-591.

56. Vittorio J, Orellana K, Martinez M, et al. Partial splenic embolization is a safe and effective alternative in the management of portal hypertension in children. *J Pediatr Gastroenterol Nutr.* 2019;68(6):793-798.

57. Watanabe Y, Todani T, Noda T. Changes in splenic volume after partial splenic embolization in children. *J Pediatr Surg.* 1996;31(2):241-244.

58. Paulino AC, Reddy SP. Splenic irradiation in the palliation of patients with lymphoproliferative and myeloproliferative disorders. *Am J Hosp Palliat Care.* 1996;13(6):32-35.

59. Peck-Radosavljevic M, Wichlas M, Zacherl J, et al. Thrombopoietin induces rapid resolution of thrombocytopenia after orthotopic liver transplantation through increased platelet production. *Blood.* 2000;95(3):795-801.

60. Rios R, Sangro B, Herrero I, et al. The role of thrombopoietin in the thrombocytopenia of patients with liver cirrhosis. *Am J Gastroenterol.* 2005;100(6):1311-1316.

61. de Sauvage FJ, Hass PE, Spencer SD, et al. Stimulation of megakaryocytopoiesis and thrombopoiesis by the c-Mpl ligand. *Nature.* 1994;369(6481):533-538.

62. Lok S, Kaushansky K, Holly RD, et al. Cloning and expression of murine thrombopoietin cDNA and stimulation of platelet production in vivo. *Nature.* 1994;369(6481):565-568.

63. McHutchison JG, Dusheiko G, Shiffman ML, et al. Eltrombopag for thrombocytopenia in patients with cirrhosis associated with hepatitis C. *N Engl J Med.* 2007;357(22):2227-2236.

64. Afdhal NH, Giannini EG, Tayyab G, et al. Eltrombopag before procedures in patients with cirrhosis and thrombocytopenia. *N Engl J Med.* 2012;367(8):716-724.

65. Moussa MM, Mowafy N. Preoperative use of romiplostim in thrombocytopenic patients with chronic hepatitis C and liver cirrhosis. *J Gastroenterol Hepatol.* 2013;28(2):335-341.

66. Tateishi R, Seike M, Kudo M, et al. A randomized controlled trial of lusutrombopag in Japanese patients with chronic liver disease undergoing radiofrequency ablation. *J Gastroenterol.* 2019;54(2):171-181.

67. Terrault N, Chen YC, Izumi N, et al. Avatrombopag before procedures reduces need for platelet transfusion in patients with chronic liver disease and thrombocytopenia. *Gastroenterology.* 2018;155(3):705-718.

68. Ramos HC, Todo S, Kang Y, et al. Liver transplantation without the use of blood products. *Arch Surg.* 1994;129(5):528-532; discussion 532-523.

69. Snook NJ, O'Beirne HA, Enright S, et al. Use of recombinant human erythropoietin to facilitate liver transplantation in a Jehovah's Witness. *Br J Anaesth.* 1996;76(5):740-743.

70. Freedman RM, Johnston D, Mahoney MJ, Pearson HA. Brief clinical and laboratory observations. *J Pediatr.* 1980;96(3 pt 1):466-468.

71. Markus HS, Toghill PJ. Impaired splenic function in elderly people. *Age Ageing.* 1991;20(4):287-290.

72. Padmanabhan J, Risemberg HM, Rowe RD. Howell-Jolly bodies in the peripheral blood of full-term and premature neonates. *Johns Hopkins Med J.* 1973;132(3):146-150.

73. Ravaglia G, Forti P, Biagi F, et al. Splenic function in old age. *Gerontology.* 1998;44(2):91-94.

74. Steinberg MH, Gatling RR, Tavassoli M. Evidence of hyposplenism in the presence of splenomegaly. *Scand J Haematol.* 1983;31(5):437-439.

75. Emond AM, Collis R, Darvill D, et al. Acute splenic sequestration in homozygous sickle cell disease: natural history and management. *J Pediatr.* 1985;107(2):201-206.

76. Looareesuwan S, Ho M, Wattanagoon Y, et al. Dynamic alteration in splenic function during acute falciparum malaria. *N Engl J Med.* 1987;317(11):675-679.

77. Lawrence S, Pussell BA, Charlesworth JA. Splenic function in primary glomerulonephritis. *Adv Exp Med Biol.* 1982;155:641-648.

78. Liote F, Angle J, Gilmore N, Osterland CK. Asplenism and systemic lupus erythematosus. *Clin Rheumatol.* 1995;14(2):220-223.

79. Webster J, Williams BD, Smith AP, et al. Systemic lupus erythematosus presenting as pneumococcal septicaemia and septic arthritis. *Ann Rheum Dis.* 1990;49(3):181-183.

80. Jarolim DR. Asplenia and rheumatoid arthritis. *Ann Intern Med.* 1982;97(4):616-617.

81. Cuthbert RJ, Iqbal A, Gates A, et al. Functional hyposplenism following allogeneic bone marrow transplantation. *J Clin Pathol.* 1995;48(3):257-259.

82. Kalhs P, Panzer S, Kletter K, et al. Functional asplenia after bone marrow transplantation. A late complication related to extensive chronic graft-versus-host disease. *Ann Intern Med.* 1988;109(6):461-464.

83. Stone RW, McDaniel WR, Armstrong EM, et al. Acquired functional asplenia in sarcoidosis. *J Natl Med Assoc.* 1985;77(11):930, 935-936.

84. Muller AF, Toghill PJ. Splenic function in alcoholic liver disease. *Gut.* 1992;33(10):1386-1389.

85. Muller AF, Toghill PJ. Functional hyposplenism in alcoholic liver disease: a toxic effect of alcohol? *Gut.* 1994;35(5):679-682.

86. Gertz MA, Kyle RA. Hepatic amyloidosis (primary [AL], immunoglobulin light chain): the natural history in 80 patients. *Am J Med.* 1988;85(1):73-80.

87. Powsner RA, Simms RW, Chudnovsky A, et al. Scintigraphic functional hyposplenism in amyloidosis. *J Nucl Med.* 1998;39(2):221-223.

88. O'Grady JG, Stevens FM, Harding B, et al. Hyposplenism and gluten-sensitive enteropathy. Natural history, incidence, and relationship to diet and small bowel morphology. *Gastroenterology.* 1984;87(6):1326-1331.

89. Robinson PJ, Bullen AW, Hall R, et al. Splenic size and function in adult coeliac disease. *Br J Radiol.* 1980;53(630):532-537.

90. Muller AF, Toghill PJ. Hyposplenism in gastrointestinal disease. *Gut.* 1995;36(2):165-167.

91. Palmer KR, Sherriff SB, Holdsworth CD, Ryan FP. Further experience of hyposplenism in inflammatory bowel disease. *Q J Med.* 1981;50(200):463-471.

92. Dailey MO, Coleman CN, Kaplan HS. Radiation-induced splenic atrophy in patients with Hodgkin's disease and non-Hodgkin's lymphomas. *N Engl J Med.* 1980;302(4):215-217.

93. Spencer RP, Sziklas JJ, Turner JW. Functional obstruction of splenic blood vessels in adults: a radiocolloid study. *Int J Nucl Med Biol.* 1982;9(3):208-211.

94. Cavenagh JD, Joseph AE, Dilly S, Bevan DH. Splenic sepsis in sickle cell disease. *Br J Haematol.* 1994;86(1):187-189.

95. Gopal V, Bisno AL. Fulminant pneumococcal infections in "normal" asplenic hosts. *Arch Intern Med.* 1977;137(11):1526-1530.

96. Torres J, Bisno AL. Hyposplenism and pneumococcemia. Visualization of Diplococcus pneumoniae in the peripheral blood smear. *Am J Med.* 1973;55(6):851-855.

97. Konradsen HB, Henrichsen J. Pneumococcal infections in splenectomized children are preventable. *Acta Paediatr Scand.* 1991;80(4):423-427.

98. Corazza GR, Ginaldi L, Zoli G, et al. Howell-Jolly body counting as a measure of splenic function. A reassessment. *Clin Lab Haematol.* 1990;12(3):269-275.

99. Holroyde CP, Oski FA, Gardner FH. The "pocked" erythrocyte. Red-cell surface alterations in reticuloendothelial immaturity of the neonate. *N Engl J Med.* 1969;281(10):516-520.

100. Reinhart WH, Chien S. Red cell vacuoles: their size and distribution under normal conditions and after splenectomy. *Am J Hematol.* 1988;27(4):265-271.

101. Rutland MD. Correlation of splenic function with the splenic uptake rate of Tc-colloids. *Nucl Med Commun.* 1992;13(11):843-847.

102. Kobel DE, Friedl A, Cerny T, et al. Pneumococcal vaccine in patients with absent or dysfunctional spleen. *Mayo Clin Proc.* 2000;75(7):749-753.

103. Castagnola E, Fioredda F. Prevention of life-threatening infections due to encapsulated bacteria in children with hyposplenia or asplenia: a brief review of current recommendations for practical purposes. *Eur J Haematol.* 2003;71(5):319-326.

104. Sumaraju V, Smith LG, Smith SM. Infectious complications in asplenic hosts. *Infect Dis Clin North Am.* 2001;15(2):551-565, x.

105. Ward KM, Celebi JT, Gmyrek R, Grossman ME. Acute infectious purpura fulminans associated with asplenism or hyposplenism. *J Am Acad Dermatol.* 2002;47(4):493-496.

106. Davies JM, Barnes R, Milligan D, British Committee for Standards in Haematology. Working Party of the Haematology/Oncology Task F. Update of guidelines for the prevention and treatment of infection in patients with an absent or dysfunctional spleen. *Clin Med (Lond).* 2002;2(5):440-443.

107. Working Party of the British Committee for Standards in Haematology Clinical Haematology Task F. Guidelines for the prevention and treatment of infection in patients with an absent or dysfunctional spleen. *BMJ.* 1996;312(7028):430-434.

CHAPTER 26
HEMOLYTIC ANEMIA RESULTING FROM IMMUNE INJURY

Charles H. Packman

SUMMARY

Autoimmune hemolytic anemia (AHA) is characterized by shortened red blood cell (RBC) survival and the presence of autoantibodies directed against autologous RBCs. Demonstration of antibody or complement on RBC membranes, usually by a positive direct antiglobulin test (DAT) result, is essential for diagnosis. Most patients (80%) with AHA exhibit warm-reactive antibodies of the immunoglobulin (Ig) G isotype on their red cells. Most of the remainder of patients exhibit cold-reactive autoantibodies. Two types of cold-reactive autoantibodies to RBCs are recognized: cold agglutinins and cold hemolysins. Cold agglutinins are generally of IgM isotype, whereas cold hemolysins usually are of IgG isotype. The DAT may detect IgG, proteolytic fragments of complement (mainly C3), or both on the RBCs of patients with warm-antibody AHA. In cold-antibody AHA, only complement is detected because the antibody dissociates from the RBCs during washing of the cells. About half of patients with AHA have no underlying associated disease; these cases are termed primary or idiopathic. Secondary cases are associated with underlying autoimmune, malignant, or infectious diseases or with administration of certain drugs.

Although most patients do not require transfusion of RBCs, transfusion should not be withheld from those with symptomatic anemia. In warm-antibody AHA, rituximab and glucocorticoids are effective in slowing the rate of hemolysis. Splenectomy is indicated for patients who are refractory to medical therapy or who require an unacceptably high maintenance dose or prolonged administration of glucocorticoids. IV immunoglobulin may provide short-term control of hemolysis. Immunosuppressive drugs and danazol have been used successfully in refractory cases. In cold agglutinin– and cold hemolysin–mediated hemolysis, keeping the patient warm and treating underlying lymphoproliferative disorders usually are effective. Rituximab alone or in combination with bendamustine has been effective in more than half of cases of cold AHA. Drug-induced immune hemolytic anemia usually is ameliorated by discontinuation of the offending drug. Glucocorticoids are effective in AHA induced by immune checkpoint inhibitors.

Acronyms and Abbreviations: AHA, autoimmune hemolytic anemia; CDC, Centers for Disease Control and Prevention; CLL, chronic lymphocytic leukemia; DAF, decay-accelerating factor; DAT, direct antiglobulin test; HLA, human leukocyte antigen; HRF, homologous restriction factor; HS, hereditary spherocytosis; IAT, indirect antiglobulin test; Ig, immunoglobulin; IGHV, immunoglobulin heavy chain variable region; LDH, lactate dehydrogenase; PNH, paroxysmal nocturnal hemoglobinuria; RBC, red blood cell; SLE, systemic lupus erythematosus.

DEFINITION AND HISTORY

The two main features of immune red blood cell (RBC) injury are (1) shortened RBC survival in vivo and (2) evidence of host antibodies reactive with autologous RBCs, most frequently demonstrated by a positive direct antiglobulin test (DAT) result, also known as the Coombs test. Most cases in adults are mediated by warm-reactive autoantibodies. A smaller proportion of patients exhibit cold-reactive autoantibodies or drug-related antibodies.

By the early 20th century, reticulocytes, spherocytes, and osmotic fragility of RBCs had been described. Clinicians could diagnose hemolytic anemia, but the distinction between congenital and acquired forms was imprecise. Some clinicians even doubted the existence of acquired hemolytic anemia.[1] The sera of some patients with hemolytic anemia directly agglutinated saline suspensions of normal or autologous human RBCs. These serum factors, later shown to be specific antibodies (largely of the immunoglobulin [Ig] M class), were termed *direct* or *saline agglutinins*. In a smaller proportion of cases, the patients' sera could mediate lysis of the test RBCs in the presence of fresh serum as a complement source. The heat-stable factors (antibodies) necessary for in vitro complement-mediated lysis were called *hemolysins*. However, in the majority of cases of hemolytic anemia, neither direct agglutinins nor hemolysins could be demonstrated. In 1945, Coombs and colleagues[2] reported that RBCs coated with nonagglutinating Rh antibodies (now known to be of the IgG isotype) could be agglutinated by rabbit antiserum to human γ-globulin. That is, the rabbit antiglobulin serum cross-linked IgG antibody-coated RBCs to produce visible agglutination. Addition of rabbit antiglobulin serum to a suspension of washed RBCs isolated from patients with suspected acquired hemolytic anemia produced agglutination in many cases, including patients lacking saline agglutinins or hemolysins. RBCs from patients with congenital hemolytic anemia did not agglutinate.[3,4] This procedure now is termed the *direct antiglobulin (Coombs) test*. Subsequent studies established that positive direct antiglobulin reactions in autoimmune hemolytic anemia (AHA) are attributable to coating of the RBCs with immunoglobulins (mainly IgG) and/or complement proteins. When the RBCs are coated chiefly with complement proteins, a positive DAT result depends on the presence of anticomplement (principally anti-C3) in the antiglobulin reagent. In warm-antibody AHA, the autoantibodies, chiefly of IgG isotype, bind optimally to RBCs at 37°C. Warm antibodies may or may not activate complement binding to RBCs.

Cryopathic hemolytic syndromes are caused by autoantibodies that bind RBCs optimally at temperatures less than 37°C and usually less than 31°C. Two major types of "cold antibody" may produce AHA. Cold agglutinins, which directly agglutinate RBCs, mediate cold agglutinin disease. The Donath-Landsteiner autoantibody, which is not an agglutinin but a potent hemolysin, mediates paroxysmal cold hemoglobinuria. In both cryopathic syndromes, the complement system plays a major role in RBC injury; as such, much greater potential exists for direct intravascular hemolysis than in warm antibody–mediated AHA.

Cold agglutinins were first described by Landsteiner[5] in 1903. However, recognition of the connection among cold agglutinins, hemolytic anemia, and Raynaud-like peripheral vascular phenomena evolved slowly. In 1918, Clough and Richter[6] detected cold agglutinins in a patient with pneumonia. In 1925 and 1926, Iwai and MeiSai[7,8] reported two patients with cold agglutinins and Raynaud phenomenon and showed that flow of blood through capillary tubes in vitro or in superficial capillaries in vivo was impeded at low temperatures. During the late 1940s and early 1950s, the observations of many investigators gradually established the pathogenic importance of cold agglutinins in RBC injury. Schubothe[9] introduced the term *cold agglutinin disease* in

1953 and clearly distinguished the disorder from other acquired hemolytic syndromes.

In current usage, cold agglutinin disease pertains to patients with chronic AHA in which the autoantibody directly agglutinates human RBCs at temperatures below body temperature, maximally at 0°C to 5°C. Fixation of complement to a patient's RBCs by cold agglutinins in vivo occurs at higher temperatures but generally less than 37°C. Cold agglutinins typically are IgM, although occasionally they may be immunoglobulins of other isotypes. The cold agglutinins in chronic cold agglutinin disease generally are monoclonal. Most cold agglutinins have specificity for oligosaccharide antigens (I or i) of the RBC (see "Origin of Cold Agglutinins" later).

Donath and Landsteiner first described the cold hemolysin that bears their names in 1904. The Donath-Landsteiner antibody is responsible for complement-mediated hemolysis in paroxysmal cold hemoglobinuria, a rare form of AHA in adults. The disorder is characterized by recurrent episodes of massive hemolysis after cold exposure.[10,11] A related form of hemolytic anemia occurs much more commonly in children (or young adults) as an acute, self-limited hemolytic process after several types of viral syndromes.[10-16] The disease was recognized during the latter half of the 19th century, when the disease was more common because of its association with congenital or tertiary syphilis. With the advent of effective therapy for syphilis, this cause of paroxysmal cold hemoglobinuria has almost disappeared. Now, recurrent paroxysmal cold hemoglobinuria occurs very rarely in a chronic idiopathic form.[10,11] An increasing proportion of Donath-Landsteiner autoantibody-mediated hemolytic anemias occurs as a single postviral episode in children, without recurrent attacks (paroxysms). The prognosis for such cases is excellent. Thus, rather than paroxysmal cold hemoglobinuria, a proposed term for this latter entity is *Donath-Landsteiner hemolytic anemia*.[13,14]

The first example of drug-related immune blood cell destruction was Ackroyd's description of sedormid purpura in 1949.[17] In 1953, Snapper and coworkers[18] described a case of immune hemolysis and pancytopenia in a patient treated with mephenytoin (Mesantoin). Hemolysis ceased upon withdrawal of the drug. In 1956, Harris[19] reported what are now classic studies of a patient who developed immune hemolytic anemia during a second course of stibophen administered for treatment of schistosomiasis. Since then, many drugs have been implicated in the production of positive DATs and accelerated RBC destruction.

CLASSIFICATION

Warm-Reactive versus Cold-Reactive Red Cell Antibody

AHA can be classified in two complementary ways (Table 26-1). The majority of cases (80%-90% in adults) are mediated by warm-reactive autoantibodies[10,11,20] or antibodies displaying optimal reactivity with human RBCs at 37°C. A smaller proportion of cases are attributable to cold-reactive autoantibodies exhibiting greater affinity for RBCs at temperatures less than 37°C. The distinction is important, not only because of differences in the pathophysiology of RBC injury but also in the therapeutic approaches required. An even smaller proportion of patients with AHA exhibit both cold-reactive and warm-reactive autoantibodies,[21,22] which apparently recognize different antigens on the RBC membrane.[23] RBC destruction is generally more severe in mixed cases.

Absence or Presence of an Associated Disease

Classification of AHA based on the presence or absence of underlying diseases also is useful (see Table 26-1). When no recognizable underlying disease is present, the AHA is termed *primary* or *idiopathic*. When AHA appears to be a manifestation or complication of an underlying disorder, the term *secondary AHA* is applied. Lymphocytic malignancies, particularly chronic lymphocytic leukemia (CLL) and lymphomas,

TABLE 26-1. Classification of Hemolytic Anemia as a Result of Immune Injury

I. Warm-Autoantibody Type: Autoantibody Maximally Active at Body Temperature (37°C)
   A. Primary or idiopathic warm autoimmune hemolytic anemia (AHA)
   B. Secondary warm AHA
      1. Associated with lymphoproliferative disorders (eg, Hodgkin lymphoma)
      2. Associated with the rheumatic disorders, particularly systemic lupus erythematosus (SLE)
      3. Associated with certain nonlymphoid neoplasms (eg, ovarian tumors)
      4. Associated with certain chronic inflammatory diseases (eg, ulcerative colitis)
      5. Associated with ingestion of certain drugs (eg, α-methyldopa)
      6. Associated with certain infections (SARS-CoV-2)
II. Cold-Autoantibody Type: Autoantibody Optimally Active at Temperatures <37°C
   A. Mediated by cold agglutinins
      1. Idiopathic (primary) chronic cold agglutinin disease (usually associated with clonal B-lymphocyte proliferation)
      2. Secondary cold agglutinin hemolytic anemia
         a. Postinfectious (eg, *Mycoplasma pneumoniae*, infectious mononucleosis, SARS-CoV-2)
         b. Associated with malignant B-cell lymphoproliferative disorder
         c. Associated with autoimmune disorders
   B. Mediated by cold hemolysins
      1. Idiopathic (primary) paroxysmal cold hemoglobinuria (very rare)
      2. Secondary
         a. Donath-Landsteiner hemolytic anemia, usually associated with an acute viral syndrome in children (relatively common)
         b. Congenital or tertiary syphilis in adults (very rare)
III. Mixed Cold and Warm Autoantibodies
   A. Primary or idiopathic mixed AHA
   B. Secondary mixed AHA
      1. Associated with autoimmune disorders, particularly SLE
IV. Drug-Immune Hemolytic Anemia
   A. Hapten or drug adsorption mechanism
   B. Ternary (immune) complex mechanism
   C. True autoantibody mechanism

account for approximately half of all secondary warm AHA cases. The majority of AHA cases mediated by cold agglutinins have a clonal lymphoproliferative disorder without clinical or radiologic evidence of malignancy; these are considered primary.[24] Systemic lupus erythematosus (SLE) and other autoimmune diseases account for a lesser but considerable proportion of secondary AHA cases. A large proportion of patients with mixed cold and warm autoantibodies have SLE.[21,22] Infectious mononucleosis and *Mycoplasma pneumoniae* occasionally are associated with AHA mediated by cold agglutinins. Both warm and cold

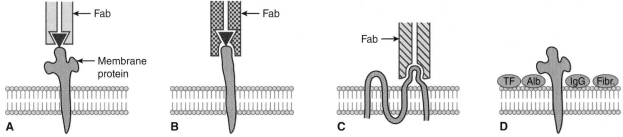

FIGURE 26–1. Effector mechanisms by which drugs mediate a positive direct antiglobulin test (DAT) result. Relationships of drug, antibody-combining site, and red blood cell (RBC) membrane protein are shown. **A, B,** and **C** show only a single immunoglobulin Fab region (bearing one combining site). **A.** Drug adsorption/hapten mechanism. The drug (▼) binds avidly to an unknown RBC membrane protein in vivo. Antidrug antibody (usually immunoglobulin [Ig] G) binds to the protein-bound drug. The membrane protein is not known to be part of the epitope recognized by the antidrug antibody. The DAT (with anti-IgG) detects IgG antidrug antibody on the patient's circulating (drug-coated) RBCs. The indirect antiglobulin test (IAT) detects antibody in the patient's serum only when the test red blood cells (RBCs) have been previously coated with the drug by incubation in vitro. **B.** Ternary complex mechanism. Drug binds loosely or in undetectable amounts to RBC membrane. However, in the presence of appropriate antidrug antibody, a stable trimolecular (ternary) complex is formed by drug, RBC membrane protein, and antibody. In general, the antibody-combining site (*Fab*) recognizes both drug and membrane protein components but binds only weakly to either drug or protein unless both are present in the reaction mixture. In this mechanism, the DAT typically detects only RBC-bound complement components (eg, C3 fragments) that are bound covalently and in large number to the patient's RBCs in vivo. The antibody itself escapes detection, possibly because of its low concentration but also because washing of the red cells (in the antiglobulin test procedure) apparently dissociates antibody and drug from the cells, leaving only the covalently bound C3 fragments. The IAT also detects complement proteins on the test RBCs when both antibody (patient serum) and a complement source (fresh patient serum or fresh normal serum) are present in the reaction mixture together with the drug. **C.** Autoantibody induction. Some drug-induced antibodies can bind avidly to RBC membrane proteins (usually Rh proteins) in the absence of the inducing drug and are indistinguishable from the autoantibodies of patients with autoimmune hemolytic anemia. The DAT detects the IgG antibody on the patient's RBCs. The IAT usually detects antibody in the serum of patients with active hemolysis. **D.** Drug-induced nonimmunologic protein adsorption. Certain drugs cause plasma proteins to attach nonspecifically to the RBC membrane. The DAT detects nonspecifically bound IgG and complement components. If special antiglobulin reagents are used, other plasma proteins, such as transferrin (TF), albumin (Alb), and fibrinogen (Fibr), also may be detected. In contrast to the other mechanisms of drug-induced RBC injury, this mechanism does not shorten RBC survival in vivo.

antibody AHA have occurred in COVID-19 patients.[25-27] Despite the frequent occurrence of immune thrombocytopenia and positive DATs in patients infected with human immunodeficiency virus (HIV), AHA is relatively rare in these patients.[28] Table 26-1 lists other associated diseases that are less-commonly reported. The etiologic and pathogenic significance of these associations is poorly understood, but most of the associated diseases involve components of the immune system, either by neoplasia or by aberrant immunopathologic responses.

Drug-Mediated Cases

Certain drugs also mediate immune injury to RBCs, and three general mechanisms are recognized (see Table 26-1 and Fig. 26-1). This classification is based on the effector mechanism of RBC injury because the induction mechanism for formation of drug-related RBC antibodies is unknown. Two of the mechanisms, hapten-drug adsorption and ternary complex formation, involve drug-dependent antibodies. In the third mechanism, the drugs in question appear to induce formation of true autoantibodies capable of reacting with human RBCs in the absence of the inciting drug. These types of drug-mediated immune injury to RBCs often are referred to collectively as *drug-immune hemolytic anemia* to distinguish them from de novo AHA. Distinguishing among the mechanisms is not always possible, and some cases involve a combination of mechanisms. In addition, drug-related nonimmunologic protein adsorption by RBCs may result in a positive DAT without actual RBC injury. This phenomenon should be distinguished from the three forms of drug-immune RBC injury. Table 26-2 lists drugs documented to cause either immune injury or a positive DAT.

●EPIDEMIOLOGY

The annual incidence of warm-antibody AHA is 1 per 75,000 to 80,000 population.[11] Estimates of the frequency of primary (idiopathic) AHA vary from 20% to 80% of all types of AHA, depending on the referral patterns of the reporting center.[11,20,111] In general, AHA is considered secondary when (1) AHA and the underlying disease occur together with greater frequency than can be accounted for by chance alone, (2) the AHA reverses simultaneously with correction of the associated disease, or (3) AHA and the associated disease are related by evidence of immunologic aberration.[11] Using these criteria, the frequency of primary warm-antibody AHA probably is closer to 50% of all cases. Careful follow-up of patients with primary AHA is essential because hemolytic anemia may be the presenting finding in a patient who subsequently develops overt evidence of an underlying disorder. For example, in one series, 18 of 107 patients with AHA developed a malignant lymphoproliferative disorder at a median of 26.5 months after diagnosis of the AHA.[112]

Warm-antibody AHA has been diagnosed in people of all ages, from infants to older adults. The majority of patients are older than 40 years, with peak incidence around the seventh decade. This age distribution probably reflects, in part, the increased frequency of lymphoproliferative malignancies in older adults, resulting in an age-related increase in the frequency of secondary AHA. Although multiple cases are occasionally observed in families,[113,114] most cases of primary AHA arise sporadically. Development of AHA does not have an apparent association with any particular human leukocyte antigen (HLA) haplotype or other genetic factor.

Cold agglutinin disease is less common than warm-antibody AHA, with a prevalence of approximately 14 per 1 million population,[24] accounting for only 10% to 20% of all cases of AHA.[10,11] Women are affected more commonly than men.[10,11] No genetic or racial factors are known to contribute to the pathogenesis of this disease.

Secondary cold agglutinin disease is seen most commonly in adolescents or young adults as a self-limited process associated with *M. pneumoniae* infections or infectious mononucleosis and, rarely, in children with chickenpox. The term is also used to describe a chronic disorder occurring in older patients with known malignant

TABLE 26–2. Association between Drugs and Positive Direct Antiglobulin Tests[a]

Drug	References	Drug	References
HAPTEN OR DRUG ADSORPTION MECHANISM			
Carbromal	29	6-Mercaptopurine	37
Cephalosporins	30–33	Oxaliplatin	38
Cianidanol	34	Penicillins	39-42
Cimetidine	35	Tetracycline	43
Hydrocortisone	36	Tolbutamide	44
TERNARY COMPLEX MECHANISM			
Amphotericin B	45	Metformin	57
Antazoline	46	Nomifensine	58
Cephalosporins	32,33,47	Oxaliplatin	38
Chlorpropamide	48,49	Pemetrexed	59
Cimetidine	35	Probenecid	60
Diclofenac	50,51	Quinidine	61
Diethylstilbestrol	52	Quinine	62
Doxepin	53	Rifampicin	63
Etodolac	54	Stibophen	19
Etoricoxib	55	Thiopental	64
Hydrocortisone	36	Tolmetin	65
Iomeprol	56	Trimethoprim-sulfa	66
AUTOANTIBODY MECHANISM: DRUGS NOT KNOWN TO MODULATE THE IMMUNE SYSTEM			
Cephalosporins	33	Mefenamic acid	72
Cianidanol	34	α-Methyl dopa	73-76
Diclofenac	51,67	Nomifensine	58
Glafenine	68	Procainamide	77
Latamoxef	68	Tolmetin	65
L-dopa	69-71		
AUTOANTIBODY MECHANISM: CHEMOTHERAPY AND IMMUNE SUPPRESSANTS			
Bendamustine	78	Oxaliplatin	38
Cladribine	79		
Efalizumab	80	Pentostatin	83
Fludarabine	81	Tacrolimus	84
Lenalidomide	82	Teniposide	68
AUTOANTIBODY MECHANISM: IMMUNE CHECKPOINT INHIBITORS			
Atezolizumab	85	Nivolumab	85
Ipilimumab	85	Pembrolizumab	85
NONIMMUNOLOGIC PROTEIN ADSORPTION			
Carboplatin	38	Cisplatin	38
Cephalosporins	86	Oxaliplatin	38
UNCERTAIN MECHANISM OF IMMUNE INJURY			
Acetaminophen	87	Melphalan	100
p-Aminosalicylic acid	88	Mesantoin	18
Apomorphine	89	Nalidixic acid	101

(continued)

TABLE 26-2. Association between Drugs and Positive Direct Antiglobulin Tests[a] (Continued)

Drug	References	Drug	References
Artesunate	90	Omeprazole	102
Cabergoline	91	Paraben	103
Chlorpromazine	92	Phenacetin	62
Efavirenz	93	*Pueraria* (Chinese herb)	104
Erythromycin	94	Quetiapine	105
5-Fluorouracil	95	Streptomycin	106
Ibuprofen	96	Sulindac	107
Insecticides	97	Temafloxacin	108
Isoniazid	98	Thiazides	109
Levofloxacin	99	Triamterene	110
Vancomycin	103		

[a]The drugs above are those that, in the author's opinion, have been documented to cause a positive direct antiglobulin test reaction, with or without immune injury. Other drugs, omitted from this list, have been alleged to cause immune injury, but laboratory confirmation is lacking. New drugs will be added to this list in the future. When an association between a drug and hemolysis is suspected, it is important to evaluate for an immune etiology and to document the mechanism by referral to a reference laboratory if necessary.

lymphoproliferative diseases. On the other hand, idiopathic (primary) chronic cold agglutinin disease has its peak incidence after age 50 years. This disorder, with its characteristic monoclonal IgM cold agglutinins, may be considered a special form of monoclonal gammopathy. Nearly all of these patients exhibit clonal B lymphocyte proliferation.[24] As with other "essential" or idiopathic monoclonal gammopathies, some patients in this group gradually develop features of a B-cell lymphoproliferative disorder resembling Waldenström macroglobulinemia, CLL, or a B-cell lymphoma. Thus, the distinction between primary and secondary types of chronic cold agglutinin disease is not absolute.

Although the majority of patients with *M. pneumoniae* have significant cold agglutinin titers, they only infrequently develop clinical hemolytic anemia.[115-117] However, subclinical RBC injury may occur. In *M. pneumoniae* infections, weakly positive direct antiglobulin reactions or mild reticulocytosis is often noted in the absence of anemia in a substantial number of cases.[115] Cold agglutinins occur in more than 60% of patients with infectious mononucleosis, but again, hemolytic anemia is rare.[118,119]

Medical centers that receive many referrals report that paroxysmal cold hemoglobinuria constitutes 2% to 5% of all cases of AHA.[10,11] Among children, however, Donath-Landsteiner hemolytic anemia accounted for 32.4% of 68 immune hemolytic syndromes diagnosed over a 4-year period.[15] Commonly, the diagnosis is missed because of lack of physician awareness or failure to perform the proper serologic studies (see "Serologic Features" later).[12,15] Thus, the true incidence may be higher. Although familial occurrence has been reported, no racial or genetic risk factors are known.[10] As noted, most childhood cases follow either specific viral infections or upper respiratory infections of undefined etiology.[10-15]

Older series report that drug-induced immune hemolytic anemia accounts for 12% to 18% of immune hemolytic anemias.[11] The disorder is much less common now that α-methyldopa and megaunit doses of penicillin rarely are used. The current incidence of drug-induced immune hemolytic anemia is estimated at 1 per 1 million population, approximately 88% of which result from the second- and third-generation cephalosporins, cefotetan, and ceftriaxone.[38] Fludarabine has replaced α-methyldopa as the most common cause of drug-induced autoantibodies.[81]

● ETIOLOGY AND PATHOGENESIS

ETIOLOGY

Warm-Antibody Autoimmune Hemolytic Anemia

The etiology of AHA is unknown. In warm-antibody AHA, the autoantibodies that mediate RBC destruction are predominantly (but not exclusively) IgG globulins possessing relatively high binding affinity for human RBCs at 37°C. As a result, the major share of plasma autoantibody is bound to the patient's circulating RBCs. Eluates prepared from the patient's washed, autoantibody-coated RBCs constitute an important source of purified autoantibody for investigation of specificity, immunoglobulin structure, or other properties. In addition, sera from patients with warm AHA often are used in blood banks for cross-matching and for general screening of antibody specificity. The quantity of such autoantibody in serum may be low and, in some cases, may not reflect the full spectrum of anti-RBC specificity revealed in concurrently prepared RBC eluates.[115]

In patients with primary AHA, erythrocyte autoantibodies are the only recognizable immunologic aberration. Furthermore, the autoantibodies of any one patient often are specific for only a single RBC membrane protein (see "Serologic Features" later). The narrow spectrum of autoreactivity suggests the mechanism underlying AHA development in such patients is not secondary to a generalized defect in immune regulation. Rather, these patients may develop warm-antibody AHA through an aberrant immune response to a self-antigen or to an immunogen that mimics a self-antigen.

In patients with secondary AHA, the disease may be associated with a fundamental disturbance in the immune system, for example, when in the setting of lymphoma, CLL, SLE, primary agammaglobulinemia (common variable immunodeficiency), or hyper-IgM immunodeficiency syndrome. In these settings, warm-antibody AHA most likely arises through an underlying defect in immune regulation, although the contribution of an aberrant immune response to self-antigen cannot be excluded. AHA seems especially frequent in patients with low-grade lymphoma or CLL treated with fludarabine[38] or 2-chlorodeoxyadenosine (cladribine).[39] The T-lymphocytopenia induced by these drugs may exacerbate the preexisting tendency of patients to form autoantibodies.

A long-recognized but poorly understood phenomenon, the development of AHA or a positive DAT result after RBC transfusion, has received renewed interest.[120,121] Although generally transient, the positive DAT result may persist for up to 300 days in some transfusion recipients, long after any transfused RBCs have disappeared.[122,123] It is not clear whether this represents true autoimmunity or some other mechanism, for example, microchimerism resulting from temporary engraftment of passenger memory lymphocytes from the RBC donor.[120]

A still unexplained observation is that certain drugs, such as α-methyldopa, can induce warm-reacting IgG anti-RBC autoantibodies in otherwise normal persons. The autoantibodies induced by α-methyldopa have Rh-related serologic and immunochemical[124] specificity similar to that of autoantibodies arising in many patients with "spontaneous" AHA. A critical difference is that the drug-associated autoantibodies subside when the drug is discontinued, suggesting that (1) the latent potential to form this type of anti-RBC autoantibody is present in many immunologically normal individuals, and (2) the steps required to generate such autoantibodies do not necessarily create a sustained autoimmune state. On the other hand, maintenance of chronic idiopathic AHA may be either secondary to a continuing (but unknown) stimulus or induced by a short stimulus to which the patient continues to respond. Immunosuppressive and chemotherapy drugs and immune checkpoint inhibitors whose primary purpose is to modulate the immune system may also induce warm reactive autoantibodies but probably by different mechanisms (see Table 26-2). Such cases may hold clues to the genesis of autoreactivity.

Normal subjects sometimes have a positive DAT result when they volunteer to donate blood.[125,126] The positive DAT result in these normal donors often results from warm-reacting IgG autoantibodies, similar in serologic specificity[127] and in IgG subclass[125] to the autoantibodies occurring in AHA. Although many of these donors remain DAT positive without developing overt hemolytic anemia, a few have been documented to develop AHA.[125,126] The prevalence of positive DATs in normal blood donors is approximately 1 in 10,000 donors.[125] Because blood donation per se likely does not contribute to an increased risk of developing autoantibodies, the 1 in 10,000 proportion probably is the approximate frequency of positive DATs in the entire population. A proportion of patients who present with clinically overt primary AHA may come from a subset of asymptomatic individuals who are DAT positive, but this notion is not established.

Of 113 patients with COVID-19 studied at a blood bank for type and cross-match, 46% exhibited a positive DAT. Of those, 88% were IgG alone pattern. In sharp contrast to what is commonly observed in cases of AHA, patient sera and eluates from RBCs of these patients did not react with either reagent RBCs or healthy donor RBCs in the indirect antiglobulin test. However, IgG containing eluates did react with RBCs from COVID-19 patients who were DAT negative.[128,129] It is unclear how many of these patients had hemolytic anemia. The finding suggests that SARS-CoV-2 somehow modifies the RBC membrane to expose a cryptic antigen. Another study has found that the RBC membrane protein Ankyrin 1 (ANK-1) shares a putative immunogenic epitope with the SARS-CoV-2 spike protein. Further studies are needed to determine whether ANK 1 is the target antigen of the IgG antibody in these patients.

Several concepts have been developed to explain immunologic tolerance to self-antigens.[131] Relevant to warm-antibody AHA, membrane-bound antigens expressed in a multivalent array at high concentration may induce tolerance by effecting clonal deletion of autoreactive B cells.[132] Both the Rh-related and the non-Rh types of RBC antigens targeted by AHA autoantibodies (see "Serologic Features" later) are expressed normally by human fetal erythrocytes, as early as 10 to 12 weeks of life.[133] However, because new B cells develop daily in the marrow throughout life and B cells may somatically mutate their Ig receptors, self-tolerance in the B-cell compartment is never assured. Analogy to observations in New Zealand black (NZB) mice[134,135] suggests the peritoneal cavity is a privileged compartment that shelters autoreactive B cells from host RBCs, allowing them to escape deletion, later to produce anti-RBC autoantibodies with appropriate T-cell help. The strong predominance of IgG antibodies in AHA suggests B-cell isotype switching, which is consistent with the idea of an antigen-driven process. Moreover, because T-cell help is necessary for inducing B-cell isotype switching, the pathway(s) to autoantibody induction in AHA also may involve an abnormal or unique mode of antigen presentation to T cells.[136]

Origin of Cold Agglutinins

Almost all patients with cold agglutinin disease display monoclonal IgM cold agglutinins (with either anti-I or anti-i specificity) whose heavy-chain variable regions are encoded by IGHV4–34 (immunoglobulin heavy chain variable region), formerly designated IGHV4.21.[131,137-140] IGHV4–34 encodes a distinct idiotype identified by the rat monoclonal antibody 9G4. This idiotype is expressed both by the cold agglutinins themselves and on the surface immunoglobulin of B cells synthesizing cold agglutinins or related immunoglobulins possessing IGHV4–34 sequences.[141] Using the 9G4 monoclonal antibody as a probe, this idiotype was found not only in a very high proportion of circulating B cells and marrow lymphoplasmacytoid cells of patients with lymphoma-associated chronic cold agglutinin disease but also in a smaller proportion of B cells in the blood and lymphoid tissues of normal adult donors and in the spleens of 15-week human fetuses.[141] These data suggest B cells expressing the IGHV4–34 gene (or a closely related sequence) are present throughout ontogeny. Therefore, chronic cold agglutinin disease may represent a marked, unregulated expansion of a subset (clone) of such B cells.

Light-chain V-region gene use in anti-I cold agglutinins is highly selective. A strong bias toward use of IgkV3-20 is observed.[138-142] Light-chain selection among anti-i cold agglutinins, however, is much more variable and includes the λ type.[138-142]

Observations that pathologic cold agglutinins are synthesized with distinct and highly selected V-region sequences must be viewed against the background of two other subsequent observations. First, IGHV4–34 or related IGHV genes also may encode the heavy-chain variable regions of other types of antibodies, such as rheumatoid factor autoantibodies and alloantibodies to a variety of blood group antigens, including polypeptide determinants such as Rh.[143] Second, normal human antibodies to an exogenous carbohydrate antigen, *Haemophilus influenzae* type b capsular polysaccharide, also are encoded by a restricted set of IGHV genes[144] and Ig light-chain V genes.[145] Thus, regulation of Ig gene use for production of anti-I or anti-i cold agglutinins may not differ fundamentally from normal antibody formation to other carbohydrate antigens.

Normal human sera generally have naturally occurring polyclonal cold agglutinins in low titer (usually 1/64 dilution or less).[10] Otherwise healthy persons may develop elevated titers of cold agglutinins specific for I/i antigens during certain infections (eg, *M. pneumoniae*, Epstein-Barr virus, cytomegalovirus). In contrast to other forms of cold agglutinin disease, hyperproduction of these postinfectious cold agglutinins is transient. Some evidence indicates postinfectious cold agglutinins may be less clonally restricted than those occurring in chronic cold agglutinin disease,[146] but this finding is not universal.[147] Whether IGHV4–34 also encodes most heavy-chain variable regions of all naturally occurring or postinfectious cold agglutinins remains to be determined.

The increased production of cold agglutinins in response to infection with *M. pneumoniae* may be secondary to the fact that the oligosaccharide antigens of the I/i type serve as specific *Mycoplasma* receptors.[148] This process may lead to altered antigen presentation involving a complex between a self-antigen (I/i) and a non–self-antigen (*Mycoplasma* spp.). Alternatively, the anti-i cold agglutinins may arise as a consequence of polyclonal B-cell activation, as occurs in infectious mononucleosis.

The mechanism(s) whereby dissimilar infectious agents (eg, spirochetes and several types of virus) induce the immune system to produce Donath-Landsteiner antibodies with specificity for the human P blood group antigen (see "Serologic Features" later) is not known.

PATHOGENESIS

Pathogenic Effects of Warm Antibodies

Warm autoantibodies to RBCs in AHA are pathogenic. In contrast to autologous RBCs, labeled RBCs lacking the antigen targeted by the autoantibodies may survive normally in patients with warm-antibody AHA.[10,149,150] Furthermore, transplacental passage of IgG anti-RBC autoantibodies from a mother with AHA to the fetus can induce intrauterine or neonatal hemolytic anemia.[151] Despite notable exceptions and differences related to IgG subclass of the autoantibody, in general, an inverse relationship between the quantity of RBC-bound IgG antibody and RBC survival is noted in serial studies performed on animals and patients.[152-157]

In warm-antibody AHA, the patient's RBCs typically are coated with IgG autoantibodies with or without complement proteins. Autoantibody-coated RBCs are trapped by macrophages in the Billroth cords of the spleen and, to a lesser extent, by Kupffer cells in the liver (Chap. 2).[149,152,153,155-158] The process leads to generation of spherocytes and fragmentation and ingestion of antibody-coated RBCs.[159,160] The macrophage has surface receptors for the Fc region of IgG, with preference for the IgG$_1$ and IgG$_3$ subclasses[161,162] and surface receptors for opsonic fragments of C3 (C3b and C3bi) and C4b.[163-165] When present together on the RBC surface, IgG and C3b/C3bi appear to act cooperatively as opsonins to enhance trapping and phagocytosis.[155,156,164-168] Although RBC sequestration in warm-antibody AHA occurs primarily in the spleen,[149,156,157] very large quantities of RBC-bound IgG[152,153,158] or the concurrent presence of C3b on the RBCs[152,155,156] may favor trapping in the liver.

Interaction of a trapped RBC with splenic macrophages may result in phagocytosis of the entire cell. More commonly, a type of partial phagocytosis results in spherocyte formation. As RBCs adhere to macrophages via the Fc receptors, portions of RBC membrane are internalized by the macrophage. Because membrane is lost in excess of contents, the noningested portion of the RBC assumes a spherical shape, the shape with the lowest ratio of surface area to volume.[159,160,169] Spherical RBCs are more rigid and less deformable than normal RBCs. As such, spherical RBCs are fragmented further and eventually destroyed in future passages through the spleen. Spherocytosis is a consistent and diagnostically important hallmark of AHA,[170] and the degree of spherocytosis correlates well with the severity of hemolysis.[10]

Direct complement-mediated hemolysis with hemoglobinuria is unusual in warm-antibody AHA, even though many warm autoantibodies fix complement. The failure of C3b-coated RBCs to be hemolyzed by the terminal complement cascade (C5-C9) has been attributed, at least in part, to the ability of complement regulatory proteins (factors I and H) in plasma and C3b receptors on the RBC surface to alter the hemolytic function of cell-bound C3b and C4b.[171] Glycosylphosphatidylinositol-linked erythrocyte membrane proteins, such as decay-accelerating factor (DAF; CD55) and homologous restriction factor (HRF; CD59), may limit the action of autologous complement on autoantibody-coated RBCs.[172-174] DAF inhibits the formation and function of cell-bound C3-converting enzyme,[172] thus indirectly limiting formation

of C5-converting enzyme. HRF, on the other hand, impedes C9 binding and formation of the C5b-9 membrane attack complex.[173]

Cytotoxic activities of macrophages and lymphocytes also may play a role in the destruction of RBCs in warm-antibody AHA. Monocytes can lyse IgG-coated RBCs in vitro independently of phagocytosis.[175,176] Cell-bound complement is neither necessary nor sufficient for such cytotoxicity, but bound C3b/C3d can potentiate the effects of IgG.[176] In one study, cytotoxicity, but not phagocytosis, was inhibited by hydrocortisone in vitro.[175] Lymphocytes also can lyse IgG antibody-coated RBCs in vitro.[177-179] The relative contribution of antibody-dependent monocyte- and lymphocyte-mediated cytotoxicity to RBC destruction in patients with warm-antibody AHA is not known.

Pathogenic Effects of Cold Agglutinins and Hemolysins

Most cold agglutinins are unable to agglutinate RBCs at temperatures higher than 30°C. The highest temperature at which these antibodies cause detectable agglutination is termed the *thermal amplitude*. The value varies considerably among patients. Generally, patients with cold agglutinins with higher thermal amplitudes have a greater risk for cold agglutinin disease.[9] For example, active hemolytic anemia has been observed in patients with cold agglutinins of modest titer (eg, 1:256) and high thermal amplitudes.[180]

The pathogenicity of a cold agglutinin depends on its ability to bind host RBCs and to activate complement.[10,166,181,182] This process is called *complement fixation*. Although in vitro agglutination of the RBCs may be maximal at 0°C to 5°C, complement fixation by these antibodies may occur optimally at 20°C to 25°C and may be significant at even higher physiologic temperatures.[10,180,181] Agglutination is not required for the process. The great preponderance of cold agglutinin molecules are IgM pentamers, but small numbers of IgM hexamers with cold agglutinin activity are found in patients with cold agglutinin disease. Hexamers fix complement and lyse RBCs more efficiently than do pentamers, suggesting that hexameric IgM plays a role in the pathogenesis of hemolysis in these patients.[183]

Cold agglutinins may bind to RBCs in superficial vessels of the extremities, where the temperature generally ranges between 28°C and 31°C, depending on ambient temperature.[184] Cold agglutinins of high thermal amplitude may cause RBCs to aggregate at this temperature, thereby impeding RBC flow and producing acrocyanosis. In addition, the RBC-bound cold agglutinin may activate complement via the classic pathway. After activated complement proteins are deposited onto the RBC surface, the cold agglutinin need not remain bound to the RBCs for hemolysis to occur. Instead, the cold agglutinin may dissociate from the RBCs at the higher temperatures in the body core and again be capable of binding other RBCs at the lower temperatures in the superficial vessels. As a result, patients with cold agglutinins of high thermal amplitude tend toward a sustained hemolytic process and acrocyanosis.[185] In contrast, patients with antibodies of lower thermal amplitude require significant chilling to initiate complement-mediated injury of RBCs. This sequence may result in a burst of hemolysis with hemoglobinuria.[185] Combinations of these clinical patterns also occur. Cold agglutinins of the IgA isotype, an isotype that does not fix complement, may cause acrocyanosis but not hemolysis.[186] Thus, the relative degree of hemolysis or impeded RBC flow is influenced significantly by the properties and quantity of the cold agglutinins in a given patient.

Complement fixation by cold agglutinins may effect RBC injury by two major mechanisms: (1) direct lysis and (2) opsonization for hepatic and splenic macrophages. Both mechanisms probably operate to varying degrees in any patient. Direct lysis requires propagation of the full C1 to C9 sequence on the RBC membrane. If this process occurs to a significant degree, the patient may experience intravascular hemolysis, leading to hemoglobinemia and hemoglobinuria. Intravascular hemolysis of this severity is relatively rare because phosphatidylinositol-linked RBC membrane proteins (DAF and HRF) protect against injury by autologous complement components. Thus, the complement sequence on many RBCs is completed only through the early steps, leaving opsonic fragments of C3 (C3b/C3bi) and C4 (C4b) on the cell surface. The fragments provide only a weak stimulus for phagocytosis by monocytes in vitro.[168,187] However, activated macrophages may ingest C3b-coated particles avidly.[188] Accordingly, RBCs heavily coated with C3b (and/or C3bi) may be removed from the circulation by macrophages either in the liver or, to a lesser extent, the spleen.[156,181,189,190] The trapped RBCs may be ingested entirely or released back into the circulation as spherocytes after losing plasma membrane.

In vivo studies of the fate of ^{51}Cr-labeled C3b-coated RBCs[155,181,189,190] indicate many of the erythrocytes trapped in the liver or spleen gradually may reenter the circulation. The released cells generally are coated with the opsonically inactive C3 fragment C3dg. Conversion of cell-bound C3b or C3bi to C3dg results from the action of the naturally occurring complement inhibitor factor I in concert with factor H or CR1 receptors.[165] The surviving C3dg-coated RBCs circulate with a near-normal life span[155,181,189,190] and are resistant to further uptake of cold agglutinins or complement.[181,189,191] However, C3dg-coated RBCs also may react in vitro with anticomplement (anti-C3) serum in the DAT. In fact, most of the antiglobulin-positive RBCs of patients with cold agglutinin disease are coated with C3dg.

In paroxysmal cold hemoglobinuria, the mechanism of hemolysis probably parallels in vitro events (see "Serologic Features" later). During severe chilling, blood flowing through skin capillaries is exposed to low temperatures. The Donath-Landsteiner antibody and early acting complement components presumably bind to RBCs at the lowered temperatures. Upon return of the cells to 37°C in the central circulation, the cells are lysed by propagation of the terminal complement sequence through C9. The Donath-Landsteiner antibody itself dissociates from the RBCs at 37°C. Donath-Landsteiner antibody is a more potent hemolysin than

cold agglutinin. Although not completely understood, it is likely related to the ability of Donath-Landsteiner antibody to rapidly initiate a large number of complement sequences that overwhelm erythrocyte membrane proteins that restrict C5b-9 assembly (eg, HRFs).

Pathogenesis of Drug-Mediated Immune Injury

Table 26-3 summarizes the three mechanisms of drug-mediated immune injury to RBCs. Drugs also may mediate protein adsorption to RBCs by nonimmune mechanisms, but RBC injury does not occur.

Hapten or Drug Adsorption Mechanism This mechanism applies to drugs that can bind firmly to proteins, including RBC membrane proteins. The classic setting is very-high-dose penicillin therapy,[39-42] which is encountered less commonly today than in previous decades.

Most individuals who receive penicillin develop IgM antibodies directed against the benzylpenicilloyl determinant of penicillin, but this antibody plays no role in penicillin-related immune injury to RBCs. The antibody responsible for hemolytic anemia is of the IgG class, occurs less frequently than the IgM antibody, and may be directed against the benzylpenicilloyl, or, more commonly, nonbenzylpenicilloyl determinants.[40,41] Other manifestations of penicillin sensitivity usually are not present.

All patients receiving high doses of penicillin develop substantial coating of RBCs with penicillin. The penicillin coating itself is not injurious. If the penicillin dose is very high ($10\text{-}30 \times 10^6$ units per day or less in the setting of renal failure) and promotes cell coating and if the patient has an IgG antipenicillin antibody, the antibody binds to the RBC-bound penicillin molecules and the DAT with anti-IgG becomes positive (see Fig. 26-1A).[39,192] Antibodies eluted from patients' RBCs or present in their sera react in the indirect antiglobulin test (IAT) only against penicillin-coated RBCs. This step is critical in distinguishing these drug-dependent antibodies from true autoantibodies.

Not all patients receiving high-dose penicillin develop a positive DAT reaction or hemolytic anemia because only a small proportion

TABLE 26-3. Major Mechanisms of Drug-Related Hemolytic Anemia and Positive Direct Antiglobulin Test Reactions				
	Hapten-Drug Adsorption	**Ternary Complex Formation**	**Autoantibody Binding**	**Nonimmunologic Protein Adsorption**
Prototype drug	Penicillin	Quinidine	α-Methyldopa	Cephalothin
Role of drug	Binds to red cell membrane	Forms ternary complex with antibody and red cell membrane component	Induces formation of antibody to native red cell antigen	Possibly alters red cell membrane
Drug affinity to cell	Strong	Weak	None demonstrated to intact red cell but binding to membranes reported	Strong
Antibody to drug	Present	Present	Absent	Absent
Antibody class predominating	Immunoglobulin (Ig) G	IgM or IgG	IgG	None
Proteins detected by direct antiglobulin test	IgG, rarely complement	Complement	IgG, rarely complement	Multiple plasma proteins
Dose of drug associated with positive antiglobulin test reaction	High	Low	High	High
Presence of drug required for indirect antiglobulin test reaction	Yes (coating test red cells)	Yes (added to test medium)	No	Yes (added to test medium)
Mechanism of red cell destruction	Splenic sequestration of IgG-coated red cells	Direct lysis by complement plus splenic–hepatic clearance of C3b-coated red cells	Splenic sequestration	None

of such individuals produce the requisite antibody. Destruction of RBCs coated with penicillin and IgG antipenicillin antibody occurs mainly through sequestration by splenic macrophages.[193] In some patients with penicillin-induced immune hemolytic anemia, blood monocytes and presumably splenic macrophages may lyse the IgG-coated RBCs without phagocytosis.[194] Hemolytic anemia resulting from penicillin typically occurs only after the patient has received the drug for 7 to 10 days and ceases a few days to 2 weeks after the patient discontinues taking the drug.

Low-molecular-weight substances, such as drugs, generally are not immunogenic in their own right. Induction of antidrug antibody is thought to require firm chemical coupling of the drug (as a hapten) to a protein carrier. In the case of penicillin, the carrier protein involved in antibody induction need not be the same as the erythrocyte membrane protein to which penicillin is coupled in the effector phase, that is, when the IgG antipenicillin antibodies bind to penicillin-coated RBCs. In contrast to evidence on the ternary complex mechanism, no evidence indicates the drug-dependent antibodies responsible for RBC injury in this hapten-drug adsorption mechanism also recognize native erythrocyte membrane structures.

Cephalosporins have antigenic cross-reactivity with penicillin[195-197] and bind firmly to RBC membranes, as do semisynthetic penicillins.[41,42] Hemolytic anemia similar to that seen with penicillin has been ascribed to cephalosporins[30-33] and some semisynthetic penicillins.[41,42] Tetracycline[43] and tolbutamide[44] also may cause hemolysis by this mechanism. Carbromal causes positive IgG antiglobulin reactions by a similar mechanism,[29] but hemolytic anemia has not been described.

Ternary Complex Mechanism: Drug–Antibody–Target Cell Interaction Many drugs can induce immune injury not only of RBCs but also of platelets or granulocytes by a process that differs in several ways from the mechanism of hapten-drug adsorption (see Table 26-3). First, drugs in this group (see Table 26-2) exhibit only weak direct binding to blood cell membranes. Second, a relatively small dose of drug is capable of triggering destruction of blood cells. Third, cellular injury appears to be mediated chiefly by complement activation at the cell surface. The cytopathic process induced by such drugs previously has been termed the *innocent bystander* or *immune complex mechanism*. The terminology reflected the prevailing notion that, in vivo, drug–antibody complexes formed first (immune complexes) and then became secondarily bound to target blood cells as "innocent bystanders," either nonspecifically or possibly via membrane receptors (eg, Fcγ receptors on platelets or C3b receptors on red cells), with the potential for subsequent activation of complement by bound complexes.

The "immune complex" and "innocent bystander" terminology now seems less appropriate because of models developed from research on analogous drug-dependent platelet injury[198-200] and a series of relevant serologic observations on drug-mediated immune hemolytic anemia. These studies suggest blood cell injury is mediated by a cooperative interaction among three reactants to generate a ternary complex (see Fig. 26-1B) involving (1) the drug (or drug metabolite in some cases), (2) a drug-binding membrane site on the target cell, and (3) antibody. For example, several patients possessed drug-dependent antibodies that exhibited specificity for RBCs bearing defined alloantigens such as those of the Rh, Kell, or Kidd blood groups. That is, even in the presence of drug, the antibodies were selectively nonreactive with human RBCs lacking the alloantigen in question.[64,68,201-203] In each case, high-affinity drug binding to cell membrane could not be demonstrated. The drug-dependent antibody is thought to bind, through its Fab domain, to a compound neoantigen consisting of loosely bound drug and a blood group antigen intrinsic to the red cell membrane. Elegant studies on quinidine- or quinine-induced immune thrombocytopenia have demonstrated the IgG antibodies implicated in this disorder bind through their Fab domains, not by their Fc domains to platelet Fcγ receptors.[204,205]

The data elucidate how one patient with quinidine sensitivity may have selective destruction of platelets and another may have selective destruction of RBCs. This process occurs because the pathogenic antibody recognizes the drug only in combination with a particular membrane structure of the RBC (eg, a known alloantigen) or of the platelet (eg, a domain of the glycoprotein Ib complex). Therefore, at least in these cases, the target cell does not appear to be purely an innocent bystander. Binding of the drug itself to the target cell membrane is weak until the attachment of the antibody to *both* drug and cell membrane is stabilized. Yet the binding of the antibody is drug-dependent. Such a three-reactant interdependent "troika" is unique to this mechanism of immune cytopenia.

The foregoing discussion depicting drugs as creating a "self + nonself" neoantigen on the target cell applies to the effector phase as opposed to the induction phase of the process. However, the same drug-binding membrane protein appears to be involved in forming the immunogen that induces the antibody, as evidenced by drug-dependent antibodies exhibiting selective reactivity with defined red cell alloantigens (carrier specificity).[64,68,201-203] How this process is accomplished in the absence of evidence for strong, covalent binding of the drugs in this group to a host membrane protein remains to be elucidated.

RBC destruction by this mechanism may occur intravascularly after completion of the whole complement sequence, resulting in hemoglobinemia and hemoglobinuria. Some destruction of intact C3b-coated RBCs may be mediated by splenic and liver sequestration via the C3b/C3bi receptors on macrophages. The DAT result is positive usually only with anticomplement reagents, but exceptions occur. Sometimes, however, the drug-dependent antibody itself can be detected on the RBCs if the offending drug (or its metabolites) is included in all steps of the antiglobulin test, including washing.[206]

Autoantibody Mechanism A variety of drugs induces the formation of autoantibodies reactive with autologous (or homologous) RBCs in the absence of the instigating drug (see Tables 26-2 and 26-3). The most studied drug in this category has been α-methyldopa, an antihypertensive agent that no longer is commonly used.[73-76] Levodopa and several unrelated drugs also have been implicated (see Table 26-2). Patients with CLL treated with pentostatin,[83] fludarabine,[81] or cladribine[79] are particularly predisposed to autoimmune hemolysis, which usually is severe and sometimes fatal. More recently, immune checkpoint inhibitors have been found to induce AHA.[85]

Positive DAT reactions (with anti-IgG reagents) in patients taking α-methyldopa vary in frequency from 8% to 36%. Patients taking higher doses of the drug develop positive reactions with greater frequency.[73,75,76] A lag period of 3 to 6 months exists between the start of therapy and development of a positive antiglobulin test reaction. The delay is not shortened when the drug is administered to patients who previously had positive antiglobulin test reactions while taking α-methyldopa.[75]

In sharp contrast to the frequent observation of positive antiglobulin reactions, fewer than 1% of patients taking α-methyldopa exhibit hemolytic anemia.[74] Development of hemolytic anemia does not depend on drug dose. The hemolysis usually is mild to moderate and occurs chiefly by splenic sequestration of IgG-coated RBCs. α-Methyldopa has been proposed to suppress splenic macrophage function in some patients, and normal survival of antibody-coated RBCs in such patients may be related, in part, to this effect of the drug.[207]

The DAT reaction usually is positive only for IgG.[11] Occasionally, weak anticomplement reactions also are encountered.[11] Patients with immune hemolytic anemia resulting from α-methyldopa therapy typically exhibit strongly positive DAT reactions and serum antibody, evidenced by the IAT reaction.[11] Antibodies in the serum or eluted from RBC membranes react optimally at 37°C with unaltered autologous or homologous RBCs in the absence of drug (see Fig. 26-1C).[74,76,208]

Frequently the autoantibodies are reactive with determinants of the Rh complex, and at least some appear to target the same 34-kDa Rh-related polypeptide targeted by the autoantibodies in many cases of "spontaneously arising" AHA.[124] Thus, distinguishing these drug-induced antibodies from similar warm-reacting autoantibodies in idiopathic AHA currently is not possible.

The mechanism by which a drug induces formation of an autoantibody is unknown. Radiolabeled α-methyldopa does not react directly with the membranes of intact human RBCs.[76,209] However, both α-methyldopa and levodopa bind to isolated RBC membranes. Binding of the drug to membranes of intact RBCs is inhibited by RBC superoxide dismutase and probably by hemoglobin.[209,210] Although not formally demonstrated, these drugs probably bind to membrane antigens of cells that are relatively hemoglobin-free, for example, cells at the early proerythroblast stage or RBC stroma. In any case, the resulting altered membrane antigens then may induce autoantibodies. The concept that a drug–membrane compound neoantigen could lead to production of an autoantibody is supported by studies of patients receiving drugs unrelated to α-methyldopa. Patients simultaneously developed a drug-dependent antibody and an autoantibody, both of which showed specificity for the same RBC alloantigen.[68] Another hypothesis is that α-methyldopa interacts with human T lymphocytes, resulting in loss of suppressor cell function.[211] Subsequent studies, however, have failed to demonstrate any evidence for such a mechanism.[212]

Patients with CLL treated with the purine analogues fludarabine,[81,213,214] pentostatin,[83] or cladribine[79] may develop AHA. Risk factors for hemolysis include previous therapy with a purine analogue, high β_2-microglobulin, a positive DAT result before therapy, and hypogammaglobulinemia. Purine analogues are potent suppressors of T lymphocytes. These drugs may accelerate the preexisting T-cell immune suppression that normally occurs during progression of CLL, exacerbating the underlying tendency to autoimmunity in CLL. However, the degree of depletion of T-cell subsets is similar in patients who develop hemolysis and in patients who do not.

Much less frequently, AHA mediated by non–drug-dependent autoantibodies has occurred in patients receiving other immunosuppressant drugs, including lenolidomide,[82] efalizumab,[80] and tacrolimus.[84] Immune checkpoint inhibitors, commonly used to treat a number of malignancies, have been increasingly recognized to induce autoantibodies to RBCs and clinical AHA. Whereas immunomodulation is a side effect of cytotoxic chemotherapy drugs previously associated with autoantibodies to RBCs, the antitumor effect of checkpoint inhibitors is mediated by upregulation of an immune response blocked by a malignancy. Nivolumab is the most common offender, but pembrolizumab, ipilimumab, and atezolizumab have also been implicated.[85] In most cases, the DAT pattern is IgG alone, but a few cases have exhibited a C alone pattern or IgG + C. Most patients respond to glucocorticoid therapy.

Nonimmunologic Protein Adsorption Fewer than 5% of patients receiving cephalosporin antibiotics develop positive antiglobulin reactions[11] as a result of nonspecific adsorption of plasma proteins to their RBC membranes.[86,215] This process may occur within 1–2 days after the drug is instituted. Multiple plasma proteins, including immunoglobulins, complement, albumin, fibrinogen, and others, may be detected on RBC membranes in such cases.[215,216] Hemolytic anemia resulting from this mechanism has not been reported. The clinical importance of this phenomenon is its potential to complicate cross-match procedures unless the drug history is considered. Cephalosporin antibiotics also may induce RBC injury by the hapten mechanism, by the ternary complex mechanism, and by the autoantibody mechanism. The latter reactions are more serious but apparently occur less frequently than nonimmunologic protein adsorption.

● CLINICAL FEATURES

WARM-ANTIBODY AUTOIMMUNE HEMOLYTIC ANEMIA

Presenting complaints of warm-antibody AHA usually are referable to the anemia itself, although occasionally jaundice is the immediate cause for the patient to seek medical advice. Symptom onset usually is slow and insidious over several months, but occasionally a patient has sudden onset of symptoms of severe anemia and jaundice over a period of a few days. In secondary AHA, the symptoms and signs of the underlying disease may overshadow the hemolytic anemia and associated features.

In idiopathic AHA with only mild anemia, results of physical examination may be normal. Even patients with relatively severe hemolytic anemia may have only modest splenomegaly. However, in very severe cases, particularly those of acute onset, patients may present with fever, pallor, jaundice, hepatosplenomegaly, hyperpnea, tachycardia, angina, or heart failure.

Clinical warm-antibody AHA may be aggravated or first become apparent during pregnancy.[151,217] Most cases are mild, however, and the prognosis for the fetus is generally good, provided the mother is treated early.[217]

COLD-ANTIBODY AUTOIMMUNE HEMOLYTIC ANEMIA

Most patients with cold agglutinin hemolytic anemia have chronic hemolytic anemia with or without jaundice. In other patients, the principal feature is episodic, acute hemolysis with hemoglobinuria induced by chilling (see the discussion of thermal amplitude in "Pathogenic Effects of Cold Agglutinins and Hemolysins" earlier). Combinations of these clinical features may occur. Acrocyanosis and other cold-mediated vasoocclusive phenomena affecting the fingers, toes, nose, and ears are associated with sludging of RBCs in the cutaneous microvasculature. Skin ulceration and necrosis are distinctly unusual. Hemolysis occurring in *M. pneumoniae* infections is acute in onset, typically appearing as the patient is recovering from pneumonia and coincident with peak titers of cold agglutinins. The hemolysis is self-limited, lasting 1–3 weeks.[11] Hemolytic anemia in infectious mononucleosis develops either at the onset of symptoms or within the first 3 weeks of illness.

Other physical findings are variable, depending upon the presence of an underlying disease. Splenomegaly, a characteristic finding in lymphoproliferative diseases or infectious mononucleosis, may be observed in idiopathic cold agglutinin disease.

In paroxysmal cold hemoglobinuria, constitutional symptoms are prominent during a paroxysm. A few minutes to several hours after cold exposure, the patient develops aching pains in the back or legs, abdominal cramps, and occasionally headaches. Chills and fever usually follow. The first urine passed after onset of symptoms typically contains hemoglobin. The constitutional symptoms and hemoglobinuria generally last a few hours. Raynaud phenomenon and cold urticaria sometimes occur during an attack; jaundice may follow.

DRUG-INDUCED IMMUNE HEMOLYTIC ANEMIA

A careful history of drug exposure should be obtained from all patients with hemolytic anemia or a positive DAT result. As in idiopathic AHA, the clinical picture in drug-induced immune hemolytic anemia is quite variable. The severity of symptoms largely depends on the rate of hemolysis. In general, patients with hapten-drug adsorption (eg, penicillin) and autoimmune (eg, α-methyldopa) types of drug-induced hemolytic anemia exhibit mild to moderate hemolysis, with insidious onset of symptoms developing over a period of days to weeks. In contrast, the ternary complex mechanism (eg, cephalosporins or quinidine) often causes sudden, severe hemolysis with hemoglobinuria. In the latter setting, hemolysis can occur after only one dose of the drug in a patient previously exposed to the drug. Acute renal failure may accompany severe hemolysis by the ternary complex mechanism.[46,47,53,55,63,64,67] Several reports indicate that second- and third-generation cephalosporins may cause severe, even fatal, hemolysis by the ternary complex mechanism.[32,33,47]

LABORATORY FEATURES

GENERAL FEATURES

By definition, patients with AHA present with anemia, the severity of which ranges from life-threatening to very mild. Patients with warm-antibody AHA may present with hematocrit levels less than 10% or may have compensated hemolytic anemia and a near-normal hematocrit. For the latter patients, the predominant laboratory features are an increased reticulocyte count and a positive DAT result. Occasionally, the patient has leukopenia and neutropenia.[10,218] Platelet counts typically are normal. Rarely, severe immune thrombocytopenia is associated with warm-antibody AHA. This constellation is termed *Evans syndrome*.[219] Neutropenia, presumably immune mediated (immune pancytopenia), may also occur. Evans syndrome may occur de novo or

as a phenomenon secondary to an autoimmune disease, lymphoma, or immunodeficiency.[220] In this syndrome, the RBC and platelet antibodies are apparently distinct.[221]

Patients with classic chronic cold agglutinin disease exhibit mild to moderate, fairly stable anemia, with hematocrit levels only occasionally as low as 15% to 20%. In contrast, patients with paroxysmal cold hemoglobinuria have hematocrit levels that decrease rapidly during a paroxysm. During a paroxysm, leukopenia is noted early followed by leukocytosis. Complement titers frequently are depressed because of consumption of complement proteins during hemolysis.

In drug-induced immune hemolytic anemia of the hapten-drug adsorption and true autoantibody types, the hematologic findings are similar to those described for spontaneously occurring warm-antibody AHA. Most patients exhibit anemia and reticulocytosis. Leukopenia and thrombocytopenia may be noted in cases of ternary complex-mediated hemolysis.

Evaluation of the blood film can reveal several features related to all types of AHA (Fig. 26-2). Polychromasia indicates a reticulocytosis, reflecting an increased rate of reticulocyte egress from the marrow. Spherocytes are seen in patients with moderate to severe hemolytic anemia. If hereditary spherocytosis (HS) can be excluded, this finding suggests an immune hemolytic process. RBC fragments, nucleated RBCs, and occasionally erythrophagocytosis by monocytes may be seen in severe cases (see Fig. 26-2). Most patients have mild leukocytosis and neutrophilia. Additionally, patients with cold-antibody AHA may

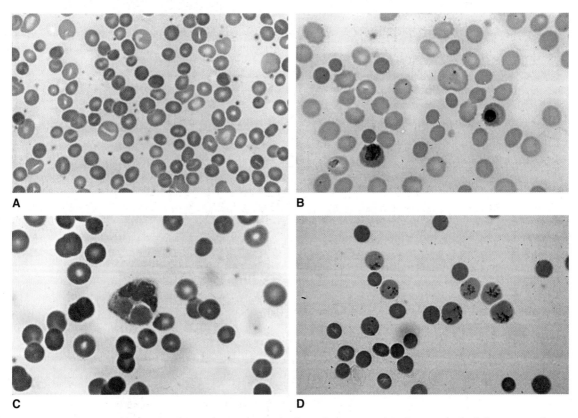

A **B** **C** **D**

FIGURE 26–2. A. Blood film showing moderately severe autoimmune hemolytic anemia (AHA). Note the high frequency of microspherocytes (small hyperchromatic RBCs) and the high frequency of macrocytes (putative reticulocytes). **B.** Blood film showing severe AHA. Note the low density of red cells on the film (profound anemia), high frequency of microspherocytes (hyperchromatic), and the large red cells (putative reticulocytes). Note the two nucleated RBCs and the Howell-Jolly body (nuclear remnant) in the macrocyte. Nucleated RBCs and Howell-Jolly bodies may be seen in AHA with severe hemolysis or after splenectomy. **C.** Blood film showing severe AHA. Monocyte engulfing two red cells (erythrophagocytosis). Note the frequent microspherocytes and scant red cell density. **D.** Reticulocyte preparation showing AHA. Note the high frequency of reticulocytes, the large cells with precipitated ribosomes. The remaining cells are microspherocytes. *(Reproduced with permission from Lichtman MA, Shafer MS, Felgar RE, et al: Lichtman's Atlas of Hematology 2016. New York, NY: McGraw Hill; 2017.)*

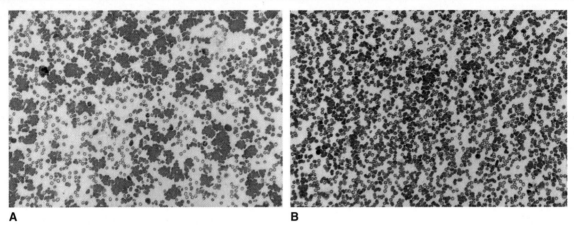

FIGURE 26–3. Blood films. **A.** Cold-reactive (IgM) antibody. Red cell agglutination at room temperature. **B.** Same blood examined at 37°C. Note the marked reduction in agglutination. *(Reproduced with permission from Lichtman MA, Shafer MS, Felgar RE, et al: Lichtman's Atlas of Hematology 2016. New York, NY: McGraw Hill; 2017.)*

exhibit RBC autoagglutination in the blood film and in chilled antico-agulated blood (Fig. 26-3). Patients with COVID-19, with or without anemia, exhibit RBC shape changes including agglutination, rouleaux, stomatocytes, and knizocytes (Chap. 1). Stomatocytes and knizocytes are unusual in other types of anemia.[222] The tendency to rouleaux formation and agglutination may contribute to the microvascular thrombosis seen in COVID-19 patients.

The reticulocyte count usually is elevated. Nevertheless, early in the course of the disease, more than one-third of all patients may have transient reticulocytopenia despite a normal or hyperplastic erythroid marrow.[223-226] The mechanism is unknown, but autoantibodies reactive against antigens on reticulocytes are speculated to lead to their selective destruction.[224] One unusual patient with warm-antibody AHA, reticulocytopenia, and marrow erythroid aplasia had a serum autoantibody that inhibited erythroid colony formation in vitro.[227] The aplastic crisis remitted after the serum IgG level was lowered by immunoadsorption. Reticulocytopenia also may be seen in patients with marrow function compromised by an underlying disease, parvovirus infection, toxic chemicals, or nutritional deficiency. Marrow examination usually reveals erythroid hyperplasia and may provide evidence of an underlying lymphoproliferative disorder.

Hyperbilirubinemia (chiefly unconjugated) is highly suggestive of hemolytic anemia, although its absence does not exclude the diagnosis. Total bilirubin is only modestly increased (up to 5 mg/dL), and with rare exceptions, the conjugated (direct) fraction constitutes less than 15% of the total. Urinary urobilinogen is increased regularly, but bile is not detected in the urine unless serum conjugated bilirubin is increased. Usually, serum haptoglobin levels are low, and lactate dehydrogenase (LDH) levels are elevated. Hemoglobinuria is encountered in rare patients with warm-antibody AHA and hyperacute hemolysis, more commonly in patients with cold agglutinin disease, and characteristically in patients with paroxysmal cold hemoglobinuria and with drug-induced immune hemolytic anemia mediated by the ternary complex mechanism.

Direct Antiglobulin Test Pattern

Diagnosis of AHA or drug-induced immune hemolytic anemia requires demonstration of immunoglobulin or complement bound to the patient's RBCs. As a screening procedure, use of a "broad-spectrum" antiglobulin (Coombs) reagent—that is, one that contains antibodies directed against human immunoglobulin and complement components (principally C3)—is customary. If agglutination is noted with a broad-spectrum reagent, antisera reacting selectively with IgG

(the γ Coombs) or with C3 (the non-γ Coombs) are used to define the specific pattern of RBC sensitization. Monospecific antisera to IgM or IgA also have been used in selected cases.

Three possible *major* patterns of direct antiglobulin reaction in AHA and drug-induced immune hemolytic anemia exist: (1) RBCs coated with only IgG, (2) RBCs coated with IgG and complement components, and (3) RBCs coated with complement components without detectable immunoglobulin.[10,228-230] In patterns 2 and 3, the complement components most readily detected are C3 fragments (mainly C3dg). Each pattern is associated with accelerated RBC destruction. Positive antiglobulin reactions with anti-IgA or anti-IgM are encountered less commonly, often in association with bound IgG, complement, or both.[231-237] Table 26-4 summarizes the diagnostic significance of each of these major patterns (see "Serologic Features" next).

SEROLOGIC FEATURES

Warm-Antibody Autoimmune Hemolytic Anemia

Free versus Bound Autoantibody The autoantibody molecules in patients with warm-antibody AHA exist in a reversible, dynamic equilibrium between RBCs and plasma.[238,239] In addition to the major portion of autoantibody bound to the patient's RBCs (detected by the DAT), "free" autoantibody may be detected in the plasma or serum of

TABLE 26–4. Major Reaction Patterns of the Direct Antiglobulin Test and Associated Types of Immune Injury

Reaction Pattern	Type of Immune Injury
Immunoglobulin (Ig) G alone	Warm-antibody autoimmune hemolytic anemia (AHA)
	Drug-immune hemolytic anemia: Hapten drug adsorption type or autoantibody type
Complement alone	Warm-antibody AHA with subthreshold IgG deposition
	Cold-agglutinin disease
	Paroxysmal cold hemoglobinuria
	Drug-immune hemolytic anemia: ternary complex type
IgG plus complement	Warm-antibody AHA
	Drug-immune hemolytic anemia: autoantibody type (rare)

these patients by the IAT. In the IAT, the patient's serum or plasma is incubated with normal donor erythrocytes at the appropriate temperature (in this case, 37°C). The cells are washed, suspended in saline solution, and then tested for agglutination by antiglobulin serum. The presence of unbound autoantibody in plasma depends on the total amount of antibody being produced and the binding affinity of the antibody for RBC antigens. In general, patients whose RBCs are heavily coated with IgG more likely exhibit plasma autoantibody. Protease-modified RBCs are more sensitive than native RBCs in detecting plasma autoantibody, but such data must be interpreted with caution because alloantibodies, naturally occurring antibodies to cryptic antigens, and other serum components may interact with enzyme-modified RBCs. Patients with a positive IAT as a result of a warm-reactive autoantibody should also have a positive DAT result. A patient with a serum anti-RBC antibody (positive IAT result) and a negative DAT result probably does not have an autoimmune process but rather an alloantibody stimulated by prior transfusion or pregnancy.

Quantity, Affinity, and Isotype of Red Blood Cell–Bound Autoantibody

Direct Antiglobulin Test–Negative Autoimmune Hemolytic Anemia Figure 55-4 relates the intensity of the direct antiglobulin reaction, using specific anti-IgG serum, to the number of IgG molecules bound per RBC. The latter was determined by a sensitive antibody-consumption method.[240] A trace-positive antiglobulin reaction (read macroscopically) detects 300 to 400 molecules of IgG per cell.[240,241] In another laboratory, a trace-positive antiglobulin reaction with anti-C3 was obtained with 60 to 115 molecules C3 per cell.[166]

Sometimes patients with warm-antibody AHA and many of its hallmarks, for example, anemia, reticulocytosis, spherocytes, elevated LDH, low or absent haptoglobin, present with a negative DAT reaction. There are three principal causes for the negative DAT reaction: (1) IgG or complement sensitization below the threshold of detection of commercial antiglobulin (Coombs) reagents; (2) low-affinity IgG sensitization with loss of cell-bound antibody during the cell washing steps before the direct antiglobulin reaction; and (3) sensitization with IgA or IgM antibodies, which many commercial DAT reagents cannot detect because they contain only anti-IgG anti-C3.

More sensitive methods for quantifying RBC-bound IgG allow identification of AHA patients having all the usual features of warm-antibody AHA but a negative DAT result with antiimmunoglobulin and anticomplement reagents.[240-242] In these cases, specialized methods (eg, anti-IgG consumption assays, automated enhanced agglutination techniques, enzyme-linked immunoassays, radioimmunoassays, flow cytometry) detect very small quantities of cell-bound IgG. In such cases, studies with highly concentrated RBC eluates confirm these IgG molecules are warm-reacting anti-RBC autoantibodies.[240] Patients generally have relatively mild hemolysis and often respond favorably to glucocorticoid therapy. By these specialized methods, subthreshold IgG also may be detected in a significant number of patients exhibiting the "complement alone" pattern of direct antiglobulin reaction in the absence of drug sensitivity or cold agglutinins. Studies with concentrated RBC eluates suggest subthreshold quantities of bound IgG antibodies are capable of fixing much larger quantities of C3 to the cell membrane.[240] In cases of low-affinity IgG sensitization, detection of IgG bound to RBCs may be accomplished by cold washing (0°C-4°C) or by use of low-ionic-strength saline in the wash steps before the DAT reaction. Cell-bound IgA and IgM may be detected by means of antisera to IgA and IgM. DAT-negative AHA has been reviewed extensively elsewhere.[243-245]

Nature of the Autoantibodies and Red Blood Cell Target Antigens In any series of warm-antibody AHA patients, the correlation between the strength of the antiglobulin reaction (IgG molecules per RBC) and the rate of RBC destruction is variable. The IgG subclass of warm autoantibodies influences the degree to which these antibodies shorten RBC survival. IgG_1 is the most commonly encountered subclass, either alone or in combination with other IgG subclasses.[230,246] IgG_1 and IgG_3 autoantibodies appear to be more effective in decreasing RBC life span than do those of the IgG_2 or IgG_4 subclass.[230,247]

The difference may result from the greater affinity of macrophage Fc receptors for IgG_1 and IgG_3[161,162] and the higher complement-fixing activity of IgG_1 or IgG_3 antibodies relative to the activity of IgG_2 or IgG_4 antibodies.[171]

Autoantibodies eluted from patients' RBCs or present in their plasma typically bind to all the common types of human RBCs represented in test panels used by blood banks and thus might appear to be nonspecific. However, the antibodies of any one patient typically recognize one or more antigenic determinants (epitopes) that are common to almost all human RBCs, that is, "public" antigens. These antibodies have been useful for evaluating RBC membrane structures and for identifying rare RBC phenotypes, namely, RBCs that lack a common blood group antigen(s). Nearly half of all AHA patients have autoantibodies specific for epitopes on Rh proteins.[10,11,127,248-250] The autoantibodies of such patients commonly do not react with human Rh$_{null}$ RBCs, which lack expression of the Rh complex. Occasionally, the anti-Rh autoantibodies have anti-e, anti-E, or anti-c (or, more rarely, anti-D) specificity. Patients who have autoantibodies with selective specificity (eg, anti-e) nearly always have other autoantibodies reactive with all human RBCs, except Rh$_{null}$. Autoantibodies with such specificity are designated collectively as Rh related.[124,250]

The remaining patients with warm-antibody AHA have IgG autoantibodies that are fully reactive with Rh$_{null}$ RBCs.[10,11,127,248-250] The exact specificity of the autoantibodies for many of these patients is undefined. However, in other instances, autoantibody specificity for serologically defined blood group antigens outside the Rh system has been identified (using RBCs of appropriate antigen-deficient phenotype), including

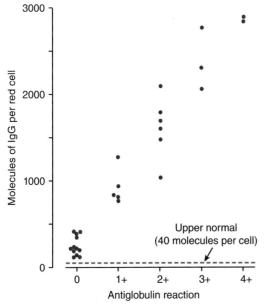

FIGURE 26–4. Comparison of direct antiglobulin reactions (with anti–immunoglobulin [Ig]G serum) with molecules of red blood cell–bound IgG determined by a quantitative antibody consumption assay (method described by Gilliland and colleagues[240]). The two assays were conducted concurrently on the same blood specimen. The antiglobulin reactions were performed manually and read macroscopically.

anti-Wr[b],[127] anti-En[a],[251] anti-LW,[252] anti-U,[253] anti-Ge,[236,254] anti-Sc1,[255] or antibodies to Kell blood group antigens.[256] For ease of reference, the entire group of autoantibodies is designated non–Rh related.[124,250]

Immunochemical studies indicate the autoantibodies from almost any AHA patient react with individual membrane proteins. The major target of Rh-related autoantibodies is a 32- to 34-kDa nonglycosylated polypeptide lacking on Rh_null RBCs.[124,257] This polypeptide is similar, if not identical, to the polypeptide expressing the Rh(e) alloantigen. Many α-methyldopa–induced autoantibodies also react with this polypeptide.[124] Autoantibodies with non-Rh serologic specificity react with the band 3 anion transporter[124,258] or with both band 3 and glycophorin A.[124] The latter autoantibodies may react with an epitope formed through the interaction of these two proteins on the RBC membrane.[259] It is interesting to note that anti-RBC autoantibodies in NZB mice exhibit anti–band 3 specificity.[260] Furthermore, naturally occurring anti–band 3 IgG autoantibodies are found in almost all humans.[261,262] These autoantibodies may play a role in the clearance of senescent RBCs by reacting with neoantigens formed on these cells by proteolytic alteration[261] or aggregation[262] of band 3 proteins. Such neoantigens are not found on younger RBCs. An important but unanswered question concerns the possible relationship between naturally occurring and pathologic anti–band 3 autoantibodies.

Cold-Antibody Hemolytic Anemia

Cold agglutinins are distinguished by their ability to directly agglutinate saline-suspended human RBCs at low temperature, maximally at 0°C to 5°C. The reaction is reversible by warming. In chronic cold agglutinin disease, serum titers are commonly 1:1000 or higher and may reach 1:512,000 or more.[11] Cold agglutinins are characteristically IgM. IgA or IgG cold agglutinins have been reported,[11,186,263] sometimes in combination with IgM.[264] In mixed warm- and cold-antibody AHA, warm-reactive IgG autoantibodies are found in association with IgM cold agglutinins.[21]

The DAT result is positive with anticomplement reagents. The antibody itself, however, is not detected by the DAT because the cold agglutinins readily dissociate from the RBCs both in vivo and during the washing steps of the standard antiglobulin procedure. In contrast, C4b and C3b are covalently bound to target RBCs via thioester linkages. In one unusual case, a low-titer IgG cold agglutinin could be detected by washing the patient's RBCs in ice-cold saline solution and performing the DAT at 4°C.[263]

The majority of cold agglutinins are reactive with oligosaccharide antigens of the I/i system, which are precursors of the ABH and Lewis blood group substances.[265-267] The I/i determinants are bound to erythrocyte membrane glycoprotein (band 3 anion transporter) or to glycolipids.[266,267] Anti-I and anti-i reportedly bind solubilized RBC glycoproteins at 37°C, suggesting the temperature dependence of cold agglutination of intact RBCs may be a function of temperature-induced conformational effects on the cell surface.[268,269]

I antigens are expressed strongly on adult RBCs but weakly on neonatal (cord) RBCs. The converse is true of i antigens, indicating I/i antigen expression is developmentally regulated.[266] The differences between adult and cord blood RBCs allow evaluation of the serologic specificity of cold agglutinins.[10,11,186] I/i antigens, or structurally related analogues, occur in human saliva, milk, amniotic fluid, and hydatid cyst fluid[186] and are expressed on human lymphocytes, neutrophils, and monocytes.[270]

Anti-I is the predominant specificity of cold agglutinins in idiopathic cold agglutinin disease, in patients with *M. pneumoniae*, and in some cases of lymphoma. Cold agglutinins with anti-i specificity are found in patients with infectious mononucleosis and in some patients with lymphoma. A small percentage of cold agglutinin-containing sera react equally well with adult and neonatal RBCs. These antibodies

recognize antigens outside the I/i system, including Pr antigens, consisting of carbohydrate epitopes of glycophorins that are inactivated by protease treatment[186] and, less commonly, the M or P blood group antigens.[271,272] Most cold agglutinins associated with chickenpox exhibit anti-Pr specificity. A single case with anti-I specificity has been observed.[273] Hemolysis resulting from a cold agglutinin with anti-Pr specificity occurred after an allogeneic marrow transplant.[274]

In hemolytic anemia associated with infectious mononucleosis, the patient's serum may contain IgM anti-i cold agglutinins or cold-reactive nonagglutinating IgG anti-i with IgM cold-reactive anti-IgG antibodies ("rheumatoid factors") that may crosslink the IgG-coated RBCs to produce agglutination.[275]

In paroxysmal cold hemoglobinuria, the direct antiglobulin reaction usually is positive during and briefly following an acute attack because of the coating of surviving RBCs with complement, primarily C3dg fragments. The Donath-Landsteiner antibody is responsible for complement deposition on the cells; it is a nonagglutinating IgG that binds RBCs only in the cold. It readily dissociates from the RBCs at room temperature. In adults subject to recurring episodes in association with cold exposure, the DAT result remains negative between attacks. The antibody is detected by the biphasic Donath-Landsteiner test, in which the patient's fresh serum is incubated with RBCs initially at 4°C, and the mixture is then warmed to 37°C.[11] Intense hemolysis occurs. Addition of fresh guinea pig serum or ABO-compatible human serum may be necessary to serve as a source of fresh complement if the patient's serum has been stored or is complement depleted. Antibody titers rarely exceed 1:16. The Donath-Landsteiner antibody typically has specificity for the P blood group antigen, a glycosphingolipid structure.[267] The P antigen also occurs on lymphocytes and skin fibroblasts.[16] The finding of P antigen on skin fibroblasts might be related in some way to the occurrence of cold urticaria in paroxysmal cold hemoglobinuria, a phenomenon that may be transferred passively by serum to normal skin.[10] Antibody specificities for RBC antigens other than the P blood group have been noted.[276]

Drug-Induced Immune Hemolytic Anemia

In the hapten-drug adsorption mechanism of immune injury associated with cephalosporins or penicillin, the patient's drug-coated RBCs bind drug-specific IgG antibody and exhibit positive DAT reactions with anti-IgG. Rarely, both anti-IgG and anti-C3d antisera produce positive DAT reactions. Such cases could have superficial resemblance to warm-antibody AHA. The key serologic difference is that, in this form of drug-induced immune hemolytic anemia, the antibodies in the patient's serum or eluted from the patient's RBCs react *only* with drug-coated RBCs. In contrast, the IgG antibodies in warm-type AHA react with unmodified human RBCs and may show preference for certain known blood groups (eg, within the Rh complex). Such serologic distinction and the history of exposure to high blood levels of penicillin or a cephalosporin should be instructive.

In hemolysis mediated by the ternary complex mechanism, the DAT result is positive with anticomplement serum. Immunoglobulins are only rarely detectable on the patient's RBCs. This pattern is similar to that encountered in AHA mediated by cold agglutinins. Moreover, the brisk type of hemolysis in the ternary complex mechanism also is seen in certain cases of cold-antibody AHA. In the drug-induced cases, however, the cold agglutinin titer and the Donath-Landsteiner test result are normal, and demonstration of serum antibody acting on human RBCs depends on the presence of the drug in the test system. Thus, the IAT reaction with anticomplement serum may be positive only if the incubation mixture permits interaction of (1) normal RBCs; (2) antidrug antibody from the patient's serum; (3) the relevant drug, either still in the patient's serum or added in vitro in appropriate concentration; and (4) a source of complement, that is, fresh normal serum or the patient's own serum if freshly obtained. A negative result does not necessarily absolve the suspected drug because the critical determinant may be a metabolite of the drug in question. In some cases, use of urine or serum (of the patient or a volunteer taking the drug) as a source of drug metabolite has permitted successful demonstration of a drug-dependent mechanism.[58,202,206,277]

In patients with true autoantibodies as a result of α-methyldopa, the DAT reaction is strongly positive for IgG, but complement only rarely is detected on the patient's RBCs. Autoantibody to RBCs is regularly present in the serum of patients and mediates a positive IAT reaction with unmodified human RBCs, often showing specificity related to the Rh complex. No presently available specific serologic test can separate idiopathic warm-reacting IgG autoantibodies with Rh-related specificities from those induced by α-methyldopa administration. The evidence must be circumstantial, with the helpful knowledge that discontinuation of α-methyldopa, without any form of immunosuppressive therapy, consistently permits a slow recovery from anemia and a gradual disappearance of anti-RBC antibodies. The DAT reaction pattern in AHA induced by chemotherapy, immunosuppressant drugs, and immune checkpoint inhibitors is more variable. IgG is almost always detected by the DAT, but IgG +C or C alone patterns are also seen.[85]

Drugs now not known to cause immune RBC injury will be implicated in the future. In any patient with a clinical picture compatible with drug-related immune hemolysis, a reasonable approach is stopping any drug that is suspect while serologic studies are being performed. The patient should be monitored for improvement in hematocrit level, decrease in reticulocytosis, and gradual disappearance of the positive DAT reaction. Repeat challenge with the suspected drug may confirm the diagnosis, but this measure is seldom necessary in patient management and may be unsafe. Therefore, rechallenge to exclude a drug-induced immune hemolytic anemia should be undertaken only for compelling reasons, such as the need to use the specific drug for the patient's illness.

● DIFFERENTIAL DIAGNOSIS

Several nonautoimmune diseases may result in spherocytic anemia, such as HS, Zieve syndrome, clostridial sepsis, and the hemolytic anemia preceding Wilson disease. Among the hereditary hemolytic anemias, HS can resemble acquired AHA most closely because the spherocytic anemia associated with HS may be detected first in adulthood (Chap. 15). In addition, splenomegaly may be prominent in both HS and AHA. Family studies of patients with HS, however, usually can identify other affected individuals. Most important, in hereditary hemolytic anemia, the DAT result is negative.

In hemolytic anemia accompanied by a positive DAT result, serologic characterization of the autoantibody may distinguish warm-antibody AHA from cold-reacting autoantibody syndromes. Diagnosis of a drug-induced immune hemolytic anemia depends on a history of appropriate drug intake supported by compatible serologic findings. In patients who recently received a transfusion, a positive DAT reaction may reflect the binding of a newly formed alloantibody to donor RBCs in the patient's circulation (delayed transfusion reaction; Chap. 30). This finding could lead to a false impression of an autoimmune process.

The venom of the brown recluse spider (*Loxosceles recluse*) may cause severe life-threatening hemolysis.[278,279] The DAT result may be positive for IgG and or complement and spherocytes and RBC fragments are present on the blood film. The diagnosis should be considered when there is history or evidence by physical examination of a spider bite. The role of IgG and complement in hemolysis is unclear, but the terminal complement inhibitor, eculizumab, inhibits lysis in vitro.

To date, the clinical use of eculizumab in this population has not been reported.

Recent recipients of allogeneic blood stem cell or solid-organ transplantations may develop autoimmune hemolysis.[280] In the former, antibodies are produced by the stem cell graft against RBCs also produced by the stem cell graft; that is, both antibodies and RBCs are of donor origin. In the case of solid-organ transplantations, the recipient's own lymphocytes make antibody against recipient RBCs. In both situations, the autoimmunity is thought to arise from immunosuppressive therapy causing delayed reconstitution or dysfunction of T-cell immunity, leading to development of antibodies autologous to the offended immune system.

Recipients of transplantations may also develop an *allo*immune hemolytic anemia that mimics warm-antibody AHA. The problem is seen in kidney, liver, or hematopoietic stem cell transplantations and usually occurs when an organ from a blood group O donor is transplanted into a blood group A or B recipient. B lymphocytes present in the donated organ or stem cell product form alloantibodies against recipient RBCs.[281-284] Patients of blood group O who receive a stem cell transplant from a donor of blood group A or B may develop a transiently positive DAT and hemolysis of RBCs made by the marrow graft because of temporary persistence of previously synthesized host anti-A or anti-B.[285] Furthermore, some group O stem cell transplantation recipients exhibit mixed hematopoietic chimerism with persistence of host B lymphocytes that can make alloantibodies directed against RBCs made by the stem cell graft.[285] In these settings, the findings of hemolysis and a positive DAT as a result of anti-A and anti-B probably are diagnostic of an alloimmune process because *auto*antibodies directed against the major blood group antigens A and B are extremely rare.

Other acquired types of hemolytic anemia are less easily confused with either warm- or cold-antibody AHA because spherocytes are not prominent on the blood film and the DAT result is negative. Patients with paroxysmal nocturnal hemoglobinuria (PNH) may complain of dark urine (hemoglobinuria). This finding is unusual in patients with warm-antibody AHA but can occur in patients with the cold-antibody syndromes. Decreased levels of CD55 and CD59 on blood cells, detected by flow analysis, are characteristic of PNH but not AHA (Chap. 8). Microangiopathic hemolytic disorders, such as thrombotic thrombocytopenic purpura and hemolytic uremic syndrome, can be distinguished from AHA by examining the blood film. In the microangiopathic hemolytic diseases, the blood film displays marked RBC fragmentation and minimal spherocytosis. In addition, microangiopathic hemolytic anemias more frequently are associated with thrombocytopenia than is either warm- or cold-antibody AHA.

The clinical and laboratory features of chronic cold agglutinin disease are sufficiently distinctive so that the diagnostic possibilities are limited. In general, a high-titer cold agglutinin (>1:512) and a positive DAT with anticomplement serum (but not with anti-IgG) are consistent with cold agglutinin disease. In many instances of drug-induced immune hemolytic anemia, the DAT result also is positive only for complement. The drug history and a low (or absent) cold agglutinin titer, however, help to distinguish drug-induced immune hemolytic anemia from cold agglutinin disease. If the patient has an elevated cold agglutinin level and a positive DAT result with both anti-IgG and anti-C3, then the patient may have a mixed-type AHA. Warm-antibody AHA, hereditary hemolytic disorders, and PNH should be excluded in cases exhibiting primarily a chronic hemolytic anemia. The pattern of antiglobulin reaction, family history, and the result of analysis of CD55/CD59 on blood cells provide additional help in difficult cases. When the hemolysis is episodic, paroxysmal cold hemoglobinuria, march hemoglobinuria, and PNH also should be considered. When cold-induced peripheral vasoocclusive symptoms are predominant, the differential diagnosis should include cryoglobulinemia and Raynaud phenomenon, with or without an associated rheumatic disease. Infectious mononucleosis, *M. pneumoniae* infection, and lymphoma can be considered in appropriate clinical settings.

Paroxysmal cold hemoglobinuria must be distinguished from the subset of cases of chronic cold agglutinin disease manifesting episodic hemolysis and hemoglobinuria. This distinction is made primarily in the laboratory. In general, patients with paroxysmal cold hemoglobinuria lack high titers of cold agglutinins. Furthermore, the Donath-Landsteiner antibody is a potent in vitro hemolysin, in contrast to most cold agglutinins, which are weak hemolysins. Warm-antibody AHA, march hemoglobinuria, myoglobinuria, and PNH can be distinguished through the history and appropriate laboratory studies.

Immune hemolysis caused by drugs should be distinguished from (1) the warm- or cold-antibody types of idiopathic AHA, (2) congenital hemolytic anemias such as HS, and (3) drug-mediated hemolysis resulting from disorders of red cell metabolism, such as glucose-6-phosphate dehydrogenase deficiency. Patients with drug-induced immune hemolytic anemia have a positive DAT result that distinguishes this group from patients with inherited RBC defects.

●THERAPY

GENERAL

There is no licensed therapy for AHA and few clinical trials to provide guidance. The rocommendations below are largely based on expert opinion and the few trials available. The First International Consensus Group reviewed the available data and has provided a set of standardized diagnostic and therapeutic approaches.[286]

Transfusion

The clinical consequences of AHA or drug-induced immune hemolytic anemia are related to the severity of the anemia and acuity of its onset. Many patients develop anemia over a period sufficient to allow for cardiovascular compensation and hence do not require RBC transfusions. However, RBC transfusions may be necessary and should not be withheld from a patient with an underlying disease complicating the anemia, such as symptomatic coronary artery disease, or a patient who rapidly develops severe anemia with signs or symptoms of circulatory failure, as in paroxysmal cold hemoglobinuria or ternary complex drug-induced immune hemolysis.

Transfusion of RBCs in immune hemolytic anemia presents two difficulties: (1) cross-matching and (2) the short half-life of the transfused RBCs (Chap. 29). Finding truly serocompatible donor blood is nearly always impossible except in rare cases when the autoantibody is specific for a defined blood group antigen (see "Serologic Features" earlier).

It is most important to identify the patient's ABO type so as to avoid a hemolytic transfusion reaction mediated by anti-A or anti-B. This part of the matching process allows for selection of either ABO-identical or -compatible blood for transfusion. With respect to compatibility, the more difficult technical issue relates to the detection of RBC alloantibodies, which may be masked by the presence of the autoantibody.

Clinicians often speak of "least incompatible" blood for transfusion, but this term has lately fallen into disrepute because it lacks a precise definition.[287,288] In fact, all units are serologically incompatible, but units that are incompatible because of the presence of autoantibody are less dangerous to transfuse than units that are incompatible because of an alloantibody.

Before transfusing an incompatible unit, the patient's serum must be tested carefully for an alloantibody that could cause a severe hemolytic transfusion reaction against donor RBCs, especially in patients with a history of pregnancy, abortion, or prior transfusion.[250,289,290] Patients who have been neither pregnant nor transfused with blood products are unlikely to harbor an alloantibody. Early consultation between the clinician and the blood bank physician is essential. An understanding of the basic aspects of blood compatibility testing coupled with the knowledge of a patient's pregnancy and transfusion history allow for informed discussion and confident transfusion of mismatched blood if the situation demands.

After selection, the packed RBCs should be administered slowly and in the case of cold hemolysis syndromes should be brought at least to room temperature. During the transfusion, the patient should be monitored for signs of a hemolytic transfusion reaction (Chap. 30). The transfused cells may be destroyed as fast as or perhaps even faster than the patient's own cells. However, the increased oxygen-carrying capacity provided by the transfused cells may be sufficient to maintain the patient during the acute interval required for other modes of therapy to become effective.

For patients with AHA who require chronic transfusion support, use of prophylactic antigen-matched donor RBCs for transfusion has been proposed as a means of preventing alloimmunization.[291] This process is feasible only in institutions with access to a good selection of phenotyped RBC units and a reference laboratory.[292]

THERAPY OF WARM-ANTIBODY AUTOIMMUNE HEMOLYTIC ANEMIA

Glucocorticoids

Therapy with glucocorticoids has reduced the mortality associated with severe idiopathic warm-antibody AHA. Glucocorticoids were first used for this disorder almost 70 years ago.[293] Glucocorticoids can cause dramatic cessation or marked slowing of hemolysis in about two-thirds of patients.[10,11,227,294,295] Approximately 20% of treated patients with warm-antibody AHA achieve complete remission. Approximately 10% show minimal or no response to glucocorticoids. The best responses are seen in idiopathic cases or in those related to SLE.

Most patients should be treated with oral prednisone at an initial daily dose of 1 to 1.5 mg/kg (eg, 50-100 mg). Critically ill patients with rapid hemolysis may receive IV methylprednisolone 100 to 200 mg in divided doses over the first 24 hours. High doses of prednisone may be required for 10 to 14 days. When the hematocrit stabilizes or begins to increase, the prednisone dose can be decreased in rapid-step dose reductions to approximately 30 mg/day. With continued improvement, the prednisone dose can be further decreased at a rate of 5 mg/day every week to a dosage of 15 to 20 mg/day. These doses should be administered for 2 to 3 months after the acute hemolytic episode has subsided, after which the patient can be weaned from the drug over 1 to 2 months or treatment switched to an alternate-day therapy schedule (eg, 20-40 mg every other day). Alternate-day therapy reduces glucocorticoid side effects but should be attempted only after the patient has achieved stable remission on daily prednisone in the range of 15 to 20 mg/day. Therapy should not be stopped until the DAT reaction becomes negative. Although many patients achieve full remission of their first hemolytic episode, relapses may occur after the glucocorticoids are discontinued. Consequently, patients should be followed for at least several years after treatment. A relapse may require repeat glucocorticoid therapy and other measures (see later).

Occasionally, patients who present with only a positive DAT reaction, minimal hemolysis, and stable hematocrit require no treatment. However, these patients should be observed for clinical deterioration because the rate of RBC destruction may increase spontaneously.

Glucocorticoids may influence hemolysis in warm-antibody AHA by several mechanisms. Earlier investigators noted that hematologic improvement was often, but not always, accompanied by reduction in the strength of the DAT.[10] The subsequent observation of a decrease in cell-bound or free serum autoantibody during stable glucocorticoid-induced remission suggested improved RBC survival after treatment with glucocorticoids resulted from a decrease in synthesis of anti-RBC autoantibodies.[154,238] However, this finding cannot explain why glucocorticoid-treated patients often improve within 24 to 72 hours, a time much shorter than the half-life of anti-RBC autoantibody. Rather, glucocorticoids may suppress RBC sequestration by splenic macrophages.[156,157,167,296] A quantitative decrease in one of the three known classes of Fcγ receptors[155,156] has been observed in the blood monocytes of patients with AHA during glucocorticoid therapy.[297]

Rituximab

Rituximab is a monoclonal antibody directed against the CD20 antigen expressed on B lymphocytes and is used for treatment of B-cell lymphoma. Its use for treatment of AHA is based on the antibody's ability to eliminate B lymphocytes, including, presumably, those making autoantibodies to RBCs. However, the mechanism of action is more complex than that, as the effect of rituximab can occur very early, before the autoantibodies can recede. In fact, sometimes in responding patients, autoantibody levels are not significantly affected.[298,299] Opsonized B lymphocytes may decoy effector monocytes and macrophages from autoantibody complexes and normalize autoreactive T-lymphocyte responses.[298]

Rituximab was used initially in refractory AHA either unresponsive to or relapsed after oral glucocorticoid therapy. In a prospective series,[300] 13 of 15 children with warm-antibody AHA responded to rituximab 375 mg/m[2] weekly for 2 to 4 weeks intravenously. Other case series support the use of similar doses of rituximab in adults, with response rates ranging from 40% to 100%.[299,301] Another prospective study in adults exhibited a 100% response using rituximab 100 mg/m[2] weekly for 4 weeks along with a short course of oral glucocorticoid as first- or second-line therapy.[302] Sustained responses were observed at 3 years in more than two-thirds of the cases.[303]

A phase 3 randomized controlled trial compared glucocorticoid monotherapy versus glucocorticoid and rituximab 375 mg/m[2] as first-line therapy in patients with warm-antibody AHA.[304] The complete and partial response rates were similar (~50%) in the two groups at 3 and 6 months. At 12 and 36 months after randomization, the relapse-free survival was superior for the combination of glucocorticoids and rituximab.

Splenectomy

Historically, nearly one-third of patients with warm-antibody AHA required prednisone chronically in doses greater than 15 mg/day to maintain an acceptable hemoglobin concentration. These patients were considered candidates for laparoscopic splenectomy. The success of rituximab and other immunosuppressive drugs (see later) has more recently relegated splenectomy to third- or fourth-line therapy.[305]

Splenectomy removes the primary site of RBC trapping. Investigations in human[154] and animal[156] subjects confirm that maintenance of a given rate of RBC destruction requires 6 to 10 times more RBC-bound IgG in splenectomized subjects than in nonsplenectomized subjects. Continuation of hemolysis after splenectomy is partly related to persisting high levels of autoantibody, favoring RBC destruction in the liver by hepatic Kupffer cells.[154,156,158]

Several investigators noted the amount of RBC-bound autoantibody decreased in AHA patients after splenectomy.[10,294,306] However, a significant proportion of patients show no change in cell-bound autoantibody after splenectomy. The processes determining the rate of autoantibody production are poorly understood. The beneficial effect of splenectomy may be related to several factors interacting in complex fashion.[307]

A patient's clinical data constitute the best selection criteria for splenectomy. Attempts to select potential responders by ^{51}Cr RBC sequestration studies have been disappointing.[10,294,308] In most cases, a reasonable approach is to continue glucocorticoids for 1 to 2 months while waiting for a maximal response. However, if no response is noted within 3 weeks, the patient's condition deteriorates, or the anemia is very severe, splenectomy should be performed sooner.

Results of splenectomy are variable. Approximately two-thirds of AHA patients have a partial or complete remission after splenectomy.[294,307] However, the relapse rate is disappointingly high. Many patients require further glucocorticoid therapy to maintain acceptable hemoglobin levels, although often at a lower dose than required before splenectomy.[10,228,294] Alternate-day therapy is preferable to daily therapy in these cases if adequate control of the anemia can be achieved.

The immediate mortality and morbidity from splenectomy depend on the presence of underlying disease and the preoperative clinical status but generally are quite low.[309,310] After splenectomy, children, more than adults, have an increased risk for developing sepsis as a result of encapsulated organisms.[310] Vaccination against *H. influenzae* type b and pneumococcal and meningococcal organisms is recommended at least 2 weeks before surgery.[311] Protocols for vaccination of splenectomy candidates are updated periodically by the Centers for Disease Control and Prevention.[311]

Other Immunosuppressive Drugs

The majority of patients with warm-antibody AHA responds to glucocorticoids or rituximab and usually are not candidates for immunosuppressive therapy. At present, immunosuppressive therapy should be reserved primarily for patients who do not respond to glucocorticoids or rituximab and for patients who are poor surgical risks.

For patients who do not respond to first- or second-line therapy, the drugs of choice are oral cyclophosphamide 50 to 100 mg daily or oral azathioprine 2 to 4 mg/kg given daily. If the patient tolerates the drug, continue treatment for at least 3 months while waiting for a response. When response occurs, the patient can be weaned slowly from the drug. If no response is observed, the alternative drug can be tried. Because cyclophosphamide and azathioprine suppress hematopoiesis, blood counts, including reticulocyte count, must be monitored with extra care during therapy. Treatment with either agent increases the risk of subsequent neoplasia. Responses occur in 60% to 70% of patients.[305] Mycophenolate mofetil and cyclosporin A are noncytotoxic immunosuppressive agents associated with response rates of 80% to 100% and 50% respectively.[305] Alemtuzumab was successfully used to treat five patients with refractory AHA associated with CLL.[312]

Another successful approach used high-dose cyclophosphamide 50 mg/kg ideal body weight per day for 4 consecutive days intravenously with granulocyte colony-stimulating factor support.[313] Of 9 patients, 8 of whom had warm autoantibodies, all became transfusion independent. All patients had prolonged severe cytopenias and required hospitalization for a median of 21 days. Cyclophosphamide may cause severe hemorrhagic cystitis, and sodium 2-mercaptoethanesulfonate (mesna) 10 mg/kg was given at 3, 6, and 8 hours intravenously, after each cyclophosphamide dose, to minimize the effect of cyclophosphamide on the bladder.

Other Therapies

For patients with chronic compensated hemolysis, treatment with oral folate at 1 mg/day is recommended to satisfy the increased demands for the vitamin because of increased red cell production. Plasma exchange or plasmapheresis has been used in patients with warm-antibody AHA.

Improvement has been reported in a few cases, but use of the method is controversial.[314,315] A patient with life-threatening warm IgG-mediated AHA refractory to glucocorticoids and splenectomy exhibited rapid clinical improvement after manual whole blood exchange.[316] A patient with severe warm IgM-mediated AHA was successfully treated with plasma-derived C1 inhibitor concentrate resulting in attenuation of complement deposition on RBCs and hemolysis, along with improved recovery of transfused RBCs.[317] Another patient with refractory warm IgM-mediated AHA responded to rituximab and eculizumab.[318] Several anecdotal reports and a case series indicate short-term successful treatment of patients with AHA using high-dose IV γ-globulin.[319-322] Uncontrolled studies indicate danazol, a nonvirilizing androgen, may be useful in patients with AHA.[323,324] In a retrospective report, all seven patients receiving erythropoiesis-stimulating agents responded with a clinically significant increase in hemoglobin.[325] Some patients with ulcerative colitis and AHA unresponsive to glucocorticoids and splenectomy may respond to colectomy.[326] In patients with AHA associated with an ovarian dermoid cyst, cyst removal produces remission of the hemolysis.[327]

THERAPY OF COLD-ANTIBODY HEMOLYTIC ANEMIA

Keeping the patient warm, particularly the patient's extremities, is moderately effective in providing symptomatic relief. This action may be the only measure required in patients with mild chronic hemolysis. Treatment directed at B lymphocytes has become standard first-line therapy for patients with cold agglutinin disease.[140] Rituximab is effective and well tolerated. In two prospective trials, approximately half the patients responded to rituximab 375 mg/m² weekly for 4 weeks.[328,329] Patients who relapsed responded to a second course of rituximab at about the same rate. In a prospective trial of rituximab and fludarabine, the response rate was 76%, including complete responses in 21% with a median response duration of 66 months.[330] In another small study, 60% of patients responded to low-dose rituximab, 100 mg/m², a rate comparable to that seen with rituximab 375 mg/m².[302] More recently, rituximab in combination with bendamustine induced a 71% response rate, 40% being complete responses.[331] A short course of bortezomib produced responses in one-third of patients refractory to previous treatments.[332] In patients with lymphoma, treatment of the underlying disorder usually results in control of the cold agglutinin disease.

Complement-directed therapies may provide temporary relief from hemolysis. Eculizumab, an inhibitor of the terminal complement sequence, induced a modest increase in hemoglobin and transfusion independence in 11 of 13 patients.[333] An inhibitor of complement C1s, sutimlimab increased hemoglobin by greater than 2 g/dL in 7 of 10 patients in a phase 1 trial. All 6 transfusion-dependent patients became transfusion independent.[334] Complement-directed therapy must be given continuously. It does not inhibit RBC agglutination, nor does it eliminate the symptoms caused by agglutination such as acrocyanosis and Raynaud phenomenon. However, such treatment may prove useful as a bridge by causing rapid cessation of hemolysis, allowing time for B cell–directed therapies to take effect.[335]

Results of splenectomy or use of glucocorticoids[10,11] generally have been disappointing, although exceptions have been reported,[10,180,263,264] particularly in atypical cases. Experimental[155] and clinical[180] bases exist for considering very high doses of glucocorticoids in seriously ill patients. RBC transfusions generally are reserved for patients with severe anemia of rapid onset who are in danger of cardiorespiratory complications. Washed RBCs often are used to avoid replenishing depleted complement components and reactivating the hemolytic process. In critically ill patients, plasma exchange (with replacement by albumin-containing saline solution) may provide transient amelioration of hemolysis.[336-338]

In a small retrospective study, 5 of 5 patients with cold agglutinin disease achieved a significant increase in hemoglobin when receiving erythropoiesis-stimulating agents.[325]

In patients with cold agglutinin disease secondary to infection, spontaneous resolution of the hemolysis is expected in all patients after resolution of the infection. RBC transfusion may be required as a temporizing measure and in severe cases, plasma exchange may be beneficial. There is little evidence to support the use of glucocorticoids or antiviral therapy.

Most contemporary cases of paroxysmal cold hemoglobinuria are self-limited. Acute attacks in both chronic and transient forms of paroxysmal cold hemoglobinuria may be prevented by avoiding cold exposure. Glucocorticoid therapy and splenectomy have not been useful. When paroxysmal cold hemoglobinuria is associated with syphilis, effective treatment of the infection may result in complete remission. Antihistaminic and adrenergic agents may relieve symptoms of cold urticaria.

THERAPY OF DRUG-INDUCED IMMUNE HEMOLYTIC ANEMIA

Discontinuation of the offending drug often is the only treatment needed. This measure is essential and may be lifesaving in patients with severe hemolysis mediated by the ternary complex mechanism.

In the past, high-dose penicillin was not necessarily discontinued because of a positive DAT result alone. A change in therapy was considered mainly in the presence of overt hemolytic anemia. For example, lowering the penicillin dose and coadministering other antibiotics sometimes allowed continuation of the drug, particularly if hemolysis was not severe. For other drugs causing only mild hemolysis by the hapten-drug adsorption mechanism, in the unlikely event that no alternatives are available, a similar approach may be effective.

In patients taking α-methyldopa in the absence of hemolysis, a positive DAT result has not necessarily been an indication for stopping the drug. However, given all the choices available, it is prudent to consider alternative antihypertensive therapy. Because less information on the natural history of autoantibodies induced by drugs other than α-methyldopa is available, discontinuation of the offending drug is advisable unless no suitable alternative exists.

Glucocorticoids are generally unnecessary, and their efficacy is questionable except in cases of AHA provoked by immune checkpoint inhibitors, in which glucocorticoids are generally effective.[85] Prednisone is effective in patients with CLL and autoimmune hemolysis caused by purine analogues,[81] as are cyclosporine, rituximab, and IV immunoglobulin.[214] For treatment of CLL, combination of cyclophosphamide with fludarabine, with or without rituximab, seems to reduce the frequency of fludarabine-induced AHA.[213,214] Transfusions should be given in the unusual circumstance of severe, life-threatening anemia. Problems with crossmatching, similar to those encountered in warm-antibody AHA, may occur in patients with a strongly positive IAT, for example, in α-methyldopa–related cases. Patients with hemolytic anemia resulting from the hapten-drug adsorption mechanism should have a compatible crossmatch because the serum antibody reacts only with drug-coated cells. However, if therapy with the offending drug is still in progress, transfused cells may be destroyed at an increased rate as they become coated with drug in vivo. Patients with ternary complex–mediated hemolysis also hemolyze transfused RBCs until the offending drug clears from the plasma.

Several cases of transfusion-associated graft-versus-host disease as a result of purine analogues have been reported in CLL patients transfused for hemolysis.[79,339,340] Such patients, who have an immunodeficiency state secondary to CLL, impairing their ability to eliminate the transfused lymphocytes, should receive irradiated blood products.

COURSE AND PROGNOSIS

Patients with idiopathic warm-antibody AHA have unpredictable clinical courses characterized by relapses and remissions. No particular feature of the illness has been a consistent predictor of outcome. Despite a rather high initial rate of response to glucocorticoids and splenectomy, the overall mortality rate was significant (up to 46%) in several older series but was much lower in more recent studies.[10,11,294,341,342] The actuarial survival rate at 10 years reportedly is 73%.[341]

Pulmonary emboli, infection, and cardiovascular collapse are causes of death. Thromboembolic episodes in the form of deep vein thrombosis or splenic infarcts are relatively common during active phases of the disease.[294,342] In one series, 8 of 30 patients with AHA developed venous thromboembolism; 19 of the patients had antiphospholipid antibodies, including 6 of the 8 patients with thromboembolism.[343] In another retrospective analysis of 36 exacerbations of severe AHA in 28 patients, only 6 of whom were tested and found negative for antiphospholipid antibodies, venous thromboembolism occurred in 5 of 15 exacerbations without anticoagulation and in 1 of 21 with anticoagulation.[344] The contribution of antiphospholipid antibodies to morbidity and mortality in AHA is not clear from these data. However, it seems prudent to consider prophylactic anticoagulation for patients with AHA and antiphospholipid antibodies or other risk factors for venous thromboembolism.[345] In a retrospective study of 4756 patients with AHA, splenectomy was associated with increased risk for thromboembolic disease in the early and late postoperative periods, but not with increased mortality.[346] It remains to be seen who among splenectomized patients needs thrombotic prophylaxis and for how long.

Infections are not only a trigger for AHA but also are a frequent complication, mostly related to treatments such as glucocorticoids, splenectomy, rituximab, other immunosuppressive agents, and in the case of secondary AHA, the underlying diseases. Reactivation of viral and bacterial diseases have also been observed in AHA patients treated with immunosuppressive drugs.[347]

The prognosis in secondary warm-antibody AHA largely depends on the course of the underlying disease. In children, warm-antibody AHA frequently follows an acute infection or immunization.[309,348,349] Most of these patients exhibit a self-limited course and respond rapidly to glucocorticoids. Those who recover from the initial hemolytic episode have a good prognosis and are unlikely to relapse, although exceptions are known. Children with chronic AHA tend to be older.[348,349] The overall mortality rate is lower than in adults, ranging from 4% to 30%,[306,348-351] with higher mortality rates in those with chronic AHA.[306,350,351] and associated autoimmune thrombocytopenia (Evans syndrome).[351,352] Evans syndrome was noted in 37% of children with AHA in one large study, a much higher frequency than observed in adults.[351]

Patients with idiopathic cold agglutinin disease often have a relatively benign course and survive for many years.[9-11] Occasionally, death results from infection or severe anemia or, commonly, from an underlying lymphoproliferative process.

The postinfectious forms of cold agglutinin disease typically are self-limited. Recovery generally occurs in a few weeks. A few cases with massive hemoglobinuria have been complicated by acute renal failure, requiring temporary hemodialysis.

Postinfectious forms of paroxysmal cold hemoglobinuria terminate spontaneously within a few days to weeks after onset,[12-15] although the Donath-Landsteiner antibody may persist in low titer for several years.[10] Most patients with chronic idiopathic paroxysmal cold hemoglobinuria survive for many years despite occasional paroxysms of hemolysis.

Immune hemolysis in response to drugs usually is mild, and the prognosis is good. Occasional episodes of exceptionally severe hemolysis with renal failure or death have been reported, usually because of drugs operating through the ternary complex mechanism or purine analogues in patients with CLL.[33,47,52,53,63,64,67,101,107] In hemolysis resulting from ternary complex or hapten-drug adsorption mechanisms, the DAT reaction becomes negative shortly after the drug is discontinued, that is, soon after the drug clears from the circulation. In addition, the hemolysis associated with α-methyldopa–induced autoantibodies ceases promptly after drug cessation. However, a positive DAT reaction of gradually diminishing intensity may remain for weeks or months.

REFERENCES

1. Packman C. Historical review: the spherocytic haemolytic anaemias. *Br J Haematol.* 2001;112:888.
2. Coombs RRA, Mourant AE, Race EE. A new test for the detection of weak and incomplete Rh agglutinins. *Br J Exp Pathol.* 1945;26:255.
3. Boorman KE, Dodd BE, Loutit JF. Haemolytic icterus (acholuric jaundice), congenital and acquired. *Lancet.* 1946;1:812.
4. Loutit JF, Mollison PL. Haemolytic icterus (acholuric jaundice), congenital and acquired. *J Pathol Bacteriol.* 46;58:711.
5. Landsteiner K. Uber Beziehungen zwischen dem Blutserum und den Körperzeller. *Munch Med Wochenschr.* 1903;50:1812.
6. Clough MC, Richter IM. A study of an autoagglutinin occurring in a human serum. *Bull Johns Hopkins Hosp.* 1918;29:86.
7. Iwai S, Mei-Sai N. Etiology of Raynaud's disease: a preliminary report. *Jpn Med World.* 1925;5:119.
8. Iwai S, Mei-Sai N. Etiology of Raynaud's disease. *Jpn Med World.* 1926;6:345.
9. Schubothe H. The cold hemagglutinin disease. *Semin Hematol.* 3:2766.
10. Dacie JV. *The Haemolytic Anaemias.* Vol 3, 3rd ed. Churchill Livingstone; 1992.
11. Petz LD, Garratty G. *Immune Hemolytic Anemias.* Churchill Livingstone; 2004.
12. Nordhagen R, Stensvold K, Winsnes A, et al. Paroxysmal cold hemoglobinuria. The most frequent autoimmune hemolytic anemia in children? *Acta Paediatr Scand.* 1984;73:258.
13. Wolach B, Heddle N, Barr RD, et al. Transient Donath-Landsteiner hemolytic anemia. *Br J Haematol.* 1981;48:425.
14. Sokol RJ, Hewitt S, Stamps BK. Autoimmune hemolysis associated with Donath-Landsteiner antibodies. *Acta Haematol.* 1982;68:268.
15. Gottsche B, Salama A, Mueller-Eckhardt C. Donath-Landsteiner autoimmune hemolytic anemia in children: a study of 22 cases. *Vox Sang.* 1990;58:281.
16. Fellous M, Gerbal A, Tessier C, et al. Studies on the biosynthetic pathway of human P erythrocyte antigens using somatic cells in culture. *Vox Sang.* 1974;26:518.
17. Ackroyd JF. The pathogenesis of thrombocytopenic purpura due to hypersensitivity to sedormid. *Clin Sci (Lond).* 1949;7:24949.
18. Snapper I, Marks D, Schwartz L, Hollander L. Hemolytic anemia secondary to mesantoin. *Ann Intern Med.* 1953;39:619.
19. Harris JW. Studies on the mechanism of drug-induced hemolytic anemia. *J Lab Clin Med.* 1956;47:760.
20. Sokol RJ, Hewitt S, Stamps BK. Autoimmune haemolysis: an 18-year study of 865 cases referred to a regional transfusion centre. *Br Med J.* 1981;282:2023.
21. Sokol RJ, Hewitt S, Stamps BK. Autoimmune haemolysis: mixed warm and cold antibody type. *Acta Haematol.* 1983;69:266.
22. Shulman IA, Branch DR, Nelson JM, et al. Autoimmune hemolytic anemias with both cold and warm autoantibodies. *JAMA.* 1985;253:1746.
23. Kajii E, Miura Y, Ikemoto S. Characterization of autoantibodies in mixed-type autoimmune hemolytical anemia. *Vox Sang.* 1991;60:45.
24. Berentsen S, Bo K, Shammas F, et al. Chronic cold agglutinin disease of the "idiopathic" type is a premalignant or low-grade malignant lymphoproliferative disease. *APMIS.* 1997;105:354.
25. Maslov, DV, Simenson V, Jain S. Badari A. COVID-19 and cold agglutinin hemolytic anemia. *TH Open.* 2020;4:e175
26. Lazarian G, Quinquenel A, Bellal M, et al. Autoimmune haemolytic anaemia associated with COVID-19 infection. *Br. J. Haematol.* 2020;190:29.
27. Lopez C, Kim J, Pandey A, et al. Simultaneous onset of COVID-19 and autoimmune haemolytic anaemia. *Br. J. Haematol.* 2020;190:31.
28. Saif M. HIV associated autoimmune hemolytic anemia: an update. *AIDS Patient Care.* 2001;15:217.
29. Steanini M, Johnson NL. Positive antihuman globulin test in patients receiving carbromal. *Am J Med Sci.* 1970;259:49.
30. Gralnick HR, McGinnis MH, Elton W, McCurdy P. Hemolytic anemia associated with cephalothin. *JAMA.* 1971;217:1193.
31. Branch DR, Berkowitz LR, Becker RL, et al. Extravascular hemolysis following the administration of cefamandole. *Am J Hematol.* 1985;18:213.
32. Chambers LA, Donovan BA, Kruskall MS. Ceftazidime-induced hemolysis patient with drug-dependent antibodies reactive by immune complex and drug adsorption mechanisms. *Am J Clin Pathol.* 1991;95:393.

33. Garratty G, Nance S, Lloyd M, Domen R. Fatal immune hemolytic anemia due to cefotetan. *Transfusion.* 1992;32:269.

34. Salama A, Mueller-Eckhardt C. Cianidanol and its metabolites bind tightly to red cells and are responsible for the production of auto- and/or drug-dependent antibodies against these cells. *Br J Haematol.* 1987;66:263.

35. Arndt PA, Garratty G, Brasfield FM, et al. Immune hemolytic anemia due to cimetidine: the first example of a cimetidine antibody. *Transfusion.* 2010;50:302.

36. Martinengo M, Ardenghi DF, Tripodi G, Reali G. The first case of drug-induced immune hemolytic anemia due to hydrocortisone. *Transfusion.* 2008;48:1925.

37. Pujol M, Fernandez F, Sancho JM, et al. Immune hemolytic anemia induced by 6-mercaptopurine. *Transfusion.* 2000;40:75.

38. Arndt P, Garratty G, Isaak E, et al. Positive direct and indirect antiglobulin tests associated with oxaliplatin can be due to drug antibody and or drug-induced nonimmunologic protein adsorption. *Transfusion.* 2009;49:711.

39. VanArsdel PP Jr, Gilliland BC. Anemia secondary to penicillin treatment: studies on two patients with non-allergic serum hemagglutinins. *J Lab Clin Med.* 1965;65:277.

40. Petz LD, Fudenberg HH. Coombs-positive hemolytic anemia caused by penicillin administration. *N Engl J Med.* 1966;274:171.

41. Seldon MR, Bain B, Johnson CA, Lennox CS. Ticarcillin-induced immune haemolytic anaemia. *Scand J Haematol.* 1982;28:459.

42. Tuffs L, Manoharan A. Flucloxacillin-induced haemolytic anaemia. *Med J Aust.* 1986;144:559.

43. Simpson MB, Pryzbylik J, Innis B, Denham MA. Hemolytic anemia after tetracycline therapy. *N Engl J Med.* 1985;312:840.

44. Bird GWG, Ecles GH, Litchfield JA, et al. Haemolytic anaemia associated with antibodies to tolbutamide and phenacetin. *Br Med J.* 1972;1:728.

45. Salama A, Burger M, Mueller-Eckhardt C. Acute immune hemolysis induced by a degradation product of amphotericin B. *Blut.* 1989;58:59.

46. Bengtsson U, Staffan A, Aurell M, Kaijser B. Antazoline-induced immune hemolytic anemia, hemoglobinuria and acute renal failure. *Acta Med Scand.* 1975;198:223.

47. Garratty G, Postoway N, Schwellenbach J, McMahill PC. A fatal case of ceftriaxone (Rocephin)-induced hemolytic anemia associated with intravascular immune hemolysis. *Transfusion.* 1991;31:176.

48. Logue GL, Boyd AE, Rosse WF. Chlorpropamide-induced immune hemolytic anemia. *N Engl J Med.* 1970;283:900.

49. Kopicky JA, Packman CH. The mechanisms of sulfonylurea-induced immune hemolysis. Case report and review of the literature. *Am J Hematol.* 1986;23:283.

50. Salama A, Kroll H, Wittmann G, Mueller-Eckhardt C. Diclofenac-induced immune haemolytic anaemia: simultaneous occurrence of red blood cell autoantibodies and drug-dependent antibodies. *Br J Haematol.* 1996;95:640.

51. Bougie D, Johnson ST, Weitekamp LA, Aster RH. Sensitivity to metabolite of diclofenac as a cause of acute immune hemolytic anemia. *Blood.* 1997;90:407.

52. Rosenfeld CS, Winters SJ, Tedrow HE. Diethylstilbestrol-associated hemolytic anemia with a positive direct antiglobulin test result. *Am J Med.* 1989;86:617.

53. Wolf B, Conradty M, Grohmann R, et al. A case of immune complex hemolytic anemia, thrombocytopenia, and acute renal failure associated with doxepin use. *J Clin Psychiatry.* 1989;50:99.

54. Cunha PD, Lord RS, Johnson ST, et al. Immune hemolytic anemia caused by sensitivity to a metabolite of etodolac, a nonsteroidal anti-inflammatory drug. *Transfusion.* 2000;40:663.

55. Pratx LB, Santoro D, Mogro BC, et al. Etoricoxib-induced immune hemolytic anemia: first case presenting acute kidney failure. *Transfusion.* 2019;59(5):1657-1660.

56. Mayer B, Leo A, Herziger A, et al. Intravascular hemolysis caused by the contrast medium iomeprol. *Transfusion.* 2013;53:2141.

57. Kashyap AS, Kashyap S. Hemolytic anemia due to metformin. *Postgrad Med J.* 2000;76:125.

58. Salama A, Mueller-Eckhardt C. Two types of nomifensine-induced immune haemolytic anaemias: drug-dependent sensitization and/or auto-immunization. *Br J Haematol.* 1986;64:613.

59. Park GM, Han KS, Chang YH, et al. Immune hemolytic anemia after treatment with pemetrexed for lung cancer. *J Thorac Oncol.* 2008;3:196.

60. Sosler SD, Behzad V, Garratty G, et al. Immune hemolytic anemia associated with probenecid. *Am J Clin Pathol.* 1985;84:391.

61. Croft JD Jr, Swisher SN, Gilliland BC, et al. Coombs test positivity induced by drugs: mechanisms of immunologic reactions and red cell destruction. *Ann Intern Med.* 68:17668.

62. Muirhead EE, Halden ER, Groves M. Drug-dependent Coombs (antiglobulin) test and anemia: observations on quinine and acetophenetidin (phenacetin). *Arch Intern Med.* 1958;101:827.

63. Pereira A, Sanz C, Cervantes F, Castillo R. Immune hemolytic anemia and renal failure associated with rifampicin-dependent antibodies with anti-I specificity. *Ann Hematol.* 1991;63:56.

64. Habibi B, Basty R, Chodez S, Prunat A. Thiopental-related immune hemolytic anemia and renal failure. *N Engl J Med.* 1985;312:353.

65. Squires JE, Mintz PD, Clark S. Tolmetin-induced hemolysis. *Transfusion.* 1985;25:410.

66. Frieder J, Mouabbi JA, Zein R, Hadid T. Autoimmune hemolytic anemia associated with trimethoprim-sulfamethoxazole use. *Am J Health-Syst Pharm.* 2017;74:894-897.

67. Kramer MR, Levene C, Hershko C. Severe reversible autoimmune haemolytic anaemia and thrombocytopenia associated with diclofenac therapy. *Scand J Haematol.* 1986;36:118.

68. Habibi B. Drug-induced red blood cell autoantibodies co-developed with drug-specific antibodies causing a hemolytic anaemia. *Br J Haematol.* 1985;61:139.

69. Cotzias GC, Papavasiliou PS. Autoimmunity in patients treated with levodopa. *JAMA.* 1969;207:1353.

70. Henry RE, Goldberg LS, Sturgeon P, Ansel RD. Serologic abnormalities associated with L-dopa therapy. *Vox Sang.* 1971;20:306.

71. Gabor EP, Goldberg LS. Levodopa-induced Coombs positive haemolytic anaemia. *Scand J Haematol.* 1973;11:201.

72. Scott GL, Myles AB, Bacon PA. Autoimmune haemolytic anaemia and mefenamic acid therapy. *Br Med J.* 1968;3:543.

73. Carstairs KC, Breckenridge A, Dollery CT, Worlledge SM. Incidence of a positive direct Coombs test in patients on alpha-methyldopa. *Lancet.* 1966;2:133.

74. Worlledge SM, Carstairs KC, Dacie JV. Autoimmune haemolytic anaemia associated with α-methyldopa therapy. *Lancet.* 1966;2:135.

75. Breckenridge A, Dollery CT, Worlledge SM, et al. Positive direct Coombs tests and antinuclear factors in patients treated with methyldopa. *Lancet.* 1967;2:1265.

76. Lo Buglio AF, Jandl JH. The nature of alpha-methyldopa red cell antibody. *N Engl J Med.* 1967;276:658.

77. Kleinman S, Nelson R, Smith L, Goldfinger D. Positive direct antiglobulin tests and immune hemolytic anemia in patients receiving procainamide. *N Engl J Med.* 1984;311:809.

78. Maverick C, Silverstein WK, Nikonov A et al. Bendamustine-induced immune hemolytic anemia: a case report and systematic review of the literature. *Blood Adv.* 2020;4:1756.

79. Chasty RC, Myint H, Oscier DG, et al. Autoimmune haemolysis in patients with B-CLL treated with chlorodeoxyadenosine (CDA). *Leuk Lymphoma.* 1998;29:391.

80. Kwan JM, Reese AM, Trafeli JP. Delayed autoimmune hemolytic anemia in efalizumab-treated psoriasis. *J Am Acad Dermatol.* 2008;58:1053.

81. Garratty G. Immune hemolytic anemia associated with drug therapy. *Blood Rev.* 2010;24:143.

82. Darabi K, Kantamnei S, Weirnik PH. Lenalidomide-induced warm autoimmune hemolytic anemia. *J Clin Oncol.* 2006;24:e59.

83. Byrd JC, Hertler AA, Weiss RB, et al. Fatal recurrence of autoimmune hemolytic anemia following pentostatin therapy in a patient with a history of fludarabine-associated hemolytic anemia. *Ann Oncol.* 1995;6:300.

84. Kaya Z, Egritas O, Dalgic B. Tacrolimus-induced autoimmune hemolytic anemia in a previously reported child with history of thrombocytopenia following liver transplant. *Exp Clin Transplant.* 2018;3:355-356.

85. Tanios GE, Doley PB, Munker R. Autoimmune hemolytic anemia associated with the use of immune checkpoint inhibitors for cancer: 68 cases from the Food and Drug Administration database and review. *Eur J Haematol.* 2019;102:157-162.

86. Gralnick HR, Wright LD, McGinnis MH. Coombs' positive reactions associated with sodium cephalothin therapy. *JAMA.* 1967;199:725.

87. Manor E, Marmor A, Kaufman S, Leiba H. Massive hemolysis caused by acetaminophen. *JAMA.* 1976;236:2777.

88. Mueller-Eckhardt C, Kretschmer V, Coburg KH. Allergic, immunohemolytic anemia due to para-aminosalicylic acid (PAS). Immunohematologic studies of three cases. *Dtsch Med Wochenschr.* 1972;97:234.

89. Venegas Pérez B, Arquero Portero T, Sánchez Fernández MS, et al. Apomorphine-induced immune hemolytic anemia. *Mov Disord Clin Pract.* 2016;4:145-147.

90. Singh S, Singh SK, Tentu AK, et al. Artesunate-induced severe autoimmune hemolytic anemia in complicated malaria. *Indian J Crit Care Med.* 2018;10:753-756.

91. Gurbuz F, Yagci-Kupeli B, Kor Y, et al. The first report of cabergoline-induced immune hemolytic anemia in an adolescent with prolactinoma. *J Pediatr Endocrinol Metab.* 2013;27:159.

92. Lindberg LG, Norden A. Severe hemolytic reaction to chlorpromazine. *Acta Med Scand.* 1961;170:195.

93. Freercks RJ, Mehta U, Stead DF, Meintjes GA. Haemolytic anaemia associated with efavirenz. *AIDS.* 2006;20:1212.

94. Wong KY, Boose GM, Issitt CH. Erythromycin-induced hemolytic anemia. *J Pediatr.* 1981;98:647.

95. Sandvei P, Nordhagen R, Michaelsen TE, Wolthuis K. Fluorouracil (5-FU) induced acute immune haemolytic anaemia. *Br J Haematol.* 1987;65:357.

96. Korsager S, Sorensen H, Jensen OH, Falk JV. Antiglobulin tests for determination of autoimmunohaemolytic anaemia during long-term treatment with ibuprofen. *Scand J Rheumatol.* 1981;10:174.

97. Muirhead EE, Groves M, Guy R, et al. Acquired hemolytic anemia, exposures to insecticides and positive Coombs' test dependent on insecticide preparations. *Vox Sang.* 1959;4:277.

98. Robinson MG, Foadi M. Hemolytic anemia with positive Coombs' test. Association with isoniazid therapy. *JAMA.* 1969;208:656.

99. Sheik-Taha M, Frenn P. Autoimmune hemolytic anemia induced by levofloxacin. *Case Rep Infect Dis.* 2014;2014:201015.

100. Eyster ME. Melphalan (Alkeran) erythrocyte agglutinin and hemolytic anemia. *Ann Intern Med.* 1967;66:573.

101. Tafani O, Mazzoli M, Landini G, Alterini B. Fatal acute immune haemolytic anaemia caused by nalidixic acid. *Br Med J.* 1982;285:936.

102. Marks DR, Joy JV, Bonheim NA. Hemolytic anemia associated with the use of omeprazole. *Am J Gastroenterol.* 1991;86:217.

103. Gniadek T, Arndt PA, Leger RM, et al. Drug-induced immune hemolytic anemia associated with anti-vancomycin complicated by a paraben antibody. *Transfusion.* 2017;58(1):181-188.

104. Chen F, Liu S, Wu J. Puerarin-induced immune hemolytic anemia. *Int J Hematol.* 2013;98:112.

105. Arici A, Altun H, Acipayam C. Quetiapine induced autoimmune hemolytic anemia in a child patient: a case report. *Clin Psychopharamcol Neurosci.* 2018;16(4):501-504.

106. Letona JM-L, Barbolla L, Frieyro E, et al. Immune haemolytic anaemia and renal failure induced by streptomycin. *Br J Haematol.* 1977;35:561.

107. Angeles ML, Reid ME, Yacob UA, et al. Sulindac-induced immune hemolytic anemia. *Transfusion.* 1994;34:255.

108. Blum MD, Graham DJ, McCloskey CA. Temafloxacin syndrome: review of 95 cases. *Clin Infect Dis.* 1994;180:946.

109. Vilal JM, Blum L, Dosik H. Thiazide-induced immune hemolytic anemia. *JAMA.* 1976;236:1723.

110. Takahashi H, Tsukada T. Triamterene-induced immune hemolytic anemia with acute intravascular hemolysis and acute renal failure. *Scand J Haematol.* 1979;23:169.

111. Chaplin H, Avioli LV. Autoimmune hemolytic anemia. *Arch Intern Med.* 1977;137:346.

112. Sallah S, Wan J, Hanrahan L. Future development of lymphoproliferative disorders in patients with autoimmune hemolytic anemia. *Clin Cancer Res.* 2001;7:791.

113. Pirofsky B. Hereditary aspects of autoimmune hemolytic anemia: a retrospective analysis. *Vox Sang.* 1968;14:334.

114. Dobbs CE. Familial auto-immune hemolytic anemia. *Arch Intern Med.* 1965;116:273.

115. Feizi T. Cold agglutinins, the direct Coombs' test and serum immunoglobulins in *Mycoplasma pneumoniae* infection. *Ann N Y Acad Sci.* 1967;143:801.

116. Jacobson LB, Longstreth GF, Edington TS. Clinical and immunologic features of transient cold agglutinin hemolytic anemia. *Am J Med.* 1973;54:514.

117. Murray HW, Masur H, Senterfit LB, Roberts RB. The protean manifestations of *Mycoplasma pneumoniae* infection in adults. *Am J Med.* 1975;58:229.

118. Rosenfield RE, Schmidt PJ, Calvo RC, McGinniss MH. Anti-i, a frequent cold agglutinin in infectious mononucleosis. *Vox Sang.* 1965;10:631.

119. Hossaini AA. Anti-i in infectious mononucleosis. *Am J Clin Pathol.* 1970;53:198.

120. Garratty G. Autoantibodies induced by blood transfusions. *Transfusion.* 2004;44:5.

121. Young PP, Uzieblo A, Trulock E, et al. Autoantibody formation after alloimmunization: are blood transfusions a risk factor for autoimmune hemolytic anemia? *Transfusion.* 2004;44:67.

122. Salama A, Mueller-Eckhardt C. Delayed hemolytic transfusion reactions: evidence for complement activation involving allogeneic and autologous red cells. *Transfusion.* 1984;24:188.

123. Ness PM, Shirey RS, Thoman SK, Buck SA. The differentiation of delayed serologic and delayed hemolytic transfusion reactions: incidence, long-term serologic findings and clinical significance. *Transfusion.* 1990;30:688.

124. Leddy JP, Falany JL, Kissel GE, et al. Erythrocyte membrane proteins reactive with human (warm-reacting) anti-red cell autoantibodies. *J Clin Invest.* 1993;91:1672.

125. Gorst DW, Rawlinson VI, Merry AH, Stratton F. Positive direct anti-globulin test in normal individuals. *Vox Sang.* 1980;38:99.

126. Bareford D, Langster G, Gilks L, Demick-Torey LA. Follow-up of normal individuals with a positive antiglobulin test. *Scand J Haematol.* 1985;35:348.

127. Issitt PD, Pavone BG, Goldfinger D, et al. Anti-Wrᵇ and other autoantibodies responsible for positive direct antiglobulin test in 150 individuals. *Br J Haematol.* 1976;34:5.

128. Berzuini A, Bianco C, Paccapelo C, et al. Red Cell-bound antibodies and transfusion requirements in hospitalized patients with COVID-19. *Blood.* 2020;136:766.

129. Hendrickson JE, Tormey CA. COVID-19 and the Coombs test. *Blood.* 2020;136:655.

130. Angileri F, Legare S, Gammazza AM, et al. Is molecular mimicry the culprit in the autoimmune hemolytic anemia affecting patients with COVID-19? *Br J Haematol.* 2020;190.

131. Leddy JP. Immune hemolytic anemia. In: Rich RR, Fleisher TA, Schwartz BD, Shearer WT, Strober W, eds. *Clinical Immunology: Principles and Practice.* Mosby; 1996:1273.

132. Hartley SB, Crosbie J, Brink R, et al. Elimination from peripheral lymphoid tissue of self-reactive B lymphocytes recognizing membrane bound antigens. *Nature.* 1991;353:765.

133. Leddy JP. Reactivity of human gamma-G erythrocyte autoantibodies with fetal, autologous and maternal red cells. *Vox Sang.* 1969;17:525.

134. Okamoto M, Murakami M, Shimizu A, et al. A transgenic model of autoimmune hemolytic anemia. *J Exp Med.* 1992;175:71.

135. Murakami M, Tsubata T, Okamoto M, et al. Antigen-induced apoptotic death of Ly-1 B cells responsible for autoimmune disease in transgenic mice. *Nature.* 1992;357:77.

136. Lin RH, Mamula MJ, Hardin JA, Janeway CA. Induction of autoreactive B cells allows priming of autoreactive T cells. *J Exp Med.* 1991;173:1433.

137. Silverman GJ, Carson DA. Structural characterization of human monoclonal cold agglutinins: evidence for a distinct primary sequence-defined Vₕ4 idiotype. *Eur J Immunol.* 1990;20:351.

138. Silberstein LE, Jefferies LC, Goldman J, et al. Variable region gene analysis of pathologic human autoantibodies to the related i and I red blood cell antigens. *Blood.* 1991;78:2372.

139. Pascual V, Victor K, Spellerberg M, et al. Vₕ restriction among human cold agglutinins: the Vₕ4-21 gene segment is required to encode anti-I and anti-i specificities. *J Immunol.* 1992;149:2337.

140. Berentsen S. New insights in the pathogenesis and therapy of cold agglutinin-mediated autoimmune hemolytic anemia. *Front Immunol.* 2020; 11:590.

141. Stevenson FK, Smith GJ, North J, et al. Identification of normal B-cell counterparts of neoplastic cells which secrete cold agglutinins of anti-I and anti-i specificity. *Br J Haematol.* 72:989.

142. Malecka A, Troen G, Tierens A, et al. Immunoglobulin heavy and light chain gene features are correlated with primary cold agglutinin disease activity. *Haematologica.* 2016;101(9):e361.

143. Thompson KM, Sutherland J, Barden G, et al. Human monoclonal antibodies against blood group antigens preferentially express a Vₕ4-21 variable region gene-associated epitope. *Scand J Immunol.* 1991;34:509.

144. Adderson EE, Shackelford PG, Quinn A, et al. Restricted immunoglobulin VH usage and VDJ combinations in the human response to *Haemophilus influenzae* type b capsular polysaccharide: nucleotide sequences of monospecific anti-*Haemophilus* antibodies and polyspecific antibodies cross-reacting with self-antigens. *J Clin Invest.* 1993;91:2734.

145. Adderson EE, Shackelford PG, Insel RA, et al. Immunoglobulin light chain variable region gene sequences for human antibodies to *Haemophilus influenzae* type b capsular polysaccharide are dominated by a limited number of V kappa and V lambda segments and VJ combinations. *J Clin Invest.* 1992;89:729.

146. Harboe M, Lind K. Light chain types of transiently occurring cold haemagglutinins. *Scand J Haematol.* 1966;3:269.

147. Feizi T. Monotypic cold agglutinins in infection by *Mycoplasma pneumoniae*. *Nature.* 1967;215:540.

148. Feizi T, Loveless W. Carbohydrate recognition by *Mycoplasma pneumoniae* and pathologic consequences. *Am J Respir Crit Care Med.* 1996;154:S133.

149. Mollison PL. Measurement of survival and destruction of red cells in haemolytic syndromes. *Br Med Bull.* 1959;15:59.

150. Hollander L. Erythrocyte survival time in a case of acquired haemolytic anaemia. *Vox Sang.* 1954;4:164.

151. Chaplin H, Cohen R, Bloomberg G, et al. Pregnancy and idiopathic autoimmune haemolytic anaemia: a prospective study during 6 months gestation and 3 months "post-partum". *Br J Haematol.* 1973;24:219.

152. Mollison PL, Crome P, Hughes-Jones NC, Rochna E. Rate of removal from the circulation of red cells sensitized with different amounts of antibody. *Br J Haematol.* 1965;11:461.

153. Mollison PL, Hughes-Jones NC. Clearance of Rh-positive red cells by low concentration of Rh antibody. *Immunology.* 1967;12:63.

154. Rosse WF. Quantitative immunology of immune hemolytic anemia: II. The relationship of cell-bound antibody to hemolysis and the effect of treatment. *J Clin Invest.* 1971;50:734.

155. Schreiber AD, Frank MM. Role of antibody and complement in the immune clearance and destruction of erythrocytes: I. In vivo effects of IgG and IgM complement-fixing sites. *J Clin Invest.* 1972;51:575.

156. Atkinson JP, Schreiber AD, Frank MM. Effects of corticosteroids and splenectomy on the immune clearance and destruction of erythrocytes. *J Clin Invest.* 1973;52:1509.

157. Atkinson JP, Frank MM. Complement independent clearance of IgG sensitized erythrocytes: inhibition by cortisone. *Blood.* 1974;44:629.

158. Jandl JH, Kaplan ME. The destruction of red cells by antibodies in man: III. Quantitative factors influencing the pattern of hemolysis in vivo. *J Clin Invest.* 1960;39:1145.

159. Abramson N, LoBuglio AF, Jandl JH, Cotran RS, The interaction between human monocytes and red cells: binding characteristics. *J Exp Med.* 1970;132:1191.

160. LoBuglio AF, Cotran RS, Jandl JH. Red cells coated with immunoglobulin G: binding and sphering by mononuclear cells in man. *Science.* 1967;158:1582.

161. Anderson CL, Looney RJ. Human leukocyte IgG Fc receptors. *Immunol Today.* 1986;7:264.

162. Ravetch JV, Kinet J-P. Fc receptors. *Annu Rev Immunol.* 1991;9:457.

163. Gigli I, Nelson RA. Complement-dependent immune phagocytosis: I. Requirements of C1, C4, C2, C3. *Exp Cell Res.* 1968;51:45.

164. Lay WF, Nussenzweig V. Receptors for complement on leukocytes. *J Exp Med.* 1968;128:991.

165. Ross GD. Opsonization and membrane complement receptors. In: Ross GD, ed. *Immunobiology of the Complement System.* Academic Press; 1986:87.

166. Fischer JT, Petz LD, Garratty G, Cooper NR. Correlations between quantitative assay of red cell bound C3, serologic reactions, and hemolytic disease. *Blood.* 1974;44:359.

167. Schreiber AD, Parsons J, McDermott P, Cooper RA. Effect of corticosteroids on the human monocyte IgG and complement receptors. *J Clin Invest.* 1975;56:1189.

168. Ehlenberger AG, Nussenzweig V. The role of membrane receptors for C3b and C3d in phagocytosis. *J Exp Med.* 1977;145:357.

169. Rosse WF, De Boisfleury A, Bessis M. The interaction of phagocytic cells and red cells modified by immune reactions: comparison of antibody and complement coated red cells. *Blood Cells.* 1975;1:345.

170. Dameshek W, Schwartz SO. Acute hemolytic anemia (acquired hemolytic icterus, acute type). *Medicine (Baltimore).* 1940;19:231.

171. Leddy JP, Rosenfeld SI. Role of complement in hemolytic anemia and thrombocytopenia. In: Ross GD, ed. *Immunobiology of the Complement System.* Academic Press; 1986:213.

172. Nicholson-Weller A, Burge J, Fearon DT, et al. Isolation of a human erythrocyte membrane glycoprotein with decay-accelerating activity for C3 convertases of the complement system. *J Immunol.* 1982;129:184.

173. Lachmann PJ. The control of homologous lysis. *Immunol Today.* 1991;12:312.

174. Packman CH. Pathogenesis and management of paroxysmal nocturnal hemoglobinuria. *Blood Rev.* 1998;12:1.

175. Fleer A, Van Schaik ML, von dem Borne AE, Engelfriet CP. Destruction of sensitized erythrocytes by human monocytes in vitro: effects of cytochalasin B, hydrocortisone and colchicine. *Scand J Immunol.* 1978;8:515.

176. Kurlander RJ, Rosse WF, Logue WL. Quantitative influence of antibody and complement coating of red cells on monocyte-mediated cell lysis. *J Clin Invest.* 1978;61:1309.

177. Urbaniak SJ. Lymphoid cell dependent (K-cell) lysis of human erythrocytes sensitized with rhesus alloantibodies. *Br J Haematol.* 1976;33:409.

178. Handwerger BS, Kay NW, Douglas SD. Lymphocyte-mediated antibody-dependent cytolysis: role in immune hemolysis. *Vox Sang.* 1978;34:276.

179. Milgrom H, Shore SL. Lysis of antibody-coated human red cells by peripheral blood mononuclear cells: altered effector cell profile after treatment of target cells with enzymes. *Cell Immunol.* 1978;39:178.

180. Schreiber AD, Herskovitz BS, Goldwein M. Low-titer cold-hemagglutinin disease. *N Engl J Med.* 1977;296:1490.

181. Evans RS, Turner E, Bingham M, Woods R. Chronic hemolytic anemia due to cold agglutinins: II. The role of C in red cell destruction. *J Clin Invest.* 1968;47:691.

182. Atkinson JP, Frank MM. Studies on *in vivo* effects of antibody: interaction of IgM antibody and complement in the immune clearance and destruction of erythrocytes in man. *J Clin Invest.* 1974;54:339.

183. Hughey CT, Brewer JW, Colosia AD, et al. Production of IgM hexamers by normal and autoimmune B cells: implications for the physiologic role of hexameric IgM. *J Immunol.* 1998;161:4091.

184. Logue GL, Rosse WF, Gockerman JP. Measurement of the third component of complement bound to red blood cells in patients with the cold agglutinin syndrome. *J Clin Invest.* 1973;52:493.

185. Evans RS, Turner E, Bingham M. Studies with radioiodinated cold agglutinins of ten patients. *Am J Med.* 1965;38:378.

186. Roelcke D. Cold agglutination: antibodies and antigens. *Clin Immunol Immunopathol.* 1974;2:266.

187. Mantovani B, Rabinovitch M, Nussenzweig V. Phagocytosis of immune complexes by macrophages: different roles of the macrophage receptor sites for complement (C3) and for immunoglobulin (IgG). *J Exp Med.* 1972;135:780.

188. Silverstein SC, Steinman RM, Cohn ZA. Endocytosis. *Annu Rev Biochem.* 1977;46:669.

189. Jaffe CH, Atkinson JP, Frank MM. The role of complement in the clearance of cold agglutinin-sensitized erythrocytes in man. *J Clin Invest.* 1976;58:942.

190. Brown DL, Nelson DA. Surface microfragmentation of red cells as a mechanism for complement-mediated immune spherocytosis. *Br J Haematol.* 1973;24:301.

191. Evans RS, Turner E, Bingham M. Chronic hemolytic anemia due to cold agglutinins: I. The mechanism of resistance of red cells to C hemolysis by cold agglutinins. *J Clin Invest.* 1967;46:1461.

192. Kerr RO, Cardamone J, Dalmasso AP, Kaplan ME. Two mechanisms of erythrocyte destruction in penicillin-induced hemolytic anemia. *N Engl J Med.* 1972;287:1322.

193. Nesmith LW, Davis JW. Hemolytic anemia caused by penicillin. *JAMA.* 1968;203:27.

194. Yust I, Frisch B, Goldsher N. Simultaneous detection of two mechanisms of immune destruction of penicillin-treated human red blood cells. *Am J Hematol.* 1982;13:53.

195. Brandriss MW, Smith JW, Steinman HG. Common antigenic determinants of penicillin G, cephalothin and 6-aminopenicillanic acid in rabbits. *J Immunol.* 1965;94:696.

196. Abraham GN, Petz LD, Fudenberg HH. Immuno-hematological cross-allergenicity between penicillin and cephalothin in humans. *Clin Exp Immunol.* 1968;3:343.

197. Petz LD. Immunologic cross reactivity between penicillins and cephalosporins: a review. *J Infect Dis.* 1978;137(suppl):S74.

198. Kunicki TJ, Russell N, Nurten AT, et al. Further studies of the human platelet receptor for quinine- and quinidine-dependent antibodies. *J Immunol.* 1981;126:398.

199. Christie DJ, Aster RH. Drug-antibody-platelet interaction in quinine-and quinidine-induced thrombocytopenia. *J Clin Invest.* 1982;70:989.

200. Berndt MC, Chong BH, Bull HA, et al. Molecular characterization of quinine/quinidine drug-dependent antibody platelet interaction using monoclonal antisera. *Blood.* 1985;66:1292.

201. Sosler SD, Behzad O, Garratty G, et al. Acute hemolytic anemia associated with a chlorpropamide-induced apparent auto-anti-Jk$_a$. *Transfusion.* 1984;24:206.

202. Salama A, Mueller-Eckhardt C.: Rh blood group-specific antibodies in immune hemolytic anemia induced by nomifensine. *Blood.* 1986;68:1285.

203. Salama A, Mueller-Eckhardt C. On the mechanisms of sensitization and attachment of antibodies to RBC in drug-induced immune hemolytic anemia. *Blood.* 1987;69:1006.

204. Christie DJ, Mullen PC, Aster RH. Fab-mediated binding of drug-dependent antibodies to platelets in quinidine- and quinine-induced thrombocytopenia. *J Clin Invest.* 1985;75:310.

205. Smith ME, Reid DM, Jones CE, et al. Binding of quinine- and quinidine-dependent drug antibodies to platelets is mediated by the Fab domain of immunoglobulin G and is not Fc dependent. *J Clin Invest.* 1987;29:912.

206. Salama A, Mueller-Eckhardt C. The role of metabolite-specific antibodies in nomifensine-dependent immune hemolytic anemia. *N Engl J Med.* 1985;313:469.

207. Kelton JG. Impaired reticuloendothelial function in patients treated with methyldopa. *N Engl J Med.* 1985;313:596.

208. Bakemeier RF, Leddy JP. Erythrocyte autoantibody associated with alpha-methyldopa: heterogeneity of structure and specificity. *Blood.* 1968;32:1.

209. Green FA, Jung CY, Rampal A, Lorusso DJ. Alpha-methyldopa and the erythrocyte membrane. *Clin Exp Immunol.* 1980;40:554.

210. Green Fa, Jung CY, Hui H. Modulation of alpha-methyldopa binding to the erythrocyte membrane by superoxide dismutase. *Biochem Biophys Res Commun.* 1980;95:1037.

211. Kirtland HH III, Mohler DN, Horwitz DA. Methyldopa inhibition of suppressor-lymphocyte function. A proposed cause of autoimmune hemolytic anemia. *N Engl J Med.* 1980;302:825.

212. Garratty G, Arndt P, Prince HE, Schulman IA. The effect of methyldopa and procainamide on suppressor cell activity in relation to red cell autoantibody production. *Br J Haematol.* 1983;84:310.

213. Dearden C, Wade R, Else M, et al. The prognostic significance of a positive direct antiglobulin test in chronic lymphocytic leukemia: a beneficial effect of the combination of fludarabine and cyclophosphamide on the incidence of hemolytic anemia. *Blood.* 2008;111:1820.

214. Borthakur G, O'Brien S, Wierda WG, et al. Immune anaemias in patients with chronic lymphocytic leukaemia treated with fludarabine, cyclophosphamide and rituximab-incidence and predictors. *Br J Haematol.* 2007;136:800.

215. Spath P, Garratty G, Petz LD. Studies on the immune response to penicillin and cephalothin in humans: II. Immunohematologic reactions to cephalothin administration. *J Immunol.* 1971;107:860.

216. Garratty G, Petz L. Drug-induced hemolytic anemia. *Am J Med.* 1975;58:398.

217. Sokol RJ, Hewitt S, Stamps BK. Erythrocyte autoantibodies, autoimmune haemolysis and pregnancy. *Vox Sang.* 1982;43:169.

218. Evans RS, Duane RT. Acquired hemolytic anemia: I. The relation of erythrocyte antibody production to activity of the disease: II. The significance of thrombocytopenia and leukopenia. *Blood.* 1949;4:1196.

219. Evans RS, Takahashi K, Duane RT, et al. Primary thrombocytopenic purpura and acquired hemolytic anemia: evidence for a common etiology. *Arch Intern Med.* 1951;87:48.

220. Michel M, Chanet V, Deschartres A, et al. The spectrum of Evans syndrome in adults: new insights into the disease based on 68 cases. *Blood.* 2009;114:3167.

221. Pegels JG, Helmerhorst FM, van Leeuwen EF, et al. The Evans syndrome: characterization of the responsible autoantibodies. *Br J Haematol.* 1982;51:445.

222. Berzuini A, Bianco C, Migliorini AC, et al. Red blood cell morphology in patients with COVID-19-related anaemia. *Blood Transfusion.* 2021;19:34.

223. Liesveld JL, Rowe JM, Lichtman MA. Variability of the erythropoietic response in autoimmune hemolytic anemia: analysis of 109 cases. *Blood.* 1987;69:820.

224. Hegde UM, Gordon-Smith EC, Worlledge SM. Reticulocytopenia and absence of red cell autoantibodies in immune haemolytic anaemia. *Br Med J.* 1977;2:1444.

225. Conley CL, Lippman SM, Ness P. Autoimmune hemolytic anemia with reticulocytopenia: a medical emergency. *JAMA.* 1980;244:1688.

226. Greenberg J, Curtis-Cohen M, Gill FM, Cohen A. Prolonged reticulocytopenia in autoimmune hemolytic anemia of childhood. *J Pediatr.* 1980;97:784.

227. Mangan KF, Besa EC, Shadduck RK, et al. Demonstration of two distinct antibodies in autoimmune hemolytic anemia with reticulocytopenia and red cell aplasia. *Exp Hematol.* 1984;12:788.

228. Eyster ME, Jenkins DE Jr. Erythrocyte coating substances in patients with positive direct antiglobulin reactions: correlation of gamma-G globulin and complement coating with underlying diseases, overt hemolysis and response to therapy. *Am J Med.* 1969;46:360.

229. Leddy JP. Immunological aspects of red cell injury in man. *Semin Hematol.* 1966;3:48.

230. Engelfriet CP, Borne AE vd, Giessen M vd, et al. Autoimmune haemolytic anaemias: I. Serological studies with pure anti-immunoglobulin reagents. *Clin Exp Immunol.* 1968;3:605.

231. Engelfriet CP, Borne AE, Beckers D, van Loghem JJ. Autoimmune haemolytic anaemia: serological and immunochemical characteristics of the autoantibodies: mechanisms of cell destruction. *Ser Haematol.* 1974;7:328.

232. Suzuki S, Amano T, Mitsunaga M, et al. Autoimmune hemolytic anemia associated with IgA autoantibody. *Clin Immunol Immunopathol.* 1981;21:247.

233. Wolf CF, Wolf DJ, Peterson P. Autoimmune hemolytic anemia with predominance of IgA autoantibody. *Transfusion.* 1982;22:238.

234. Szymanski IO, Teno R, Rybak ME. Hemolytic anemia due to a mixture of low-titer IgG lambda and IgM lambda agglutinins reacting optimally at 22°C. *Vox Sang.* 1986;51:112.

235. Reusser P, Osterwalder B, Burri H, Speck B. Autoimmune hemolytic anemia associated with IgA: diagnostic and therapeutic aspects in a case with long-term follow-up. *Acta Haematol.* 1987;77:53.

236. Göttsche B, Salama A, Mueller-Eckhardt C. Autoimmune hemolytic anemia associated with an IgA autoanti-Gerbich. *Vox Sang.* 1990;58:211.

237. Arndt P, Leger RM, Garratty G. Serologic findings in autoimmune hemolytic anemia associated with immunoglobulin M warm autoantibodies. *Transfusion.* 2009;49:235.

238. Evans RS, Bingham M, Boehni P. Autoimmune hemolytic disease: antibody dissociation and activity. *Arch Intern Med.* 1961;108:338.

239. Evans RS, Bingham M, Turner E. Autoimmune hemolytic disease: observations of serological reactions and disease activity. *Ann N Y Acad Sci.* 1965;124:422.

240. Gilliland BC, Leddy JP, Vaughan JH. The detection of cell-bound antibody on complement-coated human red cells. *J Clin Invest.* 1970;49:898.

241. Gilliland BC, Baxter E, Evans RS. Red cell antibodies in acquired hemolytic anemia with negative antiglobulin serum tests. *N Engl J Med.* 1971;285:252.

242. Gilliland BC. Coombs-negative immune hemolytic anemia. *Semin Hematol.* 1976;13:267.

243. Segel GB, Lichtman MA. Direct antiglobulin ("Coombs") test-negative autoimmune hemolytic anemia: a review. *Blood Cells Mol Dis.* 2014;52:152.

244. Kamesaki T, Toyotsuji T, Kajii E. Characterization of direct antiglobulin test-negative autoimmune hemolytic anemia: a study of 154 cases. *Am J Hematol.* 2013;88:93.

245. Leger RM, Co P, Hunt G, Garratty G. Attempts to support an immune etiology in 800 patients with direct antiglobulin test-negative hemolytic anemia. *Immunohematology.* 2010;26:156.

246. Sokol RJ, Hewitt S, Booker DJ, Bailey A. Erythrocyte autoantibodies, subclasses of IgG and autoimmune haemolysis. *Autoimmun Rev.* 1990;6:99.

247. von dem Borne AE, Beckers D, van der Meulen FW, Engelfriet CP. IgG$_4$ autoantibodies against erythrocytes, without increased hemolysis: a case report. *Br J Haematol.* 1977;37:137.

248. Weiner W, Vos GH. Serology of acquired hemolytic anemia. *Blood.* 1963;22:606.

249. Vos GH, Petz L, Funenberg HH. Specificity of acquired haemolytic anaemia autoantibodies and their serological characteristics. *Br J Haematol.* 1970;19:57.

250. Leddy JP, Peterson P, Yeaw MA, Bakemeier RF. Patterns of serologic specificity of human gamma-G erythrocyte autoantibodies. *J Immunol.* 1970;105:677.

251. Bell CA, Zwicker H. Further studies on the relationship of anti-En^a and anti-Wr^b in warm antibody hemolytic anemia. *Transfusion.* 1978;18:572.

252. Celano MJ, Levine P. Anti-LW specificity in autoimmune acquired hemolytic anemia. *Transfusion.* 1967;7:265.

253. Marsh WL, Reid ME, Scott EP. Autoantibodies of U blood group specificity in autoimmune haemolytic anaemia. *Br J Haematol.* 1972;22:625.

254. Shulman IA, Vengelen-Tyler V, Thompson JC, et al. Autoanti-Ge associated with severe autoimmune hemolytic anemia. *Vox Sang.* 1990;59:232.

255. Owen I, Chowdhury V, Reid ME, et al. Autoimmune hemolytic anemia associated with anti-Sc 1. *Transfusion.* 1992;32:173.

256. Marsh WL, Oyen R, Alicea E, et al. Autoimmune hemolytic anemia and the Kell blood groups. *Am J Hematol.* 1979;7:155.

257. Barker RN, Casswell KM, Reid ME, et al. Identification of autoantigens in autoimmune haemolytic anaemia by a non-radioisotope immunoprecipitation method. *Br J Haematol.* 1992;82:126.

258. Victoria EJ, Pierce SW, Branks MJ, Masouredis SP. IgG red blood cell autoantibodies in autoimmune hemolytic anemia bind to epitopes on red blood cell membrane band 3 glycoprotein. *J Lab Clin Med.* 1990;115:74.

259. Telen MJ, Chasis JA. Relationship of the human erythrocyte Wr^b antigen to an interaction between glycophorin A and band 3. *Blood.* 1990;76:842.

260. Barker RN, De la Sa Oliveira GG, et al. Pathogenic autoantibodies in the NZB mouse are specific for erythrocyte band 3 protein. *Eur J Immunol.* 1993;23:1723.

261. Kay MMB, Marchalonis JJ, Hughes J, et al. Definition of a physiologic aging autoantigen by using synthetic peptides of membrane protein band 3: localization of the active antigenic sites. *Proc Natl Acad Sci U S A.* 1990;87:5734.

262. Turrini F, Mannu F, Arese P, et al. Characterization of autologous antibodies that opsonize erythrocytes with clustered integral membrane proteins. *Blood.* 1993;181:3146.

263. Curtis BR, Lamon J, Roelcke D, Chaplin H. Life-threatening, antiglobulin test-negative, acute autoimmune hemolytic anemia due to a non-complement-activating IgG1 kappa cold antibody with Pr$_a$ specificity. *Transfusion.* 1990;30:838.

264. Silberstein LE, Berkman EM, Schreiber AD. Cold hemagglutinin disease associated with IgG cold reactive antibody. *Ann Intern Med.* 1987;106:238.

265. Feizi T, Kabat EA, Vicari G, et al. Immunochemical studies on blood groups. XLVII. The I antigen complex precursors in the A, B, H, Le^a, and Le^b blood group system: hemagglutination inhibition studies. *J Exp Med.* 1971;133:39.

266. Hakomori S. Blood group ABH and Ii antigens of human erythrocytes: chemistry, polymorphism, and their developmental change. *Semin Hematol.* 1981;18:39.

267. Marcus DM. A review of the immunogenic and immunomodulatory properties of glycosphingolipids. *Mol Immunol.* 1984;21:1083.

268. Rosse WF, Lauf PK. Reaction of cold agglutinins with I antigen solubilized from human red cells. *Blood.* 1970;36:777.

269. Lauf PK, Rosse WF. The reactivity of red blood cell membrane glycophorin with "cold-reacting" antibodies. *Clin Immunol Immunopathol.* 1975;4:1.

270. Pruzanski W, Shumak KH. Biologic activity of cold-reacting autoantibodies. *N Engl J Med.* 1977;297:583.

271. Chapman J, Murphy MF, Waters AH. Chronic cold hemagglutinin disease due to an anti-M-like autoantibody. *Vox Sang.* 1982;42:272.

272. von dem Borne AEG, Mol JJ, Joustra-Maas N, et al. Autoimmune hemolytic anemia with monoclonal IgM (kappa) anti-P cold autohemolysins. *Br J Haematol.* 1982;50:345.

273. Terada K, Tanaka H, Mori R, et al. Hemolytic anemia associated with cold agglutinin during chickenpox and a review of the literature. *J Pediatr Hematol Oncol.* 1998;20:149.

274. Tamura T, Kanamori H, Yamazaki E, et al. Cold agglutinin disease following allogeneic bone marrow transplantation. *Bone Marrow Transplant.* 1994;13:321.

275. Capra JD, Dowling P, Cook S, Kunkel HG. An incomplete cold-reactive gamma G antibody with i specificity in infectious mononucleosis. *Vox Sang.* 1969;16:10.

276. Shirey RS, Park K, Ness PM, et al. An anti-i biphasic hemolysin in chronic paroxysmal cold hemoglobinuria. *Transfusion.* 1986;26:62.

277. Salama A, Santoso S, Mueller-Eckhardt C. Antigenic determinants responsible for the reactions of drug-dependent antibodies with blood cells. *Br J Haematol.* 1981;78:535.

278. Gehrie EA, Nian H, Young PP. Brown recluse spider bite mediated hemolysis: clinical features, a possible role for complement inhibitor therapy and reduced RBC surface glycophorin A as a potential biomarker of venom exposure. *PLoS One.* 2013;8:e76558.

279. McDade J, Aygun B, Ware RE. Brown recluse spider (*Loxosceles reclusa*) envenomation leading to acute hemolytic anemia in six adolescents. *J Pediatr.* 2010;156:155.

280. Barcellini W, Fattizzo B, Zaninoni A. Management of refractory autoimmune hemolytic anemia after allogeneic hematopoietic stem cell transplantation: current perspectives. *J Blood Med.* 2019;10:265-278.

281. Ramsey G, Nusbacher J, Starzl TE, Lindsay GD. Isohemagglutinins of graft origin after ABO-unmatched liver transplantation. *N Engl J Med.* 1984;311:1167.

282. Mangal AK, Growe GH, Sinclair M, et al. Acquired hemolytic anemia due to "auto"-anti-A or "auto"-anti-B induced by group O homograft in renal transplant recipients. *Transfusion.* 1984;24:201.

283. Hazlehurst GR, Brenner MK, Wimperis JZ, et al. Haemolysis after T-cell depleted bone marrow transplantation involving minor ABO incompatibility. *Scand J Haematol.* 1986;37:1.

284. Solheim BG, Albrechtsen D, Egeland T, et al. Auto-antibodies against erythrocytes in transplant patients produced by donor lymphocytes. *Transplant Proc.* 1987;6:4520.

285. Sniecinski IJ, Oien L, Petz LD, Blume KG. Immunohematologic consequences of major ABO-mismatched bone marrow transplantation. *Transplantation.* 1988;45:530.

286. Jager U, Barcellini W, Broome CM, et al. *Blood Reviews* 2020;41 doi: 10.1016/j.blre.2019.100648. Epub 2019 Dec 5.

287. Petz LD: "Least incompatible" units for transfusion in autoimmune hemolytic anemia: should we eliminate this meaningless term? A commentary for clinicians and transfusion medicine professionals. *Transfusion.* 2003;42:1503.

288. Ness PM. How do I encourage clinicians to transfuse mismatched blood to patients with autoimmune hemolytic anemia in urgent situations? *Transfusion.* 2006;46:1859.

289. Wallhermfechtel MA, Pohl BA, Chaplin H. Alloimmunization in patients with warm autoantibodies: a retrospective study employing three donor alloabsorptions to aid in antibody detection. *Transfusion.* 1984;24:48284.

290. Branch DR, Petz LD. Detecting alloantibodies in patients with autoantibodies. *Transfusion.* 1999;39:6.

291. Shirey RS, Boyd JS, Parwani AV, et al. Prophylactic antigen matched donor blood for patients with warm autoantibodies: an algorithm for transfusion management. *Transfusion.* 2002;42:1435.

292. Garratty G, Petz LD. Approaches to selecting blood for transfusion to patients with autoimmune hemolytic anemia. *Transfusion.* 2002;42:1390.

293. Dameshek W, Rosenthal MC, Schwartz SO. The treatment of acquired hemolytic anemia with adrenocorticotrophic hormone (ACTH). *N Engl J Med.* 1951;244:117.

294. Allgood JW, Chaplin H Jr. Idiopathic acquired autoimmune hemolytic anemia: a review of forty-seven cases treated from 1955 to 1965. *Am J Med.* 1967;43:254.

295. Meyer O, Stahl D, Beckhove P, et al. Pulsed high-dose dexamethasone in chronic autoimmune haemolytic anaemia of warm type. *Br J Haematol.* 1997;98:860.

296. Greendyke RM, Bradley EB, Swisher SN. Studies of the effects of administration of ACTH and adrenal corticosteroids on erythrophagocytosis. *J Clin Invest.* 1965;44:746.

297. Fries LF, Brickman CM, Frank MM. Monocyte receptors for the Fc portion of IgG increase in number in autoimmune hemolytic anemia and other hemolytic states and are decreased by glucocorticoid therapy. *J Immunol.* 1983;131:1240.

298. Taylor RP, Lindorfer MA. Drug insight: the mechanism of action of rituximab in autoimmune disease—the immune complex decoy hypothesis. *Nat Clin Pract Rheumatol.* 2007;3:86.

299. Garvey B. Rituximab in the treatment of autoimmune haematological disorders. *Br J Haematol.* 2008;141:149.

300. Zecca M, Nobili B, Ramenghi U, et al. Rituximab for the treatment of refractory autoimmune hemolytic anemia in children. *Blood.* 2003;101:3857.

301. Bussone G, Ribeiro E, Dechartres A, et al. Efficacy and safety of rituximab in adults' warm antibody autoimmune hemolytic anemia: retrospective analysis of 27 cases. *Am J Hematol.* 2009;84:153.

302. Barcellini W, Zaja F, Zaninoni A, et al. Low-dose rituximab in adult patients with idiopathic autoimmune hemolytic anemia: clinical efficacy and biologic studies. *Blood.* 2012;119:3691.

303. Barcellini W, Zaja F, Zaninoni A, et al. Sustained response to low-dose rituximab in idiopathic autoimmune hemolytic anemia. *Eur J Haematol.* 2013;91:546.

304. Birgens H, Frederiksen H, Hasselbalch H, et al. A phase III randomized trial comparing glucocorticoid monotherapy versus glucocorticoid and rituximab in patients with autoimmune hemolytic anaemia. *Br J Haematol.* 2013;163:393.

305. Barcellini W, Fattizzo B, Zanioni A. Current and emerging treatment options for autoimmune hemolytic anemia. *Exp Rev Clin Immunol.* 2018;14:857-872.

306. Habibi B, Homberg JC, Schaison G, Salmon C. Autoimmune hemolytic anemia in children: a review of 80 cases. *Am J Med.* 1974;56:61.

307. Christensen BE. The pattern of erythrocyte sequestration in immunohaemolysis: effects of prednisone treatment and splenectomy. *Scand J Haematol.* 1973;10:120.

308. Parker AC, MacPherson AIS, Richmond J. Value of radiochromium investigation in autoimmune haemolytic anaemia. *Br Med J.* 1977;1:208.

309. Schwartz SI, Bernard RP, Adams JT, Bauman AW. Splenectomy for hematologic disorders. *Arch Surg.* 1970;101:338.

310. Akpek G, McAneny DD, Weintraub L. Comparative response to splenectomy in coombs-positive autoimmune hemolytic anemia without associated disease. *Am J Hematol.* 1999;61:98-102.

311. Centers for Disease Control and Prevention. General Best Practice Guidelines for Immunization. Accessed May 17, 2020. https://www.cdc.gov/vaccines/hcp/acip-recs/general-recs/index.html

312. Karlsson C, Hansson L, Celsing F, Lundin J. Treatment of severe refractory autoimmune hemolytic anemia in B-cell chronic lymphocytic leukemia with alemtuzumab (humanized CD52 monoclonal antibody). *Leukemia.* 2007;21:511.

313. Moyo VM, Smith D, Brodsky I, et al. High-dose cyclophosphamide for refractory autoimmune hemolytic anemia. *Blood.* 2002;100:704.

314. Shumak KH, Rock GA. Therapeutic plasma exchange. *N Engl J Med.* 1984;310:762.

315. Council Report. Current status of therapeutic plasmapheresis and related techniques. *JAMA.* 1985;253:819.

316. Cooling L, Boxer G, Simon R. Life-threatening autoimmune hemolytic anemia treated with manual whole blood exchange with rapid clinical improvement. *J Blood Disord Transfus.* 2013;4:163.

317. Wouters A, Stephan F, Strengers P, et al. C1-esterase inhibitor concentrate rescues erythrocytes from complement-mediated destruction in autoimmune hemolytic anemia. *Blood.* 2014;121:1242.

318. Chao MP, Hong J, Kunder C, et al. Refractory warm IgM-mediated autoimmune hemolytic anemia associated with Churg-Strauss syndrome responsive to eculizumab and rituximab. *Am J Hematol.* 2015;90:78.

319. Oda H, Honda A, Sugita K, et al. High-dose intravenous intact IgG infusion in refractory autoimmune hemolytic anemia (Evans syndrome). *J Pediatr.* 1985;107:744.

320. Bussel JB, Cunningham-Rundles C, Abraham C. Intravenous treatment of autoimmune hemolytic anemia with very high dose gammaglobulin. *Vox Sang.* 1986;41:264.

321. Besa EC. Rapid transient reversal of anemia and long-term effects of maintenance intravenous immunoglobulin for autoimmune hemolytic anemia in patients with lymphoproliferative disorders. *Am J Med.* 1988;84:691.

322. Flores G, Cunningham-Rundles C, Newland AC, Bussel JB. Efficacy of intravenous immunoglobulin in the treatment of autoimmune hemolytic anemia: results in 73 patients. *Am J Hematol.* 1993;44:237.

323. Ahn YS, Harrington WJ, Mylvaganam R, et al. Danazol therapy for autoimmune hemolytic anemia. *Ann Intern Med.* 1985;102:298.

324. Pignon J-M, Poirson E, Rochant H. Danazol in autoimmune haemolytic anaemia. *Br J Haematol.* 1993;83:343.

325. Salama A, Hartnack D, Lindemann H, et al. The effect of erythropoiesis-stimulating agents in patient with therapy-refractory autoimmune hemolytic anemia. *Transfus Med Hemother.* 2014;41:462-468.

326. Giannadaki E, Potamianos S, Roussomoustakaki M, et al. Autoimmune hemolytic anemia and positive Coombs' test associated with ulcerative colitis. *Am J Gastroenterol.* 1997;92:1872.

327. Cobo F, Pereira A, Nomdedeu B, et al. Ovarian dermoid cyst-associated autoimmune hemolytic anemia. *Am J Clin Pathol.* 1996;105:567.

328. Berentsen S, Ulvestad E, Gjertsen BT, et al. Rituximab for primary cold agglutinin disease: a prospective study of 37 courses of therapy in 27 patients. *Blood.* 2004;103:2925.

329. Schollkopf, C, Kjeldsen L, Bjerrum OW, et al. Rituximab in chronic cold agglutinin disease: a prospective study of 20 patients. *Leuk Lymphoma.* 2006;47:253.

330. Berentsen S, Randen U, Vagan AM, et al. High response rate and durable remissions following fludarabine and rituximab combination therapy for chronic cold agglutinin disease. *Blood.* 2010;116:3180.

331. Berentsen S, Rayden U, Oksman M, et al. Bendamustine plus rituximab for chronic cold agglutinin disease: results of a Nordic prospective multicenter trial. *Blood.* 2017;130:130.

332. Rossi G, Gramegna D, Paoloni F, et al. Short course of bortezomib in anemic patients with relapsed cold agglutinin disease: a phase 2 prospective GIMEMA study. *Blood.* 2018;132(5):547-550.

333. Roth A, Bommer M, Huttmann A, Herich-Terhurne D. Eculizumab in cold agglutinin disease (DECADE): an open-label, prospective, bicentric, nonrandomized phase 2 trial. *Blood Adv.* 2018;2(19):2543-2549.

334. Jager U, D'Sa S, Schorgenhofer C, Barko J. Inhibition of complement C1s improves severe hemolytic anemia in cold agglutinin disease: a first-in-human trial. *Blood.* 2019;133:893-901.

335. Berentsen S. Cold agglutinins: fending off the attack. *Blood.* 2019;133(9):885-886.

336. Taft EG, Propp RP, Sullivan SA. Plasma exchange for cold agglutinin hemolytic anemia. *Transfusion.* 1977;17:173.

337. Brooks BD, Steane EA, Sheehan RG, Frenkel EP. Therapeutic plasma exchange in the immune hemolytic anemias and immunologic thrombocytopenic purpura. *Prog Clin Biol Res.* 1982;106:317.

338. Silberstein LE, Berkman EM. Plasma exchange in autoimmune hemolytic anemia (AIHA). *J Clin Apher.* 1983;1:238.

339. Zulian GB, Roux E, Tiercy J-M, et al. Transfusion-associated graft-versus-host disease in a patient treated with cladribine (2-chlorodeoxyadenosine): demonstration of exogenous DNA in various tissue extracts by PCR analysis. *Br J Haematol.* 1995;89:83.

340. Briz M, Cabrera R, Sanjuan I. Diagnosis of transfusion-associated graft-versus-host disease by polymerase chain reaction fludarabine-treated B-chronic lymphocytic leukaemia. *Br J Haematol.* 1995;91:409.

341. Silverstein MN, Gomes MR, Elveback LR, et al. Idiopathic acquired hemolytic anemia: survival in 117 cases. *Arch Intern Med.* 1972;129:85.

342. Dausset J, Colombani J. The serology and the prognosis of 128 cases of autoimmune hemolytic anemia. *Blood.* 1959;14:1280.

343. Pullarkat V, Ngo M, Iqbal S, et al. Detection of lupus anticoagulant identifies patients with autoimmune haemolytic anaemia at increased risk of venous thromboembolism. *Br J Haematol.* 2002;118:1166.

344. Hendrick AM. Auto-immune haemolytic anaemia—a high-risk disorder for thromboembolism? *Hematology.* 2003;8:53.

345. Lecouffe-Desprets M, Neel A, Graveleau J, et al. Venous thromboembolism related to warm autoimmune hemolytic anemia: a case-control study. *Autoimmun Rev.* 2015;14:1023-1028.

346. Ho G, Brunson A, Keegan THM, Wun T. Splenectomy and the incidence of venous thromboembolism and sepsis in patients with autoimmune hemolytic anemia. *Blood Cells, Molecules and Diseases.* 2020. https://doi.org/10.1016/j.bcmd.2019.102388.

347. Giannotta JA, Fatizzo B, Cavallaro F, Barcellini W. Infectious complications in autoimmune hemolytic anemia. *J Clin Med.* 2021;10:164.

348. Buchanan GR, Boxer LA, Nathan DG. The acute and transient nature of idiopathic immune hemolytic anemia in childhood. *J Pediatr.* 1976;88:780.

349. Zupanska B, Lawkowicz W, Gorska B, et al. Autoimmune haemolytic anemia in children. *Br J Haematol.* 1976;34:511.

350. Sokol RJ, Hewitt S, Stamps BK, Hitchen PA. Autoimmune haemolysis in childhood and adolescence. *Acta Haematol.* 1984;72:245.

351. Aladjidi N, Leverger G, Leblanc T, et al. New insights into childhood autoimmune hemolytic anemia: a French national observational study of 265 children. *Haematologica.* 2011;96:655.

352. Wang WC. Evans syndrome in childhood: pathophysiology, clinical course, and treatment. *Am J Pediatr Hematol Oncol.* 1988;10:330.

CHAPTER 27
ALLOIMMUNE HEMOLYTIC DISEASE OF THE FETUS AND NEWBORN

Ross M. Fasano, Jeanne E. Hendrickson, and Naomi L.C. Luban

SUMMARY

Alloimmune hemolytic disease of the fetus and newborn (HDFN) is caused by the action of transplacentally transmitted maternal immunoglobulin (Ig) G antibodies on paternally inherited antigens present on fetal red cells but absent on the maternal red cells. Maternal IgG antibodies bind to fetal red cells, causing hemolysis or suppression of erythropoiesis. As a consequence, anemia, extramedullary hematopoiesis, and neonatal hyperbilirubinemia may result, with severe cases resulting in fetal loss or neonatal death or disability. Collaboration among maternal–fetal medicine specialists, hematologists, transfusion medicine physicians, radiologists, and neonatologists has substantially reduced perinatal mortality and morbidity resulting from hemolytic disease of the fetus and newborn. Antenatal diagnostic methods identify at risk fetuses and assess disease severity in affected fetuses. After birth, phototherapy and exchange transfusions prevent serum bilirubin from rising to levels that could produce bilirubin encephalopathy and resultant brain damage (kernicterus), remove maternal antibody, and replace circulating fetal red blood cells with those negative for the implicated antigen(s). Rho(D) immunoglobulin (RhIg) has successfully prevented alloimmune hemolytic disease resulting from rhesus D sensitization in many at risk infants, but there is not enough RhIg available to distribute to all women at risk worldwide, and no prophylactic therapy exists as of this writing to prevent alloimmune hemolytic disease resulting from other red cell antibodies. Advances in immunohematology and molecular biology may offer new avenues for prevention and treatment in the future.

Acronyms and Abbreviations: ΔOD450, change in optical density at 450 nm; AABB, American Association of Blood Banks; AMIGO, Antigen Matching Influence on Gestational Outcomes; AAP, American Academy of Pediatrics; anti-D, antibody against D antigen; CAP, College of American Pathologists; ccff-DNA, circulating cell-free fetal DNA; DAT, direct antiglobulin test; ddPCR, droplet digital polymerase chain reaction; FFP, fresh-frozen plasma; FMH, fetomaternal hemorrhage; HDFN, hemolytic disease of the fetus and newborn; HDN, hemolytic disease of the newborn; HLA, human leukocyte antigen; IAT, indirect antiglobulin test; Ig, immunoglobulin; IUT, intrauterine transfusion; IVIG, intravenous immunoglobulin G; LOTUS, Long-Term follow up after intra-Uterine transfusionS; MALDI-TOF MS, matrix-assisted laser desorption ionization/time of flight mass spectrometry; NEC, necrotizing enterocolitis; QT-PCR, quantitative polymerase chain reaction; RBC, red blood cell; Rh, rhesus; rHuEPO, recombinant human erythropoietin; RhIg, Rho(D) immunoglobulin; RT-PCR, real-time quantitative polymerase chain reaction; SGA, small for gestational age; TBV, total blood volume; TSB, total serum bilirubin; WB, whole blood.

Alloimmune hemolytic disease of the fetus and newborn (HDFN) is a disorder in which the life span of fetal and/or neonatal red cells is shortened as a result of binding of transplacentally transferred maternal immunoglobulin (Ig) G antibodies on fetal red blood cell (RBC) antigens foreign to the mother, inherited by the fetus from the father. The resulting hemolysis or suppression of erythropoiesis may cause fetal and/or neonatal anemia and significant neonatal jaundice. There are three main classes of alloimmune HDFN, based on the antigen(s) involved: Rh (rhesus), minor red cell antigens (ie, Kell, Duffy, Kidd antigens), and ABO.

Before the development of medical interventions in the 1950s, almost half of all newborn infants with Rh HDFN died or were severely disabled. Although the clinical condition was described in newborn infants as early as the 1600s, it was only in the 1930s and 1940s that the pathophysiology of Rh HDFN was uncovered. In 1932, Diamond and colleagues[1] recognized that the clinical syndromes of stillbirth with unusual erythroblastic activity in the extramedullary sites and blood, fetal hydrops, anemia in the newborn, and "icterus gravis neonatorum" were closely related and likely had the same pathophysiology in the hematopoietic system. In 1938, Ruth Darrow, a pathologist who lost a baby to kernicterus, postulated that hemolysis of fetal RBCs was a result of maternal antibody produced in response to fetal hemoglobin.[2] The discovery of the Rh factor by Landsteiner and Weiner led to elucidation of Rh HDFN by Levine and colleagues, who established that erythroblastosis fetalis was caused by immunization of an Rh-negative mother by the red cells from an Rh-positive fetus.[3] Antibodies produced by the sensitized mother crossed the placenta in the next pregnancy and coated the fetal Rh-positive erythrocytes, leading to hemolysis, anemia, hydrops, and severe neonatal jaundice.

Neonatal mortality rates from Rh HDFN decreased considerably with the development of exchange transfusion techniques to correct severe anemia and hyperbilirubinemia.[4] However, severely affected fetuses continued to die in utero before 34 weeks' gestation. In 1961, Liley demonstrated the prognostic value of amniotic fluid spectrophotometry in identifying fetuses at risk for HDFN and subsequently demonstrated that intrauterine transfusions (IUTs) were feasible and effective.[5] The most dramatic reduction in the incidence of Rh HDFN was achieved in the 1960s and 1970s with the development of postpartum and antepartum anti-D prophylaxis to prevent maternal Rh sensitization.[6]

Despite these advances, Rh HDFN has not disappeared, and cases of hemolytic disease of the newborn (HDN) resulting from red cell antibodies directed toward antigens other than the Rh blood group system are being increasingly recognized.[7-11] Furthermore, maternal Rh isoimmunization and Rh hemolytic disease still occur, particularly in developing countries where anti-RhD prophylaxis is not widely available or in infants born outside of medical facilities.[12]

⬤ EPIDEMIOLOGY

The epidemiology of HDFN varies in different ethnic and racial groups; the frequency of specific blood group alleles in a given population determines the probability of blood group incompatibility and maternal alloimmunization. Antigen-negative women may have naturally occurring antibodies to certain red cell antigens (anti-A or anti-B) or may develop antibodies as a result of exposure to foreign red cell antigens through blood transfusion or silent fetomaternal hemorrhage (FMH) during pregnancy or delivery. More than 50 different RBC antigens have been associated with maternal alloimmunization[7-11,13] and with HDFN of varying severity; however, the vast majority of clinically significant maternal alloantibodies are within the Rh (D, CE), Kell, Duffy, MNS, and Kidd systems (Table 27-1).

TABLE 27-1. Blood Group Systems Associated with Hemolytic Disease of the Fetus and Newborn

Blood Group System	Antigens
Rhesus	D, C, E, Ce, f, C^w, C^x, E^w, G, Rh29, Rh32 (R^N), Rh42, Go^a, Hr$_o$, Be^a, Evans, Tar, Sec, JAL, STEM
Kell	K, k, K$_o$, Kp^a, Kp^b, Js^a, Js^b (and others)
Duffy	Fy^a, Fy^b, Fy3
Kidd	Jk^a, Jk^b, Jk3
MNS	M, N, S, s, U, Mi^a, Mt^a, Vx, Mur, Hil, Hut, En^a, (and others)
Lutheran	Lu^a, Lu^b
Diego	Di^a, Di^b, Wr^a
Others	Co^a, Co^b, Co3, Ge3, JFV, Jones, Kg, Lan, Lsa, MAM, PPIPk, Rd (Sc^4), Vel, (and others)

Data from Moise KJ. Fetal anemia due to non-Rhesus-D red-cell alloimmunization. *Semin Fetal Neonatal Med.* 2008;13(4):207-214 and Eder AF. Update on HDFN: new information on long-standing controversies. *Immunohematology.* 2006;22(4):188-195.

Antenatal screening programs detect antibodies to clinically significant Rh or other minor RBC antigens in 0.01% to 0.4% of pregnant women,[7-11,13] though these numbers vary by country. Approximately 15% of Americans of European descent are RhD negative, compared with 7% of African Americans and Hispanics, 5% of Indians, and 0.3% of Chinese individuals.[14-16] Despite the success of Rh prophylaxis, anti-D antibodies still constitute a large proportion of clinically significant antibodies detected in Europe and the United States. When RhD is excluded, non-D Rh antibodies (c, C, e, E, cc, and Ce) and antibodies belonging to the Kell, Duffy, Kidd, and MNS systems, are most frequently involved.[7,13]

CLINICAL FEATURES OF HEMOLYTIC DISEASE OF THE FETUS AND NEWBORN

OVERVIEW

Anemia, jaundice, and hepatosplenomegaly are the hallmarks of HDN. The clinical spectrum of affected infants is highly variable. In Rh HDN, half of the infants have mild disease and do not require intervention. One-fourth of affected infants are born at term with moderate anemia and develop severe jaundice. In the days before intrauterine intervention, hydrops developed in utero in the remaining one-fourth of infants; half became hydropic before 34 weeks' gestation. Hydrops recurs in 90% of affected pregnancies, often at an earlier gestation. In Kell HDN, the clinical spectrum of hemolytic disease is less predictable, ranging from mild anemia to frank hydrops; jaundice may be less severe than that seen in Rh HDFN given that anti-Kell alloantibodies may induce erythroid suppression. Jaundice is the predominant feature of ABO HDN, but anemia and mild hepatosplenomegaly may also be seen. Severe fetal anemia and hydrops are unusual in ABO hemolytic disease.[17]

HEMOLYTIC ANEMIA

Infants with mild HDN may have cord blood hemoglobin concentrations only slightly lower than the age-related normal range. Hemoglobin values usually continue to fall after birth in all affected infants. Hemolysis continues until all incompatible red cells and circulating maternal alloantibody are eliminated from the circulation. Physical examination in infants having moderate to severe anemia reveals pallor, tachypnea, and tachycardia. In cases of severe HDFN, fetal anemia secondary to hemolysis results in compensatory extramedullary hematopoiesis in the liver, spleen, kidneys, and adrenal glands, as well as an outpouring of immature nucleated RBCs in the fetal circulation caused by increased fetal plasma erythropoietin levels.[18] The marked increase in erythropoiesis may be accompanied by downmodulation of platelet and neutrophil production.[19]

After birth, the quantity of maternal antibodies in the neonatal circulation decreases over the next 12 weeks, with a half-life of approximately 25 days. Infants with moderate to severe hemolytic disease may develop significant anemia beyond the immediate neonatal period lasting up to 8 to 12 weeks of life. Delayed anemia is related to continuing hemolysis because of persistence of maternal antibodies and a hyporegenerative component with decreased red cell production from low serum concentrations of erythropoietin.[20-22]

NEONATAL JAUNDICE

Most infants with HDN are not jaundiced at birth because the placenta effectively transports most of the lipid-soluble unconjugated fetal bilirubin. Bilirubin concentrations in amniotic fluid reflect bilirubin concentrations in fetal blood and are influenced by fetal blood and amniotic fluid albumin concentrations.[23] The mechanism of entry of bilirubin into the amniotic fluid compartment has been debated, but of the five possible pathways (excretion through the fetal kidneys, meconium, skin, fetal lung secretions, and transmembranous), transmembranous appears to be most likely.[24]

At birth, the newborn infant's immature liver is incapable of handling the large bilirubin load that results from the ongoing destruction of antibody-coated neonatal erythrocytes, and jaundice usually develops during the first day of life, often in the first few hours of life in severely affected infants. The jaundice progresses in a cephalopedal direction with rising bilirubin levels. In patients with mild disease, the serum indirect bilirubin peaks by the fourth or fifth day and then declines slowly. Premature infants may have higher levels of serum bilirubin for a longer duration because of lower hepatic glucuronyl transferase activity. Conjugated hyperbilirubinemia at birth is sometimes noted in infants who received multiple IUTs. Babies who received IUTs may still have anemia at birth and may still develop significant hyperbilirubinemia in the neonatal period.[25] As discussed later in this chapter, these infants may require intermittent transfusion therapy until 2 to 3 months of age because of persistent anemia.

KERNICTERUS

An important complication of elevated serum levels of indirect bilirubin in neonates is the development of bilirubin encephalopathy (also termed *kernicterus*), which is caused by bilirubin pigment deposition in the basal ganglia and brain stem nuclei, leading to neuronal necrosis.[26] Acute bilirubin encephalopathy is initially marked by lethargy, poor feeding, and hypotonia. With increasing severity, the infant develops a high-pitched cry, fever, hypertonia progressing to frank opisthotonos, and irregular respiration. The infants then develop any or all of the classic sequelae of kernicterus: choreoathetoid cerebral palsy, gaze abnormalities, especially in upward gaze, sensorineural hearing loss, and cognitive deficits. The clinical presentation of bilirubin encephalopathy in preterm infants may be less distinctive. Abnormal or absent brain stem auditory evoked potentials and magnetic resonance imaging scans demonstrating the characteristic bilateral lesions of the globus pallidus help confirm the clinical diagnosis of kernicterus.

Infants with HDFN are at higher risk for kernicterus than are other infants with the same bilirubin level from other causes.[27] Heme pigments produced during active hemolysis are hypothesized to inhibit bilirubin–albumin binding. Alternatively, many conditions that potentially compromise the blood–brain barrier, such as prematurity, acidosis, hypoxemia, hypothermia, and hypoglycemia, are present in severely affected infants, making them more vulnerable to bilirubin encephalopathy.

OTHER CLINICAL FEATURES

Extensive extramedullary hematopoiesis in the liver and spleen may cause portal and umbilical venous hypertension, leading to ascites, pleural effusions, and consequent pulmonary hypoplasia.[28] Trophoblastic hypertrophy and placental edema cause impaired placental function. Hypoproteinemia as a result of liver dysfunction leads to generalized edema. "Hydrops fetalis," a state of anasarca, is the end result of a combination of anemia, hypoproteinemia, cardiac failure, elevated venous pressures, increased capillary permeability, and impaired lymphatic clearance. Hepatosplenomegaly is usually present. Cholestatic liver disease, previously believed to be associated with iron overload caused by IUTs, has been shown to occur in 13% of neonates with HDFN independent of previous IUT treatment and type of alloimmunization.[29] Hydropic babies may also have respiratory distress as a result of pulmonary hypoplasia, pleural or pericardial effusions, or surfactant deficiency.

Although the pathophysiology is not entirely clear, purpura associated with thrombocytopenia is sometimes seen in infants with HDFN. Thrombocytopenia at birth has been shown to occur in 26% of neonates with HDFN independent of other comorbidities such as lower gestational age at birth, small for gestational age, and previous IUTs.[30] Severe fetal thrombocytopenia (defined as a platelet count $<50 \times 10^9$/L) has been reported in 3% of all fetal blood samplings and in 23% of severely RhD alloimmunized hydropic fetuses when fetal platelet counts were measured before IUT.[31] In addition, neutropenia is a common feature of HDN and may be prolonged up to 1 year of life, regardless of severity of HDFN, treatment received, or antibody specificity.[32]

OBSTETRIC HISTORY

The course and outcome of prior pregnancies are critically important in the initial evaluation of an alloimmunized pregnancy. A history of early fetal deaths or hydrops is ominous. In Rh alloimmunization, the severity of HDFN typically remains the same or worsens in subsequent affected pregnancies. Hydrops recurs in 90% of affected pregnancies, often at an earlier gestation in subsequent pregnancies. Alloimmunized women who report previous neonatal deaths, neonatal exchange transfusions, or IUTs should receive very close fetal surveillance.[33] Jaundice as a result of hemolysis often recurs to the same degree of severity in subsequent affected siblings. The history of prior blood transfusions may be obtained in women sensitized to antigens other than RhD, especially if Kell alloimmunization is detected. Establishment of paternity for each pregnancy is particularly relevant in both Rh and Kell alloimmunization because the fetus is at risk only if the father is positive for the antigen in question. Unlike Rh and other minor alloantibody HDFN, ABO HDN may affect the first-born ABO-incompatible infant. Although rare, severe ABO HDN may recur in subsequent ABO-incompatible pregnancies.[34]

DIFFERENTIAL DIAGNOSIS

Hydrops fetalis may result from immune (due to alloimmune HDFN) or nonimmune causes. Nonimmune causes account for approximately 85% of all affected individuals, and most commonly result from cardiac (20%), hematologic (10%), chromosomal (9%), thoracic (2%), gastrointestinal (1%), or urinary tract (1%) anomalies; lymphatic dysplasia (15%); intrauterine infections (7%); twin-to-twin transfusion syndrome (4%); and inborn errors of metabolism (1%) disorders. Other rarer congenital, placental, and idiopathic causes can also result in hydrops fetalis.[35]

Neonatal anemia caused by intrinsic red cell defects such as hereditary spherocytosis (Chap. 15), red cell enzyme deficiencies (Chap. 16), and hemoglobinopathies, notably α-thalassemia (Chap. 17), can give a similar clinical picture to HDN. The absence of maternal red cell alloantibodies, a negative direct antiglobulin test (DAT) result, and detection of the specific defect determining the disorder clarify the diagnosis. Maternal parvovirus B19 infection at any time during gestation can cause nonimmune hydrops, profound fetal anemia, and death.[36] Disorders of bilirubin metabolism can lead to unconjugated hyperbilirubinemia; however, they are not associated with anemia. Hepatitis or obstructive biliary diseases present with direct hyperbilirubinemia, most often after the first week of life.

● PATHOPHYSIOLOGY

There are three main classes of alloimmune HDFN, based on the antigen(s) involved: (1) Rh (rhesus), (2) minor red cell antigens (ie, Kell, Duffy, Kidd antigens), and (3) ABO. Factors affecting the risk to the fetus or neonate not only include the class of antigens involved but also the titer (ie, 4 vs 32) and class or subclass (ie, IgM vs IgG4 vs IgG1) of the antibody, the level of antigen expression on fetal RBCs, and the antibody's ability to suppress erythropoiesis (ie, anti-K).[37,38] Rh HDFN is discussed first because it is archetypal of this condition; however, ABO incompatibility is much more common than Rh HDFN. The distinguishing features of the three classes of HDFN are highlighted later.

RhD HEMOLYTIC DISEASE

The standard nomenclature for designation of one's blood type is ABO and Rh positive or Rh negative based on the presence or absence of the RhD antigen. However, the Rh blood system consists of numerous other antigens; the most common clinically significant include C, c, E, e, which are encoded on the paired *RHCE* gene. RhD-positive individuals may have one or two copies of *RHD* gene (heterozygous or homozygous RhD positive, respectively). More than 150 alleles have been defined for *RHD* and more are likely to be revealed as population studies expand.[39] In whites, RhD-negative individuals are most often homozygous for deletion of the *RHD* gene, which encompasses the whole of *RHD* and part of each of the flanking rhesus boxes. The resultant RhD-negative phenotype is characterized by the absence of the whole RhD protein from the red cell membrane; however, the *RHCE*-encoded antigens are present. Only 18% of RhD-negative black Africans are homozygous for *RHD* deletion. Whereas the majority (66%) of RhD-negative black Africans has an inactive *RHD* gene (RHψ), 15% have a hybrid *RHD-CE-D* gene, neither of which produces epitopes of RhD antigen.

A number of *RHD* alleles responsible for RhD protein variants with altered RhD antigen expression have been classified according to their phenotype and molecular variation as partial D, weak D, and DEL. Amino acid substitutions located in extracellular domains result in different forms of partial D phenotype. Women with partial D phenotypes may develop antibodies against D epitopes absent on their RBC membranes but present on the fetal RBCs. Amino acid substitutions located in the transmembrane or intracellular segments of the RhD protein most often result in a weak D phenotype. The expressed RhD antigen is most often reduced quantitatively but not qualitatively, so carriers are usually not susceptible to anti-D immunization. However, some types of weak D (eg, weak D type 15, weak D type 4.2 or DAR, and weak D type 7) may produce anti-D. DEL phenotypes can exhibit quantitative reductions and sometimes qualitative variation in D antigen expression. Therefore, some DEL phenotypes can result in anti-D alloimmunization upon exposure to RhD antigen through transfusion or pregnancy. The DEL phenotype is found in approximately 30% of RhD-"negative" individuals in East Asia and has been implicated in RhD HDFN.[39-42]

The current recommendation in the United States, based on a 2015 "Joint Statement on Phasing-in RHD Genotyping for Pregnant Women and Other Females of Childbearing Potential With a Serologic Weak D Phenotype" issued by the American Association of Blood Banks (AABB), America's Blood Centers, the American Red Cross, the American College of Obstetricians and Gynecologists, College of American Pathologists (CAP), and the Armed Services Blood Program,[43,44] is to order D genotyping in pregnant women who serologically test as potentially having a weak or partial D antigen. Women whose genotyping returns as being weak D types 1, 2, or 3 can be treated as being RhD positive for transfusion and pregnancy purposes. Women whose genotyping returns with any other weak D or partial D variant should be treated as RhD negative for transfusion and pregnancy purposes. Until genotyping information is obtained, women with potential weak or partial RhD should be treated as being RhD negative and, if indicated, treated with anti-D immune globulin prophylaxis.

RhD-negative pregnant women who appear to have both anti-D and anti-C, especially if at a similar strengths of reactivity serologically, require special consideration. In this instance, if the pregnant woman is lacking both RhD and RhC antigens, she is also lacking the RhG antigen, a combination antigen in the Rh Blood Group System found on RBCs containing either RhD or RhC antigens. In these situations, the laboratory must determine whether the antibodies are truly anti-D/anti-C rather than an anti-G because a patient who develops anti-C and/or anti-G antibodies but not anti-D should receive anti-D immune globulin prophylaxis.[45]

Fetomaternal Hemorrhage and Anti-D Alloimmunization

Asymptomatic transplacental passage of fetal red cells occurs in 75% of pregnant women at some time during pregnancy or during labor and delivery.[46] The incidence of FMH increases with advancing gestation: from 3% (first trimester), to 12% (second trimester), to 45% (third trimester), and 64% at delivery. The average volume of fetal blood in the maternal circulation after delivery is approximately 0.1 mL in most women and less than 1 mL in 96 % of women.[47] Intrapartum FMH of more than 30 mL may occur in up to 1% of deliveries.[48] Massive FMH may present with decreased fetal movement and sinusoidal heart rhythm (undulating wave form alternating with a flat or smooth baseline fetal heart rate); however, it also may be clinically silent, with no clinical signs differentiating such deliveries from those with minimal FMH.[48,49] FMH can also result from obstetric procedures, such as chorionic villus sampling, amniocentesis, therapeutic abortion, external cephalic version, cesarean section, and manual removal of the placenta, and from pathologic conditions such as abdominal trauma, spontaneous abortion, or ectopic pregnancy.[47,50-52]

The presence of RhD-positive red cells in an RhD-negative mother initially provokes a weak and slow primary immune response, which develops over 4 weeks and consists of transient elevation of IgM antibodies. Subsequently, approximately 5 to 15 weeks after exposure to the RhD-positive red cells, anti-D IgG antibodies capable of crossing the placenta are produced. The RhD antigen is the most immunogenic of the Rh antigens and, indeed, of all red cell antigens (after ABO).[53] The RhD protein is processed by antigen-processing cells in the spleen and lymphoid tissue of RhD-negative individuals into multiple short allogeneic linear peptides, which stimulate helper T cells, which then activate B cells to produce IgM and later IgG antibodies. Memory T and B cells that are generated after the initial immune response are long lived, and exposure to the antigen even years later results in an accelerated antibody response as a result of rapid proliferation of antigen-specific clones. Repeated exposure to RhD-positive fetal RBCs, as in a second RhD-positive pregnancy in a sensitized RhD-negative woman, produces a brisk secondary immune response marked by rapid production of large amounts of anti-D IgG antibody by maternal memory B lymphocytes.

In the absence of Rho(D) immunoglobulin (RhIg) prophylaxis, sensitization occurs in 7% to 16% of women at risk, within 6 months after delivery of the first RhD-positive ABO-compatible fetus. The relatively low rate of primary alloimmunization in RhD-negative women at risk may be a result of the low volume of FMH in most women. In fact, as little as 0.03 mL of RhD-positive RBCs has been shown to be sufficient to immunize some RhD-negative individuals.[54]

The potential for immunization of the mother is not only determined by the extent of FMH and the presence of fetomaternal blood group incompatibility but also by other factors such as the frequency of FMH and whether the mother and fetus are ABO compatible. As an example, repetitive exposure to minuscule amounts of RhD-positive red cells in RhD-negative women who abuse IV drugs and share needles with RhD-positive partners has been reported to lead to severe Rh sensitization.[55] Fetomaternal ABO incompatibility offers some protection against primary Rh immunization because incompatible fetal RBCs are destroyed rapidly by maternal anti-A and anti-B antibodies, reducing maternal exposure to RhD antigenic sites. Consequently, primary Rh immunization occurs in 2% to 4% of women at risk after delivery of an ABO-incompatible fetus (compared with the 7%-16% risk after delivery of an ABO-compatible fetus).[56] ABO incompatibility confers no protection against the secondary immune response after sensitization has occurred.[57]

Binding of transplacentally transferred maternal anti-D IgG antibodies to RhD-antigen sites on the fetal RBC membrane is followed by adherence of the coated erythrocytes to the Fcγ receptors of macrophages with rosette formation, leading to extravascular non–complement-mediated phagocytosis and lysis, predominantly in the spleen.[56] Although Rh antigens are found on fetal RBCs as early as week 6 of gestation,[41] active transport of IgG across the placenta is slow until 20 to 24 weeks of gestation. The severity of fetal anemia is influenced primarily by the anti-D IgG concentration but also by other factors, including the IgG subclass, the rate of transplacental transfer of maternal IgG, the functional maturity of the fetal mononuclear phagocyte system, and the presence of maternal human leukocyte antigen (HLA) antibodies and or maternal–fetal ABO incompatibility.[58] Although IgG anti-D consists mainly of IgG_1 and IgG_3 subclasses, the relative contribution of each of these subclasses to the severity of HDFN remains controversial.[56,59,60]

HEMOLYTIC DISEASE CAUSED BY OTHER RED CELL ANTIBODIES

Although antibodies against RhD tend to be the most clinically significant in terms of fetal outcomes, many other RBC antigens are capable of inducing alloantibodies after exposure through transfusion or pregnancy. Any alloantibody capable of inducing hemolysis or suppressing erythropoiesis may be clinically significant to developing fetuses. However, the mere presence of antibodies on screening tests may not be clinically significant because of the unique characteristics of some antibodies. For example, antibodies to Lewis antigens (Le[a], Le[b]) are IgM and do not cross the placenta. Alternatively, Lutheran (Lu[a], Lu[b]) and Chido antigens are poorly expressed on fetal and neonatal red cells and therefore are not susceptible to destruction by maternal antibodies.

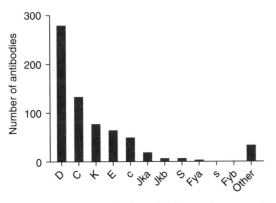

FIGURE 27–1. Red blood cell alloantibody specificities in 425 pregnancies affected by hemolytic disease of the fetus and newborn in the Blood Group Antigen Matching Influence on Gestational Outcomes (AMIGO) study. *(Data from Delaney M, Wikman A, van de Watering L, et al. Blood Group Antigen Matching Influence on Gestational Outcomes [AMIGO] study. Transfusion. 2017 Mar;57[3]:525-532.)*

Case reports may be biased toward more severe cases, and there is considerable variability in the clinical spectrum of disease produced by different alloantibodies. Figure 27-1 shows the antibody specificities associated with 425 pregnancies affected by severe HDFN requiring neonatal exchange transfusion, IUT, or both from the multinational Blood Group Antigen Matching Influence on Gestational Outcomes (AMIGO) study.[13,61,62]

Kell

The Kell blood group system consists of at least 28 discrete antigens, of which 8 are associated with HDFN. The *KEL* gene is located on chromosome 7q34, and Kell antigens are located on the red cell membrane glycoprotein CD238. Kell is unique in that it spans the RBC membrane once; it has a short N terminal domain of 47 amino acids in the cytosol and a large C terminal domain (665 amino acids) outside the membrane. The most common of the K antigens, Kell (also known as KEL1), is expressed by erythroid progenitor cells and mature erythroid cells by 9% of people of European ancestry and 1% to 2% of people of African ancestry; most KEL1-positive individuals are heterozygous. Alloimmunization to KEL1 can occur through transfusion or through pregnancy.[63,64]

Given the relatively low prevalence of the KEL1 antigen, the likelihood of KEL1 incompatibility between mother and child is less than that of RhD. However, any KEL1-positive fetus being carried by a woman alloimmunized to the KEL1 antigen is at risk of anemia. Between 2.5% and 10% of alloimmunized pregnancies result in an affected infant, with fetal hydrops and severe anemia being common presentations of Kell HDFN.[64-66] In contrast to the hemolysis observed in RhD HDFN, the severe fetal anemia observed because of maternal anti-Kell alloantibodies is caused in large part by suppression of erythropoiesis rather than brisk hemolysis. Clinical observations of inappropriately low levels of circulating reticulocytes and normoblasts for the degree of anemia have long been noted in affected fetuses, and suppression of erythropoiesis has been established by in vitro studies showing that growth of Kell-positive erythroid progenitor cells is inhibited by monoclonal IgG and IgM anti-Kell antibodies.[67] Furthermore, anti-Kell antibodies have been associated with suppression of megakaryocyte and granulocyte colony-forming units with resultant fetal and neonatal thrombocytopenia and pancytopenia.[68,69] As discussed in further detail later in this chapter, titers of maternal anti-Kell do not necessarily correlate with the severity of fetal anemia, and thus all maternal anti-Kell alloantibodies must be considered to be potentially clinically significant to antigen-positive fetuses.

Other Minor Antigens (Non-D, Non-Kell)

Many other minor RBC antigens besides RhD and Kell are immunogenic in transfusion and pregnancy settings, with some of these alloantibodies having the capacity of being detrimental to developing fetuses. The incidence and prevalence of other minor antigens contributing to HDFN depends in part on the geographical area evaluated because genetics and local transfusion practices impact alloimmunization. Any IgG that can cross the placenta is, in theory, capable of binding to cognate antigens on fetal RBCs. Antigen copy number, as well as other characteristics of the antigens or antibodies (potentially including IgG subtype), may impact the clinical significance of the alloantibodies.

ABO HEMOLYTIC DISEASE

ABO HDN occurs almost exclusively in infants with blood group A or B who are born to group O mothers, given that group O mothers have naturally occurring antibodies against the A and B antigens that are of the IgG class and are thus capable of crossing the placenta. The fetal mononuclear phagocyte system may completely remove RBCs bound with IgG, or it may remove portions of the RBCs, resulting in microspherocytes visible on blood smear. (Table 27-2 compares ABO vs RhD HDN.)

TABLE 27–2. Comparison of Rh and ABO Hemolytic Disease of the Newborn

	Rh	ABO
BLOOD GROUPS		
Mother	Negative	O
Infant	Positive	A or B
Type of antibody	IgG_1 and/or IgG_3	IgG_2
CLINICAL ASPECTS		
Occurrence in first-born child (%)	5	40–50
Predictable severity in subsequent pregnancies	Usually	No
Stillbirth or hydrops	Frequent	Rare
Severe anemia	Frequent	Rare
Degree of jaundice	+++	+ to ++
Hepatosplenomegaly	+++	+
LABORATORY FINDINGS		
Maternal antibodies	Always present	Usually present
Direct antiglobulin test (infant)	+	+ or −
Microspherocytes	−	+
TREATMENT		
Antenatal measures	Yes	No
Exchange transfusion frequency	Approximately two or three	Occasional
Donor blood type	Rh negative, group specific when possible	Group O only
Incidence of late anemia	Common	Rare

Infants with ABO HDN generally have less severe disease than those with Rh incompatibility. Hydrops fetalis caused by ABO alloimmune HDN is extremely rare. Although infants affected by ABO incompatibility may require phototherapy to treat their jaundice, fewer than 0.1% require exchange transfusion.[17,70] Unlike Rh disease, ABO HDN may affect the first-born ABO-incompatible infant because anti-A and anti-B IgG antibodies are normally present in group O adults. Antenatal testing of anti-A and anti-B levels in group O mothers has little value in predicting ABO HDN, though the number of fully developed A or B antigens on fetal RBCs may impact disease severity. A recurrence rate of 88% has been reported in siblings having the same blood type as the affected index baby, with two-thirds of the affected siblings requiring therapy.[34] A higher incidence and greater severity of jaundice caused by ABO incompatibility are reported in Southeast Asians, Hispanics, Arabs, and South African and American blacks than in whites.[17,71,72] This may be caused in part by the extent of development of A or B antigen sites on fetal RBCs, as well as to the prevalence of Gilbert syndrome in different patient populations.[73]

ANTENATAL MONITORING

The evaluation and management of patients with HDFN require close collaboration among obstetricians, maternal–fetal medicine specialists, radiologists, hematologists, transfusion medicine specialists, and neonatologists. Figure 27-2 is an algorithm for the clinical management of an alloimmunized pregnancy.

DETERMINATION OF PATERNAL ZYGOSITY AND FETAL BLOOD TYPE

When a clinically significant alloantibody is identified or if there is a history of a previous fetus or neonate affected by HDFN, the first step is

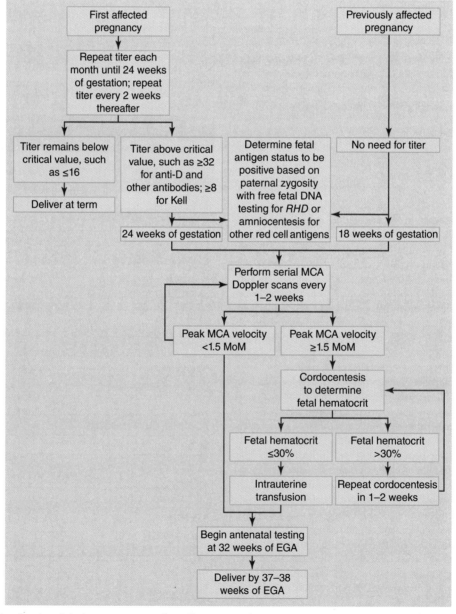

FIGURE 27–2. Algorithm for the clinical management of an alloimmunized pregnancy. EGA, estimated gestational age; MCA, middle cerebral artery; MoMs, multiples of the median. *(Reproduced with permission from Moise KJ Jr, Argoti PS. Management and prevention of red cell alloimmunization in pregnancy: a systematic review. Obstet Gynecol. 2012 Nov;120[5]:1132-1139.)*

to determine if the fetus is at risk by carrying the corresponding antigen on their red cells. If the father is homozygous for the corresponding antigen, the fetus is 100% at risk for HDFN and therefore needs further antenatal monitoring. The child of an antigen-negative mother and a heterozygous antigen-positive father has a 50% chance of being antigen positive and thus being affected by maternal allosensitization. When the father is heterozygous or paternal zygosity is unknown, determination of fetal blood type early in pregnancy allows early institution of monitoring and therapy in antigen-positive fetuses that are at risk while forestalling invasive and potentially risky procedures in antigen-negative fetuses.

Paternal zygosity can be determined using serology for most common blood group antigens implicated in HDFN except for RhD; however, serologic zygosity testing has been largely replaced by blood group genotyping for a variety of reasons. One reason is the fact that *RHD* zygosity in RhD-positive persons may only be inferred from serologic phenotyping studies based on gene frequencies in certain populations and the fact that the C/c and E/e antigens are closely linked to the *RHD* locus.[14,61] Elucidation of the genetic structure of the *RHD* locus and haplotypes responsible for RhD-negative phenotypes has led to the development of more direct and robust methods of determination of *RHD* zygosity molecularly. *RHD* zygosity testing by quantitative fluorescence polymerase chain reaction (also known as real-time PCR) is commercially available and uses *RHD* (exons 5 and 7) to *RHCE* (exon 7) amplification ratios to determine *RHD* copy number. Although suitable for use in both white and ethnic African individuals, this molecular technique has a false-positive rate of 1% because of rare *RHD* alleles that are not expressed and a false-negative rate of 1% because of rare partial D alleles (ie, DBT type 1, type II) that lack *RHD* exons 5 and 7 but still express RhD epitopes.[74,75] Droplet digital PCR (ddPCR) technology has recently been shown to provide highly accurate results to rapidly define paternal *RHD* zygosity in HDFN at-risk pregnancies.[76]

If paternal heterozygosity is suspected or confirmed, determination of fetal blood type is necessary toward planning further management. There are several sources of fetal tissue for fetal blood group genotyping. These include blood obtained by cordocentesis, chorionic villus sampling, and cervical tissue obtained by transvaginal lavage. Each of these fetal DNA sources carry risks to the fetus and have issues related to quality of sample. Cordocentesis, amniocentesis, and chorionic villus sampling for fetal genetic typing carry a risk of FMH with increased risk of augmenting maternal sensitization and of fetal loss.[50,51] The advent of noninvasive methods of prenatal diagnosis using fetal DNA extracted from maternal plasma as early as the first trimester of pregnancy has obviated those concerns and has dramatically improved the ability to perform molecular testing on fetal tissue.[77]

Circulating cell-free fetal DNA (ccff-DNA) in maternal plasma can be identified as early as 5 weeks' gestation and is derived from apoptotic syncytiotrophoblasts. Fetal DNA used for typing is extracted using real-time quantitative polymerase chain reaction (RT-PCR). Most protocols amplify three exons or more, which include *RHD* exons 4–7 and 10, and detect target Psi (ψ) pseudogene sequences in exon 4 to avoid false-positive results when the fetus has *RHDψ*.[78,79] Confirmation of detection of nonmaternal markers is required and can be accomplished by testing for the presence of the Y chromosome (in male fetuses) or housekeeping genes such as hemoglobin β chain, β actin, albumin, or chemokine receptor 5. In a meta-analysis that reviewed 37 publications describing 44 protocols reporting noninvasive *RHD* genotyping using fetal DNA obtained from more than 3000 maternal blood samples, an accuracy rate of 94.8% was reported.[78] A new method combining PCR, base extension reaction, and matrix-assisted laser desorption ionization/time of flight mass spectrometry (MALDI-TOF MS) has been shown to be an effective alternative noninvasive fetal molecular diagnostic

and is being increasingly used for noninvasive prenatal diagnostics due to several advantages over quantitative RT-PCR methodology. This MALDI-TOF MS-based assay uses PCR and extension reaction primers that detect *RHD* exons 4, 5, and 7 and the *RHDψ* pseudogene, as well as internal fetal DNA controls, and is commercially available in the United States. In a report validating this MALDI-TOF MS–based, noninvasive fetal *RHD* genotyping assay in a specialty reference laboratory, 99.5% overall test accuracy was demonstrated, with no false-negative and one false-positive result in 199 pregnant women tested at 6 to 30 weeks' gestation.[80] In a subsequent report evaluating the diagnostic accuracy of this MALDI-TOF MS *RHD* genotyping assay (SensiGene *RHD* genotyping LDT) to determine fetal *RHD* status in 120 maternal samples in each trimester, the accuracy rates for fetal *RHD* status were 99.1%, 99.1%, and 98.1%, respectively.[81] *RHD* ccff-DNA testing is commercially available, and is being increasingly used in the United States, United Kingdom, and Europe.[80,82,83]

Although there are fewer published reports on noninvasive fetal genotyping using ccff-DNA from maternal plasma to determine Rh C/c, E/e, and KEL1 status, high accuracy rates have been reported in clinical diagnostic settings. Therefore, noninvasive fetal genotyping may be used to predict whether infants of alloimmunized women carry these cognate minor RBC antigens and are thus at risk for HFDN.[84-86]

MATERNAL IMMUNOHEMATOLOGIC TESTING

The dual aims of maternal antenatal testing are to identify women who enter pregnancy already alloimmunized and to identify those at high risk of becoming alloimmunized during pregnancy. The practice guidelines and recommendations for pregnancy-associated immunohematologic and molecular testing have been established in the United States by the American Association of Blood Banks.[87]

Every obstetric patient should have samples obtained between 8 and 12 weeks' gestation and tested for ABO and RhD type; D typing discrepancies must always be investigated and resolved. These maternal samples should also be screened for the presence of red cell alloantibodies. A second sample should be obtained at 28 weeks' gestation to confirm the maternal blood type and to further evaluate the pregnant mother for other red cell alloantibodies that may have been evanescent or nonexistent earlier in pregnancy. If an unexpected antibody is identified any time during pregnancy, the specificity, titer, and likelihood of leading to HDFN must be determined. The indirect antiglobulin test (IAT), using reagent red cells expressing C, c, D, E, e, K, k, Fyᵃ, Fyᵇ, Jkᵃ, Jkᵇ, M, N, S, s, and Leᵃ, is typically used for maternal antibody screening. Blood samples from women with anti-D alloantibodies should be tested monthly until 28 weeks' gestation and every 2 weeks thereafter.[88] Antibody titers are reported as the reciprocal of the highest dilution step at which agglutination is observed. A difference of two dilutions is considered a significant change. Testing should ideally be performed in parallel with previously frozen samples to minimize the possibility that changes in the titer result from differences in technique or reagent red cell selection.[87,89] A critical titer is defined as the titer associated with significant risk of fetal anemia or hydrops and is the threshold at which the fetus will need monitoring. When the critical titer is reached and a decision is made to monitor the fetus by ultrasonography or amniocentesis, further antibody titration plays no role in assessment of fetal status. The critical titer varies from 8 to 32 in different laboratories in the United States.[88] In the United Kingdom and Europe, the level of anti-D is compared with an international standard and reported in IU/mL. Anti-D levels of 4 IU/mL or greater prompt referral to a fetomaternal specialist unit for further monitoring; at levels of 4 to 15 IU/mL, there is a potential risk of moderate HDFN; levels greater than 15 IU/mL imply a risk of severe HDN. When RhIg has been administered during pregnancy, a positive low anti-D antibody titer (usually <0.4 IU/mL) may be detected. Specific procedures may be used to manage pregnancies when anti-D has been detected in a woman's plasma for the first time after a dose of RhIg prophylaxis.[90]

The significance of titer levels for antibodies other than RhD is less defined. Maternal anti-Kell titers, in particular, correlate poorly with fetal outcome.[67] Limited data are available for anti-K and anti-c because these are the most common non-RhD minor red cell antibodies implicated in severe HDFN. In a review of 156 anti–Kell-positive pregnancies over 37 years, McKenna and colleagues found that all severely affected fetuses had a titer of at least 32.[65] Bowman and colleagues also noted that a titer of 32 or greater was present in 16 of 17 severely affected pregnancies, but 1 patient with a titer of 1:8 had a grossly hydropic fetus at 23 weeks' gestation.[66] Some recommend further testing of the fetus if a critical titer of 8 is attained and paternal red cell typing is Kell-positive.[88] In the United Kingdom, any anti-Kell identified prompts referral to a fetomaternal specialist unit regardless of antibody titer[90]; anti-Kell titers as low as two prompt referral to a perinatal center in the Netherlands.[64] In a case series of women with anti-c isoimmunization, a titer of 32 or greater was invariably associated with severe fetal or neonatal disease.[91] The British Committee for Standards in Hematology recommends referral to a fetal medicine specialist for an anti-c concentration of 7.5 IU/mL or greater in conjunction with any previous history of HDF because of a moderate risk of HDFN.[90,92]

The imperfect predictive value of serologic tests has led to the development of functional cellular assays that measure the ability of maternal antibodies to cause red cell destruction, thus providing better noninvasive differentiation of pregnancies at increased risk of fetal anemia. In these assays, RBCs sensitized with maternal antibodies are incubated with effector cells carrying Fcγ receptors, such as lymphocytes or monocytes, to measure cellular interaction, such as binding, phagocytosis, or cytotoxic lysis.[93] Some authors have reported on the superiority of the monocyte monolayer assay, the chemiluminescence test, and the antibody-dependent cell-mediated cytotoxicity assay, compared with serologic tests, in predicting severity of HDFN. However, these tests are complex, are difficult to standardize, and are not widely used in the United States.

FETAL BLOOD SAMPLING

Fetal blood sampling (also called *percutaneous umbilical blood sampling* or *cordocentesis*) allows direct measurement of blood indices to specifically evaluate the degree of severity of fetal hemolytic disease as early as 17 to 18 weeks' gestation.[94] Indications for fetal blood sampling in alloimmunized pregnancies include fetal blood typing, confirmation of severe fetal anemia suspected based on elevated peak middle cerebral artery doppler velocities, or ultrasonographic evidence of hydrops Historically, fetal blood samples were obtained when amniocentesis results returned with ΔOD_{450} measurements (assessing amniotic bilirubin level) in Liley zone 3 or in the "intrauterine death zone" in the Queenan graph.[88,95,96] Fetal blood sampling is performed under local anesthesia. A 20- to 22-gauge spinal needle is inserted into the umbilical vein at the level of cord insertion into the placenta under ultrasonographic guidance. Specimens of fetal blood are obtained for direct measurement of complete blood count, reticulocyte count, red cell antigen phenotyping, DAT, bilirubin, blood gases, and lactate to assess acid–base status. Blood should be available for immediate IUT when the procedure is being performed for suspected severe fetal anemia. Complications of fetal blood sampling include fetal loss, with procedure-related rates ranging from 0% to 4.9%, umbilical cord bleeding, chorioamnionitis, and significant risk of FMH with anamnestic maternal sensitization or the formation of additional alloantibodies.[97,98]

AMNIOTIC FLUID SPECTROPHOTOMETRY

Amniotic fluid spectrophotometry has been used for the last half century using bilirubin as an indicator to measure fetal hemolysis. Although briefly reviewed here for historical perspective, this method has been replaced by noninvasive fetal monitoring techniques.[88,99,100] In spectrophotometry, elevations of optical density at 450 nm (ΔOD_{450}) reflect the concentration of amniotic fluid bilirubin, which is derived from the fetus.[95] The original Liley chart, from 27 weeks to term, defined 3 zones: readings in zone 3, the upper zone, indicate severe fetal disease with hydrops or impending fetal death; readings in zone 1, the lowest zone, indicate mild or no hemolytic disease with a 10% risk of needing a postnatal exchange transfusion; and readings in zone 2 indicate moderate disease. The Liley chart was later modified by Queenan to include data from 14 to 40 weeks' gestation and had 4 zones, with the lowest zone representing unaffected fetuses and the highest zone associated with increased risk of intrauterine death.[95]

ULTRASONOGRAPHY

Ultrasonography is noninvasive, can be performed serially, and can be combined with other diagnostic studies to assess the fetal condition, estimate the need for further aggressive management, and obtain a biophysical profile of the fetus to determine fetal well-being. As hydrops develops in an anemic fetus, a consistent pattern may be noted on ultrasonography. Polyhydramnios appears first followed by placental enlargement, hepatomegaly, pericardial effusion, ascites, scalp edema, and pleural effusions in succession. Nevertheless, in the absence of overt hydrops, ultrasonographic parameters, such as intrahepatic and extrahepatic vein diameters, abdominal and head circumference, head-to-abdominal-circumference ratio, intraperitoneal volume, splenic size, and liver length have not been reliable in distinguishing mild from severe fetal anemia.[96]

In addition to traditional ultrasonography, measurement of fetal cerebral blood flow has become an extremely valuable technique in assessing fetal anemia. Decreased viscosity of the blood and increased cardiovascular output in anemic fetuses lead to a hyperdynamic circulation; hypoxia further increases blood flow velocity. Values greater than 1.5 multiples of the median for gestational age highly correlate with fetal anemia (Fig. 27-3).[100] Doppler measurement of peak velocity of systolic blood flow in the middle cerebral artery has been found to be more sensitive and accurate for detecting severe fetal anemia than measurement of amniotic fluid ΔOD_{450}.[99] Measurements may be initiated as early as 18 weeks of gestation and repeated at 1- to 2-week intervals until 35 weeks' gestation. After 38 weeks, a higher false-positive rate in the detection of fetal anemia necessitates amniocentesis for ΔOD_{450} and fetal lung maturity testing if elevated levels are noted.[88]

●THERAPY

ANTENATAL MANAGEMENT

Intrauterine Transfusion

Before the institution of IUTs, many severely affected fetuses died in utero or soon after birth. IUT corrects fetal anemia and reduces the risk of congestive heart failure and hydrops fetalis. Fetal bilirubin is cleared very efficiently by the placenta and the mother, so bilirubin removal is not necessary until after birth. Percutaneous intraperitoneal fetal transfusion pioneered by Liley in the 1960s[5] has been largely replaced by ultrasound-guided direct intravascular transfusion into the umbilical vein.[94,101] The intravascular technique circumvents the problem of erratic and often poor absorption of RBCs from the peritoneal cavity in such fetuses. However, intraperitoneal transfusions may be necessary

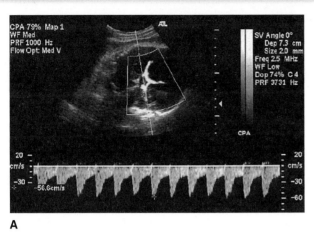

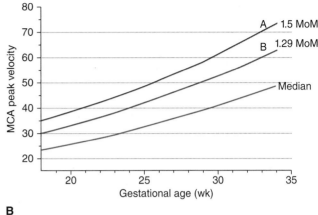

A

B

FIGURE 27–3. Peak velocity of systolic blood flow in the middle cerebral artery can be measured by ultrasound **(A)** and compared with multiples of the median (MoMs) for the prediction of fetal anemia **(B)**. MCA, middle cerebral artery. *(Part A reproduced with permission from Dukler D, et al. Noninvasive tests to predict fetal anemia: a study comparing Doppler and ultrasound parameters. Am J Obstet Gynecol. 2003 May;188[5]:1310-1314. Part B reproduced with permission from Moise KJ Jr. Management of rhesus alloimmunization in pregnancy. Obstet Gynecol. 2002 Sep;100[3]:600-611.)*

when intravascular access is difficult, as in early pregnancy when the umbilical vessels are narrow or later when increased fetal size prevents access to the umbilical cord.[102,103] The first fetal blood sampling with transfusion ideally should be performed before hydrops develops. Transfusions are typically given at fetal hematocrit levels of 25% to 30% or less or if the fetal hemoglobin is 4 to 6 standard deviations below the mean for gestational age. Generally, the hematocrit drops by 1% to 2% per day in a transfused hydropic fetus. The fall in hematocrit is rapid in fetuses with severe hemolytic disease, often necessitating a second transfusion within 7 to 14 days. The interval between subsequent transfusions varies but may be 21 to 28 days. Increased IUT frequency is often needed in hydropic fetuses.[104] Nonhydropic fetuses can tolerate rapid RBC infusions of 5 to 7 mL/min because of the capacitance of the placenta. Hydropic fetuses require slower transfusion rates and can tolerate only smaller, more frequent transfusions. Very low pretransfusion fetal hematocrit levels, rapid large increases in posttransfusion hematocrit level, and increases in umbilical venous pressure during IUTs are associated with fetal death after transfusion.[105,106]

RBCs for IUT are typically type O-negative crossmatch compatible with the mother's plasma and negative for any identified antibody; they should also be irradiated and leukoreduced.[107,108] Many centers also use RBCs negative for sickle hemoglobin to prevent sickling in the fetus at low oxygen tension and 5 to 7 days old to maximize circulatory half-life. Obtaining RBCs from a rare donor registry may be required in cases of unusual or combination of antibodies. In this circumstance, frozen, deglycerolized RBCs may be the only available product. Some centers use maternal RBCs for IUTs, supporting serial maternal donations with iron and folate therapy.[109] RBC transfusion is calculated to increase the fetal hematocrit to between 40% and 45%. The RBCs are often washed free of additive solutions and packed to a hematocrit of 70% to 85% in a volume calculation based on estimated fetal placental blood volume, fetal hematocrit, and hematocrit of donor RBCs. Various nomograms and formulas for the calculation of donor blood volume have been published.[110,111] If the hematocrit of the donor unit is approximately 75%, multiplying the estimated fetal weight in grams (estimated by ultrasonography) by a factor of 0.02 provides a fairly accurate estimate of the volume of RBCs to be transfused to achieve a fetal hematocrit increment of 10%.[112]

The largest body of IUT-related outcomes data comes from the Netherlands.[113,114] Of 1678 IUTs performed in 589 fetuses over 27 years, Zwiers and colleagues estimated procedure-related complication rates

of 6.1% per fetus and 2.1% per procedure. Complications were defined as rupture of membranes or preterm delivery within 7 days after IUT (if occurring before 34 weeks of gestation) and intrauterine infection and fetal distress resulting in either emergency cesarean section within 24 hours after IUT or fetal death. The procedure-related pregnancy loss rate was calculated to be 1.0% per procedure. Compared with IUT procedures performed between 1988 and 2001, those performed after 2001 were associated with a decrease in procedure-related perinatal loss (1.8% vs 4.7% per fetus) and procedure-related complications (3.3% vs 9.8% per fetus). Changes in transfusion techniques such as routine use of fetal paralysis, increased use of intrahepatic transfusion, and avoidance of arterial puncture were attributed to the improved outcomes.[114]

Additional RBC alloantibodies may develop in already alloimmunized women undergoing IUT. In one study, 25% (53 of 212) women treated with IUT using Rh (D, C/c, E/e)- and K-matched RBCs formed new alloantibodies, 53% of which against non-Rh and -K antigens, suggesting that extensive red cell matching should be considered for IUTs.[115]

Delivery

The decision regarding the appropriate time to deliver the baby is based on gestational age, fetal weight and lung maturity, fetal response to the IUTs, ease of performing the transfusions, and antenatal ultrasonography and Doppler studies for fetal anemia. Transfusions usually are provided up to 35 weeks so as to prolong gestation safely until the risks of preterm birth and its attendant complications are minimized, with delivery after adequate lung maturity has occurred.[88,116]

Other Therapies

In women with severe alloimmunization and with fetal losses or hydrops very early in pregnancy, a variety of methods have been used to suppress the antibody response and prolong survival of the fetus until IUT becomes technically feasible. The use of intravenous immunoglobulin G (IVIG) has shown promising results in several case series to postpone IUTs, reduce overall IUT requirements, and improve pregnancy outcome.[117-119] In this setting, a significant decrease in maternal antibody (anti-D) titers and intrauterine hemolysis has been demonstrated after IVIG treatment, especially if IVIG treatment is started before 28 weeks' gestation in women with nonhydropic fetuses. IUT with fetal IVIG has been shown to have slower hematocrit decline after IUT compared with IUT alone in a recent prospective case-control study involving 34 Rh immunized pregnant women.[120] Use of IVIG, serial plasmapheresis, or plasmapheresis combined with IVIG have been successful in some cases.[103,121-123]

POSTNATAL MANAGEMENT

Neonatal Monitoring

A sample of cord blood should be collected from all newborns at the time of delivery. However, specific testing of cord blood samples is performed only if the mother is Rh negative, if the maternal serum contains red cell alloantibodies of potential clinical significance, or if the neonate develops signs of hemolytic disease. Tests should include ABO and Rh typing and a DAT. Many birth hospitals routinely test cord blood for the infant's blood type and DAT if the mother is group O, Rh positive to predict which infants are at increased risk of hyperbilirubinemia. In severe Rh alloimmunization, high titers of maternal antibody may block Rh-antigenic sites on the neonatal red cells, leading to false-negative Rh typing. Antepartum RhIg given to the mother may cause a weakly positive DAT result in the infant at birth. Contamination of the cord blood sample with Wharton jelly during collection can also result in a false-positive DAT result. Although the DAT result usually is positive in all forms of alloimmune HDFN, the test cannot predict reliably the degree of clinical severity.[124,125] This is especially true for cases resulting from ABO sensitization. In fetomaternal ABO incompatibility, the presence of maternally derived IgG anti-A or anti-B in the infant's serum may be demonstrated by the IAT to support the diagnosis of ABO hemolytic disease. On the other hand, it is important to bear in mind that hemolysis in ABO-incompatible, DAT-negative infants may result from hematologic causes other than alloimmunization such as from red cell membrane defects (Chap. 15),[126] Elution of maternal antibody from the infant's red cells, followed by tests to determine the specificity of the antibody in the eluate, may be useful particularly when several antibodies are present in the maternal serum or when the maternal antibody screen result is negative,[87,89] Infants who received IUTs may have mild or moderate anemia with little reticulocytosis. Because most of their circulating red cells are transfused antigen-negative cells, the DAT result may be negative, but the IAT result will be strongly positive.

Cord blood hemoglobin and indirect bilirubin determinations are useful in determining disease severity. Most infants with cord hemoglobin levels within the age-adjusted normal range do not require exchange transfusion. Usually, a cord hemoglobin level less than 11 g/dL in a term newborn or a cord-indirect bilirubin level greater than 4.5 to 5 mg/dL indicate severe hemolysis and often warrants early exchange transfusion. Early exchange transfusion also may be indicated if the rate of rise of bilirubin exceeds 0.5 mg/dL per hour. The reticulocyte count usually is greater than 6% and may approach 30% to 40% in severe Rh disease. The blood film in Rh HDN is characterized by increased nucleated RBCs, polychromasia, and anisocytosis. Alternatively, the peripheral blood smear in ABO HDN is marked by microspherocytes (Fig. 27-4). Severely affected infants may also have thrombocytopenia. Low reticulocyte counts disproportionate to the low hematocrit may be noted in Kell-mediated HDN. Severely affected infants may have hypoglycemia, secondary to hyperinsulinemia. Arterial blood gas analysis may reveal metabolic acidosis or respiratory decompensation, and hypoalbuminemia is often present.

Immediate Postnatal Management

Results of antenatal monitoring and obstetric interventions during pregnancy and the history of the outcome of previous pregnancies allow the neonatal team to anticipate the needs of infants born with hemolytic disease. In infants with severe hemolytic disease without the benefit of IUTs, severe anemia and hydrops are the immediate life-threatening concerns and often are accompanied by perinatal asphyxia, surfactant deficiency, hypoglycemia, acidosis, and thrombocytopenia. Exchange transfusions and phototherapy are the mainstays of treatment. Delayed cord clamping (cord clamping at least 30 seconds after birth), historically considered controversial in cases of HDFN, has been shown to result in higher hemoglobin levels at birth with fewer postnatal exchange transfusions needed without increasing phototherapy or complication rates in non-ABO HDN.[127] However, in neonates with ABO HDN, delayed cord clamping has been shown to be associated with more phototherapy and longer hospitalization.[128] Therefore, careful monitoring of jaundice is recommended if delayed cord clamping is used in the setting of HDFN.

Resuscitation and stabilization of hydropic infants is challenging. Endotracheal intubation and positive-pressure ventilation with oxygen are usually necessary. Drainage of pleural effusions and ascites may be required to facilitate gas exchange. Metabolic acidosis and hypoglycemia

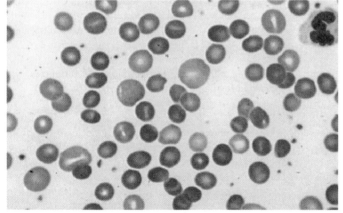

A

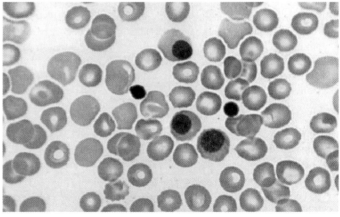

B

FIGURE 27–4. Alloimmune hemolytic disease of the newborn. Blood films. **A.** Infant with ABO blood group alloimmune hemolytic anemia. Note the high prevalence of spherocytes and the large polychromatophilic cells, indicative of reticulocytosis. **B.** Infant with Rh blood group alloimmune hemolytic anemia. Note the spherocytes, reticulocytes, and nucleated red cells. The intense erythroblastosis is characteristic of Rh blood group alloimmune hemolytic anemia and is less prominent in ABO blood group alloimmune hemolytic anemia. *(Reproduced with permission from Lichtman MA, Shafer MS, Felgar RE, et al: Lichtman's Atlas of Hematology 2016. New York, NY: McGraw Hill; 2017.)*

require correction. A partial exchange transfusion may initially be performed using packed red cells to improve hemoglobin levels and oxygenation. A double-volume exchange transfusion is considered only after the initial stabilization.

In a study of 191 infants born alive after IUTs between 1988 and 1999, the hematocrit at birth ranged from 13% to 51%.[129] Endotracheal ventilation was required more often in babies who had been severely hydropic in utero, but the requirements for exchange transfusion or simple transfusion did not differ between babies who had been hydropic in utero and those without evidence of hydrops. Although some centers report no difference in the frequency of exchange transfusions in babies who have had IUTs compared with babies who have not had IUTs,[129,130] other centers report that infants who received multiple IUTs are usually born closer to term and often require less phototherapy and fewer exchange transfusions in the neonatal period.[25,131] Nonetheless, many infants with severe HDFN require additional RBC transfusions for severe and prolonged hyporegenerative anemia secondary to suppression of fetal erythropoiesis.[21,22,130] Approximately three-quarters of term and near-term infants who had received IUT for Rh HDFN required transfusion within 6 months of age compared with 26% of infants with Rh HDFN who had not received an IUT.[130] Thus, careful monitoring of the baby and the baby's laboratory values are necessary not only during the initial hospital course but also after hospital discharge.

Exchange Transfusion

Exchange transfusion corrects anemia, removes bilirubin and free maternal antibody in the plasma, and replaces the infant's blood with antigen-negative RBCs that should have normal in vivo survival. Neonatal exchange transfusions can be performed by a continuous technique (simultaneous withdrawal and replacement) or discontinuous technique (alternating withdrawal and replacement). Regardless of the technique, the kinetics of exchange are very similar. A double-blood-volume exchange replaces approximately 85% of the infant's blood volume with antigen-negative RBCs; however, the amount of bilirubin or maternal alloantibody removed by exchange transfusion is significantly less (25%-45%), reflecting the equilibrating tissue-bound pool. Infusion of albumin before the exchange transfusion may help bilirubin binding, thus increasing the amount of bilirubin removed. Equilibration of extravascular and intravascular bilirubin and continued breakdown of red cells by persisting maternal antibodies result in a rebound of bilirubin following initial exchange transfusion, sometimes requiring repeated exchange transfusions in severe hemolytic disease.

The ideal volume for an exchange transfusion is twice the infant's blood volume. The volume needed for double-volume exchange depends on the total blood volume (TBV) recognizing differences in term and preterm infants:

- Double-blood-volume exchange volume (term) = 85 mL/kg × 2, or 170 mL/kg
- Double-blood-volume exchange volume (preterm) = 100 mL/kg × 2, or 200 mL/kg

To perform the exchange transfusion, aliquots of the reconstituted whole blood (WB) product are administered while equal amounts of the infant's blood are withdrawn. Careful attention not to exceed 2 mL/kg per minute (continuous) or 5 mL/kg at a time over 3 to 10 minutes (discontinuous technique) is required to prevent rapid fluctuations in arterial and intracranial pressure.[132]

The indications for "early" exchange transfusions performed within the first 12 hours of life have remained essentially unchanged over the past 50 years, with minor modifications. Cord hemoglobin levels of 11 g/dL or less, cord bilirubin levels of 5.5 mg/dL or greater, and rapidly rising total serum bilirubin (TSB) of 0.5 mg/dL or greater

per hour despite phototherapy are commonly used criteria for early exchange transfusions. Early exchange transfusion has the advantage of replacing sensitized RBCs with normal RBCs, thereby removing not only bilirubin but also the source of future bilirubin. Because bilirubin is distributed in the extracellular fluids, efficiency is enhanced by removing sensitized cells early in the process. Newborns who have been treated with serial IUTs until term often do not require exchange transfusions; however, late anemia is common because of IUT-induced erythropoietic suppression, which may last for many weeks after delivery.[133]

"Late" exchange transfusions are performed when serum bilirubin levels threaten to exceed approximately 20 to 22 mg/dL in term infants. The American Academy of Pediatrics (AAP) Subcommittee on Hyperbilirubinemia provides guidelines for exchange transfusion in infants 35 or more weeks' gestation.[134] In view of the fact that bilirubin levels rise steadily from birth and peak at approximately 72 to 96 hours of age, exchange transfusion should be considered if serum bilirubin levels reach 15 mg/dL in an infant of 35 weeks' gestation or 17 mg/dL in an infant of 38 weeks' gestation despite intensive phototherapy. Immediate exchange transfusion is recommended in infants showing signs of acute bilirubin encephalopathy, even if bilirubin levels are falling.[134] Conjugated or direct bilirubin values are not subtracted from total bilirubin levels when considering levels for exchange transfusions. Exchange transfusions are performed at lower bilirubin levels in premature infants, particularly those with hypoxemia, acidosis, and hypothermia, but few data are available to guide intervention in these infants. In infants with birth weights of at least 1500 g, exchange transfusions usually are performed at TSB of 13 to 16 mg/dL but may be considered even at levels as low as 8 to 9 mg/dL in sick babies of 24 weeks' gestation.[135] The bilirubin-to-albumin ratio (mg/dL:g/dL), considered to be a surrogate measure of free bilirubin, may provide additional data in determining the need for exchange transfusion in both term and preterm neonates.[136]

Blood components chosen for the exchange transfusion should be ABO and Rh compatible (Rh negative in Rh HDN), negative for offending antibody(ies), and cross-match compatible with maternal serum. In the case of ABO HDN, group O RBCs should be chosen for exchange out of concern that the more developed A or B antigens on any transfused adult donor RBCs may more avidly bind maternal anti-A or anti-B and may result in hemolysis. Either reconstituted WB (eg, RBCs plus fresh-frozen plasma) or stored whole blood if available can be used for neonatal exchange transfusions. The RBCs are reconstituted with AB or compatible plasma to a final hematocrit of 50% to 60%. Fresh (<7 days) RBCs should be used. When fresh RBC units are unavailable, some centers wash the RBCs and transfuse as soon as possible after washing to avoid hyperkalemia. Additionally, the RBC units should be leukoreduced, gamma irradiated, and sickle negative.[137]

Potential complications of exchange transfusion include hypocalcemia, hyperglycemia, hypoglycemia, thrombocytopenia, apnea and bradycardia, dilutional coagulopathy, neutropenia, disseminated intravascular coagulation, umbilical venous or arterial thrombosis, necrotizing enterocolitis (NEC), and infection. Hyperglycemia, hypocalcemia, and thrombocytopenia are reported to be the most common complications.[138-141] Thrombocytopenia results from a dilutional effect of replacing platelet rich neonatal WB with platelet deficient reconstituted WB. Infants who may be thrombocytopenic from severe HDFN or other comorbidities should be monitored closely after an exchange transfusion because they may require platelet transfusion. Hypocalcemia occurs because of the citrate load infused, which an immature neonatal liver has difficulties metabolizing. In anticipation of hypocalcemia, ionized calcium levels should be monitored throughout the exchange transfusion procedure, and IV calcium replacement may be needed in sick preterm infants. Furthermore, attempts should be made to correct conditions that may potentiate the symptoms of hypocalcemia such as alkalosis, hypothermia, hypomagnesemia, and hyperkalemia.[142]

In retrospective reviews of exchange transfusions performed in neonatal intensive care units, the risk of death or permanent serious sequelae has been reported to be as high as 12% in sick infants compared with less than 1% in healthy infants. Adverse outcomes are more frequent in exchanges done on preterm infants younger than 32 weeks of age, infants with other significant comorbidities and when umbilical venous catheters were used rather than other means of central venous access.[139,141,143,144] One center reported no increase in the number of complications and no exchange transfusion–related deaths over a 21-year period, even though there was a decline in the frequency of exchange transfusions performed over the years. In this study, a lower proportion of patients experienced an adverse event related to the exchange transfusion in recent years, which was attributed to the use of a standardized exchange transfusion protocol, more aggressive calcium replacement and platelet transfusion support, increased attending neonatologist involvement, and more experience with other neonatal advanced therapies.[139] Careful clinical judgment is required to balance the potential risk of adverse events from exchange transfusion with the risk of bilirubin encephalopathy in neonates who are premature, sick, or both.

Phototherapy

Phototherapy is the mainstay of treatment for unconjugated hyperbilirubinemia; the objective of treatment is preventing bilirubin neurotoxicity. Exposure of bilirubin to light results in structural and configurational isomerization of bilirubin to less toxic and less lipophilic products that are excreted efficiently without hepatic conjugation. The effectiveness of phototherapy is influenced by the wavelength and irradiance of light, the surface area of exposed skin, and the duration of exposure. Intensive phototherapy involves the use of high levels of irradiance ($\geq 30\ \mu W/cm^2$) in the 430- to 490-nm band, delivered to as much of the infant's surface area as possible. Intensive phototherapy effectively reduces bilirubin levels and decreases the need for exchange transfusions for hyperbilirubinemia in ABO and Rh HDN.[145,146] Early and intensive phototherapy should be initiated in infants with moderate or severe hemolysis or in infants with rapidly rising bilirubin levels (>0.5 mg/dL per hour). In full-term infants (at least 38 weeks' gestation) with HDFN, intensive phototherapy should be initiated if TSB levels are 5 mg/dL or greater at birth, 10 mg/dL at 24 hours after birth, or approximately 13 to 15 mg/dL at 48 to 72 hours after birth.[134] Phototherapy is recommended at lower levels for preterm or sick infants. Therapy often is initiated at TSB less than 5 mg/dL in preterm infants with HDFN to avoid potentially risky exchange transfusions.[134,135]

Other Therapies

A number of studies have reported on the successful administration of high-dose IVIG as an adjuvant treatment to standard therapy for HDN as way to prevent the need for exchange transfusions.[133] The decreased bilirubin levels in infants treated with IVIG is attributed to reduction in hemolysis secondary to blockade of mononuclear phagocyte Fc receptors. In 2004, the AAP published recommendations that IVIG be considered in HDN when TSB continues to rise despite aggressive phototherapy or when the TSB is within 2 to 3 mg/dL of the exchange level.[134] A 2018 Cochrane meta-analysis of 9 studies and including 658 term and preterm infants with HDN caused by Rh or ABO incompatibility (or both) demonstrated that IVIG administration decreased the use of exchange transfusion, decreased the mean number of exchange transfusions per infant, and reduced the maximum bilirubin level and duration of phototherapy. However, in this meta-analysis, no benefit of IVIG was found in the only two placebo controlled, blinded, studies, in reducing (1) the need for and number of exchange transfusions,

(2) the maximum bilirubin level, or (3) the duration of phototherapy.[147] In addition, IVIG treatment for HDN has been reported to be associated with an increase the risk of NEC in infants.[148-150] Based on the discordance of results in the meta-analysis between trials conducted with and without blinding of the intervention using a placebo and the possible association with NEC, there is currently no universal approach to the use of IVIG in patients with HDN. Therefore, careful clinical consideration is required to balance the potential risk of bilirubin encephalopathy with the adverse reactions that may result from IVIG and exchange transfusion.

In some instances but not routinely, recombinant human erythropoietin (rHuEPO) is given subcutaneously at a dose of 200 to 400 U/kg three times weekly for 2 weeks to infants in an effort to reduce or prevent transfusion for late onset anemia from HDN. Its use has been shown in some studies to decrease the need for postnatal transfusions in infants with late hyporegenerative anemia of Rh HDN and in neonates with Kell HDN.[21,151,152] In one study of 103 patients with Rh HDN, administration of 200 U/kg of rHuEPO, three times per week for 6 weeks, reduced the number of RBC transfusions to a mean of 1.5, and 55% of patients did not require any transfusions.[151] rHuEPO is more effective in decreasing future transfusion needs in neonates that never received IUTs, suggesting that IUTs may decrease the neonatal response to rHuEP.[153] Despite encouraging reports in relatively small numbers of neonates, it remains unclear whether rHuEPO or the longer-acting analog darbepoetin offers a distinct clinical benefit in regard to decreasing donor exposures or improvement of morbidity or mortality in this population. rHuEpo has been shown to lessen neurologic sequelae in term infants with hypoxic ischemic encephalopathy; therefore, it may have a role as a potential treatment for perinatal brain injury in the future.[154]

Several pharmacotherapeutic agents such as phenobarbital (via uridine diphosphate-glucuronosyl transferase induction), clofibrate (via glucuronosyl transferase induction), metalloporphyrins (via heme-oxygenase inhibition), albumin (via bilirubin scavenging), and probiotic supplementation (via enterohepatic circulation induction) have been limitedly studied as possible treatment options in neonatal hyperbilirubinemia. However, none of these agents are currently recommended as standard care in neonatal hyperbilirubinemia.[150]

●OUTCOME

Perinatal survival rates greater than 90% have been achieved with IUT in nonhydropic fetuses with severe HDFN.[113,129] The overall survival rate for hydropic fetuses is lower (78%-89%) despite IUTs.[129,131] An 11-year study (from 1988 to 1999) that examined 80 fetuses with immune-mediated hydrops reported a survival rate for fetuses with mild hydrops of 98% and an intrauterine reversal of hydrops in 88% of the fetuses. The outcome in severe fetal hydrops was poor, with reversal of hydrops in 39% of cases and a survival rate of 26% for fetuses with persistent hydrops.[129] This study underscores the importance of early diagnosis and treatment of fetal anemia, before hydrops develops. Implementation of a nationwide first trimester screening program for red cell antibodies in the Netherlands in 1998 was associated with increased referrals for suspected fetal anemia, more timely referrals, and an increase in perinatal survival in Kell HDFN from 61% to 100%.[64]

The neurodevelopmental outcome for infants saved by IUTs has generally been good, with almost 90% of survivors being free of disability, even when they have been profoundly anemic in utero.[25,131] The Long-Term follow up after intra-Uterine transfusionS (LOTUS) study evaluated 291 children at a median age of 8.2 years (range, 2-17 years) to determine the incidence and risk factors for neurodevelopmental impairment in children with HDFN treated with IUT.

The overall incidence of neurodevelopmental impairment was 4.8% with severe developmental delay seen in 3.1% of children. Cerebral palsy was detected in 2.1% and bilateral deafness in 1% of the children. Severe hydrops was identified as a strong predictor for neurodevelopmental impairment.[155]

It is estimated that kernicterus, secondary to bilirubin encephalopathy, is associated with at least 10% mortality and 70% long-term morbidity.[156] Although the preponderance of kernicterus cases occur in infants with bilirubin levels higher than 20 mg/dL, it has been shown that when treated promptly with phototherapy or exchange transfusion, peak bilirubin levels in the range of 25 and 29.9 mg/dL were not associated with adverse neurodevelopmental outcomes in term or near-term infants.[156,157] However, there was an adverse association with IQ among infants with a positive DAT result and a total serum bilirubin level of 25 mg/dL or greater, supporting the AAP recommendations to initiate treatment at lower bilirubin levels for jaundiced infants if they have a positive DAT result.[27,134,157]

● PREVENTION

Transfusion of blood phenotypically matched for D and for the Kell (K1) antigen has been advocated by some for premenopausal women to prevent primary RBC alloimmunization.[7,13,158] RhIg prophylaxis is very effective when administered to women exposed to RhD-positive RBCs either from pregnancy or from transfusion; however, after alloimmunization has occurred, RhIg is not effective for preventing or reducing the severity of HDFN. Unlike RhD, there are no commercially available immune globulin products for prevention of alloimmunization to minor RBC antigens (including non-D Rh antigens). If a nonpregnant woman is found to have an RBC alloantibody, counseling should be provided regarding the potential effects of the antibody on future pregnancies. Interventions that can be applied but are seldom offered to prevent HDFN in high risk maternal–paternal pairs include artificial insemination with sperm from an antigen-negative donor, preimplantation genetic diagnosis selecting for antigen-negative embryos, and surrogate pregnancy.[159]

Rh IMMUNOGLOBULIN

RhIg is prepared from plasma pools of screened, sensitized human donors; the plasma is tested using PCR and serologic methods for all known transfusion transmitted organisms. Several steps are taken to further inactivate potential infectious organisms, including solvent-detergent treatment, ion exchange chromatography, and nanofiltration. There are at least four formulations of RhIg, including two preparations that may be administered intravenously.[160] Use of RhIg is the standard of care for the prevention of maternal RhD immunization. Although the efficacy of RhIg is clear, its mechanism of action is not. Some of the proposed mechanisms are accelerated clearance and destruction of D-positive red cells from the circulation, antibody-mediated immune suppression, and the production of immunomodulatory cytokines.[56]

A 300-mcg (1500-IU) dose of RhIg affords protection against fetomaternal transfer of 15 mL of RhD-positive RBCs or 30 mL of RhD-positive WB. However, FMH in excess of 30 mL may occur in women without predisposing risk factors.[47,48] The blood of all RhD-negative non-immunized women should be tested for FMH approximately 1 hour after delivery of an RhD-positive baby.[87,161] Postpartum administration of RhIg to all nonsensitized RhD-negative women who deliver an RhD-positive infant decreases the incidence of Rh isoimmunization from 12% to approximately 2%. Further reduction in the incidence of Rh-isoimmunization (to 0.1%) has been achieved by antepartum RhIg prophylaxis at 28 weeks' gestation. The current recommendation in the United States for antenatal RhD allosensitization prophylaxis is 300 mcg (1500 IU) RhIg at 28 weeks' gestation.[162] In the United Kingdom and Canada, routine antenatal anti-D prophylaxis can be given as 300 mcg (1500 IU) RhIg at 28 weeks' gestation or 120 mcg (600 IU) RhIg at 28 weeks and 34 weeks' gestation.[83,163]

RhIg should be administered as soon as possible, within 72 hours of delivery of an RhD-positive baby. RhIg is thought to be ineffective once alloimmunization to RhD antigen has occurred. RhIg is also indicated after pregnancy termination, miscarriage, amniocentesis, chorionic villus sampling, abdominal trauma, or other manipulation during pregnancy. The RhD antigen is detectable on embryonic RBC membrane by 38 days from conception, and FMH has been documented in women with threatened abortion less than 20 weeks of gestation. Therefore, RhIg is recommended at 50 mcg (250 IU) or greater for women at less than 12 weeks' gestation and 300 mcg (1500 IU) for women at greater than 12 weeks' gestation for any antenatal potential sensitizing events.[163]

Screening for FMH can be performed by the rosette test, which detects as little as 2.5 mL of WB. If the rosette test result is positive, the number of fetal red cells in the maternal circulation can be quantified by the Kleihauer-Betke test, which is based on the resistance of fetal hemoglobin to acid elution unlike adult hemoglobin (Fig. 27-5)[164] or by flow cytometry evaluation for fetal hemoglobin in the maternal circulation.[165] False-positive results can be obtained in maternal conditions associated with increased fetal hemoglobin, such as hereditary persistence of fetal hemoglobin, sickle cell disease, or sickle cell trait. If a woman is exposed to more than 30 mL of D-positive blood, the dose of RhIg should be calculated to cover the volume of RhD-positive cells to prevent immunization (20 mcg of RhIg for 1 mL of RhD-positive RBCs or 2 mL of WB).[160,166]

Despite the efficacy of RhIg, RhD alloimmunization occurs in 0.1% of pregnancies. Other cases of Rh alloimmunization continue to occur because of failure to seek medical care; failure to implement immunoprophylaxis protocols; or, in some countries, lack of access to RhIg.

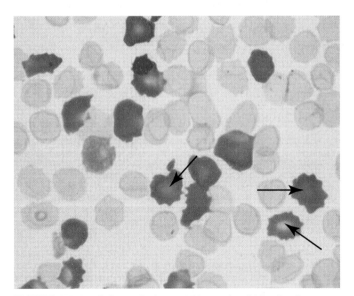

FIGURE 27–5. Kleihauer-Betke test. Maternal red blood cells appear as pale "ghost cells," whereas fetal red blood cells containing hemoglobin F are resistant to acid denaturation. Crenated red cells (*arrows*) are an artifact of the drying in preparation of the slide. (*Reproduced with permission from Lazarchick J. American Society of Hematology Image Bank. 2011-2370.*)

CONCLUSIONS

HDFN is a clinically significant problem that may potentially affect any pregnancy. Although strategies are in place to prevent RhD HDFN, few options exist to prevent the development of non-RhD HDFN. Researchers continue to investigate strategies to prevent primary maternal RBC alloimmunization to RhD and to non-RhD antigens, as well as strategies to mitigate the dangers of existing maternal RBC alloantibodies. The ability to identify pregnancies and fetuses "at risk" because of maternal RBC alloimmunization has significantly improved over time. In particular, the use of noninvasive investigations, such as evaluation of fetal RBC antigen expression using circulating cell-free fetal DNA testing and the evaluation of fetal anemia by middle cerebral artery Doppler ultrasonography, have advanced the care of fetuses at risk for HDFN. Through the continued combined efforts of maternal–fetal medicine specialists, hematologists, transfusion medicine physicians, radiologists, neonatologists, and researchers, in combination with advancements in basic science research involving alloimmunization, the care for infants at risk for HDFN and their mothers will likely continue to improve in the years to come.

REFERENCES

1. Diamond L, Blackfan K, Baty J. Erythroblastosis fetalis and its association with universal edema of the fetus, icterus gravis neonatorum and anemia of the newborn. *J Pediatr.* 1932;1:269.
2. Darrow R. Icterus gravis (erythroblastosis neonatorum, examination of etiologic considerations). *Arch Pathol.* 1938;25:378.
3. Levine P, Katzin EM, Burnham L. Isoimmunization in pregnancy: its possible bearing on the etiology of erythroblastosis fetalis. *JAMA.* 1941;116(9):825-827.
4. Diamond LK, Allen FH Jr, Thomas WO Jr. Erythroblastosis fetalis. VII. Treatment with exchange transfusion. *N Engl J Med.* 1951;244(2):39-49.
5. Liley AW. The use of amniocentesis and fetal transfusion in erythroblastosis fetalis. *Pediatrics.* 35:836-847.
6. Bowman J. Thirty-five years of Rh prophylaxis. *Transfusion.* 2003;43(12):1661-1666.
7. Poole J, Daniels G. Blood group antibodies and their significance in transfusion medicine. *Transfus Med Rev.* 2007;21(1):58-71.
8. Geifman-Holtzman O, Wojtowycz M, Kosmas E, Artal R. Female alloimmunization with antibodies known to cause hemolytic disease. *Obstet Gynecol.* 1997;89(2):272-275.
9. Gottvall T, Filbey D. Alloimmunization in pregnancy during the years 1992-2005 in the central west region of Sweden. *Acta Obstet Gynecol Scand.* 2008;87(8):843-848.
10. Koelewijn JM, Vrijkotte TG, van der Schoot CE, et al. Effect of screening for red cell antibodies, other than anti-D, to detect hemolytic disease of the fetus and newborn: a population study in the Netherlands. *Transfusion.* 2008;48(5):941-952.
11. Lee CK, Ma ES, Tang M, et al. Prevalence and specificity of clinically significant red cell alloantibodies in Chinese women during pregnancy—a review of cases from 1997 to 2001. *Transfus Med.* 2003;13(4):227-231.
12. Zipursky A, Paul VK. The global burden of Rh disease. *Arch Dis Child Fetal Neonatal Ed.* 2011;96(2):F84-F85.
13. Moise KJ. Fetal anemia due to non-Rhesus-D red-cell alloimmunization. *Semin Fetal Neonatal Med.* 2008;13(4):207-214.
14. Garratty G, Glynn SA, McEntire R. ABO and Rh(D) phenotype frequencies of different racial/ethnic groups in the United States. *Transfusion.* 2004;44(5):703-706.
15. Joseph KS. Controlling Rh haemolytic disease of the newborn in India. *Br J Obstet Gynaecol.* 1991;98(4):369-377.
16. Mak KH, Yan KF, Cheng SS, Yuen MY. Rh phenotypes of Chinese blood donors in Hong Kong, with special reference to weak D antigens. *Transfusion.* 1993;33(4):348-351.
17. Ziprin JH, Payne E, Hamidi L, et al. ABO incompatibility due to immunoglobulin G anti-B antibodies presenting with severe fetal anaemia. *Transfus Med.* 2005;15(1):57-60.
18. Thilaganathan B, Salvesen DR, Abbas A, et al. Fetal plasma erythropoietin concentration in red blood cell-isoimmunized pregnancies. *Am J Obstet Gynecol.* 1992;167(5):1292-1297.
19. Koenig JM, Christensen RD. Neutropenia and thrombocytopenia in infants with Rh hemolytic disease. *J Pediatr.* 1989;114(4 pt 1):625-631.
20. Hayde M, Widness JA, Pollak A. Rhesus isoimmunization: increased hemolysis during early infancy. *Pediatr Res.* 1997;41(5):16-21.
21. al-Alaiyan S, al Omran A. Late hyporegenerative anemia in neonates with rhesus hemolytic disease. *J Perinat Med.* 1999;27(2):112-115.
22. Pessler F, Hart D. Hyporegenerative anemia associated with Rh hemolytic disease: treatment failure of recombinant erythropoietin. *J Pediatr Hematol Oncol.* 2002;24(8):689-693.
23. Sikkel E, Pasman SA, Oepkes D, et al. On the origin of amniotic fluid bilirubin. *Placenta.* 2004;25(5):463-468.
24. Pasman SA, Sikkel E, Le Cessie S, et al. Bilirubin/albumin ratios in fetal blood and in amniotic fluid in rhesus immunization. *Obstet Gynecol.* 2008;111(5):1083-1088.
25. Janssens HM, de Haan MJ, van Kamp IL, et al. Outcome for children treated with fetal intravascular transfusions because of severe blood group antagonism. *J Pediatr.* 1997;131(3):373-380.
26. Shapiro SM. Definition of the clinical spectrum of kernicterus and bilirubin-induced neurologic dysfunction (BIND). *J Perinatol.* 2005;25(1):54-59.
27. Kuzniewicz M, Newman TB. Interaction of hemolysis and hyperbilirubinemia on neurodevelopmental outcomes in the collaborative perinatal project. *Pediatrics.* 2009;123(3):1045-1050.
28. Nicolaides KH. Studies on fetal physiology and pathophysiology in rhesus disease. *Semin Perinatol.* 1989;13(4):328-337.
29. Smits-Wintjens VE, Rath ME, Lindenburg IT, et al. Cholestasis in neonates with red cell alloimmune hemolytic disease: incidence, risk factors and outcome. *Neonatology.* 2012;101(4):306-310.
30. Rath ME, Smits-Wintjens VE, Oepkes D, et al. Thrombocytopenia at birth in neonates with red cell alloimmune haemolytic disease. *Vox Sang.* 2012;102(3):228-233.
31. Smits-Wintjens VE, Walther FJ, Lopriore E. Rhesus haemolytic disease of the newborn: postnatal management, associated morbidity and long-term outcome. *Semin Fetal Neonatal Med.* 2008;13(4):265-271.
32. Blanco E, Johnston DL. Neutropenia in infants with hemolytic disease of the newborn. *Pediatr Blood Cancer.* 2012;58(6):950-952.
33. Lobato G, Soncini CS. Relationship between obstetric history and Rh(D) alloimmunization severity. *Arch Gynecol Obstet.* 2008;277(3):245-248.
34. Katz MA, Kanto WP Jr, Korotkin JH, Recurrence rate of ABO hemolytic disease of the newborn. *Obstet Gynecol.* 1982;59(5):611-614.
35. Bellini C, Donarini G, Paladini D, et al. Etiology of non-immune hydrops fetalis: an update. *Am J Med Genet A.* 2015;167A(5):1082-1088.
36. Bascietto F, Liberati M, Murgano D, et al. Outcome of fetuses with congenital parvovirus B19 infection: systematic review and meta-analysis. *Ultrasound Obstet Gynecol.* 2018;52(5):569-576.
37. Kleinman S. Hemolytic disease of the newborn: RBC alloantibodies in pregnancy and associated serologic issues. *UpToDate.* 2014.
38. Barss VA, Moise KJ Jr. Significance of minor red blood cell antibodies during pregnancy. *UpToDate.* 2014.
39. Flegel WA. Molecular genetics of RH and its clinical application. *Transfus Clin Biol.* 2006;13(1-2):4-12.
40. Denomme GA, Wagner FF, Fernandes BJ, et al. Partial D, weak D types, and novel RHD alleles among 33,864 multiethnic patients: implications for anti-D alloimmunization and prevention. *Transfusion.* 2005;45(10):1554-1560.
41. Avent ND, Reid ME. The Rh blood group system: a review. *Blood.* 2000;95(2):375-387.
42. Wang M, Wang BL, Xu W, et al. Anti-D alloimmunisation in pregnant women with DEL phenotype in China. *Transfus Med.* 2015;25(3):163-169.
43. Practice Bulletin No. 181: prevention of Rh D Alloimmunization. *Obstet Gynecol.* 2017;130(2):e57-e70.
44. Sandler SG, Flegel WA, Westhoff CM, et al. It's time to phase in RHD genotyping for patients with a serologic weak D phenotype. College of American Pathologists Transfusion Medicine Resource Committee Work Group. *Transfusion.* 2015;55(3):680-689.
45. Shirey RS, Mirabella DC, Lumadue JA, et al. Differentiation of anti-D, -C, and -G: clinical relevance in alloimmunized pregnancies. *Transfusion.* 1997;37(5):493-496.
46. Bowman JM, Pollock JM, Penston LE. Fetomaternal transplacental hemorrhage during pregnancy and after delivery. *Vox Sang.* 1986;51(2):117-121.
47. Sebring ES, Polesky HF. Fetomaternal hemorrhage: incidence, risk factors, time of occurrence, and clinical effects. *Transfusion.* 1990;30(4):344-357.
48. Ness PM, Baldwin ML, Niebyl JR. Clinical high-risk designation does not predict excess fetal-maternal hemorrhage. *Am J Obstet Gynecol.* 1987;156(1):154-158.
49. Pourbabak S, Rund CR, Crookston KP. Three cases of massive fetomaternal hemorrhage presenting without clinical suspicion. *Arch Pathol Lab Med.* 2004;128(4):463-465.
50. Jansen MW, Brandenburg H, Wildschut HI, et al. The effect of chorionic villus sampling on the number of fetal cells isolated from maternal blood and on maternal serum alpha-fetoprotein levels. *Prenat Diagn.* 1997;17(10):953-959.
51. Bowman JM, Pollock JM. Transplacental fetal hemorrhage after amniocentesis. *Obstet Gynecol.* 1985;66(6):749-754.
52. Bowman JM, Pollock JM, Peterson LE, et al. Fetomaternal hemorrhage following funipuncture: increase in severity of maternal red-cell alloimmunization. *Obstet Gynecol.* 1994;84(5):839-843.
53. Urbaniak SJ. Alloimmunity to RhD in humans. *Transfus Clin Biol.* 2006;13(1-2):19-22.
54. Cid J, Lozano M. Risk of Rh(D) alloimmunization after transfusion of platelets from D+ donors to D- recipients. *Transfusion.* 2005;45(3):453; author reply 453-454.
55. Bowman J, Harman C, Manning F, et al. Intravenous drug abuse causes Rh immunization. *Vox Sang.* 1991;61(2):96-98.
56. Kumpel BM. On the immunologic basis of Rh immune globulin (anti-D) prophylaxis. *Transfusion.* 2006;46(9):1652-1656.
57. Bowman JM. Fetomaternal ABO incompatibility and erythroblastosis fetalis. *Vox Sang.* 1986;50(2):104-106.
58. Neppert J, v Witzleben-Schürholz E, Zupanska B, et al. High incidence of maternal HLA A, B and C antibodies associated with a mild course of haemolytic disease of the newborn. Group for the Study of Protective Maternal HLA Antibodies in the Clinical Course of HDN. *Eur J Haematol.* 1999;63(2):120-125.

59. Palfi M, Hildén JO, Gottvall T, Selbing A. Placental transport of maternal immunoglobulin G in pregnancies at risk of Rh (D) hemolytic disease of the newborn. *Am J Reprod Immunol.* 1998;39(5):323-328.

60. Lambin P, Debbia M, Puillandre P, Brossard Y. IgG1 and IgG3 anti-D in maternal serum and on the RBCs of infants suffering from HDN: relationship with the severity of the disease. *Transfusion.* 2002;42(12):1537-1546.

61. Eder AF. Update on HDFN: new information on long-standing controversies. *Immunohematology.* 2006;22(4):188-195.

62. Delaney M, Wikman A, van de Watering L, et al. Blood Group Antigen Matching Influence on Gestational Outcomes (AMIGO) study. *Transfusion.* 2017;57(3):525-532.

63. Grant SR, Kilby MD, Meer L, et al. The outcome of pregnancy in Kell alloimmunisation. *BJOG.* 2000;107(4):481-485.

64. Kamphuis MM, Lindenburg I, van Kamp IL, et al. Implementation of routine screening for Kell antibodies: does it improve perinatal survival? *Transfusion.* 2008;48(5):953-957.

65. McKenna DS, Nagaraja HN, O'Shaughnessy R. Management of pregnancies complicated by anti-Kell isoimmunization. *Obstet Gynecol.* 1999;93(5 pt 1):667-673.

66. Bowman JM, Pollock JM, Manning FA, et al. Maternal Kell blood group alloimmunization. *Obstet Gynecol.* 1992;79(2):239-244.

67. Vaughan JI, Manning M, Warwick RM, et al. Inhibition of erythroid progenitor cells by anti-Kell antibodies in fetal alloimmune anemia. *N Engl J Med.* 1998;338(12):798-803.

68. Wagner T, Bernaschek G, Geissler K. Inhibition of megakaryopoiesis by Kell-related antibodies. *N Engl J Med.* 2000;343(1):72.

69. Wagner T, Resch B, Reiterer F, et al. Pancytopenia due to suppressed hematopoiesis in a case of fatal hemolytic disease of the newborn associated with anti-K supported by molecular K1 typing. *J Pediatr Hematol Oncol.* 2004;26(1):13-15.

70. Sarici SU, Yurdakök M, Serdar MA, et al. An early (sixth-hour) serum bilirubin measurement is useful in predicting the development of significant hyperbilirubinemia and severe ABO hemolytic disease in a selective high-risk population of newborns with ABO incompatibility. *Pediatrics.* 2002;109(4):e53.

71. Lin M, Broadberry RE. ABO hemolytic disease of the newborn is more severe in Taiwan than in white populations. *Vox Sang.* 1995;68(2):136.

72. Miqdad AM, Abdelbasit OB, Shaheed MM, et al. Intravenous immunoglobulin G (IVIG) therapy for significant hyperbilirubinemia in ABO hemolytic disease of the newborn. *J Matern Fetal Neonatal Med.* 2004;16(3):163-166.

73. Kaplan M, Hammerman C, Renbaum P, et al. Gilbert's syndrome and hyperbilirubinaemia in ABO-incompatible neonates. *Lancet.* 2000;356(9230):652-653.

74. Pirelli KJ, Pietz BC, Johnson ST, et al. Molecular determination of RHD zygosity: predicting risk of hemolytic disease of the fetus and newborn related to anti-D. *Prenat Diagn.* 2010;30(12-13):1207-1212.

75. RhD Zygosity Testing. Blood Center of Wisconsin Diagnostics. http://www.bcw.edu/cs/groups/public/documents/documents/mdaw/mda0/~edisp/rhd_zygosity_desc.pdf

76. Sillence KA, Halawani AJ, Tounsi WA, et al. Rapid RHD zygosity determination using digital PCR. *Clin Chem.* 2017;63(8):1388-1397.

77. Lo YM, Bowell PJ, Selinger M, et al. Prenatal determination of fetal RhD status by analysis of peripheral blood of rhesus negative mothers. *Lancet.* 1993;341(8853):1147-1148.

78. Geifman-Holtzman O, Grotegut CA, Gaughan JP. Diagnostic accuracy of noninvasive fetal Rh genotyping from maternal blood—a meta-analysis. *Am J Obstet Gynecol.* 2006;195(4):1163-1173.

79. Daniels G, Finning K, Martin P, Massey E. Noninvasive prenatal diagnosis of fetal blood group phenotypes: current practice and future prospects. *Prenat Diagn.* 2009;29(2):101-107.

80. Bombard AT, Akolekar R, Farkas DH, et al. Fetal RHD genotype detection from circulating cell-free fetal DNA in maternal plasma in non-sensitized RhD negative women. *Prenat Diagn.* 2011;31(8):802-808.

81. Moise KJ Jr, Boring NH, O'Shaughnessy R, et al. Circulating cell-free fetal DNA for the detection of RHD status and sex using reflex fetal identifiers. *Prenat Diagn.* 2013;33(1):95-101.

82. Fasano RM. Hemolytic disease of the fetus and newborn in the molecular era. *Semin Fetal Neonatal Med.* 2016;21(1):28-34.

83. Qureshi H, Massey E, Kirwan D, et al. BCSH guideline for the use of anti-D immunoglobulin for the prevention of haemolytic disease of the fetus and newborn. *Transfus Med.* 2014;24(1):8-20.

84. Geifman-Holtzman O, Grotegut CA, Gaughan JP, et al. Noninvasive fetal RhCE genotyping from maternal blood. *BJOG.* 2009;116(2):144-151.

85. Scheffer PG, van der Schoot CE, Page-Christiaens GC, de Haas M. Noninvasive fetal blood group genotyping of rhesus D, c, E and of K in alloimmunised pregnant women: evaluation of a 7-year clinical experience. *BJOG.* 2011;118(11):1340-1348.

86. Finning K, Martin P, Summers J, et al. Fetal genotyping for the K (Kell) and Rh C, c, and E blood groups on cell-free fetal DNA in maternal plasma. *Transfusion.* 2007;47(11):2126-2133.

87. Delaney M, Svensson AM, Lieberman L. Perinatal issues in transfusion practice. In: MK Fung, et al, eds. *Technical Manual.* AABB Press; 2017:599-612.

88. Moise KJ Jr. Management of rhesus alloimmunization in pregnancy. *Obstet Gynecol.* 2008;112(1):164-176.

89. Kennedy M. Perinatal issues in transfusion practice. In: Roback J, Combs M, Grossman B, eds. *Technical Manual.* AABB Press; 2008.

90. White J, Qureshi H, Massey E, et al. Guideline for blood grouping and red cell antibody testing in pregnancy. *Transfus Med.* 2016;26(4):246-263.

91. Adeniji AA, Fuller I, Dale T, Lindow SW. Should we continue screening rhesus D positive women for the development of atypical antibodies in late pregnancy? *J Matern Fetal Neonatal Med.* 2007;20(1):59-61.

92. Kozlowski CL, Lee D, Shwe KH, Love EM. Quantification of anti-c in haemolytic disease of the newborn. *Transfus Med.* 1995;5(1):37-42.

93. Hadley AG. Laboratory assays for predicting the severity of haemolytic disease of the fetus and newborn. *Transplant Immunol.* 2002;10(2-3):191-198.

94. Daffos F, Capella-Pavlovsky M, Forestier F. Fetal blood sampling during pregnancy with use of a needle guided by ultrasound: a study of 606 consecutive cases. *Am J Obstet Gynecol.* 1985;153(6):655-660.

95. Queenan JT, Tomai TP, Ural SH, et al. Deviation in amniotic fluid optical density at a wavelength of 450 nm in Rh-immunized pregnancies from 14 to 40 weeks' gestation: a proposal for clinical management. *Am J Obstet Gynecol.* 1993;168(5):1370-1376.

96. Dukler D, Oepkes D, Seaward G, et al. Noninvasive tests to predict fetal anemia: a study comparing Doppler and ultrasound parameters. *Am J Obstet Gynecol.* 2003;188(5):1310-1314.

97. Buscaglia M, Ghisoni L, Bellotti M, et al. Percutaneous umbilical blood sampling: indication changes and procedure loss rate in a nine years' experience. *Fetal Diagn Ther.* 1996;11(2):106-113.

98. Ghidini A, Sepulveda W, Lockwood CJ, Romero R. Complications of fetal blood sampling. *Am J Obstet Gynecol.* 1993;168(5):1339-1344.

99. Oepkes D, Seaward PG, Vandenbussche FP, et al. Doppler ultrasonography versus amniocentesis to predict fetal anemia. *N Engl J Med.* 2006;355(2):156-164.

100. Mari G, Deter RL, Carpenter RL, et al. Noninvasive diagnosis by Doppler ultrasonography of fetal anemia due to maternal red-cell alloimmunization. Collaborative Group for Doppler Assessment of the Blood Velocity in Anemic Fetuses. *N Engl J Med.* 2000;342(1):9-14.

101. Oepkes D, Adama van Scheltema P. Intrauterine fetal transfusions in the management of fetal anemia and fetal thrombocytopenia. *Semin Fetal Neonatal Med.* 2007;12(6):432-438.

102. Howe DT, Michailidis GD. Intraperitoneal transfusion in severe, early-onset Rh isoimmunization. *Obstet Gynecol.* 2007;110(4):880-884.

103. Fox C, Martin W, Somerset DA, et al. Early intraperitoneal transfusion and adjuvant maternal immunoglobulin therapy in the treatment of severe red cell alloimmunization prior to fetal intravascular transfusion. *Fetal Diagn Ther.* 2008;23(2):159-163.

104. Snelgrove JW, D'Souza R, Seaward PGR, et al. Predicting intrauterine transfusion interval and perinatal outcomes in alloimmunized pregnancies: time-to-event survival analysis. *Fetal Diagn Ther.* 2019;46(6):425-432.

105. Radunovic N, Lockwood CJ, Alvarez M, et al. The severely anemic and hydropic isoimmune fetus: changes in fetal hematocrit associated with intrauterine death. *Obstet Gynecol.* 1992;79(3):390-393.

106. Hallak M, Moise KJ Jr, Hesketh DE, et al. Intravascular transfusion of fetuses with rhesus incompatibility: prediction of fetal outcome by changes in umbilical venous pressure. *Obstet Gynecol.* 1992;80(2):286-290.

107. Wong E, Luban N. Intrauterine, neonatal, and pediatric transfusion. In: Mintz PB, ed. *Transfusion Therapy: Clinical Principles and Practice.* AABB Press; 2005:159.

108. Gibson BE, Todd A, Roberts I, et al. Transfusion guidelines for neonates and older children. *Br J Haematol.* 2004;124(4):433-453.

109. Gonsoulin WJ, Moise KJ Jr, Milam JD, et al. Serial maternal blood donations for intrauterine transfusion. *Obstet Gynecol.* 1990;75(2):158-162.

110. Nicolaides KH, Clewell WH, Rodeck CH. Measurement of human fetoplacental blood volume in erythroblastosis fetalis. *Am J Obstet Gynecol.* 1987;157(1):50-53.

111. Hoogeveen M, Meerman RH, Pasman S, Egberts J. A new method to determine the fetoplacental volume based on dilution of fetal haemoglobin and an estimation of plasma fluid loss after intrauterine intravascular transfusion. *BJOG.* 2002;109(10):1132-1136.

112. Giannina G, Moise KJ Jr, Dorman K. A simple method to estimate volume for fetal intravascular transfusions. *Fetal Diagn Ther.* 1998;13(2):94-97.

113. Van Kamp IL, Klumper FJ, Oepkes D, et al. Complications of intrauterine intravascular transfusion for fetal anemia due to maternal red-cell alloimmunization. *Am J Obstet Gynecol.* 2005;192(1):171-177.

114. Zwiers C, Lindenburg ITM, Klumper FJ, et al. Complications of intrauterine intravascular blood transfusion: lessons learned after 1678 procedures. *Ultrasound Obstet Gynecol.* 2017;50(2):180-186.

115. Schonewille H, Klumper FJ, van de Watering LM, et al. High additional maternal red cell alloimmunization after Rhesus- and K-matched intrauterine intravascular transfusions for hemolytic disease of the fetus. *Am J Obstet Gynecol.* 2007;196(2):143.e1-e6.

116. Ghesquière L, Garabedian C, Coulon C, et al. Management of red cell alloimmunization in pregnancy. *J Gynecol Obstet Hum Reprod.* 2018. 47(5):197-204.

117. de la Cámara C, Arrieta R, González A, et al. High-dose intravenous immunoglobulin as the sole prenatal treatment for severe Rh immunization. *N Engl J Med.* 1988;318(8):519-520.

118. Gottvall T, Selbing A. Alloimmunization during pregnancy treated with high dose intravenous immunoglobulin. Effects on fetal hemoglobin concentration and anti-D concentrations in the mother and fetus. *Acta Obstet Gynecol Scand.* 1995;74(10):777-783.

119. Voto LS, Mathet ER, Zapaterio JL, et al. High-dose gammaglobulin (IVIG) followed by intrauterine transfusions (IUTs): a new alternative for the treatment of severe fetal hemolytic disease. *J Perinat Med.* 1997;25(1):85-88.

120. Deka D, Sharma KA, Dadhwal V, et al. Direct fetal intravenous immunoglobulin infusion as an adjunct to intrauterine fetal blood transfusion in rhesus-allommunized pregnancies: a pilot study. *Fetal Diagn Ther.* 2013;34(3):146-151.

121. Ruma MS, Moise KJ Jr, Kim E, et al. Combined plasmapheresis and intravenous immune globulin for the treatment of severe maternal red cell alloimmunization. *Am J Obstet Gynecol.* 2007;196(2):138.e1-e6.

122. Collinet P, Subtil D, Puech F, Vaast P. Successful treatment of extremely severe fetal anemia due to Kell alloimmunization. *Obstet Gynecol.* 2002;100(5 pt 2):1102-1105.

123. Nwogu LC, Moise KJ Jr, Klein KL, et al. Successful management of severe red blood cell alloimmunization in pregnancy with a combination of therapeutic plasma exchange, intravenous immune globulin, and intrauterine transfusion. *Transfusion.* 2018;58(3):677-684.

124. Dinesh D. Review of positive direct antiglobulin tests found on cord blood sampling. *J Paediatr Child Health.* 2005;41(9-10):504-507.

125. Heddle NM, Wentworth P, Anderson DR, et al. Three examples of Rh haemolytic disease of the newborn with a negative direct antiglobulin test. *Transfus Med.* 1995;5(2):113-116.

126. Herschel M, Karrison T, Wen M, et al. Isoimmunization is unlikely to be the cause of hemolysis in ABO-incompatible but direct antiglobulin test-negative neonates. *Pediatrics.* 2002;110(1 pt 1):127-130.

127. Garabedian C, Rakza T, Drumez E, et al. Benefits of delayed cord clamping in red blood cell alloimmunization. *Pediatrics.* 2016;137(3):e20153236.

128. Ghirardello S, Crippa BL, Cortesi V, et al. Delayed cord clamping increased the need for phototherapy treatment in infants with AB0 alloimmunization born by cesarean section: a retrospective study. *Front Pediatr.* 2018;6:241.

129. van Kamp IL, Klumper FJ, Bakkum RS, et al. The severity of immune fetal hydrops is predictive of fetal outcome after intrauterine treatment. *Am J Obstet Gynecol.* 2001;185(3):668-673.

130. De Boer IP, Zeestraten EC, Lopriore E, et al. Pediatric outcome in Rhesus hemolytic disease treated with and without intrauterine transfusion. *Am J Obstet Gynecol.* 2008;198(1):54.e1-e4.

131. Harper DC, Swingle HM, Weiner CP, et al. Long-term neurodevelopmental outcome and brain volume after treatment for hydrops fetalis by in utero intravascular transfusion. *Am J Obstet Gynecol.* 2006;195(1):192-200.

132. Ramasethu J. Exchange transfusions. In: MacDonald M, Ramasethu J, Rais-Bahrami K, eds. *Atlas of Procedures in Neonatology.* Lippincott, Williams & Wilkins; 2013:315-323.

133. Murray NA, Roberts IA. Haemolytic disease of the newborn. *Arch Dis Child Fetal Neonatal Ed.* 2007;92(2):F83-F88.

134. Management of hyperbilirubinemia in the newborn infant 35 or more weeks of gestation. *Pediatrics.* 2004;114(1):297-316.

135. Maisels MJ, Watchko JF. Treatment of jaundice in low birthweight infants. *Arch Dis Child Fetal Neonatal Ed.* 2003;88(6):F459-F463.

136. Hulzebos CV, Dijk PH. Bilirubin-albumin binding, bilirubin/albumin ratios, and free bilirubin levels: where do we stand? *Semin Perinatol.* 2014;38(7):412-421.

137. Fasano R, Luban N. Blood component therapy for the neonate. In: Martin R, Fanaroff A, Walsh M, eds. *Fanaroff and Martin's Neonatal-Perinatal Medicine: Diseases of the Fetus and Infant.* Elsevier; 2010:1360-1374.

138. Patra K, Storfer-Isser A, Siner B, et al. Adverse events associated with neonatal exchange transfusion in the 1990s. *J Pediatr.* 2004;144(5):626-631.

139. Steiner LA, Bizzarro MJ, Ehrenkranz RA, et al. A decline in the frequency of neonatal exchange transfusions and its effect on exchange-related morbidity and mortality. *Pediatrics.* 2007;120(1):27-32.

140. Hakan N, Zenciroglu A, Aydin M, et al. Exchange transfusion for neonatal hyperbilirubinemia: an 8-year single center experience at a tertiary neonatal intensive care unit in Turkey. *J Matern Fetal Neonatal Med.* 2015;28(13):1537-1441.

141. Murki S, Kumar P. Blood exchange transfusion for infants with severe neonatal hyperbilirubinemia. *Semin Perinatol.* 2011;35(3):175-184.

142. Fasano RM, Paul WM, Pisciotto PT. Complications of neonatal transfusion In: Popovsky M, ed. *Transfusion Reactions.* AABB Press; 2012:471-518.

143. Jackson JC. Adverse events associated with exchange transfusion in healthy and ill newborns. *Pediatrics.* 1997;99(5):E7.

144. Chen HN, Lee ML, Tsao, LY. Exchange transfusion using peripheral vessels is safe and effective in newborn infants. *Pediatrics.* 2008;122(4):e905-e910.

145. Tan KL, Lim GC, Boey KW. Phototherapy for ABO haemolytic hyperbilirubinaemia. *Biol Neonate.* 1992;61(6):358-365.

146. Ebbesen F. Evaluation of the indications for early exchange transfusion in rhesus haemolytic disease during phototherapy. *Eur J Pediatr.* 1980;133(1):37-40.

147. Zwiers C, Scheffer-Rath ME, Lopriore E, et al. Immunoglobulin for alloimmune hemolytic disease in neonates. *Cochrane Database Syst Rev.* 2018;3:CD003313.

148. Yang Y, Pan JJ, Zhou XG, et al. The effect of immunoglobulin treatment for hemolysis on the incidence of necrotizing enterocolitis—a meta-analysis. *Eur Rev Med Pharmacol Sci.* 2016;20(18):3902-3910.

149. Figueras-Aloy J, Rodríguez-Miguélez JM, Iriondo-Sanz M, et al. Intravenous immunoglobulin and necrotizing enterocolitis in newborns with hemolytic disease. *Pediatrics.* 2010;125(1):139-144.

150. Ree IMC, Smits-Wintjens VEHJ, van der Bom JG, et al. Neonatal management and outcome in alloimmune hemolytic disease. *Expert Rev Hematol.* 2017;10(7):607-616.

151. Ovaly F. Late anaemia in Rh haemolytic disease. *Arch Dis Child Fetal Neonatal Ed.* 2003;88(5):F444; author reply F445.

152. Dhodapkar KM, Blei F. Treatment of hemolytic disease of the newborn caused by anti-Kell antibody with recombinant erythropoietin. *J Pediatr Hematol Oncol.* 2001;23(1):69-70.

153. Zuppa AA, Alighieri G, Calabrese V, et al. Recombinant human erythropoietin in the prevention of late anemia in intrauterine transfused neonates with Rh-isoimmunization. *J Pediatr Hematol Oncol.* 2010;32(3):e95-e101.

154. McPherson RJ, Juul SE. Erythropoietin for infants with hypoxic-ischemic encephalopathy. *Curr Opin Pediatr.* 2010;22(2):139-145.

155. Lindenburg IT, Smits-Wintjens VE, van Klink JM, et al. Long-term neurodevelopmental outcome after intrauterine transfusion for hemolytic disease of the fetus/newborn: the LOTUS study. *Am J Obstet Gynecol.* 2012;206(2):141 e1-e8.

156. Ip S, Chung M, Kulig J, et al. An evidence-based review of important issues concerning neonatal hyperbilirubinemia. *Pediatrics.* 2004;114(1):e130-e153.

157. Newman TB, Liljestrand P, Jeremy RJ, et al. Outcomes among newborns with total serum bilirubin levels of 25 mg per deciliter or more. *N Engl J Med.* 2006;354(18):1889-1900.

158. Solheim BG. Provision of K- (KEL1-) blood to women not more than 50 years of age. *Transfusion.* 2015;55(3):468-469.

159. Moise KJ. Overview of Rhesus (Rh) alloimmunization in pregnancy. *UpToDate.* 2014.

160. Ayache S, Herman JH. Prevention of D sensitization after mismatched transfusion of blood components: toward optimal use of RhIG. *Transfusion.* 2008;48(9):1990-1999.

161. American College of Obstetrics and Gynecology. *ACOG Practice Bulletin, Prevention of Rh(D) Alloimmunization,* Number 4. 1999, Clinical Management Guidelines for Obstetricians and Gynecologists.

162. Committee on Practice Bulletins-Obstetrics. *Practice Bulletin No. 181: prevention of Rh D alloimmunization. Obstet Gynecol.* 2017;130(2):e57-e70.

163. Sperling JD, Dahlke JD, Sutton D, et al. Prevention of RhD alloimmunization: a comparison of four national guidelines. *Am J Perinatol.* 2018;35(2):110-119.

164. Kleihauer E, Braun H, Betke K. [Demonstration of fetal hemoglobin in erythrocytes of a blood smear. *Klin Wochenschr.* 1957;35(12):637-638.

165. Kim YA, Makar RS. Detection of fetomaternal hemorrhage. *Am J Hematol.* 2012;87(4):417-423.

166. Ramsey G. Inaccurate doses of R immune globulin after rh-incompatible fetomaternal hemorrhage: survey of laboratory practice. *Arch Pathol Lab Med.* 2009;133(3):465-469.

167. Moise KJ Jr, Argoti P. Management and prevention of red cell alloimmunization in pregnancy: a systematic review. *Obstet Gynecol.* 2012;120(5):1132-1139.

168. Moise KJ Jr. Management of rhesus alloimmunization in pregnancy. *Obstet Gynecol.* 2002;100(3):600-611.

Part VI **Polyclonal Erythrocytosis**

CHAPTER 28
PRIMARY AND SECONDARY ERYTHROCYTOSES (POLYCYTHEMIAS)

Josef T. Prchal

SUMMARY

Increased red cell mass has been variably termed either *erythrocytosis* or *polycythemia*; no clear consensus for either term has been achieved. Some interpret the meaning of *polycythemia* to imply that *several lineages* are increased (ie, erythrocytosis, neutrophilia, and thrombocytosis); the only form of polycythemia is *polycythemia vera (PV)*. Others, such as the late Allan Erslev, the editor and an author of earlier editions of *Williams Hematology*, argued that the proper meaning of *polycythemia is too many cells in blood*. Hence, one cannot have 6×10^9/L of leukocytes or platelets, but more than 6×10^9/L is seen in many conditions described here. Because the acceptance of first definition is increasing, this chapter reserves the term *polycythemia* only for *PV*. This may lead to initial difficulties when reviewing the literature as the entities of Chuvash polycythemia, are now designated Chuvash erythrocytosis. Similarly, the autosomal dominant erythrocytosis stemming from the germ line gain-of-function mutations of erythropoietin receptor is generally known as primary familial and congenital polycythemia but will be referred to here as erythrocytosis.

Primary polycythemias/erythrocytoses are caused by acquired or inherited mutations causing functional changes within hematopoietic stem cells or erythroid progenitors leading to an accumulation of red cells. The most common primary erythrocytosis, PV, which is a clonal disorder. The other primary erythrocytosis that is inherited from mutations in the erythropoietin receptor is discussed herein. In contrast, secondary erythrocytoses are caused by either an appropriate or inappropriate increase in the red cell mass, most often as a result of augmented levels of erythropoietin; these erythrocytoses can also be either acquired or hereditary. Some congenital disorders of hypoxia sensing share features of both primary and secondary erythrocytoses, and these are also discussed in this chapter. Although the clinical presentations of primary and secondary erythrocytoses may be similar, distinguishing among them is important for accurate diagnoses and proper management.

For example, secondary erythrocytosis states that represent an appropriate physiological compensation to tissue hypoxia should not be treated by phlebotomies. An occasional patient may experience hyperviscosity symptoms and may benefit from isovolemic reduction of hematocrit. Inappropriate erythrocytoses are caused by erythropoietin-secreting tumors; self-administration of erythropoiesis-stimulating agents, including, inherited disorders of hypoxia sensing; or, rarely, some endocrine disorders (described in Chap. 7). Correction of hypoxia, discontinuation of erythropoiesis-stimulating agents, or resection of erythropoietin-secreting tumors typically corrects the associated erythrocytosis.

Acronyms and Abbreviations: BFU-E, burst forming unit–erythroid; 2,3-BPG, 2,3-bisphosphoglycerate; CFU-E, colony forming unit–erythroid; COPD, chronic obstructive pulmonary disease; EGLN1, a gene encoding for PHD2; EPAS1, a gene encoding hypoxia-inducible factor-2 alpha (HIF2a); EPO, erythropoietin; EPOR, erythropoietin receptor (protein); FIH-1, Hbs, hemoglobins; HCP, hematopoietic phosphatase; Hct, hematocrit; HIF, hypoxia inducible factor; *HUMARA*, human androgen-receptor gene; IRE, iron-responsive element; IRP, iron-regulatory protein; JAK, Janus type tyrosine kinase; NO, nitric oxide; OSA, obstructive sleep apnea; PAI-1, plasminogen activator inhibitor; PFCP, primary familial and congenital erythrocytosis; PHD2, proline hydroxylase 2; PV, polycythemia vera; STAT, signal transducer and activator of transcription; VEGF, vascular endothelial growth factor; VHL, von Hippel Lindau syndrome.

DEFINITION AND HISTORY

The term *polycythemia*, denoting an increased amount of blood cells, has traditionally been applied to those conditions in which the mass of erythrocytes is increased. *Erythrocytosis*, the noun, or *erythrocytotic*, the adjective, are alternative terms that have also been applied to circumstances in which the increased red cell mass is the singular finding, distinguishing it from polycythemia vera (PV) in which there may be an increase in red cells, granulocytes, and platelets. Although this usage has much to recommend it, no consensus about terminology has been reached, and the term *polycythemia* is used interchangeably with *erythrocytosis* by many physicians and scientists and in publications. Here, we only use the term *polycythemia* for PV. A classification of the erythrocytoses is presented in Chap. 3 in Table 3-2.

PRIMARY ERYTHROCYTOSES

PV and *primary familial and congenital erythrocytosis/polycythemia (PFCP)* are primary polycythemic disorders that have erythroid progenitors hypersensitive to erythropoietin (EPO).[1-3] These primary disorders are due to somatic (PV) or germ-line (PFCP) mutations wherein erythroid progenitors are intrinsically hyperproliferative and have, as shown by in vitro assays, an augmented response to or independence of EPO. Some congenital erythrocytoses, as best described in Chuvash erythrocytosis, have erythroid progenitors that are hypersensitive to EPO, but also may have normal or even increased EPO levels despite the increased red cell mass.[4,5] Thus, some of these rare inherited erythrocytoses share features of both primary and secondary erythrocytoses.[6]

SECONDARY ERYTHROCYTOSES/ ERYTHROCYTOSES

The term *secondary erythrocytosis* refers to those conditions in which only erythrocytes are increased in number and describes a group of disorders characterized by an increased red cell volume brought about by enhanced stimulation of red cell production by circulating physiologic mediators, most commonly EPO. Secondary erythrocytosis may be subdivided into *appropriate erythrocytosis*, that is, responding normally to tissue hypoxia such as in pulmonary disease, Eisenmenger complex, high-altitude erythrocytosis and hemoglobins (Hbs) with increased affinity for oxygen (Chaps. 3, 18, and 19), and *inappropriate erythrocytosis* in which erythropoiesis is being stimulated by the aberrant production of EPO without regards to physiologic needs. These include EPO-secreting tumors, high levels of insulin growth factor 1, cobalt and manganese toxicities, self-administration of EPO, high levels of androgens or adrenocorticotropic hormone, and increased presence of other stimulators of erythropoiesis (as in post–renal transplant erythrocytosis).[7]

In his important monograph on barometric pressure published in 1878, Paul Bert showed that physiologic impairment observed at high altitude was caused by a reduction in the oxygen content of the air.[8] A few years earlier, his friend and mentor, Dennis Jourdanet, had observed an increase in the number of red "corpuscles" in blood of the highlanders in Mexico,[9] and Bert recognized that such an increase would tend to ameliorate the effect of atmospheric hypoxia. However, neither Bert nor Jourdanet suspected a cause-and-effect relationship. It was not until 1890, when Viault[10] observed a prompt increase in the number of his own red corpuscles after having traveled from Lima, Peru, at sea level, to Morococha, at 4570 m (~15,000 ft) above sea level, that altitude erythrocytosis was accepted as a compensatory adaptation to hypoxia.[11] At about the same time, it was observed that many patients with cyanosis were also erythrocytic. Both *cardiacos negros*,[12] with severe pulmonary failure and arterial oxygen desaturation, and children with *morbus caeruleus*, or right-to-left shunt through a congenital cardiac malformation, were found to have increased red cell counts.[13] Mechanical or neurogenic hypoventilation as a cause of cyanosis and erythrocytosis was first popularized in 1956 with the classic description of the Pickwickian syndrome by Burwell and colleagues.[14] Erythrocytosis associated with carboxyhemoglobinemia resulting in hypoxemia caused by smoking and with tissue hypoxia caused by inherited abnormal hemoglobins with high-affinity oxygen binding to Hb was recognized subsequently (Chaps. 18 and 19).[15] Erythrocytosis associated with abnormal hemoglobins with an increased affinity for oxygen also represents an appropriate response to hypoxia first noted by Charache and colleagues[15] in 1966 when they described Hb Chesapeake.

Relative erythrocytosis is the term used to depict enhanced red cell count or blood Hb values that is caused by reduced plasma volume, not increased red cell mass. The disorder is therefore not a true erythrocytosis and is designated *spurious, apparent, or relative erythrocytosis*. The cause of the reduced plasma volume and hence relative erythrocytosis is often known (eg, diuretic use, dehydration from excessive sweating). However, there are some patients with mild erythrocytosis in whom neither the cause nor the clinical significance is clear. In 1905, Gaisbock reported that a number of hypertensive patients had plethora and an elevated red cell count but no splenomegaly, a condition he termed *erythrocytosis hypertonica*, sometimes called *Gaisbock syndrome*.[16] In 1952, direct measurement of blood volume in patients with erythrocytosis led Lawrence and Berlin to identify a subgroup of patients with a normal red cell volume but reduced plasma volume. Although some members of this group were hypertensive, the authors were more impressed by their tense and anxious behavior, and they coined the term *stress erythrocytosis*.[17]

● EPIDEMIOLOGY

PRIMARY ERYTHROCYTOSES

Polycythemia Vera
PV, the prototype of primary erythrocytosis, is described in the 10th edition of *Williams Hematology*, 2021, Chap. 83.

Primary Familial and Congenital Erythrocytosis
This autosomal dominant disorder (designated PFCP) is uncommon but more prevalent than is generally appreciated because many affected subjects are initially misdiagnosed as having PV. Its prevalence is similar

to congenital erythrocytoses caused by high-oxygen-affinity Hb mutants and far more common than 2,3-biphosphoglycerate deficiency.[18]

SECONDARY ERYTHROCYTOSES

Pulmonary Disease with Hypoxia
In one study of 2524 patients with severe chronic obstructive pulmonary disease (COPD), 8.4% had a hematocrit (Hct) higher than 55%. In this study, Hct was an independent predictor of longer survival, decreased hospital admission rate, and decreased cumulative duration of hospitalization.[19] In another, smaller study of 309 subjects with COPD and chronic respiratory failure, 67% had normal Hb levels, 20% had anemia, and 18% had erythrocytosis.[20]

Obstructive Sleep Apnea
Although the evidence is largely anecdotal,[21] secondary erythrocytosis has been widely considered to be a complication of longstanding obstructive sleep apnea (OSA) and in one study was found in 5% to 10% of those with nocturnal apnea and hypopnea.[22] However, published studies remain controversial; in a study of 263 patients (189 men and 74 women), patients with severe sleep apnea had significantly higher Hct values than patients with mild to moderate sleep apnea or nonapneic control participants ($P < 0.01$).[23] In contrast, in other studies, there were no significant differences in Hb levels or Hct between participants with and without OSA.[24,25] The total number of hours of hypoxia per day may dictate whether the stimulus to EPO production is sufficient to cause erythrocytosis.

We retrospectively analyzed 527 patients in our institutions, and after excluding those OSA subjects with daytime hypoxia, the prevalence of increased Hb in OSA was only 1.7% (9 of 527 patients), and most of these participants were taking androgens.[26,27]

Erythrocytosis Associated with Smoking
Smoking clearly increases Hct in COPD compared with control participants with comparable pulmonary function. In a study of 2524 patients with severe COPD, 10.2% of patients reported as current smokers had significantly higher Hct values than ex-smokers or nonsmokers of comparable pulmonary impairment of both genders, with $P < 0.02$.[20]

Even young male smokers without pulmonary impairment have higher Hcts. In one study (age range, 18.6-22.8 years; mean, 19.4 years), 1169 participants were recruited, and 25% were smokers. Predictably, carboxyhemoglobin resulting in decreased oxygen tissue delivery (Chap. 19), was much higher in smokers than in nonsmokers ($r = 0.958$, $P < 0.001$), and both Hb and Hcts were also markedly higher in smokers (Hb, $P = 0.001$; Hct, $P = 0.004$).[28]

High Oxygen Affinity and Hemoglobins
These disorders are reviewed in detail in Chaps. 18 and 19. High-oxygen-affinity Hbs deliver less oxygen to tissues, which is appropriately compensated by increased erythropoiesis and a higher steady-state Hb concentration. The EPO of these patients is generally normal (indicating compensation of tissue hypoxia by increased red cell mass) and increases after phlebotomies, attesting to the increased tissue hypoxia and indicating that this therapeutic maneuver is misguided. Although considered rare, high oxygen affinity has been found, according to one report, in about 20% of 70 unrelated participants with otherwise idiopathic erythrocytosis.[29]

Erythrocytosis of Eisenmenger Complex
Eisenmenger syndrome, characterized by elevated pulmonary vascular resistance and right-to-left shunting of blood, is usually accompanied by erythrocytosis but not by increased thrombotic risk.[30,31] Most patients with the syndrome survive for 20 to 30 years.

Erythrocytosis of Endocrine Disorders and from Iatrogenic or Self-Administration of Androgens

Erythrocytosis has been reported in Cushing syndrome,[32] primary aldosteronism,[33] and Bartter syndrome (Chap. 7).[34] Testosterone therapy has been shown to have an eightfold increased risk of erythrocytosis compared with placebo.[35] Please refer to Chap. 7 for more details.

Cobalt and Manganese Toxicities

Cobalt-Induced Erythrocytosis Administration of cobalt was first shown to produce erythrocytosis in 1929,[36] and the mechanism was subsequently characterized in 1959 by careful studies of stimulated erythropoiesis by administration of cobalt to rats.[37] Adding cobalt to beer manufacturing decreases beer foaming, but when added in excessive concentration induces cobalt toxicity. This effect has been well publicized as *Quebec beer-drinkers' cardiomyopathy*; most of these patients had erythrocytosis.[38] Cobalt was subsequently shown to increase erythropoiesis at least in part by increasing EPO.[39] Excessive erythrocytosis (Hct >65%, reaching levels as high as 80) was reported in miners in Cerro de Pasco, Peru (altitude, 4300 m). More than half (11 of 21) of the participants with excessive erythrocytosis had high cobalt levels in plasma, but cobalt levels were undetectable in high-altitude and sea-level control participants.[40] Erythrocytosis has been repeatedly described in patients with hip replacement implanted with *metal-on-polyethylene prostheses*. The prostheses may wear down the chrome or cobalt head, resulting in a rise in blood metal ion levels, causing systemic cobalt toxicity. Other symptoms described include cognitive deterioration, cardiomyopathy, hypothyroidism, and neuropathy; all are the clinical manifestations of prosthetic cobaltism.[41]

Manganese-Induced Erythrocytosis The association of manganese and erythrocytosis was first described in rats in 1978.[42] A congenital disorder associated with manganese transport and hypermagnesemia, liver cirrhosis, erythrocytosis, and neurological defects was described in a child born to consanguineous parents.[43] Since that time, many other similar patients with a congenital neurologic disorder, erythrocytosis, and high manganese levels have been described.

Inappropriate Tissue Elaboration of Erythropoietin

The prevalence of various types of secondary erythrocytosis is a function of underlying causes, such as geographical location of the patient or presence of a causative neoplasm. About 1% to 3% of all patients with pheochromocytoma or paraganglioma have erythrocytosis.[44] Rare patients with congenital erythrocytosis develop pheochromocytoma or paraganglioma; these are most likely caused by genomic mosaicism for a gain of function of *EPAS1* (hypoxia-inducible factor [HIF] 2α)[45]; (see further). Uterine leiomyomas in premenopausal women are very common, estimated at 20% to 40% of the general population, and the occurrence of erythrocytosis ranges from 0.02% to 0.5% of cases.[46] Isolated instances of erythrocytosis have been attributed to myxoma of the atrium,[47] hamartoma of the liver,[48] and focal hyperplasia of the liver.[49] Erythrocytosis and inappropriate secretion of EPO may be found in about 15% of patients with cerebellar hemangioma.[50,51]

TEMPI Syndrome

Over 20 patients with erythrocytosis, elevated erythropoietin and monoclonal gammopathy have been described as TEMPI syndrome. It is constituted of (1) *t*elangiectasias; (2) *e*levated erythropoietin and erythrocytosis; (3) *m*onoclonal gammopathy; (4) *p*erinephric fluid collections; and (5) *i*ntrapulmonary shunting. This is an acquired erythrocytosis that is reversible with resolution of monoclonal gammopathy by plasma cell–directed therapy. Its pathophysiology is obscure.[52,53]

Self-Administration of Erythropoietin

Athletes have attempted for decades to manipulate their blood to gain a competitive advantage either by blood transfusions or EPO. This evolving, but continuous, problem has been reviewed[54]; whether the purported benefit stems from elevated red cell mass or from the stimulation of nonerythroid tissues such as the brain[55] and endothelial tissues is not clear.

Erythrocytosis of High Altitude

Elevation of red cell mass as a response to high-altitude hypoxia represents an appropriate adjustment to reduced blood oxygen content and delivery. The exponentially decreasing atmospheric oxygen pressure with altitude stimulates the body to accommodate by an increase in respiratory rate and volume. Such adaptation is possible only in the short term because the body may not always be able to adequately enhance respiration. Erythrocytosis is considered a universal, uniform adaptation response to hypoxia that arises in normal individuals, but when it is exaggerated, in some cases, it results in chronic mountain sickness with associated symptoms of fatigue, headache, and pulmonary hypertension.[56]

The evolutionary adaptation to hypoxia is discussed in Chap. 3 as well as the fact that using Hb concentration as a substitute for red cell volume may be misleading, as has been documented in Tibetan Sherpas who have a lower level of Hb concentration than other sojourners to high altitude, but their expanded red cell volume is masked by the concomitant expansion of plasma volume.[57]

Altitude above sea level should be used as an independent variable for the definition of erythrocytosis.[58,59] Appropriate adjustment values for given population, gender, age, and the altitude of the residence have been reported.[59] Even moderate altitude must also be considered when interpreting Hb levels as documented by analysis of 71,798 Swiss men aged 18 to 22 years that showed significant Hb differences with an altitude of residence between 200 and 2000 m.[60]

Post–Renal Transplant Erythrocytosis

This syndrome, defined as a persistent elevation of Hct at over 51%, is a relatively common condition found in approximately 5% to 10% of renal allograft recipients.[61,62] Post–renal transplant erythrocytosis usually develops within 8 to 24 months after transplantation, despite persistently good function of the allograft, and resolves spontaneously within 2 years in about 25% of patients.[63] Factors that increase the likelihood of its development are lack of EPO therapy before transplantation, a history of smoking, diabetes mellitus, renal artery stenosis, low serum ferritin levels, and normal or higher pretransplant EPO levels. Post–renal transplant erythrocytosis is also more frequent in patients who are not undergoing graft rejection.[64,65]

Chuvash Erythrocytosis

A Russian hematologist, Lydia A. Polyakova, described erythrocytosis in the Chuvash population (an ethnic isolate in the mid-Volga River region of Russia of Turkish descent) in the early 1960s,[66] and by 1974, 103 cases from 81 families had been described.[66] Since then, more cases have come to light; hundreds of children and adults have this condition, indicating that Chuvash erythrocytosis is the only known endemic congenital erythrocytosis in the world.[67] Outside of Chuvashia, Chuvash erythrocytosis has also been found sporadically in diverse ethnic and racial groups,[68,69] and a high prevalence of this disorder has also been reported on the Italian island of Ischia.[70] An analysis of 18 Indian patients with erythrocytosis without an obvious cause found that 11 were homozygous for the Chuvash von Hippel Lindau syndrome mutation, and 2 had a high-oxygen-affinity Hb mutant.[71]

● ETIOLOGY AND PATHOGENESIS

PRIMARY ERYTHROCYTOSES

Primary Familial and Congenital Polycythemia/ Erythrocytosis

In contrast to PV, PFCP is caused by germline rather than acquired somatic mutations. It is congenital and manifests autosomal dominant inheritance[3] and, frequently, sporadic occurrence from de novo germline mutations, attesting to its deleterious effect. Deleterious mutations keep their prevalence by de novo mutations as exemplified by the high rate of de novo mutations in hemophilia A. Similar to PV, PFCP is a primary erythrocytosis in that the defect changes intrinsic responses of erythroid progenitors, and EPO levels are low in PFCP.

To date, several mutations of the erythropoietin receptor (*EPOR*) associated with PFCP have been described (Table 28-1). Of the 12, 9 result in truncation of the EPOR cytoplasmic carboxyl terminal and are the only mutations convincingly linked with PFCP. Such truncations lead to a loss in the negative regulatory domain of the EPOR (Chap. 2). Three missense *EPOR* mutations have also been described, but these have not been linked to PFCP or any other disease phenotype (see Table 28-1).

EPO-mediated activation of erythropoiesis involves several steps (Chap. 2). First, EPO activates its receptor by inducing conformational changes of its dimers. These changes lead to initiation of an erythroid-specific cascade of events. The first signal is initiated by conformation change-induced activation of JAK (Janus type tyrosine kinase) 2 and its phosphorylation and activation of a transcription factor, signal transducer and activator of transcription (STAT) 5, which regulates erythroid-specific genes. This "on" signal is negated by dephosphorylation of EPOR by hematopoietic phosphatase (HCP), also known as SHP1 (ie, the "off" signal). EPOR truncations lead to a loss of the negative regulatory domain of the EPOR, a binding site for hematopoietic cell phosphatase HCP, explaining the gain-of-function properties of these *EPOR* mutations (Fig. 28-1). A new mechanism of augmented erythropoiesis and EPO signaling was elucidated in a study of the EPO receptor missense mutant, EPOR p.Gln434Pro. Its sequence did not result in the loss of negative signaling. However, its new C-terminal tail was shown to increase EPO receptor dimerization and stability, resulting in JAK2 constitutive signaling and hypersensitivity to EPO.[72]

SECONDARY ERYTHROCYTOSES

The morbidity of primary erythrocytoses, such as PV, is largely due to increased activated neutrophils and perhaps attendant HIF and JAK2–induced prothrombotic changes.[31] In secondary erythrocytoses, it is assumed to be related to an increase in blood viscosity and perhaps also to resulting increased cardiac work.[73] However, evidence of increased thrombotic risk in secondary erythrocytoses is lacking,[31] with the exception of secondary erythrocytoses resulting from augmented HIF signaling, in which evidence for HIF-induced prothrombotic changes in leukocytes is emerging.[74] In most instances, the etiology of morbidity or mortality, such as associated with congenital disorders of hypoxia sensing, is largely unknown.[75] The effect of blood viscosity on oxygen delivery is often oversimplified, and the emphasis on the Hct alone may lead to ill-advised therapeutic interventions. In the normovolemic state, viscosity increases in a log-linear fashion as Hct increases, and the effect is particularly pronounced when the Hct rises above 50%. The prediction is that oxygen delivery *decreases* as Hct rises significantly above 50 because the greatly increased viscosity reduces blood flow, overshadowing the increased oxygen-carrying capacity of blood with a higher concentration of Hb. However, erythrocytosis is not a normovolemic state but is accompanied by an increase in blood volume, which in turn enlarges the vascular bed and decreases peripheral resistance (Chaps. 2 and 3). Thus, hypervolemia can increase oxygen transport, and the optimum for oxygen transport occurs at higher Hct values than in normovolemic states. Consequently, despite the attendant increase in viscosity, an increase in Hct may generally be of benefit in compensatory secondary erythrocytoses. However, at some point, the high viscosity causes an increase in the work of the heart and a reduction in blood flow to most tissues and may be responsible for cerebral and cardiovascular impairment.

APPROPRIATE ERYTHROCYTOSES

High-Altitude Erythrocytosis

Adaptive adjustments of humans living at high altitude involve a series of steps that reduce the steepness of the oxygen gradient between the atmosphere and mitochondria[76] (Fig. 28-2). The initial oxygen gradient between atmospheric and alveolar air can be reduced by an increase in respiratory rate and volume. Because dead space and water vapor

TABLE 28–1. Summary of *EPOR* Gene Mutations

Type of Mutation	Mutation	Structural Defect	Association with PFCP
Deletion (7bp)	Del5985-5991	Frameshift >ter truncation	Yes
Duplication (8bp)	5968-5975	Frameshift >ter truncation	Yes
Nonsense	G6002	Trp439 > ter truncation	Yes
Nonsense	5986C>T	Gln435 >ter truncation	Yes
Nonsense	5964C>G	Tyr426 >ter truncation	Yes
Nonsense	5881C>T	Glu399 >ter truncation	Yes
Nonsense	5959G>T	Glu425 >ter truncation	Yes
Insertion (G)	5974insG	Frameshift >ter truncation	Yes
Insertion (T)	5967insT	Frameshift >ter truncation	Yes
Substitution	6148C>T	Pro 488 > ser	No
Substitution	6146A>G	Asn487 > ser	No
Substitution	2706 A>T	Unknown	No

Abbreviations: PFCP, primary familial and congenital erythrocytosis; ser, serine; ter, termination codon.

Data from Kralovics R, Indrak K, Stopka T, et al. Two new EPO receptor mutations: truncated EPO receptors are most frequently associated with primary familial and congenital polycythemias. *Blood.* 1997 Sep 1;90(5):2057-2061.

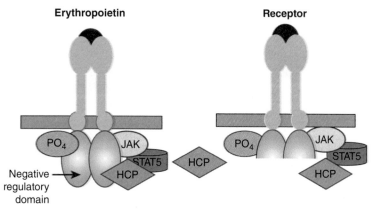

FIGURE 28–1. *Left panel,* Erythropoietin (EPO) binding to a normal EPO receptor results in interaction of a protein kinase (Janus kinase [JAK]) with the receptor. The interaction leads to phosphorylation of the receptor and initiates a cascade of signaling that ultimately results in erythroid progenitor proliferation and differentiation. This process is self-regulatory. Activated signal transduction molecules, hematopoietic cell phosphatase (Hcp) binds to the C-terminal of the erythropoietin receptor (EPOR), which is a negative regulatory domain. This interaction dephosporylates the receptor and turns off the signaling resulting in cessation of erythroid progenitor proliferation. *Right panel,* Patients with mutated gain-of-function *EPOR* gene lack the C-terminal portion of the receptor that contains the negative regulatory domain. EPO binds and the signal transduction pathway is activated by change of configuration of EPO receptor dimer, but because there is there is no structure for HCP to bind on the activated EPOR dimer, the receptor is left in the activated position, resulting in unbridled erythroid proliferation and an elevated red cell mass. PO_4, phosphate; STAT, signal transducer and activator of transcription.

pressure are constant and acclimatized individuals do not ventilate excessively, the normal sea-level gradient of about 60 mm Hg (torr) is only reduced to about 40 torr in Morococha at 4540 m (14,900 ft) above sea level.[76] Further reduction can be achieved, and at the top of Mount Everest, extreme hyperventilation reduces the gradient to less than 10 mm torr. A shift in the oxygen dissociation curve to the right, which represents decreased affinity of Hb for oxygen, may be of benefit for short-term high-altitude acclimatization,[77] but its usefulness for chronic acclimatization has probably been exaggerated.[78] In an unacclimated person exposed acutely to high altitude, hyperventilation alkalosis leads initially to a shift of the oxygen dissociation curve to the left, representing an increased affinity of Hb for oxygen, further worsening already present tissue hypoxia. The alkalosis and the hypoxia in turn promote red cell synthesis of 2,3-bisphosphoglycerate (2,3-BPG) and cause the oxygen dissociation curve to shift back to a normal or even right-shifted position (Chaps. 3 and 16). In chronic acclimatization, blood pH is slightly increased, and when this is taken into account, the

dissociation curve is shifted approximately to normal.[79] It is unlikely that a shift to the right would be to the advantage of high-altitude dwellers, except as a partial compensation for respiratory alkalosis.[80] In addition, a right-shifted curve also has a decrease in oxygen loading in the alveolar capillary, minimizing any net gain in offloading. There is a relationship between higher altitude and Hb concentration response, best studied among Andean highlanders and Europeans in the United States; Hb concentration is almost 10% higher in Andean highlanders living at 5500 m than in those living at 4355 m. Furthermore, native Andean high-altitude dwellers have a gradual increase in their Hb levels with age[81] and body weight.[82] Although it has been postulated that high Hb-oxygen affinity in the setting of extremely low ambient oxygen may be one such adaptive change,[83] increased Hb-oxygen affinity and increased fetal Hb are not adaptive phenotypes of Tibetan or Andean highlanders.[84]

In a subset of Andean high-altitude native dwellers, namely Quechuas and Aymaras, erythrocytosis becomes excessive and often results in chronic mountain sickness with its associated constitutional symptoms and pulmonary hypertension.[56,81] This excessive erythrocytosis, called Monge disease or chronic mountain sickness,[56,85] is also described in Han Chinese living in Tibet[86] and occurs in whites living at high altitudes.[87]

The erythrocytosis encountered in high-altitude dwellers is often considered to be a universal, uniform adaptation process to hypoxia that would arise in all normal individuals. In reality, there is marked variability in EPO level and subsequent erythrocytotic response to chronic hypoxia,[81,88] suggesting that some of these factors may be genetically determined; the same degree of hypoxia induces substantial differences in EPO production in response to high altitude.[83,89,90] Three distinct adaptations to high altitude appear to have evolved. Andean highlanders have higher oxygen saturation than Tibetans at the same altitudes.[83] Tibetans' mean resting ventilation and hypoxic ventilatory response are higher than those of Andean Aymaras, whereas the mean Tibetan Hb concentration is below the Andean mean. High levels of nitric oxide (NO) in the exhaled breath of Tibetans may represent increased physiological NO. This effect may improve oxygen delivery by inducing vasodilatation and increasing blood flow to tissues, thus making the compensatory increase in red cell volume unnecessary.[91] Another distinct successful pattern of human adaptation in high altitude dwellers

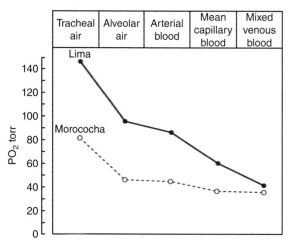

FIGURE 28–2. The oxygen gradient from atmospheric air to the tissues in individuals living at sea level and in Morococha, Peru, at 4540 m (14,900 ft) above sea level.

that contrasts with both the Andean "classic" (arterial hypoxemia with erythrocytosis) and Tibetan (arterial hypoxemia with normal venous Hb concentration) patterns evolved in Ethiopia. Although Ethiopian high-altitude dwellers have Hb concentrations that fall in the normal range (15.9 and 15.0 g/dL for males and females, respectively), they have a surprisingly, as yet unexplained high (average, 95.3%) oxygen saturation of Hb despite their hypoxic environment (reviewed by Beall[83]). Their cerebral circulation is increased but is insensitive to hypoxia, unlike Peruvian high-altitude dwellers.[92] Thus, Ethiopian highlanders maintain venous Hb concentrations and arterial oxygen saturation within the ranges of sea-level populations despite the decrease in ambient oxygen tension at high altitude.[93] Tibetans and Ethiopians have lived as mountain dwellers much longer than the Quechua or Aymara Indians,[94] suggesting that extreme elevation of red cell mass is a maladaptation which Tibetans avoided by evolving a more efficient, or less detrimental, compensatory mechanism than that which causes Monge disease.

With rapid advances in genomics, progress has been made in identification of the molecular basis of high-altitude adaptation; most of these advances have been in our understanding of Tibetan adaptation. Several studies reported evidence for positive natural selection in genomic regions in Tibetans; not surprisingly, most are haplotypes comprising genes that are components of hypoxia sensing that are mediated by HIFs (Chap. 3). Two of these selected regions include genes that have undergone the strongest genetic selection and are thus likely the most beneficial for Tibetan adaptation. These two regions encompass the *EPAS1* gene, encoding the α subunit of HIF2, and the *EGLN1* gene, encoding prolyl hydroxylase 2 (PHD2). PHD2 is the principal negative regulator of both HIF1 and HIF2. Both of these haplotypes were shown to be associated with differences in Hb concentration at high altitude by several independent studies.[95-97] Intriguingly, the *EPAS1* haplotype was previously identified as having the strongest Tibetan positive selection and was found to have an unusual haplotype structure that originated by introgression of DNA from Denisovan or Denisovan-related hominins.[98] Denisovans, a sister group to the Neanderthals, branched off from the human lineage perhaps 600,000 years ago,[99] and available evidence suggests that Denisovan and Neanderthal hominins contributed to the modern *Homo sapiens* admixture before their extinction, likely by interbreeding,[100] and that these hominin species provided genetic variations that helped humans adapt to new environments, such as extreme hypoxia associated with high altitude.[98] The first Tibetan adaptation gene mutation identified, which changes the encoded PHD2 protein within the selected haplotype, is a missense variant of the *EGLN1* gene, *c.12C>G*,[101] that is in near complete linkage disequilibrium with a previously reported missense variant, *EGLN1:c.380G>C*.[101] Both *EGLN1:c.[12C>G; 380G>C]* (PHD2^D4E,C127S) are in *cis* (ie, the constituting PHD-2^D4E,C127S locus). Analysis of Tibetans and related populations suggests that *12C>G* started on the *380G>C* variant that is not Tibetan specific,[101,102] that PHD2^D4E,C127S originated from a single individual about 8000 years ago,[102] and that now more than 80% of Tibetans carry this PHD2 variant.[102] Functional assessment of homozygous PHD2^D4E,C127S recombinant proteins showed that the variant protein has increased hydroxylase activity under hypoxic conditions. Furthermore, native homozygous PHD2^D4E,C127S erythroid progenitors have blunted erythropoietic responses to hypoxia by both EPO-specific and EPO-independent mechanisms.[102] Although this is the first identified variant that contributes to the molecular and cellular basis of Tibetan adaptation to high altitude, there are other evolutionarily selected genomic regions, and elucidation of their functional impact is, at the time of this writing, unknown.

Understanding the etiology of erythrocytosis of high altitude is made more complex by a study of inhabitants of the Peruvian mining community of Cerro de Pasco (altitude, 4280 m) with excessive erythrocytosis (mean Hct, 76%; range, 66%-91%). About half of individuals with an Hct greater than 75% had toxic serum cobalt levels,[40] suggesting that other erythropoiesis-promoting factors such as cobalt[103] can augment hypoxia induction of EPO, causing extreme erythrocytoses (Chap. 2). Most high-altitude dwellers do not have measurable levels or a history of exposure to cobalt or other heavy metals.[104]

Erythrocytosis of Pulmonary Disease

Degrees of arterial hypoxia comparable to those observed in individuals at high altitudes are observed in patients with right-to-left shunting caused by cardiac or intrapulmonary shunts or to ventilation defects, as in COPD.

Many patients with COPD are not erythrocytotic. This has been attributed to infections and inflammation often present in the lungs, resulting in anemia of chronic inflammation, and to an increase in plasma volume. Why some patients with lung disease and congenital heart disease develop erythrocytosis but others do not is not entirely clear.

Erythrocytosis of Eisenmenger Syndrome

Patients with right-to-left shunting (Eisenmenger syndrome) develop a degree of erythrocytosis comparable to that observed with similar degrees of desaturation at high altitudes.[105] The hematologic changes associated with this syndrome include hyperviscosity caused by erythrocytosis. Erythrocytosis is present in most patients, but excessive phlebotomy may cause microcytosis, and some have attributed this effect to the exacerbation of the symptoms of hyperviscosity.[30] In view of an increasing understanding of physiology of HIF regulation, it may not be the microcytosis per se that is detrimental but the induced iron deficiency that inhibits PHD2 and increases HIF, which then directly causes pulmonary vasoconstriction and enhanced pulmonary vascular pressure (Chaps. 2 and 3).

Obstructive Sleep Apnea–Induced Syndrome

In the colorfully named Pickwickian syndrome,[106] erythrocytosis is characterized by its association with extreme obesity and somnolence. Today, the more widely studied OSA is not always associated with obesity[107] but can, if severe, cause arterial hypoxemia, hypercapnia, and somnolence[108] but only rarely, if ever, secondary erythrocytosis.[26] The absence of erythrocytosis in OSA is likely mediated by marrow suppression by OSA-induced inflammatory cytokines and increased hepcidin, both suppressing erythropoiesis (Chap. 10).[109]

Smoker's Erythrocytosis

Heavy smoking results in the formation of carboxyhemoglobin, which does not transport oxygen (Chap. 11) and causes an increase in oxygen affinity of the remaining normal Hb. Carboxyhemoglobin increases in relationship to the number of cigarettes or cigars smoked each day (Table 28-2). This leads to tissue hypoxia, EPO production, and stimulation of red cell production.[110] Smoking may also cause a reduction in plasma volume.[111] Either augmentation of red cell mass or shrinkage of plasma volume could easily explain the rise in the Hct.

Erythrocytosis Secondary to High-Affinity Hemoglobins

Hbs with certain amino acid substitutions manifest an increased affinity for oxygen, producing tissue hypoxia and compensatory erythrocytosis (Chap. 18). Mutations affecting amino acids of the $\alpha_1\beta_2$ globin chain interface affect normal rotation within molecules and impair the rate of deoxygenation. Changes in the carboxyl terminal and penultimate amino acids also impair intramolecular motion and tend to keep molecules in a high-affinity state. Alterations in the amino acids lining the

TABLE 28–2. Blood Oxygen Capacity in Smokers with Erythrocytosis

Subject[a]	Hemoglobin (Hb) (g/dL)	Carboxy-Hemoglobin (COHb) (g/dL)	Hb-COHb (g/dL)	Affinity Correction (g/dL)	Adjusted Hb (g/dL)
Healthy male nonsmokers	16 (14-18)	0.16 (0.08-0.25)	15.8 (14-18)	0	16 (14.18)
Male smokers with increased Hb concentration	20 (17-23)	2 (1-3)	18 (16-21)	1.5 (0.5-2.0)	16.5 (15-19)

[a]The male smokers include 10 consecutive subjects studied with elevated hematocrit and no evidence for polycythemia vera. The hemoglobin available for O_2 binding in blood is the Hb-COHb. COHb also influences the residual hemoglobin to bind oxygen more tightly, making it less accessible to tissues. A correction for this effect has been calculated and is labeled *affinity correction*. The adjusted hemoglobin indicates the blood concentrations that would be present in the subjects in the absence of excess carbon monoxide. Thus, the blood hemoglobin in this group of smokers was increased by 3.5 g/dL on the average (from 16.5 [last column] to 20 [first column]) as a result of smoking-induced carboxyhemoglobinemia.

Data from Marshall A. Lichtman, MD.

central cavity of Hb destabilize the binding of 2,3-BPG in this cavity and lead to increased oxygen affinity (Chaps. 16 and 18). In addition, some heme pocket mutations interfere with deoxygenation. Most Hbs with a mutation involving amino acids in the heme pocket are unstable and are associated with hemolytic anemia and cyanosis. Inheritance of these disorders is autosomal dominant. High-affinity Hbs result from mutations in any of three globin genes; those from α-globin gene mutations are congenital and life-long. β-Globin gene mutations are not apparent at birth but manifest after fetal to adult Hb switching at approximately 6 months of life, whereas γ-globin gene mutations cause transient increase of Hb concentration at birth lasting only about 6 months.

Erythrocytosis Secondary to Red Cell Enzyme Deficiencies
Deficiencies of red cell enzymes in the early steps of glycolysis sometimes cause a marked decrease in the levels of 2,3-BPG (Chap. 16). Occasionally, mild erythrocytosis occurs in patients with methemoglobinemia because of cytochrome b_5 reductase (methemoglobin reductase) deficiency (Chap. 19).

The same pathophysiology as that seen in high-affinity hemoglobins is also exhibited in mutations of the *2,3-BPG* gene, resulting in low 2,3 BPG. Because these mutations are very rare, with only a single family comprehensively studied,[112] it is not clear if the mode of inheritance is recessive or dominant.

This condition, as well as other high-affinity hemoglobins, can only be conclusively confirmed by direct measurement of a Hb dissociation curve, conveniently expressed as the partial pressure of oxygen required to saturate 50% of Hb (p50 O_2); when equipment for this is not available, p50 can be estimated from pH, pO2 and Hb oxygen saturation of venous blood.[113,114]

Neonatal Erythrocytosis
Erythrocytosis at birth is a normal physiologic response to intrauterine hypoxia and to the high oxygen affinity of red cells containing very high proportions of Hb F (Chaps. 2 and 17). Hb F has a higher affinity for oxygen than does Hb A. The erythrocytosis may become excessive and even symptomatic, especially in infants of mothers with diabetes or if clamping of the cord is delayed, permitting placental blood to boost the blood volume of the infant.[115] Because it is difficult to recognize symptoms of hyperviscosity in neonates, many pediatricians perform a partial plasma exchange transfusion if the venous Hct is above 65% at birth.[116]

One study of 25,000 neonates in Utah[117] showed that the average Hct at birth would be considered "erythrocytotic" in adults but by

2 weeks later falls to "anemic" levels by a *neocytolysis* mechanism destruction of red blood cells (Chap. 2). This dramatic decrease of Hct in neonates during their first days of life contributes to neonatal jaundice (Chap. 2).[118]

INAPPROPRIATE ERYTHROCYTOSES
Chemically Induced Augmented Hypoxia Sensing by Cobalt and Manganese
Cobalt A number of chemicals have been suspected of causing histotoxic anoxia and secondary erythrocytosis, but the only elements with a predictable capacity to cause erythrocytosis are cobalt and manganese.[103] Cobalt administration increases EPO production by increasing HIFs (see later and Chaps. 2 and 3),[119] likely by inhibition of proline hydroxylase,[120] which increases HIF-1.[121]

Manganese In 1999, Bunn and Ebert demonstrated that manganese induces EPO[122] and that a manganese overdose results in erythrocytosis. The likely mechanism is blocking the negative HIFs regulator factor-inhibiting HIF (FIH) (Chap. 2) by manganese. This is expected to increase HIFs and is likely the principal molecular mechanism by which manganese causes erythrocytosis.[123]

CONGENITAL DISORDERS OF HYPOXIA SENSING
Chuvash Erythrocytosis (Polycythemia)
Chuvash erythrocytosis is the only known endemic congenital erythrocytosis. The condition is caused by an abnormality in the oxygen-sensing pathway and causes thrombotic and hemorrhagic vascular complications that lead to early mortality; survival beyond age 65 years is uncommon.[66,124] There is autosomal recessive inheritance, and affected patients tend to have normal blood gases, normal calculated p50, normal to increased EPO levels, absence of genetic linkage to *EPO* and *EPOR* loci, and no evidence of abnormal Hb.[124] In a study of five multiplex Chuvash families with Chuvash erythrocytosis, a homozygous mutation of the *VHL* gene (*598C>T*) (*VHL*[R200W]) was found in all affected individuals. This mutation impairs the interaction of pVHL with both HIF-1α and HIF-2α, thus reducing the rate of ubiquitin-mediated destruction of HIF-1α and HIF-2α (Chap. 2). As a result, the level of HIF-1 and HIF-2 heterodimers increases and leads to the increased expression of target genes, including the EPO, vascular endothelial growth factor (*VEGF*), and plasminogen activator inhibitor genes (*PAI-1*), among others.[4,5] The effect of this mutation on hypoxic sensing is depicted in Fig. 28-3.

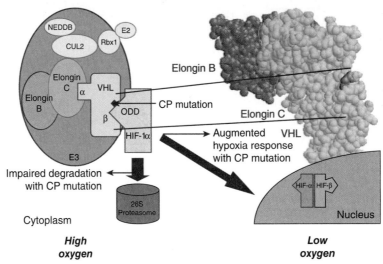

FIGURE 28–3. Elongins B, C, and proteins Rbx1, Cul2 E2, and NEDD 8 are interacting proteins that facilitate von Hippel Lindau (VHL) function. Interaction of mutated VHL protein with hypoxia-inducible factor (HIF)-1α. The Chuvash VHL mutation leads to the impaired interaction with HIF-1 and HIF-2αs, which results in impaired degradation in 26S proteasome and augmented hypoxia sensing. CP, Chuvash polycythemia.

The role of circulating EPO in the Chuvash erythrocytosis phenotype is indisputable. However, there must be other factors associated with the Chuvash erythrocytosis VHL mutation that contribute to the erythrocytotic phenotype because the erythroid progenitors of Chuvash erythrocytosis patients are hypersensitive in vitro to extrinsic EPO; the mechanism of this observation has not been fully explained.[4,5] Some but not all patients with other *VHL* mutations have EPO hypersensitive erythroid colonies[125-127]; in these patients, there is also increased expression of the *RUNX1* and *NFE1* genes, which can stimulate erythropoiesis.[6]

Despite increased expression of HIF-1α, HIF-2α, and VEGF in normoxia, patients with Chuvash erythrocytosis do not display a predisposition to tumor formation. Imaging studies of 33 patients with Chuvash erythrocytosis revealed unsuspected cerebral ischemic lesions in 45% but no tumors characteristic of VHL syndrome.[128] There also is a high prevalence of this disorder on the Italian island of Ischia.[68] The Chuvash *VHL*[R200W] mutation has also been described in whites in the United States and Europe and in people of Punjabi and Bangladeshi Asian ancestry.[129] Some patients with congenital erythrocytosis have proved to be compound heterozygotes for the *VHL*[R200W] mutation and other *VHL* mutations. Additionally, two distantly related Croatians with erythrocytosis are homozygous for *VHL*[H191D], the first example of a homozygous *VHL* germline mutation other than *VHL*[R200W] causing erythrocytosis.[69,75,130-134] Novel *VHL* mutations[135] were described that generate increased levels of a previously unrecognized cryptic *VHL* mRNA composed of a portion of intron 1 and exon 2. Increased levels of these transcripts were associated with either germline intronic mutations or synonymous germline mutations in exon 2, which facilitate alternative splicing that generates the aberrant RNA. Surprisingly, these changes were associated with either erythrocytosis or tumors, but not both, in the same family.

A small number of cases of congenital erythrocytosis that appear to have a mutation of only one *VHL* allele confound an obvious pathophysiological explanation. In a Ukrainian family, two children with erythrocytosis were heterozygotes for *VHL* 376G>T (D126Y), but the father with the same mutation was not erythrocytotic.[133] An English patient with erythrocytotic was a heterozygote for *VHL* 598C>T,[108] but the inheritance of the deletion of a *VHL* allele, or null *VHL* allele, in a trans position was not excluded. Subsequently, two erythrocytotic *VHL* heterozygous patients were described in whom a null VHL allele was

more rigorously excluded[130,131]; the molecular mechanism of their erythrocytotic phenotype remains to be elucidated.

To address the question of whether the *VHL* 598C>T substitution occurred in a single founder or resulted from recurrent mutational events, haplotype analysis of eight highly informative single nucleotide polymorphic markers covering 340 kb spanning the *VHL* gene was performed on 101 participants bearing the *VHL* 598C>T mutation and 447 normal unrelated individuals from Chuvash, Southeast Asian, European, Hispanic, and African American ethnic groups.[67] Polymorphism of the *VHL* locus in normal control participants (having a wild *VHL* 598C allele) and participant bearing Chuvash erythrocytosis *VHL* 598T were in strong linkage disequilibrium. These studies indicated that, in most individuals, the *VHL* 598C>T mutation arose in a single ancestor between 51,000 and 12,000 years ago. This observation was later extended to Afghan and Northern and Southern Indian populations.[136] However, this is not the case for a Turkish erythrocytotic family with a *VHL* 598C>T mutation wherein the *VHL* 598C>T mutation occurred independently.[131]

Chuvash erythrocytosis homozygotes have decreased survival because of thrombotic and hemorrhagic complications, mostly in the venous circulation,[128] and thus are under negative selection pressure. The high frequency of the mutation in some areas may be caused by random factors ("drift"), but it is also possible that propagation of the *VHL* 598C>T mutation is the result of a survival advantage for heterozygotes. Such an advantage might be related to a subtle improvement of iron metabolism, erythropoiesis, embryonic development, energy metabolism,[137] or some other as yet unknown effect. Indeed, heterozygotes were shown to be less likely to be anemic compared with control participants.[138] Another potential protective role of a mildly augmented hypoxic response is improved protection against bacterial infections because the hypoxia-mediated response has been reported to be essential for the bactericidal action of neutrophils.[139]

Classic von Hippel Lindau Syndrome

VHL syndrome is an autosomal dominant genetic abnormality affecting the posttranslational control of HIF-1α.[65,140,141] The syndrome is characterized by a propensity for developing renal cell carcinomas, retinal hemangioblastomas, cerebellar and spinal hemangioblastomas, pancreatic cysts, and pheochromocytomas. The tumors result

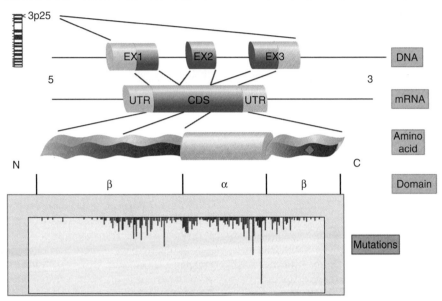

FIGURE 28–4. von Hippel Lindau (VHL) gene structure and mutation. Three exons of VHL genes are depicted encoding for UTR (untranslated portion of mRNA) and coding sequences (CDs). vHL domains β, α, β are shown. The relative number of reported VHL gene mutations are depicted in vertical lines. The location of the Chuvash polycythemia (CP) mutation is depicted by the *diamond*.

from a somatic mutation in addition to the germline mutation (ie, loss of heterozygosity). Erythrocytosis is not part of VHL syndrome, but hemangioblastomas of the central nervous system and less commonly pheochromocytoma and renal cancer have been associated with erythrocytosis mediated by paraneoplastic EPO production.[63] The schematic effect of the Chuvash erythrocytosis mutation in the context of other previously found *VHL* mutations is depicted in Fig. 28-4.

It is not clear why mutations of a single gene lead to these two diverse phenotypes. Quantitative differences in loss of activity could explain the variable phenotypes among *VHL* mutations,[142] but the *VHL* gene may also have other functions, possibly caused by interactions with other modifying factors, that can contribute to the onset of disease. These subtleties await future clarification. Another plausible explanation of erythrocytosis versus cancer predisposition syndrome is that almost all erythrocytotic subjects have germline mutations of both *VHL* alleles, but those with VHL cancer predisposition syndrome have only a single germline mutation and then acquire a somatic mutation that is essential for tumor genesis.

EGLN1 Gene Mutations, Proline Hydroxylase Deficiency

Another principal negative regulator of HIFs is PHD2 (encoded by the *EGLN1* gene), which targets the α-subunit of HIFs for degradation. The first loss-of-function mutation of PHD2 (PHD2[P317R]) was identified in a family in which heterozygotes had mild or borderline erythrocytosis.[143] Since then, many additional patients with unexplained erythrocytosis who are heterozygote carriers of different PHD2 mutations have been reported.[144] Almost all patients with PHD2-associated erythrocytosis have normal EPO levels. Whether the cause of erythrocytosis in this case is haploinsufficiency or a dominant negative effect remains to be determined.

EPAS1 (HIF-2α) Gain-of-Function Mutations

Affected patients have heterozygous missense mutations in the coding sequence of the *EPAS1* gene that encodes HIF-2α and typically have elevated EPO levels.[144,145] There is heterogeneity in these gain-of-function *HIF-2α* mutations, but their existence supports the critical role of HIF-2α in controlling the expression of EPO. Some patients with *EPAS1* mutations, similar to Chuvash erythrocytosis, have EPO

hypersensitive colonies, thus sharing features of both primary and secondary erythrocytoses.[126]

An explanation for the hypersensitivity of erythroid colonies bearing mutations that augment HIF stabilization remains to be discovered. It has been proposed that mutated VHL[R200W] protein hinders suppression of cytokine signaling SOCS1-mediated JAK2 degradation via binding of a negative regulator of erythropoiesis, SOCS1[146] to the extreme 3′ coding region of the *VHL* gene. Other observations are not consistent with this proposed mechanism: Another closely positioned VHL erythrocytosis mutation, *VHL*[H191D], is not associated with EPO hypersensitivity,[125] but other, more upstream, mutations such as *VHL*[P138L], are.[82] Furthermore, the hypersensitivity of erythroid colonies is also seen in some *HIF-2α* mutations.[88] Interestingly, in some but not all, of these families, upregulation of *NF–E2*, which enhances erythropoiesis, has been found.[6,147]

EPO Gene Mutations

A five-generation white family with autosomal dominant erythrocytosis when the propositus was 2 years old has been described. The propositus had moderately increased EPO levels, no splenomegaly, and normal leukocyte and platelet numbers.[148] His Hb oxygen dissociation curve was normal, and *HIF2A*, *HIF1A*, *EPOR*, *PHD2*, and *VHL* genes were ruled out as the cause. Exome sequencing of five affected individuals revealed a novel nucleotide change in chromosome 7 at -136nt upstream of the *EPO* gene (*EPO*-**136 G>A**) from the ATG translation initiation site. To determine the distribution of this variant and its segregation in seven affected and eight unaffected relatives, all eight unaffected relatives were negative for this *EPO* variant, but all seven affected individuals were heterozygous for this variant.[148] The mutated *EPO* cDNA introduced into the liver Hep3B EPO-producing cell line produced more *EPO* mRNA and protein when exposed to hypoxia than the liver cancer cell line transfected with wild *EPO* construct and did not generate aberrant *EPO* mRNA transcripts.[149] This mutated 5'UTR of *EPO* is a putative HIF2 binding site. Preliminary studies revealed that this mutation, *EPO*-**136 G>A**, augments interaction with HIF2, leading to increase production of EPO.[149]

In contrast, the molecular basis of erythrocytosis caused by EPO mutations was elucidated by an elegant study of the Norwegian family with autosomal dominant erythrocytosis in 2018. A genome-wide association study of this multigenerational family with the erythrocytosis phenotype segregated with the gene locus at the *EPO* gene. The exome sequencing of *EPO* revealed a single nucleotide G deletion of exon 2 causing a frameshift that would predict a loss of EPO function.[150] However, when this mutation was introduced to the liver cancer EPO-producing cell line, a peptide with biologically active EPO was produced in greater amounts than the cells transfected with wild-type cDNA. Further studies of the molecular basis revealed a complex mechanism for this observation. Two alternative *EPO* mRNA transcripts were detected. The novel transcript was found to originate from an alternative promoter in intron 1 of the *EPO* gene. The splicing mechanism of this nucleotide G deletion mutation eliminates the upstream *open reading frame* of the *EPO* gene, which inhibits translation, increasing the level of the mutant transcript. This converts an mRNA transcribed from an alternative promoter inside *EPO* intron 1 into an mRNA that produces larger amount of functional EPO protein with shortened signal peptide and a novel N-terminus.

These investigators then found a similar phenomenon in an unrelated erythrocytotic family with a deletion of nucleotide C in the same exon.[150]

Iron Responsive Protein 1 (IRP1) mutations The availability of iron is essential for normal erythropoiesis. Iron availability and erythropoiesis closely interact and this cross-regulation is indirectly mediated by hepcidin and erythroferrone (see Chap. 10). In addition, iron deficiency represses HIF-2a by the direct interaction of iron and HIF-2a (encoded by *EPAS1* gene). *EPAS1* contains at its 5′UTR an iron-responsive element (IRE) that binds to the iron-regulatory protein (IRP-1).[151] The mutations of this IRE can theoretically cause erythrocytosis but none as yet been reported.[152] However, the deletion of *Irp-1* causes erythrocytoses in mice.[153] Further, genome-wide association studies of a large number of individuals from Ireland and United Kingdom identified predicted loss-of-function mutations of *IRP-1* with elevated hemoglobin concentration and predicted gain-of-function mutations of *IRP-1* with anemia.[154]

Unexplained Congenital Erythrocytoses with Elevated or Inappropriately Normal Levels of Erythropoietin

The majority of patients with congenital erythrocytoses with inappropriately normal or elevated EPO levels do not have *VHL* mutations, *EGLN1*, *EPAS1*, *EPO* mutations, hemoglobinopathies, or 2,3-BPG deficiency, and the molecular basis of erythrocytosis in these cases remains to be elucidated. Some such families show dominant inheritance,[148] but in others, inheritance is recessive, and in some, it is sporadic. Lesions in genes linked to hypoxia independent regulation of HIF, oxygen-dependent gene regulation pathways, as well as EPO signaling, are leading candidates for mutation screening in erythrocytotic patients with normal or elevated EPO without *VHL*, *EGLN1*(proline hydroxylase 2), *EPAS1* (HIF2a), or EPO mutations.

Other Inappropriate Secondary Erythrocytoses

Renal Erythrocytosis and Post–Renal Transplant Erythrocytosis Absolute erythrocytosis has been observed in a considerable number of patients with solitary renal cysts, polycystic renal disease, or hydronephrosis. In most of these cases, EPO assays on cyst fluid, serum, or urine have disclosed the presence of EPO.[155] Patients with polycystic disease have an Hct value slightly higher than normal and definitely higher than would have been expected of patients with uremia. In some patients on prolonged dialysis treatment, cystic transformation occurs in the native kidneys. This acquired cystic disease is occasionally associated with marked erythrocytosis.[156]

In patients with pheochromocytoma or paraganglioma and erythrocytosis, EPO assays of serum and urine have disclosed higher-than-normal levels, and the erythrocytosis is most likely caused by excessive EPO secretion by the tumor. This assumption has been supported by the presence of *EPO* mRNA in tumor cells.[157] Wilms tumor[158] and paraganglioma[159] are also occasionally associated with an erythrocytosis. Many of these cases may have a somatic *VHL* gene mutation that, in combination with a germ line mutation of another allele, may constitute an unrecognized VHL syndrome. A patient with congenital erythrocytosis and recurrent paraganglioma with a PHD2 mutation was described. Tumor tissue exhibited a loss of heterozygosity of PHD2 in the tumor, suggesting that *PHD2* could be a tumor-suppressor gene.[45]

Partial obstruction of the renal artery would be expected to cause renal tissue hypoxia and a physiologic stimulation of EPO production. Nevertheless, it has proved quite difficult to induce erythrocytosis in laboratory animals by placing a Goldblatt clamp on the renal arteries.[160] Only a few of the many patients who have arteriosclerotic narrowing of the renal arteries have been reported to be erythrocytotic.[161]

Post–Renal Transplantation Erythrocytosis Although the full molecular basis of post–renal transplant erythrocytosis remains unknown, angiotensin II (Chaps. 2 and 3) plays an important role in its pathogenesis.[162] Increased activity of the angiotensin II–angiotensin receptor 1 pathway makes the erythroid progenitors hypersensitive to angiotensin II.[163,164] Furthermore, angiotensin II can modulate release of erythropoiesis stimulatory factors (Chap. 3), including EPO and IGF-1.[165,166] Studies of venous effluents have determined that the native rather than the transplanted kidneys are the source of the inappropriate production of EPO,[167] and in some patients, removal of the native kidneys has led to rapid restoration of normal Hct values.[168] The condition is rarely seen in patients with nonrenal solid-organ allografts. The role of angiotensin II in augmenting erythropoiesis was confirmed by anemia in angiotensin-converting enzyme knockout mice.[169] Before the late 1990s, when the use of angiotensin-converting enzyme inhibitors increased as a means to reduce proteinuria, the incidence of erythrocytosis in renal transplant patients was about 8% to 10% within the first 2 years after engraftment.

Erythrocytosis with Tumors of Various Tissues

Leiomyoma, Myoma, Myxoma, Hamartoma Occasionally, there is an association of erythrocytosis with large uterine myomas.[46] Usually, the tumor is huge, and extirpation results in a hematologic "cure." The suggestion that the tumor interferes with pulmonary ventilation has not been supported by the normal arterial blood gas findings in the few patients so studied. Another possible mechanism is that the large abdominal mass causes mechanical interference with the blood supply to the kidneys, resulting in renal hypoxia and EPO production. Inappropriate EPO secretion by smooth muscle cells has been demonstrated both in uterine myomas and in one case of cutaneous leiomyoma.[46,170] Rare cases of erythrocytosis attributed to a myxoma of the atrium,[47] hamartoma of the liver,[48] and focal hyperplasia of the liver[49] have been documented.

Brain Tumors In adequately studied patients with erythrocytosis and cerebellar hemangiomas, arterial blood gas tensions have been normal. That the tumors are directly responsible for the erythrocytosis can be surmised from the identification of EPO in cyst fluid and stromal cells and from a case in which *EPO* mRNA was present in the tumor.[171] Although in these cases a mutation of the *VHL* gene was not sought, it is likely that these tumors were a manifestation of an underlying VHL syndrome because cerebellar hemangiomas are an integral feature of VHL syndrome.

Hepatoma In 1958, McFadzean and coworkers reported that almost 10% of patients in Hong Kong with hepatocellular carcinoma developed erythrocytosis.[172] Since then, this association has been recognized as an important clinical clue in the diagnostic consideration of patients with liver disease.[173] The cause of erythrocytosis is probably inappropriate production of EPO by the neoplastic cells.[174] Normal hepatocytes and to a lesser degree nonparenchymal liver cells produce small amounts of EPO both constitutively and in response to hypoxia.

Endocrine Disorders (Chap. 7)

Congenital Erythrocytosis and Pheochromocytoma Pheochromocytomas have been described in association with congenital erythrocytosis.[175] In a growing number of reports, several individuals with congenital erythrocytosis have developed recurrent pheochromocytomas, paragangliomas, and sometimes somatostatinomas.[176-178] Some of these patients may also develop retinal and other ophthalmic pathology.[179] The tumors in these patients are heterozygous for gain-of-function mutations of the *EPAS1* gene (encoding HIF2-α) and *EPO*, and mutated *EPAS1* transcripts are present in tumor tissues as well as in the surrounding normal tissue (Chaps. 3 and 7). Although these tumors may occur in multiple tissues, they bear the same heterozygous mutations of the *EPAS1* gene. However, these mutations are only rarely found in leukocytes. Absence of a sufficient level of this mutation in the peripheral blood makes this syndrome particularly difficult to diagnose prior to the onset of syndrome-associated tumors. As expected, the extirpation of tumor does not cure erythrocytosis because EPO is also made by nontumor tissue. Thus, it appears that this syndrome is associated with postgonadal genetic mosaicism, wherein the *EPAS1* mutation is present in some cells in the tissue of some organs and predisposes to tumor development.[176-178] However, in one family, the *EPAS1* mutation was inherited as a germline mutation and thus detectable in the peripheral blood and was also associated with erythrocytosis in a mother and in her son and the development of recurrent pheochromocytomas and paragangliomas.[145]

Aldosterone-Producing Lesions Aldosterone-producing adenomas,[180] Bartter syndrome,[181] and dermoid cyst of the ovary[182] have been described in association with erythrocytosis. EPO levels were found to be elevated in the serum and returned to normal after extirpation of the tumors. A number of pathogenetic mechanisms have been suggested (Chaps. 3 and 7), including decreased plasma volume; mechanical interference with renal blood supply; hypertensive damage to renal parenchyma; functional interaction between aldosterone, renin, and EPO; and inappropriate secretion of EPO by the tumors. Mild erythrocytosis may be present in patients with Cushing syndrome, but its pathophysiological basis is not entirely clear (Chap. 7).

The erythropoietic effect of androgens is of considerable practical importance.[183] For many years, it was assumed that the higher red cell count in males was caused by androgens because the Hb levels of boys and girls were identical up until the time of puberty. It was not until pharmacologic doses of testosterone were administered to women with carcinoma of the breast that the full erythropoietic potency of androgens was appreciated.[184] Since then, various androgen preparations have been used in the treatment of refractory anemia, occasionally causing dramatic erythropoiesis, with Hb values climbing into the erythrocytosis range (Fig. 28-5).

Androgens The mechanism of androgen action on erythropoiesis appears to be complex, related both to their capacity to stimulate EPO production[185] and their capacity to induce differentiation of marrow stem cells directly.[183] These two effects have specific structural requirements. Whereas androgens with the 5α-H configuration stimulate renal and extrarenal EPO production, androgens with the 5β-H configuration enhance the differentiation of stem cells.[185] Testosterone administration is associated with an increase in EPO levels and a decrease in hepcidin levels.[186]

APPARENT (RELATIVE) ERYTHROCYTOSIS

Some believe that apparent erythrocytosis is merely a mild absolute erythrocytosis accentuated by a compensatory reduction in plasma volume.

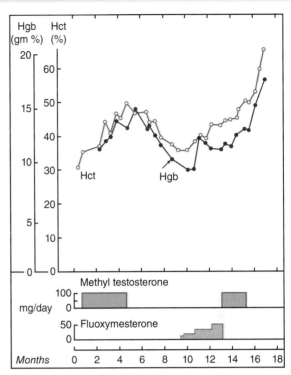

FIGURE 28–5. Erythropoietic response to testosterone derivatives in a patient with myelofibrosis. Hgb, hemoglobin; Hct, hematocrit.

Others suggest that it is caused by a primary reduction in plasma volume and have associated it with hypertension, obesity, and stress. When the red cell mass is documented to be normal, *spurious erythrocytosis* is also an appropriate term. Its clinical significance has also been disputed. The high Hct with its associated high viscosity is believed by some to be a risk factor heralding cerebral and cardiac complications, but others believe it is merely a well-tolerated anomaly. Because the designation *apparent erythrocytosis*[187] is noncommittal, it is used here.

The main clinical associations with apparent erythrocytosis are obesity, hypertension, and smoking. In obese patients, the finding of a normal red cell volume may be spurious because if the volume is expressed in terms of lean body weight, some of these patients would have a significant increase in red cell mass. In hypertensive patients, there is no adequate explanation for the apparent increase in red cell production or decrease in plasma volume. Sleep apnea (common in patients with congestive failure), excessive production of atrial natriuretic factor, increased adrenal activation, decreased aldosterone secretion, and hypoxic vasoconstriction are all factors that have been invoked[188-190] but with uncertainty. Chronic administration of diuretics to treat hypertension may be a more likely cause.[190]

● CLINICAL FEATURES

PRIMARY ERYTHROCYTOSES

For PV, refer to Chap. 83 in the 10th edition of *Williams Hematology*, 2021.

Primary Familial and Congenital Erythrocytosis

Although PFCP is uncommon, it is frequently misdiagnosed.[18] Unlike patients with PV, patients with PFCP lack splenomegaly, neutrophilia, basophilia, thrombocytosis, and a *JAK2* mutation. Unless exposed to alkylating agents or radioactive phosphorus, as many have been, these patients do not progress to acute leukemia or myelodysplastic syndrome.[191] Generally thought to be benign, this condition predisposes patients to severe cardiovascular problems perhaps caused by chronic augmented EPO signaling in all tissues bearing *EPOR*.[192,193] An increased incidence of cardiovascular disease has been observed in affected members of PFCP families.[194] Erythrocytosis may be very severe, with Hb levels that typically exceed 20 g/dL in men and 18 g/dL in women. Headaches are commonly present. Hypertension, coronary artery disease, and strokes have been reported but do not clearly appear to be related to an elevated Hct because they also occur in aggressively phlebotomized patients with normal Hct[195] and are not a constant feature of the disorder.[196]

SECONDARY CONGENITAL ERYTHROCYTOSES
Chuvash Erythrocytosis
The recessive erythrocytosis that is endemic in the Chuvash Autonomous Republic of the Russian Federation is characterized by an elevation of the Hb level to a mean of 22.6 g/L with a standard deviation of 1.4 g/L.[124] Some patients are symptomatic, with headache, fatigue hemorrhage, and peptic ulcer, and signs include clubbing. Chuvash erythrocytosis is also associated with thrombosis, relatively low blood pressure (also seen in heterozygotes), and varicose veins.[4,124,128] A matched cohort study of 155 Chuvash erythrocytosis adult and pediatric patients and 154 matched control participants was followed for a median of 11 years.[74] The details of children were reported separately with a median follow-up period of 9 years.[197] At enrollment, there was a history of 40 thrombotic events in 27 Chuvash erythrocytosis participants versus only in 3 of the control participants. During the prospective 11-year observation period, 37 new events occurred in 33 Chuvash erythrocytosis participants (9 of which were fatal), and 6 new events developed in 4 control participants. A history of therapeutic phlebotomy was associated with an increased risk of thrombosis in both univariate (hazard ratio, 2.0; $P = 0.004$) and multivariate analyses. This suggests that the thrombotic risk may be independent of elevated Hct and viscosity but rather related to the upregulated hypoxic responses associated with this congenital disorder.[74]

Because Chuvash erythrocytosis is characterized by a germline mutation in the *VHL* gene, it was expected that homozygotes for this mutation may develop certain vascular tumors similar to those associated with the classic VHL syndrome. However, tumors typical of the classic VHL syndrome, such as spinocerebellar hemangioblastomas, renal carcinomas, and pheochromocytomas/paragangliomas, were not found, indicating that increased expression of HIF1α and VEGF alone is not sufficient for tumorigenesis. Benign vertebral body hemangiomas (a distinct entity from hemangioblastoma) were found in significantly more patients with Chuvash erythrocytosis compared with control participants (55% vs 21%). Imaging studies of 33 Chuvash erythrocytosis patients revealed unsuspected cerebral ischemic lesions in 45% of patients.[128] Affected patients have elevated systolic pulmonary artery pressures as estimated by echocardiography compared to control participants, and iron deficiency associated with phlebotomy therapy may exacerbate this finding.[128]

EPAS1 (HIF-2α)
However, we studied a six-generation pedigree with dominantly inherited erythrocytosis/erythrocytosis and elevated EPO and identified a variant in *EPAS1* (c.1603A>G resulting in the missense change p.M535V in HIF2A). Over the past 2 decades, we observed a high rate of thrombotic complications (stroke, myocardial infarction, deep vein thrombosis, and Budd-Chiari syndrome).[74] Thrombotic complications occurred in five of eight participants with the p.M535V HIF2A variant compared to none of 17 HIF2A wild-type individuals. This suggests, that similar to Chuvash erythrocytosis and also erythrocytosis caused by a HIF-2α

gain-of-function mutation, the thrombotic risk may be independent of elevated Hct and viscosity and rather related to the upregulated hypoxic responses associated with these mutations.[74]

Other Congenital Disorders of Hypoxia Sensing
Because of their only recent discovery and apparent rarity, reliable clinical information about these disorders is lacking, but in view of their global deregulation of hypoxia sensing are also expected to have extra-erythroid manifestation(s). Most reports of these mutations have been in single individuals without long-term clinical follow-up.

SECONDARY ACQUIRED ERYTHROCYTOSIS
High-Altitude Erythrocytosis
Tolerance to high altitudes varies greatly, but most normal individuals have no discomfort at altitudes of up to 2130 m (7000 ft). Above this level, and especially if the ascent is rapid, some manifestations of cerebral hypoxia are common. Headaches, sleeplessness, and palpitations are frequently encountered, and weakness, nausea, vomiting, and mental dullness may be present. More severe manifestations include pulmonary and cerebral edema that may lead to death. Cheyne-Stokes respiration commonly occurs, especially during sleep. These symptoms constitute the syndrome of *acute mountain sickness*.[198]

Ruddy cyanosis and physiologic emphysema are the two characteristic features of some humans living at high altitudes. Venous and capillary engorgement can be observed readily in the conjunctiva, mucous membranes, and skin and may contribute to the remarkable capacity of Tibetan Sherpas to walk barefoot and sleep on ice and snow.[199] Asymptomatic retinal hemorrhages are seen frequently at high altitudes but rarely at altitudes of 3000 m (9000 ft) or less.[200] Splenomegaly and jaundice are unusual, although the sustained erythrocytosis is associated with an increased fractional rate of red cell destruction and bilirubin generation. It has been stated that Monge disease includes low fertility,[54,85] but this may not be universally so. High-altitude native resident Tibetans exhibit two distinct genotypes for increased oxygen affinity of Hb. Women with genotypes for high oxygen saturation have more surviving children.[201] This finding suggests that high altitude hypoxia is acting as an agent of natural selection on the locus for oxygen saturation of Hb by the mechanism of higher infant survival of Tibetan women with high oxygen saturation genotypes.[93,201-204]

Erythrocytosis Associated with Pulmonary Disease
The erythrocytosis associated with smoking is generally asymptomatic. There may be an increase in thrombotic events, but this may be caused by smoking rather than erythrocytosis.

When erythrocytosis is present in patients with COPD, with or without smoking, elevated Hct is associated with higher survival rates than anemic and normocythemic subjects.[19,20,204] Furthermore, moderate erythrocytosis has no adverse effect on vascular function in COPD[205] and is not associated with venous thromboembolism.[207]

Large studies of patients with Eisenmenger syndrome[30] and other patients with cyanotic heart disease[208] caution against routine phlebotomy for asymptomatic elevation of the Hct; in fact, thrombotic complications were not observed in these studies. Transgenic mice with extreme erythrocytosis (Hct 85%) caused by constitutive overexpression of EPO did not develop the expected thrombotic complications.[209] Adults with cyanotic congenital heart disease are at risk of having cerebrovascular events. This risk is increased in the presence of hypertension, atrial fibrillation, history of phlebotomy, and microcytosis, the latter condition having the strongest significance ($P < 0.005$). The authors of these findings endorsed a more conservative approach toward phlebotomy and more aggressive approach toward treating microcytosis with iron preparations in adults with cyanotic congenital heart disease.[210]

In a prospective cohort of United States military veteran outpatients with stable COPD ($n = 683$), erythrocytosis prevalence was low and, unlike anemia, had no association with worsened outcomes.[206]

Renal Erythrocytosis and Post–Renal Transplant Erythrocytosis

Although most patients with kidney failure are anemic, a fraction (often with polycystic kidney disease) displays erythrocytosis, which like the post–renal transplant state, can be very severe. Erythrocyte counts may be as high as 8×10^{12} cells/L and be associated with hypertension and congestive failure.[211] At higher Hct levels (usually >60 %), thrombotic events may complicate the clinical course.[60,61,212] Comorbidities that are associated with or causative of renal failure are frequently also factors predisposing to thrombosis, and the risk of erythrocytosis-associated thrombosis has not been submitted to rigorous multivariate rigorous statistical analyses. Thus, reports of increased thrombotic risks must be viewed with great caution.

Tumors

The erythrocytosis that occurs with EPO secreting tumors is generally mild,[171] and the predominating clinical manifestations are those of the tumor itself. Even moderate elevations to an Hct of 64% have been encountered without symptoms referable to the erythrocytosis.[49] Resection of the EPO-secreting tumor cures the associated erythrocytosis.[134]

In the syndrome of congenital erythrocytosis and pheochromocytoma or paraganglioma (see earlier description in the "Etiology" section), tumor resection does not lead to normalization of elevated Hct.

Neonatal Erythrocytosis

Of 55 infants with neonatal erythrocytosis, 85% had signs and symptoms attributed to this disorder. These included "feeding problems" (21.8%), plethora (20.0%), lethargy (14.5%), cyanosis (14.5%), respiratory distress (9.1%), jitteriness (7.3%), and hypotonia (7.3%). Other findings included hypoglycemia (40.0%) and hyperbilirubinemia (21.8%). In a larger group of nearly 1000 infants, six had intracranial hemorrhage,[115] but no thromboses were encountered.

●LABORATORY FEATURES

PRIMARY ERYTHROCYTOSIS

Primary Familial and Congenital Polycythemia/Erythrocytosis

Characteristic laboratory findings of PFCP are (1) increased red blood cell mass without increased leukocyte or platelet counts, (2) normal Hb-oxygen dissociation curve, (3) invariably low serum EPO levels, and (4) in vitro hypersensitivity of erythroid progenitors to EPO.[5] PFCP is often misdiagnosed as PV, although with the advent of a reliable polymerase chain reaction–based test for the $JAK2^{V617F}$ mutation, this should no longer ever happen. Whereas leukocytes are typically normal, platelet counts are often mildly decreased, presumably by dilution of the normal platelet mass by an often-dramatic increase of red cell and whole blood volumes. Some patients come to attention because of concurrent medical problems that may cause leukocytosis and secondary thrombocytosis, falsely suggesting the phenotype of PV.

Chuvash Erythrocytosis

Blood profiling in patients with Chuvash erythrocytosis indicates increased Hb and Hct and lower white blood cell and platelet counts than in controls. EPO ranges from normal (but never close to the lower limits of normal) to elevated, at times exceeding 10 times the mean normal value. In larger studies, Hb-adjusted serum EPO concentrations

were approximately 10-fold higher in *VHL* 598C>T homozygotes than in control participants.[4,5,128]

Affected subjects have lower CD4 counts, glucose and glucose and Hb A1c levels, elevated levels of both proinflammatory and antiinflammatory cytokines, and altered plasma thiol levels, with elevated homocysteine and glutathione and low cysteine concentrations compared to matched control participants.[213-215] Their serum PAI-1 and VEGF levels are also increased.[4,124,128] Circulating transferrin receptor levels are higher in Chuvash erythrocytosis homozygotes than in their unaffected relatives and spouses.[4,5,128] Ferritin-adjusted transferrin receptor concentrations were approximately threefold higher in *VHL* 598C>T homozygotes than in unaffected participants ($P < .0005$), which is consistent with upregulation by HIF-1.

Other Congenital Erythrocytoses from Augmented Hypoxia Sensing

At present, a paucity of data precludes any reliable description of other congenital erythrocytoses from augmented hypoxia sensing.

●SECONDARY ERYTHROCYTOSIS

Characteristically, only the number of erythrocytes in the blood is increased in secondary erythrocytosis. An increase in the leukocyte count, splenomegaly, or both may be present as features of the underlying disease, such as pulmonary infection in COPD with cor pulmonale or as seen in Monge's disease among Andean high-altitude dwellers or patients inheriting high-affinity Hb that is also unstable (Chaps. 2, 3, and 18).

●DIFFERENTIAL DIAGNOSIS

Also refer to Chaps. 2, 3, and 18; Table 28-3; and Fig. 28-6.

Distinguishing between PV and other polycythemic disorders used to be challenging, but discovery of the $JAK2^{V617F}$ and JAK2 exon 12 mutations has made it straightforward in most instances. Some of the clinical and laboratory features that can be helpful for differential diagnosis are summarized in Table 28-2 and in Fig. 28-6.

RED CELL MASS DETERMINATION

Determination of red cell mass is invaluable for differentiation of apparent (spurious) erythrocytosis from true erythrocytoses states. Unfortunately, determination of the red cell mass using radioisotopes is expensive and, when performed by the inexperienced, often inaccurate and furthermore, no longer generally available in United States. The carbon monoxide inhalation method is available in Europe but only in some research laboratories in the United States; this method is described in Chap. 2. Fortunately, in most cases, the diagnosis of PV and other true polycythemic states can be established with confidence without measuring the red cell mass.

ERYTHROID COLONY CULTURES

In vitro assays of erythroid progenitor cells permit the study of their responsiveness to EPO. This can be applied to PV and erythroid progenitor burst forming unit–erythroid (BFU-E) growth without added EPO,[216] referred to as "endogenous erythroid colonies." Detection of endogenous erythroid colonies in cultures of marrow or blood used to be the most specific test for PV.[68,217,218] In one study, all patients with PV, but none with secondary or other causes of erythrocytosis, had endogenous erythroid colonies.[219] EPO hypersensitive erythroid colonies are observed in PFCP, Chuvash erythrocytosis, and in a single studied

TABLE 28-3. VHL Mutations Associated with Congenital Erythrocytosis

VHL Genotype	Ethnicities	References	Clinical Features
235 C>T / 586 C>G	European	130	
598 C>T / 598 C>T	Chuvash, Danish, American (white), Bangladeshi, Pakistani, Russian, Turkish	130,131,133,134,254	Frequent thrombotic complications
598 C>T / 574 C>T	American (white)	133	
598 C>T / 562 C>G	American (white)	133	
598 C>T / 388 G>C	American (white)	134	
571 C>G / 571 C>G	Croatian	133	Failure to thrive
311 G>T / wildtype	German (?)	131	
376 G>T / wildtype	Ukranian	134	?VHL syndrome
598 C>T / wildtype	English, German	131	
523 A>G / wildtype	Portuguese	130	A-T patient
370 A.G/562 C.G	Native American	127	
376 G>A/376 G>A	Bangladeshi	255	Fatal pulmonary hypertension
413 C>T/413 C>T	Punjabi	126	

Abbreviation: A-T, ataxia-telangiectasia.

subject with the HIF-2α mutation,[220] but unlike the endogenous erythroid colonies of PV, these are abrogated by pretreatment with EPO and EPOR blocking antibodies.[6,221,222]

In experienced hands, endogenous erythroid colonies is a specific and sensitive means for detecting PV and may be useful in diagnosing patients with unusual presentations of PV, such as Budd-Chiari syndrome[223-226] wherein EPO levels may be normal or isolated thrombocytosis that may precede an eventual PV diagnosis.[227] However, this test has not been standardized, is expensive and laborious, and is generally only available in special laboratories.

ERYTHROPOIETIN LEVELS

All patients with PFCP encountered[75] have EPO below normal levels or below levels of detection. Thus, a low EPO level is not pathognomonic of PV because patients with PFCP have as low or even lower EPO levels.[18]

Because PV is distinguished by the fact that erythroid cells proliferate even in the absence of substantial levels of EPO, one would expect that at high Hct levels the production of EPO would be inhibited and serum levels consequently reduced. Older EPO assays were too insensitive to detect subnormal levels of EPO, but using improved technology, several studies have documented serum EPO levels below the normal reference range in patients with PV.[228-230] EPO levels remain low after phlebotomy in both PFCP and PV,[224] which increases EPO levels in normal individuals. However, EPO levels in Budd-Chiari syndrome in PV subjects may be normal or even increased.[231]

Patients with secondary erythrocytosis usually have normal to elevated EPO levels, which generally always increase after phlebotomies, although considerable overlap exists in the range of EPO levels.[229,232]

CLONALITY IN FEMALE SUBJECTS USING ASSAYS USING X-CHROMOSOME–BASED POLYMORPHISM ASSAYS

The principal role of the clonality assay is to differentiate PV with an incomplete phenotype or atypical presentation from idiopathic or as-yet undiagnosed erythrocytosis. PV results from an acquired mutation in a pluripotential hematopoietic stem/progenitor cell. Clonality studies based on the phenomenon of X-chromosome inactivation[233] have shown that red cells, granulocytes, platelets, monocytes, and B lymphocytes are all part of the clone.[234,235] The majority of T lymphocytes and natural killer cells are polyclonal, but a small proportion of these cells are also derived from the PV clone[236]; this is presumed to be due to the presence of long-lived normal T cells that preceded the development of the clone. Unfortunately, interpretation of publications on the applicability of X-chromosome inactivation for differential diagnosis of PV is hampered by the many methodologic and conceptual differences that have drawn conflicting conclusions.[237] Some discrepancies are due to the fact that two different approaches, which are not comparable, are used to distinguish the active from the inactive X-chromosome; one approach uses X-chromosome differential methylation,[238] typically using the polymorphic CAG repeat in the human androgen-receptor gene (*HUMARA*),[239] and the other approach uses more biologically sound but more technically demanding transcriptional analysis of the active X-chromosome.[238,240] Furthermore, the wide range of skewing of the X-chromosome allelic usage that is normally present[241] is often misinterpreted as clonality, and the potentially clonal myeloid cells are not compared with the polyclonal control cells of the same origin.[68] In a study of about 100 female PV patients, reticulocytes, platelets and granulocytes were always clonal, with the exception of a few patients who converted to polyclonal hematopoiesis after therapy with interferon-α.[68] Although it was previously reported that clonality assays based on X-chromosome inactivation are not suitable for studies of older women using the *HUMARA* assay,[242-244] that was not confirmed by studies using quantitative transcriptional analysis of active X-chromosomes.[245,246]

OTHER ERYTHROCYTOSES

Clinical history is of the utmost importance for the differential diagnosis of polycythemic states. Differentiation of an acquired from congenital disorder, and distinction between sporadic versus familial occurrence of erythrocytosis, when possible, will streamline the diagnosis. Thus, an autosomal dominant disorder is likely due to erythrocytosis from

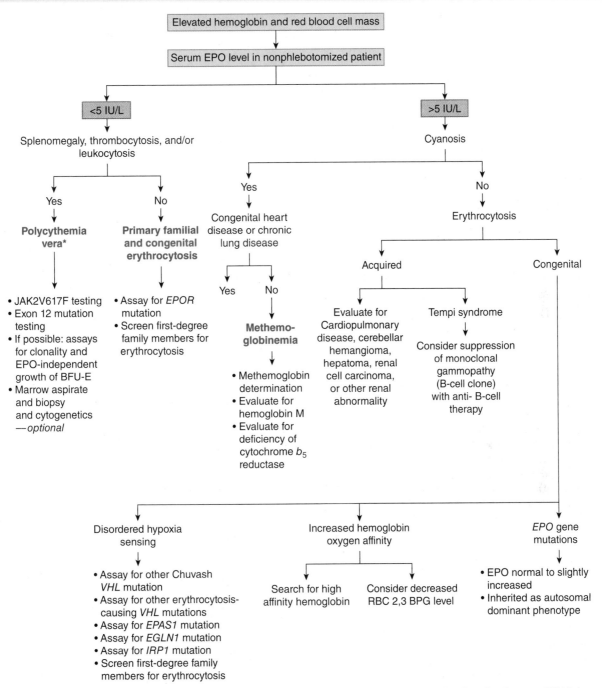

FIGURE 28–6. Diagnostic algorithm for polycythemia based on erythropoietin (EPO) level. 2,3-BPG, 2,3-bisphosphoglycerate; BFU-E, burst-forming unit–erythroid; *EPOR*, erythropoietin receptor gene; HIF2α, hypoxia-inducible factor 2α; encoded by *EPAS1* gene; PHD2, prolyl hydroxylase 2, encoded by *EGLN1* gene; *VHL*, von Hippel Lindau gene.

gain-of-function *EPOR*, *EPAS1* (HIF2a) or *EGLN1* (PHD2) mutations or a high-affinity Hb. Recessively inherited conditions may be caused by *VHL* gene mutations. Although rare patients with PV may have a history of other affected family members, PV is always an acquired condition. Many familial erythrocytoses are the result of yet-to-be-discovered genetic events.

Patients with a low level of EPO and autosomal dominant inheritance should have sequence analysis of the *EPOR* gene. This will define the defect in some patients with PFCP; if the erythrocytosis is acquired and present in multiple relatives, a diagnosis of familial clustering of PV should be pursued.[247] Patients with secondary erythrocytosis have

a genuine increase in the number of circulating erythrocytes and the red cell mass. Such patients do not typically have increased platelet or leukocyte counts or splenomegaly, which are often seen in PV. The lack of involvement of other cell lineages in hematopoietic proliferation should arouse suspicion that the patient may have erythrocytosis other than PV.

However, reactive thrombocytosis, leukocytosis, and splenomegaly may occasionally also be present in secondary erythrocytosis, which then renders the distinction from PV more difficult. In patients in whom secondary erythrocytosis is caused by lung or cardiac disease, clubbing is often present. In some cases, examination of arterial blood gases and arterial oxygen saturation or establishing presence of carboxyhemoglobin or methemoglobin (Chap. 19) will clarify the diagnosis, but modest arterial oxygen desaturation may also be present in PV.[105,248] Imaging of the kidneys may reveal a neoplasm or cyst in some patients. Determining the Hb oxygen dissociation curve (Chaps. 2, 3, 18, and 19) or estimation of p50 from venous blood[113] will detect abnormalities related to increased oxygen affinity either because of inheritance of a high affinity Hb (Chap. 18) or because of very rare 2,3-BPG depletion caused by phosphoglyceromutase deficiency (Chap. 16). The mild erythrocytosis associated with hereditary methemoglobinemia (Chap. 19) is often diagnosed because of frequent coexistent cyanosis.

In patients with elevated EPO or EPO levels inappropriately normal for the degree of Hb elevation, analysis of *VHL, EGLN1,* and *EPAS1* genes may be in order; some of these patients may have a history of autosomal recessive inheritance and have a typical history of congenital erythrocytosis. It may also be useful to determine the carboxyhemoglobin level of the blood if smoker's erythrocytosis is suspected.

SPURIOUS ERYTHROCYTOSIS

The erythrocytosis observed in patients with spurious erythrocytosis (apparent erythrocytosis, stress erythrocytosis) is the consequence of a decrease in plasma volume.[187] The observed erythrocytosis does not represent a true increase in the red cell mass. Usually, the increase in Hct is very modest. Such patients do not have an increased white blood cell count, thrombocytosis, splenomegaly, or *JAK2* mutation. The arterial oxygen study results are normal. Estimation of the red cell mass and plasma volume is required to establishing a diagnosis of spurious erythrocytosis. No treatment is required for individuals with chronic stress erythrocytosis, and fluids are all that is necessary for dehydrated individuals who present with acute increases in Hgb or Hct.

ERYTHROCYTOSES OTHER THAN POLYCYTHEMIA VERA

Treatment of patients with post–renal transplant erythrocytosis with drugs that suppress the renal–angiotensin system has virtually eliminated the need for therapeutic phlebotomy. The maximal reduction of Hb and Hct levels usually manifests by 6 months after starting therapy with either the angiotensin-converting enzyme inhibitor enalapril or the angiotensin II receptor type 1 blocker losartan.[162] Some patients are exquisitely sensitive and may become severely anemic.[249]

High-altitude erythrocytosis may be also associated with pulmonary hypertension, proteinuria, and elevated blood pressure. A prospective randomized trial of enalapril reported decreased Hb concentration, proteinuria and beneficial effects on elevated blood pressure.[250]

When erythrocytosis is secondary to a renal tumor or cyst, pheochromocytoma, myoma, or brain tumor, removal of the neoplasm usually results in disappearance of the erythrocytosis, but in the syndrome of congenital erythrocytosis with pheochromocytoma caused by *EPAS1* mutations (see earlier text on "Inappropriate Tissue Elaboration of Erythropoietin"), erythrocytosis persist after tumor resection.

No specific therapy is currently available for polycythemic subjects with *VHL, EGLN1,* or *EPAS1* mutations, but some may respond to JAK inhibitors.[249]

Lowering the Hct to a normal or near-normal level by phlebotomy is the common but empiric treatment of secondary erythrocytosis,[251,252] although it has not been proven to be beneficial.[30,208] The appropriate level is that at which the patient becomes asymptomatic. In most instances, no specific therapy is warranted unless specific therapy, such as that seen in EPO-secreting tumors or postrenal transplant erythrocytosis, is available. One should phlebotomize only those patients who are symptomatic from the elevated red cell mass and continue to do so cautiously only if symptoms respond promptly to phlebotomy.

COURSE AND PROGNOSIS

CHUVASH ERYTHROCYTOSIS

In one study, 96 patients with Chuvash erythrocytosis diagnosed before 1977 was compared with that of 65 spouses, and 79 community members of the same age, sex, and village of birth; the estimated survival to 65 years was 31% or less for Chuvash erythrocytosis patients versus 67% or more for spouses and community members ($P \leq 0.002$).[74,128,253] However, in the updated follow-up,[74] as discussed earlier under "Clinical Features" section, phlebotomy therapy was found to be detrimental. It remains to be seen if the anecdotal reports of benefit from JAK2 inhibitors[249] are confirmed by more evidence. The use of HIF inhibitors appears to be rational approach to the therapy of this and other congenital disorders of upregulation of the hypoxia sensing pathway, but at this time no such data exist.

OTHER ERYTHROCYTOSES

The clinical course of secondary erythrocytosis is largely a function of the underlying disorder. In patients with PFCP secondary to mutations of the *EPOR* gene, coronary artery disease and strokes have been reported[195] but not in all series.[196] The rarity of patients having mutations of the *EPO, EPOR, EGLN1,* and *EPAS1* genes and erythrocytoses from globin mutations and or red cell enzyme deficiencies precludes any meaningful prognostic evaluation.

REFERENCES

1. Juvonen E, Ikkala E, Fyhrquist F, et al. Autosomal dominant erythrocytosis caused by increased sensitivity to erythropoietin. *Blood.* 1991;78:3066.
2. Perrine GM, Prchal JT, Prchal JF. Study of a polycythemic family. *Blood.* 199750:134.
3. Prchal JT, Crist WM, Goldwasser E, et al. Autosomal dominant polycythemia. *Blood.* 1985;66:1208.
4. Ang SO, Chen H, Gordeuk VR, et al. Endemic polycythemia in Russia: mutation in the VHL gene. *Blood Cells Mol Dis.* 2002;28:57.
5. Ang SO, Chen H, Hirota K, et al. Disruption of oxygen homeostasis underlies congenital Chuvash polycythemia. *Nat Genet.* 2002;32:614.
6. Kapralova K, Lanikova L, Lorenzo F, et al. RUNX1 and NF-E2 upregulation is not specific for MPNs, but is seen in polycythemic disorders with augmented HIF signaling. *Blood.* 2014;123:391.
7. Prchal JT, Gregg XT. Erythropoiesis—genetic abnormalities. In: Graham, M, Foote MA, Elliott SD, eds. *Erythropoietins and Erythropoiesis.* 2nd ed. Birkhäuer-Verlag AG; 2009:61.
8. Bert P. *La Pression Barometrique.* Bailliere; 1878.
9. Jourdanet D. *De l'anemie des altitudes et de l'anemie en general dans ses rapports avec la pression l'atmorphere.* Bailliere; 1863.
10. Viault F. Sur l'augmentation considerable du nombre des globules rouges dans le sang chez les habitants des hauts plateaux de l'Amerique du Sud. *CR Acad Sci.* 1890;111:917.
11. Erslev AJ. Blood and Mountains. In: Wintrobe MM, ed. *Blood, Pure and Eloquent.* McGraw-Hill; 1980.
12. Leopold SS. The etiology of pulmonary arteriosclerosis (Ayerza's syndrome). *Am J Med.* 1950;219:152.
13. Abbott ME. *Atlas of Congenital Heart Disease.* American Heart Association; 1936.
14. Burwell CS, Robin, ED Whaley, RD, Bickelman, AG. Extreme obesity associated with alveolar hypoventilation: a Pickwickian syndrome. *Am J Med.* 1956;21:811.
15. Charache S, Weatherall DJ, Clegg JB. Polycythemia associated with a hemoglobinopathy. *J Clin Invest.* 1966;45:813.
16. Fairbanks VF, Klee GG, Wiseman GA, et al. Measurement of blood volume and red cell mass: re-examination of 51Cr and 125I methods. *Blood Cells Mol Dis.* 1996;22:169.
17. Lawrence JH, Berlin NI. Relative polycythemia—the polycythemia of stress. *Yale J Biol Med.* 1952;24:498.
18. Prchal JT. Classification and molecular biology of polycythemias (erythrocytoses) and thrombocytosis. *Hematol Oncol Clin North Am.* 2003;17:1151.
19. Chambellan A, Chailleux E, Similowski T, et al. Prognostic value of the hematocrit in patients with severe COPD receiving long-term oxygen therapy. *Chest.* 2005;128:1201.
20. Kollert F, Tippelt A, Muller C, et al. Hemoglobin levels above anemia thresholds are maximally predictive for long-term survival in COPD with chronic respiratory failure. *Respiratory care.* 2013;58:1204.

21. Hoffstein V, Mateika S. Differences in abdominal and neck circumferences in patients with and without obstructive sleep apnoea. *Eur Respir J.* 1992;5:377.

22. Carlson JT, Hedner J, Fagerberg B, et al. Secondary polycythaemia associated with nocturnal apnoea—a relationship not mediated by erythropoietin? *J Intern Med.* 1992;231:381.

23. Choi JB, Loredo JS, Norman D, et al. Does obstructive sleep apnea increase hematocrit? *Sleep Breath.* 2006;10:155.

24. Solmaz S, Duksal F, Ganidagli S. Is obstructive sleep apnoea syndrome really one of the causes of secondary polycythaemia? *Hematology.* 2015;20(2):108-111.

25. King AJ, Eyre T, Littlewood T. Obstructive sleep apnoea does not lead to clinically significant erythrocytosis. *BMJ.* 2013;347:f7340.

26. Gangaraju R, Sundar KM, Song J, et al. Polycythemia is rarely caused by obstructive sleep apnea. *Blood.* 2016;128:2444.

27. Song J, Sundar KM, Horvathova M, et al. Normal hemoglobin concentrations in obstructive sleep apnea and associated neocytolysis-mediated hemolysis and inflammation mediated suppression of expected elevated hemoglobin. *Blood.* 2019;3507.

28. Kung CM, Wang HL, Tseng ZL. Cigarette smoking exacerbates health problems in young men. *Clin Invest Med.* 2008;31:E138.

29. Bento C, Almeida H, Maia TM, et al. Molecular study of congenital erythrocytosis in 70 unrelated patients revealed a potential causal mutation in less than half of the cases (Where is/are the missing gene(s)?). *Eur J Haematol.* 2013;91:361.

30. Vongpatanasin W, Brickner ME, Hillis LD, et al. The Eisenmenger syndrome in adults. *Ann Intern Med.* 1998;128:745.

31. Gordeuk VR, Key NS, Prchal JT. Re-evaluation of hematocrit as a determinant of thrombotic risk in erythrocytosis. *Haematologica.* 2019;104:653.

32. Plotz CM, Knowlton AI, Ragan C. The natural history of Cushing's syndrome. *Am J Med.* 1952;13:597.

33. Mann DL, Gallagher NI, Donati RM. Erythrocytosis and primary aldosteronism. *Ann Intern Med.* 1967;66:335.

34. Erkelens DW, Statius van Eps LW. Bartter's syndrome and erythrocytosis. *Am J Med.* 1973;55:711.

35. Ponce OJ, Spencer-Bonilla G, Alvarez-Villalobos N, et al. The efficacy and adverse events of testosterone replacement therapy in hypogonadal men: a systematic review and meta-analysis of randomized, placebo-controlled trials. *J Clin Endocrinol Metab.* 2018, in press.

36. Waltner K. Kobalt und blut. *Klinische Wochenschrift.* 1929;8:313.

37. Berlin NI. The polycythemia produced in the rat by cobalt. *Acta Haematol.* 1951;5:30.

38. Mercier G, Patry G. Quebec beer-drinkers' cardiomyopathy: clinical signs and symptoms. *Can Med Assoc J.* 1967;97:884.

39. Thorling EB. A comparison of the cobalt, methylene blue, zinc, arsenite and amino triazole effect on erythropoietin production. *Br J Haematol.* 1973;25:55.

40. Jefferson JA, Escudero E, Hurtado ME, et al. Excessive erythrocytosis, chronic mountain sickness, and serum cobalt levels. *Lancet.* 2002;359:407.

41. Sanz Pérez MI, Rico Villoras AM, Moreno Velasco A, et al. Heart transplant secondary to cobalt toxicity after hip arthroplasty revision. *HIP Int.* 2019;29:NP1.

42. Hopfer SM, Sunderman FW Jr. Manganese inhibition of nickel subsulfide induction of erythrocytosis in rats. *Res Commun Chem Pathol Pharmacol.* 1978;19:337.

43. Tuschl K, Mills PB, Parsons H, et al. Hepatic cirrhosis, dystonia, polycythaemia and hypermanganesaemia—a new metabolic disorder. *J Inherit Metab Dis.* 2008;31:151.

44. Thorling EB. Paraneoplastic erythrocytosis and inappropriate erythropoietin production. A review. *Scand J Haematol.* 1972;17:1.

45. Ladroue C, Carcenac R, Leporrier M, et al. PHD2 mutation and congenital erythrocytosis with paraganglioma. *N Engl J Med.* 2008;359:2685.

46. LevGur M, Levie MD. The myomatous erythrocytosis syndrome: a review. *Obstetrics and gynecology.* 1995;86:1026.

47. Levinson JP, Kincaid OW. Myxoma of the right atrium associated with polycythemia. Report of successful excision. *N Engl J Med.* 1961;264:1187.

48. Josephs BN, Robbins G, Levine A. Polycythemia secondary to hamartoma of the liver. *JAMA.* 1961;179:867.

49. Sandler A, Rivlin L, Filler R, et al. Polycythemia secondary to focal nodular hyperplasia. *J Pediatr Surg.* 1997;32:1386.

50. Constans JP, Meder F, Maiuri F, et al. Posterior fossa hemangioblastomas. *Surg Neurol.* 1986;25:269.

51. Sharma RR, Cast IP, O'Brien S. Supratentorial haemangioblastoma not associated with Von Hippel Lindau complex or polycythaemia: case report and literature review. *Br J Neurosurg.* 1995;9:81.

52. Sykes DB, Schroyens W, O'Connell C. The TEMPI syndrome—a novel multisystem disease. N Engl J Med. 2011;365(5):475-477. doi:10.1056/NEJMc1106670

53. Sykes DB, O'Connell C, Schroyens W. The TEMPI syndrome. Blood. 2020;135(15):1199-1203. doi:10.1182/blood.2019004216

54. Morkeberg J. Blood manipulation: current challenges from an anti-doping perspective. *Hematology Am Soc Hematol Educ Program.* 2013;2013:627.

55. Chen ZY, Asavaritikrai P, Prchal JT, et al. Endogenous erythropoietin signaling is required for normal neural progenitor cell proliferation. *J Biol Chem.* 2007;282:25875.

56. Monge CC. Life in the Andes and chronic mountain sickness. *Science.* 1942;95:79.

57. Stembridge M, Williams AM, Gasho C, et al. The overlooked significance of plasma volume for successful adaptation to high altitude in Sherpa and Andean natives. *Proc Natl Acad Sci U S A.* 2019;116:16177.

58. Beutler E, Waalen J. The definition of anemia: what is the lower limit of normal of the blood hemoglobin concentration? *Blood.* 2006;107:1747.

59. Gassmann M, Mairbäurl H, Livshits L, et al. The increase in hemoglobin concentration with altitude varies among human populations. *Ann N Y Acad Sci.* 2019;1450:204.

60. Staub K, Haeusler M, Bender N, et al. Hemoglobin concentration of young men at residential altitudes between 200 and 2000m mirrors Switzerland's topography. *Blood.* 2020;135(13):1066-1069.

61. Dagher FJ, Ramos E, Erslev AJ, et al. Are the native kidneys responsible for erythrocytosis in renal allorecipients? *Transplantation.* 1979;28:496.

62. Kessler M, Hestin D, Mayeux D, et al. Factors predisposing to post-renal transplant erythrocytosis. A prospective matched-pair control study. *Clin Nephrol.* 1996;45:83.

63. Gaston RS, Julian BA, Curtis JJ. Posttransplant erythrocytosis: an enigma revisited. *Am J Kidney Dis.* 1994;24:1.

64. Gaston RS, Julian BA, Curtis JJ. Posttransplant erythrocytosis: an enigma revisited. *Am J Kidney Dis.* 1994;24:1.

65. Krieg M, Marti HH, Plate KH. Coexpression of erythropoietin and vascular endothelial growth factor in nervous system tumors associated with von Hippel-Lindau tumor suppressor gene loss of function. *Blood.* 1998;92:3388.

66. Polyakova LA. Familial erythrocytosis among inhabitants of the Chuvash ASSR. *Probl Gematol.* 1974;10:30.

67. Liu E, Percy MJ, Amos CI, et al. The worldwide distribution of the VHL 598C>T mutation indicates a single founding event. *Blood.* 2004;103:1937.

68. Liu E, Jelinek J, Pastore YD, et al. Discrimination of polycythemias and thrombocytoses by novel, simple, accurate clonality assays and comparison with PRV-1 expression and BFU-E response to erythropoietin. *Blood.* 2003;101:3294.

69. Percy MJ, Beard ME, Carter C, et al. Erythrocytosis and the Chuvash von Hippel-Lindau mutation. *Br J Haematol.* 2003;123:371.

70. Perrotta S, Nobili B, Ferraro M, et al. Von Hippel-Lindau-dependent polycythemia is endemic on the island of Ischia: identification of a novel cluster. *Blood.* 2006;107:514.

71. Mallik N, Sharma P, Kaur Hira J, et al. Genetic basis of unexplained erythrocytosis in Indian patients. *Eur J Haematol.* 2019;103:124.

72. Pasquier F, Marty C, Balligand T, et al. New pathogenic mechanisms induced by germline erythropoietin receptor mutations in primary erythrocytosis. *Haematologica.* 2018;103:575.

73. Chetty KG, Light RW, Stansbury DW, et al. Exercise performance of polycythemic chronic obstructive pulmonary disease patients. Effect of phlebotomies. *Chest.* 1990;98:1073.

74. Gordeuk VR, Miasnikova GY, Sergueeva AI, et al. Thrombotic risk in congenital erythrocytosis due to up-regulated hypoxia sensing is not associated with elevated hematocrit. *Haematologica.* 2019;2019.216267.

75. Gordeuk VR, Stockton DW, Prchal JT. Congenital polycythemias/erythrocytoses. *Haematologica.* 2005;90:109.

76. Hurtado A. Acclimatization of high altitudes. In: Weihe WH, ed. *Physiological Effects of High Altitude.* Macmillan; 1964.

77. Moore LG, Brewer GJ. Beneficial effect of rightward hemoglobin-oxygen dissociation curve shift for short-term high-altitude adaptation. *J Lab Clin Med.* 1981;98:145.

78. Finch CA, Lenfant C. Oxygen transport in man. *N Engl J Med.* 1972;286:407.

79. Winslow RM, Monge CC, Statham NJ, et al. Variability of oxygen affinity of blood: human subjects native to high altitude. *J Appl Physiol Respir Environ Exerc Physiol.* 1981;51:1411.

80. Eaton JW, Skelton TD, Berger E. Survival at extreme altitude: protective effect of increased hemoglobin-oxygen affinity. *Science.* 1974;183:743.

81. Leon-Velarde F, Gamboa A, Chuquiza JA, et al. Hematological parameters in high altitude residents living at 4,355, 4,660, and 5,500 meters above sea level. *High Alt Med Biol.* 2000;1:97.

82. Mejia OM, Prchal JT, Leon-Velarde F, et al. Genetic association analysis of chronic mountain sickness in an Andean high-altitude population. *Haematologica.* 2005;90:13.

83. Beall CM. Two routes to functional adaptation: Tibetan and Andean high-altitude natives. *Proc Natl Acad Sci USA.* 2007;104(suppl 1):8655.

84. Tashi T, Feng T, Koul P, et al. High altitude genetic adaptation in Tibetans: no role of increased hemoglobin-oxygen affinity. *Blood Cells Mol Dis.* 2014;53:27.

85. Maignan M, Rivera-Ch M, Privat C, et al. Pulmonary pressure and cardiac function in chronic mountain sickness patients. *Chest.* 2009;135:499.

86. Wu TY, Ding SQ, Liu JL, et al. Who should not go high: chronic disease and work at altitude during construction of the Qinghai-Tibet railroad. *High Alt Med Biol.* 2007;8:88.

87. Winslow RM, Monge CC. *Hypoxia, Polycythemia and Chronic Mountain Sickness.* Johns Hopkins University Press; 1987.

88. Chapman RF, Stray-Gundersen J, Levine BD. Epo production at altitude in elite endurance athletes is not associated with the sea level hypoxic ventilatory response. *J Sci Med Sport.* 2010;13:624.

89. Winslow RM, Chapman KW, Gibson CC, et al. Different hematologic responses to hypoxia in Sherpas and Quechua Indians. *J Appl Physiol Respir Environ Exerc Physiol.* 1989;66:1561.

90. Zhou ZN, Zhuang JG, Wu XF, et al. Tibetans retained innate ability resistance to acute hypoxia after long period of residing at sea level. *J Physiol Sci.* 2008;58:167.

91. Beall CM, Laskowski D, Erzurum SC. Nitric oxide in adaptation to altitude. *Free Radic Biol Med.* 2012;52:1123.

92. Claydon VE, Gulli G, Slessarev M, et al. Cerebrovascular responses to hypoxia and hypocapnia in Ethiopian high altitude dwellers. *Stroke.* 2008;39:336.

93. Beall CM. High-altitude adaptations. *Lancet.* 2003;362(suppl):S14.

94. Zhou D, Udpa N, Ronen R, et al. Whole-genome sequencing uncovers the genetic basis of chronic mountain sickness in Andean highlanders. *Am J Hum Genet.* 2013;93:452.

95. Simonson TS, Yang Y, Huff CD, et al. Genetic evidence for high-altitude adaptation in Tibet. *Science* 2010;329:72.

96. Yi X, Liang Y, Huerta-Sanchez E, et al. Sequencing of 50 human exomes reveals adaptation to high altitude. *Science*. 2010;329:75.

97. Beall CM, Cavalleri GL, Deng L, et al. Natural selection on EPAS1 (HIF2alpha) associated with low hemoglobin concentration in Tibetan highlanders. *Proc Natl Acad Sci U S A*. 2010;107:11459.

98. Huerta-Sanchez E, Jin X, Asan, et al. Altitude adaptation in Tibetans caused by introgression of Denisovan-like DNA. *Nature*. 2014;512:194.

99. Krause J, Fu Q, Good JM, et al. The complete mitochondrial DNA genome of an unknown hominin from southern Siberia. *Nature*. 2010;464:894.

100. Abi-Rached L, Jobin MJ, Kulkarni S, et al. The shaping of modern human immune systems by multiregional admixture with archaic humans. *Science*. 2011;334:89.

101. Lorenzo FR, Rili G, Simonson T, et al. A novel PHD2 mutation associated with Tibetan genetic adaptation to high altitude hypoxia. *ASH 52nd Annual Meeting*. Orlando, FL; 2010.

102. Lorenzo FR, Huff C, Myllymaki M, et al. A genetic mechanism for Tibetan high-altitude adaptation. *Nat Genet*. 2014;46(9):951-956.

103. Goldwasser E, Jacobson LO, Fried W, et al. Mechanism of the erythropoietic effect of cobalt. *Science*. 1957;125:1085.

104. Bernardi L, Roach RC, Keyl C, et al. Ventilation, autonomic function, sleep and erythropoietin. Chronic mountain sickness of Andean natives. *Adv Exp Med Biol*. 2003;543:161.

105. Murray JF. Classification of polycythemic disorders. With comments on the diagnostic value of arterial blood oxygen analysis. *Ann Intern Med*. 1966;64:892.

106. Kuhl W. History of clinical research on the sleep apnea syndrome. The early days of polysomnography. *Respiration*. 1997;64(suppl 1):5.

107. Block AJ, Boysen PG, Wynne JW, et al. Sleep apnea, hypopnea and oxygen desaturation in normal subjects. A strong male predominance. *N Engl J Med*. 1979;300:513.

108. Moore-Gillon JC, Treacher DF, Gaminara EJ, et al. Intermittent hypoxia in patients with unexplained polycythaemia. *Br Med J*. 1986;293:588.

109. Song J, Sundar KM, Horvathova M, et al. Normal hemoglobin concentrations in obstructive sleep apnea and associated neocytolysis-mediated hemolysis and inflammation mediated suppression of expected elevated hemoglobin. *Blood*. 2019;134:3507.

110. Smith JR, Landaw SA. Smokers' polycythemia. *N Engl J Med*. 1978;298:6.

111. Stonesifer LD. How carbon monoxide reduces plasma volume. *N Engl J Med*. 1978;299:311.

112. Cartier P, Labie D, Leroux JP, et al. [Familial diphosphoglycerate mutase deficiency: hematological and biochemical study]. *Nouv Rev Fr Hematol*. 1972;12:269.

113. Lichtman MA, Murphy MS, Adamson JW. Detection of mutant hemoglobins with altered affinity for oxygen. A simplified technique. *Ann Intern Med*. 1976;84:517.

114. Agarwal N, Mojica-Henshaw MP, Simmons ED, et al. Familial polycythemia caused by a novel mutation in the beta globin gene: essential role of P50 in evaluation of familial polycythemia. *Int J Med Sci*. 2007;4:232.

115. Wiswell TE, Cornish JD, Northam RS. Neonatal polycythemia: frequency of clinical manifestations and other associated findings. *Pediatrics*. 1986;78:26.

116. Black VD, Lubchenco LO, Koops BL, et al. Neonatal hyperviscosity: randomized study of effect of partial plasma exchange transfusion on long-term outcome. *Pediatrics*. 1985;75:1048.

117. Jopling J, Henry E, Wiedmeier SE, et al. Reference ranges for hematocrit and blood hemoglobin concentration during the neonatal period: data from a multihospital health care system. *Pediatrics*. 2009;123:e333.

118. Christensen RD, Lambert DK, Henry E, et al. Unexplained extreme hyperbilirubinemia among neonates in a multihospital healthcare system. *Blood Cells Mol Dis*. 2013;50:105.

119. Xia W, Huang T, Sun Y, et al. Identification of chemical compounds that induce HIF-1 alpha activity. *Toxicol Sci*. 2009;112(1):153-163.

120. Smith RJ, Fisher JW. Effects of cobalt on the renal erythropoietic factor and kidney hydrolase activity in the rat. *Blood*. 1973;42:893.

121. Wang GL, Semenza GL. Desferrioxamine induces erythropoietin gene expression and hypoxia-inducible factor 1 DNA-binding activity: implications for models of hypoxia signal transduction. *Blood*. 1993;82:3610.

122. Ebert BL, Bunn HF. Regulation of the erythropoietin gene. *Blood*. 1999;94:1864.

123. Fandrey J, Gorr TA, Gassmann M. Regulating cellular oxygen sensing by hydroxylation. *Cardiovasc Res*. 2006;71:642.

124. Sergeeva A, Gordeuk VR, Tokarev YN, et al. Congenital polycythemia in Chuvashia. *Blood*. 1997;89:2148.

125. Tomasic NL, Piterkova L, Huff C, et al. The phenotype of polycythemia due to Croatian homozygous VHL (571C>G:H191D) mutation is different from that of Chuvash polycythemia (VHL 598C>T:R200W). *Haematologica*. 2013;98:560.

126. Lanikova L, Lorenzo F, Yang C, et al. Novel homozygous VHL mutation in exon 2 is associated with congenital polycythemia but not with cancer. *Blood*. 2013;121:3918.

127. Lorenzo FR, Yang C, Lanikova L, et al. Novel compound VHL heterozygosity (VHL T124A/L188V) associated with congenital polycythaemia. *Br J Haematol*. 2013;162:851.

128. Gordeuk VR, Sergueeva AI, Miasnikova GY, et al. Congenital disorder of oxygen sensing: association of the homozygous Chuvash polycythemia VHL mutation with thrombosis and vascular abnormalities but not tumors. *Blood*. 2004;103:3924.

129. Percy MJ, McMullin MF, Jowitt SN, et al. Chuvash-type congenital polycythemia in 4 families of Asian and Western European ancestry. *Blood*. 2003;102:1097.

130. Bento MC, Chang KT, Guan Y, et al. Congenital polycythemia with homozygous and heterozygous mutations of von Hippel-Lindau gene: five new Caucasian patients. *Haematologica*. 2005;90:128.

131. Cario H, Schwarz K, Jorch N, et al. Mutations in the von Hippel-Lindau (VHL) tumor suppressor gene and VHL-haplotype analysis in patients with presumable congenital erythrocytosis. *Haematologica*. 2005;90:19.

132. Collins TS, Arcasoy MO. Iron overload due to X-linked sideroblastic anemia in an African American man. *Am J Med*. 2004;116:501.

133. Pastore Y, Jedlickova K, Guan Y, et al. Mutations of von Hippel-Lindau tumor-suppressor gene and congenital polycythemia. *Am J Hum Genet*. 2003;73:412.

134. Pastore YD, Jelinek J, Ang S, et al. Mutations in the VHL gene in sporadic apparently congenital polycythemia. *Blood*. 2003;101:1591.

135. Lenglet M, Robriquet F, Schwarz K, et al. Identification of a new VHL exon and complex splicing alterations in familial erythrocytosis or von Hippel-Lindau disease. *Blood*. 2018;132:469.

136. Min C, Song J, Goethert JR, et al. Chuvash polycythemia patients from Afghanistan and Southern India share a common VHL gene haplotype. Support for its origin before Asians and Europeans diverged. *Blood*. 2017;130:930.

137. Semenza GL. HIF-1 and mechanisms of hypoxia sensing. *Curr Opin Cell Biol*. 2001;13:167.

138. Miasnikova GY, Sergueeva AI, Nouraie M, et al. The heterozygote advantage of the Chuvash polycythemia VHLR200W mutation may be protection against anemia. *Haematologica*. 2011;96:1371.

139. Cramer T, Yamanishi Y, Clausen BE, et al. HIF-1alpha is essential for myeloid cell-mediated inflammation. *Cell*. 2003;112:645.

140. Friedrich CA. Von Hippel-Lindau syndrome. A pleomorphic condition. *Cancer*. 1999;86:2478.

141. Haase VH, Glickman JN, Socolovsky M, et al. Vascular tumors in livers with targeted inactivation of the von Hippel-Lindau tumor suppressor. *Proc Natl Acad Sci U S A*. 2001;98:1583.

142. Couvé S, Ladroue C, Laine E, et al. Genetic evidence of a precisely tuned dysregulation in the hypoxia signaling pathway during oncogenesis. *Cancer Res*. 2014;74(22):6554-6564.

143. Percy MJ, Zhao Q, Flores A, et al. A family with erythrocytosis establishes a role for prolyl hydroxylase domain protein 2 in oxygen homeostasis. *Proc Natl Acad Sci U S A*. 2006;103:654.

144. Bento C, Percy MJ, Gardie B, et al. Genetic basis of congenital erythrocytosis: mutation update and online databases. *Hum Mutat*. 2014;35:15.

145. Lorenzo FR, Yang C, Ng Tang Fui M, et al. A novel EPAS1/HIF2A germline mutation in a congenital polycythemia with paraganglioma. *J Mol Med*. 2013;91:507.

146. Russell RC, Sufan RI, Zhou B, et al. Loss of JAK2 regulation via a heterodimeric VHL-SOCS1 E3 ubiquitin ligase underlies Chuvash polycythemia. *Nat Med*. 2011;17:845.

147. Kaufmann KB, Grunder A, Hadlich T, et al. A novel murine model of myeloproliferative disorders generated by overexpression of the transcription factor NF-E2. *J Exp Med*. 2012;209:35.

148. Lorenzo F, Margraf R, Swierczek S, et al. A novel EPO gene mutation in a family with autosomal dominant polycythemia. *Blood*. 2013;122(Supplement 11) 950.

149. Lanikova L, Song J, Babosova O, et al. Mutation of EPO 5'UTR Facilitates Interaction with HIF-2 and Causes Autosomal Dominant Erythrocytosis. *Blood*. 2020; 136 (Supplement 1): 28.

150. Zmajkovic J, Lundberg P, Nienhold R, et al. A gain-of-function mutation in EPO in familial erythrocytosis. *N Engl J Med*. 2018;378:924.

151. Sanchez M, Galy B, Muckenthaler MU, Hentze MW. Iron-regulatory proteins limit hypoxia-inducible factor-2alpha expression in iron deficiency. *Nat Struct Mol Biol*. 2007, 14:420.

152. Percy MJ, Sanchez M, Swierczek S, et al. Is congenital secondary erythrocytosis/polycythemia caused by activating mutations within the HIF-2 alpha iron-responsive element? *Blood*. 2007, 110:2776.

153. Ghosh MC, Zhang DL, Jeong SY, et al. Deletion of iron regulatory protein 1 causes polycythemia and pulmonary hypertension in mice through translational derepression of HIF2alpha. *Cell Metab*. 2013;17:271.

154. Oskarsson, G.R., Oddsson, A., Magnusson, M.K. et al. Predicted loss and gain of function mutations in *ACO1* are associated with erythropoiesis. *Commun Biol*. 2020;3(189):1.

155. Hammond D, Winnick S. Paraneoplastic erythrocytosis and ectopic erythropoietins. *Ann N Y Acad Sci*. 1974;230:219.

156. Navarro J, Aguilera A, Liano F, et al. Phlebotomy for polycythemia associated with acquired cystic renal disease in a patient on hemodialysis. *Nephron*. 1992;62:110.

157. Da Silva JL, Lacombe C, Bruneval P, et al. Tumor cells are the site of erythropoietin synthesis in human renal cancers associated with polycythemia. *Blood*. 1990;75:577.

158. Lal A, Rice A, al Mahr M, et al. Wilms tumor associated with polycythemia: case report and review of the literature. *J Pediatr Hematol Oncol*. 1997;19:263.

159. Grignon DJ, Eble JN. Papillary and metanephric adenomas of the kidney. *Semin Diagn Pathol*. 1998;15:41.

160. Fisher JW, Samuels AI. Relationship between renal blood flow and erythropoietin production in dogs. *Proc Soc Exp Biol Med*. 1967;125:482.

161. Beebe HG, Chesebro K, Merchant F, et al. Results of renal artery balloon angioplasty limit its indications. *J Vasc Surg*. 1988;8:300.

162. Mrug M, Julian BA, Prchal JT. Angiotensin II receptor type 1 expression in erythroid progenitors: implications for the pathogenesis of postrenal transplant erythrocytosis. *Semin Nephrol*. 2004;24:120.

163. Danovitch GM, Jamgotchian NJ, Eggena PH, et al. Angiotensin-converting enzyme inhibition in the treatment of renal transplant erythrocytosis. Clinical experience and observation of mechanism. *Transplantation*. 1995;60:132.

164. Mrug M, Stopka T, Julian BA, et al. Angiotensin II stimulates proliferation of normal early erythroid progenitors. *J Clin Invest.* 1997;100:2310.

165. Glicklich D, Burris L, Urban A, et al. Angiotensin-converting enzyme inhibition induces apoptosis in erythroid precursors and affects insulin-like growth factor-1 in posttransplantation erythrocytosis. *J Am Soc Nephrol.* 2001;12:1958.

166. Gossmann J, Burkhardt R, Harder S, et al. Angiotensin II infusion increases plasma erythropoietin levels via an angiotensin II type 1 receptor-dependent pathway. *Kidney Int.* 2001;60:83.

167. Thevenod F, Radtke HW, Grutzmacher P, et al. Deficient feedback regulation of erythropoiesis in kidney transplant patients with polycythemia. *Kidney Int.* 1983;24:227.

168. Friman S, Nyberg G, Blohme I. Erythrocytosis after renal transplantation; treatment by removal of the native kidneys. *Nephrol Dial Transplant.* 1990;5:969.

169. Cole J, Ertoy D, Lin H, et al. Lack of angiotensin II-facilitated erythropoiesis causes anemia in angiotensin-converting enzyme-deficient mice. *J Clin Invest.* 2000;106:1391.

170. Venencie PY, Puissant A, Boffa GA, et al. Multiple cutaneous leiomyomata and erythrocytosis with demonstration of erythropoietic activity in the cutaneous leiomyomata. *Br J Dermatol.* 1982;107:483.

171. Trimble M, Caro J, Talalla A, et al. Secondary erythrocytosis due to a cerebellar hemangioblastoma: demonstration of erythropoietin mRNA in the tumor. *Blood.* 1991;78:599.

172. McFadzean AJS, Todd D, Tsang, KC. Polycythemia in primary carcinoma of the liver. *Blood.* 1958;13:427.

173. Davidson CS. Hepatocellular carcinoma and erythrocytosis. *Semin Hematol.* 1976;13:115.

174. Muta H, Funakoshi A, Baba T, et al. Gene expression of erythropoietin in hepatocellular carcinoma. *Intern Med.* 1994;33:427.

175. Shulkin BL, Shapiro B, Sisson JC. Pheochromocytoma, polycythemia, and venous thrombosis. *Am J Med.* 1987;83:773.

176. Zhuang Z, Yang C, Lorenzo F, et al. Somatic HIF2A gain-of-function mutations in paraganglioma with polycythemia. *N Engl J Med.* 2012;367:922.

177. Pacak K, Jochmanova I, Prodanov T, et al. New syndrome of paraganglioma and somatostatinoma associated with polycythemia. *J Clin Oncol.* 2013;31:1690.

178. Yang C, Sun MG, Matro J, et al. Novel HIF2A mutations disrupt oxygen sensing, leading to polycythemia, paragangliomas, and somatostatinomas. *Blood.* 2013;121:2563.

179. Därr R, Nambuba J, Del Rivero J, et al. Novel insights into the polycythemia-paraganglioma-somatostatinoma syndrome. *Endocr Relat Cancer.* 2016;23:899.

180. Mann DL, Gallagher NI, Donati RM. Erythrocytosis and primary aldosteronism. *Ann Intern Med.* 1967;66:335.

181. Erkelens DW, Statius van Eps LW. Bartter's syndrome and erythrocytosis. *Am J Med.* 1973;55:711.

182. Ghio R, Haupt E, Ratti M, et al. Erythrocytosis associated with a dermoid cyst of the ovary and erythropoietic activity of the tumour fluid. *Scand J Haematol.* 1981;27:70.

183. Shahani S, Braga-Basaria M, Maggio M, et al. Androgens and erythropoiesis: a review. *J Endocrinol Invest.* 2009;32(8):704-716.

184. Gardner FH, Nathan DG, Piomelli S, et al. The erythrocythaemic effects of androgen. *Br J Haematol.* 1968;14:611.

185. Besa EC. Hematologic effects of androgens revisited: an alternative therapy in various hematologic conditions. *Semin Hematol.* 1994;31:134.

186. Bachman E, Travison TG, Basaria S, et al. Testosterone induces erythrocytosis via increased erythropoietin and suppressed hepcidin: evidence for a new erythropoietin/hemoglobin set point. *J Gerontol A Biol Sci Med Sci.* 2014;69:725.

187. Pearson TC. Apparent polycythaemia. *Blood reviews.* 1991;5:205.

188. Chrysant SG, Frohlich ED, Adamopoulos PN, et al. Pathophysiologic significance of "stress" or relative polycythemia in essential hypertension. *Am J Cardiol.* 1976;37:1069.

189. Isbister JP. The contracted plasma volume syndromes (relative polycythaemias) and their haemorheological significance. *Bailliere Clin Haematol.* 1987;1:665.

190. Leth A. Changes in plasma and extracellular fluid volumes in patients with essential hypertension during long-term treatment with hydrochlorothiazide. *Circulation.* 1970;42:479.

191. Prchal JT. Personal communication and direct experience with about 100 affected subjects; 2009.

192. Queisser W, Heim ME, Schmitz JM, et al. [Idiopathic familial erythrocytosis. Report on a family with autosomal dominant inheritance]. *Dtsch Med Wochenschr.* 1988;113:851.

193. Filser M, Aral B, Airaud F. Low incidence of EPOR mutations in idiopathic erythrocytosis. *Haematologica.* 2021;106(1):299-301.

194. Prchal JT, Semenza GL, Prchal J, et al. Familial polycythemia. *Science.* 1995;268:1831.

195. Kralovics R, Sokol L, Prchal JT. Absence of polycythemia in a child with a unique erythropoietin receptor mutation in a family with autosomal dominant primary polycythemia. *J Clin Invest.* 1998;102:124.

196. Arcasoy MO, Degar BA, Harris KW, et al. Familial erythrocytosis associated with a short deletion in the erythropoietin receptor gene. *Blood.* 1997;89:4628.

197. Sergueeva AI, Miasnikova GY, Polyakova LA, et al. Complications in children and adolescents with Chuvash polycythemia. *Blood.* 2015;125:414.

198. Zafren K, Honigman B. High-altitude medicine. *Emerg Med Clin North Am.* 1997;15:191.

199. Bishop BC. Wintering in the high Himalayas. *Natl Geogr.* 1962;122:503

200. Botella de Maglia J, Martinez-Costa R. [High altitude retinal hemorrhages in the expeditions to 8,000 meter peaks. A study of 10 cases]. *Med Clin.* 1998;110:457.

201. Beall CM, Song K, Elston RC, et al. Higher offspring survival among Tibetan women with high oxygen saturation genotypes residing at 4,000 m. *Proc Natl Acad Sci U S A.* 2004;101:14300.

202. Beall CM. Oxygen saturation increases during childhood and decreases during adulthood among high altitude native Tibetans residing at 3,800-4,200m. *High Alt Med Biol.* 2000;1:25.

203. Beall CM. Tibetan and Andean contrasts in adaptation to high-altitude hypoxia. *Adv Exp Med Biol.* 2000;475:63.

204. Beall CM, Decker MJ, Brittenham GM, et al. An Ethiopian pattern of human adaptation to high-altitude hypoxia. *Proc Natl Acad Sci U S A.* 2002;99:17215.

205. Cote C, Zilberberg MD, Mody SH, et al. Haemoglobin level and its clinical impact in a cohort of patients with COPD. *Eur Respir J.* 2007;29:923.

206. Boyer L, Chaar V, Pelle G, et al. Effects of polycythemia on systemic endothelial function in chronic hypoxic lung disease. *J Appl Physiol.* 2011;110:1196.

207. Nadeem O, Gui J, Ornstein DL. Prevalence of venous thromboembolism in patients with secondary polycythemia. *Clin Appl Thromb Hemost.* 2013;19(4):363-366.

208. Thorne SA. Management of polycythaemia in adults with cyanotic congenital heart disease. *Heart.* 1998;79:315.

209. Shibata J, Hasegawa J, Siemens HJ, et al. Hemostasis and coagulation at a hematocrit level of 0.85: functional consequences of erythrocytosis. *Blood.* 2003;101:4416.

210. Ammash N, Warnes CA. Cerebrovascular events in adult patients with cyanotic congenital heart disease. *J Am Coll Cardiol.* 1996;28:768.

211. Stefenelli T, Silberbauer K, Ulrich W, et al. Cardial decompensation caused by hypertension and polyglobulia associated with multiple renal oncocytomas. *Clin Nephrol.* 1985;23:307.

212. Lezaic V, Biljanovic-Paunovic L, Pavlovic-Kentera V, et al. Erythropoiesis after kidney transplantation: the role of erythropoietin, burst promoting activity and early erythroid progenitor cells. *Eur J Med Res.* 2001;6:27.

213. Bushuev VI, Miasnikova GY, Sergueeva AI, et al. Endothelin-1, vascular endothelial growth factor and systolic pulmonary artery pressure in patients with Chuvash polycythemia. *Haematologica.* 2006;91:744.

214. Niu X, Miasnikova GY, Sergueeva AI, et al. Altered cytokine profiles in patients with Chuvash polycythemia. *Am J Hematol.* 2009;84:74.

215. Sergueeva AI, Miasnikova GY, Okhotin DJ, et al. Elevated homocysteine, glutathione and cysteinylglycine concentrations in patients homozygous for the Chuvash polycythemia VHL mutation. *Haematologica.* 2008;93:279.

216. Prchal JF, Axelrad AA. Letter: bone-marrow responses in polycythemia vera. *N Engl J Med.* 1974;290:1382.

217. Kralovics R, Buser AS, Teo SS, et al. Comparison of molecular markers in a cohort of patients with chronic myeloproliferative disorders. *Blood.* 2003;102:1869.

218. Weinberg RS. In vitro erythropoiesis in polycythemia vera and other myeloproliferative disorders. *Semin Hematol.* 1997;34:64.

219. Shih LY, Lee CT, See LC, et al. In vitro culture growth of erythroid progenitors and serum erythropoietin assay in the differential diagnosis of polycythaemia. *Eur J Clin Invest.* 1998;28:569.

220. Prchal JT. Personal communication; 2009.

221. Fisher MJ, Prchal JF, Prchal JT, et al. Anti-erythropoietin (EPO) receptor monoclonal antibodies distinguish EPO-dependent and EPO-independent erythroid progenitors in polycythemia vera. *Blood.* 1994;84:1982.

222. Kralovics R, Indrak K, Stopka T, et al. Two new EPO receptor mutations: truncated EPO receptors are most frequently associated with primary familial and congenital polycythemias. *Blood.* 1997;90:2057.

223. Acharya J, Westwood NB, Sawyer BM, et al. Identification of latent myeloproliferative disease in patients with Budd-Chiari syndrome using X-chromosome inactivation patterns and in vitro erythroid colony formation. *Eur J Haematol.* 1995;55:315.

224. De Stefano V, Teofili L, Leone G, et al. Spontaneous erythroid colony formation as the clue to an underlying myeloproliferative disorder in patients with Budd-Chiari syndrome or portal vein thrombosis. *Semin Thromb Hemost.* 1997;23:411.

225. Pagliuca A, Mufti GJ, Janossa-Tahernia M, et al. In vitro colony culture and chromosomal studies in hepatic and portal vein thrombosis—possible evidence of an occult myeloproliferative state. *Q J Med.* 1990;76:981.

226. Valla D, Casadevall N, Lacombe C, et al. Primary myeloproliferative disorder and hepatic vein thrombosis. A prospective study of erythroid colony formation in vitro in 20 patients with Budd-Chiari syndrome. *Ann Intern Med.* 1985;103:329.

227. Shih LY, Lee CT. Identification of masked polycythemia vera from patients with idiopathic marked thrombocytosis by endogenous erythroid colony assay. *Blood.* 1994;83:744.

228. Birgegard G, Wide L. Serum erythropoietin in the diagnosis of polycythaemia and after phlebotomy treatment. *Br J Haematol.* 1992;81:603.

229. Messinezy M, Westwood NB, El-Hemaidi I, et al. Serum erythropoietin values in erythrocytoses and in primary thrombocythaemia. *Br J Haematol.* 2002;117:47.

230. Mossuz P, Girodon F, Donnard M, et al. Diagnostic value of serum erythropoietin level in patients with absolute erythrocytosis. *Haematologica.* 2004;89:1194.

231. Thurmes PJ, Steensma DP. Elevated serum erythropoietin levels in patients with Budd-Chiari syndrome secondary to polycythemia vera: clinical implications for the role of JAK2 mutation analysis. *Eur J Haematol.* 2006;77:57.

232. Remacha AF, Montserrat I, Santamaria A, et al. Serum erythropoietin in the diagnosis of polycythemia vera. A follow-up study. *Haematologica.* 1997;82:406.

233. Beutler E, Yeh M, Fairbanks VF. The normal human female as a mosaic of X-chromosome activity: studies using the gene for C-6-PD-deficiency as a marker. *Proc Natl Acad Sci U S A.* 1962;48:9.

234. Adamson JW, Fialkow PJ, Murphy S, et al. Polycythemia vera: stem-cell and probable clonal origin of the disease. *N Engl J Med.* 1976;295:913.

235. Prchal JT. Pathogenetic mechanisms of polycythemia vera and congenital polycythemic disorders. *Semin Hematol.* 2001;38:10.

236. Kralovics R, Guan Y, Prchal JT. Acquired uniparental disomy of chromosome 9p is a frequent stem cell defect in polycythemia vera. *Exp Hematol.* 2002;30:229.

237. Chen GL, Prchal JT. X-linked clonality testing: interpretation and limitations. *Blood.* 2007;110:1411.

238. Curnutte JT, Hopkins PJ, Kuhl W, et al. Studying X inactivation. *Lancet.* 1992;339:749.

239. Allen RC, Zoghbi HY, Moseley AB, et al. Methylation of HpaII and HhaI sites near the polymorphic CAG repeat in the human androgen-receptor gene correlates with X chromosome inactivation. *Am J Hum Genet.* 1992;51:1229.

240. Prchal JT, Guan YL, Prchal JF, et al. Transcriptional analysis of the active X-chromosome in normal and clonal hematopoiesis. *Blood.* 1993;81:269.

241. Prchal JT, Prchal JF, Belickova M, et al. Clonal stability of blood cell lineages indicated by X-chromosomal transcriptional polymorphism. *J Exp Med.* 1996;183:561.

242. Busque L, Mio R, Mattioli J, et al. Nonrandom X-inactivation patterns in normal females: lyonization ratios vary with age. *Blood.* 1996;88:59.

243. Champion KM, Gilbert JG, Asimakopoulos FA, et al. Clonal haemopoiesis in normal elderly women: implications for the myeloproliferative disorders and myelodysplastic syndromes. *Br J Haematol.* 1997;97:920.

244. Gale RE, Fielding AK, Harrison CN, et al. Acquired skewing of X-chromosome inactivation patterns in myeloid cells of the elderly suggests stochastic clonal loss with age. *Br J Haematol.* 1997;98:512.

245. Swierczek SI, Agarwal N, Nussenzveig RH, et al. Hematopoiesis is not clonal in healthy elderly women. *Blood.* 2008;112:3186.

246. Swierczek SI, Piterkova L, Jelinek J, et al. Methylation of AR locus does not always reflect X chromosome inactivation state. *Blood.* 2012;119:e100.

247. Kralovics R, Stockton DW, Prchal JT. Clonal hematopoiesis in familial polycythemia vera suggests the involvement of multiple mutational events in the early pathogenesis of the disease. *Blood.* 2003;102:3793.

248. Lertzman M, Frome BM, Israels LG, et al. Hypoxia in polycythemia vera. *Ann Intern Med.* 1964;60:409.

249. Zhou AW, Knoche EM, Engle EK, et al. Clinical improvement with JAK2 inhibition in Chuvash polycythemia. *N Engl J Med.* 2016;375:494.

250. Plata R, Cornejo A, Arratia C, et al. Angiotensin-converting-enzyme inhibition therapy in altitude polycythaemia: a prospective randomised trial. *Lancet.* 2002;359:663.

251. Manglani MV, DeGroff CG, Dukes PP, et al. Congenital erythrocytosis with elevated erythropoietin level: an incorrectly set "erythrostat"? *J Pediatr Hematol Oncol.* 1998;20:560.

252. Piccirillo G, Fimognari FL, Valdivia JL, et al. Effects of phlebotomy on a patient with secondary polycythemia and angina pectoris. *Int J Cardiol.* 1994;44:175.

253. Gordeuk VR, Sergueeva AI, Miasnikova GY, et al. Congenital disorder of oxygen sensing: association of the homozygous Chuvash polycythemia VHL mutation with thrombosis and vascular abnormalities but not tumors. *Blood.* 2004;103:3924.

254. Hultberg B, Sjoblad S, Ockerman PA. Properties of five acid hydrolases in human skin fibroblast cultures. Possible use in the diagnosis of inborn lysosomal diseases. *Acta Paediatr Scand.* 1973;62:474.

255. Sarangi S, Lanikova L, Kapralova K, et al. The homozygous VHL(D126N) missense mutation is associated with dramatically elevated erythropoietin levels, consequent polycythemia, and early onset severe pulmonary hypertension. *Pediatr Blood Cancer.* 2014;61(11):2104-2106.

Part VII **Red Cell Transfusion**

CHAPTER 29
ERYTHROCYTE ANTIGENS AND ANTIBODIES

Christine Lomas-Francis

SUMMARY

Blood group antigens are structures on the outer surface of human red blood cells (RBCs) that can be recognized by the immune system of individuals who lack that particular structure. Identification of RBC antigens and antibodies is the basis of pretransfusion compatibility testing and the safe transfusion practices used today and provides insights into understanding the etiology of hemolytic disease of the fetus and the newborn. Biochemical and molecular studies have led to definition of the biologic functions of molecules expressing blood group antigens. These molecules play a critical role in susceptibility to infection by malarial parasites, some viruses, and bacteria. Alteration of RBC antigen expression is associated with many molecular backgrounds, and some play a role in the clinical manifestations of certain diseases. Erythrocytes, far from being inert containers of hemoglobin, are active in a variety of physiologic processes.

● DEFINITIONS AND HISTORY

A *blood group system* consists of a group of antigens encoded by alleles at a single gene locus or at gene loci so closely linked that crossing over does not occur or is very rare. An *antigen collection* consists of antigens that are phenotypically, biochemically, or genetically related, but the genes encoding them have not been identified.[1] Placement of a blood group antigen into a system or collection begins with the discovery of an antibody, usually in the serum of a multiparous woman or a multiply-transfused recipient, with a unique pattern of reactivity. The antibody can be used to study basic biochemical properties of the corresponding antigen, to enable recognition of the pattern of inheritance of the antigen in families and in populations, to identify red blood cells

Acronyms and Abbreviations: 2-ME, 2-mercaptoethanol; ABC, ATP-binding cassette; AET, 2-aminoethylisothiouronium bromide; AQP1, aquaporin 1; AUG, antigens of the Augustine; CD, cluster of differentiation; CGD, chronic granulomatous disease; DTT, dithiothreitol; EDTA, ethylenediaminetetraacetic acid; EKLF, erythroid Krüppel-like factor; EMP3, epithelial membrane protein 3; EtNP, ethanolamine phosphate; Fuc, fucose; Gal, galactose; GalNac, N-acetylglucosamine; GPA, glycophorin A; GPB, glycophorin B; GPC, glycophorin C; GPD, glycophorin D; GlcNAc, N-acetylglucosamine; GPI, glycosylphosphatidylinositol; HDFN, hemolytic disease of the fetus and newborn; HEMPAS, hereditary erythroblastic multinuclearity with a positive acidified serum test; HNA-3, human neutrophil antigen-3; Ig, immunoglobulin; ISBT, International Society of Blood Transfusion; LAD, leukocyte adhesion deficiency; MRP, multidrug resistance protein; NeuAc, N-acetylneuraminic acid; PNH, paroxysmal nocturnal hemoglobinuria; RBC, red blood cell.

(RBCs) that lack the antigen, and to search for an antithetical antigen. Identified characteristics, such as prevalence of positive reactions or sensitivity or resistance to specific enzymes, are compared with antigens in known systems and collections. A newly recognized antigen is also evaluated using biochemical and molecular genetic methods. Orphan antigens of low or high prevalence are placed in "holding tanks" until the gene that encodes them is established.

The majority of genes encoding blood group antigens have been cloned and sequenced,[2] and the molecular bases of most blood group antigens have been determined.[3-6] Details on the alleles associated with blood group antigens and phenotypes can be obtained from the International Society of Blood Transfusion (ISBT) website (www.isbtweb.org/working-parties/red-cell-immunogenetics-and-blood-group-terminology/) or from www.bloodantigens.com and www.erythrogene.com.

RBC antigens are inherited carbohydrate or protein structures located on the outside surface of the RBC membrane (Fig. 29-1). Although most of the protein blood group antigens are carried on integral transmembrane proteins (either single-pass type I or type II, or multipass; Fig. 29-1), a few are carried on glycosylphosphatidylinositol (GPI)-linked proteins or adsorbed from plasma. Some carbohydrate antigens are attached to proteins or lipids and some require a combination of a specific portion of protein and carbohydrate. Blood group antigens have revealed that certain transmembrane proteins interact with other transmembrane proteins (eg, band 3 and glycophorin A [GPA]; Kell and Kx; Rh and RhAG), with lipids (eg, Rh), or with proteins in the membrane skeleton (eg, band 3 and ankyrin, glycophorin C [GPC], and protein 4.1 and p55); (Chap. 15). Many of the proteins carrying blood group antigens reside in the erythrocyte membrane as complexes.[7-10] Many components carrying blood group antigens have been assigned cluster of differentiation (CD) numbers (Table 29-1). In human blood grouping, agglutination of RBCs usually serves as the detectable end point, but it also can be detectable by hemolysis.[11] Our ability to detect and identify blood group antigens and antibodies has contributed significantly to current safe blood transfusion practice, reducing death from hemolytic disease of the fetus and newborn (HDFN) from 40% to less than 2%, and supporting patients receiving chemotherapy or organ transplantation.

The naming of blood group antigens usually does not follow the classic convention wherein dominant traits are given capital letters and recessive traits are designated with lowercase letters. For example, in the ABO blood group system, A and B are codominant and the recessive O phenotype is encoded by a gene designated *O*, whereas in the MNS system the genes *S* and *s* are codominant. To standardize terminology used to describe RBC blood groups, ISBT Working Party for Terminology for Red Cell Surface Antigens recommended using the traditional name for an antigen for verbal communication and a numerical system in computer databases (see the blood group terminology website: www.isbtweb.org). The working party has placed blood group antigens into four categories: (1) genetically discrete blood group systems; (2) serologically, biochemically, or genetically related antigens in blood group collections; (3) series of low-incidence antigens; and (4) series of high-incidence antigens. Each system and collection have been given a number and letter designation, and each antigen within the system is numbered sequentially in order of discovery. As of this writing, 43 blood group systems and five antigen collections are defined (see Table 29-1; www.isbtweb.org).[1,5,6,12-14] Over time, notations devised to describe blood group antigens have changed. A single letter (eg, A, D, K), a symbol with a superscript (eg, Fy^a, Jk^b, Lu^a), a symbol with a number (eg, Fy3, Lu4, K12), and three to four letters (eg, Vel, JMH, ELO, FPPT) are all used, sometimes within the same blood group system. The ISBT Blood Group Terminology Working Party name has changed to ISBT Working Party on Red Cell Immunogenetics and Blood Group Terminology,

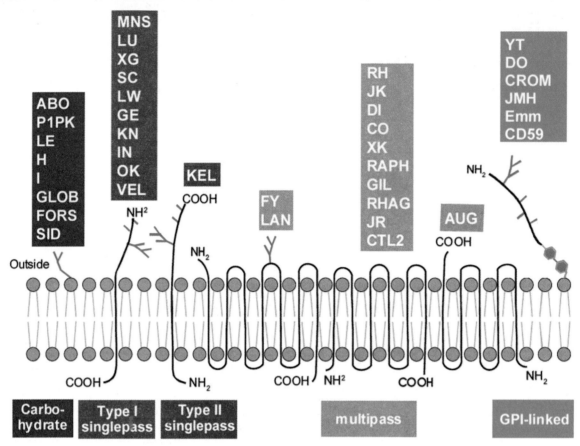

FIGURE 29–1. Membrane structures carrying blood group antigens.

which reflects that DNA testing is now often used to predict a blood group. The original aim of the working party to develop and maintain guidelines for blood group antigens has expanded to include allele nomenclature for use in transfusion medicine and related sciences.

BLOOD GROUP SYSTEMS

Tables 29-1 and 29-2 summarize the characteristics of common blood group antigens. The following sources provide more detail: Issitt and Anstee[5]; Reid, Lomas-Francis, and Olsson[6]; Reid and Lomas-Francis[15]; Mollison and colleagues[16]; Daniels[4]; and Cohn and associates.[11] In the interest of space, reviews or books are referenced in place of original reports.

ABO BLOOD GROUP SYSTEM

The ABO blood group system was the first system described and remains the most significant in transfusion medicine. A mismatch of ABO may be fatal, whereas a mismatch of other blood groups, initially, is mostly harmless. This situation occurs because anti-A and anti-B antibodies usually are present in the blood of all people (except for newborns) lacking the corresponding antigen. These antibodies are stimulated by the ubiquitous distribution of the antigen that forms part of the membrane structure of many bacteria, plants, and animals. For this reason, all donor blood for transfusion is tested and labeled with the ABO group. The four main phenotypes are A, B, AB, and O, the latter indicating a lack of A and B antigens. The sugars defining A and B antigens are added to carbohydrate chains carrying the H antigen (fucose), which is "hidden" by the A (GalNAc) or B (Gal) sugar. Thus, group A or B erythrocytes appear to have less H antigen than group O cells. Nonetheless,

H is found on all human erythrocytes except those from rare individuals of the O_h (Bombay) phenotype.

Anti-A or anti-B immunoglobulins can cause intravascular hemolysis when ABO-incompatible RBCs are transfused. Because A and B antigens also are expressed on most tissue cells, ABO compatibility is a significant consideration in solid-organ transplantation. However, ABO incompatibility only rarely causes severe HDFN because antibodies directed against A and B antigens are predominantly immunoglobulin (Ig) M, which do not cross the placenta; in addition, A and B antigens are not fully developed on RBCs from a fetus (Chap. 27).

Although the ABO blood group system has only four phenotypes, hundreds of alleles have been identified by DNA analyses. The ABO gene was cloned in 1990 after purification of A transferase.[17,18] A and B transferases have only four amino acid differences in the catalytic domain, two of which (Leu266Met and Gly268Ala) are primarily responsible for substrate specificity.[19] The group O phenotype results from nucleotide changes in A and/or B alleles that cause loss of glycosyltransferase activity. The most common group O (O_1) results from a single nucleotide deletion near the 5′ end of the gene that causes a frameshift and early termination with no active enzyme production.[20] The *ABO* gene has seven exons, and A or B subgroups (with only few exceptions) result from a variety of nucleotide changes in exon 7 that cause alterations in the catalytic domain of the glycosyltransferase (reviewed by Chester and Olsson[21]). The rare B(A), A(B), and *cis*-AB phenotypes expressing both A and B antigens result from variant glycosyltransferases that have a combination of A- and B-specific residues.[21] Numerous common and rare ABO alleles have been reported, and current information is available at: http://www.isbtweb.org/working-parties/red-cell-immunogenetics-and-blood-group-terminology/). In addition to nucleotide changes, recombinations and gene rearrangements can result in

TABLE 29–1. Characteristics of International Society of Blood Transfusion Defined Blood Group Systems and Antigen Collections

Conventional Name	ISBT Symbol (No.)	Chromosome Location	Gene Name*	Associated Antigens [Null Phenotype]	Function of RBC Membrane Component (CD No.)	Disease Association
BLOOD GROUP SYSTEMS						
ABO	ABO (001)	9q34.2	ABO	A, B, A, B, A1 [group O]	Glycocalyx	Altered expression in some hematologic disorders
MNS	MNS (002)	4q31.21	GYPA, GYPB	M, N, S, s, U, and 45 more [En(a–); U–; M^{k}M^k]	Binds microbes, glycocalyx, complement regulation, chaperone for band 3 (CD235a/235b)	Decreased *Plasmodium falciparum* invasion, may be receptor for *Escherichia coli*
P1PK	P1PK (003)	22q13.2	A4GALT	P1, P^k, NOR [p phenotype (PP1P^k–)]	Glycocalyx (CD77)	
Rh	RH (004)	1p36.11	RHD, RHCE	D, C, E, c, e, and 50 more [Rh$_{null}$]	Possibly transports CO_2 or NH_3 (CD240)	Hemolytic anemia, hereditary stomatocytosis, hematologic malignancies
Lutheran	LU (005)	19q13.32	BCAM	Lu^a, Lu^b, Lu3, and 24 more [recessive Lu(a–b–)]	Binds laminin (CD239)	Increased expression possibly involved in vaso-occlusion in sickle cell disease
Kell	KEL (006)	7q34	KEL	K, k, Kp^a, Kp^b, Js^a, Js^b, and 30 more [K$_0$ or K$_{null}$]	Cleaves big endothelin-3 to ET-3, a potent vasoconstrictor (CD238)	
Lewis	LE (007)	19p13.3	FUT3	Le^a, Le^b, and 4 more [Le(a–b–)]	Glycocalyx, Le^b is receptor for *Helicobacter pylori*	Increased expression in fucosidosis, Lewis antibodies may be important in graft rejection
Duffy	FY (008)	1q23.2	ACKR1	Fy^a, Fy^b, Fy3, Fy5, Fy6 [Fy(a–b–)]	Chemokine, *P. vivax* receptor (CD234)	Resistance to *P. vivax* invasion
Kidd	JK (009)	18q12.3	SLC14A1	Jk^a, Jk^b, Jk3 [Jk(a–b–)]	Urea transporter	Impaired urea transport, urine-concentrating defect
Diego	DI (010)	17q21.31	SLC4A1	Di^a, Di^b, Wr^a, Wr^b, and 18 more	Anion exchanger (CD233), Band 3 cytoskeletal protein	Southeast Asian ovalocytosis, hereditary spherocytosis, renal tubular acidosis
Yt	YT (011)	7q22.1	ACHE	Yt^a, Yt^b, YTEG, YTLI, YTOT	Acetylcholinesterase	Absent from PNH III RBCs
Xg	XG (012)	Xp22.32	XG, MIC2	Xg^a, CD99	Adhesion molecules (CD99)	
Scianna	SC (013)	1p34.2	ERMAP	Sc1, Sc2, Sc3, and 6 more [SC: –1, –2, –3]	Possible adhesion	
Dombrock	DO (014)	12p12.3	ART4	Do^a, Do^b, Gy^a, Hy, Jo^a and 5 more [Gy(a–)]	Enzymatic (CD297)	Absent from PNH III RBCs
Colton	CO (015)	7p14.3	AQP1	Co^a, Co^b, Co3, Co4 [Co(a–b–)]	Water transport	Monosomy 7, inability to maximally concentrate urine, congenital dyserythropoietic anemia
Landsteiner-Wiener	LW (016)	19p13.2	ICAM4	LW^a, LW^{ab}, LW^b [LW(a–b–)]	Binds CD11/CD18, ligand for integrins (CD242)	Depressed in pregnancy and some malignant diseases
Chido/Rogers	CH/RG (017)	6p21.32	C4A, C4B	CH1, RG1, and 7 more [C4 deficient RBCs]	Complement components	Certain phenotypes have increased susceptibility to certain autoimmune conditions and infections

(continued)

TABLE 29–1. Characteristics of International Society of Blood Transfusion Defined Blood Group Systems and Antigen Collections (Continued)

Conventional Name	ISBT Symbol (No.)	Chromosome Location	Gene Name*	Associated Antigens [Null Phenotype]	Function of RBC Membrane Component (CD No.)	Disease Association
H	H (018)	19q13.33	FUT1	H [Bombay, O$_h$]	Glycocalyx (CD 173)	Decreased in some tumor cells, increased in hematopoietic stress
Kx	XK (019)	Xp21.1	XK	Kx [McLeod]	Possible neurotransmitter, function in RBCs not known	Acanthocytosis, muscular dystrophy, hemolytic anemia; McLeod syndrome sometimes associated with CGD, peripheral neuropathy, cardiomyopathy seizures, a late-onset dementia, and behavioral changes
Gerbich	GE (020)	2q14.3	GYPC	Ge2, Ge3, Ge4, and 10 more [Leach phenotype]	Membrane attachment; interacts with 4.1R and p55 (CD236)	Hereditary elliptocytosis, hemolytic anemia, decreased 4.1R and p55
Cromer	CROM (021)	1q32.2	CD55	Cr^a, Tc^a, Tc^b, Tc^c, Dr^a, and 15 more [Inab phenotype]	Complement regulation, binds C3b, disassembles C3/C5 convertase (CD55)	Absent from PNH III RBCs, Dr^a is the receptor for uropathogenic E coli
Knops	KN (022)	1q32.2	CR1	Kn^a, Kn^b, McC^a, Sl^a, Yk^a, and 7 more [Helgeson phenotype]	Complement regulation, binds C3b and C4b, mediates phagocytosis (CD35)	Antigens depressed in certain autoimmune and malignant conditions
Indian	IN (023)	11p13	CD44	In^a, In^b, INFI, INJA, INRA, INSL	Binds hyaluronic acid, mediates adhesion of leukocytes (CD44)	Depressed in pregnancy, congenital dyserythropoietic anemia
Ok	OK (024)	19p13.3	BSG	Ok^a, OKGV, OKVM	Possible adhesion (CD147)	
Raph	RAPH (025)	11p15.5	CD151	MER2 [RAPH$_{null}$]	Adhesion molecule involved in kidney function (CD151)	Renal disease, associated with pretibial epidermolysis bullosa and sensorineural deafness
John Milton Hagen	JMH (026)	15q24.1	SEMA7A	JMH, and 7 more	Adhesion molecule, function in RBCs not known (CD108)	Absent from PNH III RBCs
I	I (027)	6p24.2	GCNT2	I [I–; i adult]	Glycocalyx	Congenital cataracts in Asians
GLOB	Globoside (028)	3q25	β3GALNT1	P, PX2 [P–]	Glycocalyx	Receptor E. coli and parvovirus B19
Gil	GIL (029)	9p13.3	AQP3	GIL [GIL–]	Glycerol/water/urea transporter	
Rh-associated glycoprotein	RHAG (030)	6p12.3	RHAG	Duclos, Ol^a, DSLK, Kg	Possibly transports CO$_2$, or NH$_3$ (CD241)	Hemolytic anemia, hereditary stomatocytosis
FORS	FORS (031)	9q34.2	GBGT1	FORS1	Glycocalyx	
JR	JR (032)	4q22.1	ABCG2	Jr^a [Jr(a–)]	ATP-dependent transporter (CD338)	
Lan	LAN (033)	2q36	ABCB6	Lan [Lan–]	ATP-dependent transporter	
Vel	VEL (034)	1p36.32	SMIM1	Vel [Vel–]		
CD59	CD59 (035)	1p13.33	CD59	CD59.1 [CD59–]	Complement regulation (CD59)	Absent from PNH III RBCs
Augustine	AUG (36)	6p21.1	SLC29A1	AUG1, At^a, ATML, ATAM	Equilibrative nucleoside transporter 1; facilitates diffusion of hydrophilic nucleosides across plasma membrane	Multiple small calcifications around the joints in the hand and ectopic calcification or mineralization in hips, feet, pubic symphysis, and lumbar discs

(continued)

TABLE 29–1. Characteristics of International Society of Blood Transfusion Defined Blood Group Systems and Antigen Collections (Continued)

Conventional Name	ISBT Symbol (No.)	Chromosome Location	Gene Name*	Associated Antigens [Null Phenotype]	Function of RBC Membrane Component (CD No.)	Disease Association
KANNO	KANNO (37)	20p13	PRNP	KANNO1	Antigen expressed on Prion Protein (CD230)	
Sid	SID (38)	17q21.32	B4GALNT2	Sd^a	Sd^a inhibits invasion of malaria parasites into RBCs Implicated in pathogen invasion, cancer, xenotransplantation	Expressed on Tamm-Horsfall glycoprotein in urine that prevents adherence of pathogenic bacteria to urothelial cells
CTL2	CTL2 (39)	19p13.2	SLC44A2	CTL2.1, Rif	Choline transporter	Deafness, choline deficiency disease
PEL	PEL (40)	13q32.1	ABCC4	Pel [Pel–]	ATP-dependent transporter	Lack impairs platelet aggregation Variants may increase toxicity or cause resistance to cancer drugs
MAM	MAM (41)	19q13. 3	EMP3	MAM [MAM–]	Possible function for EMP3 in regulating the level and stabilizing CD44 at the cell surface of erythroid progenitors	A purported tumor suppressor in various solid tumors. No evidence that MAM– (EMP3null) individuals have an increased risk of cancer.
EMM	EMM (42)	4p16.3	PIGG	Emm [Emm–]	Component of GPI anchor Ethanolamine phosphate (EtNP) absent from second mannose of GPI-anchor	Absent from PNH III RBCs Various inherited GPI deficiency (IGD) disorders PIGG mutations may be implicated in neurological phenotypes including seizures, developmental delay/intellectual disability, cerebral atrophy and hypotonia.
ABCC1	ABCC1 (43)	16p13.11	ABCC1	ABCC1 [ABCC1–]	Exporter of glutathione-S-conjugates and ATP	Multidrug resistance protein 1 Possible role in protection of kidney epithelial cells
ANTIGEN COLLECTIONS						
Cost	COST (205)	—	—	Cs^a, Cs^b		
Ii	I (207)	—	—	i		
Er	ER (208)	—	—	Er^a, Er^b, Er3		
	Unnamed (210)	—	—	Le^c, Le^d		
	MN CHO (213)	—	—	Hu, M$_1$, Tm, Can, Sext, Sj		
Low-incidence series	— (700)	—	—	16		
High-incidence series	— (901)	—	—	AnWj,, ABTI, LKE		

CGD, chronic granulomatous disease; PNH, paroxysmal nocturnal hemoglobinuria; RBC, red blood cell.

*As defined by the HUGO Gene Nomenclature Committee: http://www.genenames.org/

Data from Daniels GL, Anstee DJ, Cartron J-P, et al. Blood group terminology 1995. ISBT, International Society of Blood Transfusion Working Party on Terminology for Red Cell Surface Antigens. *Vox Sang.* 1995;69:265; Issitt PD, Anstee DJ. *Applied Blood Group Serology.* 4th ed. Montgomery Scientific; 1998; Reid ME, Lomas-Francis C, Olsson ML. *Blood Group Antigen FactsBook.* 3rd ed. Academic Press; 2012; Reid ME, Lomas-Francis C. *Blood Group Antigens & Antibodies: A Guide to Clinical Relevance & Technical Tips.* Star Bright Books; 2007; www.isbt-web.org.

TABLE 29–2. Summary of Common Blood Group Systems or Collections and Their Antigens

Blood Group (Year Reported)	Common Phenotypes	Frequency White/ Black (%)	No. Antigen Copies on Adult RBC × 10³	Dosage (See Text)	Cord Cell Expression	Biochemistry	Antigen Distribution in Blood, Fluids, and Tissues	Comments
ABO (1900)	A B AB	40/27 11/20 4/4	AB: ~800–1000	A/B: not evident	Weak: ~1/3 adult expression	Carbohydrate on types 1, 2, 3, and 4 precursor chains	RBC, lymphs, plts	Most significant antigens in transfusion and transplantation
H (1948)	O	45/49	H: ~1700	H expression depends on ABO: $O>A_2>B>A_2B>A_1>A_1B$	Weak Main RBC carrier: bands 3 and 4.5	Attached to lipids in plasma and protein in secretions	Plasma, secretions; broad tissue distribution; most epithelial/ endothelial cells	Weak subgroups result from variant transferases
Rh (1939)	R_1 Dce r ce R_2 DcE R_0 Dce r'Ce r" cE	42/17 37/26 14/11 4/44 2/2 1/0	D on R_2R_2: 15–33 R_1R_1: 14–19 R_0r: 12–20 R_1r: 9–14 c on cc: 70–85	D: not evident C and c: yes E and e: yes	Normal adult	Multipass, nonglycosylated protein: 30–32 kDa; 417 aa C: serine 103/c: proline 103 E: proline 226/e: alanine 226	Erythroid specific Possible cation transport Possible role in RBC membrane integrity	D most significant antigen after A and B Three causes for weak D expression (see text) Nulls: amorphic type and regulator type
	R_z DCE r^y CE	<1 <1	Cc: 37–53 e on ee: 18–24 Ee: 13–14			Forms "Rh complex" with LW, GPB, and Rh-related glycoprotein (chromosome 6)		
Lewis (1946)	Le(a+b–) Le(a–b+) Le(a–b–) Le(a+b+)	22/23 72/55 6/22 Rare in European populations; found in Australasian populations; 10 in Japanese	Leª: ~3	Not evident	Weak: adult expression at age 2 years	Carbohydrate on type 1 precursor chains only Attached to lipids in plasma and protein in secretions	Plasma and secretion antigen; on RBC, lymphs, plts only by adsorption of plasma antigen	Le antigens depend on *Le/Se* interaction; *Le/Se* = Le(a–b+), ABH secretor; *lele/sese* = Le(a+b–), ABH nonsecretor; *lele* = Le(a–b–), Sese status not apparent Le(a–b+) express some Leª, do not make anti-Leª. Women may test Le(a–b–) during pregnancy
I (1956)	I adult(↑↑I↓i) i cord (↓I↑i) i adult (↓I↑↑i)	Common Common <1:10,000	I: ~500	Not evident	Strong i; weak I. Adult expressions at age 2 years	Carbohydrate on ABH active chains; lipid on RBC; protein in plasma	Broad tissue distribution; RBCs, plts, lymphs, granules, monos; also in plasma, secretions (eg, milk, saliva, urine)	I and i expression are inversely proportional but not products of alleles

(continued)

TABLE 29–2. Summary of Common Blood Group Systems or Collections and Their Antigens (Continued)

Blood Group (Year Reported)	Common Phenotypes	Frequency White/ Black (%)	No. Antigen Copies on Adult RBC × 10³	Dosage (See Text)	Cord Cell Expression	Biochemistry	Antigen Distribution in Blood, Fluids, and Tissues	Comments
P1PK and GLOB								
P1 (1927) GLOB (1951)	P_1: P_2: p: $P^k-P-P1-$	79/94 21/6 Rare	P1: ~500 Globoside: ~15,000	Not evident, but inherited variations exist; eg, P1 may be normal, strong, or weak	Weak: adult expression by 7 years	Carbohydrate on RBC and plasma glycolipids; not in secretions	RBC, lymphs, plts, monos, fibroblasts, uroepithelial cells	P1-like antigen is associated with pigeon and earthworm protein and parasitic infections
MNS (M: 1927) (S: 1947)	M+N– M+N+ M–N+ S+s– S+s+ S–s+ S–s–U–	28/26 50/44 22/30 11/3 44/28 45/69 0/<1	GPA: ~800 GPB: ~200	Yes	Normal adult	Single-pass sialoglycoprotein type 1 GPA: 43 kDa, 131 aa, carries MN GPB: 25 kDa, 72 aa, carries SsU; part of Rh complex	RBCs plus renal capillary epithelial/ endothelium	GPA and GPB carry multiple antigens and many hybrids of GPA–GPB Can have absence of GPA, GPB, or both
Kell (1946)	K–k+	91/98	Kell: 2–6	Yes	Normal adult	Single-pass glycoprotein type II highly folded: 93kDa, 732 aa	Kell: RBC plus marrow and fetal liver tissue; not on brain, kidney, adult liver	System of high- and low-frequency antigens
Kpª/Jsª: (1957)	K+k+ K+k– Kp(a–b+) Kp(a+b+) Kp(a+b–) Js(a–b+) Js(a+b+) Js(a+b–)	8.8/2 0.2/rare 97.7/100 2.3/rare Rare/0 100/80 Rare/19 0/1				K/k Met 193 Thr Kpª/Kpᵇ: Trp 281 Arg Jsª/Jsᵇ: Pro 597 Leu	Kx: RBC plus skeletal/heart muscle, neurologic tissues	Common phenotype: k, Kpᵇ, Jsᵇ Kell antigen expression depends on both Kell and Xk genes K_{null} lacks Kell antigens, has Kx Kx_{null} lacks Kx, has poor Kell antigen expression (McLeod phenotype) Other causes of poor Kell expression: *cis* Kpª, Ge-, K_{mod}, autoantibody
Duffy (1950)	Fy(a+b–) Fy(a+b+) Fy(a–b+) Fy(a–b–)	17/9 49/1 34/22 Rare/68	Fyª: 6–13	Yes, but not always evident because of *Fy* gene	Normal: adult levels at 12 weeks	Multipass glycoprotein: 35–45 kDa, 338 aa Fyª/Fyᵇ Gly 42Asp	RBC plus brain, colon, lung, spleen, thyroid, thymus, kidney, endothelium; not in liver or placenta tissue	Fy(a–b–) blacks do not express Fyᵇ on their RBC, but express it on other tissues and seldom make anti-Fyᵇ

(continued)

TABLE 29–2. Summary of Common Blood Group Systems or Collections and Their Antigens (Continued)

Blood Group (Year Reported)	Common Phenotypes	Frequency White/Black (%)	No. Antigen Copies on Adult RBC × 10³	Dosage (See Text)	Cord Cell Expression	Biochemistry	Antigen Distribution in Blood, Fluids, and Tissues	Comments
Kidd (1951)	Jk(a+b−)	28/57	Jkª: ~14	Yes	Normal adult	Multipass protein: ~43 kDa, 391 aa 1 potential *N*-glycan Jkª/Jkᵇ: Asp284 Asn	RBC specific	Important cause of DHTR
	Jk(a+b+)	49/34						Nulls are unable to fully concentrate urine; dominant inhibitor *In(Jk)* has weak Jk antigen
	Jk(a−b+)	23/9						
	Jk(a−b−)	<1% Polynesians						
Lutheran (1951)	Lu(a+b−)	0.15/−	Luᵇ: 1.5–4	Yes, but family variations exist	Weak: adult level at 15 years	Single-pass glycoprotein type I: 85 kDa, 597 aa 78 kDa	RBC plus brain, heart, kidney, lung, pancreas, placenta, skeletal muscle	System of high- and low-frequency antigens
	Lu(a+b+)	7.5/0				5 Ig superfamily domains: two variable, three constant		Dominant inhibitor *In(Lu)* and X-linked inhibitor *(XS2)* cause greatly reduced Lu expression
	Lu(a−b+)	92.3/−				B-CAM		
	Lu(a−b−)	Very rare				Luª/Luᵇ: His77Arg		First known autosomal linkage to *Se*

aa, amino acids; B-CAM, B-cell adhesion molecule; DHTR, delayed hemolytic transfusion reactions; GPA, glycophorin A; GPB, glycophorin B; granulos, granulocytes; Ig, immunoglobulin; ISBT, International Society of Blood Transfusion; lymphs, lymphocytes; monos, monocytes; plts, platelets; RBC, red blood cell.

hybrid alleles that encode for unexpected transferase activity. This situation makes typing of ABO by DNA analysis difficult to interpret.[22] The function of the ABO system is not known, although several disease associations are well established.[23]

Rh BLOOD GROUP SYSTEM

The Rh (*not* Rhesus) system is the second most important blood group system in transfusion medicine because antigen-positive RBCs frequently immunize antigen-negative individuals through transfusion and pregnancy.

Inheritance of Rh antigens is determined by a complex of two closely linked genes: one encodes the protein-carrying D antigen (RhD); the other encodes the protein carrying C or c and E or e antigens (RhCE). RBCs from Rh-positive people have both RhD and RhCE, whereas Rh-negative RBCs have only RhCE. In the Rh system, eight common antigen combinations or haplotypes are possible: Dce (R₀, Rh₀), DCe (R₁, Rh₁), DcE (R₂, Rh₂), DCE (R_z, Rh_z), ce (r, rh), Ce (r′, rh′), cE (r″, rh″), and CE (rʸ, rhʸ). The letter "d" is commonly used to designate the lack of D, but there is no d antigen or anti-d.

Several nomenclatures can be used to describe Rh genes and antigens. The Fisher-Race nomenclature, which uses CDE terminology, is more commonly used for antigens; the Wiener nomenclature, which uses Rh/rh (or R/r) designations, is favored for haplotypes and gene complexes; and the Rosenfield and Rubinstein nomenclature, which uses numerical designations, was introduced to allow interpretation without bias.[24]

The Rh blood group system has 55 antigens at the time of this writing (the ABO system has four). By far, the most important and immunogenic antigen is D (Rh₀ in Wiener terminology, referring to Wiener's discovery that a rhesus monkey injected with human RBCs would produce antibody that agglutinated the RBCs of 85% of white New Yorkers). For most clinical purposes, testing individuals for the D antigen and

classifying them as D+ (or Rh-positive), or D− (or Rh-negative) is sufficient. Approximately 85% of the white population is Rh-positive, and 15% is Rh-negative. Most Rh-negative recipients produce anti-D if they receive Rh-positive blood. Anti-D can cause hemolysis in adults after an Rh-mismatched transfusion and in the newborn (HDFN) if antibodies were made by the mother from a prior transfusion or pregnancy. Thus, donors and recipients are routinely typed and matched for D. The risk of anti-D sensitization by transfusion is essentially eliminated by matching. The risk of anti-D sensitization in pregnancy is minimized by passive immunization of mothers at risk against D.

The antigens C, c, E, and e are less immunogenic and become important for patient care only after the corresponding antibody develops or when the basic Rh haplotype must be determined. The remaining 50 antigens are other Rh protein epitopes whose corresponding antibodies are seldom encountered. Some are encoded by variant Rh alleles and appear as antithetical antigens to C, c, E, or e, or as related "extra" antigens. Others are referred to as *compound* antigens or *cis* gene products. For example, the protein produced by *RHCE*ce* encodes c and e antigens, and the compound f (or ce) antigen. Other compound antigens include Ce, cE, and CE. Still other Rh antigens are related to the complex "mosaic" nature of D and e, and less commonly C, c, and E antigens. If immunized, individuals who lack a part of an antigen and who make antibody to the portion they lack, can present with a challenging serologic picture. For example, the D+ person who lacks part of the D antigen and makes an antibody to the missing portion appears to make alloanti-D because normal D+ RBCs carry all D epitopes.[25]

Some, but not all, individuals who lack part of the D antigen (partial D) have weak expression of D on their red cells that is detected only by the antiglobulin test. Having a RHCE*C gene in trans position to an RHD gene (eg, Dce/Ce or DCe/Ce genotypes) also can weaken expression of D in some individuals. A third type of weak D expression results from inheriting an RHD gene that encodes all epitopes of D, but in less-than-normal quantity.

DNA analyses have revealed the molecular basis underlying antigens and phenotypes. A list of the RH alleles that have been described as of this writing is available at: http://www.isbtweb.org/working-parties/red-cell-immunogenetics-and-blood-group-terminology/) and at https://www.bloodgroupgenomics.org/rhce/isbt-allele-tables/. Rh blood group orthologs are present in nonhuman primates and other species on the evolutionary tree.[26] The RhD and RhCE proteins complex with the Rh-associated glycoprotein (RhAG) in the membrane. RhAG acts as a transporter of gases, most likely for ammonium, nitrous oxide, CO_2, and/or O_2, but confirmation is needed as to which it is.

OTHER BLOOD GROUP SYSTEMS

In terms of transfusion and HDFN, the other blood group systems and their antigens become clinically relevant only when antibody develops. Transfusion service laboratories identify (*antibody identification*) the specificity and characterize the reactivity of antibodies detected in routine testing (*antibody screening*). Once this information is known, the blood bank assesses the clinical significance of the antibody and selects the most appropriate blood for transfusion. Tables 29-1 and 29-2 summarize the number of antigens in each blood group system and other relevant information. A detailed description of all the blood group antigens is beyond the scope of this chapter. Because the molecular bases of most blood group antigens and phenotypes are known,[6] DNA analysis can be used to predict the type of transfused patients and to identify the fetus at risk for HDFN.[27]

GENERAL IMMUNOLOGY OF BLOOD GROUP ANTIGENS

An *antigen* is a substance that can evoke an immune response when introduced into an immunocompetent host and react with the antibody produced from that immune response. An antigen can have several *epitopes*, which together are called an *antigenic determinant*, each of which can elicit an antibody response.

The ability of an antigen to stimulate an immune response is called *immunogenicity*, and its ability to react with an antibody is called *antigenicity*. These primary characteristics are affected by antigen size, shape, rigidity, and the number and location of the determinants on the red cell membrane.

IMMUNOGENICITY

Immunogenicity depends on many antigen characteristics, not just the number of antigen sites. Relative immunogenicity is estimated by comparing the actual observed incidence of an antibody with the calculated likelihood of a possible immunizing event. After A and B, the D antigen is most immunogenic (early work suggested that approximately 80% of Rh-negative individuals produce anti-D after receiving a single Rh-positive RBC component, but more recent studies indicate it is more like 20%-30%[4]), followed by K, which stimulates anti-K in approximately 10% of cases.[16] Giblett's original calculation ranked immunogenicity as K>E/c>Fyᵃ>Jkᵃ.[28] Stack and Tormey[29] refined Giblett's calculation to correct for transfusion exposures and ranked immunogenicity as: K>Jkᵃ> E>>c>C>Fyᵃ>S. Immunogenicity does not always correlate with the hemolytic potential of an antibody specificity; for example, K is more immunogenic than Jkᵃ but anti-Jkᵃ is more likely to cause hemolysis.

● ANTIGEN EXPRESSION

NUMBER OF ANTIGEN SITES

The number of antigen sites per RBC has been estimated by measuring the uptake of ¹²⁵I-labeled antibody or of ferritin-conjugated anti-IgG.

Numbers vary widely among blood group systems from a few hundred to over 1 million (see Table 29-2). Also, estimates for any given antigen can vary greatly.

ANTIGEN DEVELOPMENT ON FETAL ERYTHROCYTES

Most RBC antigens can be detected early in fetal development (A, B, and H antigens can be detected at 5 to 6 weeks of gestation), but not all are fully developed at birth. A, B, H, I, P1, Luᵃ, Luᵇ, Ytᵃ, Xgᵃ, Vel, Bg, Doᵃ, Doᵇ, and Knᵃ antigen expression is considerably weaker on cord RBCs than on RBCs from adults. Leᵃ—sometimes Leᵇ, Ch/Rg, AnWj, and Sdᵃ—are not readily detectable, although 50% of cord samples type Le(a+) with more sensitive test methods. Full expression of A, B, H, I, and Lewis antigens usually is present by age 3 years, whereas full expression of P1 and Lutheran antigens may not occur until age 7 years.

VARIATION IN ANTIGEN EXPRESSION

RBCs from individuals who are homozygous for an allele typically have a greater number of antigen sites than do RBCs from individuals who are heterozygous. Consequently, their RBCs can react more strongly with antibody. This difference in expression and antigen–antibody reactivity because of zygosity is known as *dosage*. For example, RBCs from a homozygous *MM* individual carry a double dose of M antigen and react more strongly with anti-M than do RBCs from an *MN* heterozygous individual carrying only a single dose of M. Antithetical antigens C/c, E/e, M/N, S/s, and Jkᵃ/Jkᵇ commonly show dosage effect. Dosage is less obvious with D, K/k, and Luᵃ/Luᵇ antigens. It typically is more apparent within a family than between families. Dosage within the Duffy system also may not be serologically obvious because Fy(a+b–) or Fy(a–b+) phenotypes are seen in either homozygous (*FyᵃFyᵃ* or *FyᵇFyᵇ*) or hemizygous (*FyᵃFy* or *FyᵇFy*) individuals.

Some blood group antigens are inherited as closely-linked genes or haplotypes. Haplotype pairings and gene interaction (either *cis* or *trans*) also can affect phenotypic expression. For example, the pairing of *RHCE*C* in *trans* position to *RHD* can result in weak expression of D (see "Rh Blood Group System" earlier), whereas *RHCE*E* in *cis* position with *RHD* is associated with strong expression of D. Among the common phenotypes, R₂R₂ RBCs carry the strongest expression of D. In the Kell system, *Kpᵃ* is associated with weakened expression of *in cis* k and Jsᵇ antigens.

Still other antigens are affected by regulator genes.[30] The dominant type of the Lu(a–b–) phenotype [In(Lu)] results from heterozygosity for an allele of the *KLF1* gene, the gene that encodes erythroid Krüppel-like factor. The dominant inhibitor gene *KLF1* suppresses expression of Lutheran, P1, i, and many other antigens.[31] The dominant inhibitor *In(Jk)* is the result of a zinc-finger deletion at ZNF850[32] and suppresses expression of Jkᵃ and Jkᵇ antigens.[4] Rare variants of the *RHAG* gene depress or prevent expression of the Rh antigens (see "Rh_null Syndrome" further).

● BIOCHEMISTRY OF ERYTHROCYTE ANTIGENS

An antibody typically recognizes an epitope consisting of four to five amino acids on linear proteins or one to seven sugars. Alternatively, the antibody-binding site may encompass a more complex three-dimensional structure with branches or folds, and recognition may depend on both amino acids and sugars. Tables 29-2 and 29-3 and Fig. 29-1 summarize blood group biochemistry and antigen structure.[4,6,16]

TABLE 29–3. Biochemistry of Common Carbohydrates and Antigens on Glycophorin A and Glycophorin B

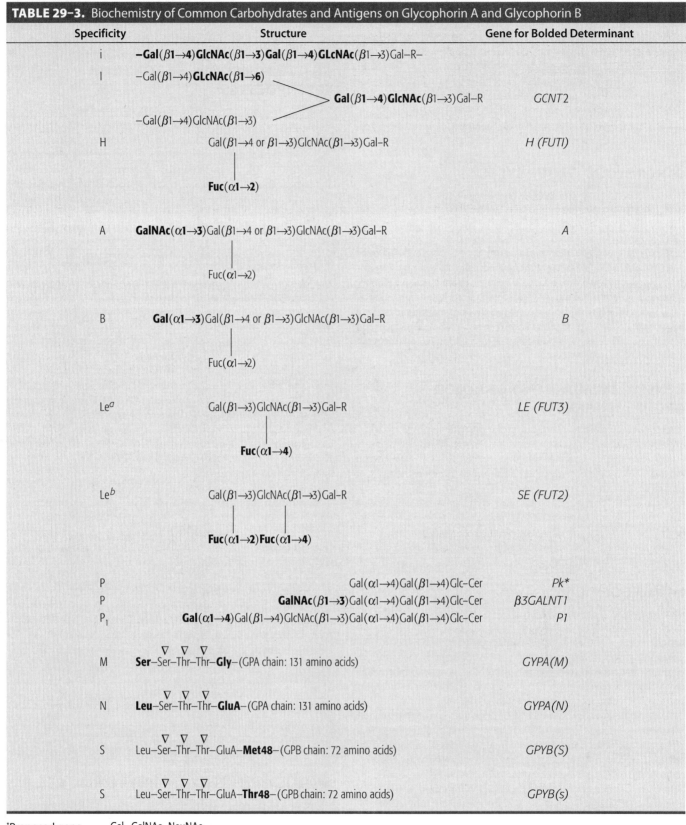

Specificity	Structure	Gene for Bolded Determinant
i	**−Gal**(β1→4)**GlcNAc**(β1→3)**Gal**(β1→4)**GlcNAc**(β1→3)Gal−R−	
I	−Gal(β1→4)**GlcNAc**(β1→6) ⟩ **Gal**(β1→4)**GlcNAc**(β1→3)Gal−R / −Gal(β1→4)GlcNAc(β1→3)	GCNT2
H	Gal(β1→4 or β1→3)GlcNAc(β1→3)Gal−R | **Fuc**(α1→2)	H (FUTI)
A	**GalNAc**(α1→3)Gal(β1→4 or β1→3)GlcNAc(β1→3)Gal−R | Fuc(α1→2)	A
B	**Gal**(α1→3)Gal(β1→4 or β1→3)GlcNAc(β1→3)Gal−R | Fuc(α1→2)	B
Le^a	Gal(β1→3)GlcNAc(β1→3)Gal−R | **Fuc**(α1→4)	LE (FUT3)
Le^b	Gal(β1→3)GlcNAc(β1→3)Gal−R | | **Fuc**(α1→2)**Fuc**(α1→4)	SE (FUT2)
P	Gal(α1→4)Gal(β1→4)Glc−Cer	Pk*
P	**GalNAc**(β1→3)Gal(α1→4)Gal(β1→4)Glc−Cer	β3GALNT1
P$_1$	**Gal**(α1→4)Gal(β1→4)GlcNAc(β1→3)Gal(α1→4)Gal(β1→4)Glc−Cer	P1
M	∇ ∇ ∇ **Ser**−Ser−Thr−Thr−**Gly**−(GPA chain: 131 amino acids)	GYPA(M)
N	∇ ∇ ∇ **Leu**−Ser−Thr−Thr−**GluA**−(GPA chain: 131 amino acids)	GYPA(N)
S	∇ ∇ ∇ Leu−Ser−Thr−Thr−GluA−**Met48**−(GPB chain: 72 amino acids)	GPYB(S)
S	∇ ∇ ∇ Leu−Ser−Thr−Thr−GluA−**Thr48**−(GPB chain: 72 amino acids)	GPYB(s)

*Proposed gene

∇, −Gal−GalNAc−NeuNAc \| NeuNac .

GPA, glycophorin A; GPB, glycophorin B; R, primary glycolipid attachment Glc-Ger, primary glycoprotein attachment GlcNAc-Asp;∇, Immunodominant sugars and amino acids are indicated in bold.

CARBOHYDRATE ANTIGENS

Polysaccharides with blood group activity are made by sequential addition of specific sugars (or sugar derivatives) to specific precursors in specific linkages by specific transferases. Sugars commonly involved are galactose (Gal), N-acetyl-D-galactosamine (GalNAc), N-acetylglucosamine (GlcNAc), fucose (Fuc), and N-acetylneuraminic acid (NeuAc).

Antigens in ABO, LE, P1PK, and GLOB blood group systems depend on an immunodominant sugar, usually terminally located, the polysaccharide to which the sugar is attached, and the type of linkage involved. The basis of the Sd^a antigen of the newly defined Sid blood group system depends on GalNAcβ1-4(NeuAcα2-3)Galβ, a terminal trisaccharide on ganglioside or RBC glycoproteins, or on Tamm-Horsfall glycoprotein in urine.[33] I/i specificity is defined by a series of sugars on the inner portion of ABH saccharide chains. The presence of at least two repeating Gal(β1–4)GlcNAc(β1–3)Gal units in a linear structure defines i activity. I activity involves these same sugars in branched form (see Table 29-3). The gene for I (GCNT2) encodes the transferase responsible for branching (β(1–6) glucosaminyltransferase). During the first years of a child's life, linear chains are modified into branched chains, resulting in the appearance of I antigens.[34] The I antigen is reduced on RBCs from fetuses and infants. A rare i phenotype occurs in adults (see "I-Negative Phenotype [i Adult]" further).

Polysaccharide chains are attached to glycoproteins in secretions (on type 2 chains), to glycolipids in plasma (on type 1 chains), and to both on the RBC membrane. Approximately 70% of A, B, H, and I antigens on the RBC membrane are carried on glycoproteins, primarily on the anion transporter, but also on the glucose transporter, the RhAG, and others. Approximately 10% of these antigens are on NeuAc-rich glycoproteins, 5% on simple glycolipids, and the remainder on polyglycosylceramide.[16] P1, P^k, and P antigens are found on glycolipids both on the membrane and in plasma.[35]

Lewis antigens are unique because they occur only on type 1 polysaccharide chains, which are found in plasma and secretions but not made by RBCs. Hence, they exist on RBCs only by adsorption of Lewis substance from plasma. The FUT3 (or LE) gene encodes an α(1–4)fucosyltransferase. Whether the resulting antigen is Le^a or Le^b depends on the secretor gene FUT2 (or SE), which encodes an α(1–2) fucosyltransferase.

PROTEIN ANTIGENS

Protein structures that carry blood group antigens can be grouped into three categories: (1) those that make a single pass through the erythrocyte membrane, (2) those that make multiple passes through the membrane, and (3) those that are attached to the membrane through a covalent linkage to lipid (GPI-linked; see Fig. 29-1).

Single-pass proteins include GPA with M and N antigens; glycophorin B (GPB) with S, s, and U antigens; GPC and glycophorin D (GPD) with Gerbich antigens; and the Lutheran, LW, Indian, Knops, Xg, Ok, and Scianna proteins (see Fig. 29-1). These proteins have an extracellular amino-terminus and an intracellular carboxyl-terminus (referred to as type I). In contrast, the Kell glycoprotein has an extracellular carboxyl-terminus and an intracellular amino-terminus (referred to as type II).

Most proteins that carry blood group antigens and make multiple passes through the erythrocyte membrane have both carboxyl- and amino-terminal ends that are intracellular, are hydrophobic, and have a transport function. Rh, RhAG, Diego, Colton, Kidd, Kx, GIL, Raph, PEL, MAM and ABCC1[36-38] proteins are included in this category. Duffy and Lan are multipass proteins, but they have an extracellular amino-terminus whereas ENT1, the Augustine antigen carrier, has an extracellular carboxyl-terminus. Duffy has homology with a family of cytokine receptors, and the Lan protein belongs to the family of ATP-binding cassettes.[4,6,39,40]

Lipid-linked proteins have their carboxyl-terminus attached to the lipid GPI and are said to be GPI-linked or anchored. Cromer, Yt, Dombrock, JMH, CD59[41], KANNO[42] and EMM[43,44] proteins belong to this category. GPI-linked proteins are of special interest to hematologists because defective synthesis of the GPI anchor is responsible for paroxysmal nocturnal hemoglobinuria (PNH), (Chap. 8).[45] Thus, PNH-III RBCs lack all proteins attached by a GPI anchor, including those carrying blood groups.

EFFECT OF ENZYMES AND OTHER CHEMICALS ON ERYTHROCYTE ANTIGENS

Expression of an RBC antigen is determined by its exposure as a result of its position on the cell surface and its biochemical structure. Expression can be modified with treatment of RBCs by enzymes and other chemicals. These reagents are used to help identify complex mixtures of antibodies and to help characterize antibody specificity when identity is not readily apparent.

Proteolytic enzymes, such as ficin, papain, bromelin, trypsin, and α-chymotrypsin, cleave proteins from the erythrocyte membrane at specific amino acids. Enzyme treatment of RBCs cleaves certain protein antigens and allows carbohydrate and other resistant protein antigens to react more strongly with their antibody. The reactivity of antibodies with antigens in ABO, I, P1PK, LE, RH, and JK systems is enhanced after enzyme treatment of the RBCs, whereas reactivity of antibodies to M, N, Fy^a, Fy^b, and many minor antigens (Xg^a, Ch, Rg, JMH, In^b, Ge2, Ge4, Pr, Tn, and some examples of Yt^a) is reduced or eliminated. S and s are variably affected by enzyme treatment, and Kell and Scianna antigens are relatively unaffected.[4-6]

Reagents that reduce disulfide bonds, such as 2-mercaptoethanol, dithiothreitol (DTT), and 2-aminoethylisothiouronium bromide, denature Kell blood group antigens but enhance Kx. Reducing reagents also denature antigens in LW, SC, IN, JMH, and YT systems and weaken antigens in LU, DO, CROM, KN, and RAPH systems and the AnWj antigen.[4-6]

Acid treatment of RBCs (ethylenediaminetetraacetic acid/glycine/acid reagent), which is frequently used to remove IgG from RBCs, can weaken or completely denature antigens in the KEL blood group system and those of the ER collection. Chloroquine treatment of erythrocytes (also sometimes used to remove IgG from RBCs) at room temperature has little effect on most antigens. However, treatment for 30 minutes at 37°C can weaken expression of many antigens, including Fy^b, Lu^b, Yt^a, JMH, and those in the RH, DO, and KN systems.

GENETICS OF ERYTHROCYTE ANTIGENS

Protein antigens are direct gene products: The gene encodes a protein that expresses one or more antigens. Carbohydrate antigens, made by transferase action, are indirect gene products. Most blood group genes are located on autosomes; only two, Xg and XK, are located on the X chromosome (see Table 29-1 for locations of genes on chromosomes).

Most genes that encode blood groups have two or more alleles. Individuals who inherit two identical alleles are homozygous and make a double dose of a single gene product, whereas those who inherit two different alleles are heterozygous and make a single dose of each of two gene products. Males are hemizygous for the genes located on their single X chromosome and make a single gene product. In contrast, women produce a double dose of the *Xg* and *XK* gene products, because X-chromosome inactivation does not involve Xg^a or Kx antigens. The molecular basis of the Xg(a–) phenotype was shown to be due to the disruption of a GATA1-binding motif upstream of the *XG/PBDX* locus.[46]

ALLELES

Alleles encoding blood group antigens commonly arise from only a single or a few nucleotide changes. For example, A and B alleles differ by only seven DNA base substitutions, which result in four amino acid substitutions in their respective transferases.[4-6] The common O allele is similar to *A* except for a single base deletion at nucleotide 261 that shifts the reading frame during RNA translation. The resulting protein is truncated and has no transferase activity. Another variant O allele encodes a transferase identical to that of B except it has arginine instead of alanine at amino acid position 268, which blocks the enzyme activity. A comprehensive listing of blood group alleles is available at: http://www.isbtweb.org/working-parties/red-cell-immunogenetics-and-blood-group-terminology/.

GENE COMPLEXES

Some blood group genes are complexes of several closely linked genes or loci that evolved through duplication of an ancestral gene. The antigens they encode are inherited as a haplotype with no or few crossovers. Blood group examples include the Rh system with genes *RHD* and *RHCE*, and the MNS system with genes *GYPA*, *GYPB*, and *GYPE*.

RHD and *RHCE* show remarkable homology between them and with *RHAG*, which encodes the RhAG. *GYPA* and *GYPB* probably arose by duplication of an ancestral GYPA gene encoding the N antigen.[47] The most common MNS complex is Ns, followed by Ms, MS, and NS.

In both RH and MNS systems, other antigens arose by further nucleotide changes, deletions, or rearrangements within the gene complex. Unequal pairing of *GYPA* and *GYPB* during meiosis, with subsequent recombination, resulted in several hybrids, such as *GYP(A-B)* (called Lepore type, by analogy with a similar hemoglobin hybrid (Chaps. 17 and 18), which encodes a protein with the amino-terminal end of GPA but the carboxyl-terminal end of GPB. Anti–Lepore-type hybrids, *GYP(B-A)* (amino-terminal end of GPB and carboxyl-terminal end of GPA), and other rearrangements (eg, *GYP[B-A-B]* and *GYP[A-B-A]*) are known. Within the Rh complex, numerous hybrids of *RH(D-CE-D)* and *RH(CE-D-CE)* have been identified. Such hybrids can result in altered antigen expression and new antigens.[4-6]

Kell and Lutheran proteins are single-gene products that carry multiple antigens. The most common alleles in humans are $kKp^bJs^bK^{11}$ and $Lu^bLu^6Lu^8Au^a$. Antigens of lower prevalence (K, Kp^a/Kp^c, or Js^a; and Lu^a, Lu9, Lu14, or Au^b) arise from separate nucleotide changes.

SILENT ALLELES

Some blood group alleles are amorphs, or silent; that is, they do not produce a recognizable antigen, although they may encode a product that is simply not detected with standard test methods. As discussed with regard to the ABO system, A and B genes produce transferases that add GalNAc or Gal, respectively, to the same precursors, but *O* produces no active enzyme. *AB* individuals express both A and B antigen, but *AA* and *AO* individuals express A, and *BB* and *BO* individuals express B. Amorphic alleles are recognized only in a homozygous state, and the result is a "null" phenotype. Null phenotypes exist in most blood group systems (see Table 29-1). Group O is the most common, followed by Fy(a–b–) and Le(a–b–) in Africans. Other null phenotypes are rare.

The Fy(a–b–) phenotype is especially interesting. Fy(a–b–) Africans have *Fyᵇ* genes that express normal Fy^b glycoprotein on tissue cells but not on RBCs. A nucleotide change that disrupts the GATA-1 binding site for RBC transcription is present in these individuals,[4] which helps explain why many Fy(a–b–) or Fy(a+b–) Africans do not make anti-Fy^b despite exposure to antigen-positive RBCs from transfusion.

GENE FREQUENCIES

Gene and phenotype frequencies vary widely with race and geographical boundaries.[6,11,16,48] This information is useful when estimating the availability of compatible blood and the probability of HDFN.

● RED CELL ANTIGENS IN HEALTH AND DISEASE

EXPRESSION OF RED CELL ANTIGENS IN OTHER BODY TISSUES AND FLUIDS

Antigens in the RH and JK blood group systems are present only on RBCs and have not been detected on platelets, lymphocytes, or granulocytes or in plasma, other body tissues, or secretions (saliva, milk, amniotic fluid).[4-6,16] Antigens in MNS, LU, KEL, and FY systems are found on RBCs and other body tissues (see Table 29-2).

ABH antigens have broad tissue distribution. In embryos, A, B, and H antigens are detectable on all endothelial cells and all epithelial cells except those of the CNS. Antigens in ABO, P1PK, LE, H, and I systems are in plasma and on platelets and lymphocytes. Granulocytes carry I antigen but no ABH. ABH on platelets and lymphocytes may be acquired at least in part by adsorption from plasma. Lewis antigen is acquired by RBCs by adsorption. Secretions (saliva, milk, sweat, semen, and urine, but not cerebrospinal fluid) contain soluble A, B, H, I, and Le^a and Le^b antigens but no P1PK or GLOB system antigens. Sd^a antigen is found in most body secretions, with the greatest concentration in urine.[5,16]

● ASSOCIATIONS OF RED CELL ANTIGENS WITH DISEASE

ANTIGENS ASSOCIATED WITH POSSIBLE SUSCEPTIBILITY TO DISEASE

Some blood groups are statistically associated with medical conditions or disease (Table 29-4).[4-6,16] For example, blood group A is more common in persons with cancer of the salivary glands, stomach, colon, or ovary, and with thrombosis (because of higher levels of coagulation factors VIII, V, and IX). Blood group O is more common in patients with duodenal and gastric ulcers, rheumatoid arthritis, and von Willebrand disease.

Associations with infection arise when microorganisms carry structures homologous with blood group activity. The presence of blood group antibody and/or soluble blood group antigen in secretions may help confer protection. Having anti-B may offer protection against *Salmonella*, *Shigella*, *Neisseria gonorrhoeae*, and some *Escherichia coli* infections. An association exists between nonsecretion of ABH antigen and susceptibility to *Candida albicans*, *N. meningitidis*, *Streptococcus pneumoniae*, and *Haemophilus influenzae*.[6]

Several disease associations with globoside have been identified. *S. suis*, which can cause meningitis and septicemia in humans, binds exclusively to P^k antigen. A class of toxins secreted by *Shigella dysenteriae*, *Vibrio cholerae*, and *V. parahaemolyticus* have binding specificity for

TABLE 29–4. Blood Group Antigens and Antibodies Associated with Disease

PHENOTYPES ASSOCIATED WITH DISEASE SUSCEPTIBILITY

Group A	Carcinoma of the salivary glands, stomach, colon, rectum, ovary, uterus, cervix, bladder (T1 and T2 tumors); idiopathic thrombocytopenic purpura, coronary thrombosis, thrombosis (oral contraceptives), pernicious anemia, giardiasis, meningococcal meningitis infections
Group B	*Escherichia coli* urinary tract infection, gonorrhea
Group O	Duodenal and gastric ulcers, rheumatoid arthritis, von Willebrand disease, typhoid, paratyphoid, cholera
ABH nonsecretors	Duodenal ulcers, spondyloarthropathies; increased susceptibility to *Candida albicans*, *Neisseria meningitidis*, *Streptococcus pneumoniae*, *Haemophilus influenzae*
Le(a–b–)	Sjögren syndrome
Group O, Le(a–b+)	*Helicobacter pylori*
Globoside	Parvovirus

PHENOTYPES ASSOCIATED WITH DISEASE RESISTANCE

p (PP1P^k–)	Pyelonephritogenic infections of *E. coli*, parvovirus B
Fy(a–b–)	*Plasmodium vivax*, *P. knowlesi*
Tn–, Cad–, En(a–), U–, Ge–	*P. falciparum*

DISEASES ASSOCIATED WITH ALTERED ANTIGEN EXPRESSION

Weakened AB	Leukemia, myelodysplastic syndrome, Hodgkin lymphoma and non-Hodgkin lymphomas, aplastic anemia, bacterial infections
Weakened MN	Bacterial infections, myelodysplastic syndrome, leukemia (Tn, T, Tk activation)
Enhanced i	Thalassemia, sickle cell disease, HEMPAS, Diamond-Blackfan anemia, myeloblastic or sideroblastic erythropoiesis, refractory anemia
Acquired A (Tn)	Myelodysplastic syndrome, acute myelogenous leukemia
Acquired B	Bacterial infections, gastrointestinal lesions or malignancies
Acquired T, Tk	Bacterial infections
Acquired K antigens	*Enterococcus faecium*
Acquired Jk^b antigen	*E. faecium* or *Micrococcus* infection
Absent Cromer, Yt, Dombrock, JMH, CD59, Emm antigens	Paroxysmal nocturnal hemoglobinuria
Weakened target antigens (Rh, Kell, Kidd, LW)	Autoimmune hemolytic anemia
LW	Hodgkin disease, lymphoma, leukemia, sarcoma
Weakened I, Rh, S, s, U, Kp^b, Jk^a, Xg^a, or En^a	Stomatocytic hereditary elliptocytosis

DISEASES ASSOCIATED WITH NULL PHENOTYPES

Rh$_{null}$ (D–C–E–c–e–)	Hereditary stomatocytosis, mild hemolytic anemia
McLeod phenotype (Kx–)	Hereditary acanthocytosis, mild hemolytic anemia, see text
GE$_{null}$ (Leach type)	Hereditary elliptocytosis, mild hemolytic anemia
Bombay (O$_h$)	Leukocyte adhesion deficiency II (some)
I– (i Adult)	Congenital cataracts in Asians (some)
CO$_{null}$	Inability to maximally concentrate urine
RAPH$_{null}$	Kidney disease
Jk(a–b–) [In(Jk)]	Mood and/or anxiety disorder with increased suicidal risk (7.4-fold)
AUG$_{null}$ (AUG:–1,–2)	Multiple small calcifications around joints in the hand; ectopic calcification or mineralization in hips, feet, pubic symphysis, and lumbar discs
ABCC1$_{null}$ (ABCC1–)	Possible impact on renal function

(continued)

TABLE 29–4. Blood Group Antigens and Antibodies Associated with Disease (Continued)

DISEASES ASSOCIATED WITH ANTIBODY PRODUCTION	
Anti-I, -IH, -i, -H, -Pr	Cold agglutinin disease
Anti-"Rh," –"Kell," -U, -Wr[b]	Warm autoimmune hemolytic anemia
Anti-I	*Mycoplasma pneumoniae*, chronic lymphocytic leukemia, Hodgkin lymphoma and non-Hodgkin lymphomas
Anti-i	Infectious mononucleosis, reticuloendothelial diseases
Anti-I[T]	Hodgkin lymphoma and non-Hodgkin lymphomas
Anti-K	Enterocolitis, bacterial infections (*E. coli* 0125:B15, *Campylobacter jejuni, E. coli*)
Anti-P1	Parasitic infections: hydatid cyst disease, liver flukes
Anti-PP1P[k]	Early spontaneous abortions
Anti-P	Paroxysmal cold hemoglobinuria, early spontaneous abortions, lymphoma
Anti-NF	Renal dialysis (formaldehyde exposure)
Anti-Forssman	Neoplastic disorders
Anti-Rx	Virally induced hemolysis
Decreased anti-A or -B	Agammaglobulinemia or hypogammaglobulinemia
"NULL" PHENOTYPES ASSOCIATED WITH BIOLOGIC DIFFERENCES BUT NO OR MILD DISEASE	
Group O	Lack GalNAc or Gal on terminal Gal
Bombay (O$_h$)	Lack Fuc on terminal Gal
Le(a–b–)	Lack Fuc on terminal GlcNAc
M–N– or En(a–)	Lack or have altered GPA
S–s–U–	Lack or have altered GPB
Wr(a–b–)	Lack or have altered GPA
M[k] phenotype	Lack GPA and GPB
K$_0$	Lack Kell glycoprotein
Jk(a–b–)	Lack or have altered Jk protein, reduced ability to concentrate urine
Lu(a–b–)	Lack or have reduced or altered Lu glycoprotein; RBC may show poikilocytosis, potassium loss, increased hemolysis during storage
LW(a–b–)	Lack or have altered LW glycoprotein
Do(a–b–), Gy(a–)	Lack a GPI-linked protein (Do glycoprotein)
SC:–1,–2,–3	Lack or have altered Sc glycoprotein

Fuc, fucose; GlcNAc, *N*-acetylglucosamine; GPA, glycophorin A; GPB, glycophorin B; GPI, glycosylphosphatidylinositol; HEMPAS, hereditary erythroblastic multinuclearity with positive acidified serum lysis test.

Data from Issitt PD, Anstee DJ. *Applied Blood Group Serology*. 4th ed. Montgomery Scientific; 1998; Daniels G. *Human Blood Groups*. 3rd ed. Blackwell Science; 2013; Reid ME, Lomas-Francis C, Olsson ML. *Blood Group Antigen FactsBook*, 3rd ed. Academic Press; 2012; Reid ME, Lomas-Francis C. *Blood Group Antigens & Antibodies: A Guide to Clinical Relevance & Technical Tips*. Star Bright Books; 2007.

Gal(α1–4)-Gal(β1–4). In addition, globoside is the receptor of human parvovirus B19. Some strains of *E. coli* use the disaccharide receptor Gal(α1–4)-Galβ on uroepithelial cells to gain entry to the urinary tract receptors associated with P1, P^k, and P antigens.[5,35] People with the rare p phenotype lack this disaccharide and are not susceptible to acute pyelonephritis from such *E. coli* strains or to infection by human parvovirus B19 (Chap. 5).

PHENOTYPES ASSOCIATED WITH DISEASE RESISTANCE

Erythrocytes lacking Fy^a and Fy^b antigens are not infected by the malarial parasite *Plasmodium vivax* or by the simian malarial parasite *P. knowlesi* (Chap. 24) These parasites attach to the Fy(a–b–) RBC

membrane, but penetration does not take place. The Fy6 antigen is the critical receptor for *P. vivax* attachment.[5] *P. falciparum* attaches to RBC glycophorins and their *O*-linked oligosaccharides (carrying NeuAc). RBCs with the following phenotypes have a decreased rate of infection: M–N– (GPA-deficient), S–s–U– (GPB-deficient), Ge– (Leach type or GPC/GPD-deficient), and Cad-positive and Tn-positive RBCs (which have abnormal *O*-linked sugars).

DISEASES ASSOCIATED WITH ALTERED ANTIGEN EXPRESSION

Antigen expression can be altered with inherited or acquired disease. Inherited changes are fixed and consistent; acquired changes can disappear with remission or recovery. In some diseases, antigen expression weakens; in others, antigen expression increases, or new antigens appear.

Weakened ABH expression on RBCs has been noted in acute myeloid leukemias and may result from reduced transferase activity.[5,16] Normal antigen expression returns with disease remission. Transient weakened expression of target antigen also occurs in some cases of autoimmune hemolytic anemia. Weak Rh, Kell, Kidd, LW, and AnWj blood group activity has been reported with concurrent autoantibody.[5,16,49]

Increased expression of i on RBCs is associated with inherited disorders, such as thalassemia (Chap. 17), sickle cell disease (Chap. 18), Diamond-Blackfan syndrome (Chap. 4), and hereditary erythroblastic multinuclearity with a positive acidified serum test (HEMPAS) (Chap. 14). Increased i expression also is noted with acquired conditions that decrease the red cell maturation time in the marrow, such as myeloblastic or sideroblastic myeloblastic erythropoiesis, refractory anemia, and excessive phlebotomy.[16,23] Expression of the de novo antigen Tn is caused by a galactosyltransferase deficiency acquired by somatic mutation in a population of stem cells. The antigen is present on RBCs, platelets, and granulocytes arising from these stem cells. This condition (seen as persistent mixed-field agglutination because of the presence of both normal and abnormal cells) causes other RBC changes, such as depressed MN expression, enhanced H, and reduced NeuAc content. Tn antigen exposure is associated with myelodysplastic syndrome and acute myelomonocytic leukemia.[16] Other antigens (T, Tk) occur as a result of infection when microbes produce enzymes that remove some sugars (NeuAc) and expose new ones. Group A individuals can appear to acquire a B antigen when bacterial deacetylase removes the acetyl group on GalNAc.[4,16] This phenomenon is associated with severe infection, gastrointestinal lesions, and malignancies.

RBCs may acquire blood group activity when they adsorb material from certain microorganisms. Group B activity has been associated with *E. coli*[86] and *Proteus vulgaris* infection, and K antigen with *Enterococcus faecium*. Acquired Jk[b]-like activity has been associated with *E. faecium* and *Micrococcus* infections, although the mechanism is not clear.[50]

DISEASES ASSOCIATED WITH ABSENT ANTIGENS OR NULL PHENOTYPES

Rh_null Syndrome

The Rh_null phenotype is associated with hereditary stomatocytosis, hemolytic anemia (usually mild and well compensated), and a lack of proteins carrying Rh antigens. The Rh protein resides in the RBC membrane, interacts with other membrane proteins and possibly the membrane skeleton, and may help regulate or organize the lipids within the red cell membrane bilayer (see Chap. 15).[9,10] Hence, it is an important determinant of membrane shape and expression of other antigens. Rh_null cells have depressed expression or absence of S, s, U, LW, and Fy5 antigens.

Most Rh_null red cells are stomatocytes, or occasionally spherocytes, and demonstrate increased osmotic fragility, increased potassium permeability, and higher potassium pump activity. They have reduced cation and water content and a relative deficiency of membrane cholesterol. Although these abnormalities are assumed to contribute to shortened in vivo survival, Rh_null RBCs survive normally in splenectomized patients, suggesting their removal is related more to splenic clearance because of shape rather than some other intrinsic factor (Chap. 2).

Two genetic mechanisms account for the Rh_null phenotype. Persons with the amorphic type are homozygous for the silent *RHCE* gene on a deleted *RHD* background. Individuals with the more common regulator type of Rh_null have normal RH genes but an altered (silenced) *RHAG* gene. RhAG is required for expression of Rh antigens. Individuals

with the Rh_mod phenotype have similar membrane and clinical anomalies associated with Rh_null syndrome but demonstrate some Rh antigen expression. The reduced expression of Rh antigens results from the presence of an altered form of RhAG.[4,24,26]

McLeod Phenotype

Numerous males (but no females) with the McLeod phenotype have been identified. These individuals have acanthocytosis (Chap. 15), decreased RBC survival, very weak expression of Kell blood group antigens, lack of Kx antigen on RBCs, and a well-compensated hemolytic anemia.[51]

Kx antigen is carried on the Xk protein encoded by the XK gene on the X chromosome, which interacts with the RBC membrane skeleton and helps stabilize the membrane. The absence of Kx is associated with a lipid deficiency in the membrane bilayer that may be critical to the Kell glycoprotein and general RBC discoid shape. RBCs with the McLeod phenotype show a defect in water transport, increased mobility of phosphatidylcholine across the membrane, and increased phosphorylation of protein band 3 and β-spectrin.[51]

After age 40 years, patients with the McLeod phenotype develop a slowly progressive form of muscular dystrophy that is associated with areflexia, choreiform movements, and cardiomegaly, leading to cardiomyopathy. They have elevated levels of serum creatine kinase and carbonic anhydrase III. Some patients with the McLeod phenotype and X-linked chronic granulomatous disease (CGD) have a deletion of both the XK and Phox-91 genes. The McLeod phenotype results from deletions or nucleotide changes in the XK gene.[52]

Gerbich-Negative Phenotype

The *GYPC* on chromosome 2 encodes two proteins: GPC, with antigens Ge3 and Ge4 (the Ge2 portion is "hidden" by the Ge4-bearing terminal end); and its shorter partner, GPD, with antigens Ge2 (now exposed) and Ge3. GPC and GPD interact with membrane skeleton proteins 4.1 and p55, which are involved in cell deformability and membrane stability. Gerbich-negative RBCs of the Leach type (Ge:−2,−3,−4) lack both GPC and GPD, have reduced protein 4.1, and elliptocytosis (Chap. 15), but exhibit normal survival in vivo.[6,10]

Bombay (O_h) Phenotype

Rare people lack A, B, and H antigens and have naturally occurring anti-A, anti-B, and anti-H in their plasma. Such people are said to have the Bombay (O_h) phenotype. In rare people with the Le(a−b−) Bombay phenotype, the gene that encodes the Fuc transporter is silenced. As a consequence, all cells lack Fuc. Without Fuc, neutrophils lack sialyl Le[X] and thus cannot roll and ingest bacteria. These patients have a high white blood cell count and severe recurrent infections. The condition is called *leukocyte adhesion deficiency II* or *congenital disorder of glycosylation II*.[53,54]

In(Jk) Phenotype

A zinc-finger deletion at ZNF850 defines the dominant Kidd-null red blood cell phenotype, In(Jk), that was identified in five families from the Subbetic area of Southern Spain. Most In(Jk) Kidd-null individuals (80.77%) fulfilled criteria for mood and/or anxiety disorder, with increased suicidal risk in the families (7.4-fold), Reduced ability to concentrate urea in the urine was documented in two cases.[32]

I-Negative Phenotype (i Adult)

The gene encoding the I-branching β-1,6-N-acetylglucosaminyltransferase (GCNT2) has three alternative forms of exon 1, with common exons 2 and 3. Mutations in exon 2 or 3 silence GCNT2 and give rise to the form of I-negative phenotype associated with congenital cataracts in Asians.[55,56] Mutations in exon 1C (*IGnTC* or *IGnT3*) silence the gene in RBCs but not in other tissues, and lead to the I-negative phenotype (i adult) without cataracts.[57]

CO~null~ Phenotype

Antigens of the Colton blood group system are carried on the water transporter (aquaporin 1 [AQP1]). Although an absence of this protein from the RBC membrane was thought to be incompatible with life, these rare individuals have been shown only to be unable to maximally concentrate urine.[58]

RAPH~null~ Phenotype

The MER2 antigen in the RAPH blood group system is carried on CD151. Rare individuals who lack CD151 have chronic renal failure, skin ulcers, and deafness.[59]

CD59~null~ Phenotype

Absence of CD59 protein is associated with hemolytic anemia, thrombosis, and other autoimmune diseases such as systemic lupus erythematosus.[41]

AUG~null~ Phenotype

Antigens of the Augustine (AUG) blood group system are carried on the erythrocyte protein, equilibrative nucleoside transporter 1. People with the rare AUG~null~ phenotype were found to have multiple small calcifications around the joints in the hand and ectopic calcification or mineralization also in hips, feet, pubic symphysis, and lumbar discs.[40]

CTL2~null~ Phenotype

Lack of the choline transporter–like 2 protein (encoded by *SLC44A2*) has been associated with hearing impairment, especially in the upper frequency range, in both humans and (knockout) mice. CTL2 is highly expressed on neutrophils and carries the human neutrophil antigen-3 (HNA-3). HNA-3 has been associated with transfusion-related acute lung injury.[60]

PEL~null~ Phenotype

A large deletion in the *ABCC4/MRP4* gene encoding the ATP-binding cassette (ABC) transporter ABCC4 results in the PEL~null~ phenotype. ABCC4 is a member of the multidrug resistance protein (MRP4) subfamily involved in multidrug resistance. People with the rare PEL– blood type are the first reported humans with no expression of ABCC4, indicating that it is not a life-essential protein. Although ABCC4 is an important cyclic nucleotide exporter, RBCs from ABCC4null/PEL– people exhibit normal cGMP level, suggesting a compensatory mechanism by other erythroid ABC transporters. No mutual symptoms or diseases were identified in a study of 12 PEL– people from within four families but PEL– individuals did show an impaired platelet aggregation, confirming a role for ABCC4 in platelet function. Studies have suggested that ABCC4 variants may increase toxicity or cause resistance for cancer drugs.[36]

MAM~null~ Phenotype

Whole exome sequencing of MAM– individuals showed that all had inactivating mutations in *EMP3*, the gene encoding the transmembrane protein EMP3 (epithelial membrane protein 3) and that EMP3 is expressed in erythroid cells. Although EMP3 is a purported tumor suppressor in various solid tumors, no evidence was found that MAM– (EMP3null) individuals have an increased risk of cancer.[37] An interaction of EMP3 with the cell surface signaling molecule CD44 showed that EMP3 participates in a cell-to-cell interaction. An important finding of their study was that cultured erythroid progenitor cells from

MAM– individuals showed markedly increased proliferation and higher reticulocyte yields (average of fivefold increase), suggesting an important regulatory role for EMP3 in erythropoiesis and control of cell production.

EMM~null~ Phenotype

PIGG encodes the EMM blood group system and the Emm– phenotype is associated with deficiency of a transferase enzyme, PIGG, potentially defining a new blood group antigen composed of ethanolamine phosphate (EtNP) bound to mannose in the GPI-anchor.[43] The absence of Emm on PNH type III cells had strongly suggested that Emm antigen was expressed on a GPI-anchored protein, but the finding that Emm is a component of the anchor itself was unexpected.

The association of the Emm– phenotype and *PIGG* loss of function mutations may have important biological relevance. *PIGG* loss of function mutations have been reported to be responsible for neurologic phenotypes including seizures, developmental delay, intellectual disability, and hypotonia.[61,62] The diagnosis and medical histories of several of the Emm– patients are largely unknown inherited glycosylphosphatidylinositol defects cause the rare Emm– RBC phenotype and developmental disorders.[44]

ABCC1~null~ Phenotype

An unidentified antibody to a high-prevalence antigen resulted in the identification of a null allele of *ABCC1* encoding ABCC1 (also known as the multidrug resistance protein 1) and in the discovery of a novel blood group system.[38] ABCC1 allows for the transport of various substrates involved in oxidative stress homeostasis, inflammation and nucleotide metabolism (efflux pump). In RBCs, ABCC1 is an exporter of glutathione-S-conjugates and ATP. ABCC1 plays a role in the protection of kidney epithelial cells and the original proband died at the age of 26 from severe chronic renal failure. Two younger brothers, also with the ABCC1 null phenotype, had no apparent clinical signs or abnormalities in standard blood hematological and biochemical analysis, except for varying amounts of calcium oxalate crystals in urine, especially prevalent in the older of the two brothers. Whether or not this finding represents an early marker for a potential future renal disease is still unknown.

Other Null Phenotypes

Patients with null phenotypes can develop RBC antibodies that make it difficult to find compatible blood to avoid the otherwise serious hemolytic transfusion reactions. For example, people with the Bombay phenotype (O~h~ or H~null~) demonstrate no red cell abnormality but make potent hemolytic anti-H as well as anti-A and anti-B. These antibodies are incompatible with all RBCs except those from other persons with the Bombay phenotype. Likewise, p individuals (PP1P^k^-negative) or P^k^ individuals (P-negative) can make hemolytic antibodies to the antigens they lack. Anti-PP1P^k^ and anti-P also are associated with spontaneous abortions in the first trimester.[16] Women with such antibodies (notably IgG anti-P), even those with a history of spontaneous abortions, have delivered viable infants after plasmapheresis.[63]

Null phenotypes in the MNS and Lutheran systems are interesting because several types of null phenotypes are known. Within the MNS blood group system, people may lack GPA [En(a–) or MN-negative], GPB (SsU-negative), or both GPA and GPB (M^k^M^k^ phenotype). The rare Lu(a–b–) phenotype is caused by a dominant inhibitor called *In(Lu)*, by homozygous pairing of the silent allele *Lu*, or by a nucleotide change in *GATA-1*, resulting in X-linked inheritance of the phenotype.[31] Only the *LuLu*-type null (recessive Lu[a–b–]) is associated with antibody production because the inhibitor type nulls produce small amounts of Lutheran antigen. *In(Lu)* type, Lu(a–b–) RBCs have low expression of CD44 and AnWj, and have varying degrees of poikilocytosis and acanthocytosis. RBCs of this type tend to hemolyze more quickly during storage, even though they demonstrate normal osmotic fragility.[64] Inactivating nucleotide changes in *KLF1*, which encodes an altered transcription factor, cause the In(Lu) phenotype.[31]

The Jk(a–b–) phenotype is caused by the silent alleles *JkJk* or the dominant inhibitor *In(Jk)*. RBCs having the Jk(a–b–) phenotype resist lysis in 2*M* urea,[4] a reagent commonly used in automated platelet counting systems, resulting in erroneously high platelet counts. Jk(a–b–) individuals have reduced ability to concentrate urine[65] and mood and/or anxiety disorders occur in people with the In(Jk) phenotype.[32]

The following diagnoses are made easily by simply typing the RBCs with appropriate antisera: Rh syndrome, McLeod syndrome, and leukocyte adhesion deficiency (LAD) II.

⬤ ERYTHROCYTE ANTIBODIES

IMMUNOLOGY OF RED CELL ANTIBODIES

Blood group antibodies are classified as *alloantibodies* if they only react with antigens present on the RBCs of other people and as *autoantibodies* if they react with *self-antigens* present on the patient's own RBC. Alloantibodies also can be classified according to their mode of sensitization as *naturally occurring* (no apparent sensitization) or *immune* (after sensitization). Table 29-5 summarizes the common antierythrocyte antibodies.[4,6,15,16]

IMMUNOGLOBULIN CLASSES ASSOCIATED WITH BLOOD GROUP ACTIVITY

Immunoglobulin G

IgG is the predominant antibody made in an immune response and constitutes approximately 80% of total serum Ig.[16] These antibodies, when specific for RBC antigens, can attach to or induce hemolysis of transfused antigen-positive RBCs. Receptors on macrophages in the liver and spleen allow the macrophages to remove IgG-coated RBCs from the circulation (Chaps. 25 and 26). IgG blood group antibodies also are capable of fixing complement, although some subclasses do so less efficiently than others: $IgG_3 > IgG_1 > IgG_2 > IgG_4$. How well an IgG erythrocyte antibody binds complement depends on the surface density and location of the recognized antigen. This situation occurs because C1q, the initiator of the classic complement cascade, requires binding of at least two IgG molecules to the RBC within a span of 20 to 30 nm to initiate the complement cascade.[16] For example, IgG anti-D rarely binds complement, presumably because most D sites are spaced too far apart.[16] Most IgG blood group antibodies do not agglutinate saline-suspended RBCs, presumably because the IgG molecule is too small to span the distance between RBCs, although some exceptions are known (ie, potent IgG examples of anti-A, anti-B, anti-M, and anti-K). Some IgG anti-D can directly agglutinate RBCs with the D– – phenotype. Most IgG antibodies sensitize RBCs at 37°C and are detected with an antiglobulin reagent.[11]

Immunoglobulin M

IgM is a pentamer of five basic units (having μ heavy chains plus a short J, or joining, chain) and makes up only approximately 4% of total serum Ig.[16] IgM is the first class of Ig produced by the fetus and is the predominant antibody in a primary immune response, but it does not cross the placenta. Because of their pentameric structure, even low-affinity IgM blood group antibodies can agglutinate RBCs and activate complement. Both hemolyzing and agglutinating abilities of IgM molecules are destroyed by reducing reagents, such as 2-mercaptoethanol and DTT.

IgM antibodies of low affinity may agglutinate RBCs only at temperatures below 37°C. Such antibodies still may fix complement onto the RBC membrane in vivo, at the lower temperatures in the extremities, and activate the complement cascade in the core of the body. Because such IgM antibodies dissociate from RBCs at higher temperatures, their reactivity may be detected in routine antiglobulin tests (using polyspecific antiglobulin) by virtue of the complement components that remain bound to the red cell membrane.[11,16]

Immunoglobulin A

IgA is the primary Ig in body secretions, where it exists predominantly as a dimer with a secretory component.[16] IgA does not cross the placenta or fix complement, but aggregated IgA can activate the alternative pathway of complement, and IgA can trigger cell-mediated events. Multimeric IgA antibodies in serum are seen as hemagglutinins in blood bank tests and most often are associated with anti-A or anti-B.

IMMUNOGLOBULIN IN THE FETUS AND NEWBORN

Initially, the fetus acquires low levels of maternal IgG, probably by diffusion across the placenta. These levels rise significantly between 20 and 33 weeks of gestation as a selective transport system matures and maternal IgG is actively transported across the placenta. Thus, almost all blood group antibodies detected in the fetus and newborn originate from the mother and disappear within the first few months of life.

Actual fetal antibody production begins shortly before birth with low levels of IgM, followed by IgG and IgA several weeks after birth. Anti-A and anti-B usually are readily detected by age 2 to 6 months.

Because of this late immune response in the newborn and because maternal antibody is so predominant at birth, blood bank standards permit abbreviated testing on neonates younger than 4 months.[66] If available, the mother's serum is used (and preferred) for identifying antibodies in a newborn and for crossmatching RBC components.

NATURALLY OCCURRING ANTIBODIES

Naturally Occurring Antibodies in Development

An antibody is said to be *naturally occurring* when it is found in the serum of an individual who has not been exposed to the antigen through transfusion or pregnancy. These antibodies most likely are heteroagglutinins produced in response to substances in the environment that are similar to those on RBC antigens.

Evidence supporting this concept has come from studies on the formation of anti-B in chickens.[16] Chicks raised in a normal environment made anti-B within the first 30 days of life, whereas chicks raised in a germ-free environment, did not make anti-B by day 60. Naturally occurring anti-A and anti-B in humans, also called *isoagglutinins*, can increase in titer following ingestion or inhalation of suitable bacteria.[16]

However, a great many antigens that likely are not present in the environment have been associated with naturally occurring antibodies, so the stimulus for naturally occurring antibodies is not clearly known.

Blood Group Associations and Presence of Naturally Occurring Antibodies

Naturally occurring alloantibodies are commonly associated with the carbohydrate antigens of the ABO, H, LE, and P1PK blood group systems. Anti-A and anti-B are expected in people who lack the corresponding antigens, as are antibodies specific for H, PP1P^k, or P antigens. Naturally occurring antibodies reactive with A1, Le^a, Le^b, or P1 determinants also are seen frequently. Carbohydrate antigens, especially those with repetitive epitopes, can stimulate B cells to make specific antibody

TABLE 29-5. Summary of Selected Erythrocyte Antibodies

Blood Group	Antibody	Ig Class		Serologic Activity			Activates Complement	HTR	Implicated in HDFN	Antigen Frequency (%)		Comments
		IgM	IgG	RT	37°C AHG	ENZ/DTT				Whites	Blacks	
ABO	A	Most	Some	Most	Most	I/nc	Yes	Yes	Mild	40	27	A/B: very clinically significant, sometimes IgA
	B	Most	Some	Most	Most	I/nc	Yes	Yes	Mild	11	20	
	A1	Most	Rare	Most	Rare	I/nc	Rare	Rare	No	30	—	A1: usually not clinically significant
	H	Most	Rare	Most	Rare	I/nc	Rare	Rare	—	>99.9	—	H: usually weak autoantibody, but strong alloantibody in O_h
Rh	D	Some	Most	Some	Most	I/nc	No	Yes	Mild to Sev	85	92	D: most common immune antibody
	C	Few	Most	—	Most	I/nc	No	Yes	Mild to Sev	70	33	C: often found with D
	E	Some	Most	Some	Most	I/nc	No	Yes	Mild	30	21	E/C or E/c: often found together
	c	—	Most	—	Most	I/nc	No	Yes	Mild to Sev	80	97	All alloantibodies: clinically significant
	e	—	Most	—	Most	I/nc	No	Yes	Mild	98	99	Autoantibodies commonly directed against Rh protein
	f (ce)	—	Most	—	Most	I/nc	No	Yes	Mild	64	—	
	C^w	Some	Most	—	Most	I/nc	No	Yes	Mild to Mod	2	—	
	VS/V	—	Most	—	Most	I/nc	No	Yes	No	<1	30	
Lewis	Le^a	Most	Rare	Most	Some	I/nc	Yes	Rare	No	22	23	Common in pregnancy
	Le^b	Most	Rare	Most	Some	I/nc	Yes	No	No	72	55	Not clinically significant; Le(a–b–) individuals commonly make anti-Le^a but can simultaneously make anti-Le^a and anti-Le^b
Ii	I	Most	—	Most	Some	I/nc	Yes	Rare	No	>99.9	>99.9	I: common autoantibody, rare significant alloantibody
	i	Most	—	Most	Some	I/nc	Yes	No	Rare (mild)	100	100	i: rare autoantibody
P1PK	P1	Most	Rare	Most	Some	I/nc	Few	Rare	No	79	94	P1: usually not clinically significant
GLOB	P	Most	Few	Most	Some	I/nc	Yes	Yes	No – Mild	>99.9	>99.9	P: Donath-Landsteiner antibody in PCH
	PP1Pk	Most	Few	Most	Some	I/nc	Yes	Yes	No – Sev	>99.9	>99.9	
MNSs	M	Some	Some	Most	Few	D/nc	No	Rare	Rare	78	70	M: common, usually not clinically significant
	N	Some	Some	Most	Rare	D/nc	No	Rare	(Rare)	72	74	N: rare, usually not clinically significant
	S	Some	Some	Some	Most	V/nc	Some	Yes	Mild to Sev	55	31	
	s	Few	Most	Few	Most	V/nc	Rare	Yes	No – Sev	89	97	

System	Antigen											Comments
	U	—	Most	—	Most	nc/nc	Rare	Yes	Mild to Sev	100	99.7	SsU: clinically significant autoantibody specificities reported
Kell	K	Some	Most	Few	Most	nc/D	Rare	Yes	Mild to Sev	9	2	K: very common immune antibody
	k	—	Most	Rare	Most	nc/D	No	Yes	Mild to Sev	99.9	—	
	Kpa	—	Most	Rare	Most	nc/D	No	Yes	Mild to Sev	2.3	—	
	Kpb	—	Most	Rare	Most	nc/D	No	Yes	Mild to Mod	>99.9	100	Autoantibodies reported
	Jsa	—	Most	Rare	Rare	nc/D	No	Yes	Mild to Sev	—	20	
	Jsb	—	Most	—	—	nc/D	No	Yes	Mild to Sev	>99.9	99	
Duffy	Fya	—	Most	Rare	Most	D/nc	Rare	Yes	Mild to Sev	66	10	Fya: common immune antibody
	Fyb	—	Most	Rare	Most	D/nc	Rare	Yes	Mild	83	23	
Kidd	Jka	Few	Most	Rare	Most	I/nc	Yes	Yes	Mild to Mod	77	92	Jka: associated with delayed HTR; hemolytic; disappears quickly from serum
	Jkb	Few	Most	Rare	Most	I/nc	Yes	Yes	No – Mild	72	41	Jkb: associated with delayed HTR; hemolytic; disappears quickly from serum
Lutheran	Lua	Some	Few	Most	Few	nc(V)/D	No	No	No – Mild	7.7	—	Mild RBC destruction
	Lub	Some	Some	Few	Most	nc(V)/D	No	Yes	Mild	99.9	—	Lu glycoprotein on placental tissue may adsorb maternal Lu antibodies
Xg	Xga	Some	Most	Rare	Most	D/nc	Some	No	No	64(m) 89(f)	—	Xga: poor immunogen
Yt	Yta	—	Most	No	Most	D(V)/D(V)	No	No – Mod	No	99.7	—	Yt: some antibody examples clinically significant, others not
	Ytb	—	Most	No	Most	D(V)/D	No	No	No	8	—	
Ch/Rg	Ch	Rare	Most	—	Most	D/nc	No	No	No	96	—	Ch/Rg: associated with C4 complement, clinically insignificant antibodies
	Rg	—	Most	—	Most	D/nc	No	No	No	98	—	
Colton	Coa	—	Most	Some	Most	nc/nc	Some	No – Mod	No – Mod	99.9	—	
	Cob	—	Most	Some	Most	nc/nc	Rare	No – Mod	Mild	10	—	
Cromer	General group	Most	Most	Most	Most	nc/V	No	No	No	>99.9	>99.9	CD55 on apical surface of trophoblasts in placenta may absorb maternal antibody
Diego	Dia	—	Most	Some	Most	nc/nc	Rare	Yes	Mild to Sev	Rare	—	Dia: antigen found in South Native Americans and Asians
	Dib	—	Most	No	Most	nc/nc	No	No – Mod	Mild	100	—	
Dombrock	Doa	—	Most	No	Most	nc/D(V)	No	Yes	+DAT	67	—	Doa Dob: poor immunogens
	Dob	—	Most	No	Most	nc/D(V)	No	Yes	+DAT	83	—	
	Hy	—	Most	—	Most	nc(I)/D(V)	No	No – Mod	+DAT	>99	—	Hy– found only in blacks

(continued)

TABLE 29-5. Summary of Selected Erythrocyte Antibodies (Continued)

Blood Group	Antibody	Ig Class		Serologic Activity			Activates Complement	Implicated in		Antigen Frequency (%)		Comments
		IgM	IgG	RT	37°C AHG	ENZ/DTT		HTR	HDFN	Whites	Blacks	
	Gy^a	—	Most	—	Most	nc(I)/D(V)	No	No – Mod	+DAT	>99	—	Gy(a−) (Do_null) found in eastern Europeans and Japanese
	Jo^a	—	Most	—	Most	nc(I)/D(V)	No	No – Mod	No	>99	—	Jo(a−): found only in blacks
Gerbich	General group	—	Most	—	Most	D/nc	Yes	No – Mod	Yes for some Ge specificities	>99.9	>99.9	Ge: located on glycophorins C and D
Indian	In^a	—	Most	—	Most	D/D	No	Yes	(+DAT)	<0.1	<0.1	In: located on CD44 adhesion protein
	In^b	—	Most	—	Most	D/D	No	No – Sev	(+DAT)	99	96	
Knops	Kn^a	—	Most	—	Most	D/D/V	No	No	No	98	99	Knops antigens associated with CR1 (complement) receptor, clinically insignificant antibodies
	McC^a	—	Most	—	Most	D/D	No	No	No	98	94	
	Yk^a	—	Most	—	Most	D/D	No	No	No	92	98	
Scianna	Sc1	—	Most	—	Most	nc/nc	Yes	No	+DAT	>99.9	—	Sc1: some antibodies react in serum but not plasma
	Sc2	—	Most	—	Most	nc/-V	No	No	+DAT	1	—	
	Sc3	—	Most	—	Most	nc(I)/nc	No	No – Mild	Mild	>99.9	—	
JMH	JMH	—	Most	—	Most	D/D	No	No	No	>99.9	>99.9	JMH: carrier protein CDw108

D, destroyed; DTT, dithiothreitol; ENZ, enzyme (papain/ficin); I, increased; nc, no change; V, variable.

without the aid of helper T cells. Such thymus-independent immune responses typically result in antigen-specific antibodies of the IgM class.

Within other systems,[16] anti-Sd[a], anti-Vw, and anti-Wr[a] are found in up to 2% of normal people. Other, less common antibody specificities in approximate order of descending occurrence are anti-M, S, N, Ge, K, Lu[a], Di[a], and Xg[a]. Rh antigens are thought to reside only on RBCs, but apparent naturally occurring anti-D has been reported in 0.15% of Rh-negative donors and anti-E in more than 0.1% of Rh-positive donors when more sensitive enzyme detection methods are used. Examples of naturally occurring anti-C, anti-C[W], and anti-C[X] also have been described.[4-6]

Some naturally occurring antibodies exist as autoagglutinins (eg, anti-H and anti-I). Patients with autoimmune hemolytic anemia can produce many antibodies to low-prevalence antigens with no specific stimulus, in addition to autoantibody.[5,6,16,49]

Characteristics of Naturally Occurring Alloantibodies

Most naturally occurring antibodies are IgM, but some have an IgG component, and a few are predominantly IgG. Some anti-A or anti-B may even be of the IgA class. Antibodies that cause direct agglutination of saline-suspended RBCs most commonly are of the IgM class. However, even IgG antibodies may cause agglutination of RBCs when they bind antigens that are present at high density on the RBC membrane, such as the ABO or MN antigens. Except for anti-A and anti-B, most common naturally occurring antibodies do not react at body temperature and are considered clinically insignificant. However, if they are found to react at 37°C, providing crossmatch-compatible blood for transfusion is prudent.

ANTIBODIES GENERATED IN RESPONSE TO IMMUNIZATION: IMMUNE ANTIBODIES

Blood Group Associations and Occurrence of Immune Antibodies

Immune antibodies are produced after exposure to foreign RBC antigens through pregnancy or transfusion. The primary immune response is seen several weeks to several months after the first exposure to antigen. IgM usually is associated with early primary responses, but whether it is always the first antibody class made is unclear. In most individuals, IgG soon predominates. This process is characteristic of a thymus-dependent immune response, where T cells help induce B cells to undergo isotype switching from IgM to IgG.

In a secondary or anamnestic response, antibody concentration starts to increase several days to several weeks after exposure, and IgG may rise to very high levels. Some IgG antibodies remain detectable for decades after a stimulus. Others, especially Kidd (antibodies, can disappear after several months and are more commonly associated with delayed hemolytic transfusion reactions.[5,6,16]

Immune antibodies are found more commonly in individuals who have been multiply transfused than in multiparous women. This situation occurs because in pregnancy the immunizing dose of red cells often is too small to elicit a primary response and the foreign antigens are limited to those of the father.[16]

Anti-D used to be the most common immune antibody, but with the advent of Rh matching of donors and recipients in the late 1940s and use of RhIg prophylaxis since the 1970s, its incidence has sharply decreased. Anti-D is present in 0.27% to 0.56% of transfusion recipients, 0.10% to 0.20% of pregnant women, and 0.16% to 0.25% of healthy blood donors.[16]

In contrast, the occurrence of immune antibodies other than anti-D has increased. Specificities other than anti-D have been reported in approximately 0.6% of transfusion recipients, 0.14% of pregnant

women, and 0.19% of healthy blood donors. Pooled data from three 5-year periods and approximately 300,000 patients suggest the absolute occurrence of Rh antibodies other than anti-D is 0.22%, other than anti-K is 0.19%, other than anti-Fy[a] is 0.05%, and other than anti-Jk[a] is 0.04%.[16] The rate of alloimmunization in patients with sickle cell anemia was 18.6% in one survey, and 55% of the immunized patients made more than one antibody. The most common specificities were anti-C, anti-E, and anti-K.[16]

Characteristics of Immune Antibodies

Immune antibodies most often are IgG but may be IgM and sometimes are IgA. Most immune antibodies react at body temperature and are considered clinically significant, except those directed against Bg, Knops, Cs[a], JMH, and sometimes Yt[a] and Lutheran antigens.

⬤ CLINICAL SIGNIFICANCE OF ERYTHROCYTE ANTIBODIES

Information about the clinical significance of alloantibodies is available at www.nybc.org and in publications.[11,67,68]

HEMOLYTIC TRANSFUSION REACTIONS

Clinically significant antibodies can destroy transfused RBCs. The severity of the reaction varies with antigen density and antibody characteristics.

Antibodies commonly associated with intravascular hemolysis include anti-A, anti-B, anti-Jk[a], and anti-Jk[b]. ABO incompatibility is the most potent cause of immediate hemolytic reactions because A and B antigens are strongly expressed on RBCs and the antibodies so efficiently bind complement. Kidd antibodies (recognizing JK antigens) are associated more often with delayed hemolytic reactions because they typically are difficult to detect and can disappear quickly from the circulation. IgG anti-Jk[a] appears to bind complement only when traces of IgM anti-Jk[a] are present.[16] Anti-PP1P[k], anti-Vel, and anti-Le[a] have been associated with hemolysis, but such examples are rare.

Extravascular hemolysis occurs with IgG_1 and IgG_3 antibodies that react at body temperature; that is, immune antibodies reactive with Rh, Kidd, Kell, Duffy, or Ss antigens. These antibodies make up the bulk of clinically significant antibodies. Antibodies not expected to cause RBC destruction are those that react only at temperatures below 37°C and IgG antibodies of the IgG_2 or IgG_4 subclass.[16]

HEMOLYTIC DISEASE OF THE FETUS AND NEWBORN

HDFN is caused by blood group incompatibility between a sensitized mother and her antigen-positive fetus (Chap. 27). The antibodies most significant in HDFN are those that cross the placenta (IgG_1 and IgG_3), react at body temperature to cause red cell destruction, and are directed against well-developed RBC antigens. ABO incompatibility most commonly is seen, but ABO HDFN is clinically mild, presumably because the antigens are not fully expressed at birth. Antibodies directed against the D antigen can cause severe HDFN, and fetal health should be carefully monitored when anti-D titers are greater than 16. The severity of HDFN is less predictable with other blood group antibodies and can vary from mild to severe. For example, anti-K and anti-Ge3 not only cause red cell hemolysis but also may suppress erythropoiesis.[4,6]

AUTOIMMUNE HEMOLYTIC ANEMIA

Autoimmune hemolytic anemia is caused by the production of "warm-" or "cold-" reactive autoantibodies directed against RBC antigens (Chap. 26).[49]

Production can be triggered by disease, viral infection, or drugs; from breakdown in immune system tolerance to self-antigens; or from exposure to foreign antigens that induce antibodies that cross-react with self-RBC antigens. Autologous specificity is not always obvious because antigen expression can be depressed when autoantibody is present.[49]

Warm autoantibodies react best at 37°C and are primarily IgG (rarely IgM or IgA). Most are directed against the Rh protein, but Wr^b, Kell, Kidd, and U blood group specificities have been reported.[49]

Cold-reactive autoantibodies are primarily IgM. They react best at temperatures below 25°C but can agglutinate RBCs or activate complement at or near 37°C, causing hemolysis or vascular occlusion upon exposure to cold.[16] Patients with cold agglutinin disease often have C3d on their RBCs, which can provide some protection from hemolysis. Most cold-reactive autoantibodies have anti-I activity. Reactivity with i, H, Pr, P, or other antigenic specificities is much less common.

The biphasic cold-reactive IgG antibody associated with paroxysmal cold hemoglobinuria ("Donath-Landsteiner" antibody) typically reacts with the high-prevalence antigen P (GLOB). It attaches to RBCs in the cold and very efficiently activates complement before it dissociates at warmer temperatures.

DISEASES ASSOCIATED WITH ANTIBODY PRODUCTION

Table 29-4 lists diseases associated with specific antibody production. These antibodies cause autoimmune hemolytic anemia only if the patient carries the corresponding antigen.

● SEROLOGIC DETECTION OF ERYTHROCYTE ANTIGENS AND ANTIBODIES

ABO

ABO grouping is the single most important test performed in the transfusion service because it is the fundamental basis for determining blood compatibility. ABO grouping is determined by testing RBCs with licensed antisera to identify the A or B antigens they carry (forward, or cell, grouping) and by testing the corresponding serum or plasma with known A and B cells to identify the antibodies present (reverse, or serum, grouping). Positive reactions are seen as hemagglutination or hemolysis, and the results of one test should confirm the results of the other.

If results are discrepant or reactions are weaker than expected, the cause must be investigated before the ABO group can be interpreted with confidence. Discrepancies can be related to RBC anomalies, serum anomalies, or both, and they may be associated with disease.[5,11,16] Table 29-6 lists common causes, excluding clerical and technical error. If the ABO group of a patient cannot be determined, group O blood can be used for transfusion.

Rh

The D type is the next most important test performed for blood compatibility. Individuals whose RBCs type D+ are called *Rh-positive*, and those who type D– are called *Rh-negative*, provided controls are acceptable. Blood donors who type D– using standard typing sera are tested further for weak D expression using more sensitive methods, such as an indirect antiglobulin test. Donors with weak D antigen are considered Rh-positive. Testing for weak D is optional for transfusion recipients and pregnant women.[66]

TABLE 29–6. Common Causes of ABO Discrepancies

RED CELLS MAY APPEAR TO HAVE	
Weak or missing antigens	Weak subgroup of A or B antigen
	Excess soluble A or B antigen in plasma
	Disease-associated loss (leukemia)
	ABO nonidentical marrow transplantation
	ABO nonidentical red blood cell (RBC) transfusions
	Chimera
Extra antigens	Positive direct antiglobulin test
	Antibody to reagent additive or dye
	Rouleaux or cold agglutinin on cells
	Disease-associated acquisition (polyagglutination)
SERUM MAY APPEAR TO HAVE	
Weak or missing antibody	Age related (newborns or geriatric adults)
	Disease-associated immunosuppression
	Congenital hypogammaglobulinemia
	ABO nonidentical marrow transplantation
Extra antibody	Alloantibodies (A$_1$, Le^a, Le^b, P$_1$, M, N)
	Autoantibodies (I, i, H, Pr, P)
	Rouleaux
	Antibodies to additives in reagent RBCs
	Passive antibody acquisition from transfusion or from passenger lymphocytes in organ transplantation

EXTENDED ANTIGEN PHENOTYPING

Reagent antisera to detect other common antigens (eg, CcEe, MNSs, Kk, Fy^{a}Fy^b, Jk^{a}Jk^b) are available and used when identification of the red cell phenotype is essential to antibody identification, blood compatibility, determination of zygosity, or paternity or forensic issues. Extended phenotyping is especially important to patients who are at high risk for alloimmunization from chronic blood transfusion, for example, those with sickle cell anemia or thalassemia. Ideally, an extended RBC phenotype of patients who are likely to be chronically transfused should be determined before initiation of transfusion therapy. Prediction of a blood group antigen can be made by testing DNA of a patient, even in the presence of transfused RBCs.[27]

ANTIBODY SCREEN

The antibody screen, or indirect antiglobulin test, detects "atypical" or "unexpected" antibodies in the serum (ie, other than anti-A and anti-B) using group O reagent red cells that are known to carry various combinations of antigens. The methods used must be able to detect clinically significant antibodies. Typically, serum or plasma and screening cells are incubated at 37°C with an additive to potentiate antibody–antigen reactions, then an indirect antiglobulin test is performed. Hemagglutination or hemolysis at any point is a positive reaction, indicating the presence of naturally occurring or immune alloantibody or autoantibody. The antibody screen will not detect all atypical antibodies in serum, such as antibodies to low-prevalence antigens not present on screening cells and antibodies that are not apparent at 37°C and in the antiglobulin phase.

DIRECT ANTIGLOBULIN TEST

The direct antiglobulin test (often referred to as the direct Coombs test, a term discouraged by Robin Coombs because he said that Race and Mourant were also key to the description of the test) detects antibody or complement bound to RBCs in vivo. Red cells are washed free of serum and then mixed with an antiglobulin reagent that agglutinates RBCs coated with IgG or the C3 component of complement.

Positive direct antiglobulin test results are associated with the following: (1) transfusion reactions, in which recipient alloantibody coats transfused donor RBCs or transfused donor antibody coats recipient RBCs; (2) HDFN, in which maternal antibody crosses the placenta and coats fetal RBCs; (3) autoimmune hemolytic anemias, in which autoantibody coats the patient's own RBCs; (4) drug or drug–antibody complex interactions with RBCs that sometimes lead to hemolysis; (5) passenger lymphocyte syndrome, in which transient antibody produced by passenger lymphocytes from a transplanted organ coats recipient RBCs; and (6) hypergammaglobulinemia, in which Ig nonspecifically adsorb onto circulating RBCs.

A positive direct antiglobulin test result does not always indicate decreased red cell survival. As many as 10% of hospital patients and 0.1% of blood donors have a positive direct antiglobulin test result with no clinical indication of hemolysis.[11]

COMPATIBILITY TESTING

Compatibility testing refers to a set of donor and recipient tests that are performed before red cell transfusion. The collecting facility tests donors for ABO, Rh, and unexpected antibody. However, transfusing hospitals retest the ABO (and D on Rh-negative units) to verify the accuracy of the blood label.[66] Routine recipient testing includes an ABO, D, and antibody screening on a blood sample collected within three days of the intended transfusion. Results are checked against historical records to verify ABO, D, and antibody status.[66]

If the recipient has a negative antibody screening test result and no history of clinically significant antibodies, a serologic immediate spin cross-match between recipient serum and donor red cells or a "computer crossmatch" (wherein computer software compares the ABO test results of both donor and recipient) is required to confirm ABO compatibility.[11]

If clinically significant antibodies are detected in a recipient's serum or previously were identified, red cell components should test negative for the corresponding antigens and be crossmatch compatible at 37°C by the antiglobulin test. The chance of finding compatible units usually reflects the antigen prevalence in the population, that is, 91% of units should be compatible with a patient making anti-K because 9% of the population is K+. This reasoning will not be valid if the local donor population varies significantly from the general population. When more than one antibody is present, the probability of finding compatible blood is the product of the prevalence (probability) of each independent antigen tested. For example, only 21% of units will be compatible for the recipient having both anti-K and anti-Jk[a]: (0.91 for K–) × (0.23 for Jk[a–]) = 0.21.

When multiple clinically significant antibodies or an antibody directed against a high-prevalence antigen are present, finding compatible RBC components can be extremely difficult. Such antibody producers should be encouraged to give autologous donations before their elective blood needs. If the patient is not a candidate for autologous donation, compatible units may be found by testing the patient's siblings or by asking regional blood suppliers to check their rare donor inventories and files. Such procurement requires additional time.

Repeat donor testing and crossmatching are not performed for plasma and platelet components, but the recipient's ABO and Rh

TABLE 29–7. ABO-Rh Compatibility Guidelines

			Compatible Blood Groups	
	Antigen on Red Cells	Antibody in Serum	Donor Red Cells	Donor Plasma
IF RECIPIENT BLOOD GROUP IS				
A	A	Anti-B	A, O	A, AB
B	B	Anti-A	B, O	B, AB
O	O	Anti-A, anti-B	O	O, A, B, AB
AB	A, B	None	AB, A, B, O	AB
Rh-positive	D	None	Rh-positive, Rh-negative	Rh not considered
Rh-negative	None	Anti-D only if immunized	Rh-negative	Rh not considered

Whole blood must be identical to recipient's blood group. Red blood cell (RBC) products must be compatible with recipient's serum. Plasma products should be compatible with recipient's RBCs. Platelet and cryoprecipitate products should be compatible with recipient's RBCs, but any ABO group can be given if compatible products are not available.

phenotypes must be known for appropriate selection of components. Table 29-7 gives general ABO-D compatibility guidelines.

ANTIBODY IDENTIFICATION

All unexpected antibodies should be investigated. Those detected in serum or plasma as an ABO discrepancy, a positive antibody screening result, or an incompatible crossmatch are identified using a panel of 8 to 16 different group O red cells that have been typed for antigens corresponding to clinically significant antibodies. Serum reactions with these RBCs are compared with their antigen typing to determine specificity.[11] For example, an antibody that reacts with all K+ RBCs but not with K– cells most likely is anti-K.

A control of autologous RBCs and serum is tested concurrently with panel RBCs. Absence of reactivity with autologous cells implies the antibody is an alloantibody, whereas a positive result suggests autoantibody or a positive direct antiglobulin test result. Once antibody specificity is identified, the patient's RBCs are tested for the corresponding antigen. If the alloantibody is anti-K, the cells should type K–. Such antigen typing helps to confirm serum findings.

When antibody is detected both on red cells (a positive direct antiglobulin test result) and in serum, only the antibody in serum is identified unless a review of the medical, pregnancy, and transfusion history offers evidence that the antibodies might be different. When antibody is detected only on RBCs and in vivo hemolysis is suspected, the antibody can be eluted from the patient's RBCs and tested against panel RBCs to identify the specificity.

REFERENCES

1. Lewis M, Anstee DJ, Bird GWG, et al. Blood group terminology 1990. ISBT working party on terminology for red cell surface antigens. *Vox Sang.* 1990;58:152.
2. Lögberg L, Reid ME, Zelinsky T. Human blood group genes 2010: chromosomal locations and cloning strategies revisited. *Transfus Med Rev.* 2011;25:36.
3. Cartron JP, Bailly P, Le Van Kim C, et al. Insights into the structure and function of membrane polypeptides carrying blood group antigens. *Vox Sang.* 1998;74(suppl 2):29.

4. Daniels G. *Human Blood Groups*. 3rd ed. Blackwell Science; 2013.

5. Issitt PD, Anstee DJ. *Applied Blood Group Serology*. 4th ed. Montgomery Scientific; 1998.

6. Reid ME, Lomas-Francis C, Olsson ML. *Blood Group Antigen FactsBook*. 3rd ed. Academic Press; 2012.

7. Telen MJ. Erythrocyte blood group antigens: not so simple after all. *Blood*. 1995;85:299.

8. Cartrine JP, Colin Y. Structural and functional diversity of blood group antigens. *Transfus Clin Biol*. 2001;8:163.

9. Bruce LJ, Ghosh S, King MJ, et al. Absence of CD47 in protein 4.2-deficient hereditary spherocytosis in man: an interaction between the Rh complex and the band 3 complex. *Blood*. 2002;100:1878.

10. Reid ME, Mohandas N. Red blood cell blood group antigens: structure and function. *Semin Hematol*. 2004;41:93.

11. Cohn CS, Delaney M, Johnson ST, Katz LM, editors. *Technical Manual, 20th ed.* American Association of Blood Banks, Bethesda, MD, 2020.

12. Storry JR, Banch Clausen F, Castilho L, Chen Q, et al. International Society of Blood Transfusion Working Party on Red Cell Immunogenetics and Blood Group Terminology: report of the Dubai, Copenhagen and Toronto meetings. *Vox Sang*. 2019;114:95.

13. Daniels GL, Anstee DJ, Cartron J-P, et al. Blood group terminology 1995. ISBT working party on terminology for red cell surface antigens. *Vox Sang*. 1995;69:265.

14. Garratty G, Dzik WH, Issitt PD, et al. Terminology for blood group antigens and genes: historical origins and guidelines in the new millennium. *Transfusion*. 2000;40:477.

15. Reid ME, Lomas-Francis C. *Blood Group Antigens & Antibodies: A Guide to Clinical Relevance & Technical Tips*. Star Bright Books; 2007.

16. Klein HG, Anstee DJ. *Mollison's Blood Transfusion in Clinical Medicine*. 12th ed. Wiley-Blackwell; 2014.

17. Clausen H, White T, Takio K, et al. Isolation to homogeneity and partial characterization of a histo-blood group A defined Fuca1—>2Gala1—>3-N-acetylglucosaminyltransferase from human lung tissue. *J Biol Chem*. 1990;265:1139.

18. Yamamoto F, Marken J, Tsuji T, et al. Cloning and characterization of DNA complementary to human UDP-GalNAc: Fuca1—>2Gala1—>3GalNAc transferase (histoblood group A transferase) mRNA. *J Biol Chem*. 1990;265:1146.

19. Yamamoto F, Hakomori S. Sugar-nucleotide donor specificity of histo-blood group A and B transferases is based on amino acid substitutions. *J Biol Chem*. 1990;265:19257.

20. Yamamoto F, Clausen H, White T, et al. Molecular genetic basis of the histo-blood group ABO system. *Nature*. 1990;345:229.

21. Chester MA, Olsson ML. The ABO blood group gene: a locus of considerable genetic diversity. *Transfus Med Rev*. 2001;15:177.

22. Olsson ML, Chester MA. Polymorphism and recombination events at the *ABO* locus: a major challenge for genomic ABO blood grouping strategies. *Transfus Med*. 2001;11:295.

23. Garratty G. Association of blood groups and disease: do blood group antigens and antibodies have a biological role? *Hist Philos Life Sci*. 1996;18:321.

24. Avent ND, Reid ME. The Rh blood group system: A review. *Blood*. 2000;95:375.

25. Westhoff CM. The structure and function of the Rh antigen complex. *Semin Hematol*. 2007;44:42.

26. Huang C-H, Liu PZ, Cheng JG. Molecular biology and genetics of the Rh blood group system. *Semin Hematol*. 2000;37:150.

27. Reid ME, Denomme GA. DNA-based methods in the Immunohematology Reference Laboratory. *Transfus Apher Sci*. 2011;44:65.

28. Giblett ER. A critique of the theoretical hazard of inter vs. intra-racial transfusion. *Transfusion*. 1961;1:233.

29. Stack G, Tormey CA. Estimating the immunogenicity of blood group antigens: a modified calculation that corrects for transfusion exposures. *Br J Haematol*. 2016;175:154.

30. Tippett P. Regulator genes affecting red cell antigens [review]. *Transfus Med Rev*. 1990;4:56.

31. Singleton BK, Burton NM, Green C, et al. Mutations in EKLF/KLF1 form the molecular basis of the rare blood group In(Lu) phenotype. *Blood*. 2008;112:2081.

32. García-Sánchez F, Krause D, Pérez-García D, et al. A zinc-finger deletion at ZNF850 defines the dominant Kidd-Null red blood cell phenotype (INJK) with familiar mood disorder. *Vox Sang*. 2017;112(suppl 1);4B-S22-01.

33. Stenfelt L, Hellberg, Möller M, et al. Missense mutations in the C-terminal portion of the B4GALNT2-encoded glycosyltransferase underlying the Sd(a−) phenotype. *BB Reports*. 2019;19:100659.

34. Hakomori S. Blood group ABH and Ii antigens of human erythrocytes: chemistry, polymorphism, and their developmental change. *Semin Hematol*. 1981;18:39.

35. Hellberg Å, Westman JS, Olsson ML. An update on the GLOB blood group system and collection. *Immunohematology*. 2013;29(1):19.

36. Azouzi S, Mikdar M, Hermand P, et al. Lack of the multidrug transporter MRP4/ABCC4 defines the PEL-negative blood group and impairs platelet aggregation. *Blood* 2020;135:441.

37. Thornton N, Karamatic Crew V, Tilley L, et al. Disruption of the tumour-associated EMP3 enhances erythroid proliferation and causes the MAM-negative phenotype. *Nat Commun* 2020;11:3569.

38. Sugier H, Vrignaud C, Duval R, et al. Null allele of ABCC1 encoding the Multidrug Resistance Protein 1 defines a novel human blood group system. (Abstract 1352) The 36th International ISBT Congress, Virtual meeting, 12–16 December 2020.

39. Pogo AO, Chaudhuri A. The Duffy protein: A malarial and chemokine receptor. *Semin Hematol*. 2000;37:122.

40. Daniels G, Ballif BA, Helias V, et al. Lack of the nucleoside transporter ENT1 results in the Augustine-null blood type and ectopic mineralization. *Blood*. 2015;125:3651.

41. Anliker M, von Zabern I, Höchsmann B, et al. A new blood group antigen is defined by anti-CD59, detected in a CD59-deficient patient. *Transfusion*. 2014;54:1817.

42. Omae Y, Ito S, Takeuchi M, et al. Integrative genome analysis identified the KANNO blood group antigen as prion protein. *Transfusion*. 2019;59:2429.

43. Lane W, Aeschlimann J, Vege S, et al. PIGG Defines the Emm Blood Group System. ISBT Congress virtual meeting of the working Party on blood group terminology and Immunogenetics, 2020.

44. Duval R, Gaël N, Willemetz A, et al. Inherited glycosylphosphatidylinositol defects cause the rare Emm-negative blood phenotype and developmental disorders. Blood. 2020; 2021 Mar 24;blood.2020009810. doi: 10.1182/blood.2020009810.

45. Araten DJ, Swirsky D, Karadimitris A, et al. Cytogenetic and morphological abnormalities in paroxysmal nocturnal haemoglobinuria. *Br J Haematol*. 2001;115:360.

46. Möller M, Lee YQ, Vidovic K, et al. Disruption of a GATA1-binding motif upstream of XG/PBDX abolishes Xg^a expression and resolves the Xg blood group system. *Blood*. 2019;132:334.

47. Cartron J-P, Rahuel C. Human erythrocyte glycophorins: protein and gene structure analyses. *Transfus Med Rev*. 1992;6:63.

48. Mourant AE, Kopec AC, Domaniewska-Sobczak K. *Distribution of the Human Blood Groups and Other Polymorphisms*. 2nd ed. Oxford University Press; 1976.

49. Petz LD, Garratty G. *Acquired Immune Hemolytic Anemias*. 2nd ed. Churchill Livingstone; 2003.

50. Moulds JM, Moulds JJ. Blood group associations with parasites, bacteria, and viruses. *Transfus Med Rev*. 2000;14:302.

51. Lee S, Russo D, Redman CM. The Kell blood group system: Kell and XK membrane proteins. *Semin Hematol*. 2000;37:113.

52. Danek A, Rubio JP, Rampoldi L, et al. McLeod neuroacanthocytosis: genotype and phenotype. *Ann Neurol*. 2001;50:755.

53. Luhn K, Wild MK, Eckhardt M, et al. The gene defective in leukocyte adhesion deficiency II encodes a putative GDP-fucose transporter. *Nat Genet*. 2001;28:69.

54. Etzioni A, Tonetti M. Leukocyte adhesion deficiency II-from A to almost Z. *Immunol Rev*. 2000;178:138.

55. Yu L-C, Twu Y-C, Chang C-Y, Lin M. Molecular basis of the adult i phenotype and the gene responsible for the expression of the human blood group I antigen. *Blood*. 2001;98:3840.

56. Inaba N, Hiruma T, Togayachi A, et al. A novel I-branching beta-1,6-N-acetylglucosaminyltransferase involved in human blood group I antigen expression. *Blood*. 2003;101:2870.

57. Yu LC, Twu YC, Chou ML, et al. The molecular genetics of the human I locus and molecular background explaining the partial association of the adult i phenotype with congenital cataracts. *Blood*. 2003;101:2081.

58. Agre P, King LS, Yasui M, et al. Aquaporin water channels—from atomic structure to clinical medicine. *J Physiol*. 2002;542:3.

59. Crew VK, Burton N, Kagan A, et al. CD151, the first member of the tetraspanin (TM4) superfamily detected on erythrocytes, is essential for the correct assembly of human basement membranes in kidney and skin. *Blood*. 2004;104:2217.

60. Vrignaud C, Mikdar M, Koehl B, et al. Alloantibodies directed to the SLC44A2/CTL2 transporter define two new red cell antigens and a novel human blood group system. *Transfusion*. 2019;59(suppl 3).

61. Makrythanasis P, Kato M, Zaki MS, et al. Pathogenic Variants in PIGG Cause Intellectual Disability with Seizures and Hypotonia. *Am J Hum Genet* 2016;98:615.

62. Zhao JJ, Halvardson J, Knaus A, et al. Reduced cell surface levels of GPI-linked markers in a new case with PIGG loss of function. *Hum Mutat* 2017;38:1394.

63. Rock JA, Shirey RS, Braine HG, et al. Plasmapheresis for the treatment of repeated early pregnancy wastage associated with anti-P. *Obstet Gynecol*. 1985;66:57S.

64. Udden MM, Umeda M, Hirano Y, Marcus DM. New abnormalities in the morphology, cell surface receptors, and electrolyte metabolism of In(Lu) erythrocytes. *Blood*. 1987;69:52.

65. Sands JM. Molecular mechanisms of urea transport. *J Membr Biol* 2003;191:149.

66. Standards Committee of American Association of Blood Banks. *Standards for Blood Banks and Transfusion Services*. 32nd ed. American Associations of Blood Banks; 2020.

67. Reid ME, Øyen R, Marsh WL. Summary of the clinical significance of blood group alloantibodies. *Semin Hematol*. 2000;37:197.

68. Poole J, Daniels G. Blood group antibodies and their significance in transfusion medicine. *Transfus Med Rev*. 2007;21:58.

CHAPTER 30
BLOOD PROCUREMENT AND RED CELL TRANSFUSION

Claudia S. Cohn, Jeffrey McCullough, and Xiangrong He

SUMMARY

Blood procurement is a vital national priority that is met in the United States (U.S.) by volunteer donors and a pluralistic blood collection program that includes the American Red Cross, independent community blood centers, and hospitals. Approximately 12 million units of whole blood are collected from approximately 9 million donors annually.[1,2] Recruitment of donors is preceded by a medical history and limited physical examination. The donated blood is subjected to tests of blood type, red cell antibodies, and infectious agents that may be transmitted by blood transfusion. In some cases, collection of red cells, platelets, leukocytes, or plasma is achieved by hemapheresis. Plasma for the subsequent manufacture of derivatives such as albumin and intravenous immunoglobulin (IVIG) is obtained from paid donors by for-profit organizations different from those that collect whole blood and prepare blood components. The meticulous attention to donor risk characteristics and the use of sensitive assays to detect infectious agents that may be transmitted by blood have greatly improved the safety of blood.

It is widely accepted that red blood cell (RBC) transfusions save lives and prevent ischemic-related morbidity in severely hemorrhaging patients and those with acute anemia (hemoglobin [Hb] <60 g/L). When a patient's Hb level exceeds 100 g/L, oxygen delivery and consumption do not necessarily increase with RBC transfusions. For patients in the 60 to 100 g/L Hb "gray zone," the benefit of a transfusion will depend on a patient's clinical status, and should be weighed against the inherent risks of allogeneic blood, but primarily these patients do not benefit from transfusion (see later in this chapter).

These risks include adverse reactions, which occur in up to 3% of transfusions. Transfusion-associated circulatory overload (TACO) is the number one cause of transfusion-related fatalities, and new pathogens causing transfusion-transmitted infections continue to pose a threat to the blood supply. TACO overload is often not recognized but has been associated with increased morbidity and prolonged lengths of hospital stay.

As the older population grows in the U.S., the demand for blood will increase, even as the donor population declines. Patient blood management efforts are growing in popularity as hospitals grapple with the risks and costs associated with transfusion. The implementation of evidence-based practice is the best way to benefit patients and minimize the risks of transfusion.

Acronyms and Abbreviations: AABB, American Association of Blood Banks; AHTR, acute hemolytic transfusion reactions; APACHE II, Acute Physiology and Chronic Health Evaluation II; ARDS, acute respiratory distress syndrome; ARV, antiretroviral; ATRs, allergic transfusion reactions; BCHS, British Committee for Standards in Haematology; BNP, B-type natriuretic peptide; CI, confidence interval; CMV, cytomegalovirus; DAT, direct antiglobulin test; DHTRs, delayed hemolytic transfusion reactions; ESAs, erythropoiesis-stimulating agents; FDA, Food and Drug Administration; FFP, fresh frozen plasma; FNHTRs, febrile non-hemolytic transfusion reactions; FOCUS, Functional Outcomes in Cardiovascular Patients Undergoing Surgical Hip Fracture Repair; FP, frozen plasma; GI, gastrointestinal; GVHD, graft-versus-host disease; Hb, hemoglobin; Hct, hematocrit; HLA, human leukocyte antigen; HPC-A, hematopoietic progenitor cells are obtained by apheresis; HPC-C, hematopoietic progenitor cells obtained from umbilical cords; HR, hazard ratio; HSCT, hematopoietic stem cell transplantation; Ig, immunoglobulin; IL, interleukin; IVIG, intravenous immunoglobulin; MINT, Myocardial Ischemia and Transfusion; MODS, multiple organ dysfunction syndrome; NT-pro BNP, N terminal-propeptide BNP; PBM, patient blood management; PINT, Premature Infants in Need of Transfusion; PLS, passenger lymphocyte syndrome; PRCA, pure red cell aplasia; PrEP, pre-exposure prophylaxis; RBC, red blood cell; RR, relative risk; SCD, sickle cell disease; TACO, transfusion-associated circulatory overload; TA-GVHD transfusion-associated graft-versus-host disease; TRACS, Transfusion Requirements After Cardiac Surgery; TRALI, transfusion-related acute lung injury; TRICC, Transfusion Requirements in Critical Care; TRIPICU, Transfusion Strategies for Patients in Pediatric Intensive Care Unit; U.S. United States.

OVERVIEW OF THE BLOOD SUPPLY SYSTEM IN THE UNITED STATES

The United States (U.S.) has a pluralistic rather than a single national system of blood collection that exists in other developed countries. During 2017, approximately 12.2 million units of blood were available for use in the U.S. (Table 30-1). This was a 3.3% decrease from 2015. Approximately 96% of the blood was collected in regional blood centers, and hospitals collected 4%.[1] Less than 1% of the units donated in the U.S. were autologous donations or directed donations—that is, blood given by family or friends for a specific patient. Although autologous donations increased slightly, directed donations decreased substantially from 2015.[2] Of red cells collected, about 4% of allogeneic red cells are not used and the nonutilization rates are much higher for autologous and directed donor red cells.

Nearly all whole blood for transfusion in the U.S. is donated by unpaid volunteers; however, costs are incurred in the collection, testing, production, and distribution of blood components. Blood banks pass on these costs to hospitals. Some areas of the U.S. are able to collect more blood than is needed locally and other areas are unable to collect enough blood to meet their local needs. Several inventory-sharing systems are used to move blood around the U.S. to alleviate the shortages.

Blood is considered a drug and all aspects of the selection of donors, collection, processing, testing, preservation, and dispensing are regulated by the Food and Drug Administration (FDA). The FDA requirements in the code define the procedures, record-keeping, staff proficiency, specific testing, and donor medical requirements that blood banks must follow. Blood banks meet these requirements using the FDA-defined good manufacturing practices similar to those used by pharmaceutical manufacturers. Additional standards are formulated by the AABB (formerly the American Association of Blood Banks), a voluntary organization that accredits blood banks.

INTERNATIONAL PRACTICES

Approximately 112.5 million units of blood are collected annually worldwide.[3] Considerable differences in the availability of blood and blood components throughout the world are related to the extent of

TABLE 30–1. United States Blood Supply System in 2017*

	Number	Percent
Total units whole blood	12,275,000	100
Blood centers	11,713,000	96
Hospitals	502,000	4
Red blood cell transfusions	10,575,000	100
Allogeneic	10,491,000	99
Autologous	21,000	<1
Directed	56,000	<1
Platelets – total dose	2,559,000	100
SDP collected	2,338,000	91
WB platelet concentrates	221,000	9
Total platelets transfused*	1,936,000	
Fresh-frozen plasma	3,210,000	—
Fresh-frozen plasma transfused	2,318,000	—
Cryoprecipitate	2,156,000	
Cryoprecipitate transfused	1,068,000	

SDP, single-donor platelet concentrate prepared by plateletpheresis (1 SDP is equivalent to 5 platelet concentrates); WB, whole-blood–derived platelet concentrate (usually 5 units are pooled to obtain a therapeutic dose).

*Data from Jones J. Blood collection and utilization in the United States 2017 Centers for Disease Control and Prevention. cdcinfo@cdc.gov; www.cdc.gov; and Raybhandary S, Whitaker B, Perez G. The 2015-2015 National Blood Collection and Utilization Survey Report. Bethesda, MD: AABB; 2018.

development in the country and the country's health care system.[3] The amount of blood collected in relation to the population ranges from 50 donations per 1000 population in industrialized countries to 5 to 15 per 1000 in developing countries and 1 to 5 per 1000 in the least-developed countries.[3] Thus, industrialized countries use transfused blood products far more commonly. In developed countries, especially Western Europe and parts of Asia, a governmental agency usually oversees the blood collection activities, although the extent to which the government sets requirements and monitors or inspects the blood collection system varies. In developed countries, the basic processes of donor medical screening, blood collection, laboratory testing, and preparation of blood components are similar to the system found in the U.S. In virtually all developed countries, blood is donated by volunteers because paid donors are associated with a higher risk of disease transmission.[4] The basic blood components—red cells, platelets, and plasma—usually are available in developed countries, and apheresis instruments are used to collect some platelets. Plasma derivatives such as albumin, coagulation factor VIII, other plasma protein concentrates (coagulation factors or inhibitors, or complement factor-1 inhibitor) and immune globulins are available.

However, in the developing world, the blood supply is very limited, and components are often not available. Patients may be required to arrange for the blood they need so donors may be friends or family members of patients or even individuals who have been paid by the patient's family to donate the blood needed. Donor screening may not be as extensive,[3] transmissible disease testing may be lacking, and equipment may be reused. These difficulties may be compounded by the presence of endemic transfusion-transmissible diseases for which

screening is difficult or expensive and thus not performed as extensively as in more developed countries. Great strides have been made primarily from the U.S.-funded President's Emergency Plan for AIDS Relief (PEPFAR) program.[5] Thus, the availability of blood and its components around the world varies widely, from inadequate supplies and uncertain safety to sophisticated supply systems and component availability equal to or surpassing those of the U.S.

● PROCUREMENT OF PLASMA DERIVATIVES

The plasma industry is separate from the blood banking system described above. Plasma can be subjected to a fractionation process to produce several medically valuable products referred to as *plasma derivatives*. Plasma fractionation is performed in manufacturing plants in batches of up to 10,000 liters involving the pooling of plasma from a large number of donors. Plasma for manufacture or fractionation into derivatives can be obtained from units of whole blood, but this amount of plasma is inadequate to meet the needs for plasma derivatives. Consequently, large amounts of plasma are obtained by plasmapheresis in which only the plasma and not red cells or platelets are retained from the donor. Individuals can donate plasma up to two times per week and usually are paid because of the more extensive time commitment. This plasma collection system usually is operated by for-profit organizations and functions separately from the system for whole-blood donation.

In 2018, approximately 48.7 million liters of plasma were collected in the U.S. Twenty-six plasma derivatives are approved for licensure by the FDA. Disruption in the sources of plasma or in one manufacturer's plant can have serious consequences and create shortages of certain derivatives. The large increase in use of intravenous immunoglobulin (IVIG) has caused a substantial increase in plasma collection.

The remainder of this chapter describes the blood collection system operated by voluntary community organizations to provide cellular and whole blood–derived components.

● RECRUITMENT OF BLOOD DONORS

Although most Americans will require a blood transfusion at some time in their lives, about two-thirds of the U.S. population is eligible to donate blood,[6] but only a small portion of those actually donate. Blood donors are more likely than the general population to be male, between ages 30 and 50 years, white, employed, and have more education and higher income.[7] It is generally believed that the most effective way to get someone to donate blood is to ask him or her personally. Factors such as the convenience of donation, peer pressure, receipt of blood by a family member, and perceived community needs are important factors that are superimposed onto the individual's basic social commitments.[7]

● WHOLE-BLOOD DONOR SCREENING

The approach to the selection of blood donors is designed to: (1) ensure the safety of the donor and (2) obtain a high-quality blood component that is as safe as possible for the recipient. Some specific steps that are taken to ensure that blood is as safe as possible are the use of only volunteer blood donors; questioning of donors about their general health before their donation is scheduled; obtaining a medical history, including specific risk factors, before donation; conducting a brief physical examination before donation; laboratory testing of donated blood; checking the donor's identity against a donor deferral registry; and providing a method by which the donor can confidentially designate the unit as unsuitable for transfusion after the donation is completed.

HEALTH HISTORY, PHYSICAL EXAMINATION, AND LABORATORY TESTING OF DONATED BLOOD

The health history is usually done by a computer-assisted self-interview. The questions designed to protect the safety of the donor include whether the donor is under the care of a physician or has a history of cardiovascular or lung disease, seizures, present or recent pregnancy, recent donation of blood or plasma, recent major illness or surgery, unexplained weight loss, unusual bleeding, or is taking medication(s). Some medications may make the donor unsuitable because of the condition requiring the medication, whereas other medications may be potentially harmful to the recipient. Questions designed to protect the safety of the recipient include those related to the donor's general health, history of receipt of growth hormone, and occurrence of or exposure to patients with hepatitis or other liver disease, or a previous diagnosis of HIV or AIDS (or symptoms of AIDS), Chagas disease, or babesiosis. A history also is obtained regarding the injection of drugs, receipt of coagulation factor concentrates, blood transfusion, tattoos, acupuncture, body piercing, receipt of an organ or tissue transplant, recent travel to areas endemic for malaria or Zika virus, recent immunizations, ingestion of medications (especially aspirin), presence of a major illness or surgery, and previous notice of a positive test for a transmissible disease. In addition, several questions are related to AIDS risk behavior, including whether the potential donor has had sex with anyone with AIDS, given or received money or drugs for sex, (for males) had sex with another male, or (for females) had sex with a male who has had sex with another male.

The physical examination includes determination of the temperature, pulse, blood pressure, weight, and blood hemoglobin (Hb) concentration. The donor's general appearance is assessed for any signs of illness or the influence of drugs or alcohol. The skin at the venipuncture site is examined for signs of IV drug abuse, and local lesions that would make disinfecting the skin difficult and thus lead to contamination of the blood unit during venipuncture.

COLLECTION OF WHOLE BLOOD

BLOOD CONTAINERS, ANTICOAGULANTS, AND PRESERVATIVES

Blood must be collected into single-use, sterile, FDA-licensed containers. The containers are made of plasticized material that is biocompatible with blood cells and allows diffusion of gases to provide optimal cell preservation. These blood containers are combinations of bags and integral tubing that allow separation of the whole blood into its components in a closed system, thus minimizing the chance of bacterial contamination while making storage of the components for days or weeks possible. Plasticizers from the bags accumulate in red cell components during storage and can be found in tissues of multitransfused patients but also in healthy nontransfused individuals.[8] Although no evidence indicates that transfusion of this material causes clinical problems, containers without plasticizers are now used in some countries.

Citrate solutions are used for anticoagulation. These comprise various concentrations of sodium citrate, citric acid, and dextrose. Some have additional adenine and sodium phosphate. Because most whole blood is separated into components, when the plasma has been removed, the remaining RBCs are resuspended in what is referred to as an "additive solution." In addition to citrate and dextrose, these additive solutions contain adenine, mannitol, and phosphate. The additive solutions enable storage of RBCs for up to 42 days at 1°C to 6°C.

VENIPUNCTURE AND BLOOD COLLECTION

The blood should be drawn from an area free of skin lesions and the phlebotomy site should be decontaminated. The site is scrubbed with a soap solution, followed by the application of tincture of iodine or iodophor complex solution. The venipuncture is done with a needle that should be used only once to prevent contamination. The blood must flow freely and be mixed with anticoagulant frequently as the blood fills the container to prevent the development of small clots. The actual time for collection of 450 to 500 mL usually is approximately 7 minutes and almost always is less than 10 minutes. During blood donation, cardiac output falls slightly but heart rate changes little. A slight decrease in systolic blood pressure results with a rise in peripheral resistance and diastolic blood pressure.[9]

Usually 500 mL is collected. The blood is mixed with 63 to 70 mL of anticoagulant composed of citrate, phosphate, and dextrose. The amount of blood withdrawn must be within prescribed limits to maintain the proper ratio with the anticoagulant; otherwise, the blood cells may be damaged and/or anticoagulation may be unsatisfactory.

An untoward reaction after blood donation occurs in approximately 2% to 5% of donors, but, fortunately, most of the reactions are not serious. Donors who have reactions are more likely to be younger, unmarried, have a higher predonation heart rate and lower diastolic blood pressure, have a lower weight, are female, and are first-time or infrequent donors.[10] Donors who experience a reaction are less likely to donate in the future.

The most common reactions to blood donation are weakness, cool skin, and diaphoresis.[10] More extensive, but still moderate, reactions are dizziness, pallor, hypertension, and bradycardia.[9,11] Bradycardia usually is considered a sign of a vasovagal reaction rather than hypotensive or cardiovascular shock, where tachycardia would be expected. In a more severe form, a vasovagal reaction may progress to loss of consciousness, convulsions, and involuntary passage of urine or stool. Other reactions include nausea and vomiting; hyperventilation, sometimes leading to twitching or muscle spasms; hematoma at the venipuncture site; convulsions; and serious cardiac difficulties. Such serious reactions are rare. Injury of the brachial nerve and resulting pain and/or paresthesia may occur as a result of needle puncture of the nerve or compression from a hematoma.

Donors are advised to drink extra fluids to replace lost blood volume and to avoid strenuous exercise for the remainder of the day of donation. The latter advice is given to prevent fainting and to minimize the possibility of hematoma development at the venipuncture site. Some donors are subject to lightheadedness or even fainting if they change position quickly. Therefore, donors are advised not to return to work for the remainder of the day if they have an occupation where fainting would be hazardous to themselves or others.

BLOOD COMPONENTS

Within a few hours of collection, whole blood is separated into the components of RBCs, plasma and occasionally platelets. The components are produced in large high-speed centrifuges using multiple plastic bag systems to allow the separation of the components in a closed system to maintain sterility.

RED BLOOD CELLS

RBCs are those remaining after the plasma has been removed. This component has a final hematocrit of about 80% and is often called packed red cells. A unit of packed red cells has a volume of around 300 mL and will contain about 190 mL of red cells. The fluid portion of the

TABLE 30-2. Established or Potential Adverse Effects of Leukocytes in Blood Components

Immunologic effects	Alloimmunization
	Febrile nonhemolytic transfusion reactions
	Refractoriness to platelet transfusion
	Rejection of transplanted organs
	Graft-versus-host disease
	Transfusion-related acute lung injury
Immunomodulation	Increased bacterial infections
	Increased recurrence of malignancy
Infectious disease transmission	Cytomegalovirus infection
	Human T-cell leukemia virus type I infection
	Epstein-Barr virus infection

unit is the additive solution mentioned earlier. About 20 mL of plasma remains from the original unit of whole blood. This red cell component can be stored at 1°C to 6°C for up to 42 days. Most packed red cells are depleted of the leukocytes, usually by filtration, which spares essentially all the red cells. There has been considerable discussion over the value of leukocyte depletion, but there is general agreement of the advantages summarized in Table 30-2. As of this writing, about 95% of packed red cells in the U.S. are leukocyte reduced.

PLASMA

When whole blood is separated, about 200 to 250 mL of plasma are removed. If this is frozen within eight hours of collection it is referred to as fresh frozen plasma (FFP) and contains essentially all of the hemostatic capacity of fresh plasma. Occasionally plasma is not frozen until about 24 hours after collection and this has become known as frozen plasma (FP)-24. FP-24 has some value in hemostasis but lacks all of the levels of coagulation factors found in FFP. Plasma products are stored at −18°C or below for up to 1 year.

PLATELETS

Platelets can be prepared from whole blood, although currently only about 10% of platelets in the U.S. are made this way. In the U.S., most platelets are prepared by plateletpheresis. When platelets are prepared from whole blood, four or five units from whole blood are pooled to obtain a therapeutic dose of platelets. Such a pool of whole blood–derived platelets will contain about the same number of platelets as a unit of platelets prepared by plateletpheresis. The therapeutic benefit is essentially similar between these two different kinds of platelets. Whole blood–derived platelets are stored at 20°C to 24°C, similar to apheresis platelets.

● SPECIAL BLOOD DONATIONS

AUTOLOGOUS DONOR BLOOD

Autologous blood for transfusion can be obtained by preoperative donation, acute normovolemic hemodilution, intraoperative salvage, and postoperative salvage, but only preoperative donation is discussed here. Most commonly this situation occurs with elective surgery.

Autologous blood accounts for a very low level (<1%) of the U.S. blood supply (see Table 30-1).[1] If patient candidates for autologous blood donation meet the usual FDA criteria for blood donation, their blood can be used for other patients if the original autologous donor has no need for the blood. However, this practice is not allowed by AABB standards and is usually not relevant because most patients do not meet the FDA donation criteria. If the autologous donor does not meet the FDA criteria for blood donation, the blood must be specially labeled, segregated during storage, and discarded if it is not used by that specific patient. Thus, the autologous blood donation should be collected only for procedures with a substantial likelihood that the blood will be used. Without this type of planning, a very high rate of wastage of autologous blood is observed, estimated at 59% in 2011.[1] Thus, the cost of autologous blood is high.

No age or weight restrictions exist for autologous donation. Pregnant women can donate, but this practice is not recommended because these patients rarely require transfusion. The autologous donor's Hb may be lower (110 g/L) than that required for routine donors (125 g/L), although usually only 2 to 4 units of blood can be obtained before the Hb falls below 110 g/L. Autologous blood donors can be given erythropoietin and iron to increase the number of units of blood they can donate,[12,13] although this strategy has not been shown to reduce the need for allogeneic donor blood. Reactions in autologous donors are similar to allogeneic donors and are related to first-time donation, female gender, lower age, and lower weight.

Autologous blood must be typed for ABO and Rh antigens. If the unit is to be shipped to another facility for transfusion, it must be tested for transmissible diseases, similar to allogeneic blood. If any of the transmissible disease tests are positive, the unit must be labeled with a biohazard label.

DIRECTED DONOR BLOOD

Directed donors are friends or relatives who wish to give blood for a specific patient because the patient hopes those donors will be safer than the regular blood supply. However, directed donors do not have a lower incidence of transmissible disease markers[14] and thus do not support a realistic rationale for these donations. Because the blood becomes part of the community's general blood supply if it is not used for the originally intended patient, directed donors must meet all the usual FDA requirements for routine blood donation. The practice of directed donation is rarely done.

PATIENT-SPECIFIC DONATION

In a few situations, appropriate transfusion therapy involves collecting blood from a particular donor for a particular patient. Examples are past use of donor-specific transfusions before kidney transplantation, maternal platelets for a fetus projected to have neonatal alloimmune thrombocytopenic purpura, or family members of a patient with a rare blood type. Usually, these donors must meet all the usual FDA requirements, except that they may donate as often as every 3 days as long as the Hb remains above the normal donor minimum of 125 g/L. An exception is donation of maternal platelets for a neonate with neonatal alloimmune thrombocytopenic purpura. Patient-specific donated units must undergo all routine laboratory testing.

THERAPEUTIC BLEEDING

Blood can be collected as part of the therapy of diseases such as polycythemia vera or primary hemochromatosis. Usually such blood is not used for transfusion because the donors do not meet the FDA standards for donor health. As the genetic basis of hemochromatosis has become better understood, blood removed from these patients appears to be safe and red cells from patients with hemochromatosis are normal during blood bank storage,[15] and although a blood collection program can operate successfully, this has not gained general acceptance.

COLLECTION AND PRODUCTION OF BLOOD COMPONENTS BY APHERESIS

Blood components can be obtained by apheresis rather than prepared from whole blood. In apheresis, the donor's anticoagulated whole blood is passed through an instrument in which centrifugation is used to separate the blood components. Red cells, platelets, granulocytes, blood stem cells, mononuclear cells, or plasma can be obtained by apheresis.

PLATELETPHERESIS

In the U.S., about 91% of platelet concentrates are produced by plateletpheresis (see Table 30-1). Plateletpheresis requires approximately 90 minutes, during which approximately 4000 to 5000 mL of the donor's blood is processed through the blood cell separator. The process results in a platelet concentrate with a volume of approximately 250 mL and containing approximately 3.5×10^{11} platelets and less than 0.5 mL red cells. Currently, blood cell separators produce a platelet concentrate that contains less than 5×10^6 leukocytes and thus can be considered leukocyte reduced. After plateletpheresis, the donor's platelet count declines by approximately 30% but returns to pre-plateletpheresis levels in approximately 4 days.[16]

COLLECTION OF RED CELLS BY APHERESIS

Chronic shortages of group O red cells stimulated interest in the use of apheresis for collecting the equivalent of two units of red cells from some donors, especially group O.[17] In 2017, approximately 1.7 million units or about 15% of all red cells were collected by apheresis.[1] The collection procedure is similar to other apheresis procedures, except that red cells are retained rather than returned to the donor. The red cells usually have a very high hematocrit (Hct) count as they are removed from the instrument, but an additive solution is incorporated, and the red cells can be stored for the usual 42 days. Red cells obtained by apheresis have the same characteristics as those produced from whole blood. Because two units of red cells are removed, donors may donate only every 4 months.

LEUKAPHERESIS

Leukapheresis has been used to produce a granulocyte concentrate for transfusion therapy of infections unresponsive to antibiotics. Because the efficiency of granulocyte extraction from whole blood is less than for platelets, the leukapheresis procedure involves processing 6500 to 8000 mL of donor blood for approximately 3 hours. To increase the separation of granulocytes from other blood components, hydroxyethyl starch is added to the blood-cell–separator flow system. In addition, glucocorticoids and granulocyte colony-stimulating factor have been administered to granulocyte donors to increase the granulocyte count and the granulocyte yield.[18]

PLASMAPHERESIS

Plasmapheresis is used to obtain plasma for manufacture of derivatives but not plasma for transfusion. Plasmapheresis usually can be performed in approximately 30 minutes and produces up to 750 mL of plasma. Because few red cells are removed, the procedure can be repeated up to two times per week, so theoretically a donor could provide a large amount of plasma. Because of the nature and possible frequency of plasma donation, special donor criteria apply. This plasma is the starting material for the manufacture of derivatives. Because of the large and rapidly increasing use of IVIG, plasmapheresis is widely used and the donors are paid.

SELECTION OF APHERESIS DONORS

The selection of donors for apheresis uses the same criteria as for whole-blood donation, with some additional donor requirements. No more than 15% of the donor's blood should be extracorporeal during apheresis; thus, the donor's size is considered when making decisions about specific apheresis procedures or instruments to be used. The platelet count must be monitored for frequent platelet donors. Because a plateletpheresis concentrate would be the sole source of platelets for a transfusion, the donor must not have taken aspirin for at least 3 days.

The amount of blood components removed from apheresis donors must be monitored. Not more than 200 mL of red cells per 2 months or approximately 1500 mL of plasma per week can be removed. The laboratory testing of donors and apheresis components for transmissible diseases is the same as for whole-blood donation. Thus, the likelihood of disease transmission from apheresis components is the same as from whole blood.

REACTIONS IN APHERESIS DONORS

Apheresis donors can experience the same kind of reactions as whole-blood donors. In addition, apheresis donors experience a higher incidence of paresthesias, probably because of the infusion of citrate (that may affect calcium levels) used to anticoagulate the donor's blood while it is in the cell separator. This type of reaction is managed by slowing the blood flow rate through the instrument, which slows the rate of citrate infusion. When granulocyte colony-stimulating factor and glucocorticoids are used in leukapheresis to obtain a granulocyte concentrate, approximately 60% of donors experience side effects—usually myalgia, arthralgia, headache, or flulike symptoms.[18] The major side effect of hydroxyethyl starch is blood volume expansion manifested by headache and/or hypertension.

LABORATORY TESTING OF DONATED BLOOD

Each unit of whole blood or each apheresis component undergoes a standard battery of tests, including those for blood type, red cell antibodies (including ABO, Rh, minor antigens), and transmissible diseases (Table 30-3). Additional tests, such as those for cytomegalovirus (CMV) antibodies may be done. During the last few years, testing for West Nile virus, Trypanosoma cruzi, Babesia,[19] and, more recently, Zika have been added.

SAFETY OF THE BLOOD SUPPLY

Ironically, the improvements in blood safety have occurred at a time of the public's increased fear of transfusion and the more cautious use of blood components by physicians. Each step in the overall process of donor evaluation and testing adds to blood safety in important ways, and the donor medical history is important as illustrated by the 90% reduction in HIV infectivity from the use of donor-selection criteria identifying HIV risk behavior.[20] for transmissible diseases further

TABLE 30–3. Laboratory Tests for Transmissible Agents of Donated Blood

Agent/Test	Disease
Treponema	Syphilis
Hepatitis B surface antigen	Hepatitis B
Hepatitis B core antibody	Hepatitis B
HBV nucleic acid	Hepatitis B
Hepatitis C antibody	Hepatitis C
Hepatitis C nucleic acids	Hepatitis C
HIV-1 and HIV-2 antibody	AIDS
HIV nucleic acids	AIDS
West Nile virus nucleic acids	West Nile infection
Bacterial culture[a]	Sepsis
HTLV-I antibody	Leukemia
	Lymphoma
	Tropical paresis
HTLV-II antibody	Disease unknown
Trypanosoma cruzi[b]	Chagas disease
Zika virus	Central nervous system infection
CMV antibody[c]	CMV disease

CMV, cytomegalovirus; HBV, hepatitis B virus; HTLV, human T-cell lymphotropic virus.

[a]Only platelet concentrates tested.

[b]Only first-time donors are tested.

[c]Of use for immunodeficient recipients.

reduce the proportion of infectious donors.[21] Donor deferral registries detect individuals who previously were deferred as blood donors but who for various reasons attempt to donate again. Currently, the risk of acquiring a transfusion-transmitted disease is very low (Table 30-4). However, new threats to the blood supply may come from unexpected sources; The antiretroviral (ARV) drugs and pre-exposure prophylaxis (PrEP) are effective tools to help reduce the burden of HIV, however, ARV and PrEP may hinder the detection of HIV in donated blood. A study found that approximately 15% of HIV-positive individuals who donated blood took ARVs within days of donation, and nearly 5% of men who have sex with men who donated blood reported taking PrEP

within the same period as blood donation.[22] Nonetheless, the residual risk of HIV remains extremely low, and the most problematic infections transmitted currently are caused by bacteria from infected platelet concentrates that are stored at room temperature.[23] When contaminated, these concentrates usually become infected by contaminants at the venipuncture site and can cause serious, even fatal, septic reactions in the recipient.[24] A mitigation strategy for reduction of this risk has been published by the FDA (Guidance) and is in the process of being adopted. Thus, although the blood supply is safer than ever, transfusion is not risk free and should be undertaken only after careful consideration of the patient's clinical situation and specific blood component needs.

● RED CELL TRANSFUSIONS

Anemia becomes symptomatic when there is an imbalance between oxygen delivery and tissue consumption. Oxygen delivery equals the product of cardiac output and the arterial oxygen content, which is mainly found bound to Hb. Oxygen delivery in most anemic patients can generally be compensated by increasing cardiac output. However, in patients with underlying comorbidities such as cardiovascular diseases, oxygen delivery becomes more dependent on arterial oxygen content and Hb level. Therefore, red cell transfusions are indicated to increase oxygen-carrying capacity in anemic patients, particularly in critically ill patients with cardiovascular comorbidities.

It had been common practice to maintain critically ill patients at a Hb of 100 g/L; however, data in favor of this target level are lacking. Instead, multicenter randomized controlled trials indicate that compared with a target Hb of 100 g/L, target hemoglobin values of 70 to 80 g/L are associated with equivalent or better outcomes in most patient populations.

RED CELL TRANSFUSION THRESHOLDS

Red cell transfusions were previously given routinely for Hb levels below 100 g/L. This practice was based mainly on unproven clinical assumptions. An Hb concentration of less than 70 g/L became the accepted threshold after the multicenter Transfusion Requirements in Critical Care (TRICC) trial in 1999. The TRICC trial was the first adequately powered study to compare a restrictive transfusion threshold (Hb <70 g/L) versus liberal threshold (Hb <100 gdL) for red cell transfusions in critically ill patients.[25] A total of 838 ICU patients were randomly assigned to either a liberal or restrictive transfusion group. The exclusion criteria included age under 16 years, active blood loss at the time of enrollment, admission after a routine cardiac procedure, chronic anemia, imminent death, and others. Primary outcome measure was the 30-day mortality from all causes. Secondary outcomes included 60-day mortality, death during hospitalization, and multiple-organ dysfunction.

TABLE 30–4. Incidence of Transfusion-Transmitted Diseases

	Data from Strong and Katz (2002)[115]	Data from Dodd, Notari, and Stramer (2002)[21]	Data from Tabor and Epstein (2002)[117]	Total U.S. Cases[a]
Hepatitis C	1/1,200,000	1/1,935,000	1/625,000	8
Hepatitis B	1/150,000	—	1/150,000	80[b]
HTLV-I/HTLV-II	1/641,000	—	—	20[b]
HIV	1/1,400,000	1/2,135,000	1/769,230	7

HTLV, human T-cell lymphotropic virus.

[a]Calculated based on transfusion of 15,000,000 units of blood annually and Dodd[21] incidence figures.

[b]Calculations based on data from Strong and Katz.[115]

TABLE 30–5. Major Randomized Controlled Trials for Safe Hemoglobin Thresholds in Adults

Trial	Patient Population	Number Enrolled	Hb (g/L) or Hct (%) Thresholds (Restrictive/Liberal)	Primary End Point	Conclusions
TRICC[24]	ICU	838	Hb 70/100 g/L	30-day all-cause mortality	Restrictive strategy as effective and possibly superior to liberal strategy
FOCUS[31]	History or risk factor for CV disease after hip fracture surgery	2016	Hb 80/100 g/L	60-day all-cause mortality or inability to walk 10 ft.	Liberal strategy did not reduce death rates or inability to walk
TRACS[32]	Cardiac surgery	502	Hct 24/30%	30-day all-cause mortality and severe morbidity	Restrictive strategy was noninferior to liberal strategy
Upper GI Bleed[116]	Severe acute upper GI bleed	921	Hb 70/90 g/L	45-day all-cause mortality	Restrictive strategy improved outcomes compared with liberal

CV, cardiovascular; FOCUS, Functional Outcomes in Cardiovascular Patients Undergoing Surgical Hip Fracture Repair; GI, gastrointestinal; Hb, hemoglobin; Hct, hematocrit; TRACS, Transfusion Requirements After Cardiac Surgery; TRICC, Transfusion Requirements in Critical Care.

The severity of a patient's illness was classified using the Acute Physiology and Chronic Health Evaluation II (APACHE II) scores. The study found the restrictive transfusion strategy decreased hospital mortality rates among patients who were less acutely ill (APACHE II ≤20) (8.7 vs 16.1%; P = .03) or who were younger than 55 years (5.7 vs 13.0%; P = .02). It also reduced 30-day mortality. These findings also have been confirmed in subsequent metaanalysis of trials examining transfusion threshold.[26,27] Lower transfusion thresholds are also supported for specific subgroups of critically ill patients (Table 30-5). These studies have focused on patients with upper gastrointestinal (GI) bleeding, cardiovascular risk factors, orthopedic surgery, and other populations that usually require a large number of red cell transfusions. All studies followed the basic structure of the TRICC trial, randomizing patients into a restrictive versus liberal transfusion arm. Most studies also used mortality or end-organ dysfunction as end points.

A 2018 systematic review and meta-analysis of 37 randomized clinical trials comparing liberal versus restrictive transfusion thresholds in 19,049 medical and surgical patients (adults and children) found restrictive strategies decreased transfusion frequency (41% decrease; relative risk [RR], 0.59; 95% confidence interval [CI], 0.53-0.66). Between the two groups, there were no differences in 30-day mortality (RR, 1.0; 95% CI, 0.86-1.16), infection rate (RR, 0.97; 95% CI, 0.88-1.07), functional recovery, or hospital or ICU length of stay.[28]

Based on these results, the current consensus follows a restrictive strategy with a threshold Hb of 70 to 80 g/L for most hemodynamically stable medical and surgical patients. Evidence developed for specific patient populations is presented below.

RED CELL TRANSFUSIONS FOR PATIENTS WITH GASTROINTESTINAL BLEEDING

An important trial was conducted with 921 patients who had acute upper GI bleeding. They were randomized to either the restrictive arm of Hb lower than 70 g/L versus 90 g/L for the liberal arm.[29] Patients with massive exsanguinating bleeding were excluded from the trial. Mortality within the first 45 days was the primary outcome, and the rate of further bleeding and in-hospital complications were used as secondary outcomes. The two patient groups had similar characteristics, including equivalent numbers and grades of cirrhosis. The results of this study also favored a restrictive transfusion strategy. The probability of survival at 6 weeks was higher in the restrictive strategy group

(P = 0.02) and the risk of further bleeding was lower (P = 0.01). Overall adverse events were lower in the restrictive transfusion group as well (P = 0.02). As with the TRICC trial, a significant difference in transfusion frequency was also reported. In the restrictive transfusion arm, 51% of patients did not receive any transfusion, compared with 15% of patients in the liberal arm (P < 0.001).

RED CELL TRANSFUSIONS FOR CARDIOVASCULAR PATIENTS

The optimal transfusion threshold for patients having acute myocardial ischemia is controversial, because most large clinical trials excluded such patients. Generally, a transfusion threshold of 80 g/L is supported by subgroup analysis of three randomized transfusion trials that included patients with coronary artery disease. A subgroup analysis of the TRICC trial found that patients with ischemic cardiovascular disease had improved outcomes in the liberal transfusion arm (<100 g/L), although the improvement was not statistically significant. However, the rate of patients with acute pulmonary edema was significantly higher in the liberal transfusion arm.[30]

The Transfusion Trigger Trial for Functional Outcomes in Cardiovascular Patients Undergoing Surgical Hip Fracture Repair (FOCUS trial) compared a liberal transfusion strategy of less than 100 g/L versus less than 80 g/L in patients with preexisting coronary artery disease who were status post hip repair.[31] A total of 2016 patients older than 50 years were enrolled and randomly assigned to restrictive or liberal transfusion threshold groups. The primary outcome was death or an inability to walk across a room without human assistance on 60-day follow-up. Secondary outcomes included in-hospital myocardial infarction, unstable angina, or death for any reason. The study found that a restrictive transfusion strategy of 80 g/L was not associated with worse outcomes, with the exception of an increase in myocardial infarction that was marginally statistically significant.

The Transfusion Requirements After Cardiac Surgery (TRACS) trial randomly assigned patients who underwent cardiac surgery with cardiopulmonary bypass into a liberal (maintaining Hct ≥30%) or restrictive (Hct ≥24%) strategy for red cell transfusions.[32] This noninferiority study found similar rates of 30-day all-cause mortality and severe morbidity between the two groups. However, the number of transfused red cell units was found to be an independent risk factor for complications or death at 30 days (hazard ratio [HR], 1.2 for each unit transfused).

Taken together, the evidence points to a Hb threshold of 80 g/L as the safe level to maintain for most asymptomatic patients with a history of cardiovascular disease.

Patients with acute coronary syndrome continue to be an important exception for which current data are insufficient to support any guideline. The 2013 Myocardial Ischemia and Transfusion (MINT) pilot trial suggested the liberal transfusion strategy (<100 g/L) was associated with fewer major cardiac events and deaths.[33] The pilot trial enrolled 110 patients and found the primary outcome of death, myocardial infarction, or unscheduled revascularization within 30 days occurred in 6 (10.9%) patients in the liberal transfusion strategy and 14 (25.5%) in the restrictive transfusion strategy (<80 g/L), $P = 0.054$. Death at 30 days was less frequent with liberal transfusion of one death (1.8%) compared with restrictive transfusion of 7 deaths (13.0%), $P = 0.032$. The pilot trial results led to the 2016 MINT clinical trial which is a multicenter randomized trial randomly assigning 3500 hospitalized adult patients with acute myocardial infarctions and significant anemia to receive either a restrictive or a liberal red cell transfusion strategy. The primary outcome measures the composite of all-cause mortality or recurrent nonfatal myocardial infarction within 30 days after randomization. The estimated study completion date is April 2021.

RED CELL TRANSFUSIONS FOR ORTHOPEDIC PATIENTS

Results of the FOCUS trial, discussed above (see "Red Blood Cell Transfusions for Cardiovascular Patients"), suggest a lower threshold of 80 g/L for asymptomatic patients who have undergone orthopedic surgery, even in older patients (mean, 82 years) with underlying cardiovascular disease or cardiovascular risk factors.[31] A 2018 systematic review that included the FOCUS trial and nine others in patients who underwent hip or knee surgery actually found a higher risk of cardiovascular complications with the restrictive transfusion strategy (RR, 1.51; 95% CI, 1.16-1.98). However, there were no differences in mortality and other morbidity events.[34]

There are other studies on orthopedic patients that looked at more general outcomes such as ability to ambulate after hip surgery. One prospective study found a significant association between anemia and a decreased ability to walk independently after recovering from surgical procedures.[35] Another prospective study found no differences in postoperative mobility and length of hospital stay when comparing patients on a restrictive (80 g/L) versus liberal (100 g/L) transfusion strategy.[36] Furthermore, the liberal transfusion group had fewer cardiovascular complications and lower mortality. The authors concluded that a liberal transfusion strategy does not increase ambulation scores.

Although the transfusion threshold of 80 g/L may not be generalizable to the lower-risk orthopedic patient populations, until adequately powered studies are conducted, maintaining Hb lower than 80 g/L is generally considered the right approach for orthopedic patients. In addition, quality-of-life studies do indicate that a higher Hb level allows for faster recovery.

RED CELL TRANSFUSIONS FOR NEUROLOGICALLY IMPAIRED PATIENTS

A 2014 randomized clinical trial is the only large-scale, prospective randomized trial that has addressed the safety and efficacy of transfusion practice in neurologically impaired patients. It compared two Hb transfusion thresholds (70 and 100 g/L) on neurologic recovery after traumatic brain injury. A total of 200 patients with closed head trauma were enrolled within 6 hours of injury. The Glasgow Outcome Scale score was dichotomized as favorable (good recovery and moderate disability) or unfavorable (severe disability, vegetative, or dead) at 6 months post injury. The authors found, in this patient population, that maintaining Hb concentration of greater than 100 g/L did not result in improved neurologic outcome at 6 months. On the contrary, the transfusion threshold of 100 g/L was associated with a higher incidence of thromboembolic events.[37]

A systematic review of six studies with a combined total of 537 neurologically impaired patients compared the Hb triggers ranging from 70 to 100 g/L in restrictive transfusion groups, to 93 to 115 g/L in liberal groups. Although some studies reported a shorter hospital stay in the restrictive transfusion groups, the systematic review found insufficient evidence to recommend a restrictive strategy for neurologically impaired patients.[38]

RED CELL TRANSFUSIONS IN VASCULAR SURGERY PATIENTS

A small (n = 58) randomized feasibility trial was done in patients undergoing vascular surgery. In contrast to most of the other studies as of this writing, the evidence developed in this pilot trial suggests potential harm from using a lower threshold in this population.[39]

Patients undergoing lower-limb bypass or open repair of abdominal aortic aneurysm were randomly assigned, if their hemoglobin dropped below 97 g/L, to a red cell transfusion threshold of either Hb less than 80 g/L or Hb less than 97 g/L. The primary outcome was mean Hb for 15 days after surgery, which demonstrated a statistically significant hemoglobin separation of the two groups (94.6 g/L in the low-trigger group vs 103.3 g/L in the high-trigger group; $P = 0.022$). Regarding secondary outcomes, the evidence showed greater cerebral desaturation in the low trigger group, but no difference in muscular desaturation using near-infrared spectroscopy. The clinical significance of these findings is unknown. Vascular complications were increased in the low-trigger group (18 vs 8 in the high-trigger group; $P = 0.007$), primarily a result of vascular reoperations and amputations. Because this is a small pilot trial, the optimal transfusion threshold for vascular surgery patients is unknown at this time.

RED CELL TRANSFUSIONS FOR PEDIATRIC PATIENTS

The principles for red cell transfusion in children are similar to those used in adults—to provide a sufficient Hb level to prevent or reverse tissue hypoxia caused by limited oxygen delivery. Basically, clinical trials of transfusion triggers for pediatric patients fall into two categories: general studies of critically ill pediatric patients and studies focused on high-risk neonates (Table 30-6). The Transfusion Strategies for Patients in Pediatric Intensive Care Units (TRIPICU) trial and its affiliated subanalyses represent the major dataset covering the pediatric population ranging from 3 days old to 14 years of age.[40] The trial enrolled 626 patients who had Hb less than or equal to 95 g/L during their first 7 days in the pediatric ICU. The restrictive arm used an Hb threshold of 70 g/L, versus a liberal threshold of 95 g/L. The restrictive group received significantly fewer transfusions, yet multiple organ dysfunction syndrome (MODS) and mortality were almost identical in the two arms. Thus, the authors concluded that for critically ill children, an Hb threshold of 70 g/L could decrease transfusion requirements without increasing the incidence of adverse outcomes.

Similar comparisons were also conducted on different subpopulations of the TRIPICU trial, including postoperative patients,[41] patients after cardiac surgery,[42] and patients with sepsis.[43] No significant differences in new or progressive MODS or 28-day mortality were identified between the restrictive and liberal arms. However, all three subanalyses

TABLE 30–6. Major Randomized Controlled Trials for Safe Hemoglobin Thresholds in Children

Trial	Patient Population	Number Enrolled	Hb (g/L)	Primary End Point	Conclusions
TRIPICU[40]	PICU (age from 3 days to 14 years)	626	70/95 g/L	New or progressive multiple organ dysfunction syndrome	In stable, critically ill children, a Hb threshold of 70 g/L can decrease transfusions without increasing adverse outcomes
PINT[33]	ELBW	451	68-115 g/L (low) 77-135 g/L (high)	Death before home discharge or survival with severe retinopathy, bronchopulmonary dysplasia, or brain injury	In ELBW infants, maintaining a higher Hb results in more transfusions but confers little evidence of benefit
Higher or lower hemoglobin transfusion thresholds for preterm infants[44]	Preterm infants	1824	Hemoglobin transfusion thresholds in both groups were determined according to postnatal age and according to the use of respiratory support.	A composite of death or neurodevelopmental impairment at 22-26 months of age	In ELBW infants, a higher Hb threshold for red-cell transfusion did not improve survival without neurodevelopmental impairment at 22-26 months of age, corrected for prematurity.

ELBW, extremely low-birth-weight infants; Hb, hemoglobin; Hct, hematocrit; PICU, pediatric intensive care unit; PINT, Premature Infants In Need of Transfusion; TRIPICU, Transfusion Strategies for Patients in Pediatric Intensive Care Unit.

were limited by small sample size, so no definitive conclusions could be drawn because of insufficient power.

Trials in the neonate population have focused on premature babies and infants of very low birth weight. Unlike the clinical trials in adults, where most studies found that a restrictive transfusion approach was as good as, or possibly superior to, a liberal transfusion strategy, the results from clinical trials in premature infants were mixed. The most recent trial randomized infants with a birth weight of 1000 g or less and a gestational age between 22 weeks 0 days and 28 weeks 6 days to receive red-cell transfusions at higher or lower hemoglobin thresholds until 36 weeks of postmenstrual age or discharge, whichever occurred first.[44] Primary outcome data—a composite of death or neurodevelopmental impairment at 22 to 26 months of age, corrected for prematurity—were available for 1692 infants. Of 845 infants in the higher-threshold group, 423 (50.1%) died or survived with neurodevelopmental impairment, as compared with 422 of 847 infants (49.8%) in the lower-threshold group (relative risk adjusted for birth-weight stratum and center, 1.00; 95% CI, 0.92-1.10; $P = 0.93$). Similar findings were made at 2-year follow-up, with similar incidences of death (16.2% and 15.0%) and neurodevelopmental impairment (39.6% and 40.3%) in the higher- and lower-threshold groups, respectively. The researchers concluded that for extremely-low-birth-weight infants, a higher Hb threshold for red-cell transfusion did not improve survival without neurodevelopmental impairment.

The Iowa Trial was a single-center randomized clinical trial to test whether using lower Hct thresholds for red cell transfusion would reduce the number of transfusions received by preterm infants with birth weights of 500 to 1300 g. The transfusion thresholds varied with the level of respiratory support needed and age.[45] The Hct transfusion thresholds varied from 22% to 34% in the restrictive arm and 30% to 46% in the liberal arm. They found infants in the restrictive transfusion group were more likely to develop parenchymal brain hemorrhage or periventricular leukomalacia; they also had more frequent episodes of apnea. The Iowa Trial also found a reduction in the number of transfusions but not the number of donor exposures in the restrictive transfusion arm. However, the lack of difference in donor exposure most

likely resulted from the use of a single-donor transfusion program. The authors suggested a more liberal transfusion practice in the neonatal population, especially in preterm infants.

The 2006 Premature Infants in Need of Transfusion (PINT) study was a multicenter randomized clinical trial designed to examine the impact of transfusion strategy on the incidence of a composite outcome—death, retinopathy of prematurity, bronchopulmonary dysplasia, or abnormal brain ultrasound—in infants with birth weight below 1000 g.[46] A total of 451 infants were randomized into restrictive (Hb 68-115 g/L) or liberal (Hb 77-135 g/L) transfusion arms. Using the same strategy as the Iowa Trial, the actual transfusion threshold was determined by a combination of age and level of respiratory support. The study found the mean number of transfusions triggered by a Hb threshold was significantly lower in the restrictive group. However, this difference was offset by a small but statistically significant difference in transfusions given for clinical reasons, many of which were for bleeding or surgery. The authors concluded that in extremely-low-birth-weight infants, maintaining a higher Hb level results in more infants receiving transfusions but confers little evidence of benefit.

A 2011 meta-analysis based on four trials with 614 premature infants found that the restrictive transfusion group received fewer transfusion and donor exposures, but they were more likely to be transfused at a later age. More importantly, the rate of mortality between the two groups was comparable (RR, 1.23; 95% CI, 0.86-1.76). There were no differences in the composite outcome of death and serious morbidity at the time of discharge (RR, 1.07; 95% CI, 0.96-1.2).[47]

In addition, a 2016 systematic review of the literature that included both randomized clinical trials and nonrandomized studies reported similar findings of no differences in morbidity and mortality between restrictive and liberal transfusion groups.[48]

The Transfusion of Prematures trial is an ongoing randomized clinical trial to determine whether higher transfusion thresholds for extremely-low-body-weight infants lead to improved outcome of survival and rates of neurodevelopmental impairment, using standardized assessments. It is scheduled to complete around 2020. The trial data should provide us with useful insights into transfusion strategies in pediatric patients.

HEMOGLOBINOPATHIES

SICKLE CELL DISEASE

Transfusion therapy is indicated for patients with sickle cell disease (SCD) who experience stroke, acute chest syndrome, acute exacerbations of anemia, and other complications. Regular transfusions also significantly reduce the recurrence of cerebral infarcts in children with SCD.[49] Transfusions are usually not necessary to correct baseline anemia or alleviate vasoocclusive crises. Because transfusion also carries significant risks, such as iron overload, transfusion reactions, alloimmunization, and delayed hemolytic transfusion reactions, clinicians should take particular care when considering transfusions for patients with SCD.

Chronic transfusion can lead to a high rate of red cell alloimmunization in patients with SCD, which can lead to difficulty in future crossmatching and, in turn, reduces eligibility for chronic transfusion therapy. The rate of alloimmunization in SCD ranged from 18% to 47%, which is significantly higher than the rate of the general U.S. population (0.5%-1.5%)[50] or the highly transfused hematology-oncology population (9%-15%). The reasons for this high rate include number of transfusions, age at first transfusion, the inflammatory milieu created by SCD,[51] and the different RBC antigens present in donors of mostly European descent versus patients with SCD of African ancestry.

The multiple antibodies specific for RBC antigens can cause delayed hemolytic transfusion reactions (DHTRs).[52] In SCD, DHTRs can be more serious and difficult to diagnose. The direct antiglobulin test (DAT) may be borderline or weak without specificity. Some DHTRs occur without any detectable antibody present.[53] In addition, some DHTRs even occur without obvious clinical signs of hemolysis.[52] Severe cases of DHTR result in the hyperhemolysis syndrome, defined by a drop in the patient's Hb to a level lower than the pretransfusion value. This steep decline in Hb suggests hemolysis of autologous cells, as well as the transfused allogeneic RBCs.

Transfusion services may attempt to ameliorate the alloimmunization rate by prophylactically matching donor and patient for Rh (antigens D, C, c, E, e) and Kell antigens. A few will also provide an extended phenotype match for the common Kidd, Duffy, and S antigens. Both strategies reduce alloimmunization; yet even with matched transfusions, patients with SCD continue to form RBC antibodies at rates up to 58% of chronically transfused and 15% of episodically transfused patients with SCD.[52] Most of these antibodies were made against Rh antigens, and more than half occurred in patients who received RBCs phenotypically matched for the corresponding Rh antigen. The likely explanation for this seeming paradox is that patients with SCD have variant *RH* genes. In fact, high-resolution *RH* genotyping showed variant alleles in 87% of the subjects.[52,54]

Red blood cell exchange transfusions remain an effective but underused therapy in the treatment of SCD. The advantage of RBC exchange transfusion is that the sickle cells can be removed and normal cells supplied without significantly increasing the Hb and iron levels, and the viscosity of the blood. Conversely, exchange transfusion often requires extra resources not available at all hospitals and can result in increased donor exposures.

THALASSEMIA

Patients with thalassemia major are chronically transfusion dependent. Over time, this will lead to iron overload and RBC alloimmunization. No clinical trial has been staged to find the optimal transfusion threshold for patients with thalassemia; however, the consequences of anemia can be severe and must be balanced with the risks of transfusion. Transfusing to maintain a Hb of 100 g/L is considered sufficient to suppress extramedullary erythropoiesis, thereby averting the bone deformities and other sequelae of this disease; however, some transfusion regimens call for a pretransfusion minimum of greater than 100 g/L, with a posttransfusion goal of more than 150 g/L. Patients with thalassemia intermedia have more varied transfusion requirements, in keeping with the wide clinical presentation of this disease. If transfusion therapy is clinically indicated, the transfusion recommendations are similar to those for thalassemia major (Chap. 17).

HEMATOPOIETIC STEM CELL TRANSPLANT

TRANSFUSION SUPPORT

Virtually all hematopoietic stem cell transplantation (HSCT) recipients require blood product support in the form of RBC and platelet transfusions until the transplanted marrow cells engraft sufficiently to support hematopoiesis. The duration and specificity of transfusion support for HSCT recipients depends on the disease, the source of the stem cells, the preparative regimen applied before transplant, and patient factors during the posttransplant recovery period. Human leukocyte antigen (HLA) matching remains an important predictor of success with HSCT. As a result, the ABO barrier is often crossed when searching for the best HLA match between donor and patient. Crossing the ABO barrier has little or no effect on overall outcomes; however, transfusion difficulties can arise because of antigenic incompatibility between the transplanted cells and the patient.

Transfusion support can be divided into the pre- and posttransplantation periods. Before an HSCT, an immunocompetent patient (eg, aplastic anemia, hemoglobinopathies) is capable of mounting an immune response to transfusions, leading to alloimmunization against HLA antigens present on the surface of leukocytes. Leukoreduction reduces alloimmunization rates, but sufficient white blood cells remain in the unit for alloimmunization to occur. Antibodies against HLA contribute to delayed engraftment and graft rejection in some patient populations.[55] As a result, pretransplantation transfusions in immunocompetent patients should be avoided, because they are associated with increased graft failure rates.[56,57] RBC transfusions can be minimized by using a Hb trigger of 80 g/L for stable patients.[58]

Patients who are immunocompromised, either because of their disease, or from chemotherapy, are less likely to become immunized to foreign antigens. Nonetheless, using leukoreduced products to minimize the risk of alloimmunization is still recommended. Extra care must also be taken if the stem cell donation comes from a blood relative. In this situation, family members should not give directed blood donations before transplantation, because this may lead to alloimmunization against major and/or minor HLA antigens that are present in the transplant organ. In addition, all RBC and platelet transfusions should be irradiated because the risk for transfusion-associated graft-versus-host disease (TA-GVHD) is high in HSCT recipients (see "Transfusion-Associated Graft-versus-Host Disease" below for more in-depth discussion of TA-GVHD).

RBC engraftment is difficult to assess but may be defined by the appearance of 1% reticulocytes in the blood, or as the day of the last RBC transfusion, with no transfusion given in the following 30 days. In general, engraftment time is shortest when hematopoietic progenitor cells are obtained by apheresis (HPC-A), and greatest when hematopoietic progenitor cells obtained from umbilical cords (HPC-C) are used; however, considerable patient-to-patient variability exists. Prolonged engraftment directly translates into higher transfusion rates for RBCs and platelets.

When an ABO incompatible transplant is used, group O red cells are used to avoid incompatibility issues. The ABO type of plasma products may be different from the red cell type. Once the patient begins to produce "donor-type" erythrocytes, their blood type should be reassessed. The decision to switch a patient's blood type is highly variable across institutions. In our hospital, when a patient is RBC-transfusion independent for 120 days, molecular studies indicate appropriate engraftment and no incompatible isohemagglutinins against the new RBC phenotype can be detected in two consecutive blood samples, so the patient's native blood type is switched to the donor type for future transfusions.

TRANSFUSION-RELATED COMPLICATIONS

There are transfusion-related complications that are specific to, or more frequently seen, in the HSCT population. Some of these complications arise when lymphocytes within the transplant are activated against the recipient; these include TA-GVHD and passenger lymphocyte syndrome (PLS). Another complication, pure red cell aplasia (PRCA), occurs when the patient's residual antibodies attack the transplanted red cells. Standard transfusion reactions, such as allergic or febrile nonhemolytic reactions, are frequently seen in this heavily transfused patient population; however, these "standard" transfusion reactions are discussed more fully later in this chapter in the section "Adverse Effects of Red Cell Transfusions."

Major and Minor ABO Mismatches

Complications from ABO incompatibility depend on whether a major or minor ABO mismatch is present (Table 30-7). A major mismatch

TABLE 30–7. Component Type Selection for HSCTs That Cross the ABO Barrier

Mismatch	Transplant Donor Type	Transplant Recipient Type	RBC	Transfuse Platelets[a]/ Plasma
Major mismatch	A	O	O	A, AB
	B	O	O	B, AB
	AB	O	O	AB
	AB	A	A, O	AB
	AB	B	B, O	AB
Minor mismatch	O	A	O	A, AB
	O	B	O	B, AB
	O	AB	O	AB
	A	AB	A, O	AB
	B	AB	B, O	AB
Bidirectional mismatch	A	B	O	AB
	B	A	O	AB

[a]Platelets stored in additive solution (periodic acid-Schiff) reduce the volume of incompatible plasma transfused.

Modified with permission from Cohn CS. Transfusion support issues in hematopoietic stem cell transplantation. *Cancer Control.* 2015 Jan;22(1):52-59.

occurs when the transplant contains RBCs that are incompatible with the recipient's plasma. Conversely, a minor mismatch is present when the donor plasma contains isohemagglutinins against the recipient's RBCs. Bidirectional transplants (eg, group A transplant into group B recipient) carry both major and minor mismatches.

Major ABO Mismatch When a major ABO-mismatched transplant is given, immediate hemolysis may occur during the infusion. This complication is more commonly seen when the HSCT is derived from marrow, because more RBCs are present; however, RBC depletion techniques have effectively eliminated this complication. Because HPC-A units contain a minimal volume of RBCs (8-15 mL), clinically significant cases of immediate hemolysis have not been identified.[59] Most HPC-C units are RBC-depleted before cryopreservation, and the residual erythrocytes lyse during cryopreservation, thus immediate hemolysis is not a problem with cord blood transplants.

Preformed antibodies against non-ABO RBC antigens can remain in a recipient's peripheral circulation for many weeks after transplantation. These antibodies may cause lysis when engrafted cells begin to produce new RBCs. Also, chimeric patients may develop antibodies against ABO or non-ABO RBC antigens, resulting in delayed hemolysis. When recipients have isohemagglutinins specific for the ABO type of the transplant, delayed erythrocyte engraftment and PRCA may ensue. This is seen most frequently when group O patients receive a group A transplant, or with bidirectional mismatches. PRCA develops when anti-ABO antibodies destroy erythrocyte progenitor cells in the marrow.

Minor Mismatches When lymphocytes within the HSCT recognize the recipient RBCs as foreign, antibodies may be produced that are specific for ABO or minor RBC antigens. This PLS usually presents 7 to 14 days after the transplant with the abrupt onset of hemolysis. The hemolysis ranges from mild to severe, and may be intra- or extravascular, depending on the nature of the antibody involved. These "passenger lymphocytes" are reported most frequently in transplants that use a group O donor with a group A recipient.[60] Antibodies against minor RBC antigens are less frequently reported and cause less severe hemolysis.[60]

In cases involving the ABO system, the Hb level may drop precipitously. The laboratory signs of intravascular hemolysis, that is, hemoglobinemia, hemoglobinuria, and an elevated lactate dehydrogenase should be used to follow the course of disease. In most cases, a DAT will be positive, unless all antibody-bound cells have already been lysed. The hemolysis can persist as long as incompatible RBCs are present, but usually subsides within 5 to 10 days.[60]

Nonmyeloablative conditioning regimens carry a greater risk for PLS than when full ablation is used. Because HPC-A preparations carry a greater lymphocyte load when compared with hematopoietic cell concentrate-marrow and HPC-C collections, recipients of peripheral blood stem cells are at an increased risk of developing PLS. The authors are not aware of a case of PLS that has been reported with an umbilical cord stem cell transplant. Maintaining graft-versus-host disease (GVHD) prophylaxis with only a T-cell inhibitor, such as cyclosporine, without an accompanying B-cell inhibitor, is also considered a risk factor.

Transfusion-Transmitted CMV

Cytomegalovirus infection continues to be a serious complication after HSCTs. Most CMV infections are likely the result of reactivation of virus from a previous infection rather than acquisition of a new strain. However, in CMV antibody–negative patients, there is a risk of development of a transfusion-transmitted de novo CMV infection. To reduce this risk, one may use CMV antibody–negative blood, or leukocyte-reduced components. A large controlled trial and a meta-analysis from 2007 showed that leukocyte-reduced components are as effective as antibody-negative components in preventing transfusion-transmitted CMV.[61,62] Two additional studies support the safety of using only leukoreduced blood in preventing transfusion transmission of CMV.[63,64] Both studies found 0% risk of transfusion-transmitted CMV infection. Nonetheless, the overall risk of transfusion transmission of CMV in leukoreduced components is not zero. CMV DNA was found in 44% of newly seropositive blood donors, and the overall prevalence of CMV DNA was 0.13% in nearly 32,000 donations.[65] Although blood products could be obtained from donors with a longstanding history of CMV-positive serology, a more practical approach is to screen donated blood for CMV DNA or immunoglobulin (Ig) M antibodies, although we believe that the use of leukoreduced blood components is adequate.

Transfusion-Associated Graft-versus-Host Disease

All HSCT patients should receive irradiated components from the time of initiation of conditioning chemotherapy, and for at least one year after transplantation to prevent TA-GVHD. However, many centers continue to provide irradiated products for the life of the patient. The British Committee for Standards in Haematology (BCSH) recommends that allogeneic transplant recipients should receive irradiated components for six months post transplantation, or until the patient's lymphocyte count is greater than 1×10^9/L; however, if chronic GVHD is present, then irradiated products should be given indefinitely.[66] Autologous transplant patients should begin receiving irradiated components from the time of initiation of conditioning chemotherapy, but can revert to nonirradiated components three months after transplantation. If autologous transplant patients received total-body irradiation, then the BCSH recommends extending the use of irradiated products for six months after transplantation.

● SOLID-ORGAN TRANSPLANT

Patients awaiting a solid organ transplant should have minimal exposure to allogeneic blood products to reduce the risk of alloimmunization. Leukoreduced components contain sufficient white blood cells to immunize a patient against class I and class II HLA molecules. The risk of sensitization from a blood transfusion ranges from 2% to 21%.[67] Sensitization may increase the extent of alloimmunization, which contributes to delays in finding a compatible organ for transplantation. In fact, patients who have been transfused have an 11% reduction in the likelihood of ever receiving a renal transplant.[67] Attempts to reduce alloimmunization by matching blood donors and patients[68] or matching for the DR locus have shown no consistent reduction.[69] Using a Hb of 70 g/L as a safe threshold for transfusions can minimize exposure. In some patients, the use of erythropoiesis-stimulating agents (ESAs) may help decrease the number of RBC transfusions; however, ESAs are contraindicated in patients with a history of malignancy or stroke.

● ADVERSE EFFECTS OF TRANSFUSIONS

The precise risk of an adverse reaction is difficult to estimate; many reactions may be wrongly attributed to the patient's underlying illness, and approximately half of all transfusions are given to anesthetized patients in the operating rooms, where reactions may be blunted or more difficult to recognize. The incidence of some adverse reactions has fallen in the past decade because of changes in component handling, such as leukoreduction. Adverse reactions may occur soon after a transfusion begins, as seen with acute hemolytic reactions or acute lung injury, or within days to weeks of a transfusion, as seen with delayed hemolytic reactions.[70] Management of a transfusion reaction usually consists of

supportive measures, although a more in-depth understanding of specific management measures is helpful.[71] Fortunately, the majority of acute transfusion reactions are mild and manageable. Many of the reported transfusion-related fatalities involve human errors, which may be as much as 1:18,000 transfusions.

IMMEDIATE TRANSFUSION REACTIONS

In general, immediate transfusion reactions are more dangerous than delayed reactions. Severe complications, including death, can on rare occasions develop within a few minutes of initiating transfusion. Close attention and early vital sign assessments are recommended at the beginning and within 15 minutes of starting a transfusion.

Acute Hemolytic Transfusion Reactions

Case A 46-year-old man presents with a GI bleed. He has a Hb of 63 g/L, tachycardia, and feels uncomfortable. You decide to transfuse one unit of packed red cells to increase his Hb above 70 g/L. After 50 mL is transfused, he is hypotensive, feels anxious, complains of low back pain, becomes febrile, and a new onset of red urine is noted in his Foley catheter.

Acute hemolytic transfusion reactions (AHTRs) are almost always caused by the immune-mediated destruction of ABO-incompatible transfused blood. ABO incompatible transfusions are estimated to occur in one in 38,000 to one in 70,000 RBCs transfusions.[72] Isohemagglutinins can activate the complement and coagulation systems. C3a and C5a can activate white blood cells to release inflammatory cytokines (interleukin [IL]-1, IL-6, IL-8, and tumor necrosis factor-α), contributing to fever, hypotension, wheezing, chest pain, nausea, and vomiting.[73] The presence of antigen-antibody complexes and activated complement on donor RBCs may lead to bradykinin generation. This can increase capillary permeability and arteriolar dilation, causing a fall in systemic blood pressure. Activation of factor XII may initiate the coagulation cascade, with formation of thrombin, and lead to disseminated intravascular coagulation. Renal failure may also develop as a result of ischemia, hypotension, antigen-antibody complex deposition, and thrombosis. Although rare, AHTRs can be caused by other blood group antibodies, particularly those in the Kidd blood group system.

Clinical Features The most common presenting symptom is fever with or without chills or rigors. In mild cases, this may be accompanied with abdominal, chest, flank, or back pain, whereas in severe cases, dyspnea, hypotension, hemoglobinuria, and eventually shock can be seen. Bleeding as a result of the consumptive coagulopathy can occur. Hematuria can be the first sign of intravascular hemolysis, particularly in anesthetized or unconscious patients. The severity of AHTR is extremely variable and usually depends on the rate and total volume of blood administered. Approximately 47% of the recipients of ABO-incompatible blood show no effects, even after receiving a whole unit; 41% showed symptoms of AHTR; and mortality was approximately 2%.[70,72]

Laboratory evaluation involves checking for technical and identification errors, examination of a post-transfusion specimen for hemolysis, and performing a DAT to detect antibody-coated red cells. If AHTR is strongly suspected, repeat ABO and Rh typing of the patient and the transfused blood, and repeat antibody screen and cross match may be helpful. A negative DAT occurs in rare cases when all transfused RBCs are lysed.

Management Immediate discontinuation of transfusion should always be the first step in any transfusion reaction. Maintaining vascular access with slow infusion of normal saline, monitoring vital signs, and assessing urine output are key early steps. A blood specimen should be collected immediately for laboratory evaluation. The component bag should be returned to the blood bank. If severe hemolysis has occurred, therapy focuses on management of hypotension, coagulation disorders, and renal function. A urine output of approximately 100 mL/hour for 24 hours should be maintained in adults without contraindications. In simple cases, normal saline infusion may be sufficient; however, diuretics may be necessary in some cases. Intravenous administration of furosemide (40-80 mg) promotes diuresis and improves blood flow to the renal cortex. In severe cases of hypotension, dopamine, which dilates renal vasculature and increases cardiac output, can be used at a dosage of 1 mcg/kg of body weight per hour. Patients with coagulopathy and active bleeding may require administration of platelets, FFP, or cryoprecipitate.

Prevention The most common cause of AHTRs is clerical and human errors resulting from mistakes in identifying the patient, labeling the pretransfusions sample, or identifying the correct red cell unit for the patient.[72-74] A careful safety check comparing the unit tag and the patient's wristband is worth the extra time to prevent this reaction.

Febrile Nonhemolytic Transfusion Reactions

Case A 17-year-old female patient is undergoing HSCT for acute myeloid leukemia. While receiving a platelet transfusion, she develops chills/rigors and her temperature rises from 37.0°C (98.6°F) to 38.9°C (102.0°F). You stop the transfusion and initiate a transfusion reaction.

The workup in the blood bank shows a clerical check is correct, there is no evidence of hemolysis, and a Gram stain on the unit is negative.

An febrile non-hemolytic transfusion reaction (FNHTR) is defined, arbitrarily, as a temperature increase of 1°C (1.8°F) or more during or up to 4 hours after transfusion. Other possible symptoms include increases in respiratory rate and, more unusually, nausea or vomiting.

FNHTRs are one of the most commonly encountered transfusion reactions occurring in approximately 0.12% to 0.5% of RBC units transfused and are more likely to occur after transfusion of platelets than RBCs. Leukocyte reduction decreases the incidence of FNHTRs with both whole blood–derived and apheresis platelets.

Fever is triggered by the action of cytokines (eg, IL-1, IL-6, tumor necrosis factor-α). This may be the result of activation of donor leukocytes by anti-HLA or other antibodies in the recipient, activation of recipient leukocyte and endothelial cells by transfused donor leukocytes or plasma constituents, or passive transfer of cytokines or CD40 ligand (CD154) that accumulated in the unit during storage.

Clinical Features Fever should not be solely attributed to FNHTR until other potential life-threatening transfusion reactions or patient-related factors have been excluded. All associated blood components must be placed in quarantine until a septic transfusion reaction has been ruled-out. Past transfusion reaction history should be reviewed to determine whether additional measures should be implemented for future transfusions.

The laboratory investigation should concentrate on ruling out a septic transfusion reaction. A Gram stain is not a highly sensitive technique in this setting but may be used to rule-in bacterial contamination. Rapid qualitative immunoassay tests (eg, Verax or BacTx) are highly sensitive for most commonly encountered bacterial contaminants and may be used in lieu of Gram stain to screen implicated platelet units. In cases with a high index of suspicion, the unit should be cultured. If all results are negative and the patient's presentation is consistent with a mild FNHTR, no additional testing is required.

Management FNHTRs are typically benign, and usually resolve completely within 1 to 2 hours after the transfusion is discontinued. The remainder of the transfused unit and a posttransfusion blood sample from the patient should be sent to the laboratory for investigation. Antipyretics may be administered to shorten the duration of the fever and provide analgesia. Acetaminophen for adults (325-650 mg orally) or children (10-15 mg/kg/dose orally) is effective for this purpose.

Prevention Transfusing leukoreduced red cells and/or platelets stored in additive solution (periodic acid-Schiff) will significantly reduce the risk of FNHTRs.[75] Premedication with antipyretics (acetaminophen) is not helpful.[76]

Allergic Transfusion Reactions

Case A 55-year-old woman with breast cancer is undergoing chemotherapy. Her platelet count is 8×10^9/L and you decide to transfuse a unit of platelets before having a central line placed. Five minutes after starting the transfusion, she feels itchy. The nurse notices red raised lesions forming on her arms and face. The transfusion is stopped and you are called to the room. When you arrive, the patient is having trouble breathing (you can hear her wheezing across the room) and is becoming hypotensive. What should you do?

This patient is experiencing an allergic transfusion reaction (ATR). An ATR is a common adverse reaction of transfusion therapy, ranging from a mild form characterized by localized pruritus and/or urticaria, to a severe anaphylactic or anaphylactoid reaction. The mild forms of ATR occur in 1% to 3% of transfusions of plasma-rich components (ie, platelets/FFP) and in 0.1% to 0.3% for red cells. Severe anaphylactic reactions are much less frequent and estimated at 1:20,000 to 1:50,000 transfusions.[77]

The majority of ATRs are immediate (Type 1) hypersensitivity reactions, mediated by preformed IgE antibodies binding to soluble proteins present within donor plasma.[78] Severe anaphylactic transfusion reactions have been historically attributed to antibodies against IgA found in patients with complete IgA deficiency (<0.05 mg/dL). A review of international hemovigilance data has shown that most anaphylactic reactions occur in IgA-replete individuals, and that the underlying cause for the majority of reactions remains unknown.[79] Anaphylactoid reactions are similar to anaphylaxis but clinically less severe and caused by non–IgE-mediated activation of mast cells.

Clinical Features ATRs usually begin during or within an hour of starting a transfusion but may not become evident until several hours later. Common findings include urticaria, rash, pruritus, and flushing. More severe reactions occur sooner and may include angioedema, chest tightness, dyspnea, cyanosis, hoarseness, stridor, or wheezing. In addition, GI symptoms such as abdominal pain, nausea, vomiting, and diarrhea may also occur. Unlike other acute transfusion reactions, fever is usually absent. Anaphylaxis occurs immediately after starting the transfusion. Symptoms can include bronchospasm, angioedema, respiratory distress, nausea, vomiting, abdominal cramps, diarrhea, shock, and loss of consciousness. There is no need for laboratory investigation with simple urticarial and/or localized pruritus. However, the incident should be reported to the blood bank to update the patient's record for any future transfusions. Patients with a history of anaphylactic reactions receive washed red cells and platelets. Attempts should be made to avoid plasma transfusions whenever possible; however, if transfusion is needed, pooled, solvent-detergent–treated plasma can mitigate the risk of a reaction.

Management Most ATRs are mild, self-limited, and respond well to transfusion discontinuation and, if indicated, administration of antihistamine (diphenhydramine hydrochloride, usually orally). In cases limited to urticaria, the transfusion may be resumed immediately after symptoms resolve. However, transfusion should never be resumed when there is a severe reaction. In acute anaphylaxis, fluid resuscitation may be needed to maintain blood pressure followed by administration of subcutaneous epinephrine (0.3 mL of 1:1000 dilution), as well as airway management and intensive care. In case of shock, a higher concentration of IV epinephrine (3-5 mL of a 1:10,000 dilution) can be administered. Glucocorticoids are usually not helpful in acute crises.

Prevention Patients with a history of mild ATRs should not be premedicated with an antihistamine, because this does not reduce the overall risk of ATRs.[76] Washing cellular components to remove residual plasma or using platelets stored in periodic acid-Schiff can reduce the risk of a reaction.[75]

Transfusion-Associated Circulatory Overload

Case A 78-year-old frail female with heart disease, history of a coronary artery bypass graft, atrial fibrillation for which she is taking warfarin, diabetes mellitus, hyperlipidemia, and obesity presents to the hospital with her husband, who noticed the patient could not walk or move her left arm for the past 3 hours. Imaging confirms she has an acute hemorrhagic stroke. Her international normalized ratio is 10.2 and you order 4 units of plasma to start to reverse her warfarin. During the transfusion of the third unit, the patient is noted to be tachypneic and her oxygen saturation has decreased to 80%. What is the cause of her respiratory distress? What laboratory studies should you order to rule in and rule out likely diagnoses?

TACO occurs when patients are unable to effectively process the expansion in intravascular volume from a blood transfusion. Circulatory overload may be caused by the infusion rates, the volume of infused blood product, and/or an underlying cardiac, renal, and/or pulmonary pathology. The fluid volume transfused may be less important than the infusion flow rate and the patient's ability to process the fluid.

TACO has become the number one cause of transfusion-related fatalities in the U.S. The increase in TACO is likely related to increased recognition and reporting. Using international hemovigilance data, the incidence of TACO is 10 to 29 per 100,000 blood components transfused.[80] A 100-fold higher incidence of TACO has been reported when active surveillance is compared with voluntary reporting (passive surveillance) systems.[81]

TACO is seen more in younger and advanced age patients.[82] Additional risk factors include female sex, a history of congestive heart failure, hemodialysis, mechanical ventilation, recent use of vasopressors, and positive fluid balance.[83]

Clinical Features The symptoms of TACO may include dyspnea, orthopnea, cough, headache, and hypoxemia, which are not specific. An international panel published a revised and validated definition for TACO in 2019. The revised surveillance definition classifies transfusion-related adverse events as TACO during or up to 12 hours after transfusion when a patient has three of the following criteria, with at least one from the required criteria (1 and 2): (1) acute or worsening respiratory compromise, (2) evidence of pulmonary edema, (3) evidence of cardiovascular system changes not explained by the patient's underlying medical condition, (4) evidence of fluid overload, and (5) supportive result of a relevant biomarker (eg, an increase of B-type natriuretic peptide level [BNP] or N terminal-propeptide BNP [NT-pro BNP]).[80]

Management Once TACO is suspected, IV fluids should be restricted followed by the administration of supplemental oxygen and a diuretic, if not contraindicated. Placing the patient in a sitting position also can be helpful. In severe cases, mechanical ventilation may be required. A chest radiograph should be ordered as well as an NT-pro BNP, unless the level is already elevated in the patient.

Prevention If a patient is at risk for TACO and blood transfusion is imperative, blood should be administered slowly (1-4 mL/kg/h). Most blood banks can also reduce the transfusion volume by splitting the blood product into smaller volumes if the transfusion is going to last longer than 4 hours. Close monitoring of the patient's vital signs throughout the transfusion may also help in decreasing the development of TACO.

Transfusion-Related Acute Lung Injury

Transfusion-related acute lung injury (TRALI) is a syndrome of acute hypoxia caused by noncardiogenic pulmonary edema that occurs after a transfusion. TRALI has been the leading cause of transfusion-related fatalities for several years. A recent consensus conference reviewed and revised the definition of TRALI by separating diagnoses into TRALI Types I and II based on whether the patient has preexisting risk factors for acute respiratory distress syndrome (ARDS).[84] TRALI Type I patients with no risk factors for ARDS must meet the following criteria: acute onset; hypoxemia (paO_2/FiO_2 ≤300 or SpO_2 <90% on room air); clear evidence of bilateral pulmonary edema on imaging; and no evidence of left atrial hypertension, or if left atrial hypertension is present, it is judged not to be the main contributor to the hypoxemia. To meet criteria for TRALI Type I, the onset must be during or within 6 hours of transfusion and there should be no temporal relationship to an alternative risk factor for ARDS. TRALI Type II is reserved for patients who have risk factors for ARDS or have existing mild ARDS (paO_2/FiO_2 of 200-300), but whose respiratory status deteriorates secondary to a transfusion. For TRALI Type II, the following criteria must be met: acute onset and hypoxemia (paO_2/FiO_2 ≤300 or SpO_2 <90% on room air). In addition, the patient must have a stable respiratory status in the 12 hours before transfusion. In this new system, the diagnosis of "possible TRALI" has been dropped and patients with ARDS diagnostic criteria who show respiratory deterioration 12 hours before a transfusion should be classified as ARDS. A final diagnostic category has been proposed that includes patients with TACO complicated by TRALI, or TACO/TRALI.

There are two main hypotheses regarding the capillary leak seen in TRALI. The two-hit hypothesis states that underlying patient factors act as a necessary first hit, leading to adherence of primed neutrophils to the pulmonary endothelium. The second hit is caused by mediators within the transfused component, which activate pulmonary neutrophils, which in turn damage the endothelium.[85] The mediators are often antibodies specific for either class II HLA, or for human neutrophil antigens. There are also cases in which no antibody was detected, which are thought to be caused by proinflammatory mediators' bioactive lipids and CD40 ligand that accumulate in the blood product during storage.[86] Despite reports of a direct correlation between storage time of cellular blood components and TRALI, this mechanism remains controversial.

Specific patient factors (first hits) that are associated with a greater risk of TRALI include: patients on mechanical ventilation, sepsis, chronic alcohol abuse, severe liver disease, hematologic malignancy, and others. It is not known whether the risk is determined by the patient's condition or by a greater transfusion requirement. The two-hit hypothesis accounts for critically ill patients who develop TRALI; however, there are reports of TRALI in reasonably healthy patients. This observation led to the threshold model of TRALI.[87] In this paradigm, a threshold, or tipping point, must be surpassed to induce TRALI. A healthy patient may develop TRALI when transfused with a high titer of antibody. Conversely, a critically ill patient with primed neutrophils can be tipped into TRALI with a lower titer of antibody.

Clinical Features It is often impossible to fully distinguish TRALI from other causes of respiratory distress. The typical presentation of TRALI is the sudden development of dyspnea, severe hypoxemia (O_2 saturation <90% on room air), hypotension, and fever that develop within 6 hours of transfusion and usually resolve with supportive care within 48 to 96 hours. Although hypotension is considered one of the important signs in diagnosing TRALI, hypertension can occur in some cases.

In addition to new or worsening oxygen desaturation, TRALI is characterized by chest radiograph findings of bilateral diffuse patchy pulmonary densities without cardiac enlargement. TRALI can be ruled out as the sole cause of pulmonary failure by the presence of rales and jugular venous distension on physical examination and/or dilated pulmonary arteries on chest radiograph, which are evidence of congestive heart failure with or without TACO. Transient leukopenia, which follows the reaction within few hours, can also distinguish TRALI from TACO.

Management Supportive care is the mainstay of therapy in TRALI. Oxygen supplementation and aggressive respiratory support, IV fluid for hypotension support, and vasopressors, if indicated. It has been suggested that diuretics, which are indicated in TACO management, are not efficacious and should be avoided in TRALI. Corticosteroids may provide benefit.

Prevention HLA alloimmunization has been directly correlated with the number of times a woman is pregnant, and plasma from multiparous women has been implicated as a risk factor in TRALI. To reduce this risk, blood banks attempt to collect plasma from males, nulliparous females, and/or females tested and found to be negative for HLA antibodies. After blood collection centers implemented TRALI mitigation strategies, the incidence of TRALI dropped from an estimate of 1:4000 transfusions to approximately 1:12,000.[88] Nonetheless, TRALI continues to be one of the leading causes of transfusion-related fatalities.

Pooled plasma also may be used for TRALI mitigation because antibody titers drop as a result of dilution. No cases of TRALI resulting from transfusion of pooled solvent-detergent–treated plasma have been reported.[89,90]

Transfusion-Related Sepsis

Case A 15-year-old girl who is undergoing HSCT for Hodgkin disease presents with new-onset epistaxis. She is transfused one unit of apheresis platelets for a platelet count of 5×10^9/L. Within 15 minutes of starting the transfusion, the nurse calls you because the patient is having chills and rigors, and fever and hypotension have developed. Her pretransfusion vital signs are as follows: blood pressure 120/80 torr, pulse 67 beats/minute, respiration rate 20 breaths/minute, and temperature 37.0°C (98.6°F). The posttransfusion vital signs are concerning for hypotension, tachycardia, an elevated respiratory rate, and new onset of fever: blood pressure 90/50 torr, pulse 104 beats/minute, respiration rate 28 breaths/minute, temperature 38.9°C (102.1°F).

Transfusion-related sepsis usually occurs from platelet units that are stored at room temperature; however, the introduction of pathogen-reduction technology for platelets should mitigate this risk. RBCs, stored at refrigerator temperatures, are very rarely contaminated by unusual cold-growing organisms (eg, *Yersinia, Serratia, Pseudomonas*). The rate of fatal transfusion-transmitted bacteremia from RBCs has been estimated to be 0.13 per 1 million units transfused in the U.S.[91]

Clinical Features The infusion of large numbers of gram-negative microorganisms may lead to fever (>38.5°C [101.3°F]), rigors, marked hypotension, abdominal pain, vomiting, diarrhea, and the development of profound shock. Gram-positive contaminants may cause fever and rigors but are not associated with the severe symptoms produced by gram-negative toxins. Although the onset of fever and other symptoms is often rapid, symptoms may present as late as 24 hours after the transfusion.[92] Rapid diagnosis usually may be made via Gram stain of the residual donor blood; however, a culture of the transfused component is necessary.

Management A blood culture should be drawn before antibiotics are started. Septic shock from transfusion of contaminated blood should be managed as for septic shock from other causes.

DELAYED TRANSFUSION REACTIONS

Delayed Hemolytic Transfusion Reactions

DHTRs occur when a previously immunized patient receives RBCs containing the corresponding antigen but are compatible in the crossmatch because of a low titer of circulating alloantibody. DHTRs occur in 0.2% to 2.6% of patients. It is vanishingly rare in infants younger than 4 months of age, and more common in chronically transfused patients.

Approximately 30% to 40% of alloantibodies become undetectable months to years after their initial identification. However, a patient previously immunized by transfusion or pregnancy may have a secondary immune response after reexposure to a blood-group antigen. Decreasing Hct or failure to see the typical 10 g/L Hb/3% Hct increment after transfusion may be noted within several days to weeks of a blood transfusion, as well as an unexplained fever. Hemolysis from DHTR is typically extravascular, without dramatic clinical symptoms and signs, although some classes of IgG bind complement and will cause intravascular hemolysis. Hemolysis in DHTRs is usually mild and gradual; however, when antibodies are produced against antigens in the Kidd blood system, the hemolysis may be rapid, intravascular, and severe.

The usual evidence of hemolysis is seen, including: the appearance of spherocytes and reticulocytes on peripheral smear, increases in total and unconjugated bilirubin, and increased lactate dehydrogenase. The DAT is usually positive, but may be negative if all the transfused RBCs have been eliminated from the circulation. The antibody screen is usually positive, and the antibody can be identified. No specific management is usually needed because these reactions are usually subtle and clinically silent. In cases of intravascular hemolysis, clinical support measures are similar to those described for an acute hemolytic transfusion reaction. If transfusion is necessary donor red cells negative for the offending antigen may be selected.

Posttransfusion Purpura

Description Posttransfusion purpura is a rare immune-mediated disorder directed against platelet alloantigens.

Iron Overload

Description One of the most common complications of chronic RBC transfusion is iron overload, which is further discussed in the chapters on congenital hemoglobinopathies (Chaps. 14, 17, and 18).

TA-GVHD

Most cases of TA-GVHD are associated with HSCT. TA-GVHD is a very rare complication that occurs when a susceptible patient is exposed to viable lymphocytes introduced in a blood transfusion. This can occur when transfusions from close relatives or other unintentionally genetically matched donors are administered to severely immunocompromised recipients. The immunocompromised recipient is incapable of "rejecting" or mounting an attack against the lymphocytes in the transfused blood. In addition, cases of TA-GVHD have been reported in recipients with an intact immune system.[93,94]

TA-GVHD may present with maculopapular rash, fever, watery diarrhea, liver dysfunction, and bone marrow failure within 8 to 10 days of transfusion. The mortality rate in TA-GVHD is approximately 90% and rapid clinical deterioration.

RBC, platelet, and granulocyte units all contain some lymphocytes and therefore carry a risk of TA-GVHD; plasma and cryoprecipitate are acellular and therefore pose no risk. To prevent TA-GVHD, lymphocytes within a blood component must be eliminated or disabled. Leukoreduction is not sufficient because it reduces, but does not completely eliminate, white blood cells. Frozen units may also carry a risk, because the lymphocytes may survive. Gamma and x-ray irradiation of components are effective prophylaxis for TA-GVHD.[95] A dose of at least 2500 sGy to the center of a cellular blood component and 1500 cGy throughout the unit leaves lymphocytes intact but unable to proliferate. This simple precaution prevents TA-GVHD.

Irradiation at the indicated dose appears to damage the red cell membrane. The damage does not affect the oxygen-carrying capacity of the erythrocyte, but does allow potassium to leak from the cell. The level of extracellular potassium has been shown to increase with storage time. As a result, RBCs may be stored for only 28 days after irradiation.

POTENTIAL EFFECT OF AGE OF RED CELLS ON TRANSFUSION OUTCOME

In the U.S., RBCs may be stored in additive solution for up to 42 days. The criteria used to determine storage limits are based on in vivo recovery and in vitro hemolysis data. During storage, RBC units develop a progressive "storage lesion." Some of these changes include: an increase in free Hb, which acts as a nitric oxide scavenger; a reduction in 2,3-diphosphoglycerate, which leads to increased oxygen affinity/ decreased oxygen delivery; an increase in hydrogen ions in the supernatant, causing a drop in the pH; an increase in microvesicles in the supernatant, creating a procoagulant effect; a release in free iron, which could support the growth of some infectious organisms; and reduced RBC membrane deformability. Each of these changes is a dynamic process, with some occurring on the first day of blood storage, and others taking days or weeks to be evident. Some of these changes, such as the decreased 2,3-diphosphoglycerate level, are reversed after transfusion; however, RBC deformability continues to be reduced, which could potentially reduce perfusion in microvascular beds.

Although preclinical studies have found evidence that the storage lesion could have negative effects, several large randomized clinical trials encompassing over 30,000 adult and pediatric patients have found no evidence that prolonged storage of RBCs is associated with poorer outcomes when compared with RBCs stored for a shorter duration.[96-99] Although each trial was conducted with different patient populations—slightly different definitions of "older" versus "younger" units and different outcome measures—meta-analyses of the data found that there was no statistically significant difference in clinical outcomes when older versus younger units were compared (RR, 1.04; 95% CI, 0.98-1.12).[100] It is worth noting that the outcome measures for most of these trials were mortality at 7-day or 30-day follow-up.

The outcome measure of death on short-term follow-up is informative for an overall effect, but trials with narrower outcome measures have begun to detect possibly smaller but clinically relevant effects of the storage lesion. One trial found that patients receiving younger RBCs did not have a statistically significant difference in the rate of postoperative infections when compared with those receiving RBCs stored for more than 14 days (22% vs 25%, respectively; RR, 1.17; 95% CI, 0.71-1.93), although wound infections occurred more frequently with older RBC transfusions (15% vs 5%; RR, 3.09; 95% CI, 1.17-8.18). Patients receiving older units had a higher rate of acute kidney injury (24% vs 6%; $P < 0.001$) and longer lengths of stay (mean difference, 3.6 days; 95% CI, 0.6-7.5 in an "as-treated" analysis).[101] In another study, a subset of patients enrolled in the Age of Blood Evaluation study had coagulation and immune factors tested. This study found that transfusion of fresh versus standard-issue RBCs units does not result in substantial changes in coagulation or immune parameters.[102]

The data from two recent trials in neonate and pediatric populations also found no significant difference in outcomes in patients transfused with blood stored for longer or shorter durations.[103,104] In premature very-low-birth-weight infants, the primary outcome was a composite measure of major neonatal morbidities, including necrotizing enterocolitis, retinopathy of prematurity, bronchopulmonary dysplasia, and intraventricular hemorrhage, as well as death. The rate of nosocomial infection was a secondary outcome. Overall, the use of fresh RBCs compared with standard blood bank practice did not improve outcomes in this patient population.[105] A trial with pediatric patients in Kampala, Uganda enrolled six 60-month-old subjects, most with malaria or SCD, who presented to the hospital with a Hb level of 50 g/L or lower and a lactate level of 5 mmol/L or higher. The primary outcome was the proportion of patients with a lactate level of 3 mmol/L or lower at 8 hours after transfusion with either RBCs of shorter (7-9 days) or longer (30-34 days) storage periods. The proportion achieving the primary end point was 0.61 (95% CI, 0.52-0.69) in the longer-storage group versus 0.58 (95% CI, 0.49-0.66) in the shorter-storage group (between-group difference, 0.03 [95% CI, −0.07 to ∞], $P < 0.001$), meeting the prespecified margin of noninferiority of 25%. Mean lactate levels were not statistically different between the two groups at up to 24 hours after transfusion. Other secondary end points, such as cerebral oxygen saturation, electrolyte abnormalities, adverse events, and 30-day recovery, were also not significantly different between the groups, supporting the conclusion that transfusion of longer-storage versus shorter-storage RBCs did not result in inferior results for the study end points in this pediatric population.[103] A Cochrane meta-analysis of these and older studies of RBC storage age in pediatric and neonate populations reached no strong conclusion because they found the quality of evidence to be low or very low.[106]

PATIENT BLOOD MANAGEMENT

Patient blood management (PBM) is an evidence-based, systematic, and multifaceted approach to optimizing the care of patients who might need transfusion. The risks associated with unnecessary transfusions, coupled with the rising cost of blood have helped fuel the growth of PBM efforts. PBM was recently adopted by the World Health Organization as the new standard of care, and the AABB has issued guidelines and other tools designed to help hospitals implement a PBM program. A comprehensive PBM program includes: (1) hospital-wide guidelines for evidence-based use of blood components, (2) early assessment and correction of preoperative anemia, and (3) application of a variety of techniques to minimize perioperative blood loss.

Guidelines for transfusion have been published by multiple medical professional societies and can serve as a useful starting point for hospitals; however, the evidence for Hb thresholds was developed in selected patient populations and does not apply in all clinical situations. Combining evidence with a clinical assessment is necessary when deciding whether a transfusion is indicated. Adding decision support tools into computerized physician order entry systems can remind clinicians of guidelines and safety considerations when ordering blood.[107] These systems have been shown to reduce blood use and decrease costs associated with transfusions.[108] Auditing transfusion orders may reveal patterns of blood utilization that can be corrected with education. Prospective audits of orders are most useful; however, this practice requires an intensive effort by blood bank staff and/or transfusion physicians. Because this level of effort is not always feasible because of staffing constraints, a semiautomated retrospective review of transfusions can be implemented.[108]

Preoperative anemia is associated with adverse outcomes in surgery.[109] Anemia levels act as an inverted sliding scale, with higher mortality seen in patients with lower preoperative Hb. The effect of blood loss on mortality was also more pronounced in patients with lower versus higher preoperative Hb values. When preexisting comorbidities and other confounders were considered, preoperative anemia continued to be independently associated with adverse outcomes after cardiac and noncardiac surgeries. Even relatively mild preoperative anemia was shown to be an independent risk factor for higher early mortality in cardiac surgical procedures,[110] and for 30-day morbidity and mortality in patients undergoing major noncardiac surgery.[111]

Given the risks of preoperative anemia, both patients and hospitals may benefit from a preoperative anemia assessment program for all surgical patients. When possible, this assessment should be undertaken 28 days before surgery, to correct anemia with oral iron when possible, and IV iron or erythropoietin when necessary and not contraindicated. Hematologists should be consulted for cases of refractory anemia.

Perioperative blood management is the third pillar of a strong PBM program. Blood-sparing surgical techniques and anesthesiology-based blood conservation tools should be used whenever possible. Minimizing perioperative blood loss reduces the need for RBC transfusion and the length of hospital stay.[112] The combination of a restrictive transfusion strategy, preoperative anemia correction, and perioperative blood management has been shown to reduce RBC transfusions, decrease adverse events, and reduce hospital costs.[112]

A systematic review and meta-analysis of PBM studies looked at the efficacy of a PBM program in terms of preoperative anemia, RBC transfusion thresholds, and implementation of PBM programs in adults.[113] The authors issued strong recommendations to detect and manage preoperative anemia before major elective surgery, and to use restrictive RBC transfusion thresholds in critically ill but clinically stable patients (Hb <70 g/L) and in patients undergoing cardiac surgery (Hb <75 g/L). They issued several conditional recommendations, including implementation of PBM programs to improve appropriate RBC utilization and use of electronic clinical decision support as a tool to help achieve this goal. These measures can help hospitals limit inappropriate blood transfusions and promote patient safety.

REFERENCES

1. Jones J. Blood collection and utilization in the United States 2017 Centers for Disease Control and Prevention. http://www.cdc.gov
2. Raybhandary S, Whitaker B, Perez G. *The 2015-2015 National Blood Collection and Utilization Survey Report.* American Association of Blood Banks; 2018.
3. Global status report on blood safety and availability 2016. Geneva: World Health Organization; 2017.
4. Eastlund T. Monetary blood donation incentives and the risk of transfusion-transmitted infection. *Transfusion.* 1998;38:874-882.
5. Dybul M. Partnerships for blood safety in Africa: the U.S. President's Emergency Plan for AIDS Relief. *Transfusion.* 2008;48:1044-1046.
6. To L, Dunnington T, Thomas C, Love K, McCullough J, Riley W. The United States' potential blood donor pool: updating the prevalence of donor-exclusion factors on the pool of potential donors. *Transfusion.* 2020;60(1):206-215.
7. McCullough J. *Transfusion Medicine.* 4th ed. John Wiley & Sons; 2017.
8. Rubin RJ, Ness PM. What price progress? An update on vinyl plastic bags. *Transfusion.* 1989;29:358-361.
9. Wiltbank TB, Giordano GF, Kamel H, Tomasulo P, Custer B. Faint and prefaint reactions in whole-blood donors: an analysis of predonation measurements and their predictive value. *Transfusion.* 2008;48:1799-1808.
10. Eder AF, Dy BA, Kennedy JM, et al. The American Red Cross donor hemovigilance program: complications of blood donation reported in 2006. *Transfusion.* 2008;48:1809-1819.
11. Goldman M, Osmond L, Yi QL, Cameron-Choi K, O'Brien SF. Frequency and risk factors for donor reactions in an anonymous blood donor survey. *Transfusion.* 2013;53:1979-1984.
12. Goodnough LT, Rudnick S, Price TH, et al. Increased preoperative collection of autologous blood with recombinant human erythropoietin therapy. *N Engl J Med.* 1989;321:1163-1168.
13. Spivak JL. Recombinant human erythropoietin and its role in transfusion medicine. *Transfusion.* 1994;34:1-4.
14. Starkey NM, MacPherson JL, Bolgiano DC, et al. Markers for transfusion-transmitted disease in different groups of blood donors. *JAMA* 1989;262:3452-3454.
15. Luten M, Roerdinkholder-Stoelwinder B, Rombout-Sestrienkova E, de Grip WJ, Bos HJ, Bosman GJ. Red cell concentrates of hemochromatosis patients comply with the storage guidelines for transfusion purposes. *Transfusion.* 2008;48:436-441.
16. Lasky LC, Lin A, Kahn RA, McCullough J. Donor platelet response and product quality assurance in plateletpheresis. *Transfusion.* 1981;21:247-260.
17. Shi PA, Ness PM. Two-unit red cell apheresis and its potential advantages over traditional whole-blood donation. *Transfusion.* 1999;39:218-225.
18. McCullough J, Clay M, Herr G, Smith J, Stroncek D. Effects of granulocyte-colony-stimulating factor on potential normal granulocyte donors. *Transfusion.* 1999;39:1136-1140.
19. Herwaldt BL, Linden JV, Bosserman E, Young C, Olkowska D, Wilson M. Transfusion-associated babesiosis in the United States: a description of cases. *Ann Intern Med.* 2011;155:509-519.
20. Busch MP, Young MJ, Samson SM, Mosley JW, Ward JW, Perkins HA. Risk of human immunodeficiency virus (HIV) transmission by blood transfusions before the implementation of HIV-1 antibody screening. The Transfusion Safety Study Group. *Transfusion.* 1991;31:4-11.
21. Dodd RY, Notari EP, Stramer SL. Current prevalence and incidence of infectious disease markers and estimated window-period risk in the American Red Cross blood donor population. *Transfusion.* 2002;42:975-979.
22. Custer B, Quiner CA, Haaland R, et al. HIV antiretroviral therapy and prevention use in US blood donors: a new blood safety concern. *Blood.* 2020;136(11):1351-1358.
23. Food and Drug Administration. Fatalities reported to FDA following blood collection and transfusion annual summary. Accessed July 8, 2020. https://www.fda.gov/media/124796/download
24. Benjamin RJ. Transfusion-related sepsis: a silent epidemic. *Blood.* 2016;127:380-381.
25. Hébert PC, Wells G, Blajchman MA, et al. A multicenter, randomized, controlled clinical trial of transfusion requirements in critical care. Transfusion Requirements in Critical Care Investigators, Canadian Critical Care Trials Group. *N Engl J Med.* 1999;340:409-417.
26. Salpeter SR, Buckley JS, Chatterjee S. Impact of more restrictive blood transfusion strategies on clinical outcomes: a meta-analysis and systematic review. *Am J Med.* 2014;127:124-131.e3.
27. Holst LB, Petersen MW, Haase N, Perner A, Wetterslev J. Restrictive versus liberal transfusion strategy for red blood cell transfusion: systematic review of randomised trials with meta-analysis and trial sequential analysis. *BMJ.* 2015;350:h1354.
28. Carson JL, Stanworth SJ, Alexander JH, et al. Clinical trials evaluating red blood cell transfusion thresholds: an updated systematic review and with additional focus on patients with cardiovascular disease. *Am Heart J* 2018;200:96-101.
29. Villanueva C, Colomo A, Bosch A, et al. Transfusion strategies for acute upper gastrointestinal bleeding. *N Engl J Med.* 2013;368:11-21.
30. Hébert PC, Yetisir E, Martin C, et al. Is a low transfusion threshold safe in critically ill patients with cardiovascular diseases? *Crit Care Med.* 2001;29:227-234.
31. Carson JL, Terrin ML, Noveck H, et al. Liberal or restrictive transfusion in high-risk patients after hip surgery. *N Engl J Med.* 2011;365:2453-2462.
32. Hajjar LA, Vincent JL, Galas FR, et al. Transfusion requirements after cardiac surgery: the TRACS randomized controlled trial. *JAMA.* 2010;304:1559-1567.
33. Carson JL, Brooks MM, Abbott JD, et al. Liberal versus restrictive transfusion thresholds for patients with symptomatic coronary artery disease. *Am Heart J* 2013;165:964-971.e1.
34. Gu WJ, Gu XP, Wu XD, et al. Restrictive versus liberal strategy for red blood-cell transfusion: a systematic review and meta-analysis in orthopaedic patients. *J Bone Joint Surg Am.* 2018;100:686-695.
35. Foss NB, Kristensen MT, Kehlet H. Anaemia impedes functional mobility after hip fracture surgery. *Age Ageing.* 2008;37:173-178.
36. Foss NB, Kristensen MT, Jensen PS, Palm H, Krasheninnikoff M, Kehlet H. The effects of liberal versus restrictive transfusion thresholds on ambulation after hip fracture surgery. *Transfusion.* 2009;49:227-234.
37. Robertson CS, Hannay HJ, Yamal JM, et al. Effect of erythropoietin and transfusion threshold on neurological recovery after traumatic brain injury: a randomized clinical trial. *JAMA.* 2014;312:36-47.
38. Desjardins P, Turgeon AF, Tremblay MH, et al. Hemoglobin levels and transfusions in neurocritically ill patients: a systematic review of comparative studies. *Crit Care.* 2012;16:R54.
39. Moller A, Nielsen HB, Wetterslev J, et al. Low vs high hemoglobin trigger for transfusion in vascular surgery: a randomized clinical feasibility trial. *Blood.* 2019;133:2639-2650.
40. Lacroix J, Hébert PC, Hutchison JS, et al. Transfusion strategies for patients in pediatric intensive care units. *N Engl J Med.* 2007;356:1609-1619.
41. Rouette J, Trottier H, Ducruet T, et al. Red blood cell transfusion threshold in postsurgical pediatric intensive care patients: a randomized clinical trial. *Ann Surg.* 2010;251:421-427.
42. Willems A, Harrington K, Lacroix J, et al. Comparison of two red-cell transfusion strategies after pediatric cardiac surgery: a subgroup analysis. *Crit Care Med.* 2010;38:649-656.
43. Karam O, Tucci M, Ducruet T, et al. Red blood cell transfusion thresholds in pediatric patients with sepsis. *Pediatr Crit Care Med.* 2011;12:512-518.
44. Kirpalani H, Bell EF, Hintz SR, et al. Higher or lower hemoglobin transfusion thresholds for preterm infants. *NEJM.* 2020;383:2639-2651.
45. Bell EF, Strauss RG, Widness JA, et al. Randomized trial of liberal versus restrictive guidelines for red blood cell transfusion in preterm infants. *Pediatrics.* 2005;115:1685-1691.
46. Kirpalani H, Whyte RK, Andersen C, et al. The Premature Infants in Need of Transfusion (PINT) study: a randomized, controlled trial of a restrictive (low) versus liberal (high) transfusion threshold for extremely low birth weight infants. *J Pediatr.* 2006;149:301-307.
47. Whyte R, Kirpalani H. Low versus high haemoglobin concentration threshold for blood transfusion for preventing morbidity and mortality in very low birth weight infants. *Cochrane Database Syst Rev.* 2011;CD000512.
48. Keir A, Pal S, Trivella M, et al. Adverse effects of red blood cell transfusions in neonates: a systematic review and meta-analysis. *Transfusion.* 2016;56:2773-2780.

49. DeBaun MR, Gordon M, McKinstry RC, et al. Controlled trial of transfusions for silent cerebral infarcts in sickle cell anemia. *N Engl J Med.* 2014;371:699-710.

50. Lasalle-Williams M, Nuss R, Le T, et al. Extended red blood cell antigen matching for transfusions in sickle cell disease: a review of a 14-year experience from a single center (CME). *Transfusion.* 2011;51:1732-1739.

51. Hendrickson JE, Desmarets M, Deshpande SS, et al. Recipient inflammation affects the frequency and magnitude of immunization to transfused red blood cells. *Transfusion.* 2006;46:1526-1536.

52. Chou ST, Jackson T, Vege S, Smith-Whitley K, Friedman DF, Westhoff CM. High prevalence of red blood cell alloimmunization in sickle cell disease despite transfusion from Rh-matched minority donors. *Blood.* 2013;122:1062-1071.

53. de Montalembert M, Dumont MD, Heilbronner C, et al. Delayed hemolytic transfusion reaction in children with sickle cell disease. *Haematologica.* 2011;96:801-807.

54. Reid ME, Halter Hipsky C, Hue-Roye K, Hoppe C. Genomic analyses of RH alleles to improve transfusion therapy in patients with sickle cell disease. *Blood Cells Mol Dis.* 2014;52:195-202.

55. Storb R, Prentice RL, Thomas ED. Marrow transplantation for treatment of aplastic anemia. An analysis of factors associated with graft rejection. *N Engl J Med.* 1977;96:61-66.

56. Champlin RE, Horowitz MM, van Bekkum DW, et al. Graft failure following bone marrow transplantation for severe aplastic anemia: risk factors and treatment results. *Blood.* 1989;73:606-613.

57. Patel SR, Zimring JC. Transfusion-induced bone marrow transplant rejection due to minor histocompatibility antigens. *Transfus Med Rev.* 2013;27:241-248.

58. Webert KE, Cook RJ, Couban S, et al. A multicenter pilot-randomized controlled trial of the feasibility of an augmented red blood cell transfusion strategy for patients treated with induction chemotherapy for acute leukemia or stem cell transplantation. *Transfusion.* 2008;48:81-91.

59. Rowley SD. Hematopoietic stem cell transplantation between red cell incompatible donor-recipient pairs. *Bone Marrow Transplant.* 2001;28:315-321.

60. Petz LD. Immune hemolysis associated with transplantation. *Semin Hematol.* 2005;42:145-155.

61. Vamvakas EC. White-blood-cell-containing allogeneic blood transfusion and postoperative infection or mortality: an updated meta-analysis. *Vox Sang.* 2007;92:224-232.

62. Bowden RA, Slichter SJ, Sayers M, et al. A comparison of filtered leukocyte-reduced and cytomegalovirus (CMV) seronegative blood products for the prevention of transfusion-associated CMV infection after marrow transplant. *Blood.* 1995;86:3598-3603.

63. Nash T, Hoffmann S, Butch S, Davenport R, Cooling L. Safety of leukoreduced, cytomegalovirus (CMV)-untested components in CMV-negative allogeneic human progenitor cell transplant recipients. *Transfusion.* 2012;52:2270-2272.

64. Thiele T, Krüger W, Zimmermann K, et al. Transmission of cytomegalovirus (CMV) infection by leukoreduced blood products not tested for CMV antibodies: a single-center prospective study in high-risk patients undergoing allogeneic hematopoietic stem cell transplantation (CME). *Transfusion.* 2011;51:2620-2626.

65. Ziemann M, Krueger S, Maier AB, Unmack A, Goerg S, Hennig H. High prevalence of cytomegalovirus DNA in plasma samples of blood donors in connection with seroconversion. *Transfusion.* 2007;47:1972-1983.

66. Treleaven J, Gennery A, Marsh J, et al. Guidelines on the use of irradiated blood components prepared by the British Committee for Standards in Haematology blood transfusion task force. *Br J Haematol.* 2011;2011;152:35-51.

67. Obrador GT, Macdougall IC. Effect of red cell transfusions on future kidney transplantation. *Clin J Am Soc Nephrol.* 2013;8:852-860.

68. Reed A, Pirsch J, Armbrust MJ, et al. Multivariate analysis of donor-specific versus random transfusion protocols in haploidentical living-related transplants. *Transplantation.* 1991;51:382-384.

69. Christiaans MH, van Hooff JP, Nieman F, van den Berg-Loonen EM. HLA-DR matched transfusions: development of donor-specific T- and B-cell antibodies and renal allograft outcome. *Transplantation.* 1999;67:1029-1035.

70. Pineda AA, Brzica SM, Taswell HF. Hemolytic transfusion reaction. Recent experience in a large blood bank. *Mayo Clin Proc.* 1978;53:378-390.

71. Delaney M, Wendel S, Bercovitz RS, et al. Transfusion reactions: prevention, diagnosis, and treatment. *Lancet.* 2016;88:2825-2836.

72. Linden JV, Wagner K, Voytovich AE, Sheehan J. Transfusion errors in New York State: an analysis of 10 years' experience. *Transfusion.* 2000;40:1207-1213.

73. Davenport RD. The role of cytokines in hemolytic transfusion reactions. *Immunol Invest.* 1995;24:319-331.

74. Sazama K. Reports of 355 transfusion-associated deaths: 1976 through 1985. *Transfusion.* 1990;30:583-590.

75. Martí-Carvajal AJ, Solà I, González LE, Leon de Gonzalez G, Rodriguez-Malagon N. Pharmacological interventions for the prevention of allergic and febrile non-haemolytic transfusion reactions. *Cochrane Database Syst Rev.* 2010;CD007539.

76. Tobian AA, King KE, Ness PM. Prevention of febrile nonhemolytic and allergic transfusion reactions with pretransfusion medication: is this evidence-based medicine? *Transfusion.* 2008;8:2274-2276.

77. American Association of Blood Banks. Cohn CS, Delaney M, Johnson ST, Katz LM, eds. *Technical Manual.* 20th ed. American Association of Blood Banks; 2020.

78. Savage WJ, Tobian AA, Savage JH, Wood RA, Schroeder JT, Ness PM. Scratching the surface of allergic transfusion reactions. *Transfusion.* 2013;53:1361-1371.

79. Sandler SG, Eder AF, Goldman M, Winters JL. The entity of immunoglobulin A-related anaphylactic transfusion reactions is not evidence based. *Transfusion.* 2015;55:199-204.

80. Wiersum-Osselton JC, Whitaker B, Grey S, et al. Revised international surveillance case definition of transfusion-associated circulatory overload: a classification agreement validation study. *Lancet Haematol.* 2019;6:e350-e358.

81. Roubinian NH, Hendrickson JE, Triulzi DJ, et al. Incidence and clinical characteristics of transfusion-associated circulatory overload using an active surveillance algorithm. *Vox Sang.* 2017;112:56-63.

82. Robillard P, Nawej K, Chapdelaine A. Transfusion-associated circulatory overload (TACO): current leading cause of transfusion-associated fatalities reported to the Quebec hemovigilance system. *Transfus Med.* 2009;19:280-281.

83. Li G, Rachmale S, Kojicic M, et al. Incidence and transfusion risk factors for transfusion-associated circulatory overload among medical intensive care unit patients. *Transfusion.* 2011;51:338-343.

84. Vlaar APJ, Toy P, Fung M, et al. A consensus redefinition of transfusion-related acute lung injury. *Transfusion.* 2019;59:2465-2476.

85. Marik PE, Corwin HL. Acute lung injury following blood transfusion: expanding the definition. *Crit Care Med.* 2008;36:3080-3084.

86. Silliman CC, Voelkel NF, Allard JD, Elzi DJ, Tuder RM, Johnson JL, Ambruso DR. Plasma and lipids from stored packed red blood cells cause acute lung injury in an animal model. *J Clin Invest.* 1998;101:1458-1467.

87. Bux J, Sachs UJ. The pathogenesis of transfusion-related acute lung injury (TRALI). *Br J Haematol.* 2007;36:788-799.

88. Eder AF, Dy BA, Perez JM, Rambaud M, Benjamin RJ. The residual risk of transfusion-related acute lung injury at the American Red Cross (2008-2011): limitations of a predominantly male-donor plasma mitigation strategy. *Transfusion.* 2013;53:1442-1449.

89. Report of the US Department of Health and Human Services. The 2010 national blood collection and utilization survey report. US Department of Health and Human Services; 2011.

90. Flesland O. A comparison of complication rates based on published haemovigilance data. *Intensive Care Med.* 2007;33(suppl 1):S17-S21.

91. Kuehnert MJ, Roth VR, Haley NR, et al. Transfusion-transmitted bacterial infection in the United States, 1998 through 2000. *Transfusion.* 2001;41:1493-1499.

92. Hong H, Xiao W, Lazarus HM, Good CE, Maitta RW, Jacobs MR. Detection of septic transfusion reactions to platelet transfusions by active and passive surveillance. *Blood.* 2016;127:496-502.

93. Triulzi D, Duquesnoy R, Nichols L, Clark K, Jukic D, Zeevi A, Meisner D. Fatal transfusion-associated graft-versus-host disease in an immunocompetent recipient of a volunteer unit of red cells. *Transfusion.* 2006;46:885-888.

94. Petz LD, Calhoun L, Yam P, et al. Transfusion-associated graft-versus-host disease in immunocompetent patients: report of a fatal case associated with transfusion of blood from a second-degree relative, and a survey of predisposing factors. *Transfusion.* 1993;33:742-750.

95. Moroff G, Luban NL. The irradiation of blood and blood components to prevent graft-versus-host disease: technical issues and guidelines. *Transfus Med Rev.* 1997;1997;11:15-26.

96. Lacroix J, Hébert PC, Fergusson DA, et al. Age of transfused blood in critically ill adults. *N Engl J Med.* 2015;372:1410-1418.

97. Steiner ME, Ness PM, Assmann SF, et al. Effects of red-cell storage duration on patients undergoing cardiac surgery. *N Engl J Med.* 2015;372:1419-1429.

98. Heddle NM, Cook RJ, Arnold DM, et al. Effect of short-term vs. long-term blood storage on mortality after transfusion. *N Engl J Med.* 2016;375:1937-1945.

99. Cooper DJ, McQuilten ZK, Nichol A, et al. Age of red cells for transfusion and outcomes in critically ill adults. *N Engl J Med.* 2017;377:1858-1867.

100. Chai-Adisaksopha C, Alexander PE, Guyatt G, et al. Mortality outcomes in patients transfused with fresher versus older red blood cells: a meta-analysis. *Vox Sang.* 2017;112:268-278.

101. Spadaro S, Taccone FS, Fogagnolo A, et al. The effects of storage of red blood cells on the development of postoperative infections after noncardiac surgery. *Transfusion.* 2017;57:2727-2737.

102. Norris PJ, Schechtman K, Inglis HC, et al. Influence of blood storage age on immune and coagulation parameters in critically ill transfused patients. *Transfusion.* 2019;59:1223-1232.

103. Dhabangi A, Ainomugisha B, Cserti-Gazdewich C, et al. Effect of transfusion of red blood cells with longer vs shorter storage duration on elevated blood lactate levels in children with severe anemia: the TOTAL Randomized Clinical Trial. *JAMA.* 2015;314:2514-2523.

104. Fergusson DA, Hébert P, Hogan DL, et al. Effect of fresh red blood cell transfusions on clinical outcomes in premature, very low-birth-weight infants: the ARIPI randomized trial. *JAMA.* 2012;308:1443-1451.

105. Chasse M, Fergusson DA. Blood donor characteristics on transfusion outcomes-should obesity be assessed in future clinical trials? [Reply] *JAMA Intern Med.* 2017;177:599-600.

106. Shah A, Brunskill SJ, Desborough MJ, Doree C, Trivella M, Stanworth SJ. Transfusion of red blood cells stored for shorter versus longer duration for all conditions. *Cochrane Database Syst Rev.* 2018;12:CD010801.

107. Fernández Pérez ER, Winters JL, Gajic O. The addition of decision support into computerized physician order entry reduces red blood cell transfusion resource utilization in the intensive care unit. *Am J Hematol.* 2007;82:631-633.

108. Cohn CS, Welbig J, Bowman R, Kammann S, Frey K, Zantek N. A data-driven approach to patient blood management. *Transfusion.* 2014;54:316-322.

109. Carson JL, Duff A, Poses RM, Berlin JA, Spence RK, Trout R, Noveck H, Strom BL. Effect of anaemia and cardiovascular disease on surgical mortality and morbidity. *Lancet.* 1996;348:1055-1060.

110. van Straten AH, Hamad MA, van Zundert AJ, Martens EJ, Schönberger JP, de Wolf AM. Preoperative hemoglobin level as a predictor of survival after coronary artery bypass grafting: a comparison with the matched general population. *Circulation.* 2009;120:118-125.

111. Musallam KM, Tamim HM, Richards T, et al. Preoperative anaemia and postoperative outcomes in non-cardiac surgery: a retrospective cohort study. *Lancet.* 2011;378:1396-1407.

112. Spahn DR. Anemia and patient blood management in hip and knee surgery: a systematic review of the literature. *Anesthesiology.* 2010;2113:482-495.

113. Mueller MM, Van Remoortel H, Meybohm P, et al. Patient blood management recommendations from the 2018 Frankfurt Consensus Conference. *JAMA.* 2019;321:983-997.

114. Cohn CS. Transfusion support issues in hematopoietic stem cell transplantation. *Cancer Control.* 2015;22:52-59.

115. Strong DM, Katz L. Blood-bank testing for infectious diseases: how safe is blood transfusion? *Trends Mol Med.* 2002 Jul;8(7):355-358.

116. Jairath V, Kahan BC, Gray A, et al. Restrictive versus liberal blood transfusion for acute upper gastrointestinal bleeding (TRIGGER): a pragmatic, open-label, cluster randomised feasibility trial. *Lancet* 2015;386:137-144.

117. Tabor E, Epstein JS. NAT screening of blood and plasma donations: evolution of technology and regulatory policy. *Transfusion.* 2002;42(9):1230-1237.

INDEX

Note: Page numbers followed by *f* and *t* indicate figures and tables, respectively.